ELSEVIER

NETTER:

It's How You Know Anatomy.

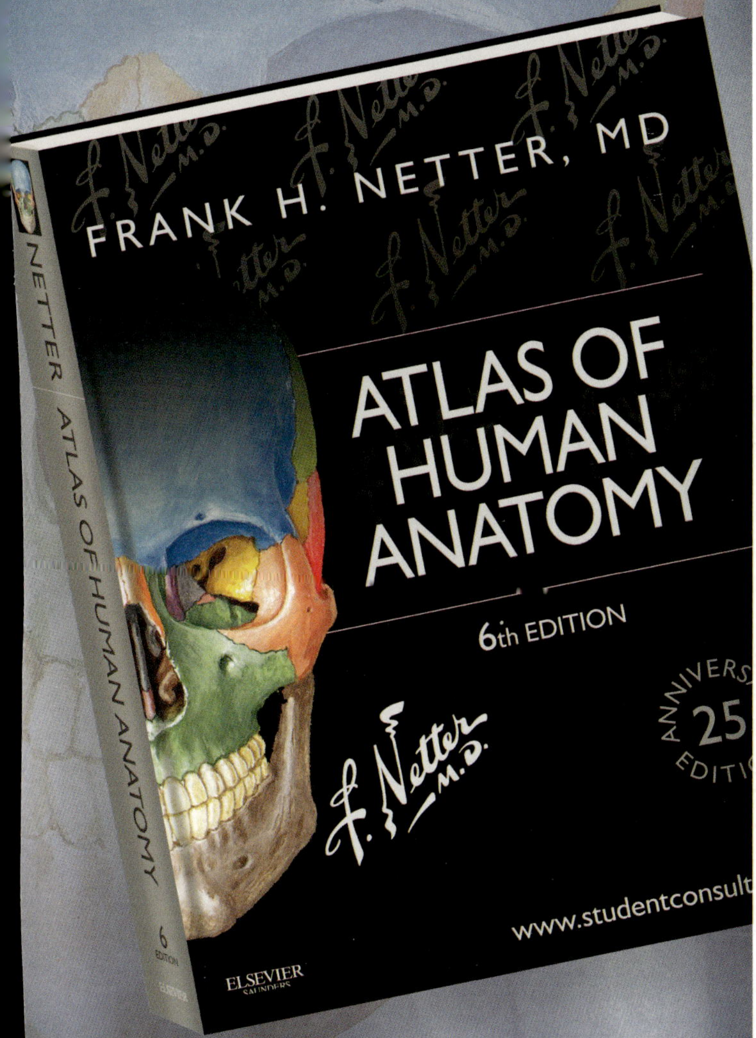

Master anatomy the **NETTER** way with these great companion resources!

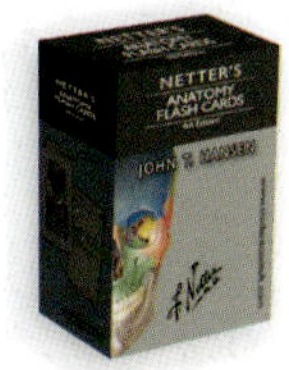

Netter's Anatomy Flashcards
With **Student Consult** Access
By John T. Hansen, PhD
A convenient and portable way to review anatomy on the go!

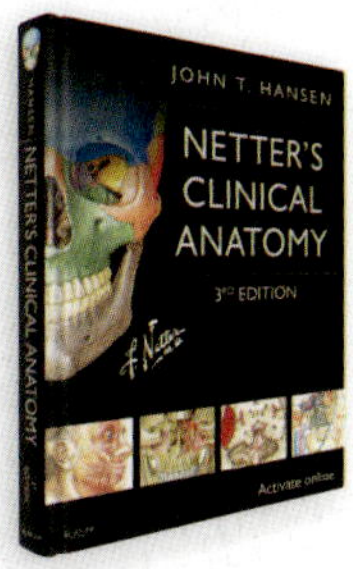

Netter's Clinical Anatomy
With **Online** Access
By John T. Hansen, PhD
Gain a comprehensive understanding of complex clinical anatomical concepts.

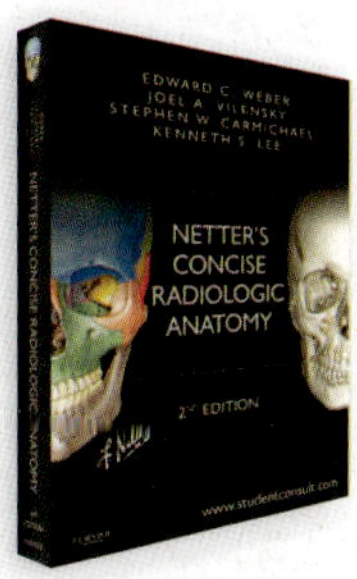

Netter's Concise Radiologic Anatomy
With **Student Consult** Access
By Edward C. Weber, DO et al.
Easily understand the clinical context of anatomy through vivid illustrations and modern imaging.

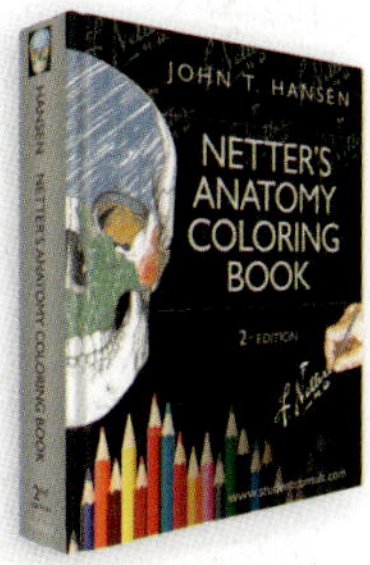

Netter's Anatomy Coloring Book
With **Student Consult** Access
By John T. Hansen, PhD
An interactive coloring workbook that helps you master anatomy *and* have fun!

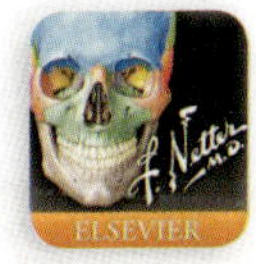

Netter's Anatomy Atlas App
Use Dr. Netter's most famous illustrations of human anatomy as your intuitive and interactive study guide!

Learn more at MyNetter.com!

Atlas of Human Anatomy

Sixth Edition

Frank H. Netter, MD

SAUNDERS
ELSEVIER

SAUNDERS
ELSEVIER

1600 John F. Kennedy Blvd.
Ste. 1800
Philadelphia, PA 19103-2899

ATLAS OF HUMAN ANATOMY
SIXTH EDITION

Standard Edition: 978-1-4557-0418-7
Professional Edition: 978-1-4557-5888-3
IE: 978-0-8089-2451-7
Enhanced IE Edition: 978-0-323-39009-5

Notices

Senior Content Strategist: Elyse O'Grady
Senior Content Development Specialist: Marybeth Thiel
Publishing Services Manager: Patricia Tannian
Senior Project Manager: John Casey
Senior Design Manager: Lou Forgione
Illustration Buyer: Karen Giacomucci

Printed in the United States of America

Last digit is the print number: 9 8 7 6 5 4 3 2
Standard Edition: 9 8 7 6 5 4 3 2
Enhanced IE: 9 8 7 6 5 4 3 2 1

Contributing Medical Illustrator

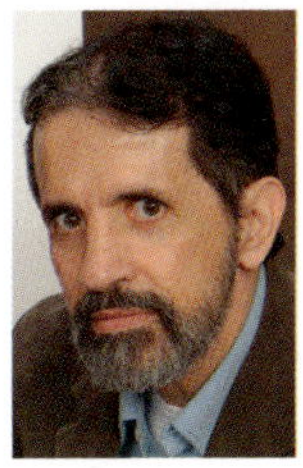

Carlos A. G. Machado, MD

Consulting Editors

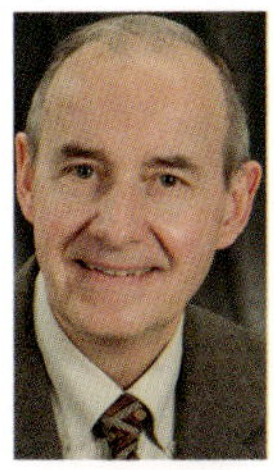

John T. Hansen, Ph.D.
Lead Editor
Associate Dean for Admissions
Professor of Neurobiology and Anatomy
University of Rochester Medical Center
Rochester, New York

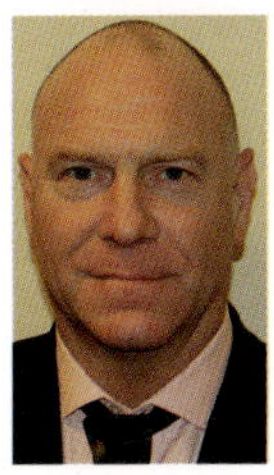

Brion Benninger, MD, MS
Professor, Chair Medical Anatomical Sciences, Family Medicine,
and Neuromuscular Medicine College of Dental Medicine,
Western University of Health Sciences Lebanon, Oregon;
Orthopaedic and General Surgery Residency Program
Samaritan Hospital Corvallis, Oregon;
Surgery, Orthopedics & Rehabilitation,
and Oral Maxillofacial Surgery
Oregon Health & Science University
Portland, Oregon

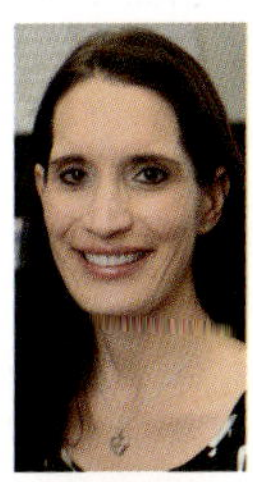

Jennifer Brueckner-Collins, PhD
Professor and Vice Chair of Educational Programs
Anatomical Sciences and Neurobiology
University of Louisville School of Medicine
Louisville, Kentucky

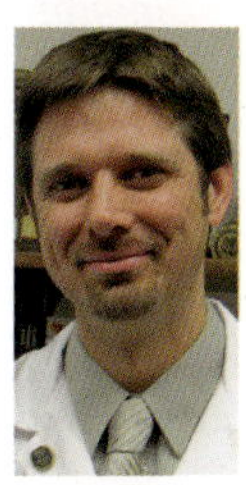

Todd M. Hoagland, PhD
Associate Professor
Department of Cell Biology, Neurobiology, and Anatomy
Medical College of Wisconsin
Milwaukee, Wisconsin

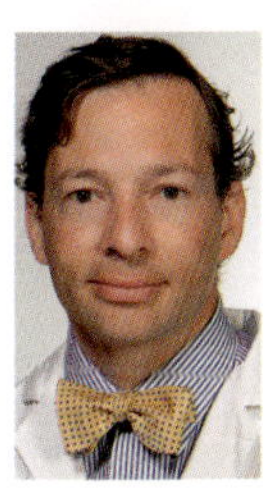

R. Shane Tubbs, MS, PA-C, PhD
Pediatric Neurosurgery
Children's Hospital of Alabama
Birmingham, Alabama
Professor of Anatomy
Department of Anatomical Sciences, St. George's University,
Grenada Centre of Anatomy and Human Identification,
Dundee University, United Kingdom

Editors of Previous Editions

First Edition
Sharon Colacino, PhD

Second Edition
Arthur F. Dalley II, PhD

Third Edition
John T. Hansen, PhD

Fourth Edition
John T. Hansen, PhD
Jennifer K. Brueckner, PhD
Stephen W. Carmichael, PhD, DSc
Thomas R. Gest, PhD
Noelle A. Granger, PhD
Anil H. Waljii, MD, PhD

Fifth Edition
John T. Hansen, PhD
Brion Benninger, MD, MS
Jennifer K. Brueckner, PhD
Stephen W. Carmichael, PhD, DSc
Noelle A. Granger, PhD
R. Shane Tubbs, MS, PA-C, PhD

International Advisory Board

Netter's Atlas of Human Anatomy – Celebrating 25 Years

"Anatomy, of course, does not change, but our understanding of anatomy and its clinical significance does."

– **Frank H. Netter, MD**

Whether you're using this 6th edition of ***Atlas of Human Anatomy*** in print, as an e-Book, online, or in the Netter's Anatomy Atlas for iPad app—Dr. Netter's paintings of the intricacies of the human form remain as relevant today as at first launch. The publication of the 6th edition marks the silver anniversary of the first release of Frank H. Netter's *Atlas of Human Anatomy*—when its vibrant colors and unique clinical perspective made it a must-have companion in anatomy classes, dissection labs, and clinical professional offices worldwide—solidifying his legacy to so many as one of the world's most influential medical educators.

Anatomy remains a cornerstone of healthcare education. It is often one of the first topics taught in medical or healthcare curricula. Anatomy is also central to so much in clinical practice, from physical examination and radiologic imaging to surgery and physical rehabilitation. However, changes in anatomy education and its clinical application over these past 25 years have been significant. Medical and healthcare curricula increasingly integrate anatomy throughout and dedicated gross-anatomy hours have decreased. Some programs have discontinued full-body dissection. Advances in imaging technology have provided increasingly clearer views of living anatomy, and 3D models of anatomy continue to evolve. Likewise, the *Atlas* has evolved. Thanks to the tremendous guidance of leading clinical anatomists and expert anatomy educators, as well as the contributions of talented medical illustrators, the 6th edition features newly created illustrations and modern radiologic images that provide students with views of current clinical significance and perspectives that elucidate complex anatomic relationships. This edition also includes the illustrations from older editions of the *Atlas*, like Dr. Netter's depictions of common anatomic variations (in electronic editions and print+electronic packages) as bonus plates to help provide more comprehensive coverage that dissection lab hours may not allow. For the first time, the *Atlas* incorporates muscle tables as quick look-up appendices at the end of each section for the convenience of the clinician, student, or educator with little time. StudentConsult.com and NetterReference.com electronic resources include some 3D models extracted from Netter's 3D Interactive Anatomy, dissection video selections from Netter's Online Dissection Modules by UNC at Chapel Hill, and other supporting resources. In addition, all text throughout the Atlas has been meticulously updated to be in line with the most recent version of *Terminologia Anatomica* by the Federal International Program for Anatomical Terminology (FIPAT) of the International Federation of Associations of Anatomists (IFAA).

The unique visual perspective of Frank H. Netter is unsurpassed. Dr. Netter brought the hand of a master medical illustrator, the brain of a physician, and the soul of an artist to his depictions of the human body. This 25th anniversary edition celebrates the lasting impact of his work that continues to teach and inspire.

We want to hear from you—about the history and future of anatomy education and medicine and the Netter legacy and invite you to share your thoughts, inspirations, memories, tributes, and feedback with us through email: NetterAppFeedback@elsevier.com and on Facebook: www.facebook.com/NetterImages

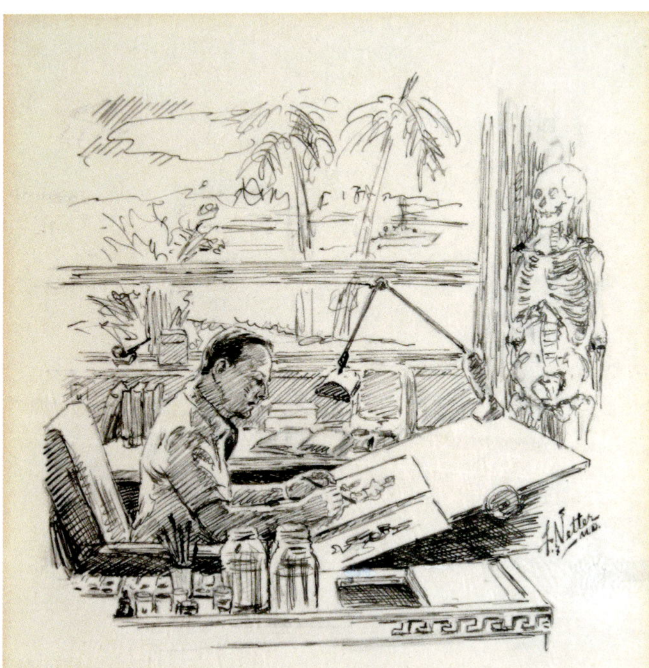

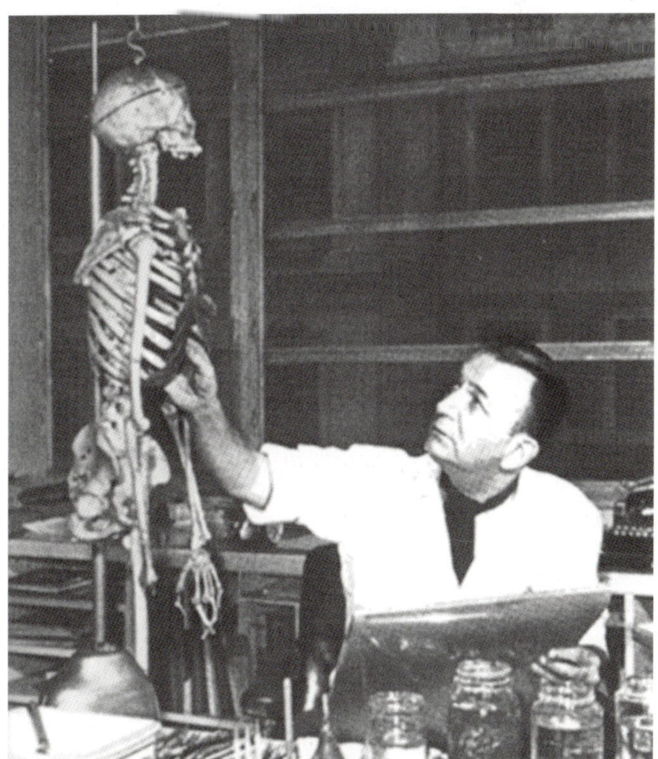

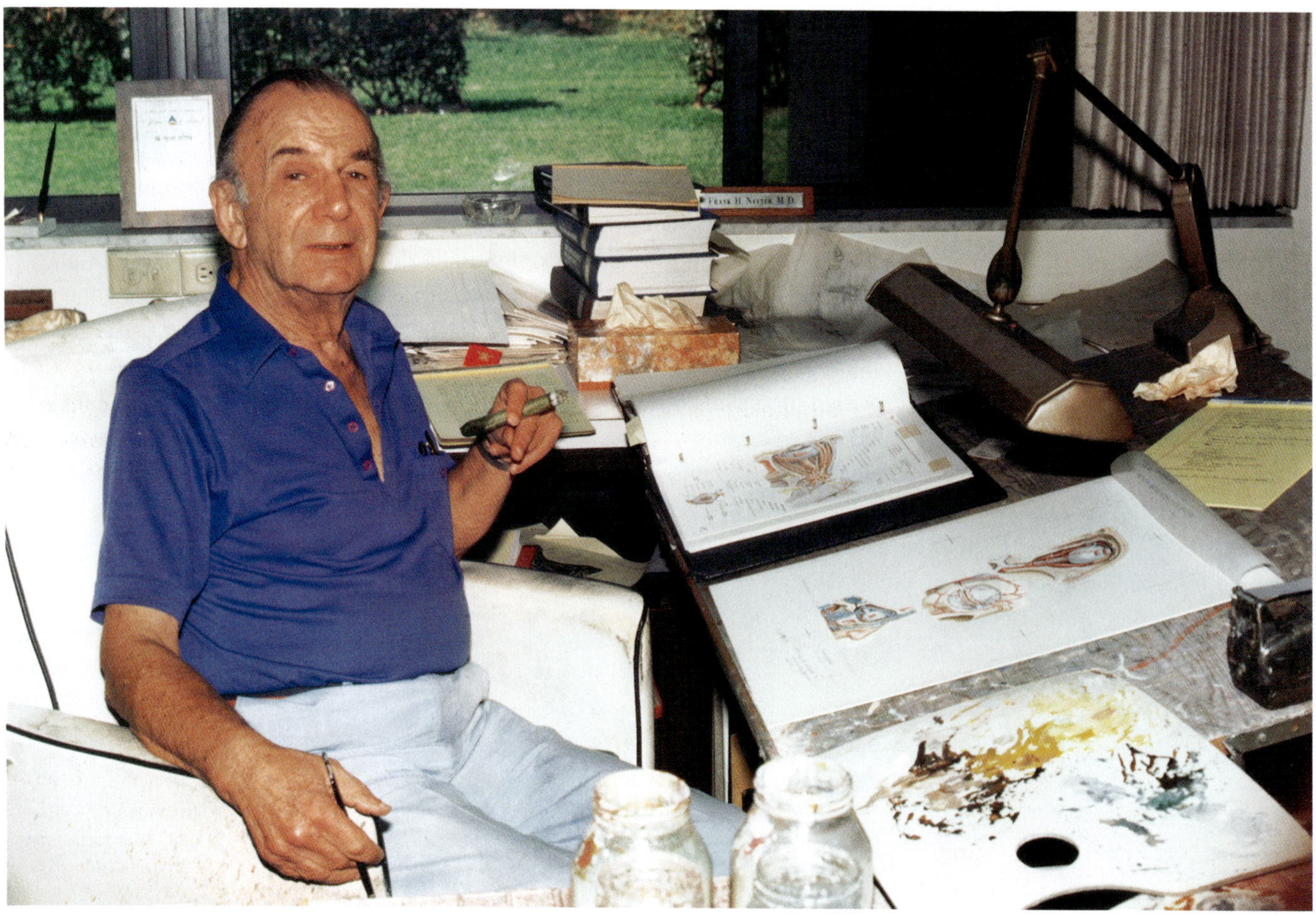

Frank H. Netter, MD

Photograph by James L. Clayton

To my dear wife, Vera

Preface to the First Edition

I have often said that my career as a medical artist for almost 50 years has been a sort of "command performance" in the sense that it has grown in response to the desires and requests of the medical profession. Over these many years, I have produced almost 4,000 illustrations, mostly for *The CIBA* (now *Netter*) *Collection of Medical Illustrations* but also for *Clinical Symposia*. These pictures have been concerned with the varied subdivisions of medical knowledge such as gross anatomy, histology, embryology, physiology, pathology, diagnostic modalities, surgical and therapeutic techniques, and clinical manifestations of a multitude of diseases. As the years went by, however, there were more and more requests from physicians and students for me to produce an atlas purely of gross anatomy. Thus, this atlas has come about, not through any inspiration on my part but rather, like most of my previous works, as a fulfillment of the desires of the medical profession.

It involved going back over all the illustrations I had made over so many years, selecting those pertinent to gross anatomy, classifying them and organizing them by system and region, adapting them to page size and space, and arranging them in logical sequence. Anatomy of course does not change, but our understanding of anatomy and its clinical significance does change, as do anatomical terminology and nomenclature. This therefore required much updating of many of the older pictures and even revision of a number of them in order to make them more pertinent to today's ever-expanding scope of medical and surgical practice. In addition, I found that there were gaps in the portrayal of medical knowledge as pictorialized in the illustrations I had previously done, and this necessitated my making a number of new pictures that are included in this volume.

In creating an atlas such as this, it is important to achieve a happy medium between complexity and simplification. If the pictures are too complex, they may be difficult and confusing to read; if oversimplified, they may not be adequately definitive or may even be misleading. I have therefore striven for a middle course of realism without the clutter of confusing minutiae. I hope that the students and members of the medical and allied professions will find the illustrations readily understandable, yet instructive and useful.

At one point, the publisher and I thought it might be nice to include a foreword by a truly outstanding and renowned anatomist, but there are so many in that category that we could not make a choice. We did think of men like Vesalius, Leonardo da Vinci, William Hunter, and Henry Gray, who of course are unfortunately unavailable, but I do wonder what their comments might have been about this atlas.

Frank H. Netter, MD
(1906–1991)

Frank H. Netter, MD

Frank H. Netter was born in New York City in 1906. He studied art at the Art Students League and the National Academy of Design before entering medical school at New York University, where he received his Doctor of Medicine degree in 1931. During his student years, Dr. Netter's notebook sketches attracted the attention of the medical faculty and other physicians, allowing him to augment his income by illustrating articles and textbooks. He continued illustrating as a sideline after establishing a surgical practice in 1933, but he ultimately opted to give up his practice in favor of a full-time commitment to art. After service in the United States Army during World War II, Dr. Netter began his long collaboration with the CIBA Pharmaceutical Company (now Novartis Pharmaceuticals). This 45-year partnership resulted in the production of the extraordinary collection of medical art so familiar to physicians and other medical professionals worldwide.

Icon Learning Systems acquired the Netter Collection in July 2000 and continued to update Dr. Netter's original paintings and to add newly commissioned paintings by artists trained in the style of Dr. Netter. In 2005, Elsevier Inc. purchased the Netter Collection and all publications from Icon Learning Systems. There are now over 50 publications featuring the art of Dr. Netter available through Elsevier Inc.

Dr. Netter's works are among the finest examples of the use of illustration in the teaching of medical concepts. The 13-book *Netter Collection of Medical Illustrations,* which includes the greater part of the more than 20,000 paintings created by Dr. Netter, became and remains one of the most famous medical works ever published. *The Netter Atlas of Human Anatomy,* first published in 1989, presents the anatomic paintings from the Netter Collection. Now translated into 16 languages, it is the anatomy atlas of choice among medical and health professions students the world over.

The Netter illustrations are appreciated not only for their aesthetic qualities, but, more importantly, for their intellectual content. As Dr. Netter wrote in 1949 "clarification of a subject is the aim and goal of illustration. No matter how beautifully painted, how delicately and subtly rendered a subject may be, it is of little value as a *medical illustration* if it does not serve to make clear some medical point." Dr. Netter's planning, conception, point of view, and approach are what inform his paintings and what make them so intellectually valuable.

Frank H. Netter, MD, physician and artist, died in 1991.

Acknowledgments

Brion Benninger, MD, MS

I would like to thank my wife, Alison, and our son, Jack, for their wit, caring, and the love they provide me daily. I want to thank Elsevier, especially Marybeth Thiel, for her insight and direction, enabling John Hansen, my fellow coeditors, and Carlos Machado to work in such a rich environment. I particularly want to thank my early clinical anatomy mentors, Gerald Tressidor and Harold Ellis (Guy's Hospital); Dean P. Crone and the University Board for continuous support; all my past and future patients and students; and clinical colleagues who keep anatomy dynamic. Special thanks to Jim McDaniel and Bill Bryan and all who represent what is good in teaching. Lastly, I thank my mother for her love of education and my father for his inquisitive mind.

Jennifer Brueckner-Collins, PhD

I am very grateful to the wonderful Elsevier team, particularly Marybeth Thiel and Elyse O'Grady, for their guidance and expertise during our preparation of the sixth edition. It is always privilege to collaborate with Carlos Machado, whose artistic talent brings our anatomical visions from concept to reality. Sincere thanks to Mark Sturgill, DO, who most generously provided us with updated images for abdominal MRCP, axial and coronal CT with contrast, as well as CT angiography. Finally, I am eternally indebted to my parents, John and Rheba, and to my husband, Kurt, for their support, encouragement, love, and inspiration; they are my raison d'etre.

John T. Hansen, PhD

At Elsevier I would like to thank Marybeth Thiel, Senior Development Editor, Elyse O'Grady, Senior Content Strategist, John Casey, Senior Project Manager, and Madelene Hyde, Publishing Director, for their continuous support and meticulous attention to detail during the development of this sixth edition of the *Atlas of Human Anatomy.* They, along with the entire Editorial, Production, Design, and Marketing team at Elsevier have been a delight to work with and to know. I am also indebted to Carlos Machado for his superb artistic skill in producing and updating plates appearing in the *Atlas*. His renderings of human anatomy are the perfect complement to the Netter images. In addition to my fellow editors of this edition, I wish to express my thanks to my faculty colleagues at Rochester and to all my past and present students who have provided generous and constructive feedback and have enriched my life. Finally, I am indebted to my entire family for their continued support and especially to my wife, Paula. Their love and encouragement sustains me and is the source of all the happiness and joy I know.

Todd M. Hoagland, PhD

It is a privilege to teach clinical human anatomy and I am eternally grateful to all the body donors and their families for enabling healthcare professionals to train in the dissection laboratory. It is my honor to work with outstanding medical students and colleagues at the Medical College of Wisconsin. I am grateful to John Hansen and the professionals of the Elsevier team for the opportunity to be a steward of the incomparable *Netter Atlas*. Marybeth Thiel and Elyse O'Grady were especially helpful and a pleasure to work with. It was an honor to collaborate with the brilliant Carlos Machado and all the consulting editors. I thank Joe Besharse for being an outstanding mentor. I am deeply appreciative of Stan Hillman and Jack O'Malley for inspiring me with masterful teaching and rigorous expectations. I am indebted to Richard Hoyt, Jr., for helping me become a competent anatomist, and to Rob Bouchie for his support. I am most grateful to my brother, Bill, for his unwavering optimism and gregarious nature. I thank my mother, Liz, for her dedication and love and for instilling a strong work ethic. Finally, I am humbled by my two awesome children, Ella and Caleb, for helping me redefine love, wonder, and joy.

R. Shane Tubbs, MS, PA-C, PhD

First and foremost, I would like to thank Elsevier and in particular, Madelene Hyde, Marybeth Thiel, and Elyse O'Grady for all of their hard work in making this edition come to life. The evolution of the current atlas continues with the superb skills of Dr. Carlos Machado and his works of art. I would like to thank Dr. Satinder Singh for his kind assistance in providing radiographic images of the heart. I thank my beautiful wife, Susan, and son, Isaiah, for their patience and guidance during the editing of the sixth edition. Without the continued support of my mentor, friend, and colleague, Dr. W. Jerry Oakes, I could not fulfill all of my academic endeavors. I dedicate my efforts in this edition to my late brother-in-law, Nelson Jones, whose appetite for inquisitiveness inspires me today.

Contents

Section 1 HEAD AND NECK

Topographic Anatomy 1
Superficial Head and Neck 2–3
Bones and Ligaments 4–23
Superficial Face 24–25
Neck 26–34
Nasal Region 35–55
Oral Region 56–63
Pharynx 64–75
Thyroid Gland and Larynx 76–82
Orbit and Contents 83–93
Ear 94–100
Meninges and Brain 101–116
Cranial and Cervical Nerves 117–136
Cerebral Vasculature 137–149
Regional Scans 150–151
Muscle Tables Table 1-1–Table 1-6

Section 2 BACK AND SPINAL CORD

Topographic Anatomy 152
Bones and Ligaments 153–159
Spinal Cord 160–170
Muscles and Nerves 171–175
Cross-Sectional Anatomy 176–177
Muscle Tables Table 2-1–Table 2-2

Section 3 THORAX

Topographic Anatomy 178
Mammary Gland 179–182
Body Wall 183–192
Lungs 193–207
Heart 208–226
Mediastinum 227–236
Regional Scans 237
Cross-Sectional Anatomy 238–241
Muscle Table Table 3-1

Section 4 ABDOMEN

Topographic Anatomy 242
Body Wall 243–262
Peritoneal Cavity 263–268
Viscera (Gut) 269–276
Viscera (Accessory Organs) 277–282
Visceral Vasculature 283–296
Innervation 297–307

Kidneys and Suprarenal Glands 308–320
Sectional Anatomy 321–328
Muscle Table Table 4-1

Section 5 PELVIS AND PERINEUM

Topographic Anatomy 329
Bones and Ligaments 330–334
Pelvic Floor and Contents 335–345
Urinary Bladder 346–348
Uterus, Vagina, and Supporting Structures 349–353
Perineum and External Genitalia: Female 354–357
Perineum and External Genitalia: Male 358–365
Homologues of Genitalia 366–367
Testis, Epididymis, and Ductus Deferens 368
Rectum 369–374
Regional Scans 375
Vasculature 376–386
Innervation 387–395
Cross-Sectional Anatomy 396–397
Muscle Tables Table 5-1–Table 5-2

Section 6 UPPER LIMB

Topographic Anatomy 398
Cutaneous Anatomy 399–403
Shoulder and Axilla 404–416
Arm 417–421
Elbow and Forearm 422–438
Wrist and Hand 439–458
Neurovasculature 459–466
Regional Scans 467
Muscle Tables Table 6-1–Table 6-4

Section 7 LOWER LIMB

Topographic Anatomy 468
Cutaneous Anatomy 469–472
Hip and Thigh 473–492
Knee 493–499
Leg 500–510
Ankle and Foot 511–524
Neurovasculature 525–529
Regional Scans 530–531
Muscle Tables Table 7-1–Table 7-4

References 577

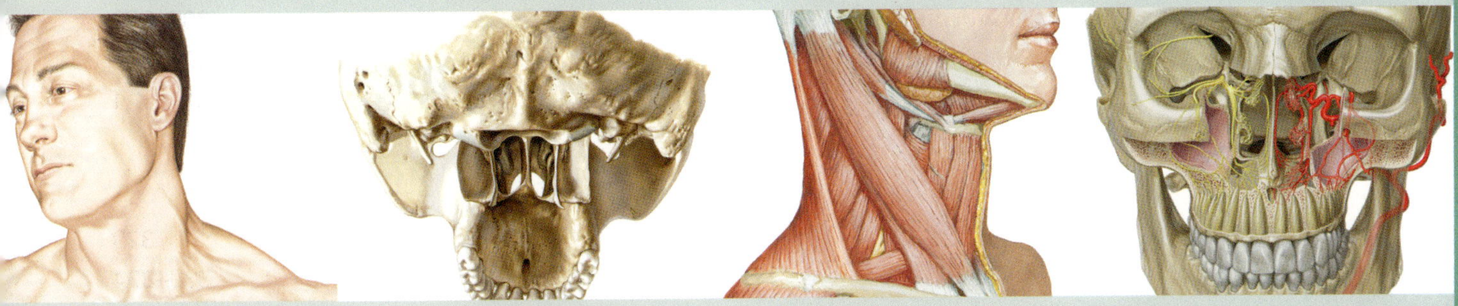

Section 1 HEAD AND NECK

Topographic Anatomy

Plate 1

1 Head and Neck: Surface Anatomy

Superficial Head and Neck

Plates 2–3

2 Cutaneous Nerves of Head and Neck

3 Superficial Arteries and Veins of Face and Scalp

Bones and Ligaments

Plates 4–23

4 Skull: Anterior View

5 Skull: Anteroposterior Radiograph

6 Skull: Lateral View

7 Skull: Lateral Radiograph

8 Skull: Midsagittal Section

9 Calvaria

10 Cranial Base: Inferior View

11 Cranial Base: Superior View

12 Foramina and Canals of Cranial Base: Inferior View

13 Foramina and Canals of Cranial Base: Superior View

14 Skull of Newborn

15 Bony Framework of Head and Neck

16 Pterygoid Fossae: Posterior and Inferolateral Views

17 Mandible

18 Temporomandibular Joint
19 Cervical Vertebrae: Atlas and Axis
20 Cervical Vertebrae (continued)
21 Cervical Vertebrae: Uncovertebral Joints
22 External Craniocervical Ligaments
23 Internal Craniocervical Ligaments

Superficial Face

Plates 24–25

24 Facial Nerve Branches and Parotid Gland
25 Muscles of Facial Expression: Lateral View

Neck

Plates 26–34

26 Fascial Layers of Neck
27 Muscles of Neck: Anterior View
28 Infrahyoid and Suprahyoid Muscles
29 Muscles of Neck: Lateral View
30 Scalene and Prevertebral Muscles
31 Superficial Veins and Cutaneous Nerves of Neck
32 Nerves and Vessels of Neck
33 Nerves and Vessels of Neck (continued)
34 Carotid Arteries

Nasal Region

Plates 35–55

35 Nose
36 Lateral Wall of Nasal Cavity
37 Lateral Wall of Nasal Cavity (continued)
38 Medial Wall of Nasal Cavity (Nasal Septum)
39 Nerves of Nasal Cavity
40 Arteries of Nasal Cavity: Nasal Septum Turned Up
41 Nerves of Nasal Cavity: Nasal Septum Turned Up
42 Nose and Maxillary Sinus: Transverse Section
43 Paranasal Sinuses
44 Paranasal Sinuses (continued)
45 Paranasal Sinuses: Changes with Age
46 Salivary Glands
47 Tongue and Salivary Glands: Sections
48 Muscles Involved in Mastication
49 Muscles Involved in Mastication (continued)
50 Mandibular Nerve (V_3)
51 Maxillary Artery
52 Ophthalmic (V_1) and Maxillary (V_2) Nerves
53 Autonomic Innervation of Nasal Cavity
54 Pterygopalatine Fossa
55 Orientation of Nerves and Vessels of the Cranial Base

Oral Region

Plates 56–63

56 Inspection of Oral Cavity
57 Roof of Oral Cavity
58 Floor of Oral Cavity
59 Tongue
60 Tongue (continued)
61 Afferent Innervation of Oral Cavity and Pharynx
62 Teeth
63 Teeth (continued)

Pharynx

Plates 64–75

64 Pharynx: Median Section
65 Muscles of Pharynx: Sagittal Section
66 Pharynx: Opened Posterior View
67 Muscles of Pharynx: Partially Opened Posterior View
68 Fauces
69 Pharyngoesophageal Junction
70 Muscles of Pharynx: Lateral View
71 Nerves of Oral and Pharyngeal Regions
72 Arteries of Oral and Pharyngeal Regions
73 Veins of Oral and Pharyngeal Regions
74 Lymph Vessels and Nodes of Head and Neck
75 Lymph Vessels and Nodes of Pharynx and Tongue

Thyroid Gland and Larynx

Plates 76–82

76 Thyroid Gland: Anterior View
77 Thyroid Gland and Pharynx: Posterior View
78 Parathyroid Glands
79 Cartilages of Larynx
80 Intrinsic Muscles of Larynx
81 Action of Intrinsic Muscles of Larynx
82 Nerves of Larynx

Orbit and Contents

Plates 83–93

83 Eyelids
84 Lacrimal Apparatus
85 Fasciae of Orbit and Eyeball
86 Extrinsic Eye Muscles
87 Arteries and Veins of Orbit and Eyelids
88 Nerves of Orbit
89 Eyeball
90 Anterior and Posterior Chambers of Eye
91 Lens and Supporting Structures
92 Intrinsic Arteries and Veins of Eye
93 Vascular Supply of Eye

Ear

Plates 94–100

94 Pathway of Sound Reception
95 External Ear and Tympanic Cavity
96 Tympanic Cavity
97 Bony and Membranous Labyrinths
98 Bony and Membranous Labyrinths (continued)
99 Orientation of Labyrinths in Skull
100 Pharyngotympanic (Auditory, Eustachian) Tube

Meninges and Brain

Plates 101–116

101 Meninges and Diploic Veins
102 Meningeal Arteries
103 Meninges and Superficial Cerebral Veins
104 Dural Venous Sinuses
105 Dural Venous Sinuses (continued)
106 Cerebrum: Lateral Views
107 Cerebrum: Medial Views
108 Cerebrum: Inferior View
109 Ventricles of Brain
110 Circulation of Cerebrospinal Fluid
111 Basal Nuclei (Ganglia)
112 Thalamus
113 Hippocampus and Fornix
114 Cerebellum
115 Brainstem
116 Fourth Ventricle and Cerebellum

Cranial and Cervical Nerves

Plates 117–136

117 Cranial Nerve Nuclei in Brainstem: Schema
118 Cranial Nerve Nuclei in Brainstem: Schema (continued)
119 Cranial Nerves (Motor and Sensory Distribution): Schema
120 Olfactory Nerve (I): Schema
121 Optic Nerve (II) (Visual Pathway): Schema
122 Oculomotor (III), Trochlear (IV), and Abducent (VI) Nerves: Schema
123 Trigeminal Nerve (V): Schema
124 Facial Nerve (VII): Schema
125 Vestibulocochlear Nerve (VIII): Schema
126 Glossopharyngeal Nerve (IX): Schema
127 Vagus Nerve (X): Schema
128 Accessory Nerve (XI): Schema
129 Hypoglossal Nerve (XII): Schema
130 Cervical Plexus: Schema
131 Autonomic Nerves in Neck
132 Autonomic Nerves in Head
133 Ciliary Ganglion: Schema
134 Pterygopalatine and Submandibular Ganglia: Schema
135 Otic Ganglion: Schema
136 Taste Pathways: Schema

Cerebral Vasculature

Plates 137–149

137 Arteries to Brain and Meninges

138 Internal Carotid Artery in Petrous Part of Temporal Bone

139 Arteries to Brain: Schema

140 Arteries of Brain: Inferior Views

141 Cerebral Arterial Circle (of Willis)

142 Arteries of Brain: Frontal View and Section

143 Arteries of Brain: Lateral and Medial Views

144 Arteries of Posterior Cranial Fossa

145 Veins of Posterior Cranial Fossa

146 Deep Veins of Brain

147 Subependymal Veins of Brain

148 Hypothalamus and Hypophysis

149 Arteries and Veins of Hypothalamus and Hypophysis

Regional Scans

Plates 150–151

150 Cranial Imaging (MRV and MRA)

151 Cranial Imaging (MRI)

Muscle Tables

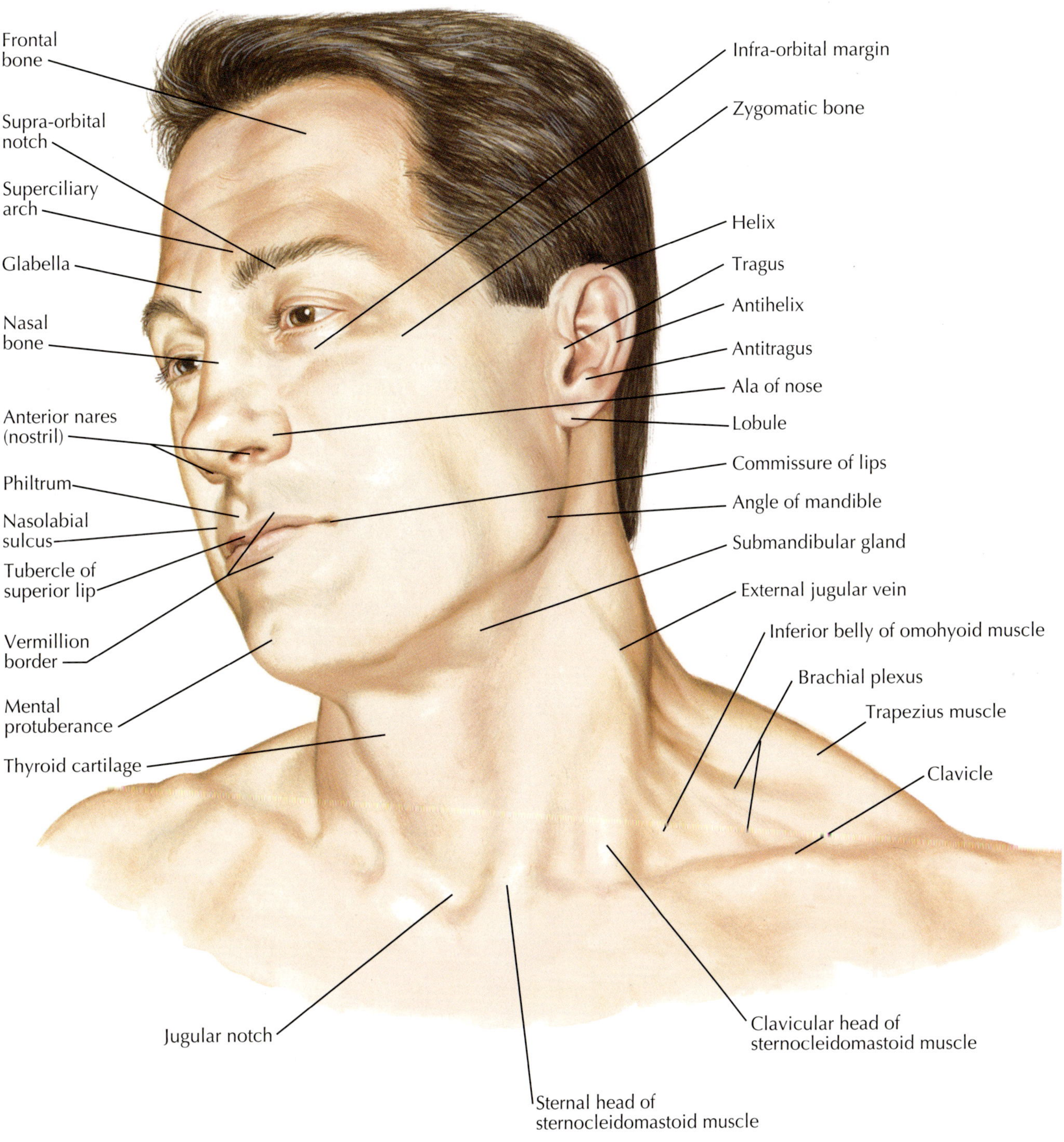
Frontal bone
Supra-orbital notch
Superciliary arch
Glabella
Nasal bone
Anterior nares (nostril)
Philtrum
Nasolabial sulcus
Tubercle of superior lip
Vermillion border
Mental protuberance
Thyroid cartilage
Jugular notch
Infra-orbital margin
Zygomatic bone
Helix
Tragus
Antihelix
Antitragus
Ala of nose
Lobule
Commissure of lips
Angle of mandible
Submandibular gland
External jugular vein
Inferior belly of omohyoid muscle
Brachial plexus
Trapezius muscle
Clavicle
Clavicular head of sternocleidomastoid muscle
Sternal head of sternocleidomastoid muscle
C. Machado M.D.

See also Plates 32, 35, 52

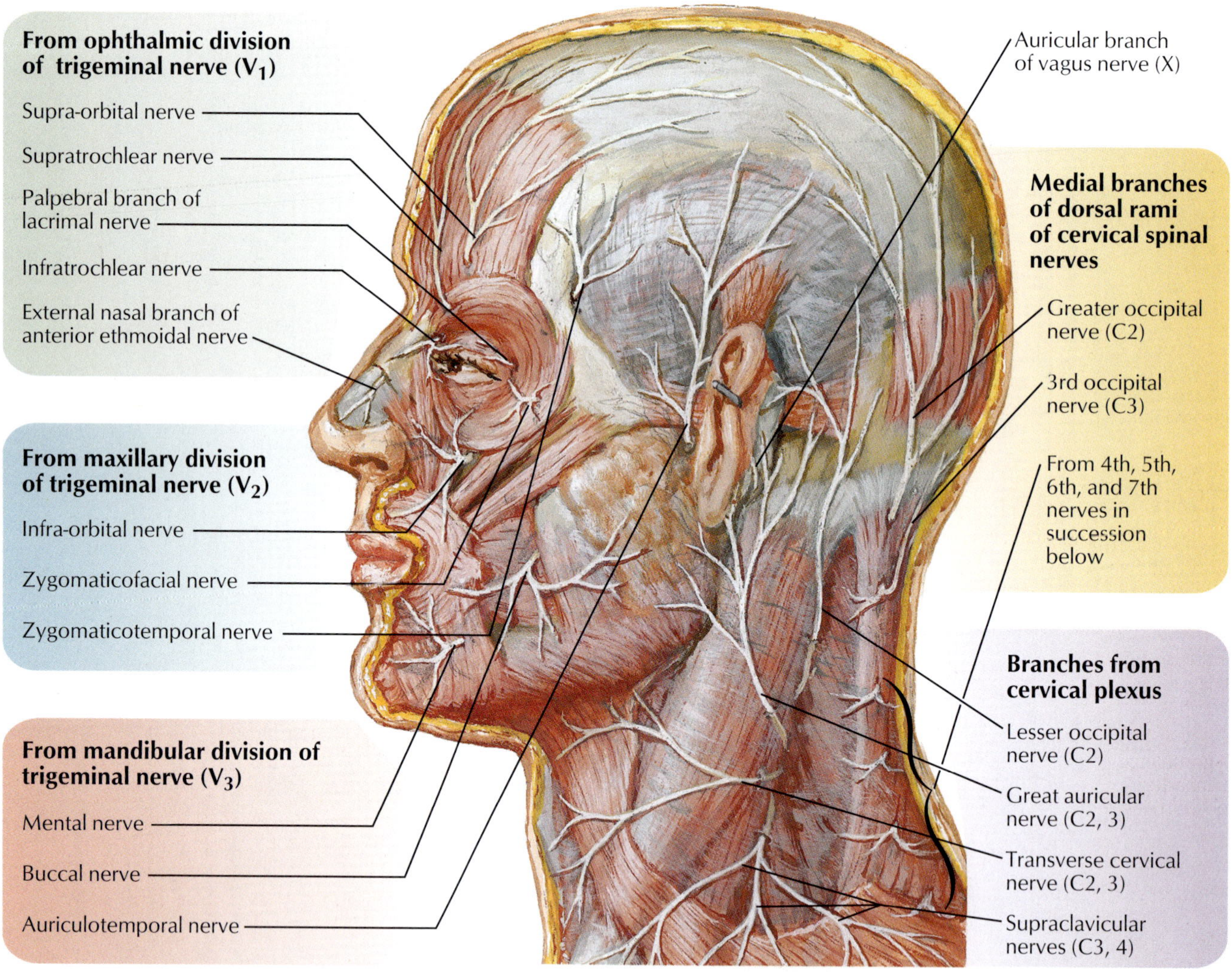

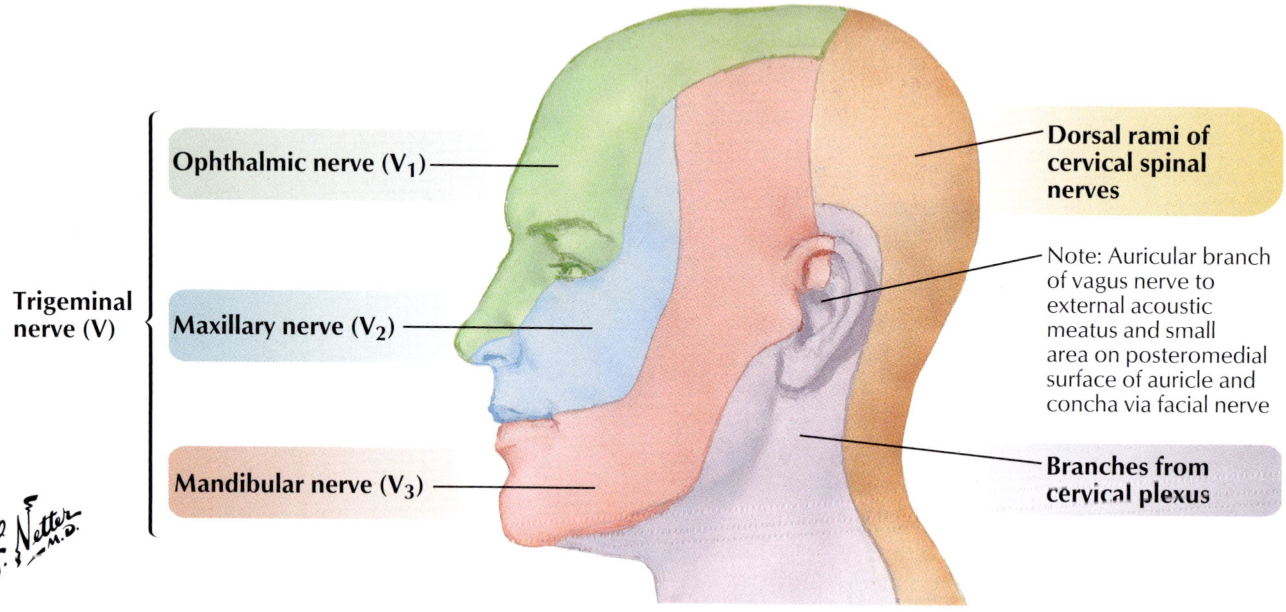

Superficial Arteries and Veins of Face and Scalp

See also Plates 51, 72, 73

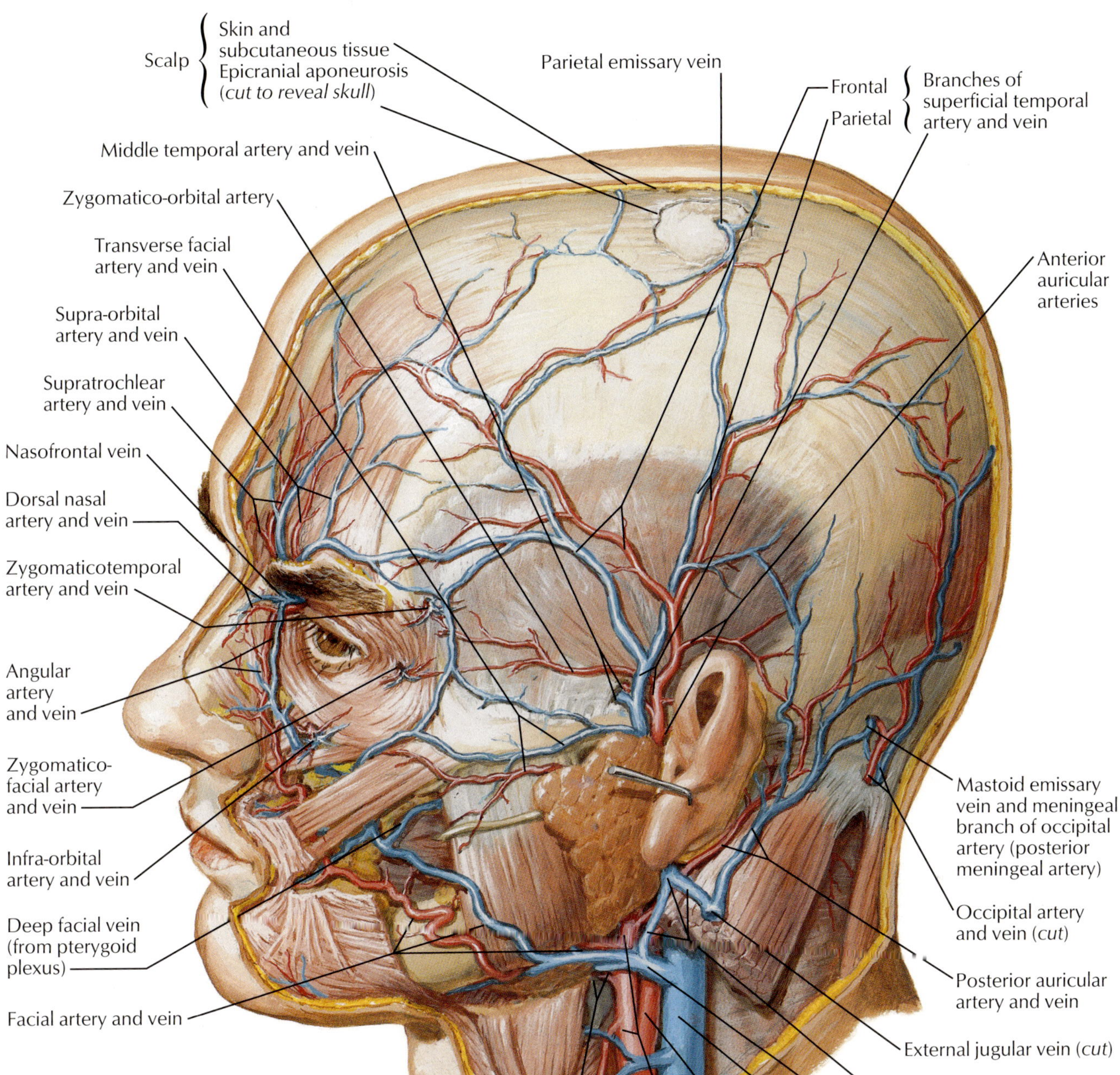

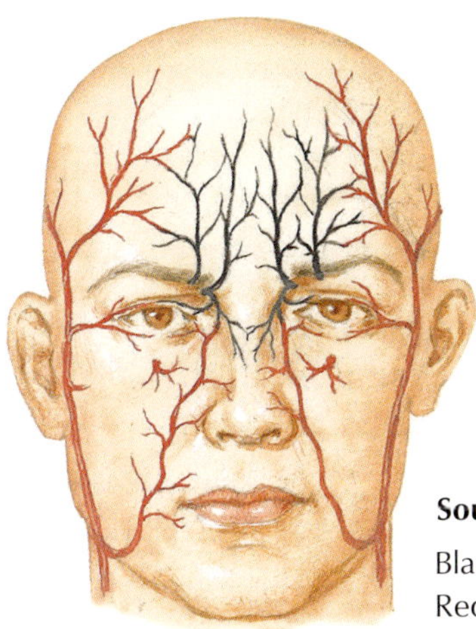

Sources of arterial supply of face

Black: from internal carotid artery (via ophthalmic artery)

Red: from external carotid artery

Skull: Anterior View

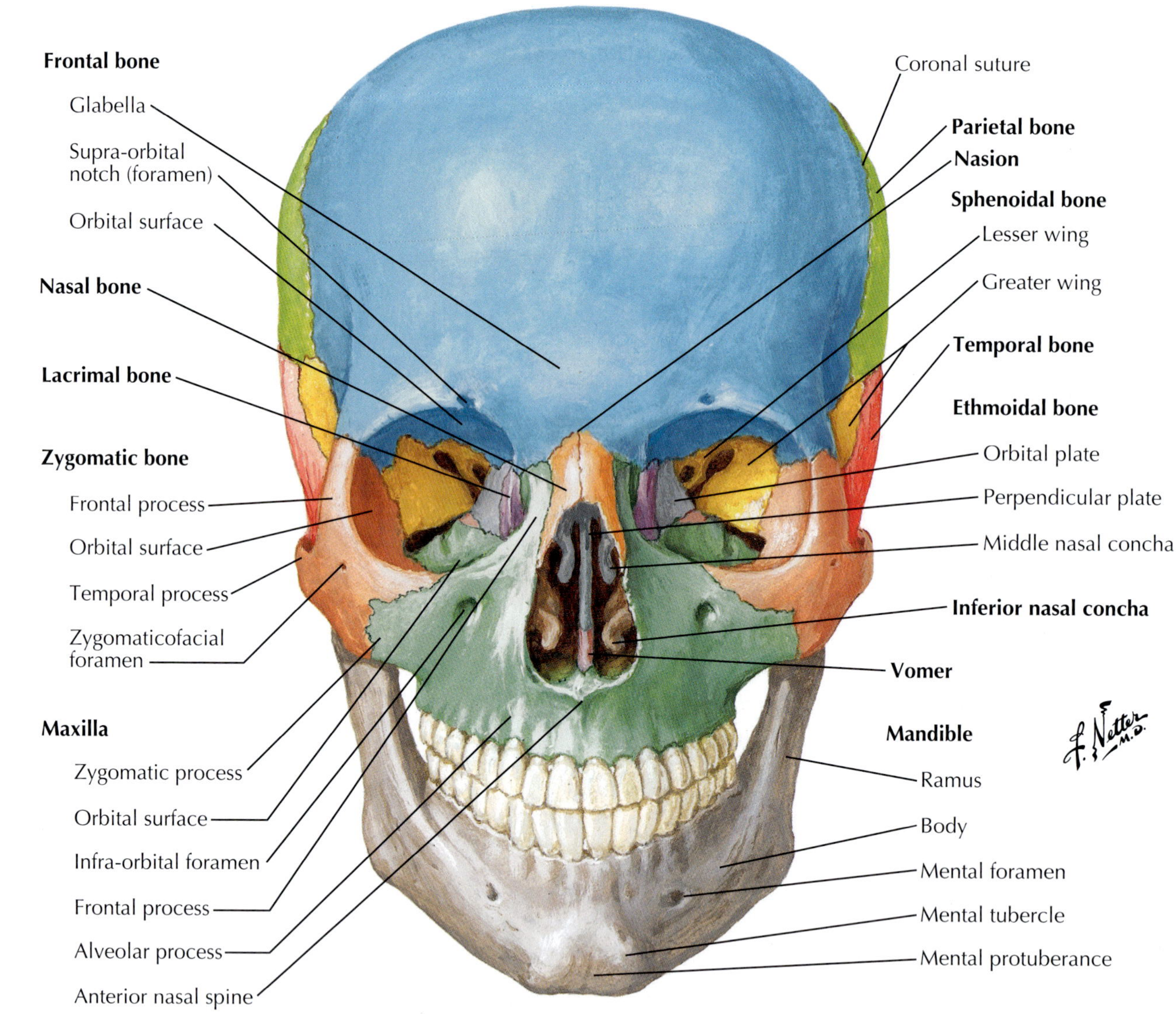

Right orbit: frontal and slightly lateral view

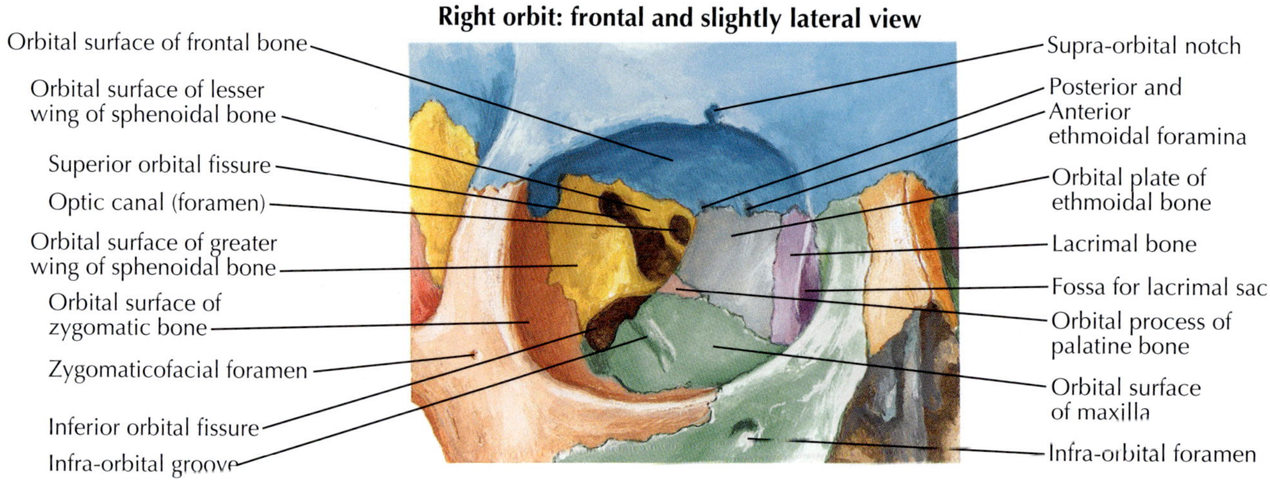

Skull: Anteroposterior Radiograph

See also Plate 4

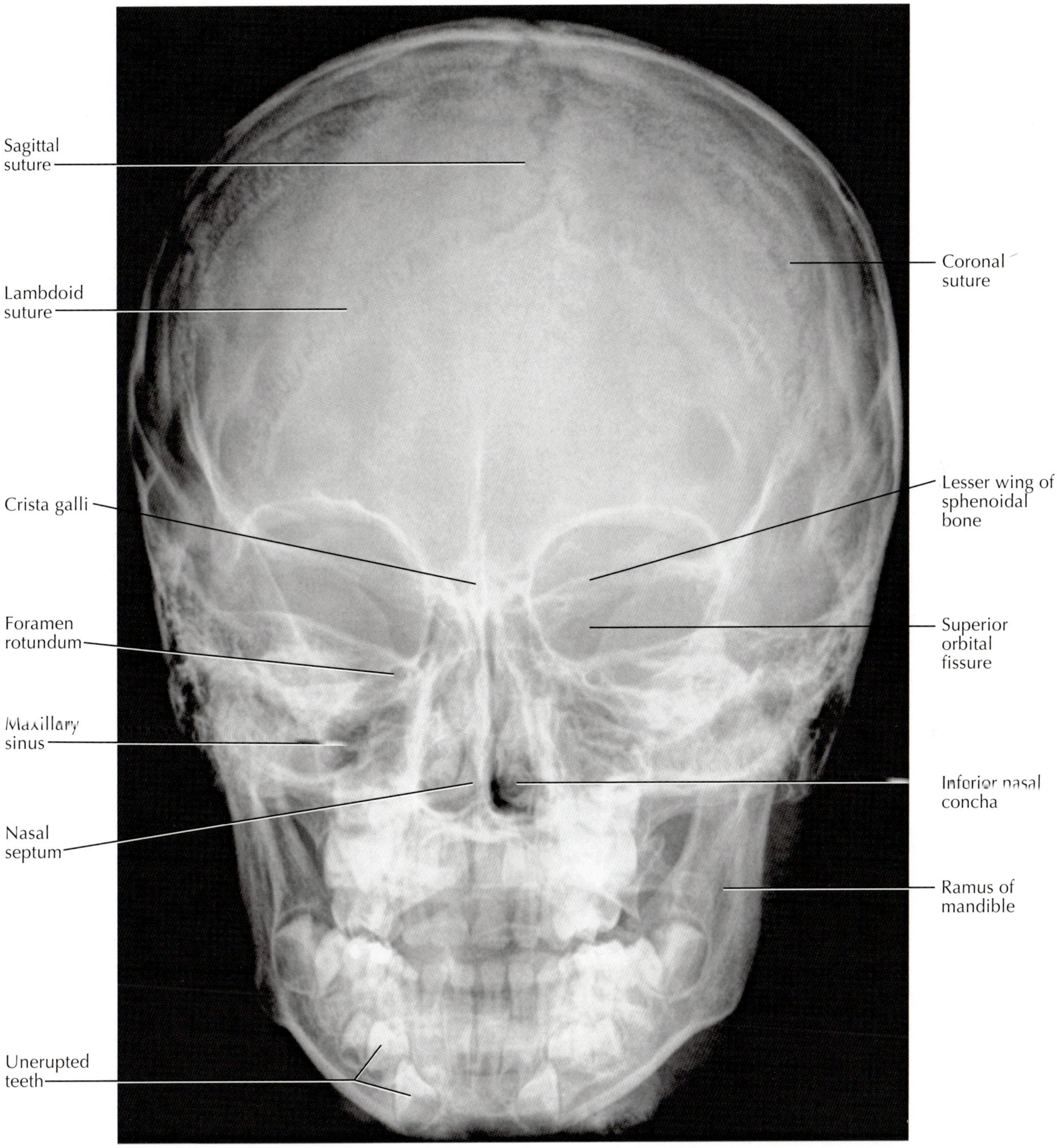

Skull: Lateral View

See also Plates 7, 8, 15

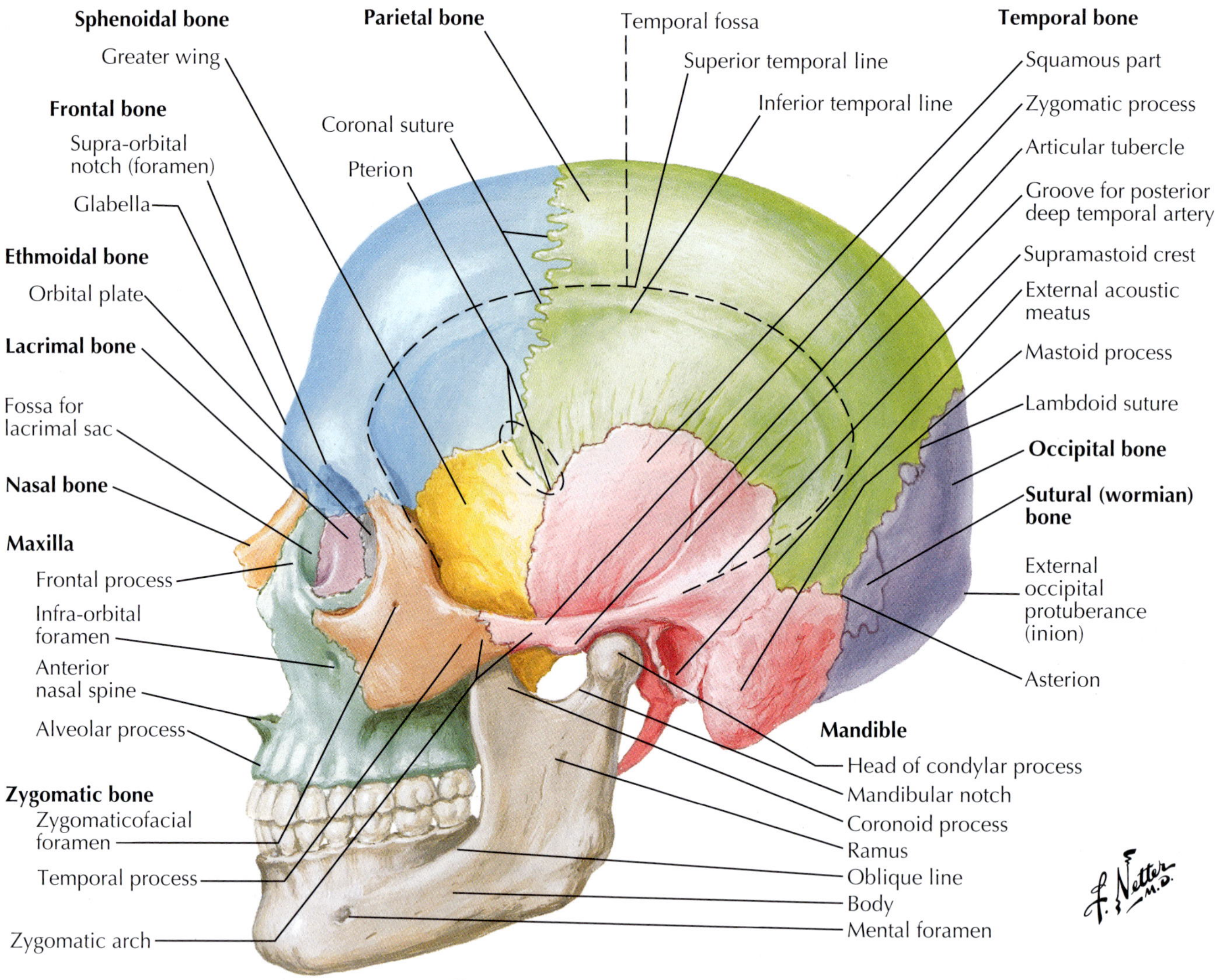

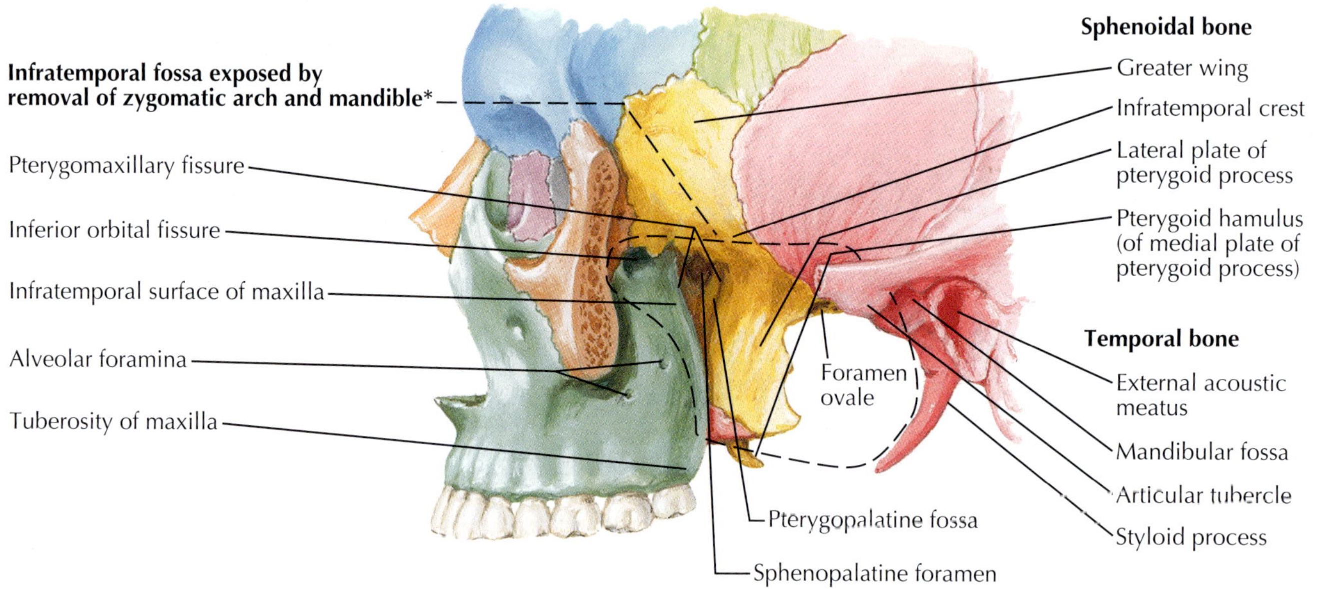

*Superficially, mastoid process forms posterior boundary.

Skull: Lateral Radiograph

See also Plate 8

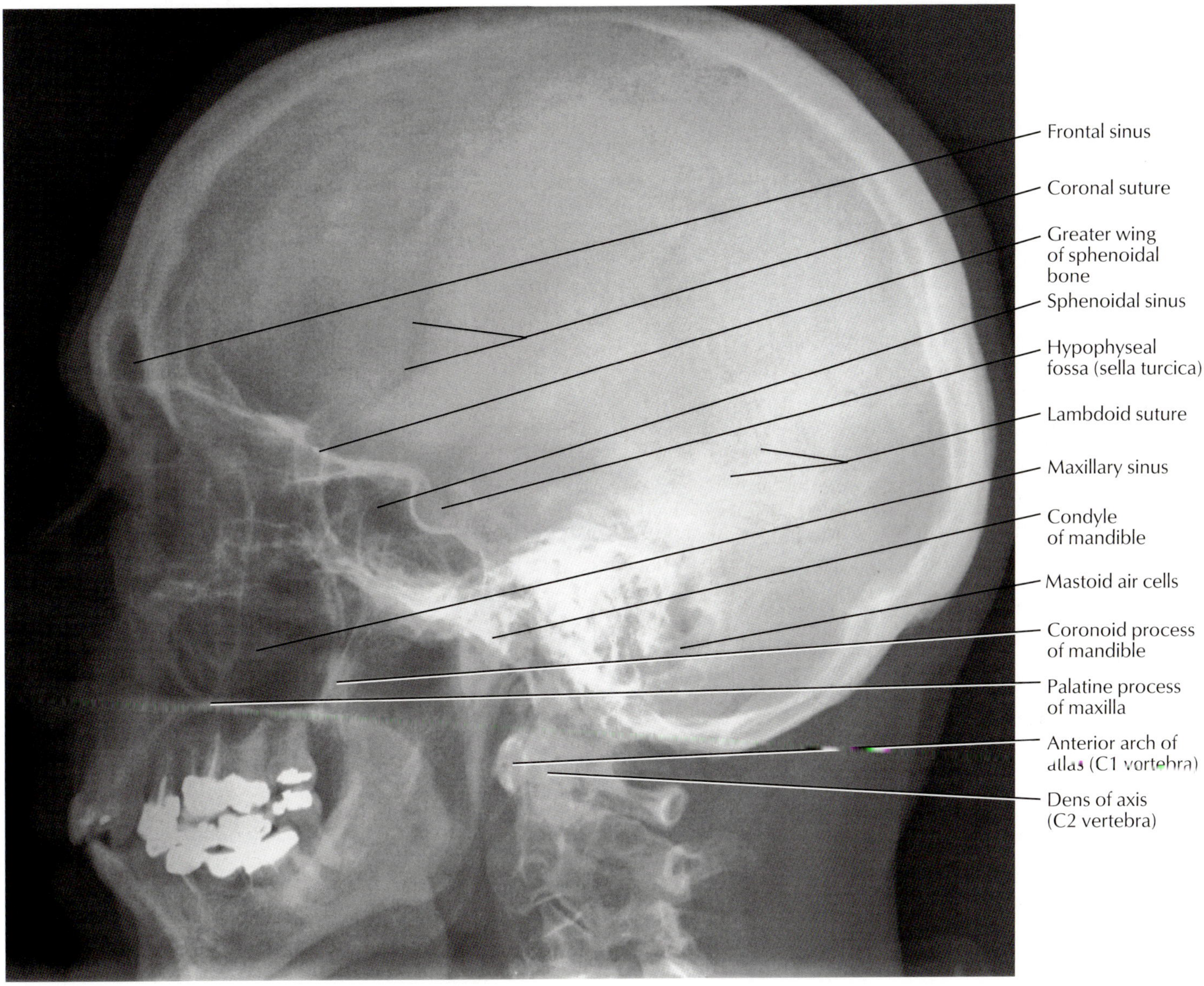

See also Plates 37, 39

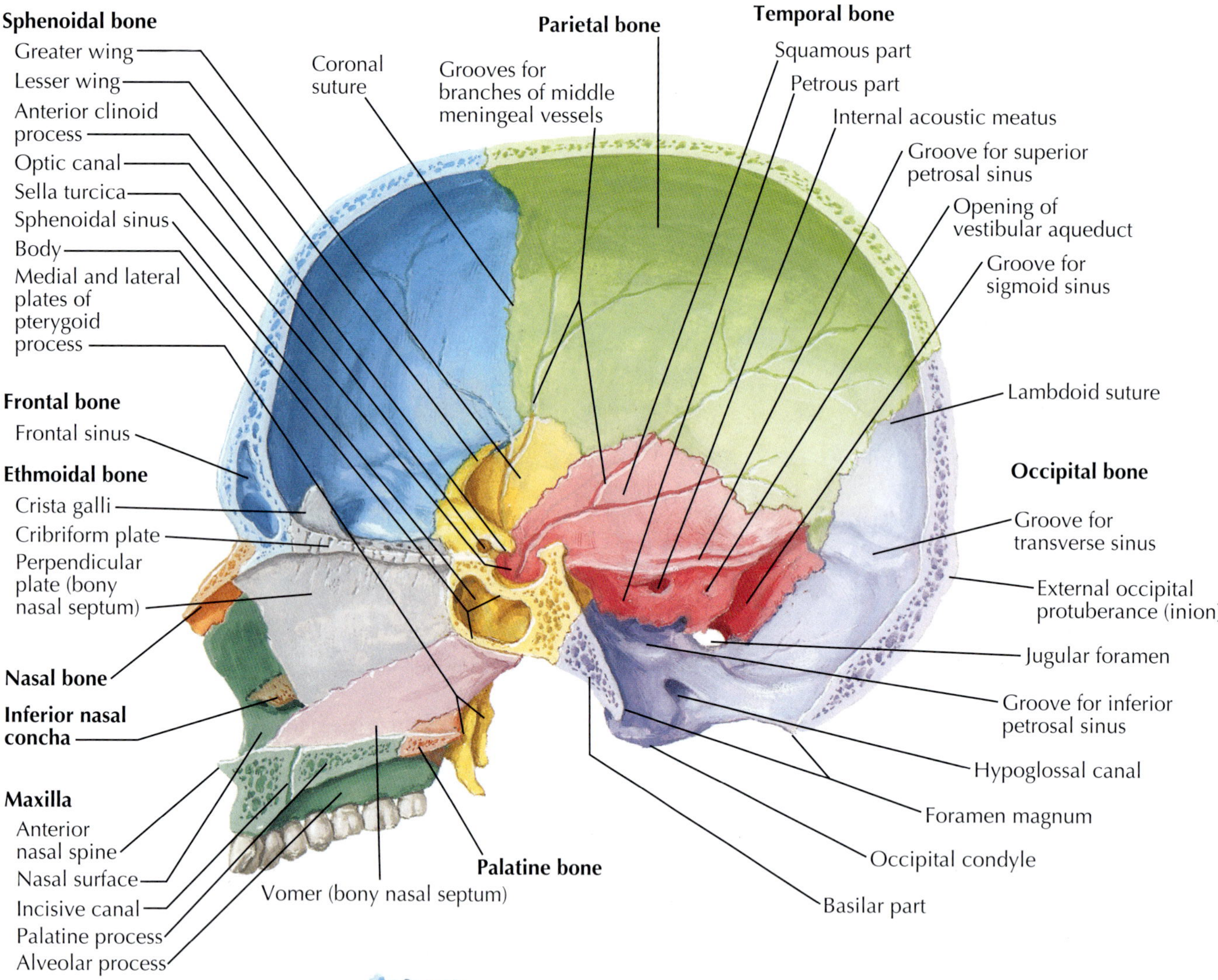

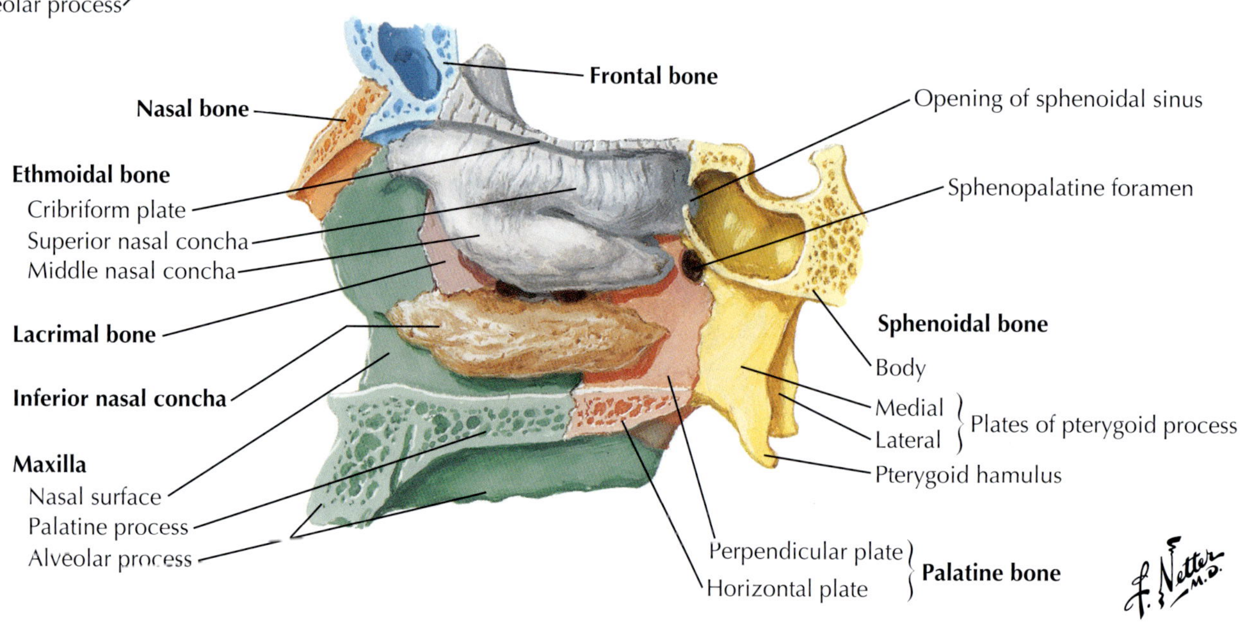

View of lateral nasal wall with nasal septum removed

Superior view

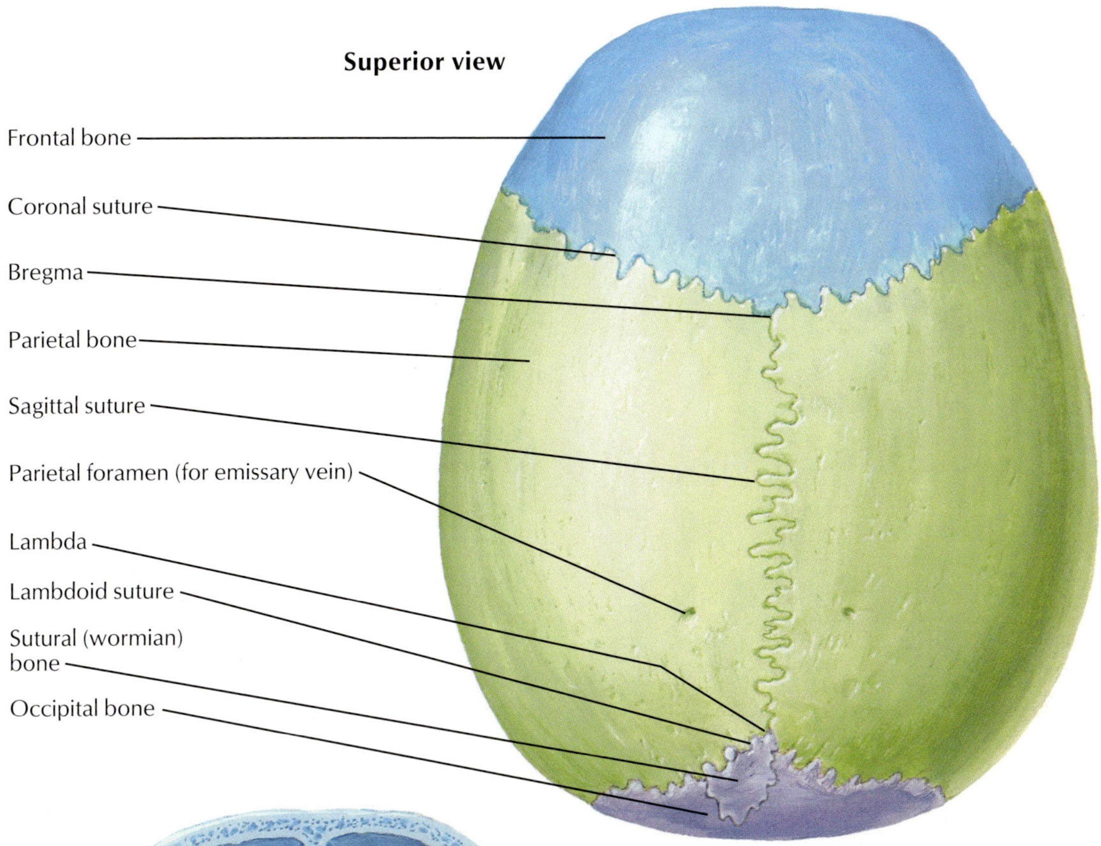

Inferior view

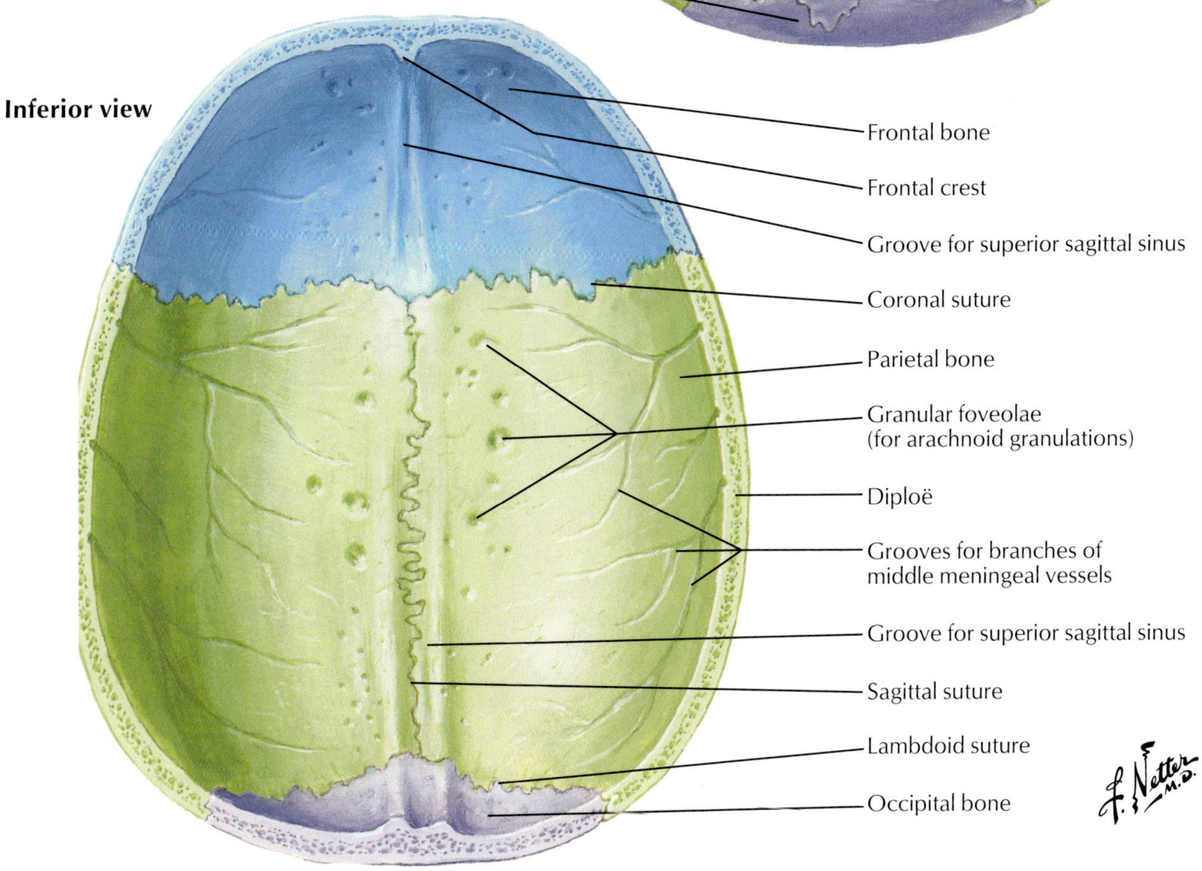

Cranial Base: Inferior View

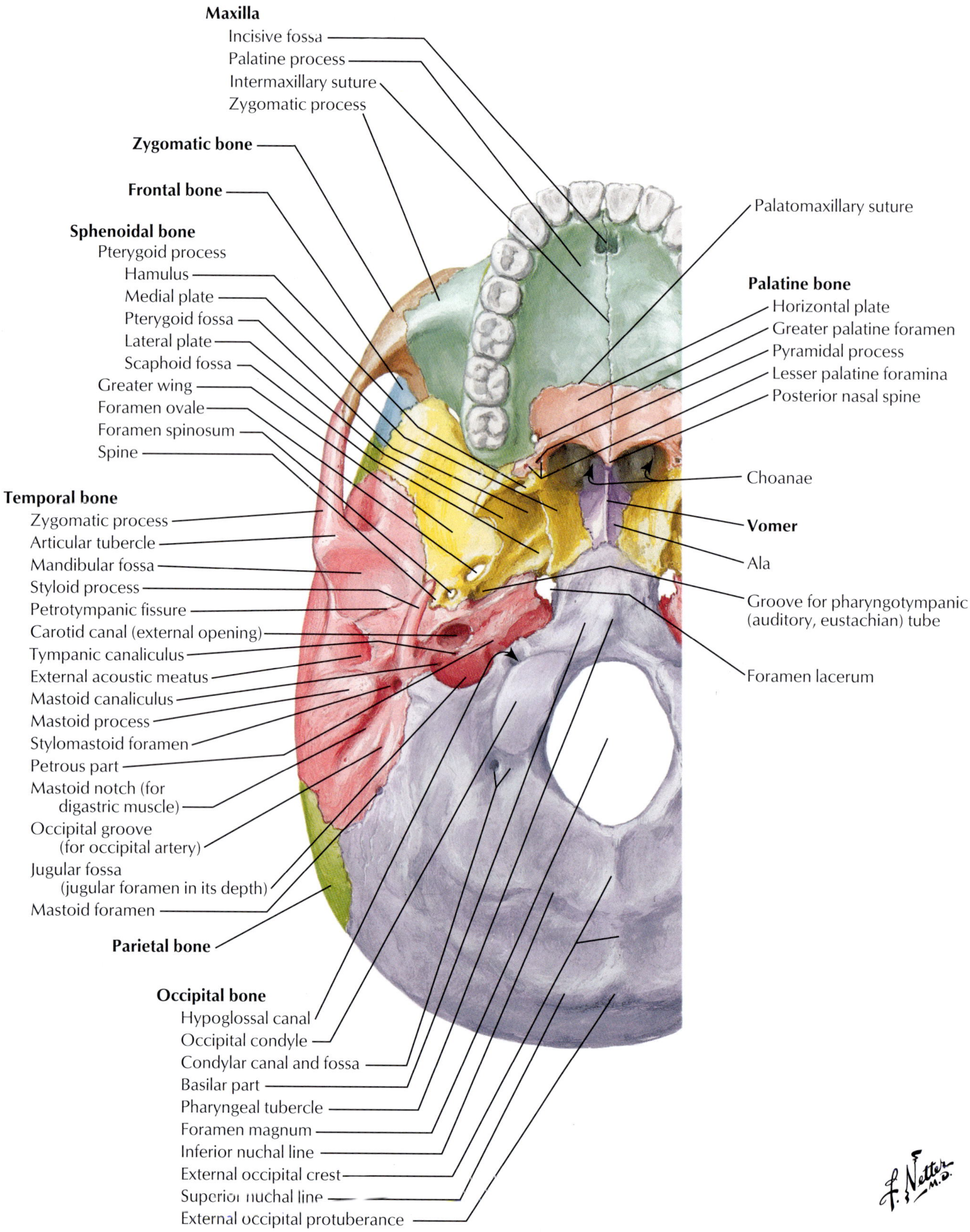

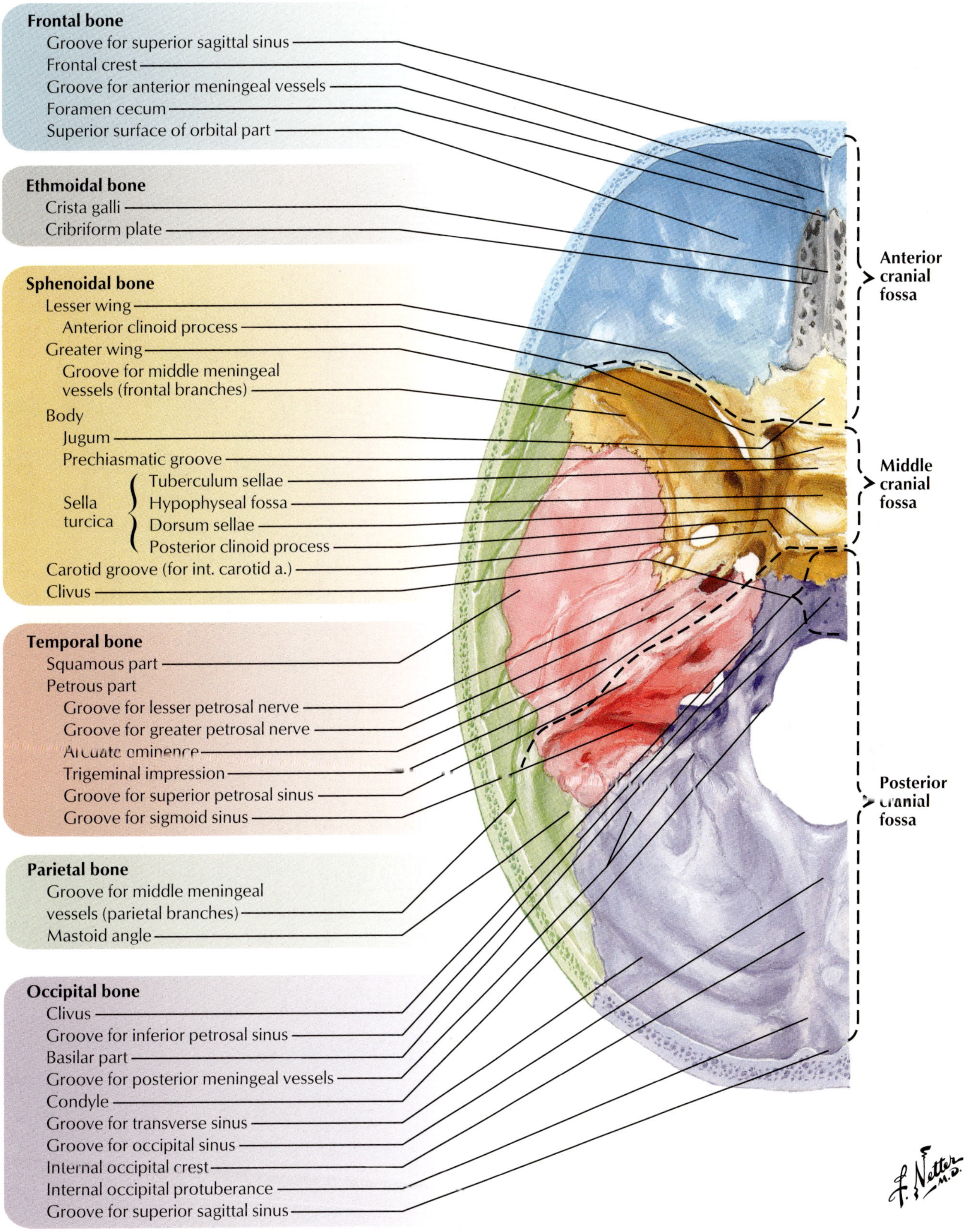

Frontal bone
Groove for superior sagittal sinus
Frontal crest
Groove for anterior meningeal vessels
Foramen cecum
Superior surface of orbital part
Ethmoidal bone
Crista galli
Cribriform plate
Sphenoidal bone
Lesser wing
Anterior clinoid process
Greater wing
Groove for middle meningeal vessels (frontal branches)
Body
Jugum
Prechiasmatic groove
Sella turcica
Tuberculum sellae
Hypophyseal fossa
Dorsum sellae
Posterior clinoid process
Carotid groove (for int. carotid a.)
Clivus
Temporal bone
Squamous part
Petrous part
Groove for lesser petrosal nerve
Groove for greater petrosal nerve
Arcuate eminence
Trigeminal impression
Groove for superior petrosal sinus
Groove for sigmoid sinus
Parietal bone
Groove for middle meningeal vessels (parietal branches)
Mastoid angle
Occipital bone
Clivus
Groove for inferior petrosal sinus
Basilar part
Groove for posterior meningeal vessels
Condyle
Groove for transverse sinus
Groove for occipital sinus
Internal occipital crest
Internal occipital protuberance
Groove for superior sagittal sinus
Anterior cranial fossa
Middle cranial fossa
Posterior cranial fossa
F. Netter M.D.

Foramina and Canals of Cranial Base: Inferior View

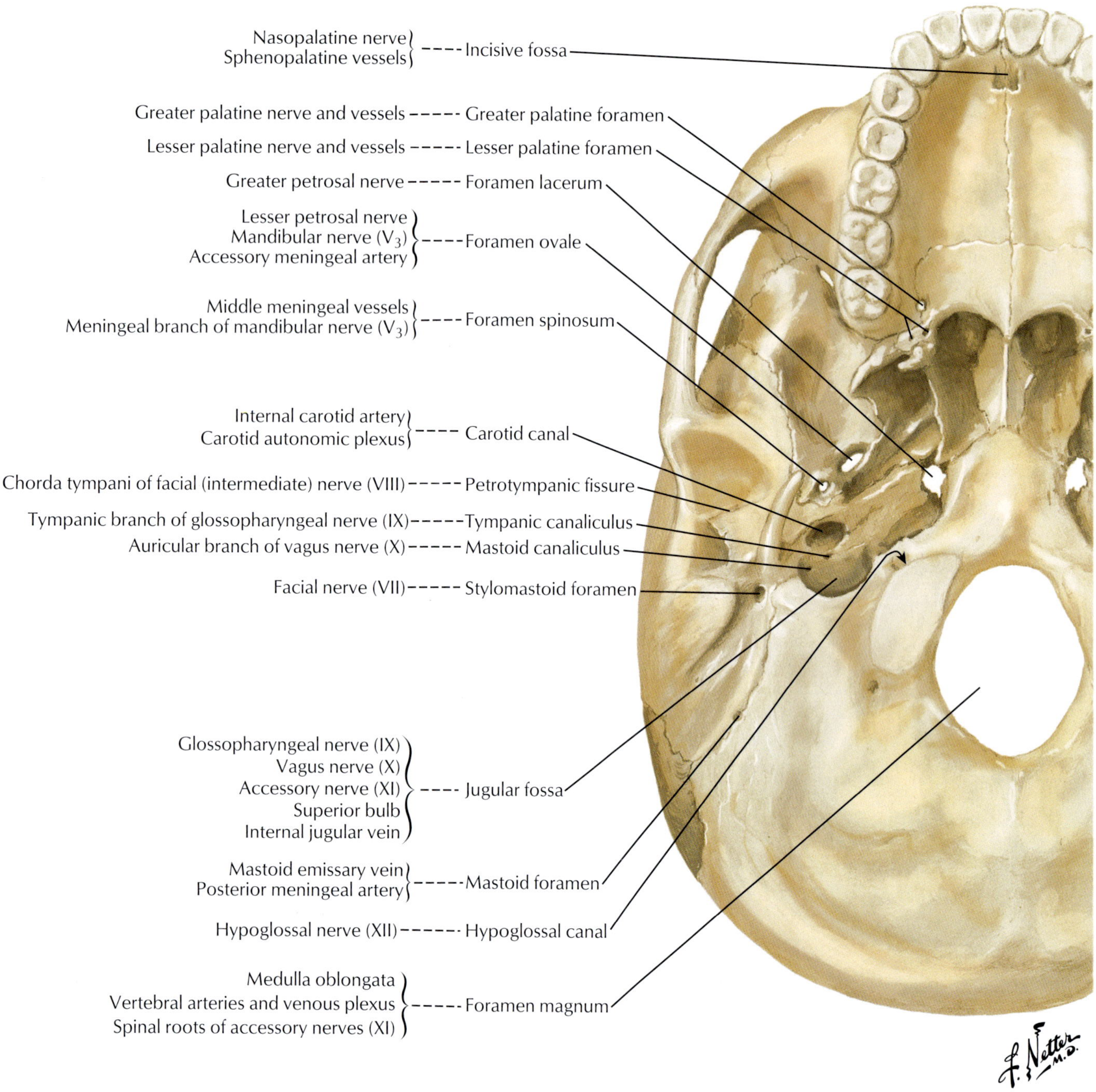

Foramina and Canals of Cranial Base: Superior View

See also Plate 11

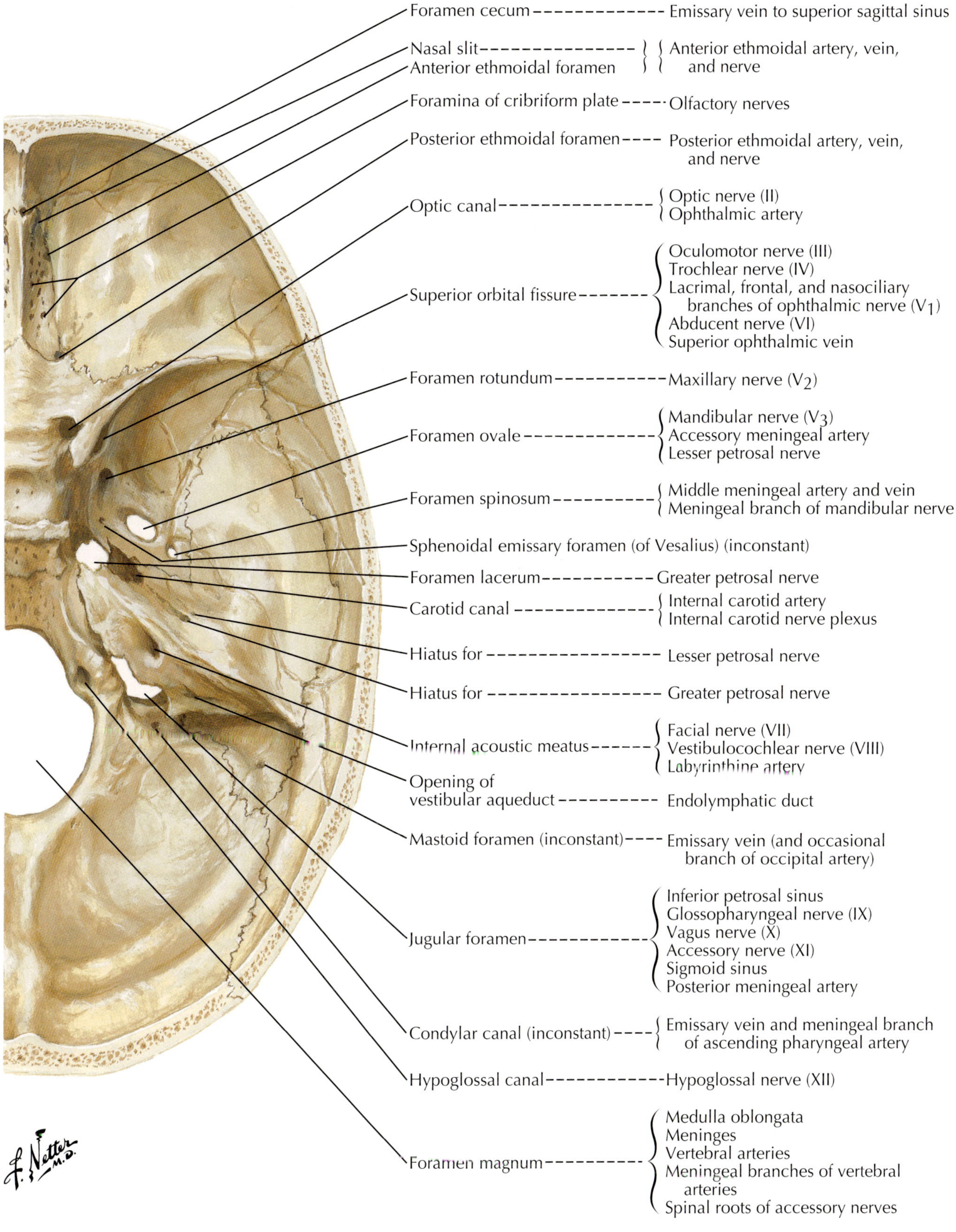

Skull of Newborn

See also Plate 6

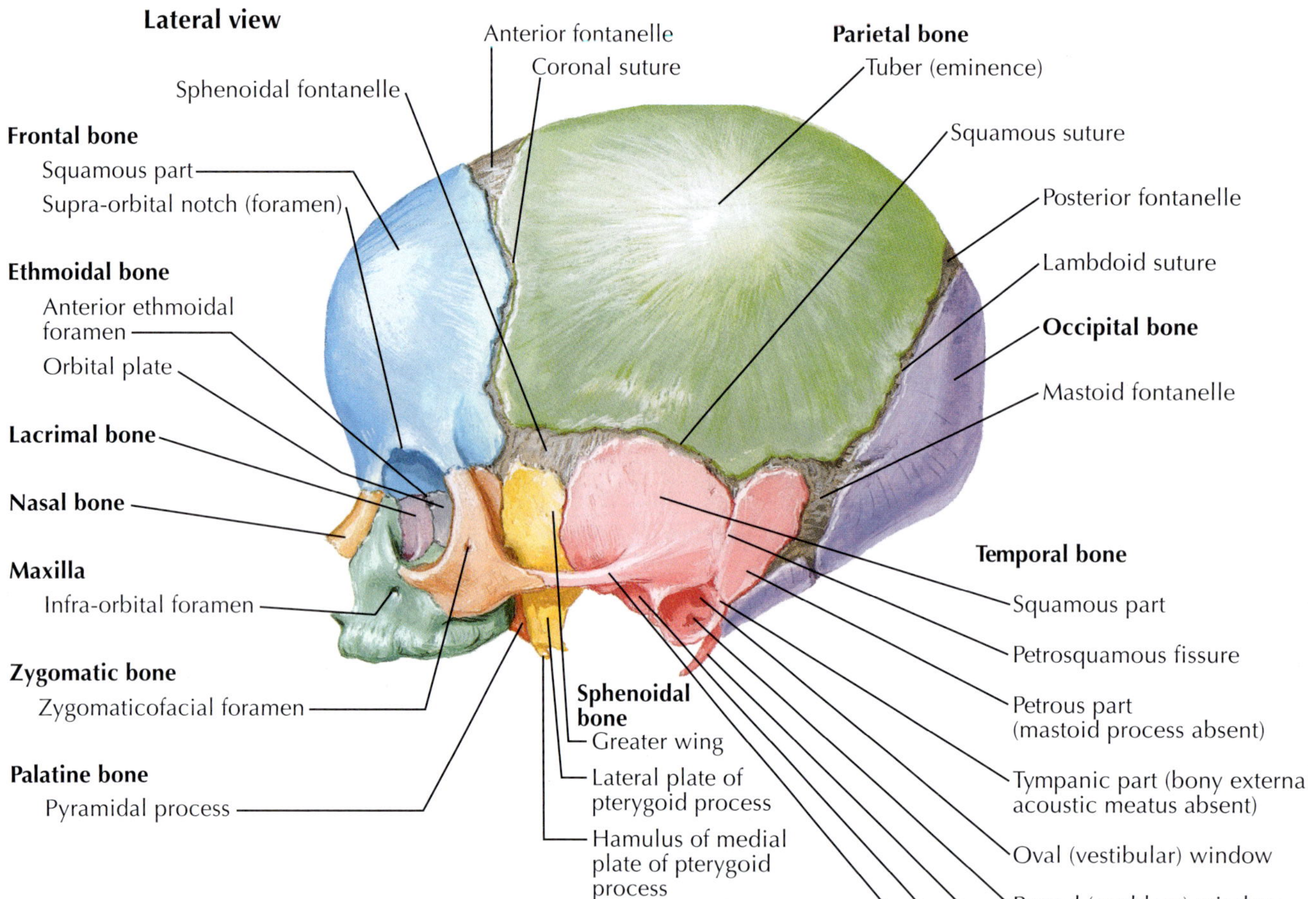

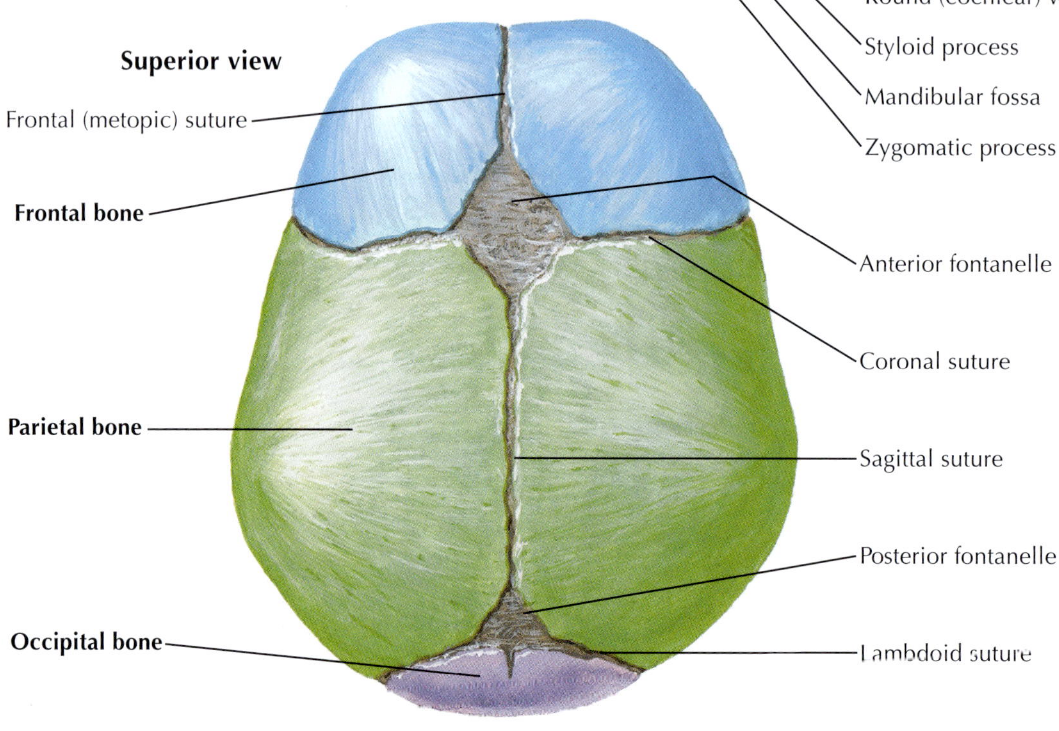

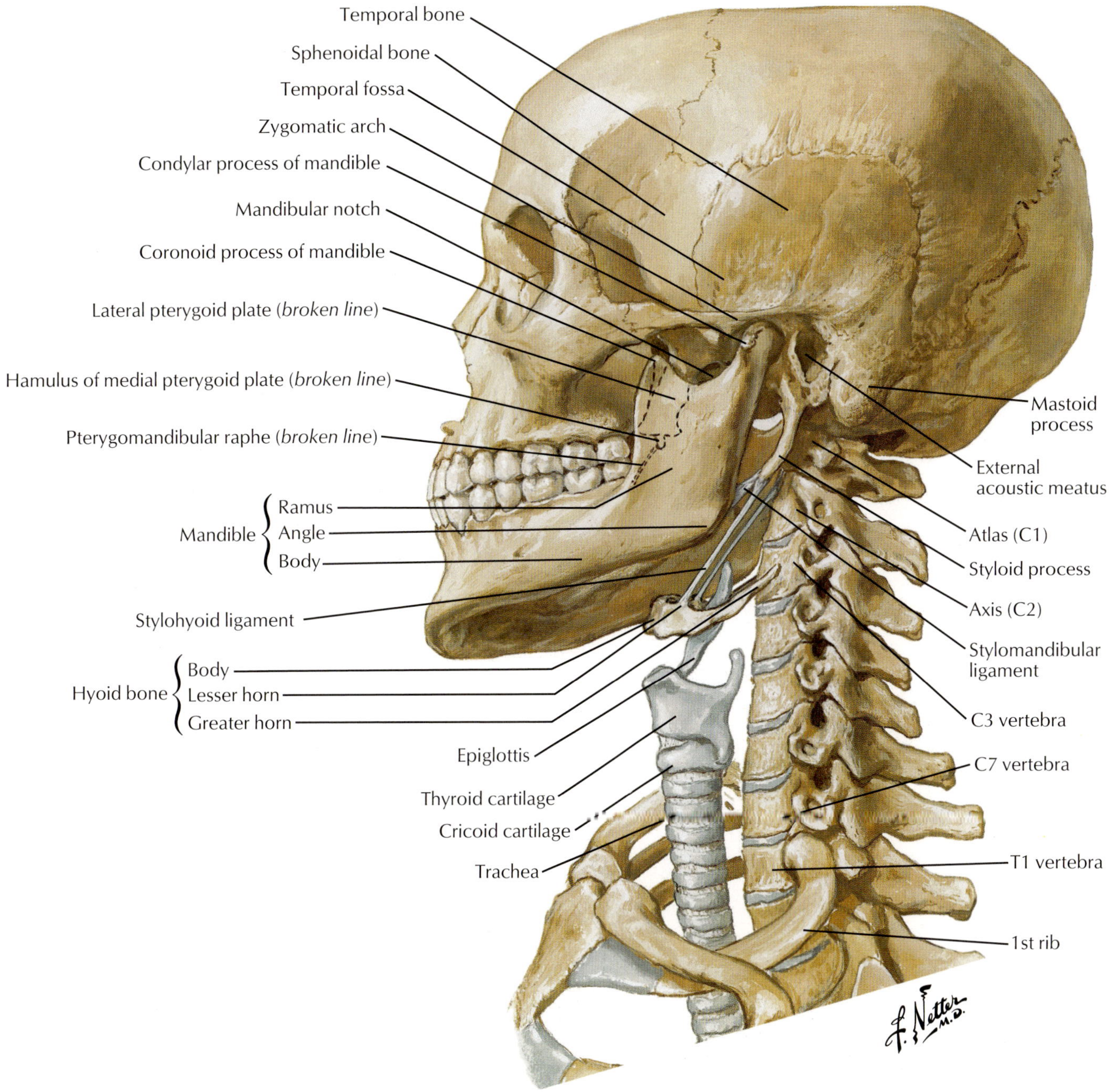
Temporal bone
Sphenoidal bone
Temporal fossa
Zygomatic arch
Condylar process of mandible
Mandibular notch
Coronoid process of mandible
Lateral pterygoid plate (broken line)
Hamulus of medial pterygoid plate (broken line)
Pterygomandibular raphe (broken line)
Mandible
Ramus
Angle
Body
Stylohyoid ligament
Hyoid bone
Body
Lesser horn
Greater horn
Epiglottis
Thyroid cartilage
Cricoid cartilage
Trachea
Mastoid process
External acoustic meatus
Atlas (C1)
Styloid process
Axis (C2)
Stylomandibular ligament
C3 vertebra
C7 vertebra
T1 vertebra
1st rib

Pterygoid Fossae: Posterior and Inferolateral Views

See also **Plates 39, 40, 41**

Posterior view

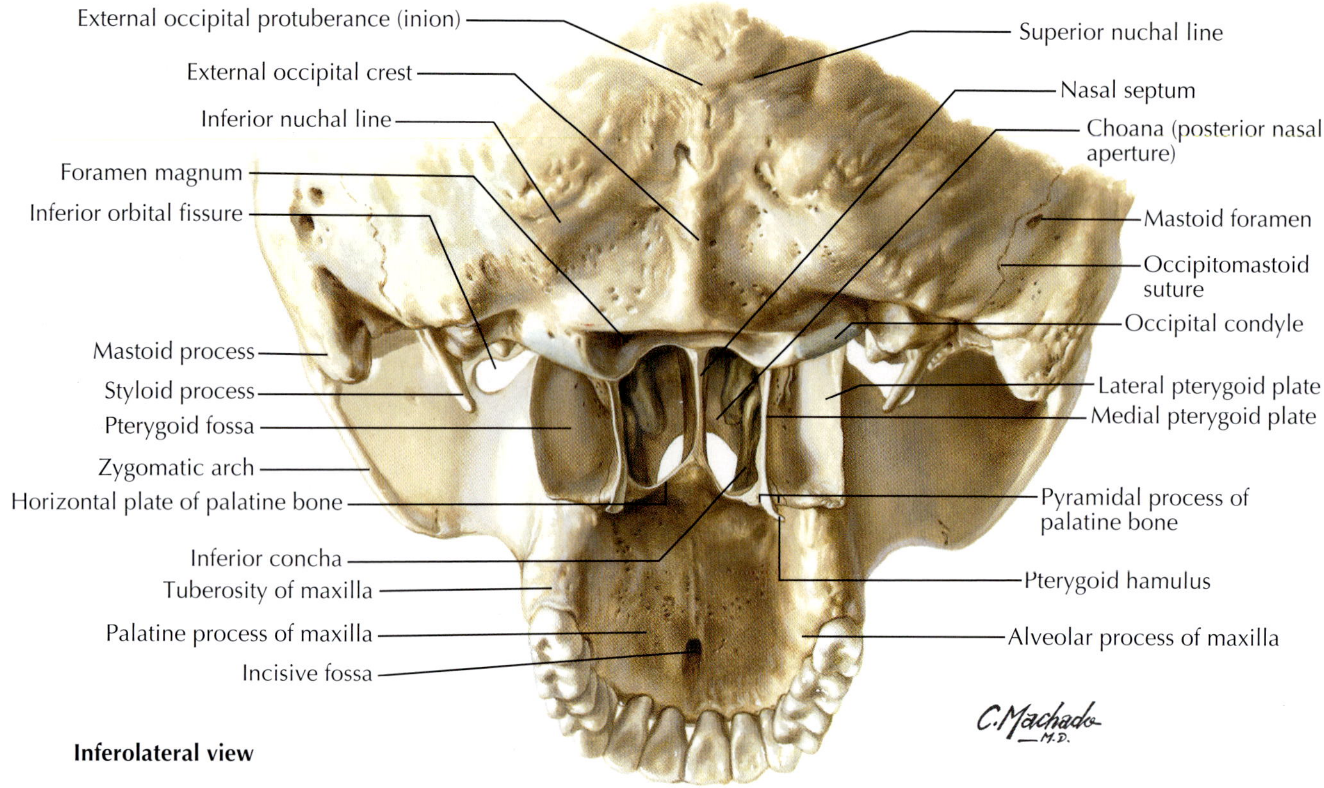

Inferolateral view

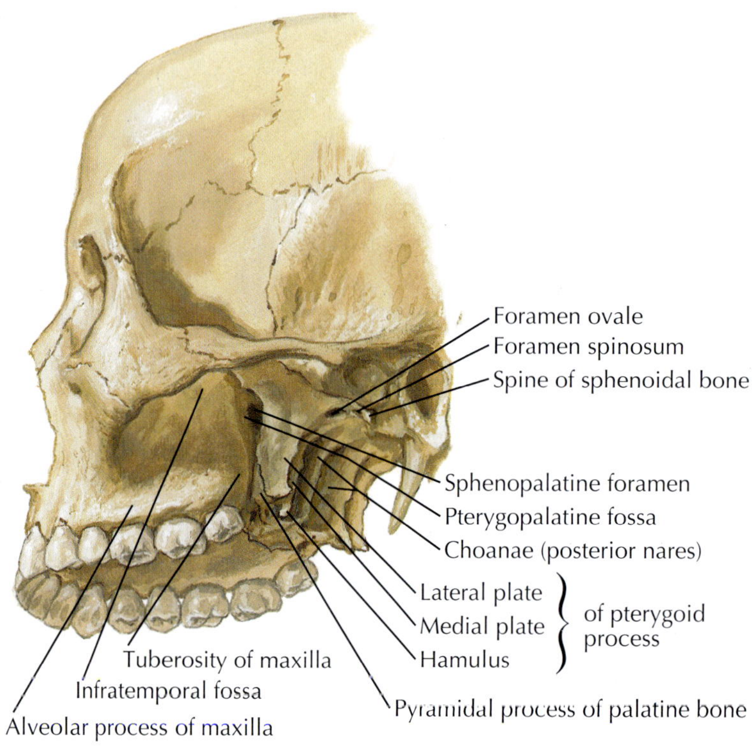

Mandible

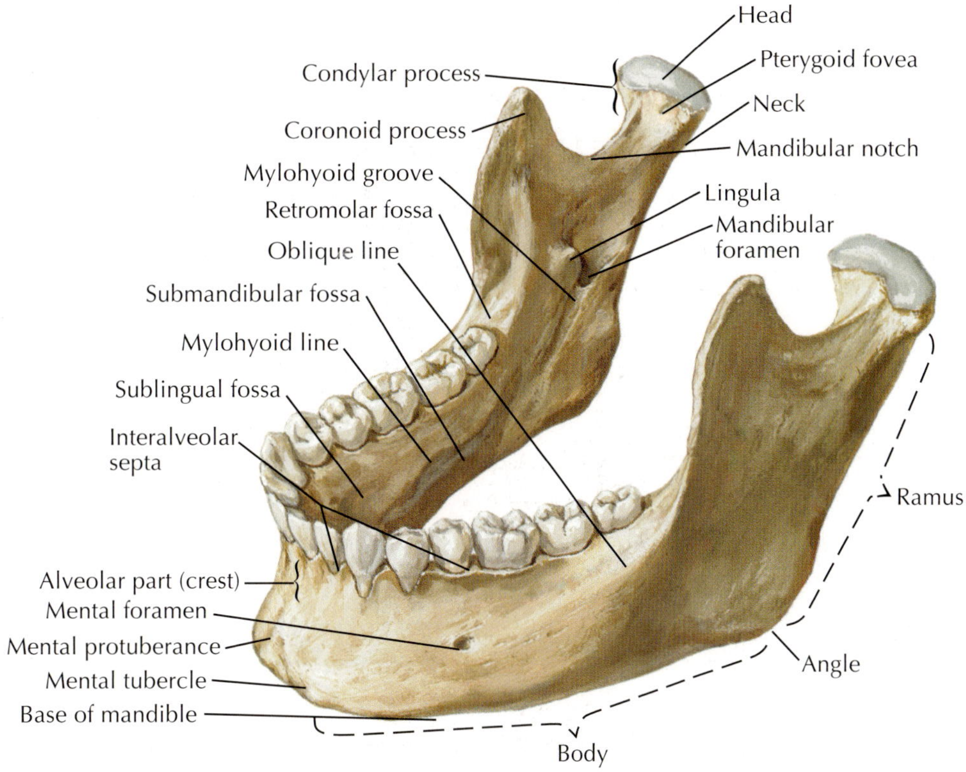

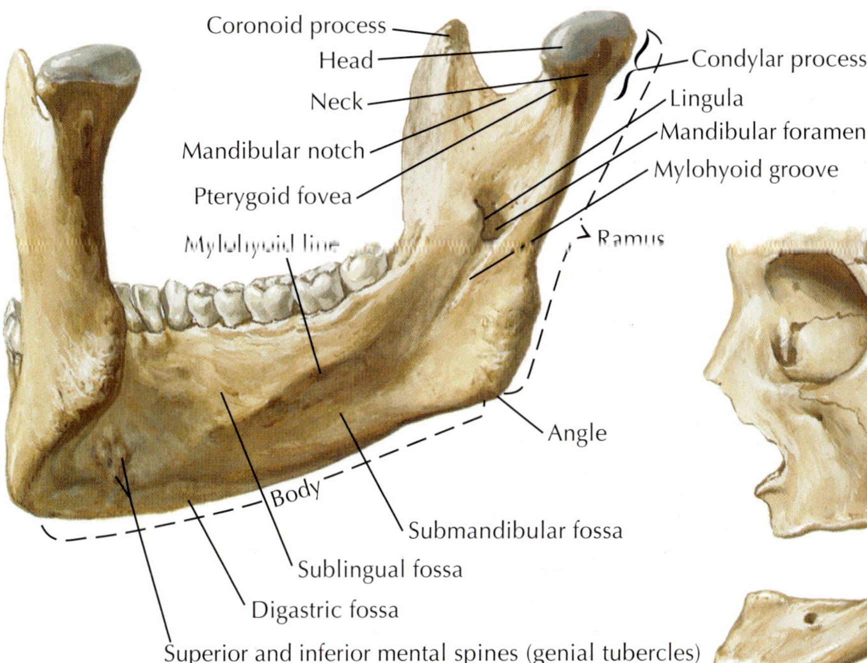

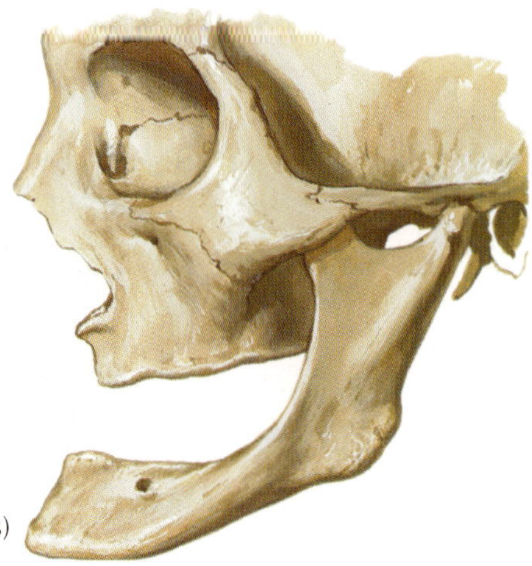

Mandible of aged person (edentulous)

Temporomandibular Joint

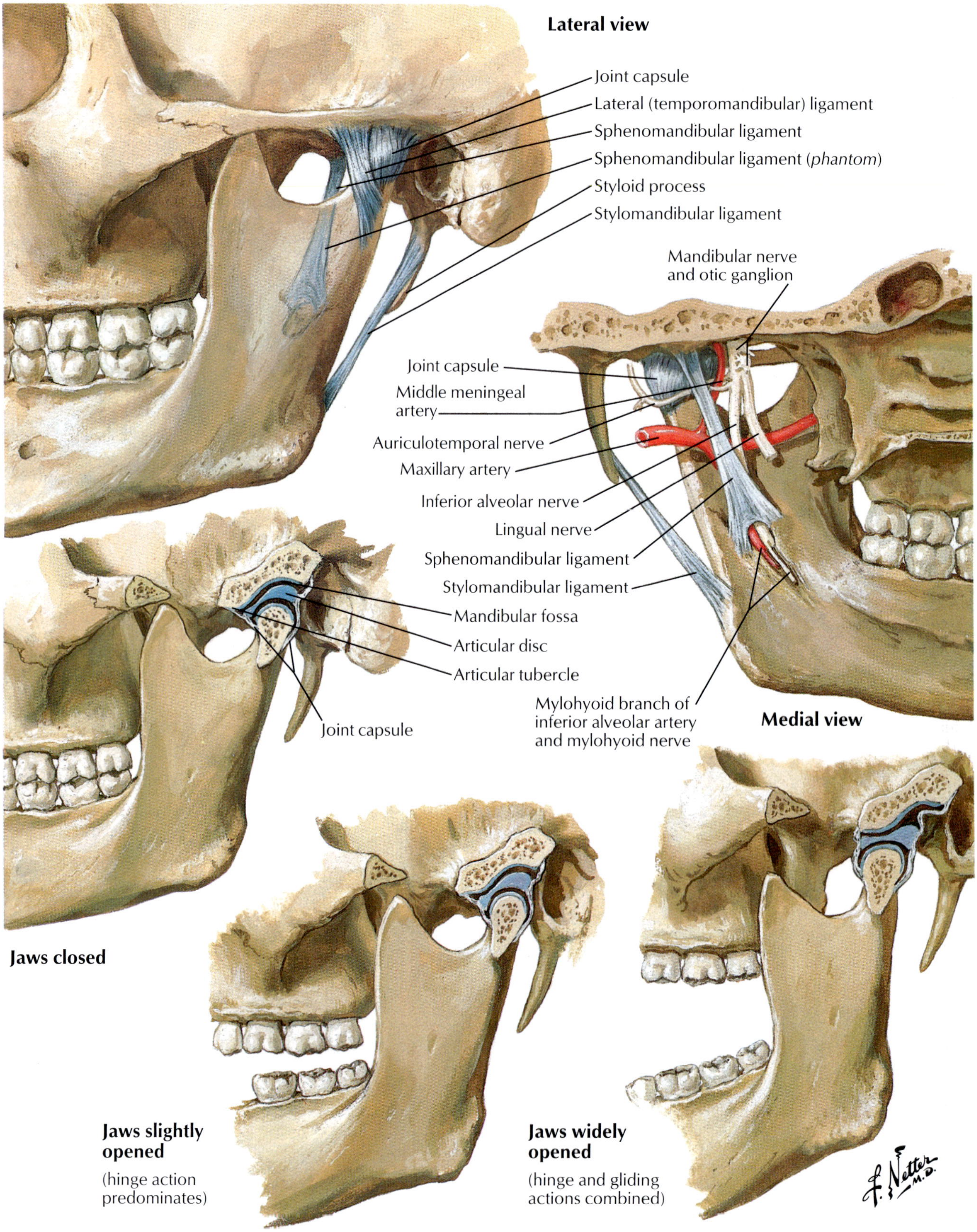

Cervical Vertebrae: Atlas and Axis

See also Plates 21, 22

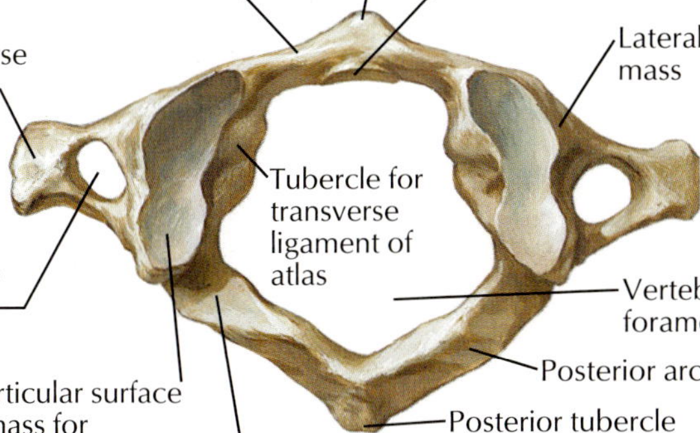

Atlas (C1): superior view

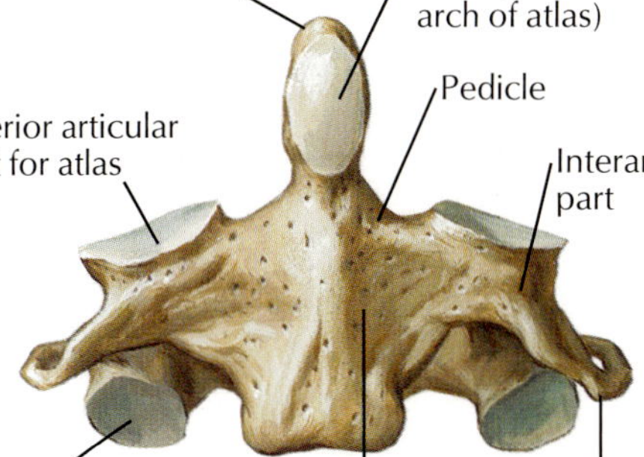

Axis (C2): anterior view

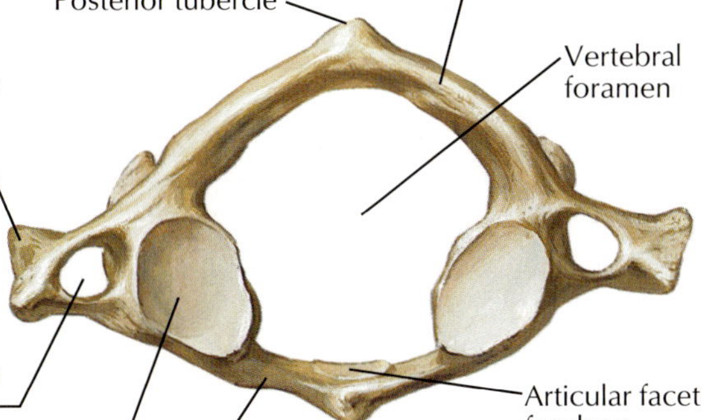

Atlas (C1): inferior view

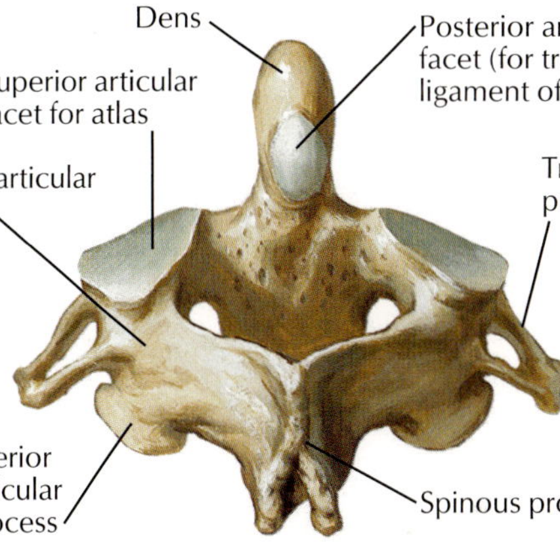

Axis (C2): posterosuperior view

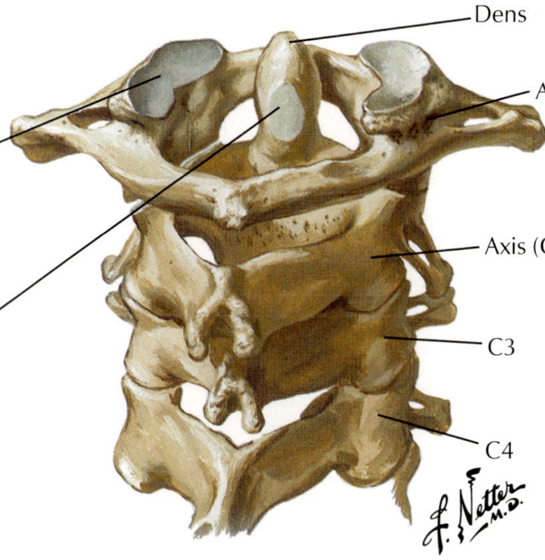

Upper cervical vertebrae, assembled: posterosuperior view

See also Plates 21, 22

Inferior aspect of C3 and superior aspect of C4 showing the sites of the facet and uncovertebral articulations

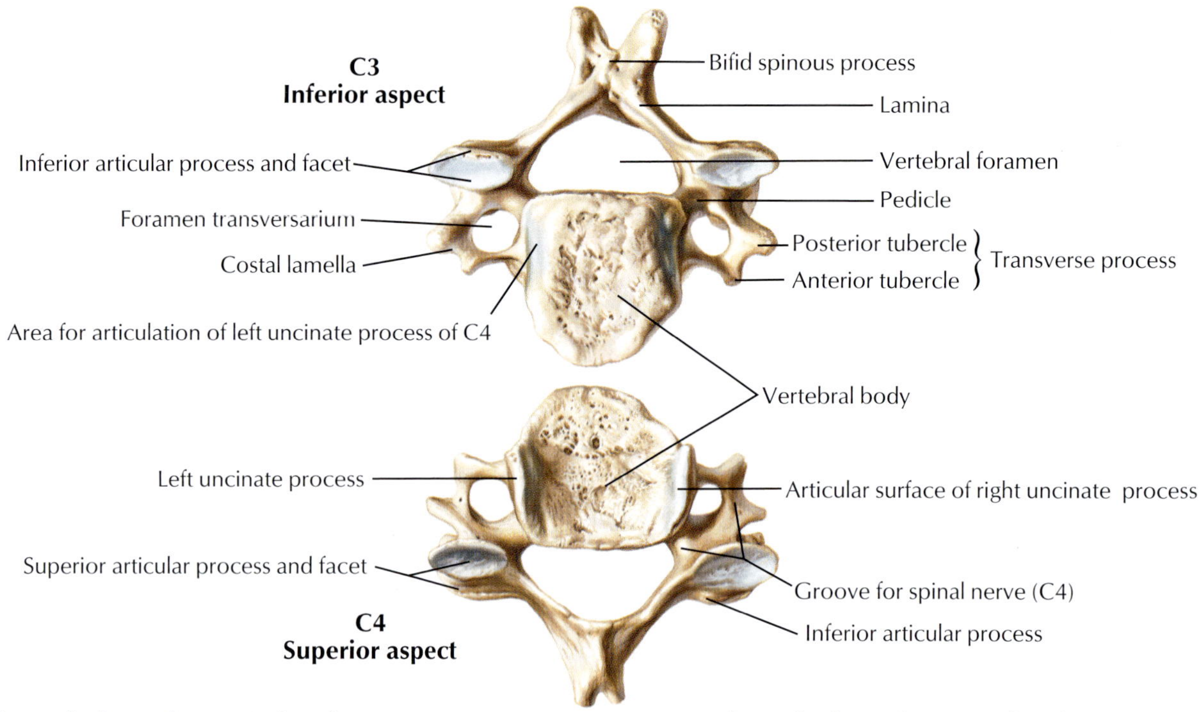

4th cervical vertebra: anterior view

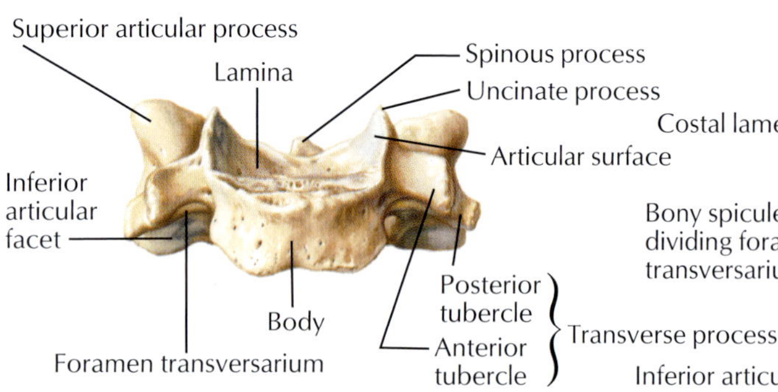

7th cervical vertebra: anterior view

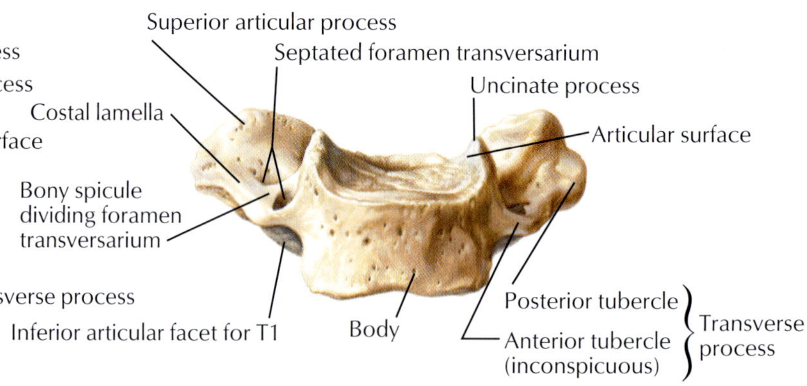

7th cervical vertebra (vertebra prominens): superior view

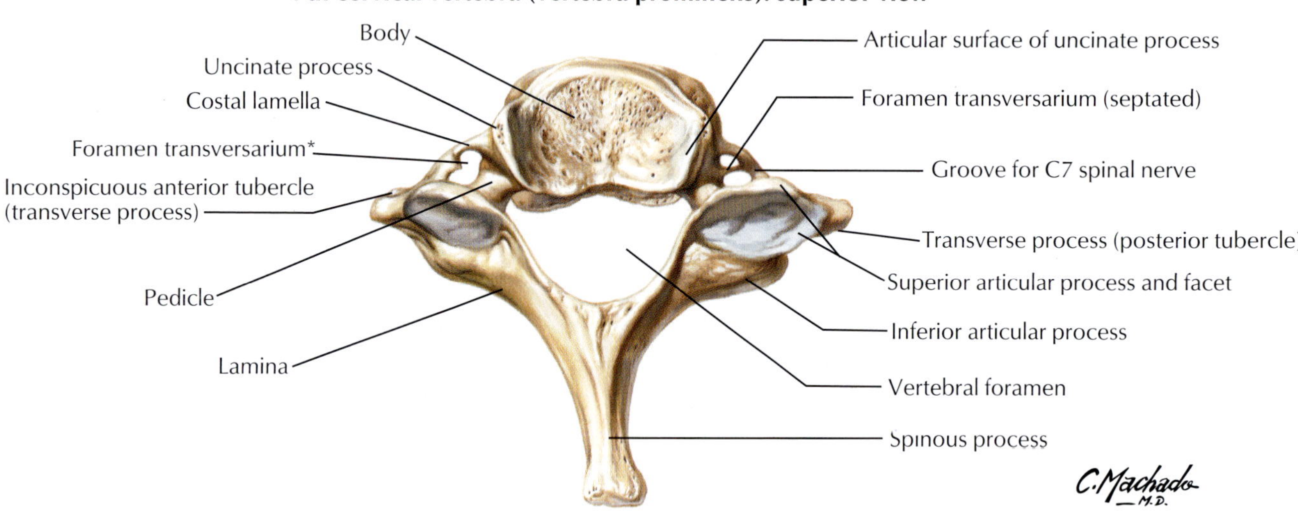

**The foramina transversaria of C7 transmit vertebral veins, but usually not the vertebral artery, and are asymmetrical in this specimen.*

Cervical vertebrae: anterior view

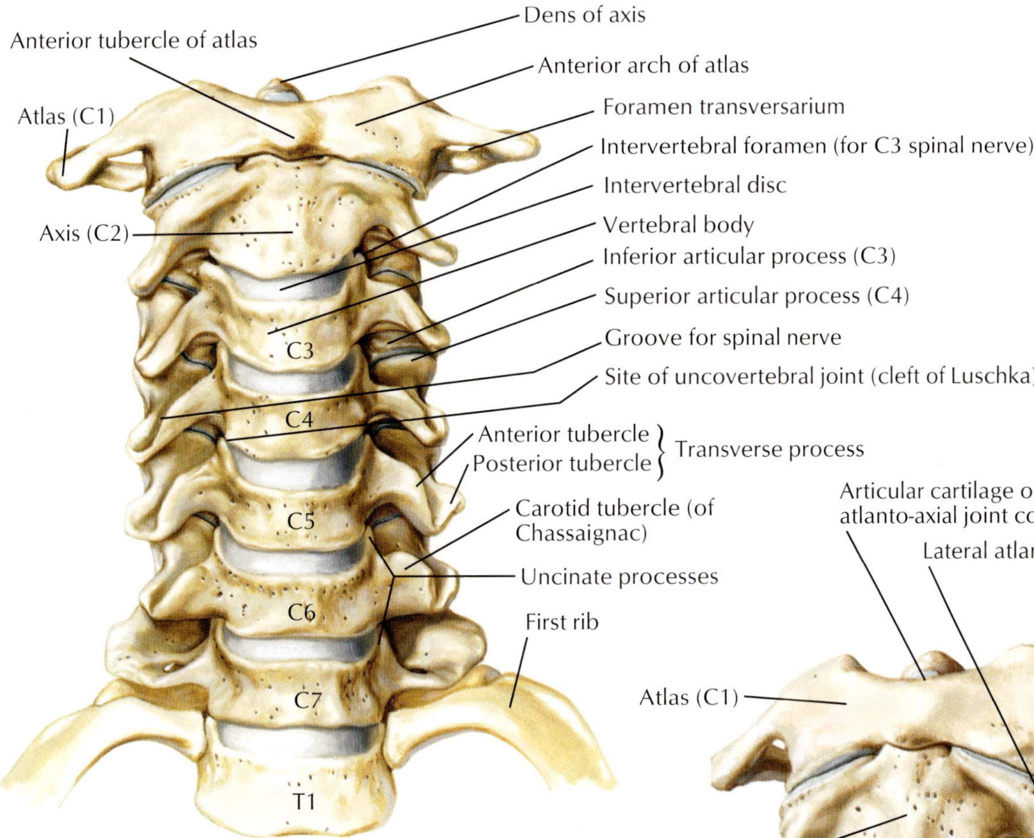

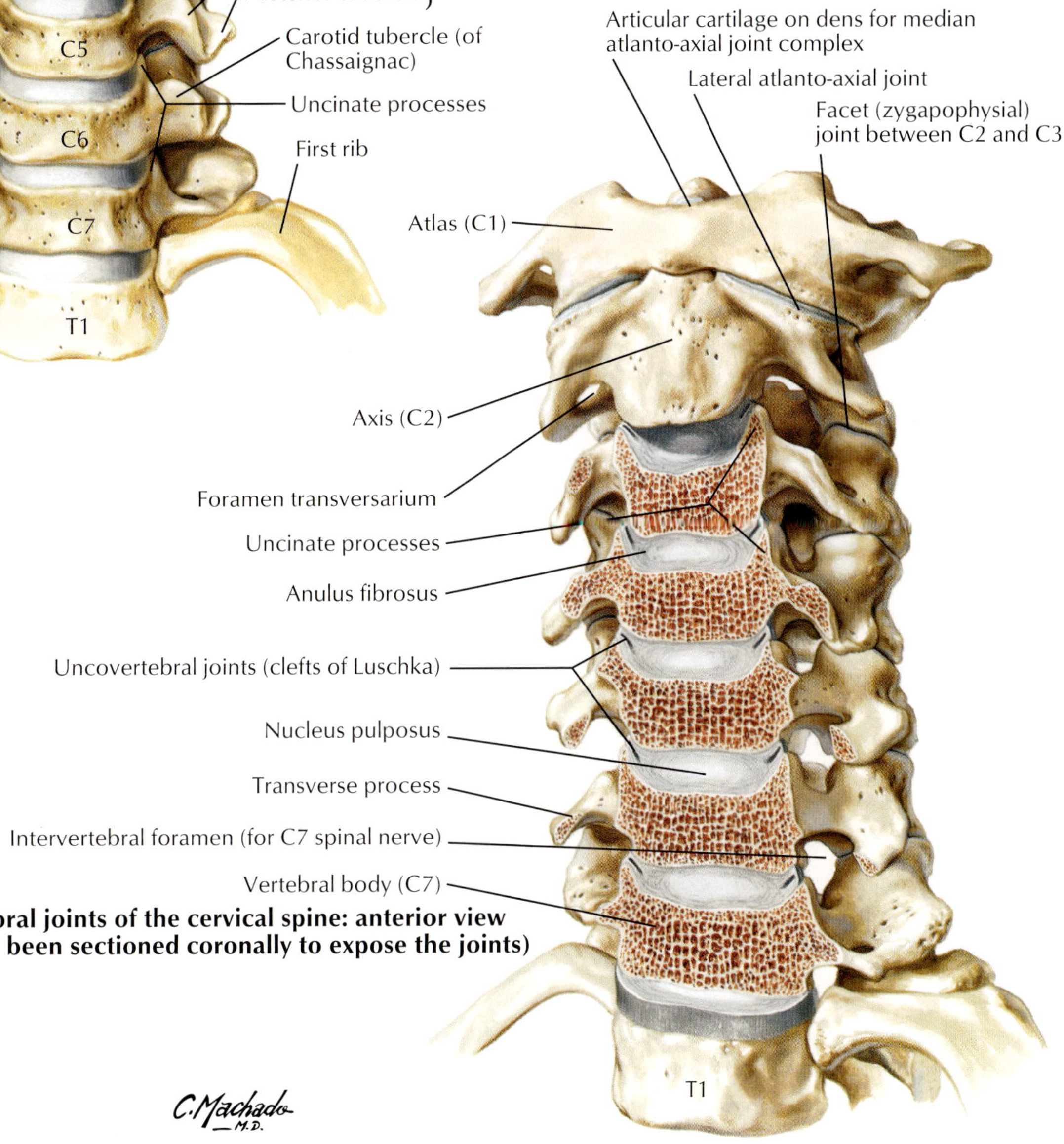

The uncovertebral joints of the cervical spine: anterior view (C3 to C7 have been sectioned coronally to expose the joints)

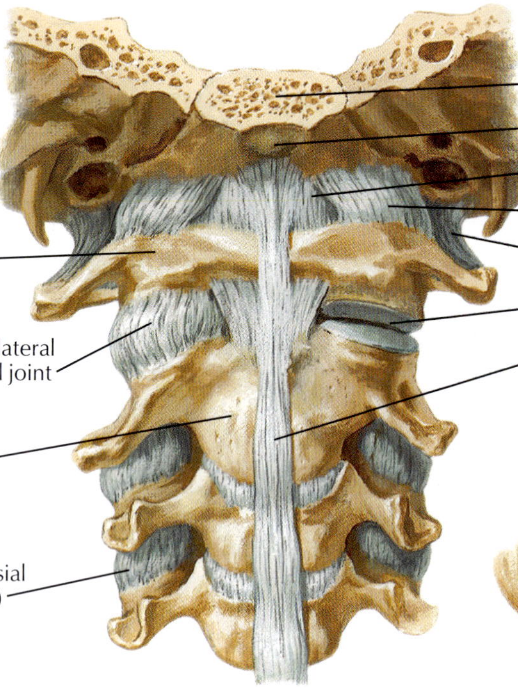

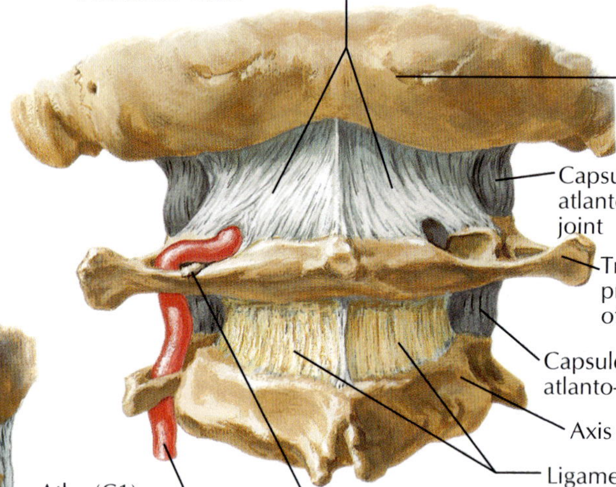

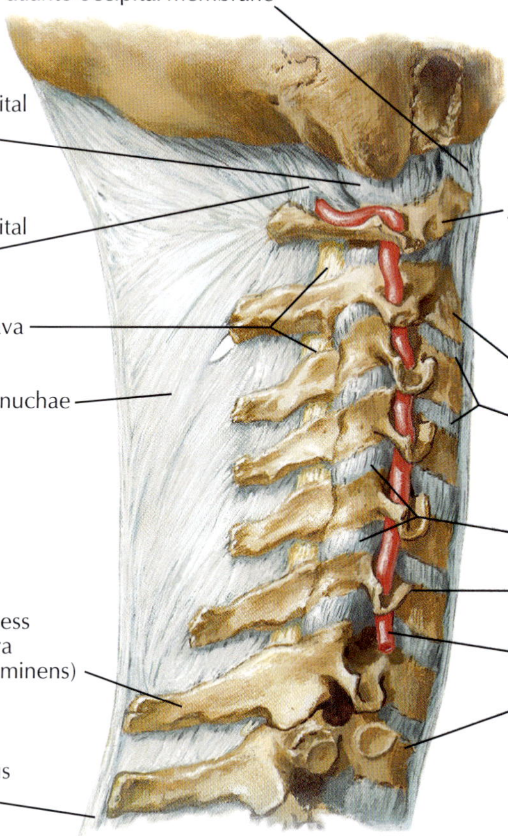

Right lateral view

Upper part of vertebral canal with spinous processes and parts of vertebral arches removed to expose ligaments on posterior vertebral bodies: posterior view

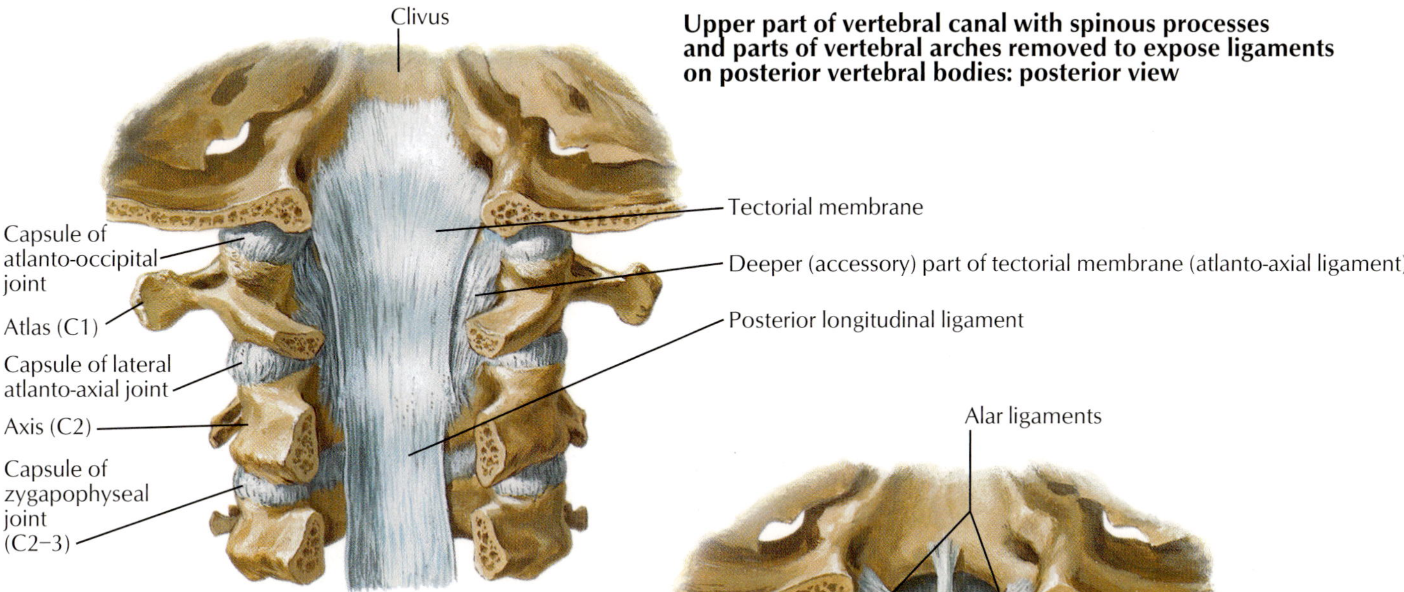

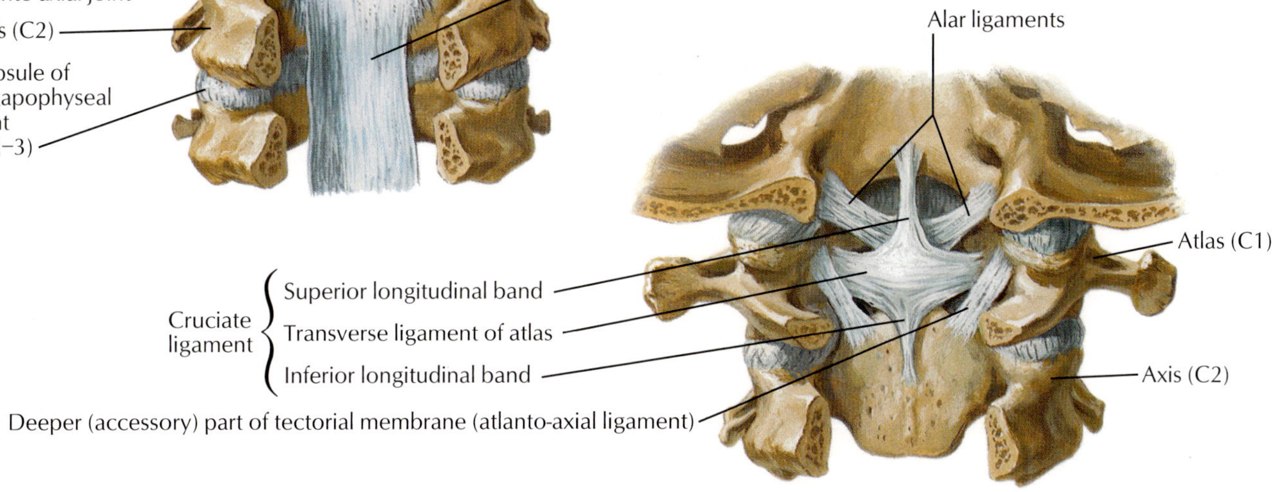

Principal part of tectorial membrane removed to expose deeper ligaments: posterior view

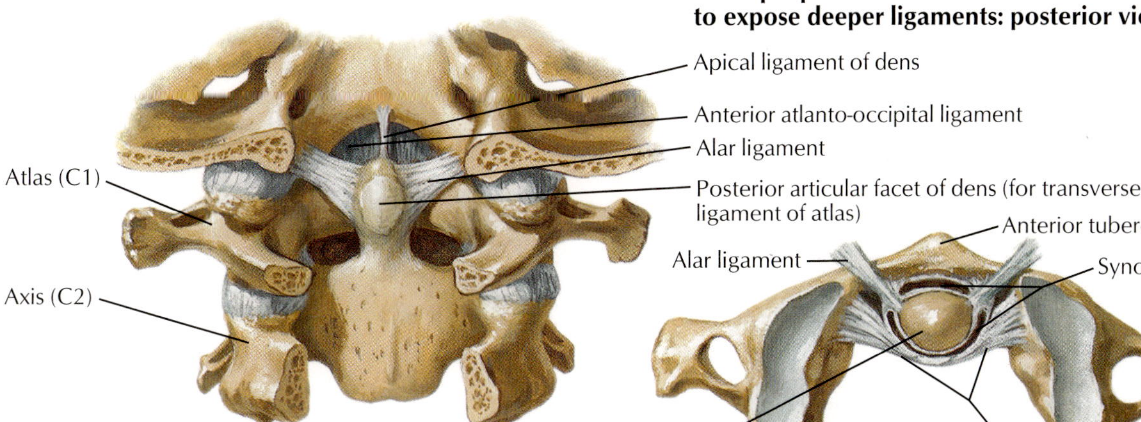

Cruciate ligament removed to show deeper ligaments: posterior view

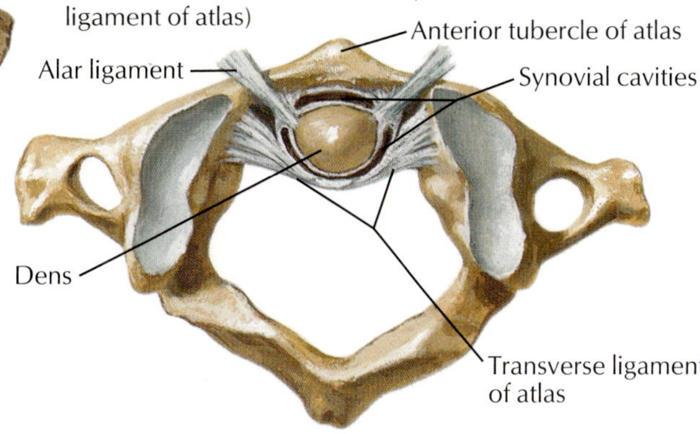

Median atlanto-axial joint: superior view

Facial Nerve Branches and Parotid Gland

See also Plates 46, 124

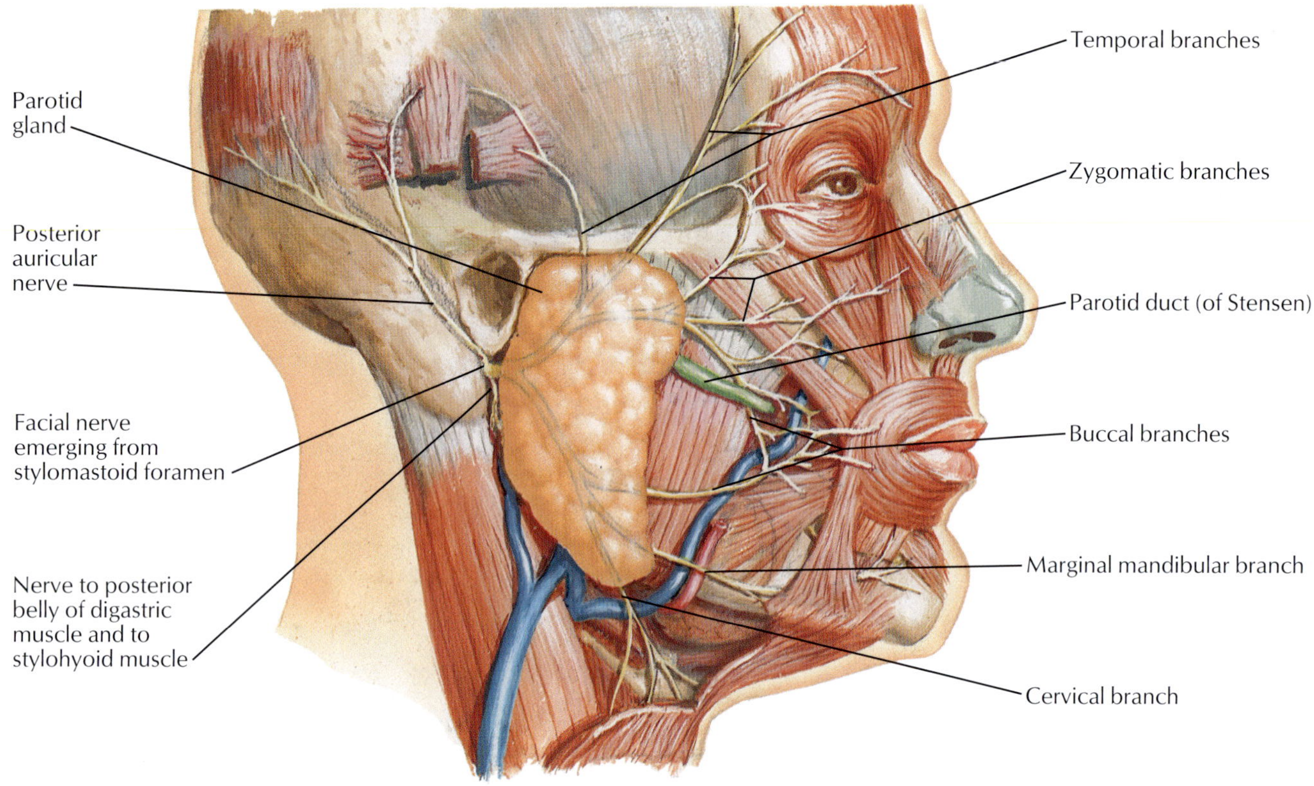

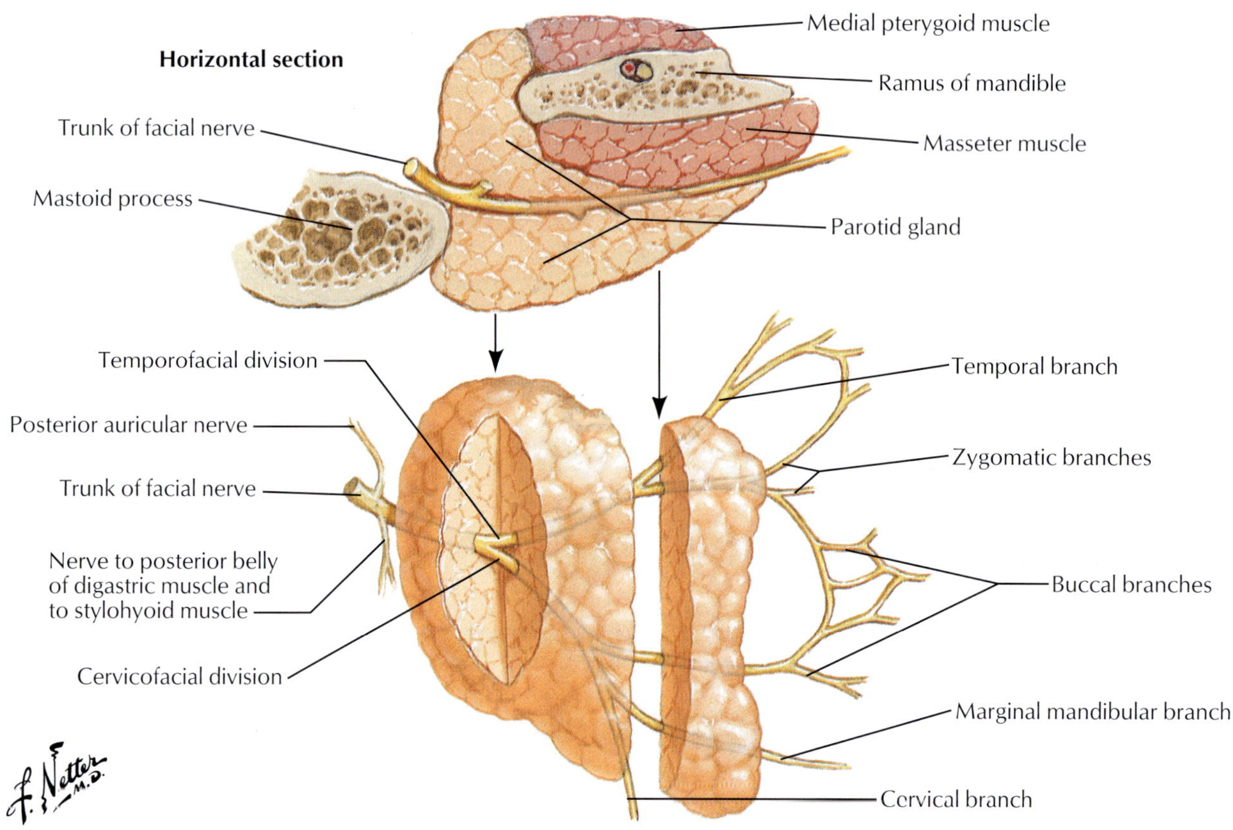

Muscles of Facial Expression: Lateral View

See also **Plates 48, 49**

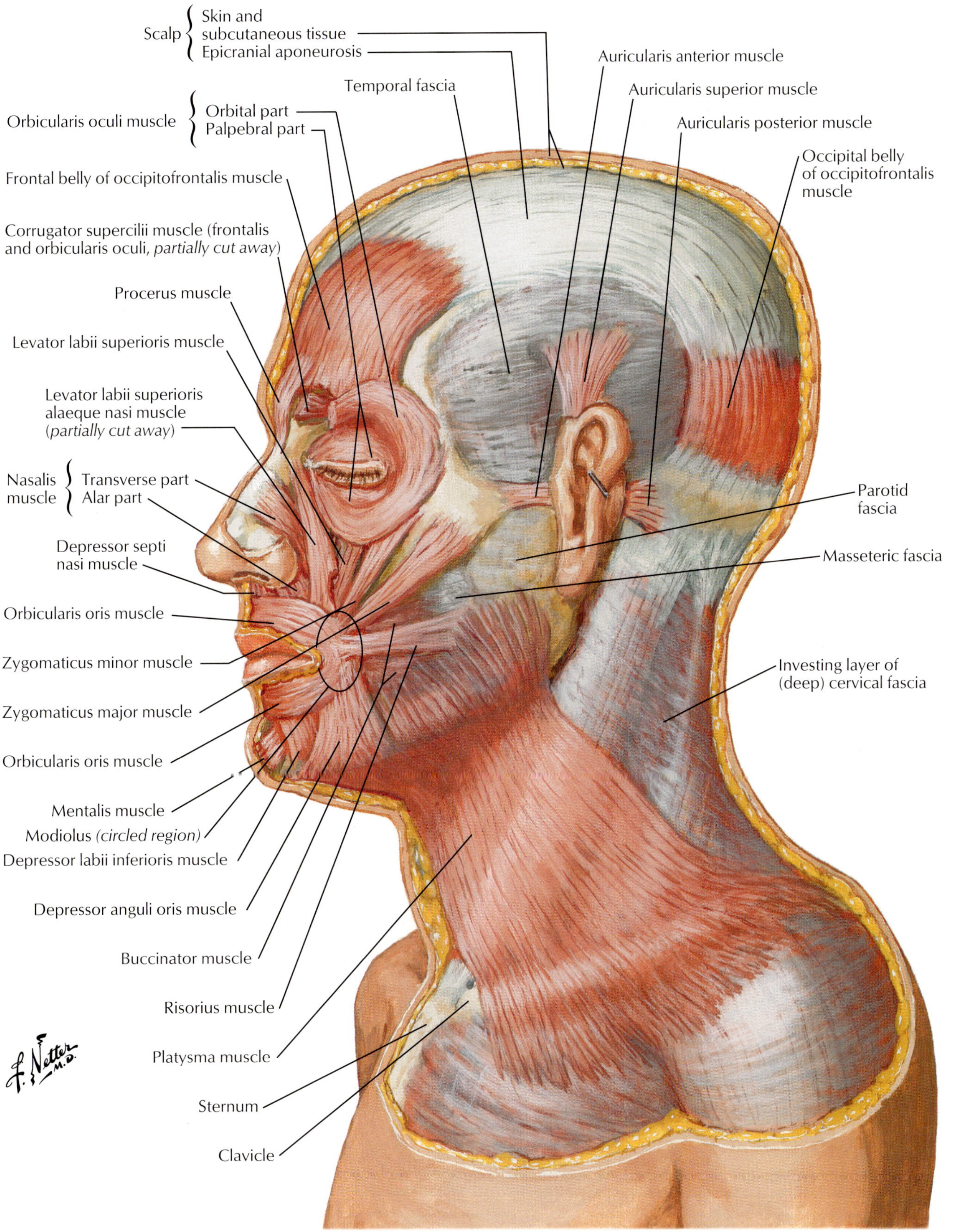

See also Plate 27

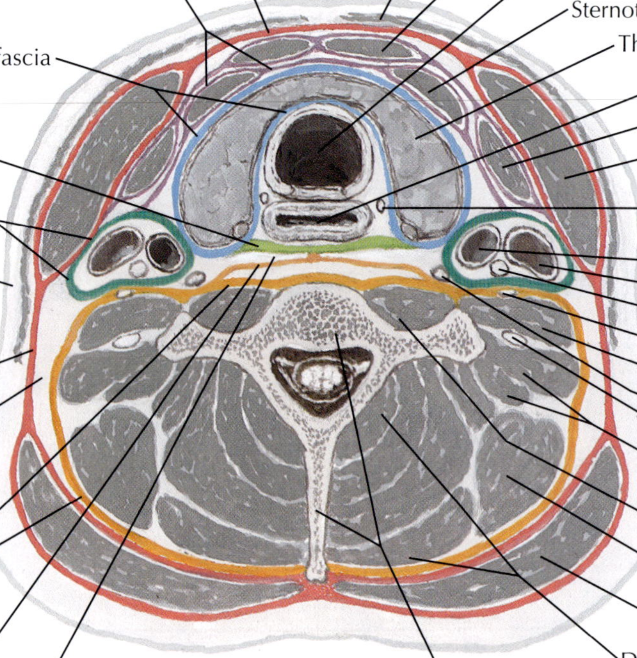

Cross section

Sagittal section

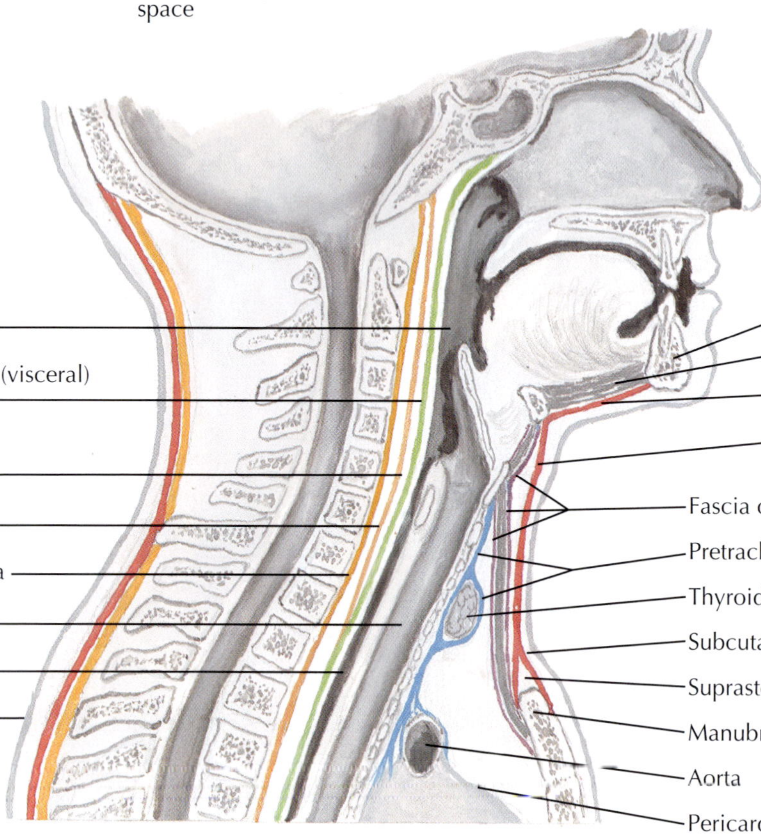

Muscles of Neck: Anterior View

See also **Plates 26, 28, 31**

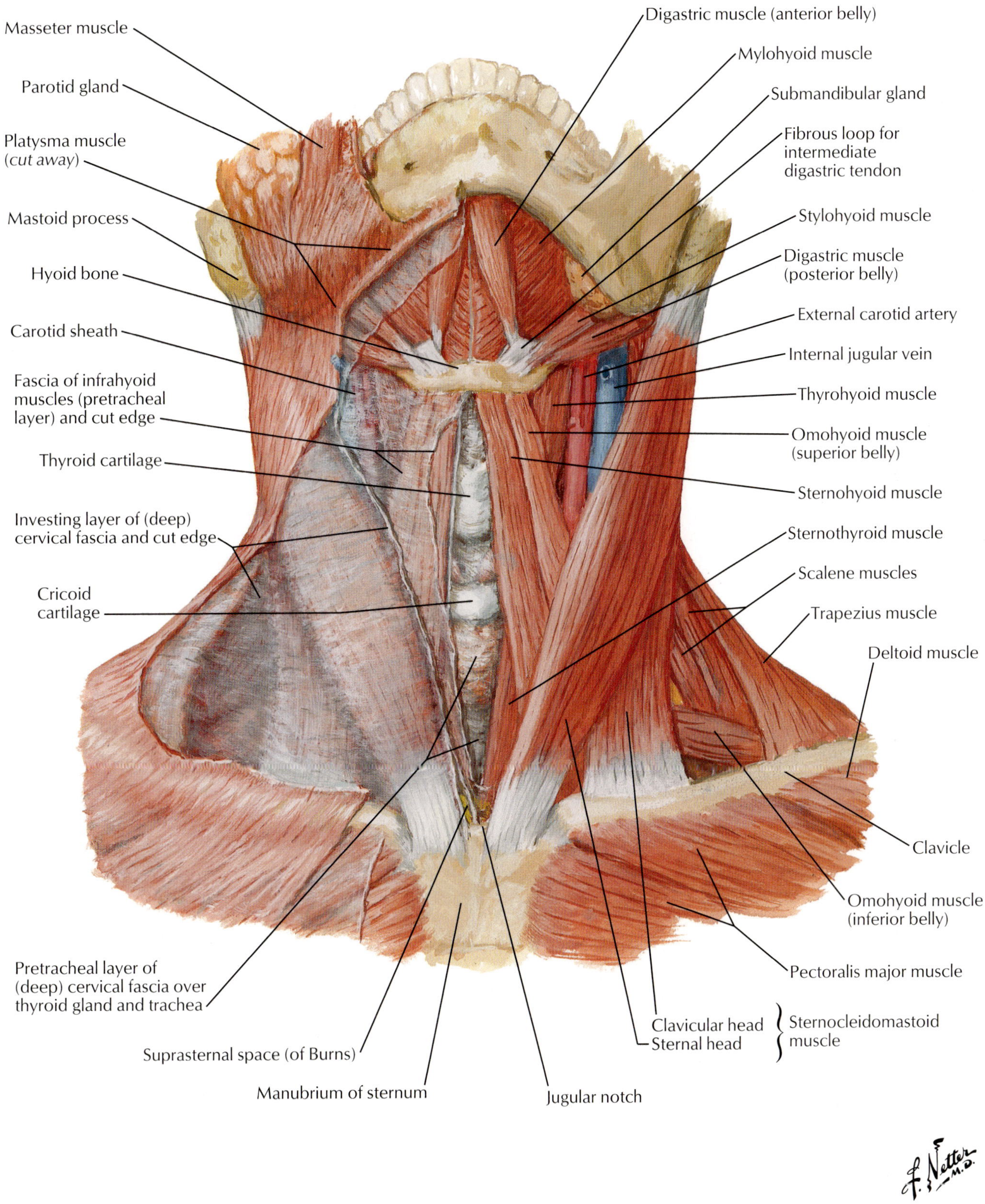

Infrahyoid and Suprahyoid Muscles

See also **Plates 27, 29, 58**

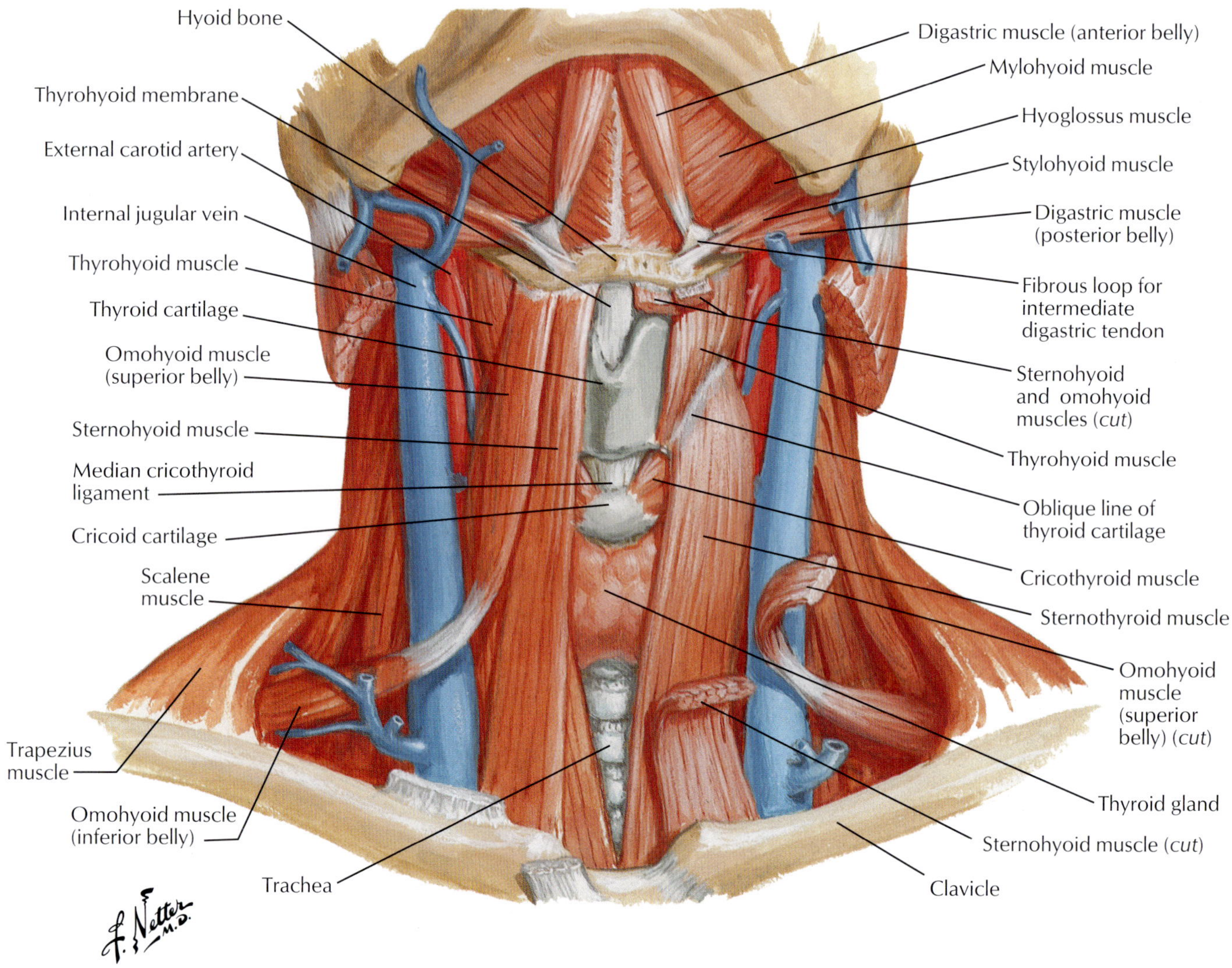

Muscles of Neck: Lateral View

See also **Plates 27, 28, 31**

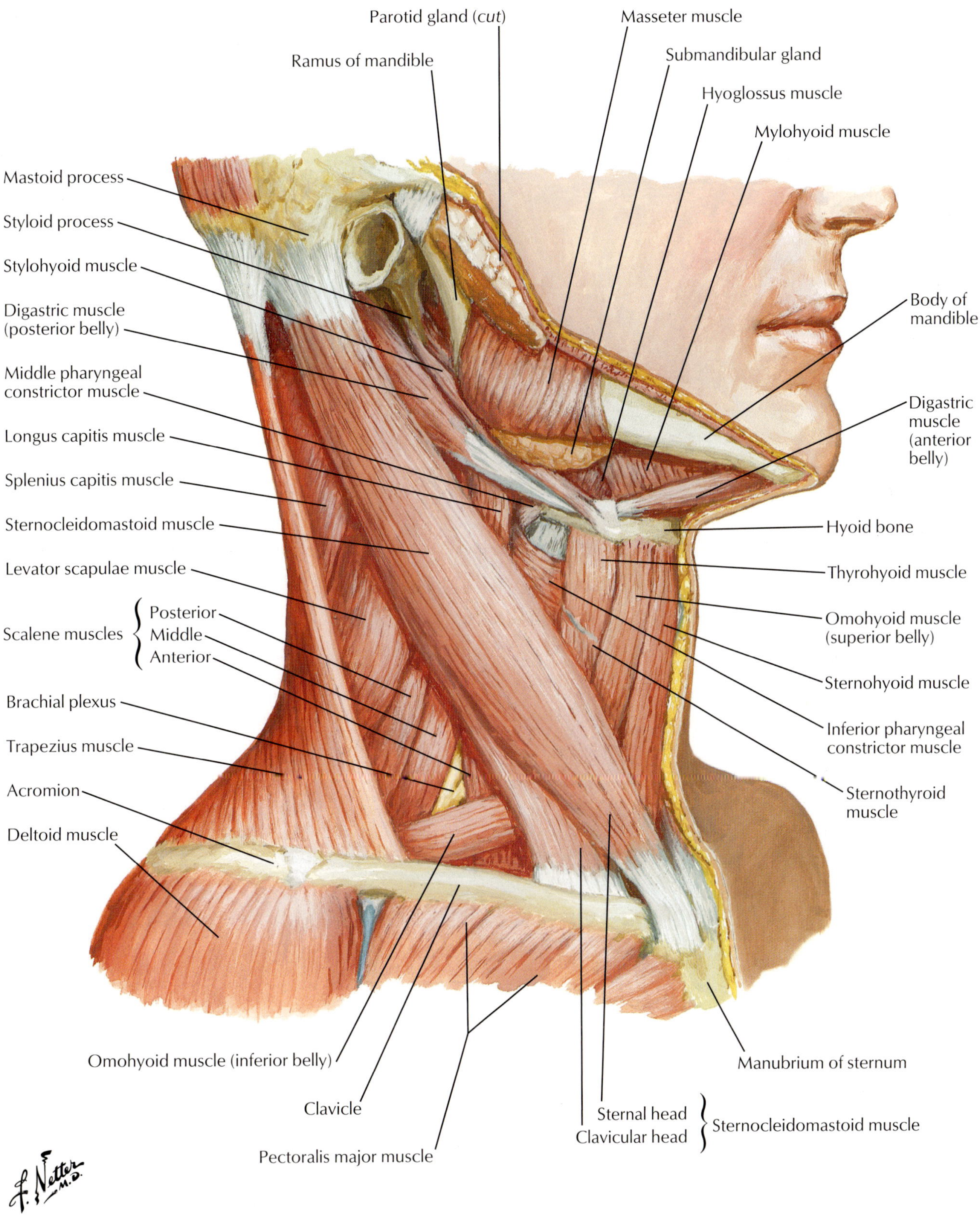

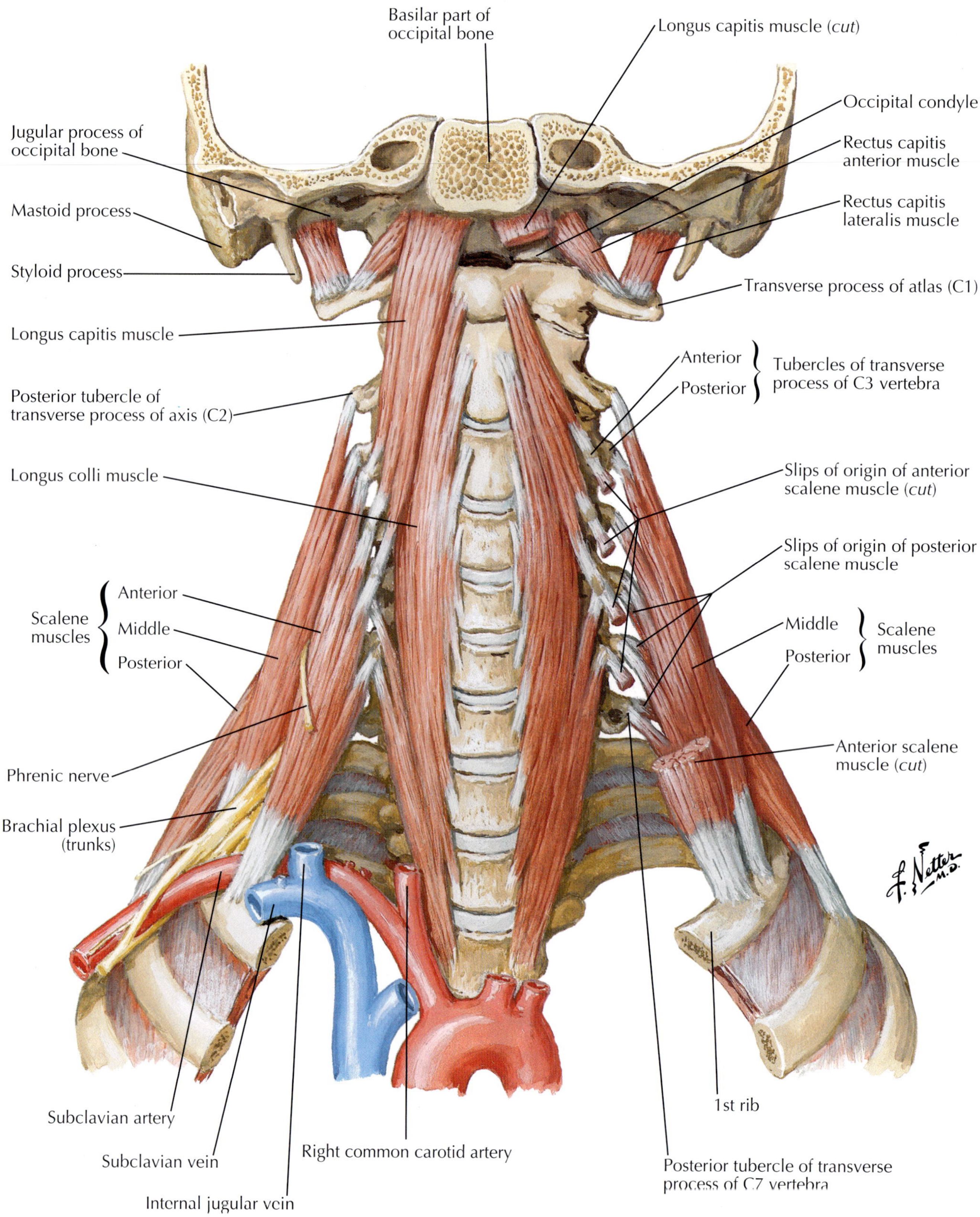
Basilar part of occipital bone
Longus capitis muscle (cut)
Occipital condyle
Rectus capitis anterior muscle
Rectus capitis lateralis muscle
Jugular process of occipital bone
Mastoid process
Styloid process
Transverse process of atlas (C1)
Longus capitis muscle
Anterior
Posterior
Tubercles of transverse process of C3 vertebra
Posterior tubercle of transverse process of axis (C2)
Longus colli muscle
Slips of origin of anterior scalene muscle (cut)
Slips of origin of posterior scalene muscle
Scalene muscles
Anterior
Middle
Posterior
Middle
Posterior
Scalene muscles
Phrenic nerve
Anterior scalene muscle (cut)
Brachial plexus (trunks)
Subclavian artery
Subclavian vein
Internal jugular vein
Right common carotid artery
1st rib
Posterior tubercle of transverse process of C7 vertebra

Superficial Veins and Cutaneous Nerves of Neck

For deep veins of neck see **Plate 73**

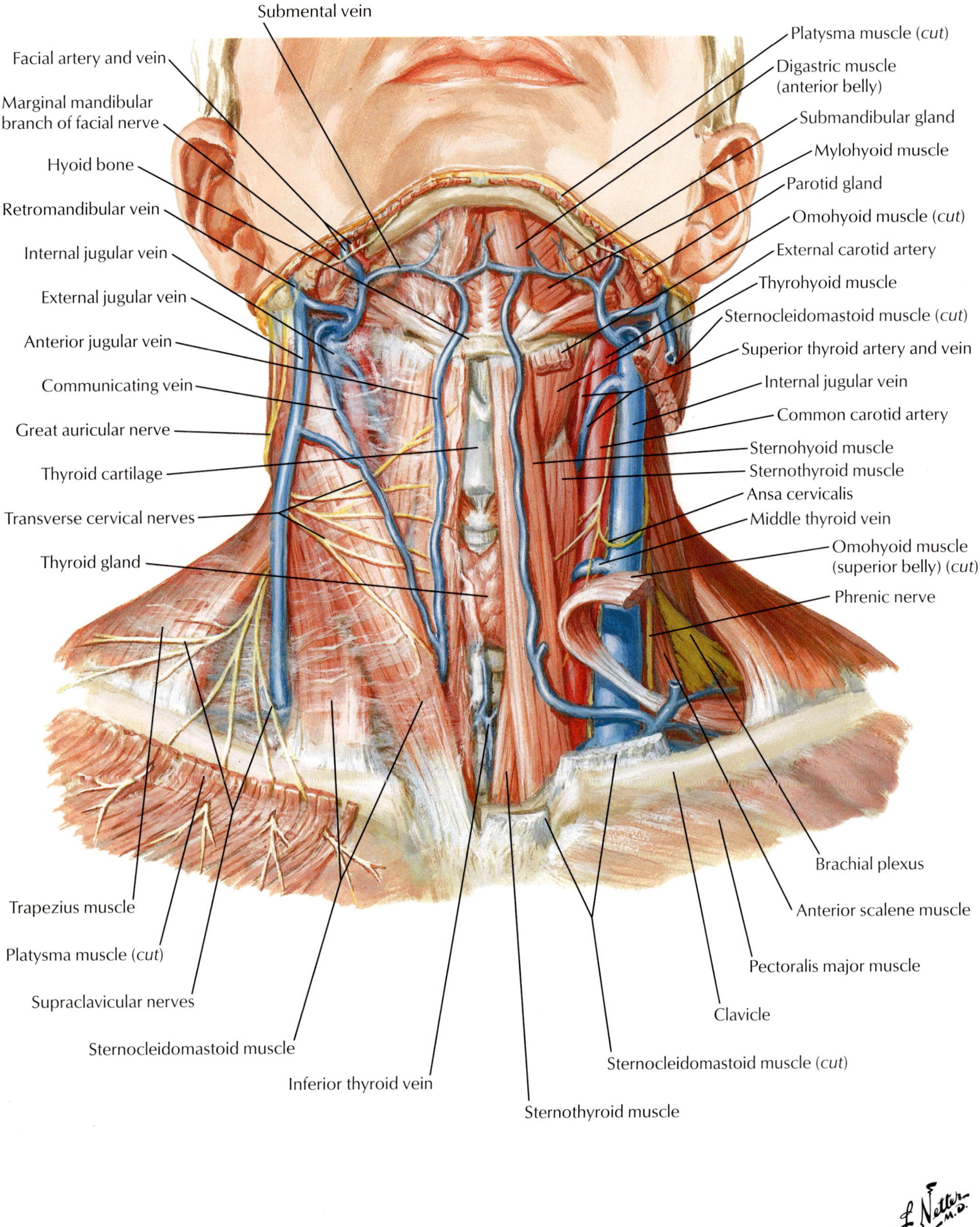

Nerves and Vessels of Neck

See also Plates 128–130

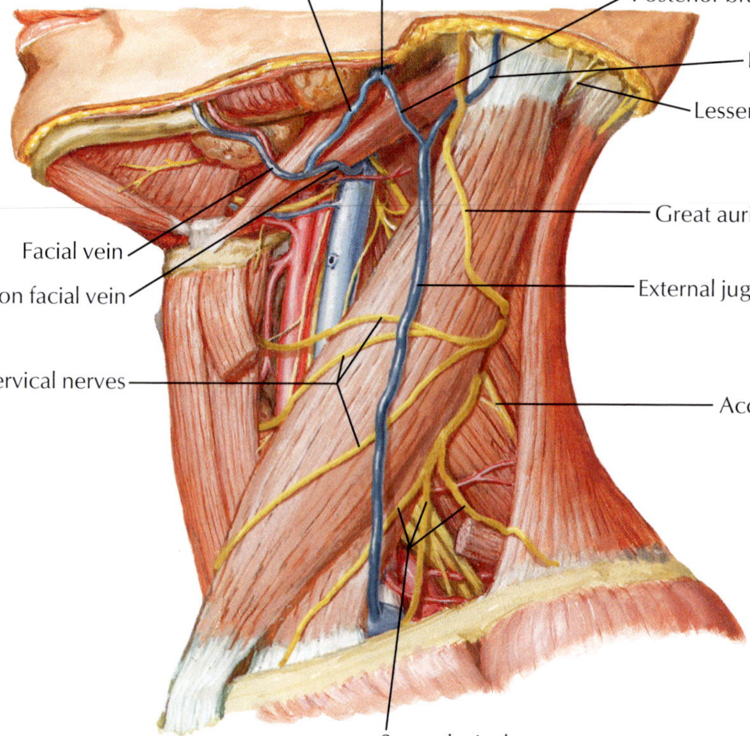

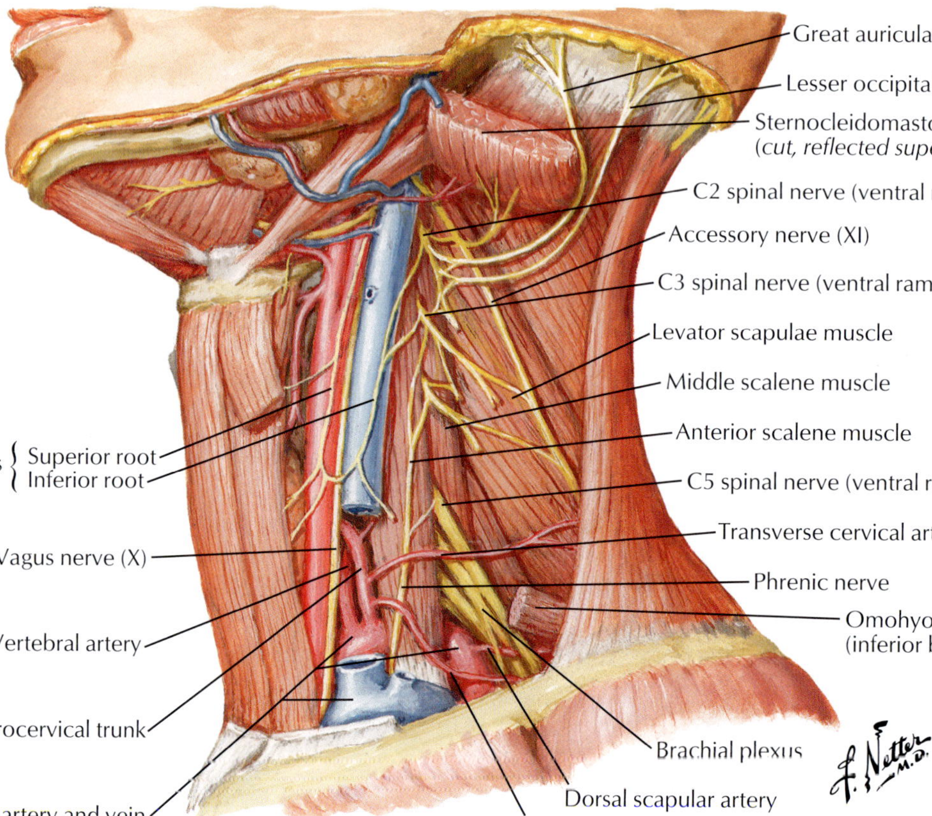

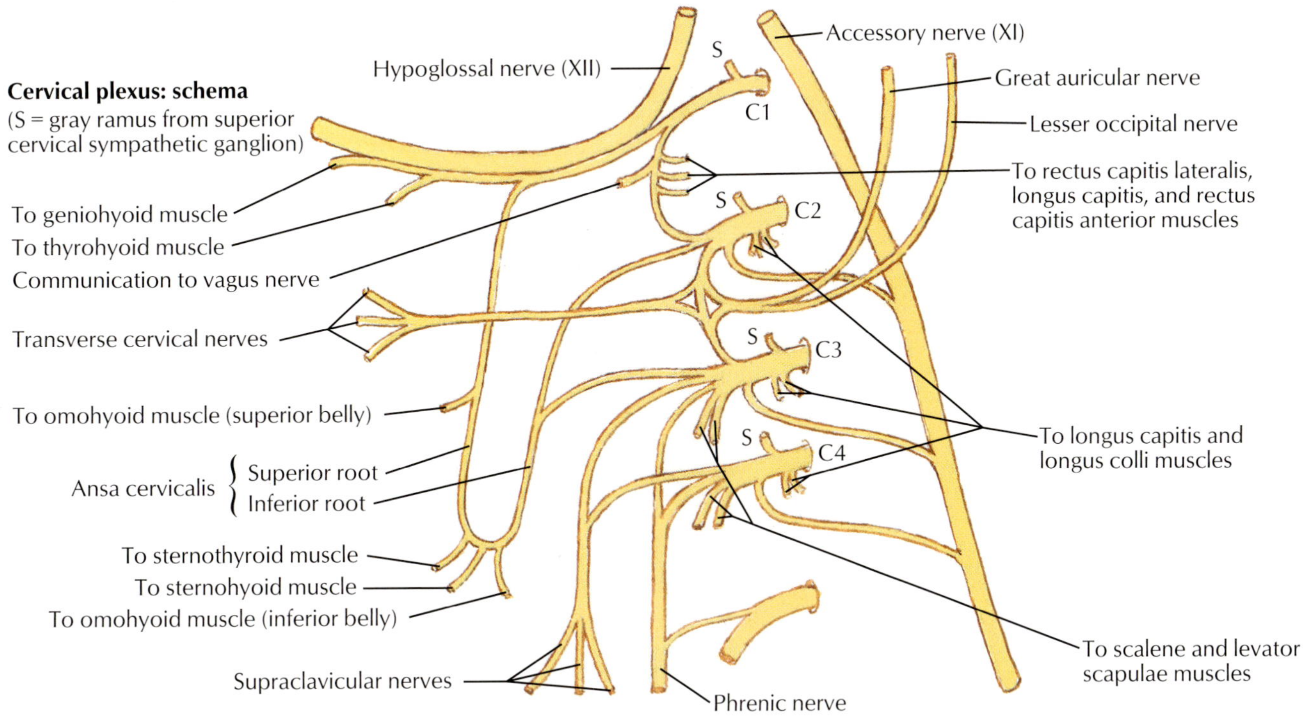
Cervical plexus: schema
(S = gray ramus from superior cervical sympathetic ganglion)
Hypoglossal nerve (XII)
S
C1
Accessory nerve (XI)
Great auricular nerve
Lesser occipital nerve
To rectus capitis lateralis, longus capitis, and rectus capitis anterior muscles
To geniohyoid muscle
To thyrohyoid muscle
Communication to vagus nerve
S
C2
Transverse cervical nerves
S
C3
To omohyoid muscle (superior belly)
S
C4
To longus capitis and longus colli muscles
Ansa cervicalis
Superior root
Inferior root
To sternothyroid muscle
To sternohyoid muscle
To omohyoid muscle (inferior belly)
To scalene and levator scapulae muscles
Supraclavicular nerves
Phrenic nerve

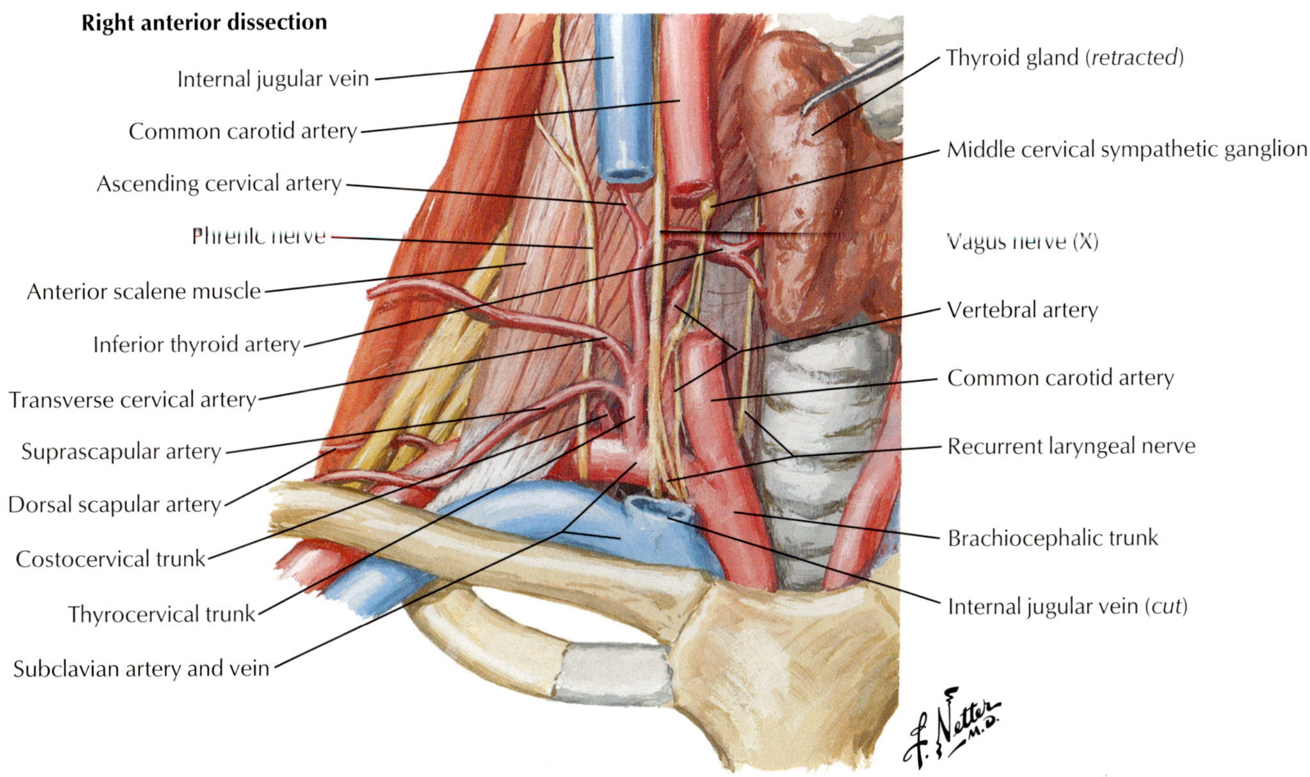
Right anterior dissection
Internal jugular vein
Common carotid artery
Ascending cervical artery
Phrenic nerve
Anterior scalene muscle
Inferior thyroid artery
Transverse cervical artery
Suprascapular artery
Dorsal scapular artery
Costocervical trunk
Thyrocervical trunk
Subclavian artery and vein
Thyroid gland (retracted)
Middle cervical sympathetic ganglion
Vagus nerve (X)
Vertebral artery
Common carotid artery
Recurrent laryngeal nerve
Brachiocephalic trunk
Internal jugular vein (cut)
F. Netter M.D.

See also **Plates 3, 137, 139**

Parotid space (bed): right lateral dissection

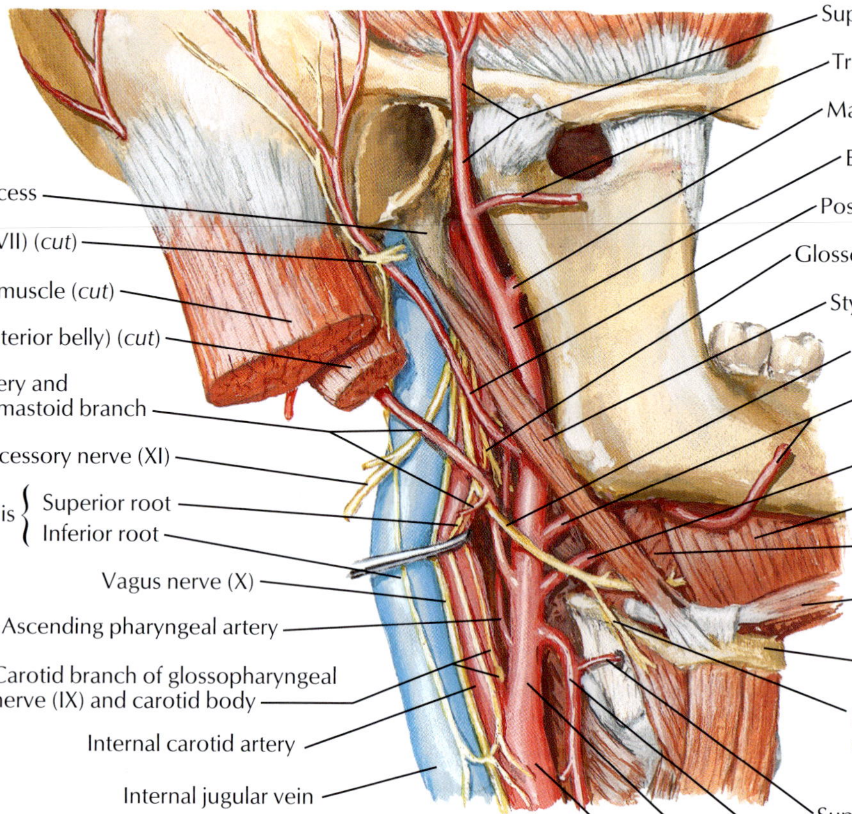

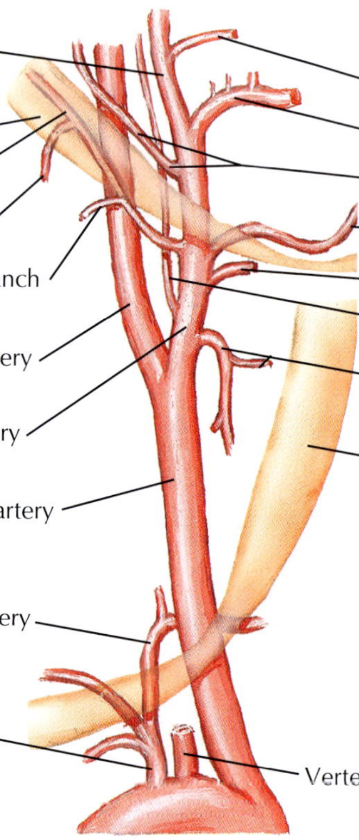

Right external carotid artery branches: schema

Anterolateral view

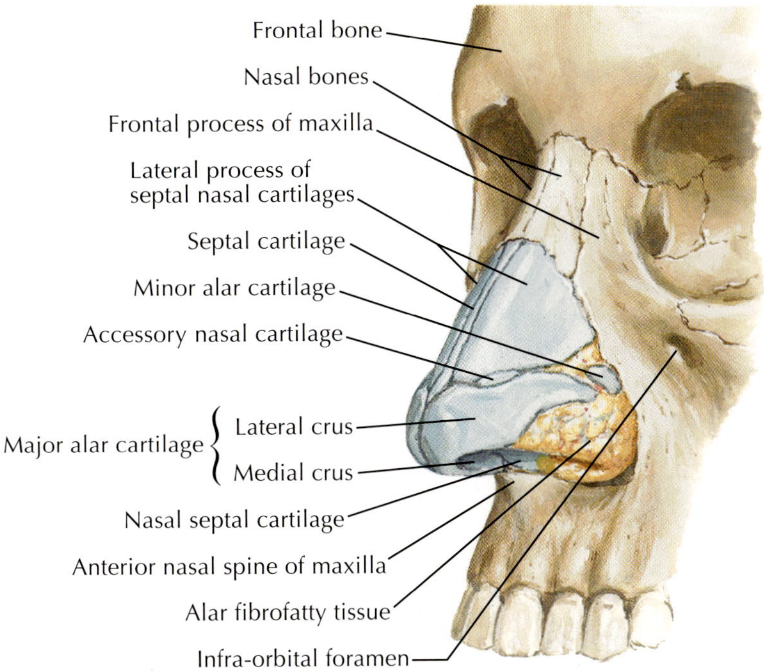

Inferior view

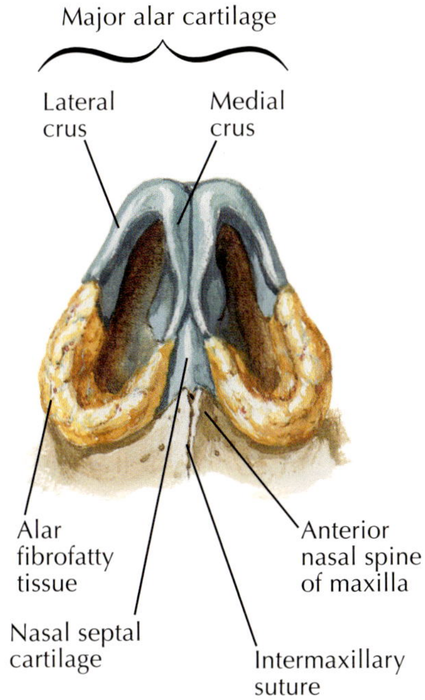

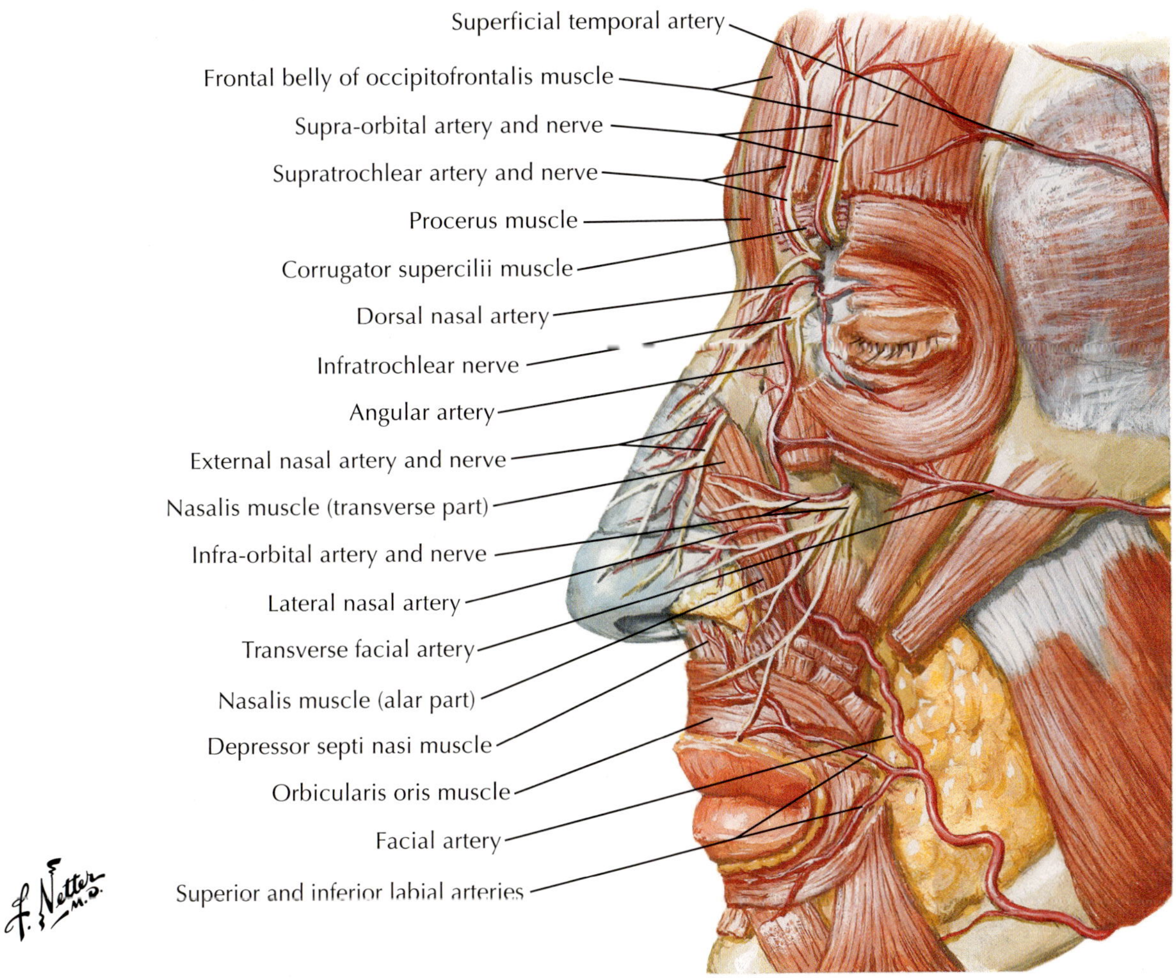

Lateral Wall of Nasal Cavity

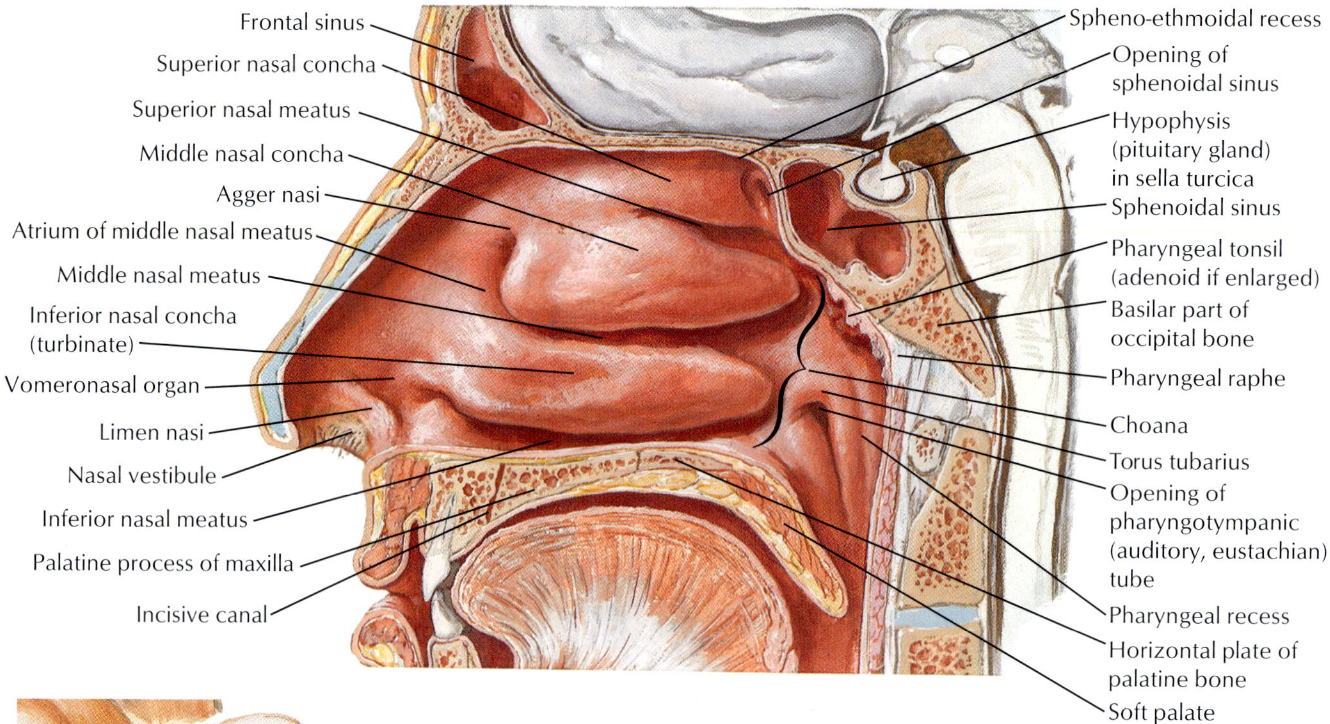

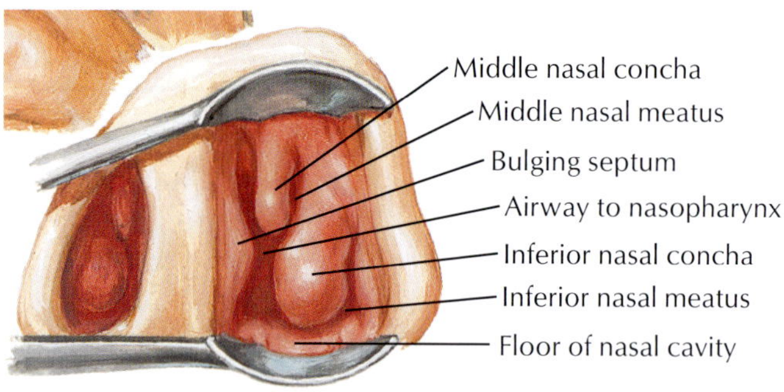

Speculum view

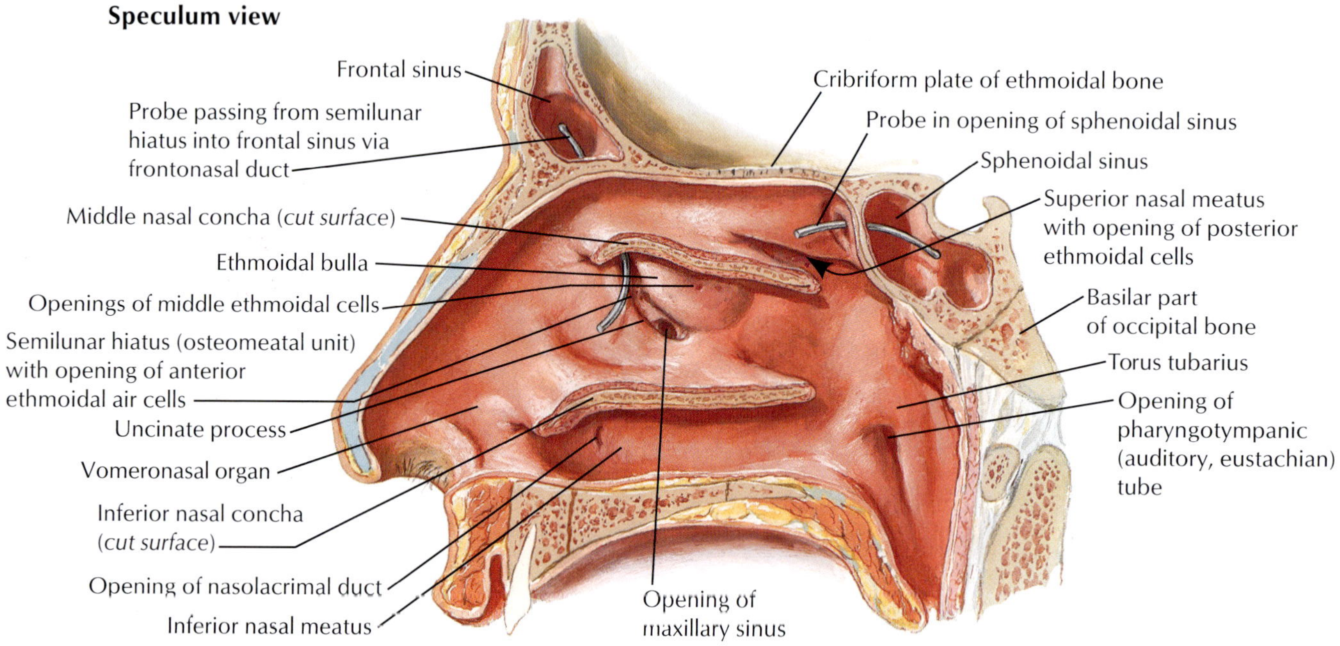

Lateral Wall of Nasal Cavity (continued)

See also Plate 36

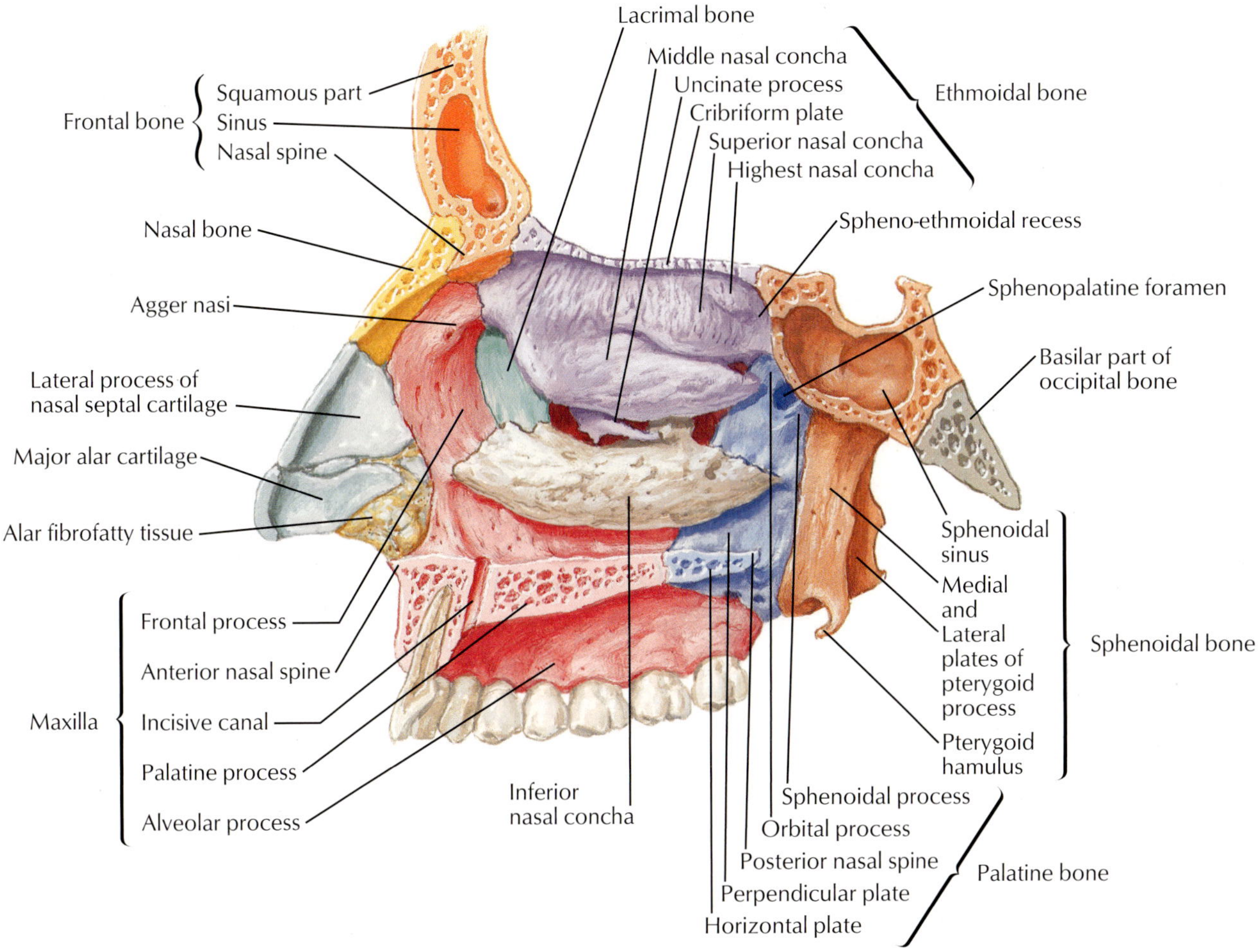

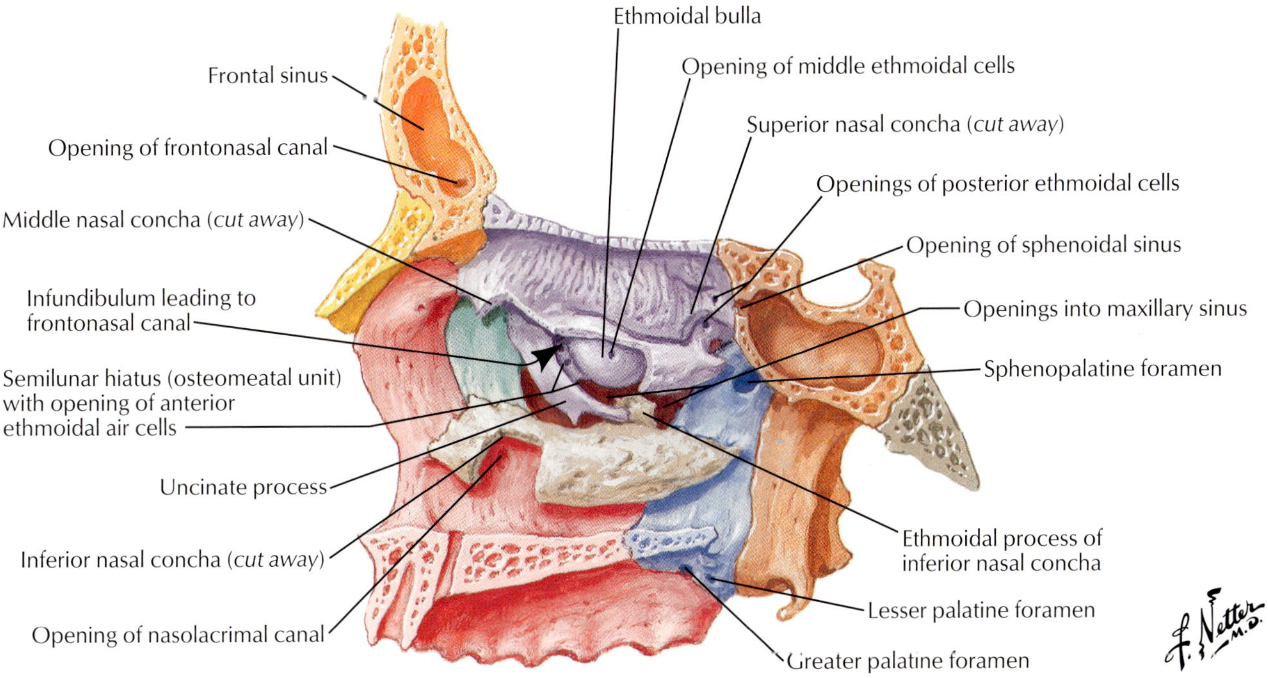

Medial Wall of Nasal Cavity (Nasal Septum)

See also Plate 8

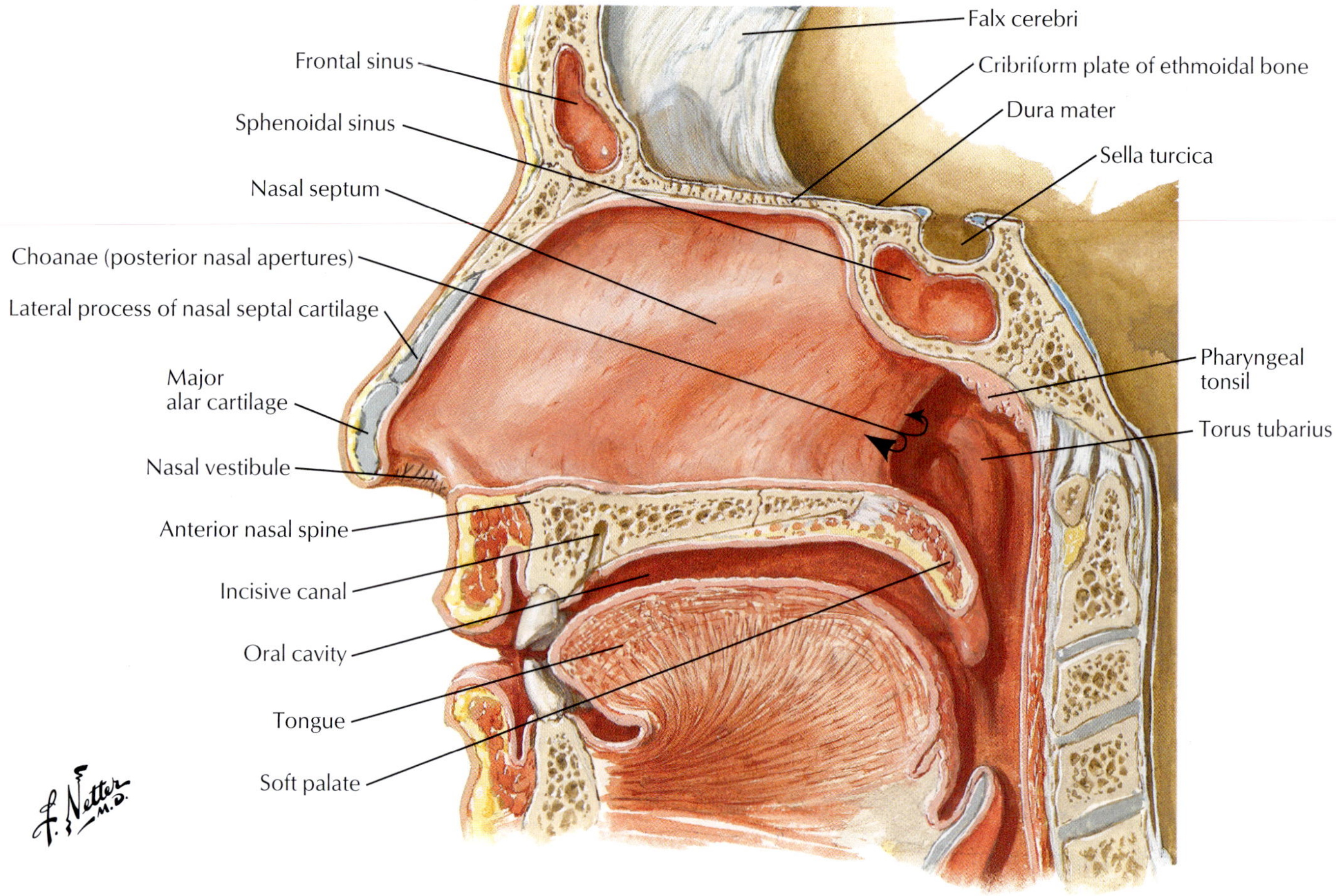

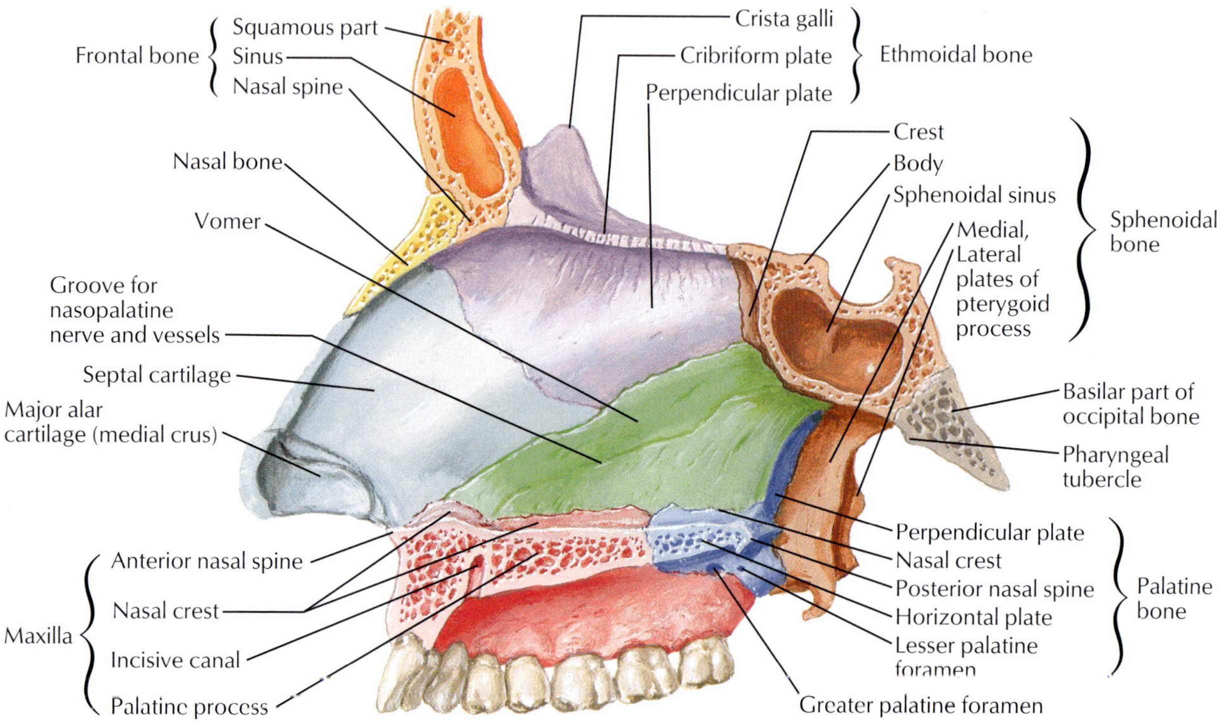

Nerves of Nasal Cavity

See also **Plates 54, 62, 120**

Distribution of olfactory mucosa (*shaded blue*)

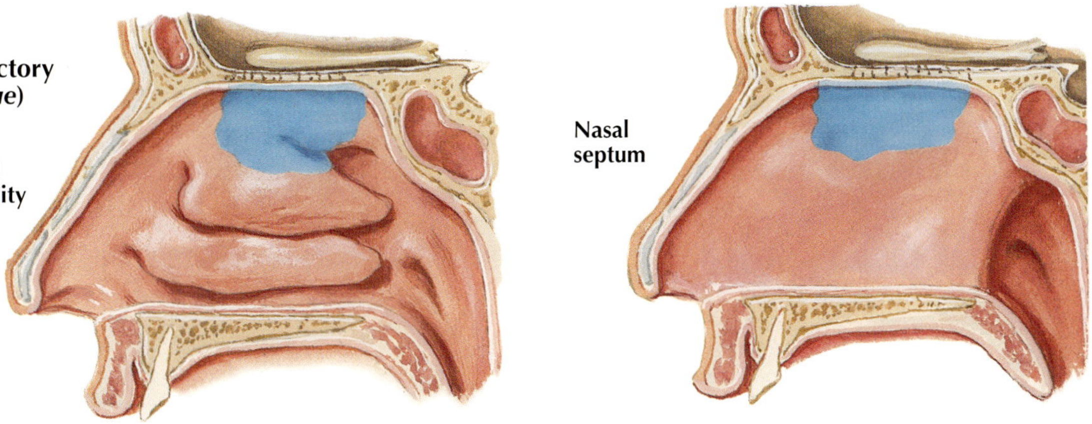

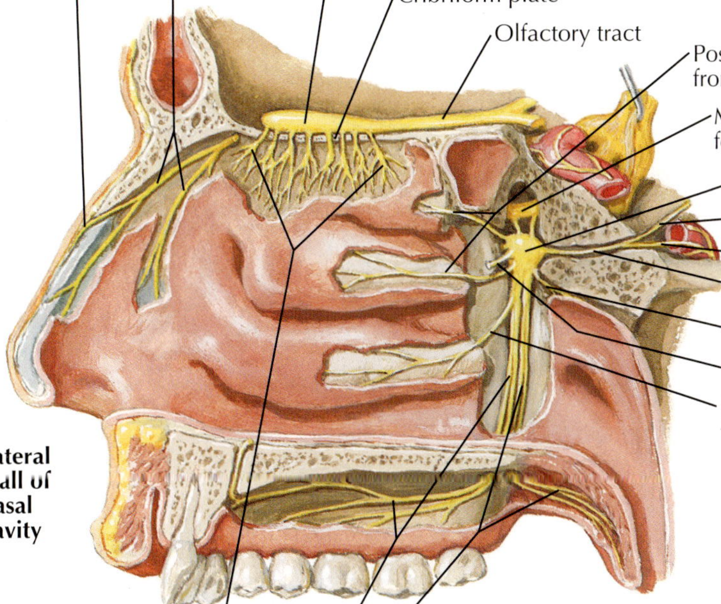

Lateral wall of nasal cavity

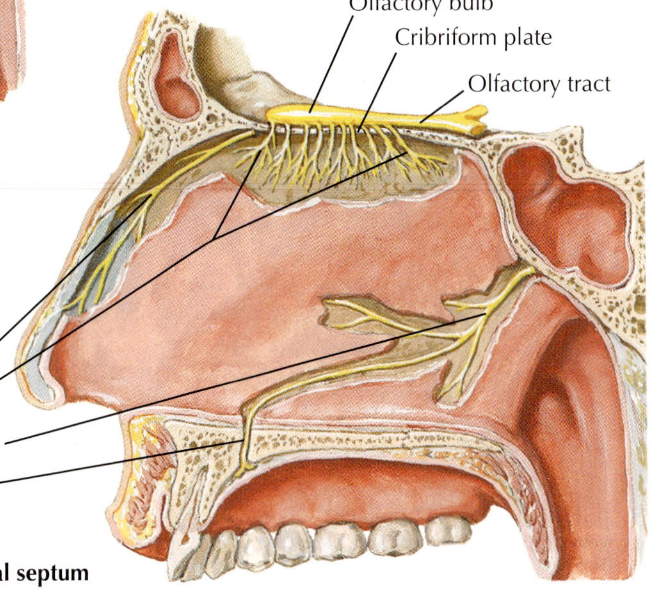

Nasal septum

F. Netter M.D.

Arteries of Nasal Cavity: Nasal Septum Turned Up

See also **Plate 57**

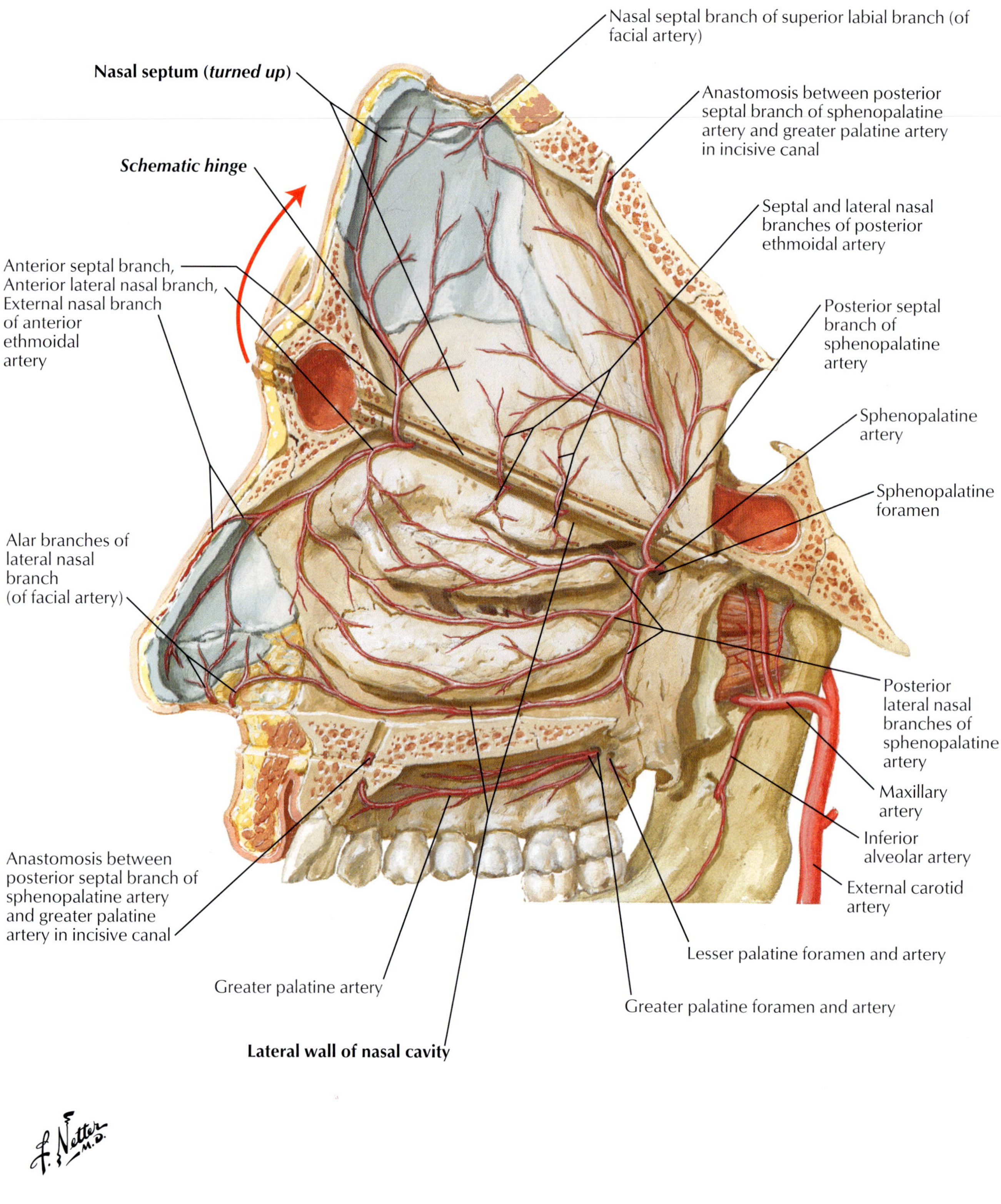

Nerves of Nasal Cavity: Nasal Septum Turned Up

See also Plates 52, 53

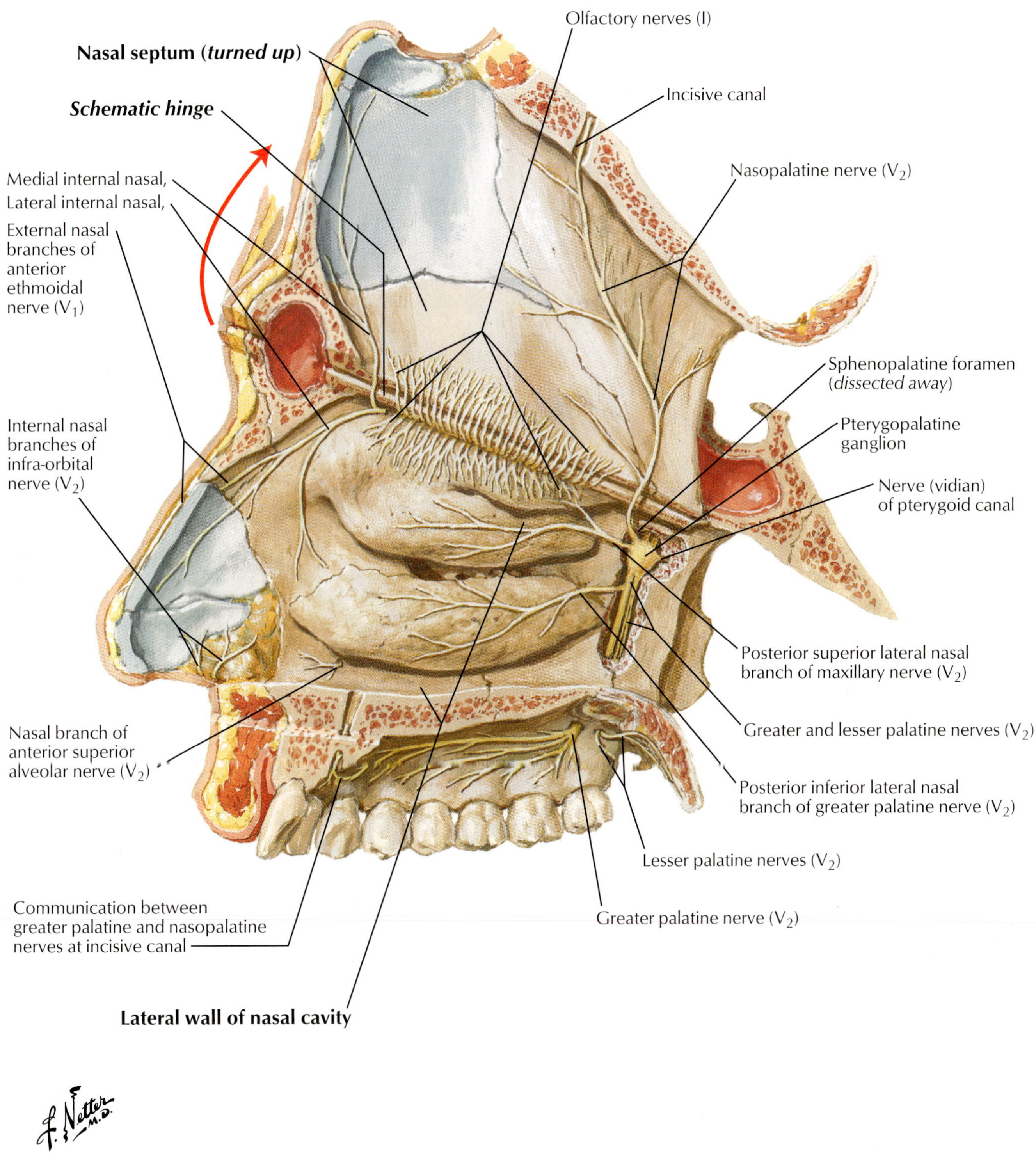

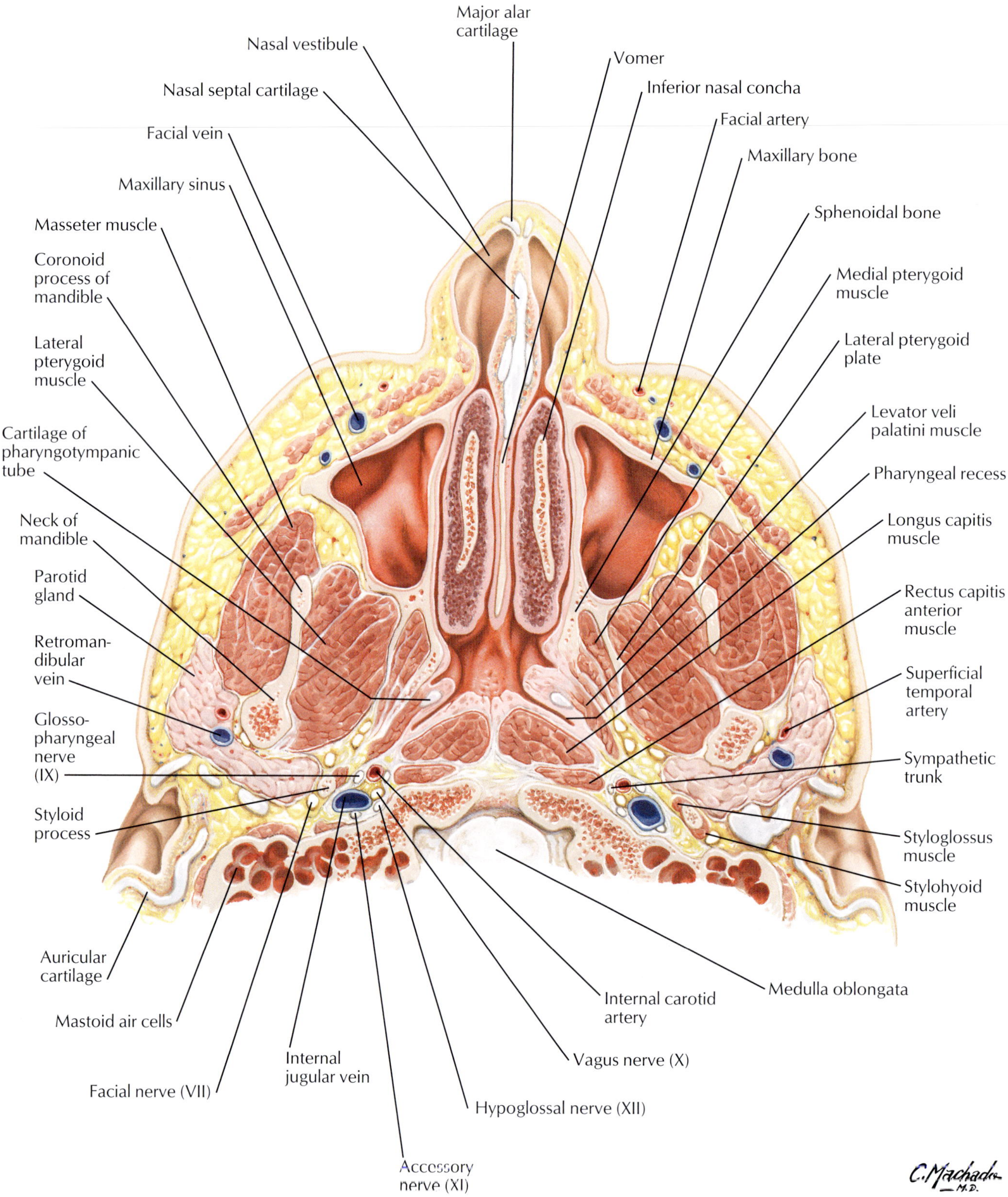
Major alar cartilage
Nasal vestibule
Vomer
Inferior nasal concha
Nasal septal cartilage
Facial artery
Facial vein
Maxillary bone
Maxillary sinus
Sphenoidal bone
Masseter muscle
Medial pterygoid muscle
Coronoid process of mandible
Lateral pterygoid plate
Lateral pterygoid muscle
Levator veli palatini muscle
Cartilage of pharyngotympanic tube
Pharyngeal recess
Neck of mandible
Longus capitis muscle
Parotid gland
Rectus capitis anterior muscle
Retromandibular vein
Superficial temporal artery
Glossopharyngeal nerve (IX)
Sympathetic trunk
Styloid process
Styloglossus muscle
Stylohyoid muscle
Auricular cartilage
Medulla oblongata
Mastoid air cells
Internal carotid artery
Vagus nerve (X)
Facial nerve (VII)
Internal jugular vein
Hypoglossal nerve (XII)
Accessory nerve (XI)
C. Machado M.D.

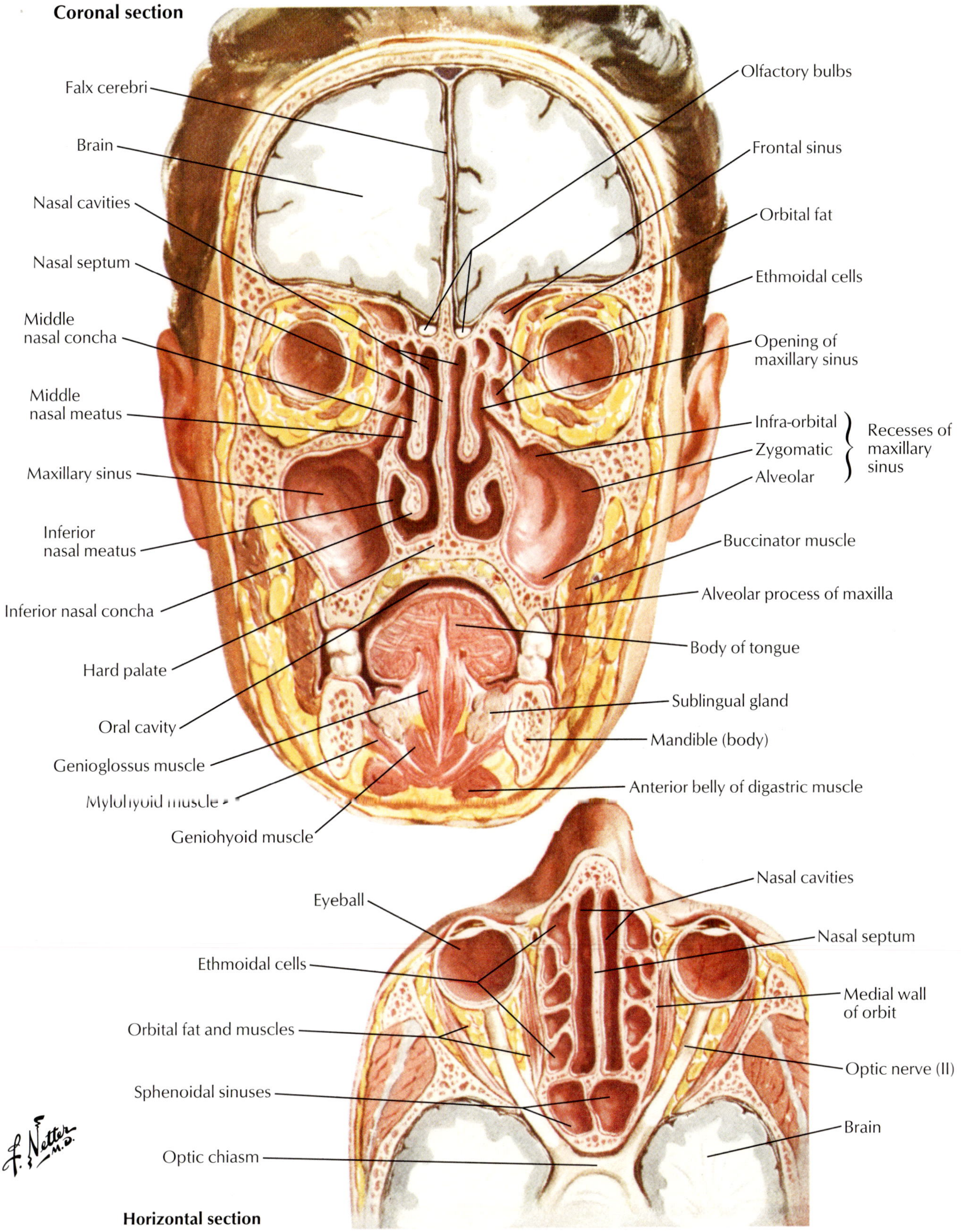
Coronal section
Falx cerebri
Brain
Nasal cavities
Nasal septum
Middle nasal concha
Middle nasal meatus
Maxillary sinus
Inferior nasal meatus
Inferior nasal concha
Hard palate
Oral cavity
Genioglossus muscle
Mylohyoid muscle
Geniohyoid muscle
Olfactory bulbs
Frontal sinus
Orbital fat
Ethmoidal cells
Opening of maxillary sinus
Infra-orbital
Zygomatic
Alveolar
Recesses of maxillary sinus
Buccinator muscle
Alveolar process of maxilla
Body of tongue
Sublingual gland
Mandible (body)
Anterior belly of digastric muscle
Eyeball
Ethmoidal cells
Orbital fat and muscles
Sphenoidal sinuses
Optic chiasm
Nasal cavities
Nasal septum
Medial wall of orbit
Optic nerve (II)
Brain
Horizontal section
F. Netter M.D.

See also **Plate 52**

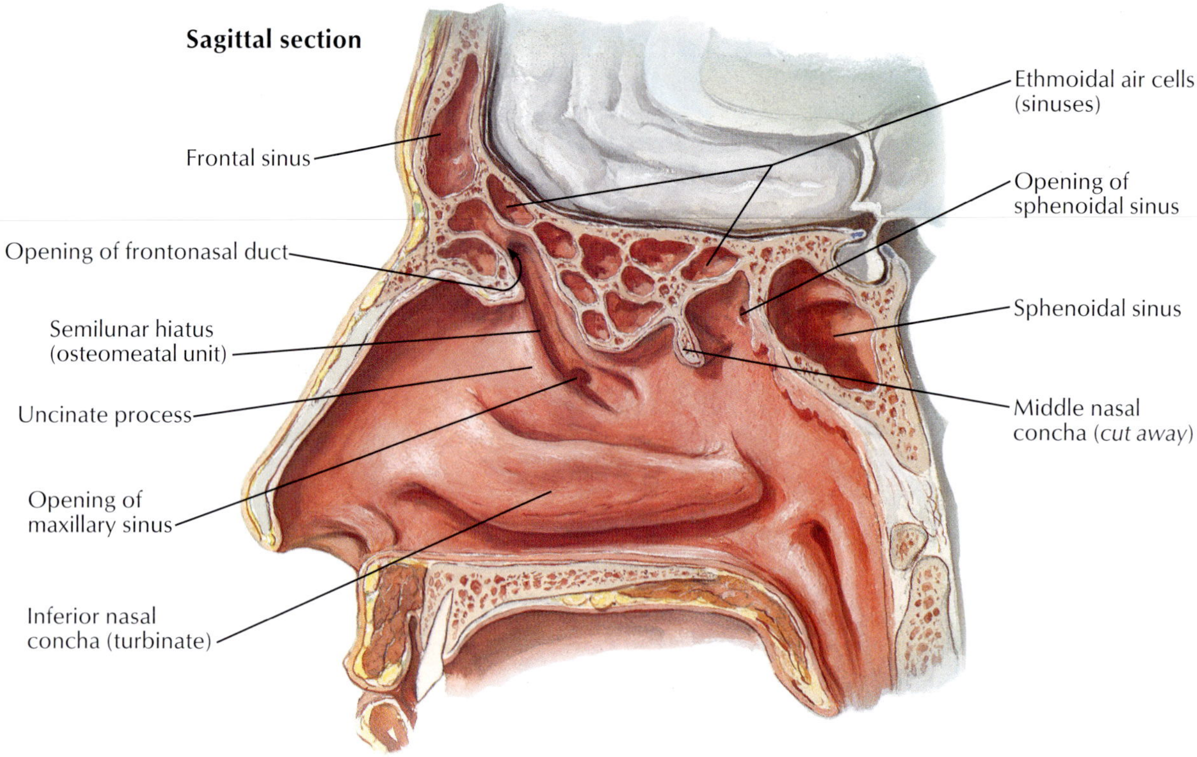

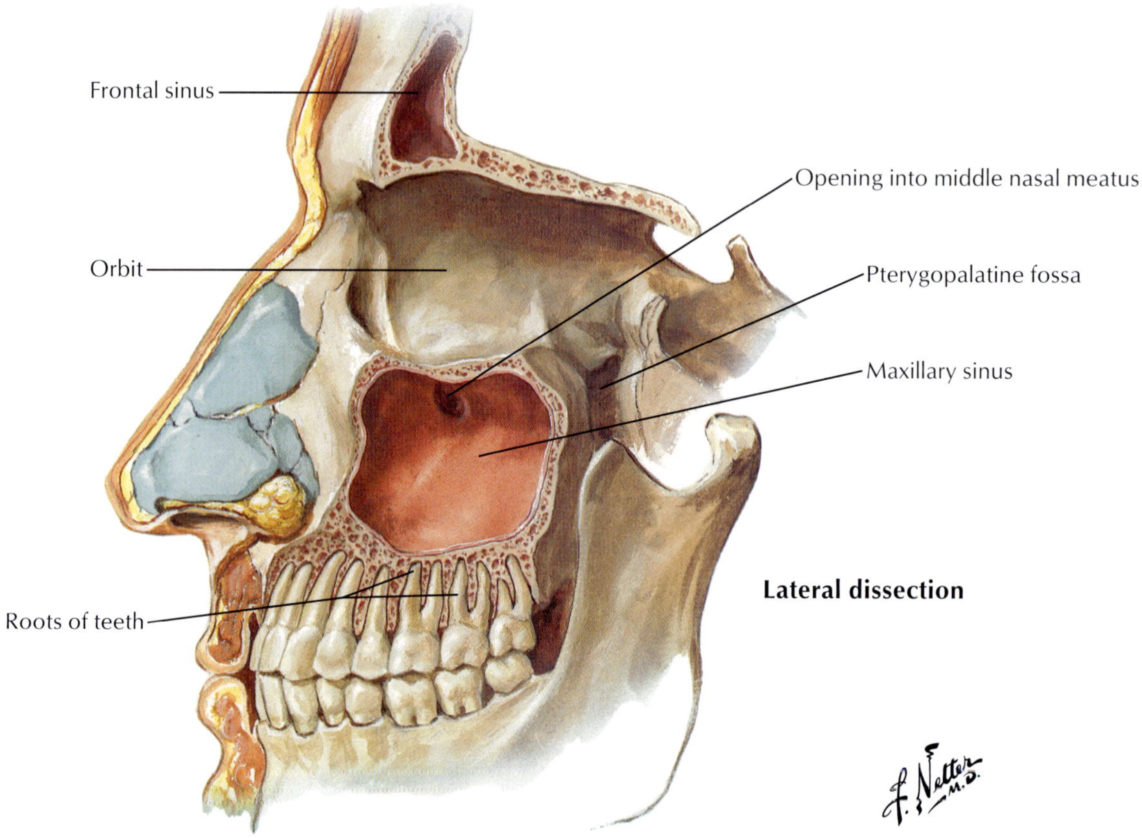

Bones of nasal cavity and paranasal sinuses at birth

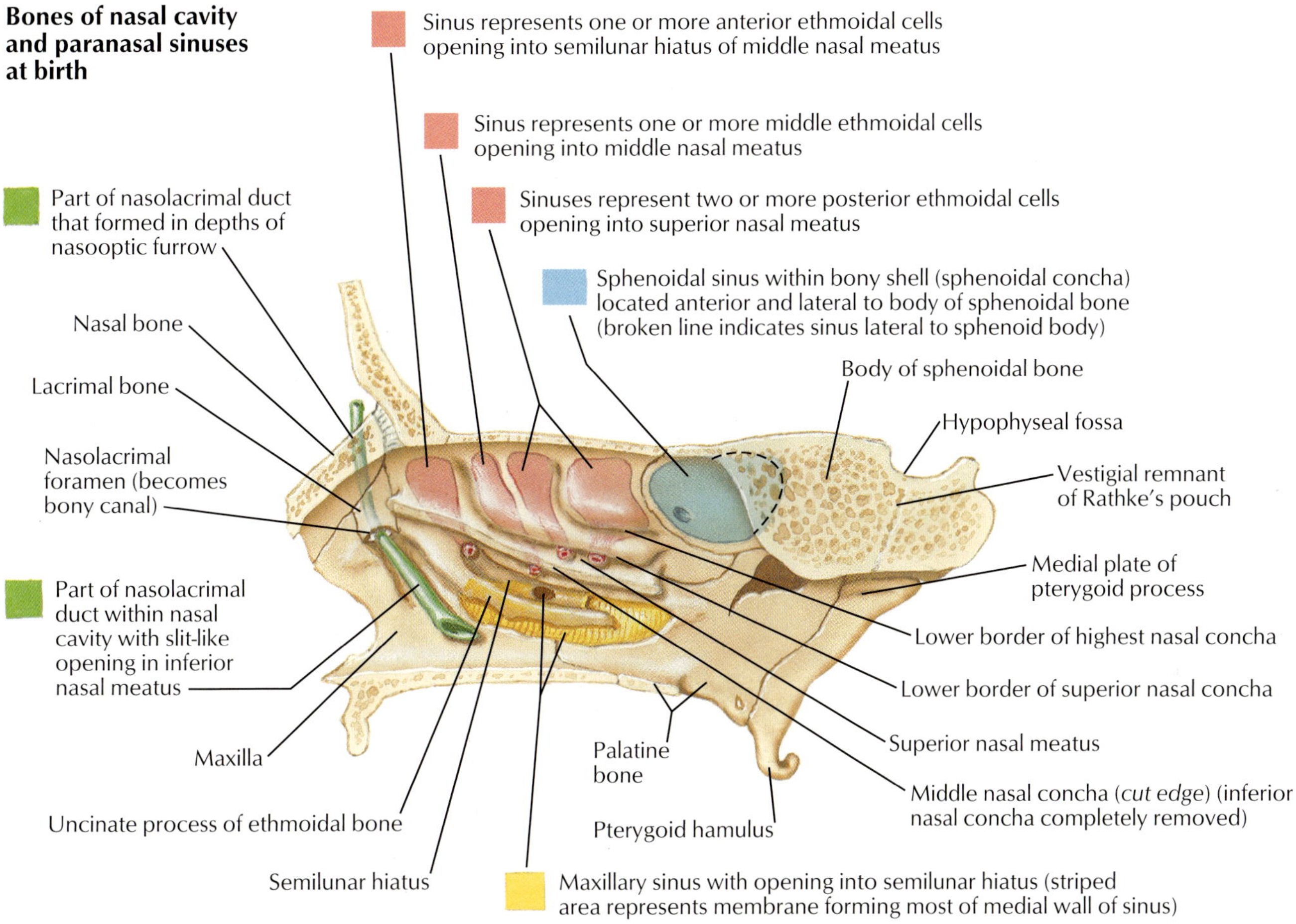

Growth of frontal and maxillary sinuses throughout life

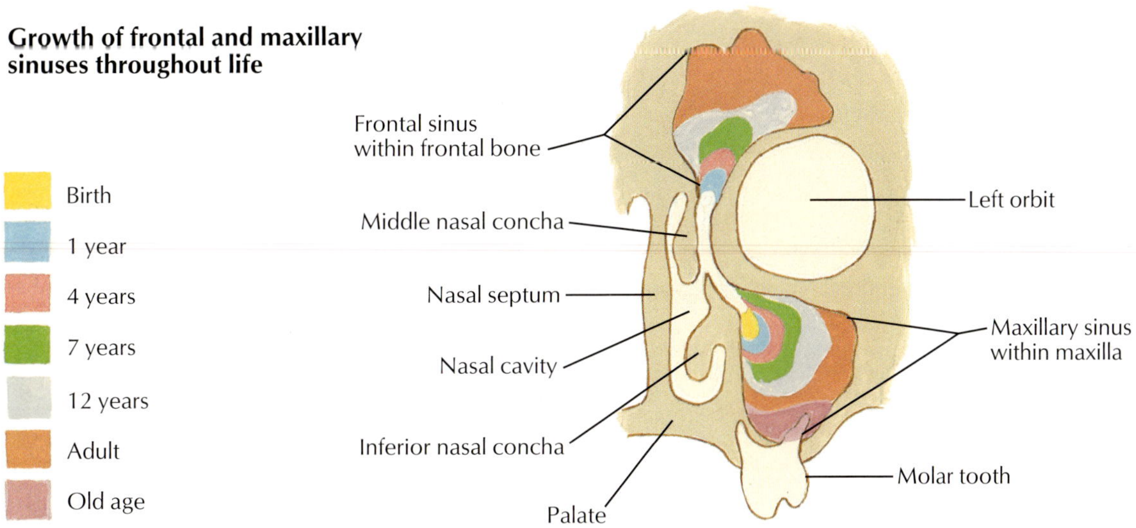

Salivary Glands

See also Plates 24, 134, 135

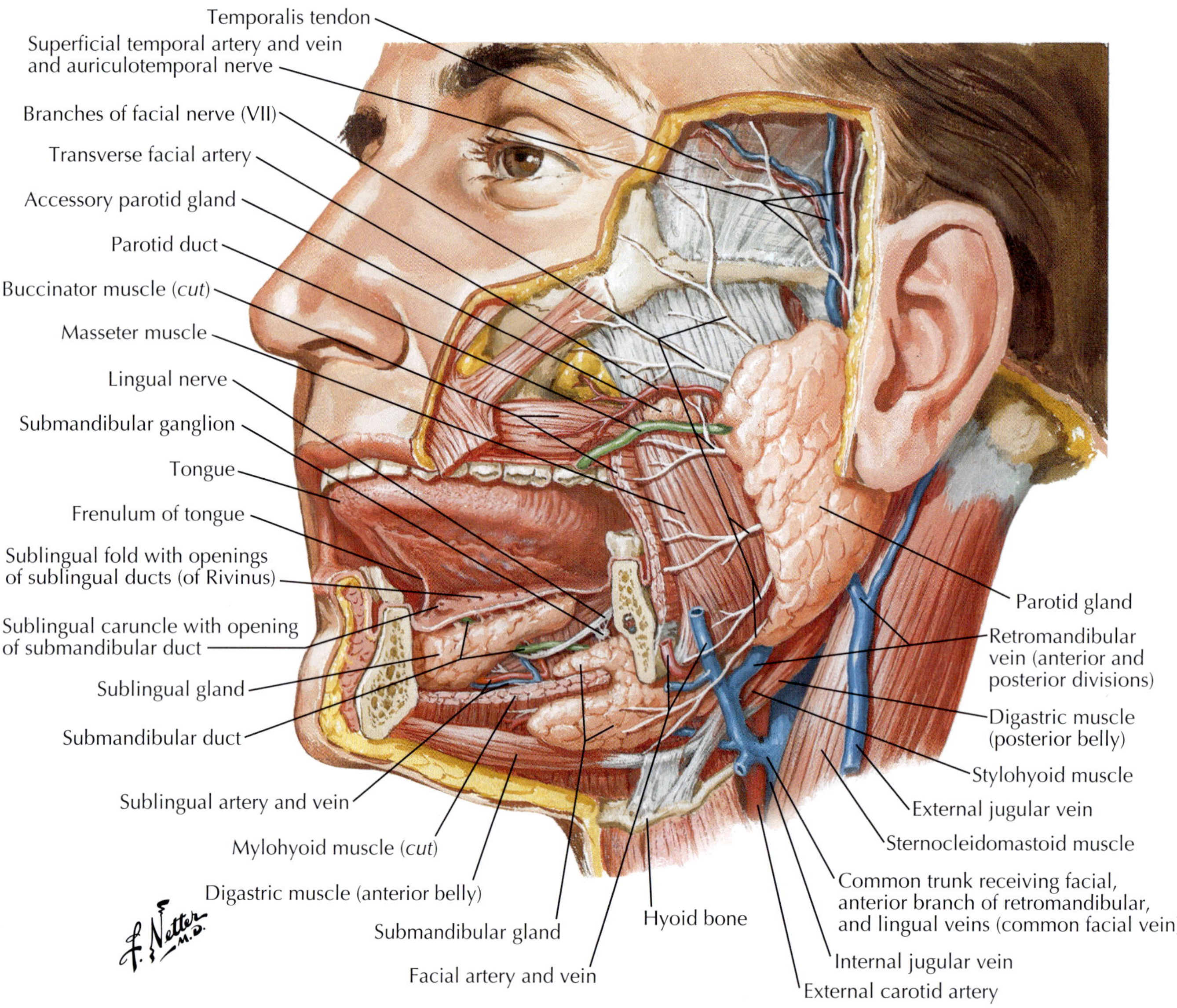

Horizontal section below lingula of mandible (superior view) demonstrating bed of parotid gland

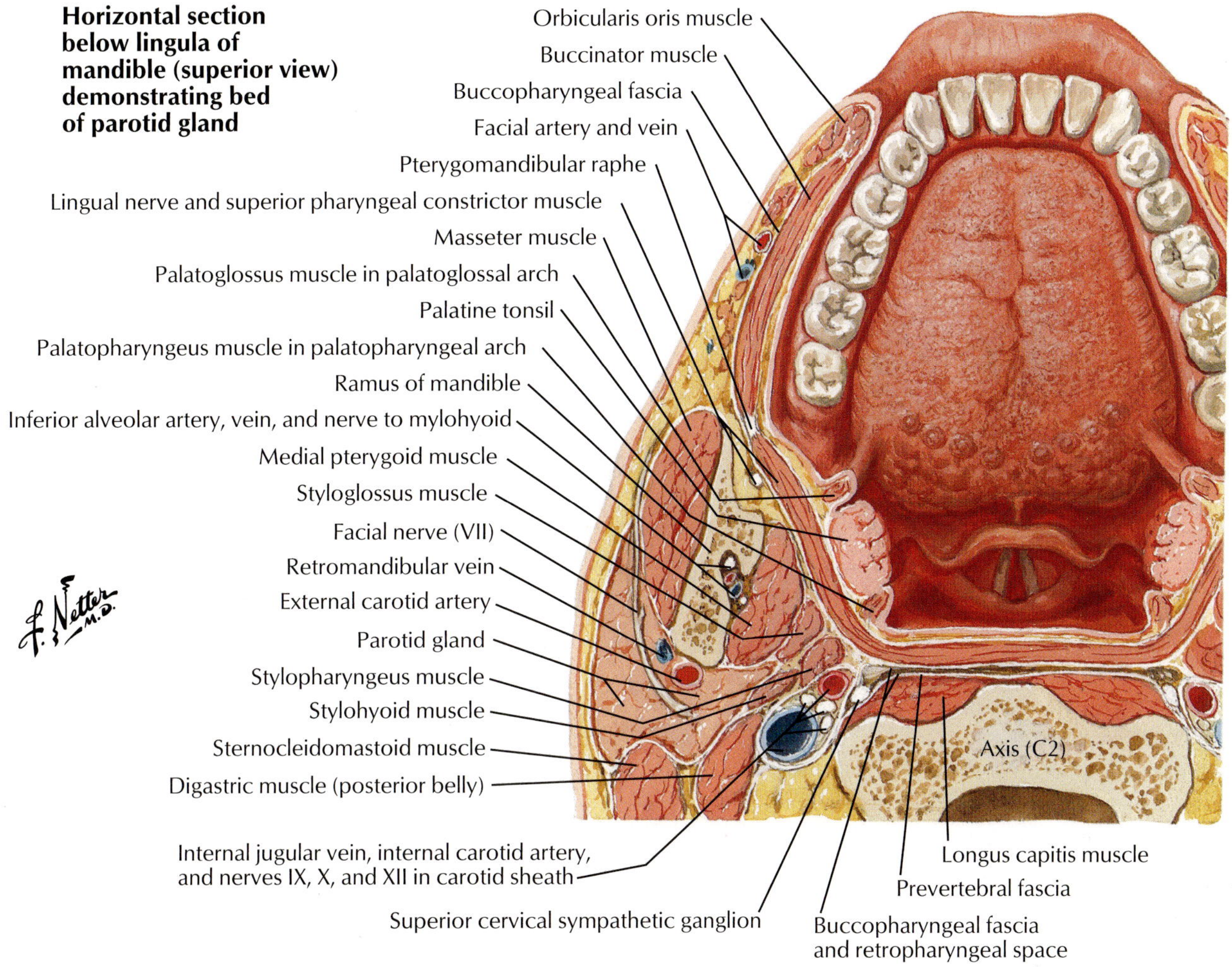

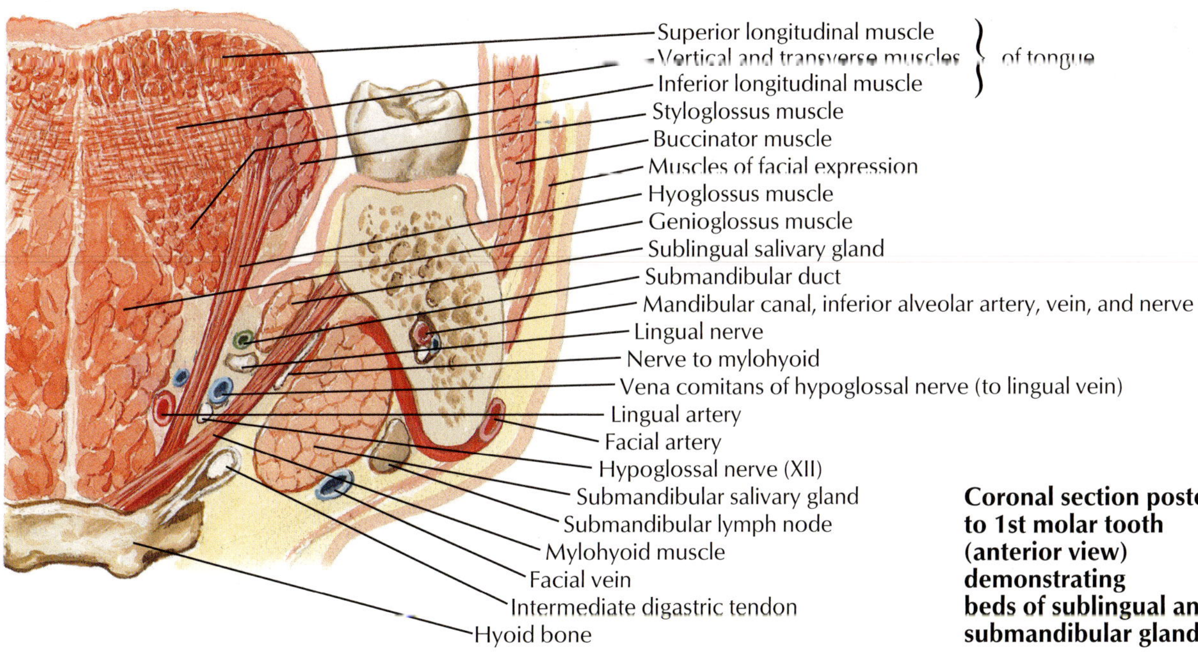

Coronal section posterior to 1st molar tooth (anterior view) demonstrating beds of sublingual and submandibular glands

Muscles Involved in Mastication

For facial muscles see **Plate 25**

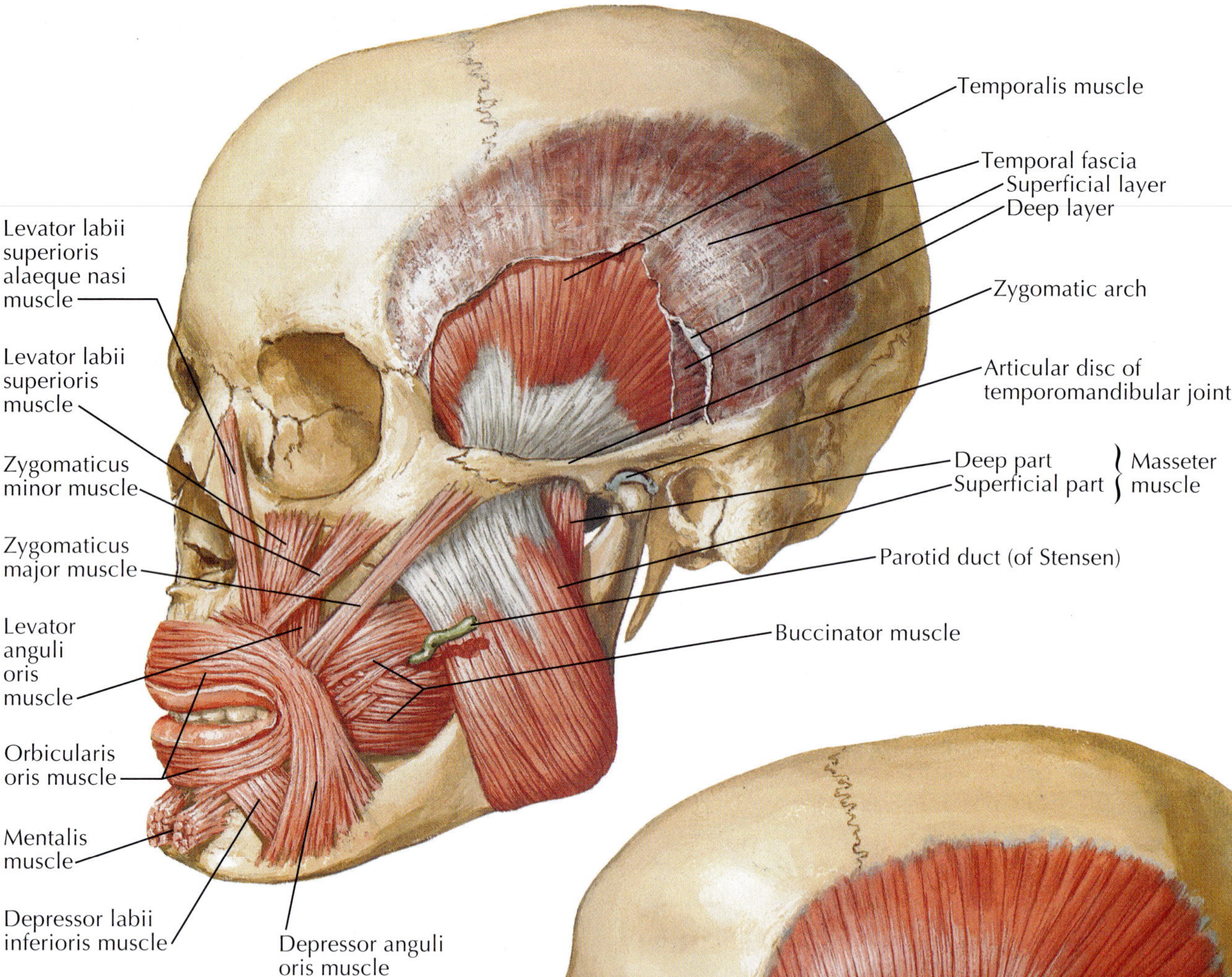

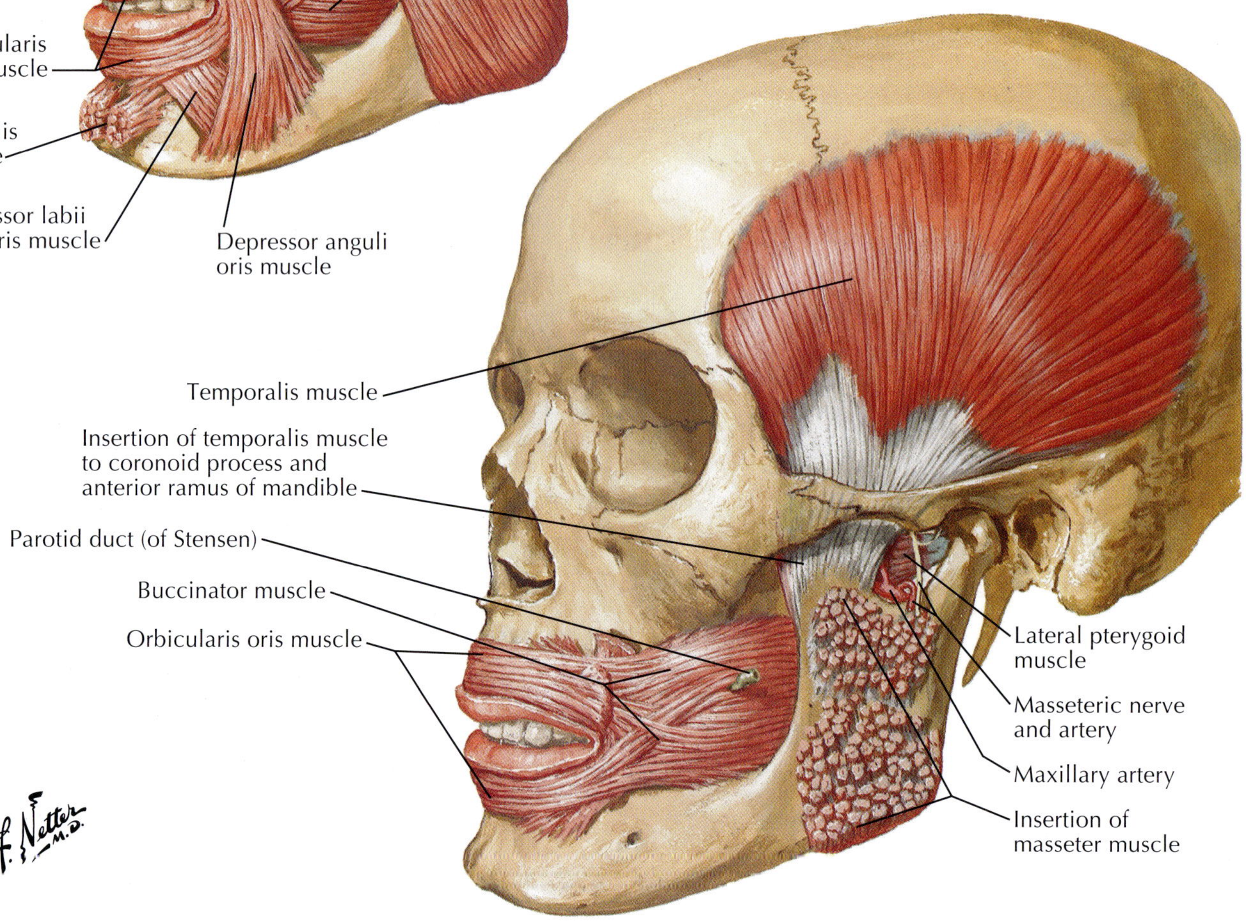

Muscles Involved in Mastication (continued)

See also Plates 18, 68

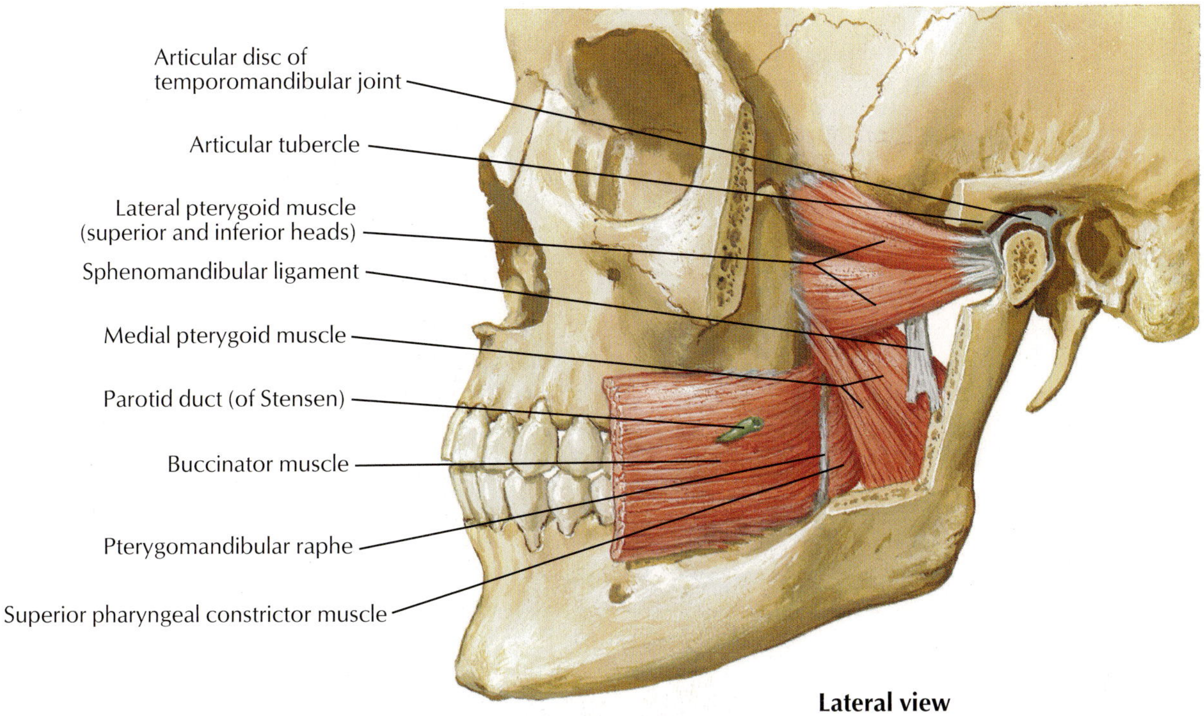

Lateral view

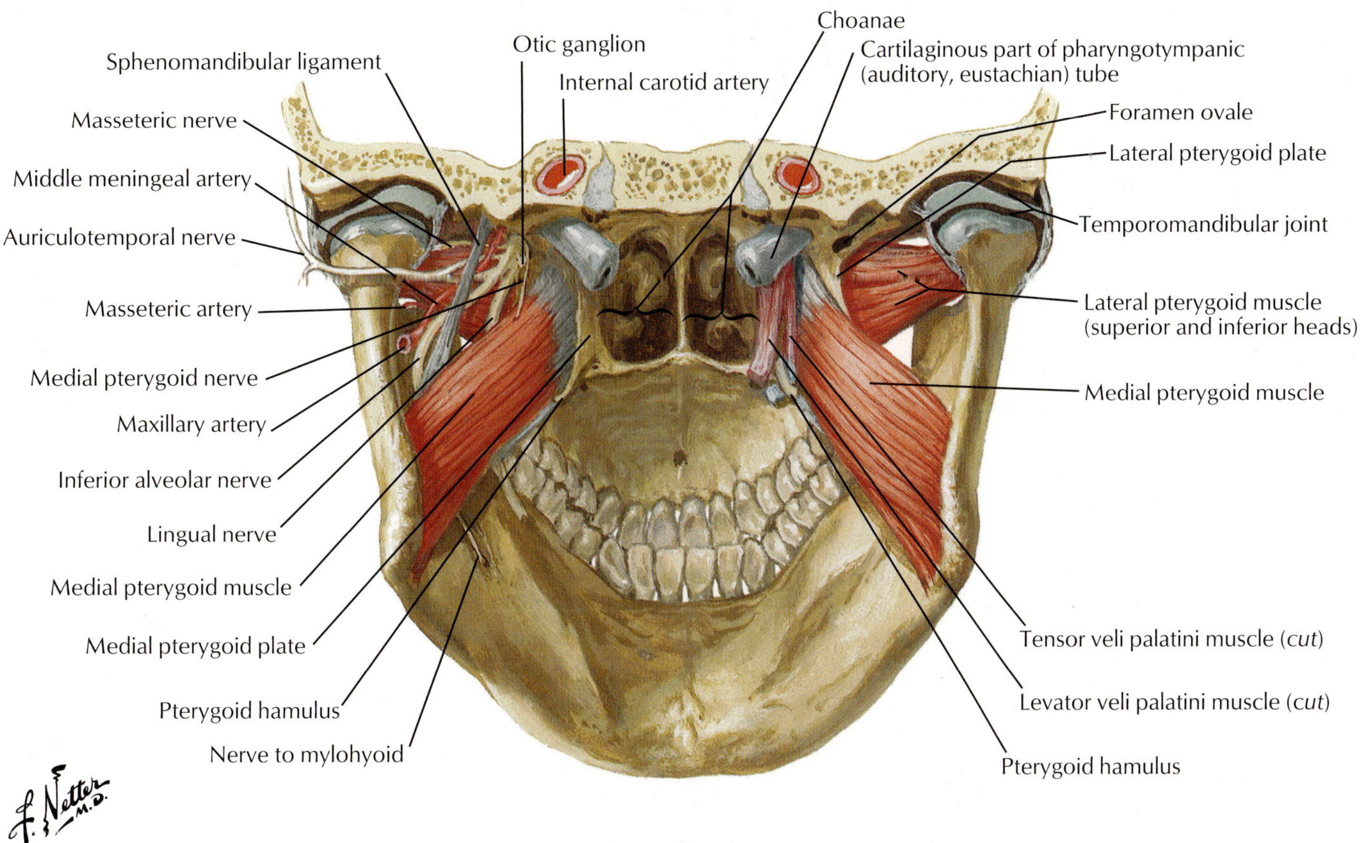

Posterior view

See also Plates 71, 123

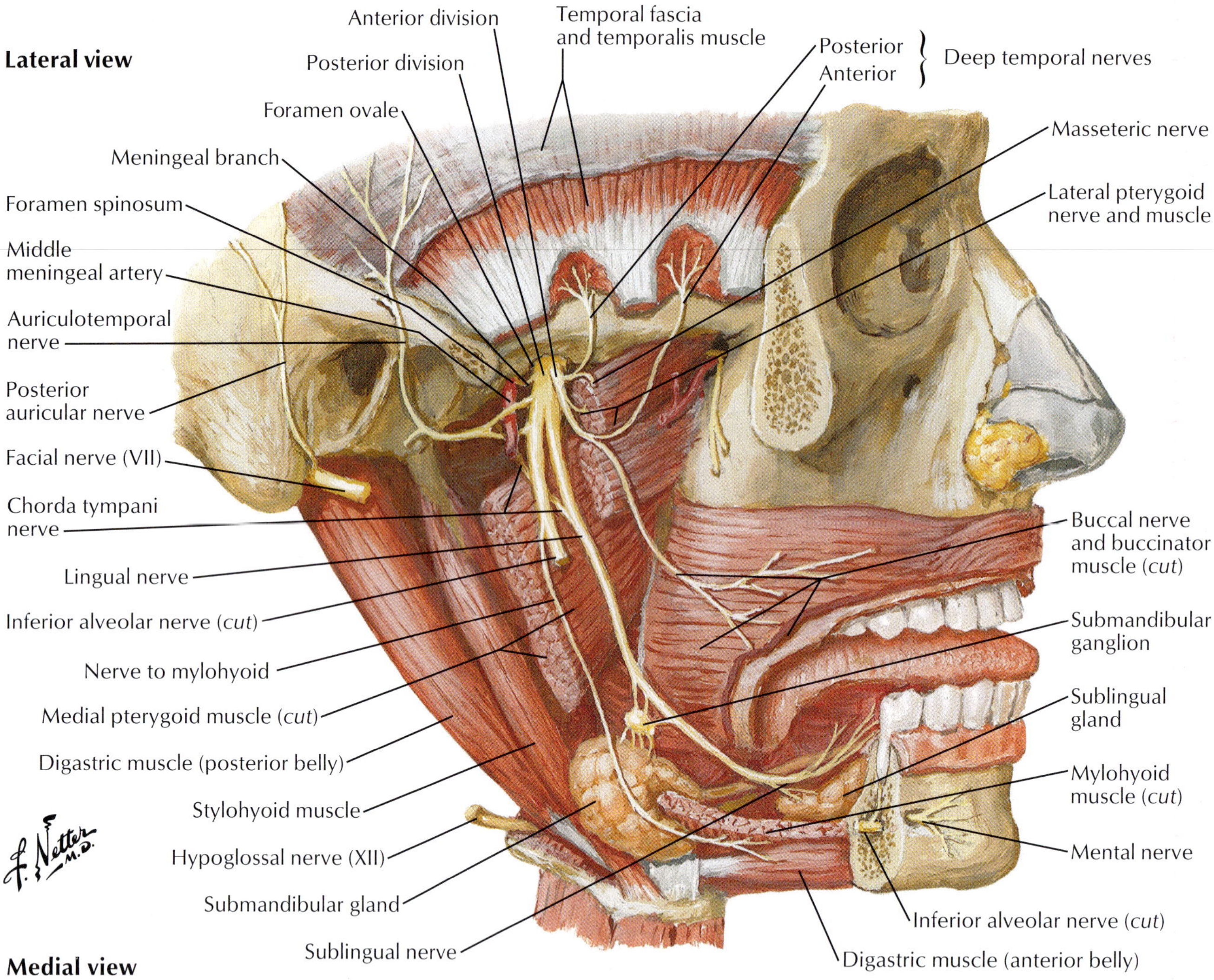

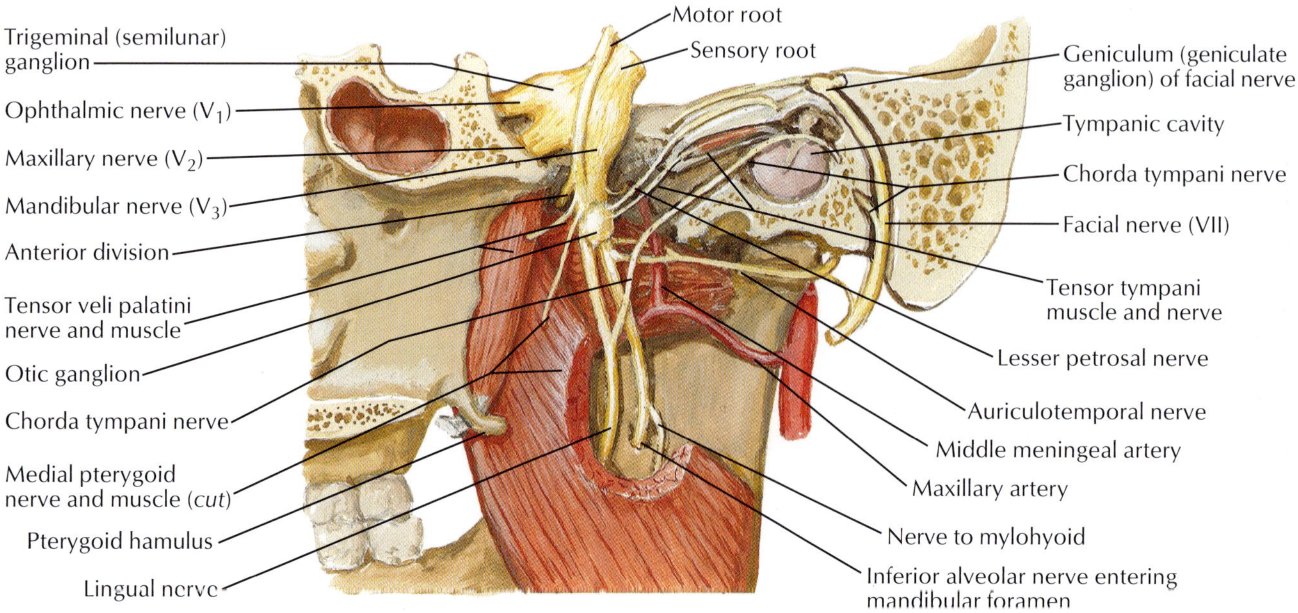

Maxillary Artery

See also Plates 34, 72

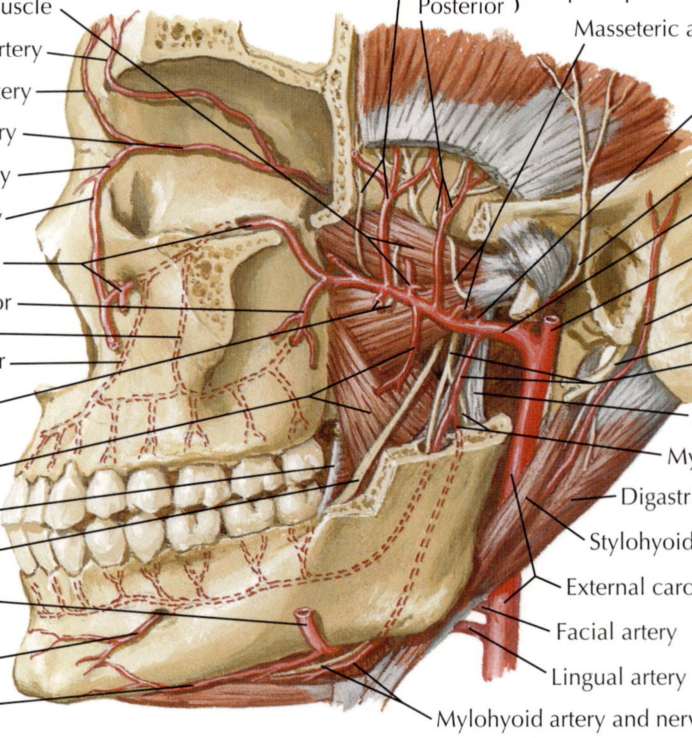

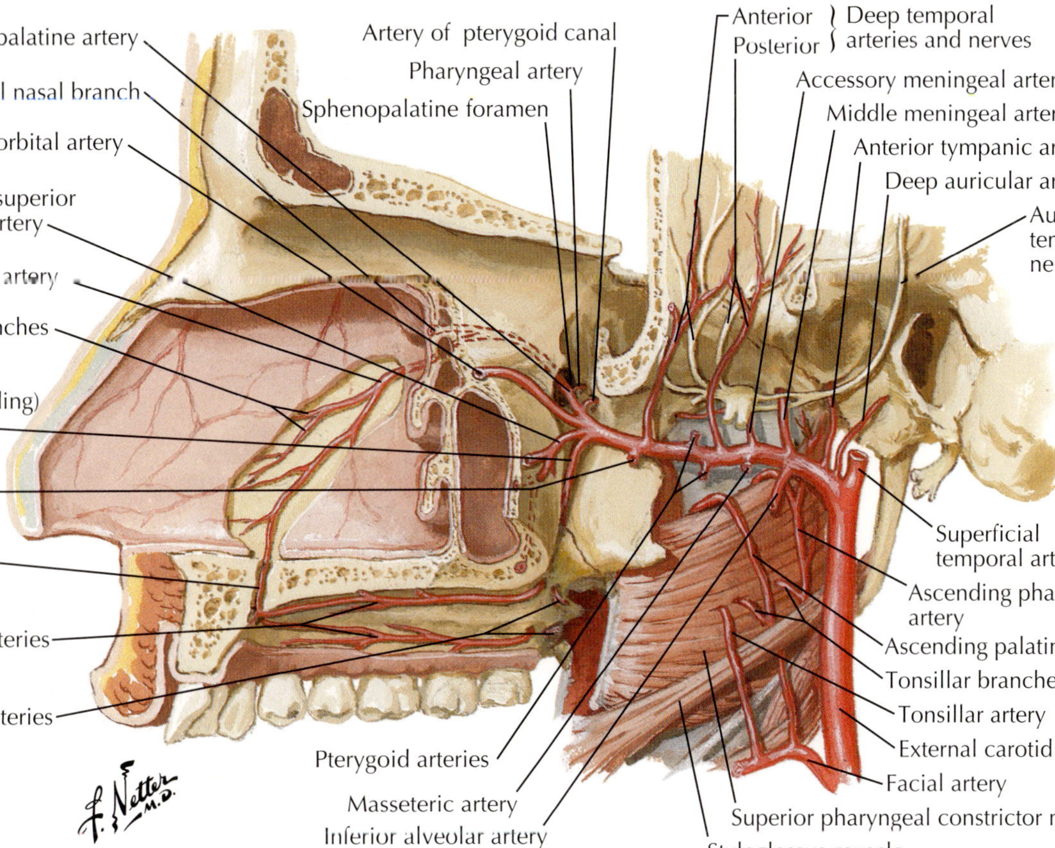

See also Plate 44

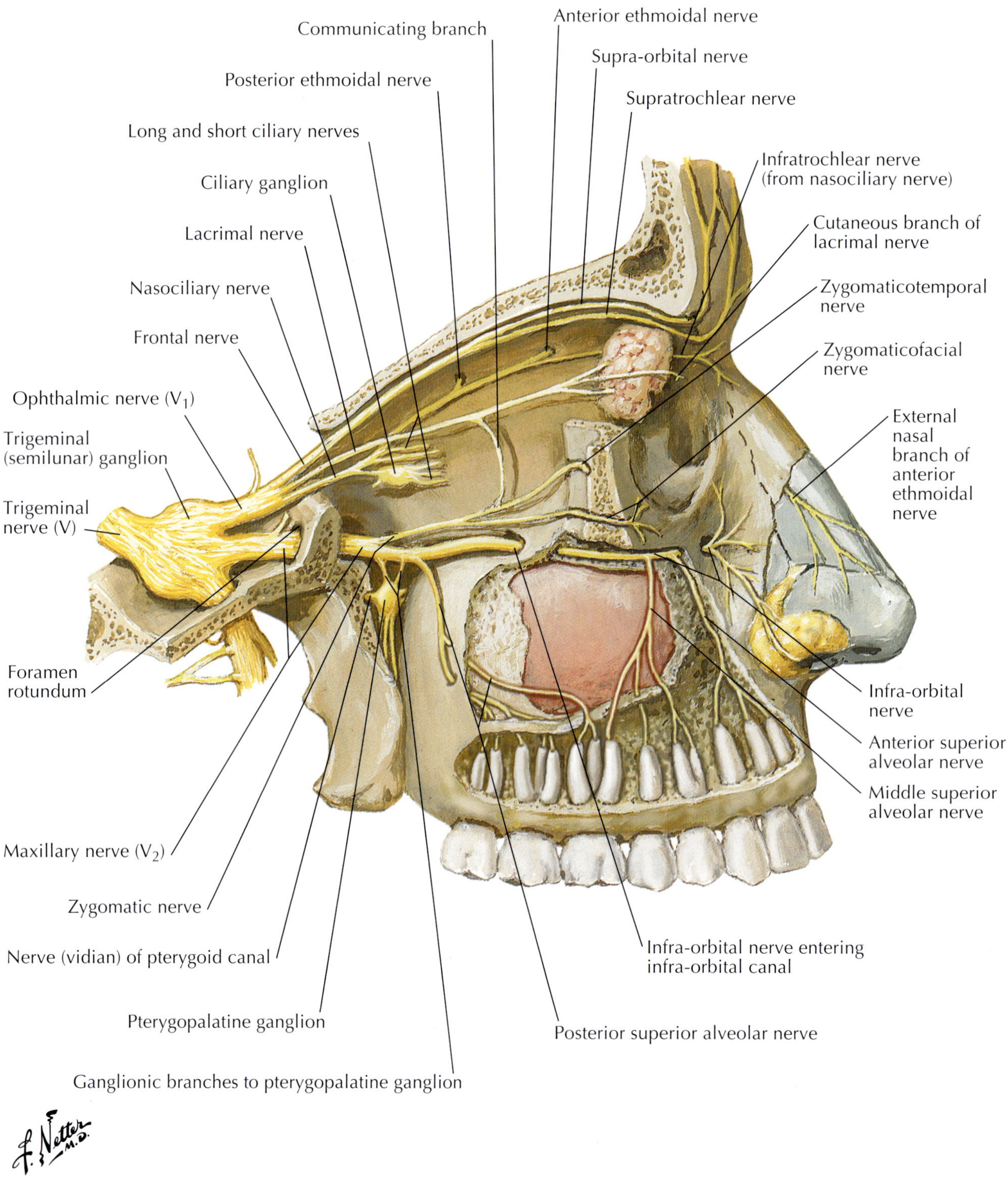

Autonomic Innervation of Nasal Cavity

See also Plates 123, 132, 134

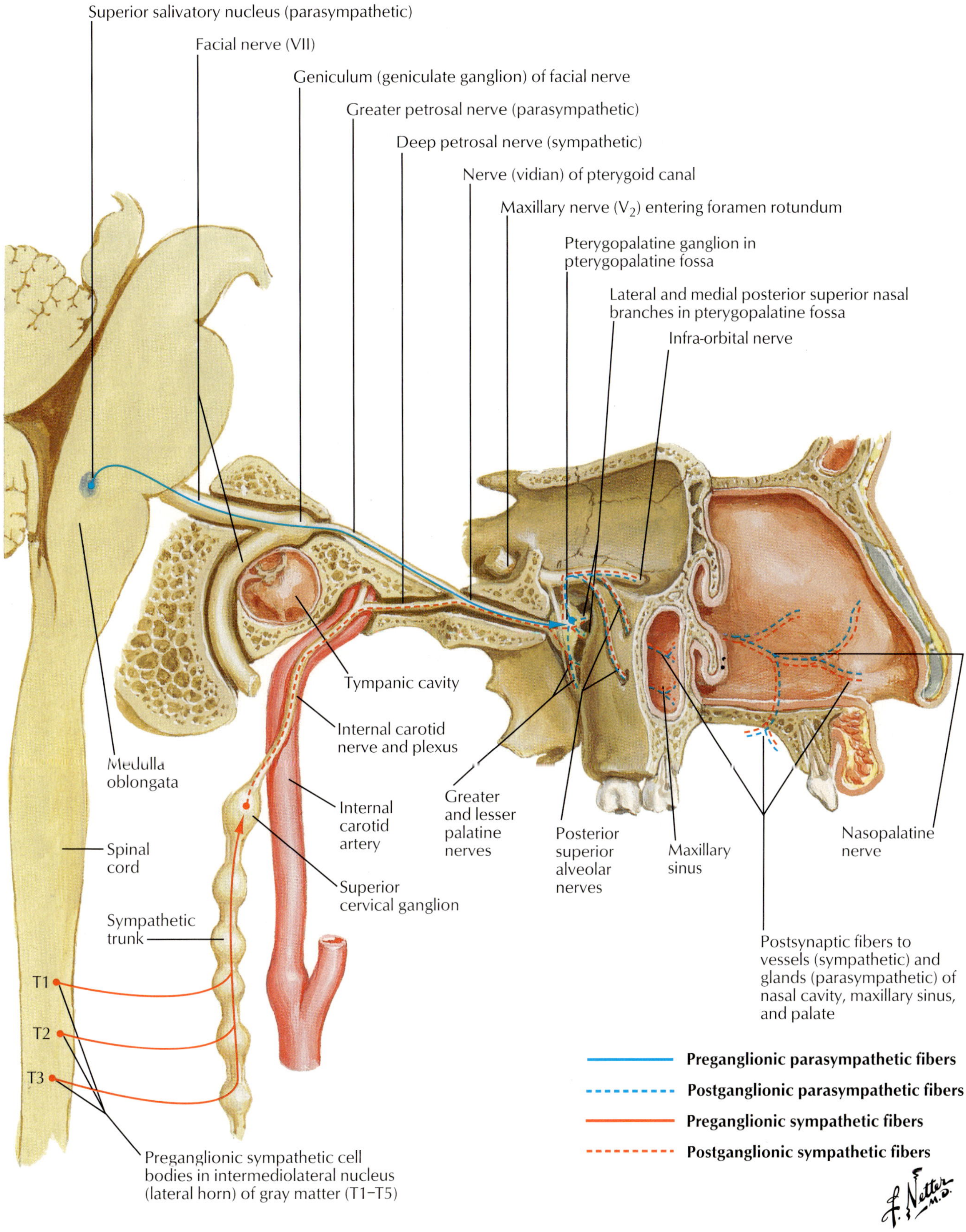

See also Plates 39, 41, 52

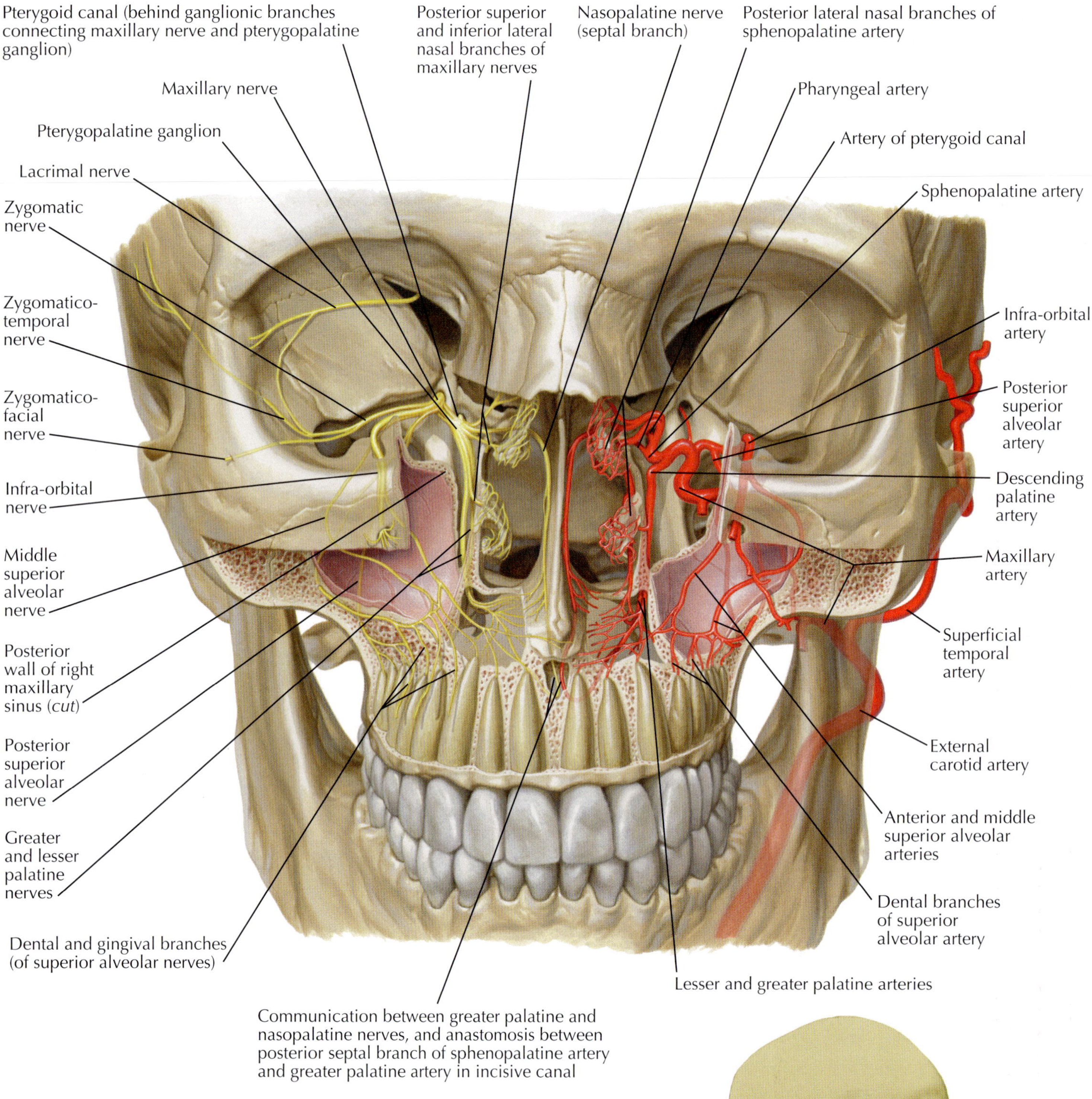

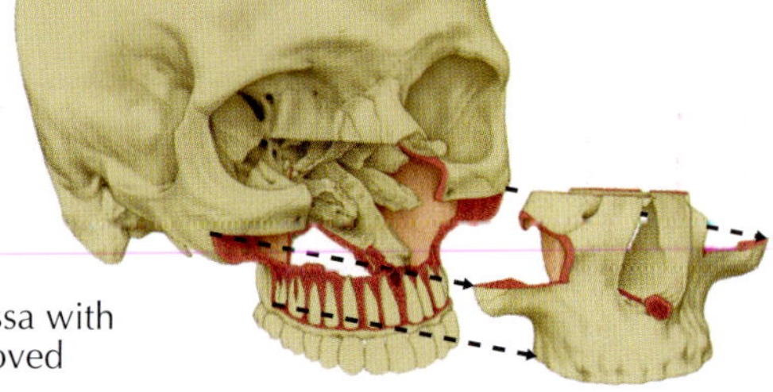

Anterior perspective of fossa with lower facial skeleton removed

Orientation of Nerves and Vessels of the Cranial Base

See also Plates 105, 132, 137

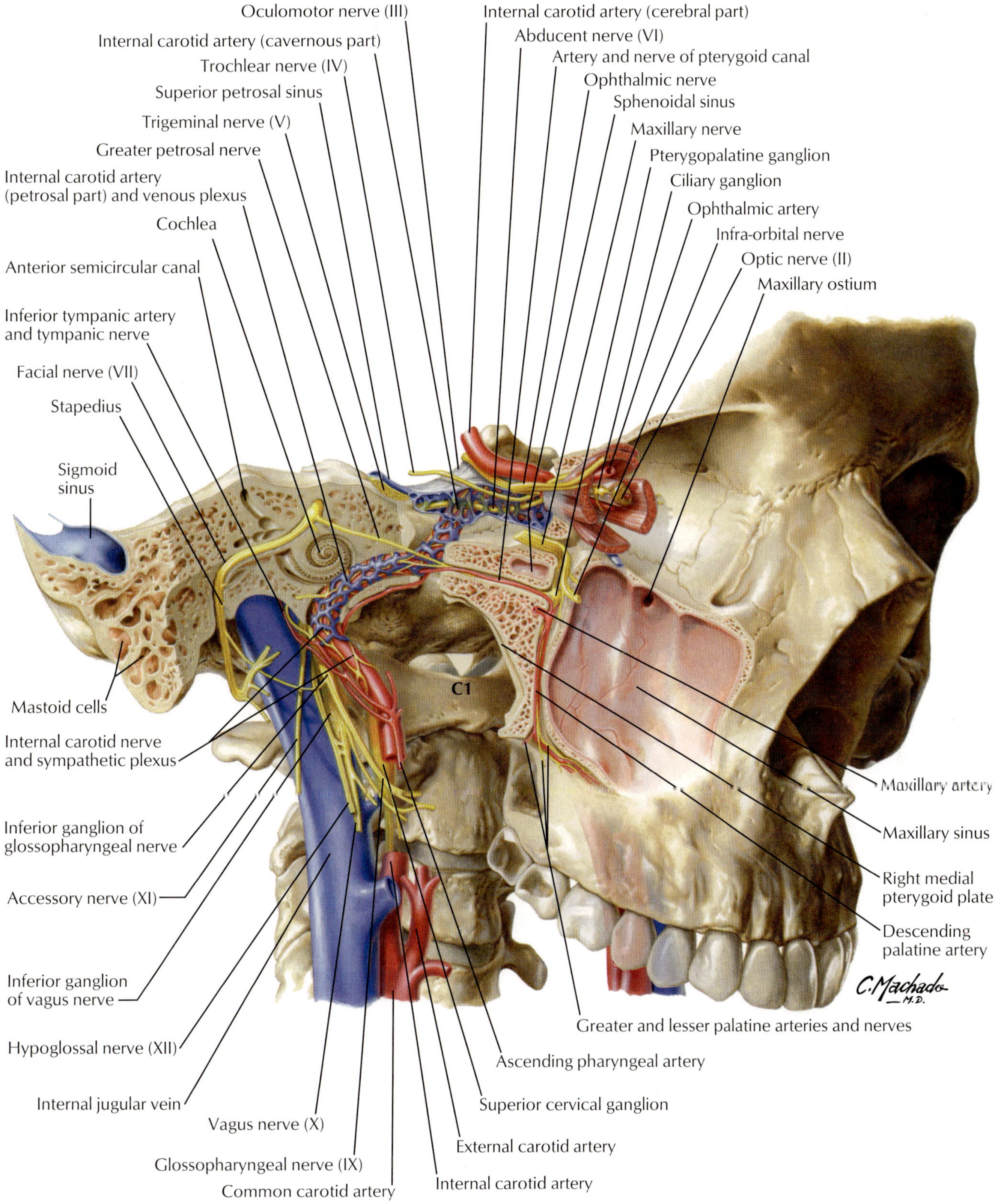

Inspection of Oral Cavity

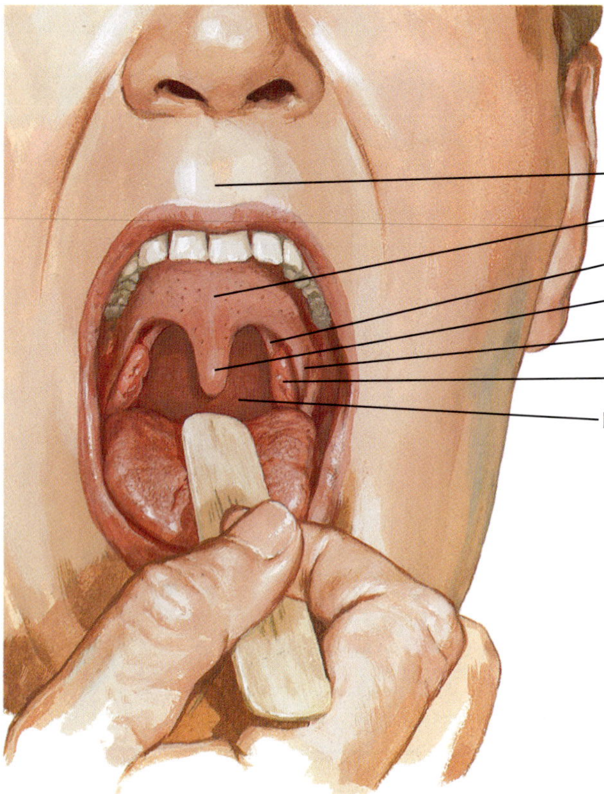

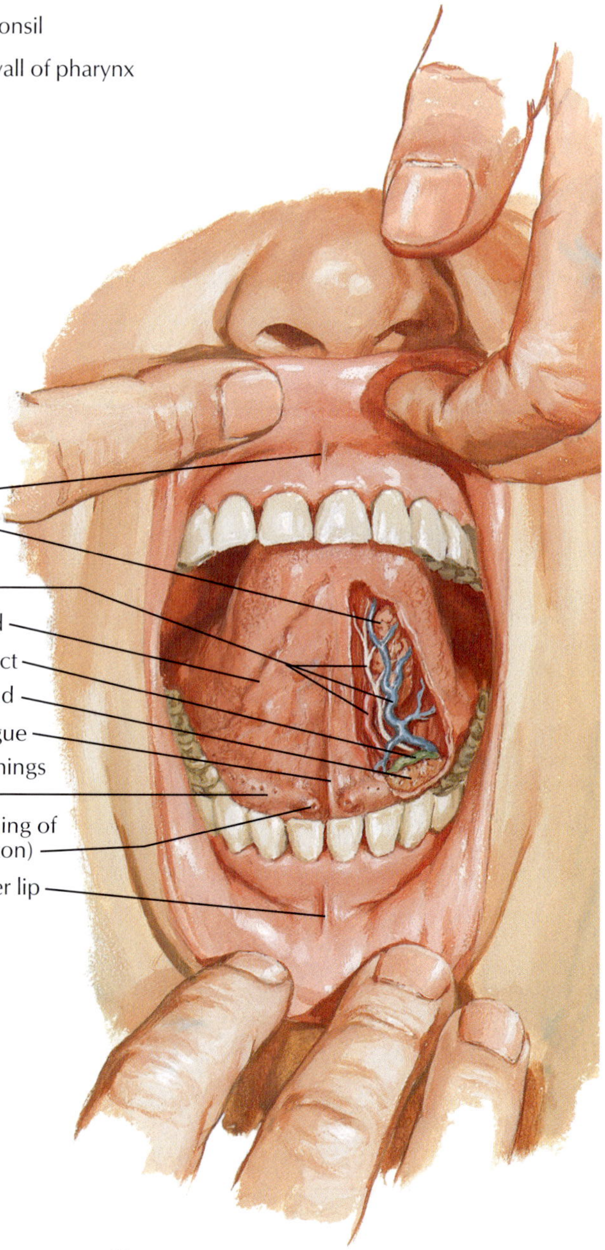

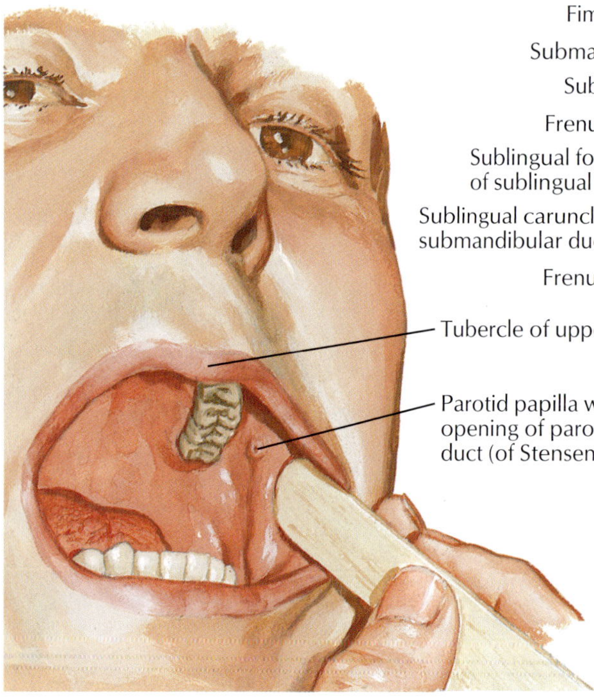

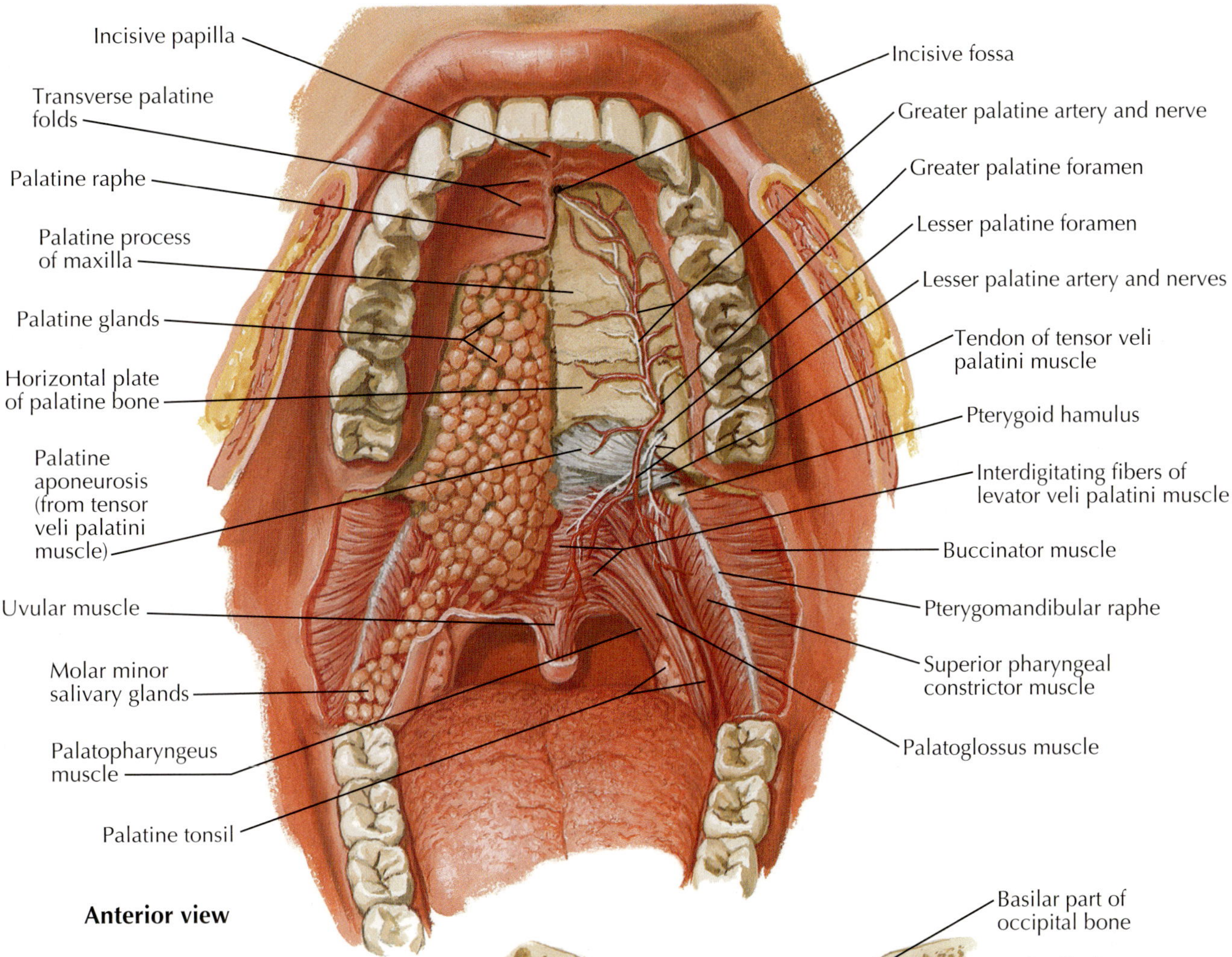

Anterior view

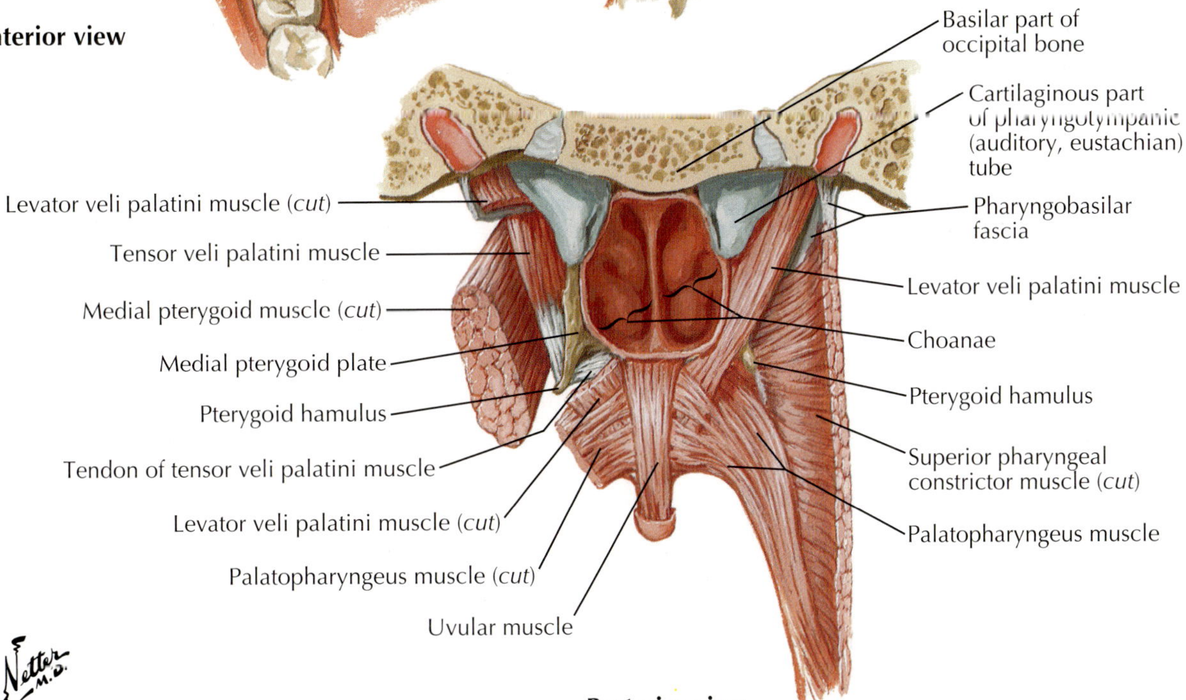

Posterior view

See also Plate 28

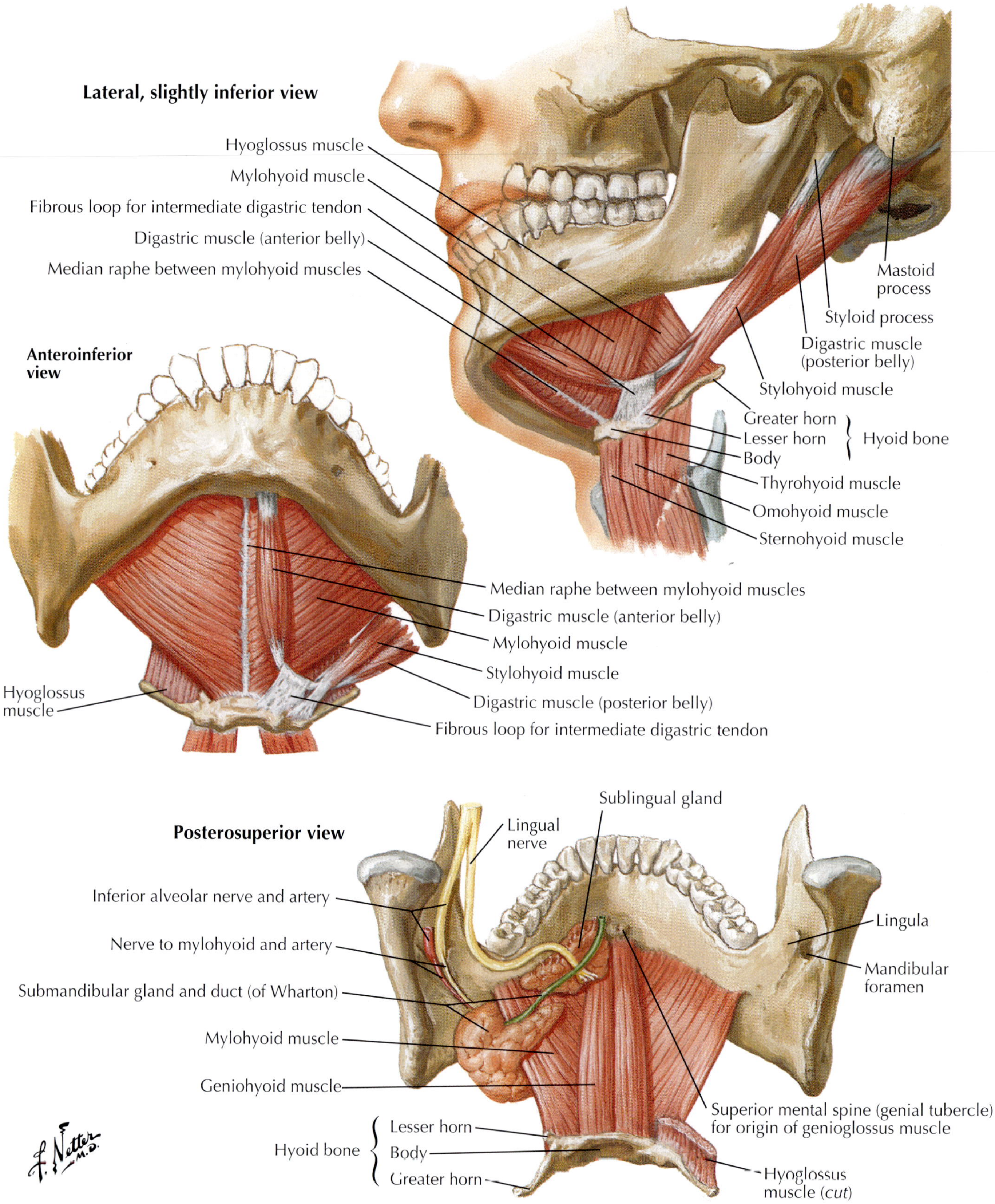

See also Plates 58, 129

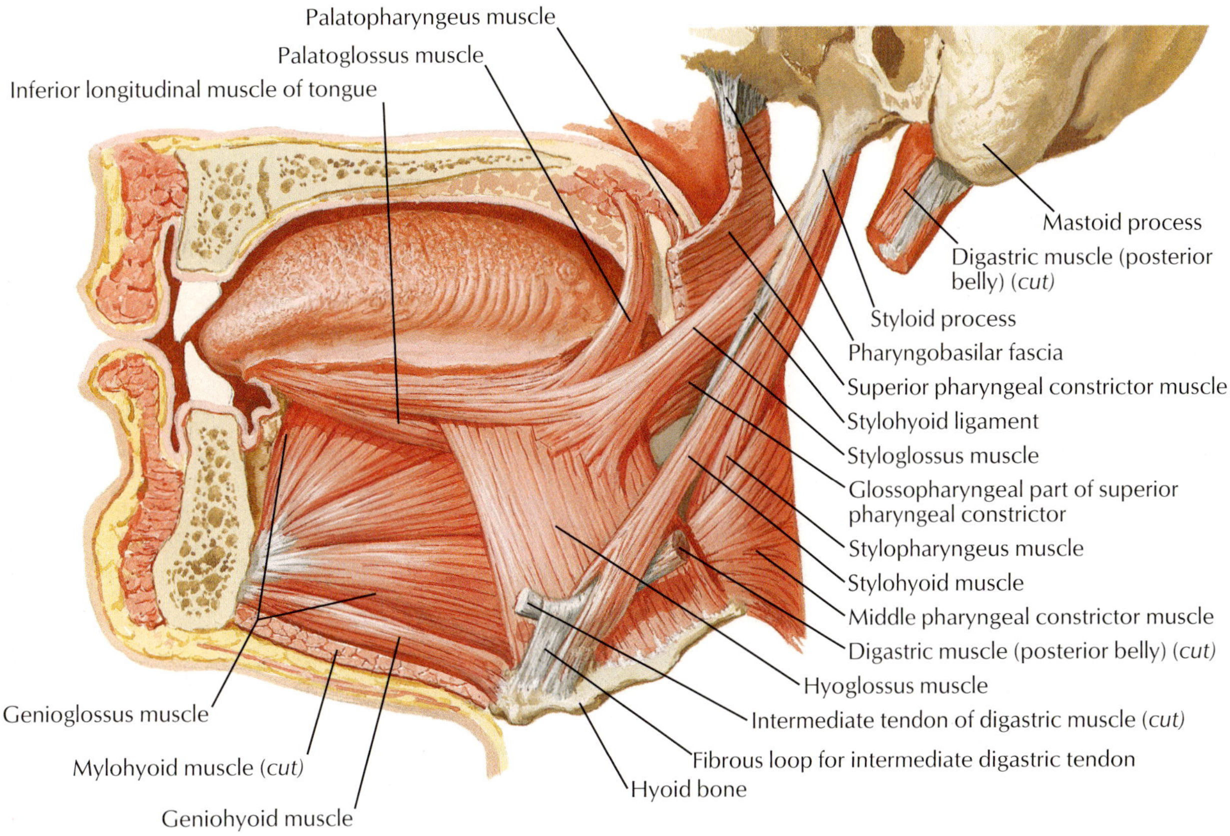

Lateral view

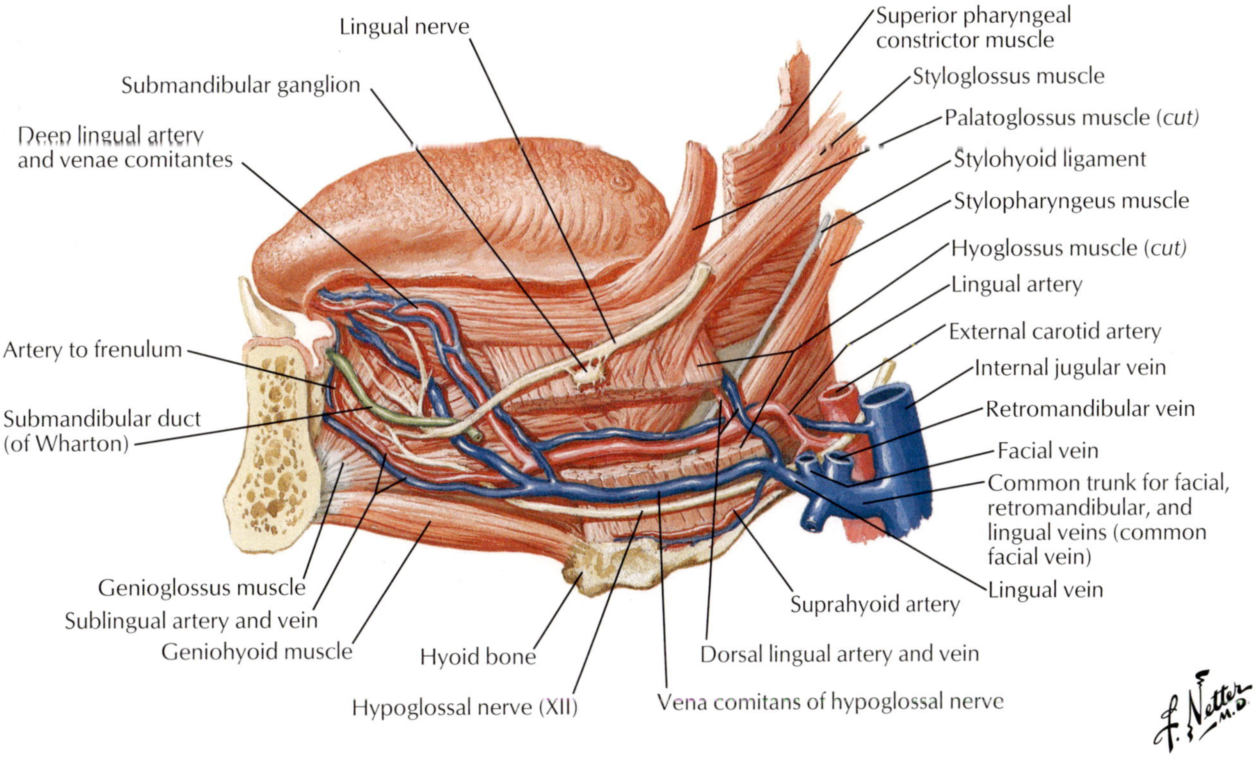

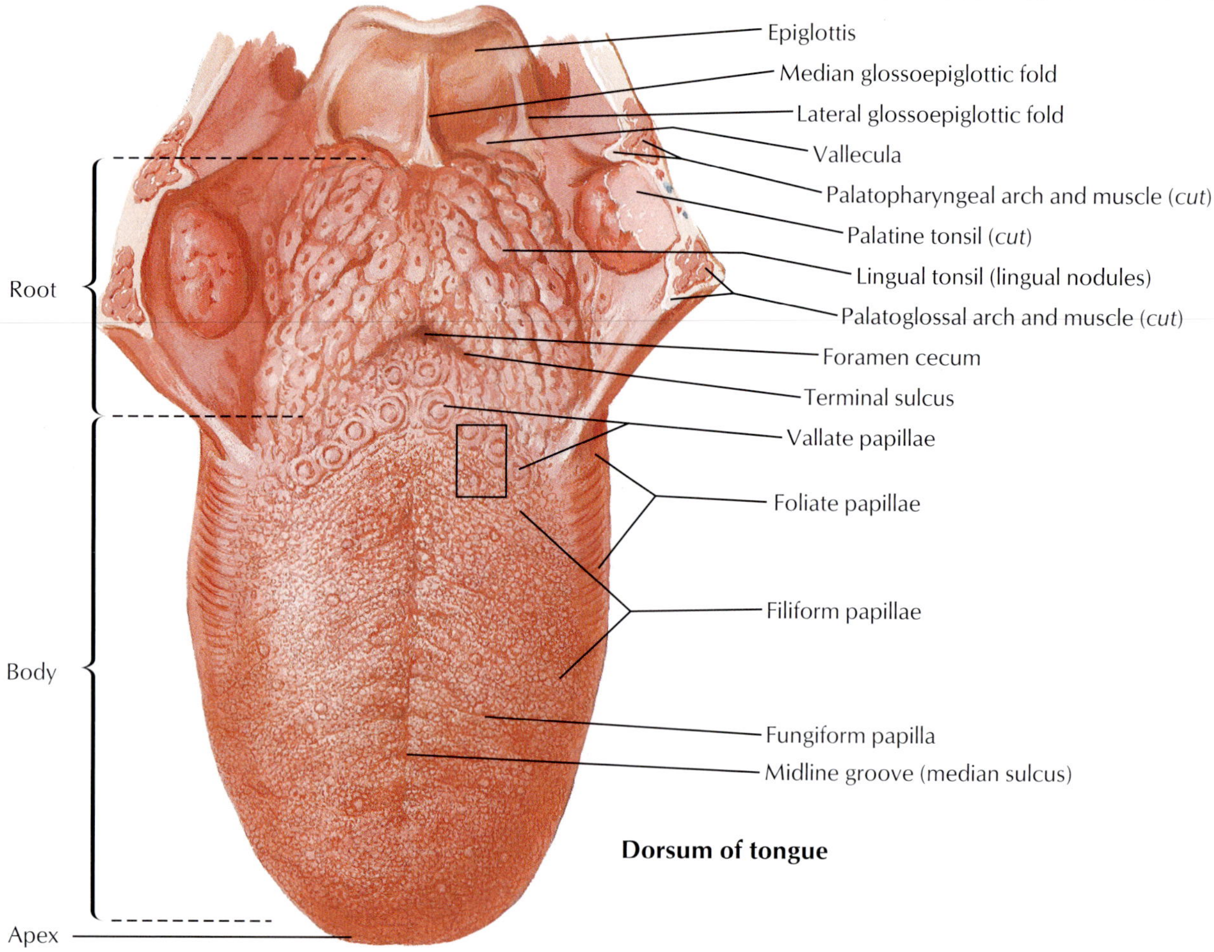

Dorsum of tongue

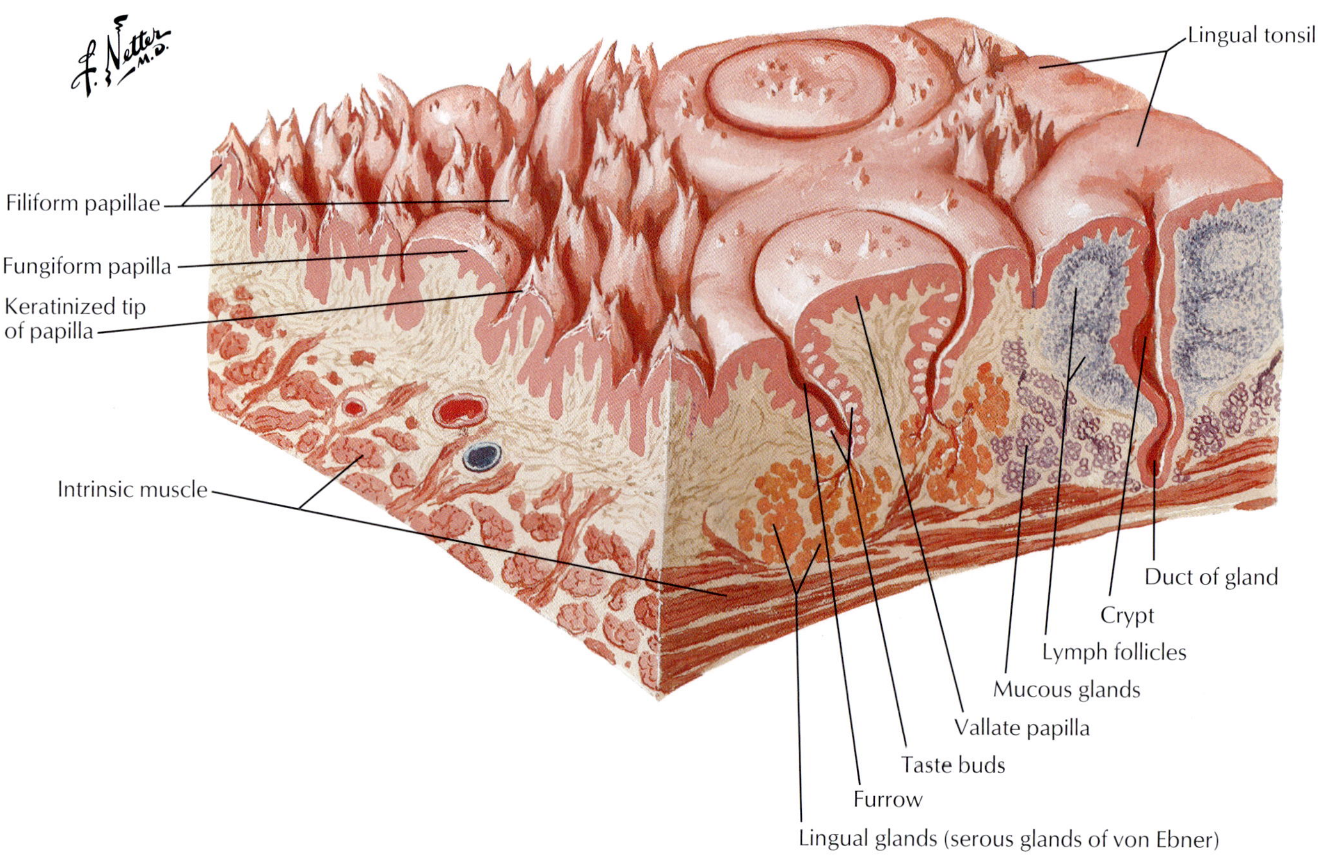

Schematic stereogram: area indicated above

Afferent Innervation of Oral Cavity and Pharynx

See also **Plates 126, 134, 136**

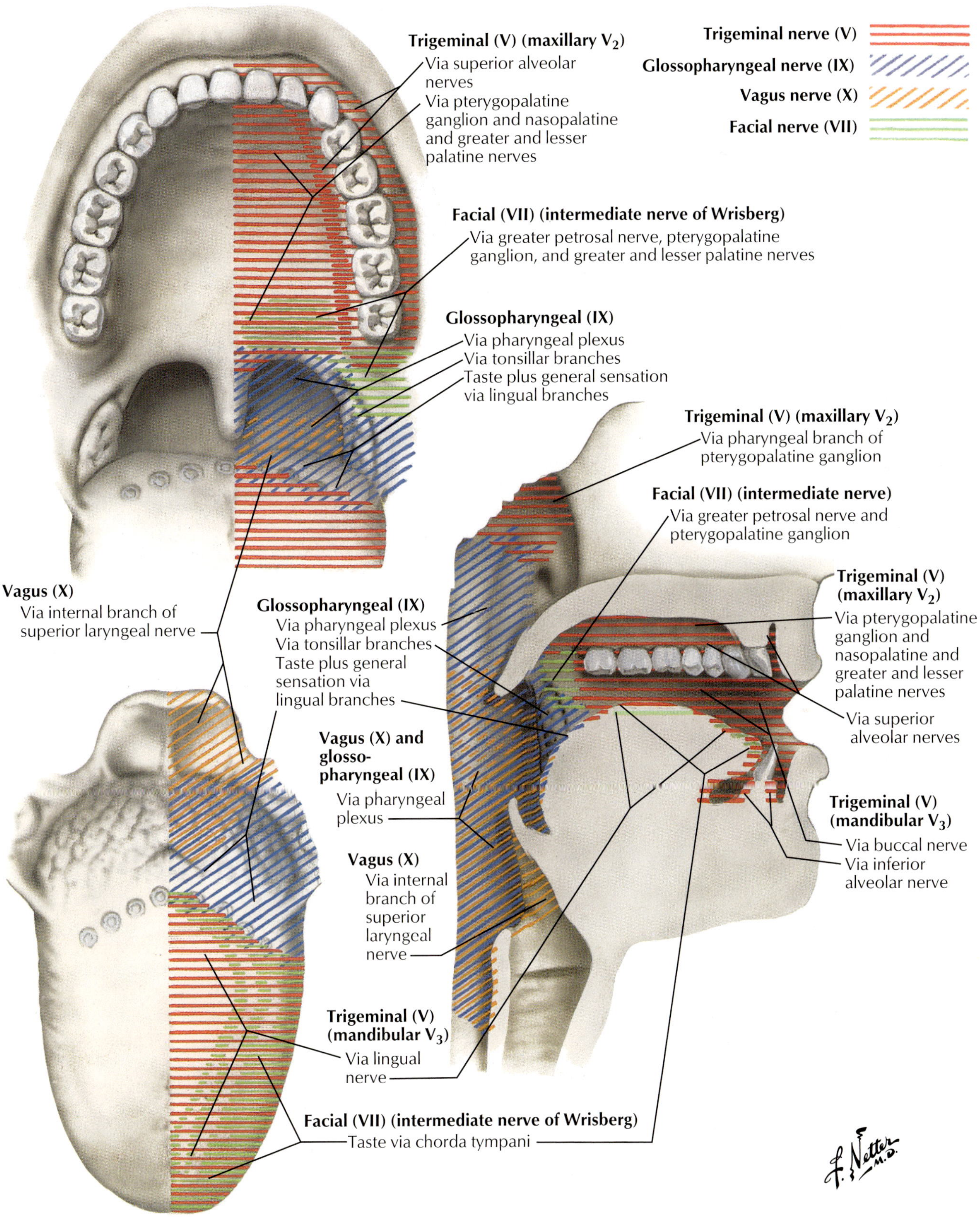

See also Plates 40, 41, 57

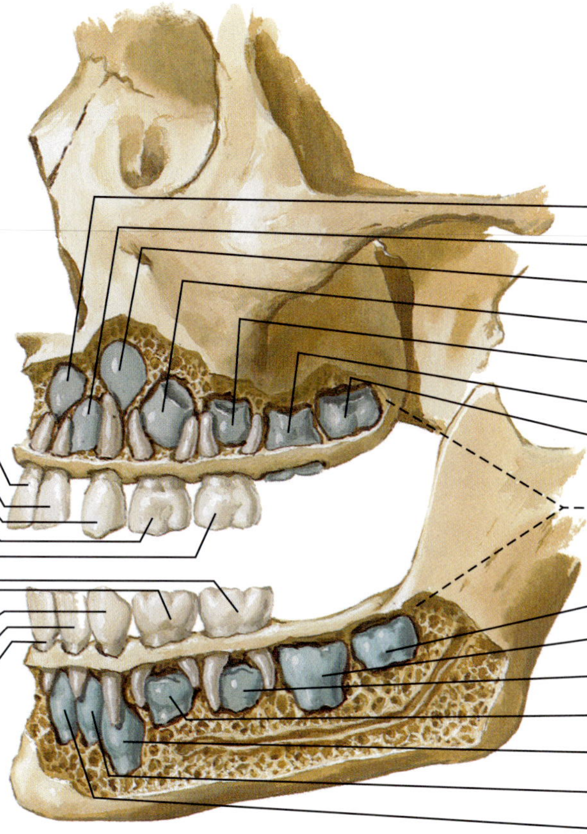

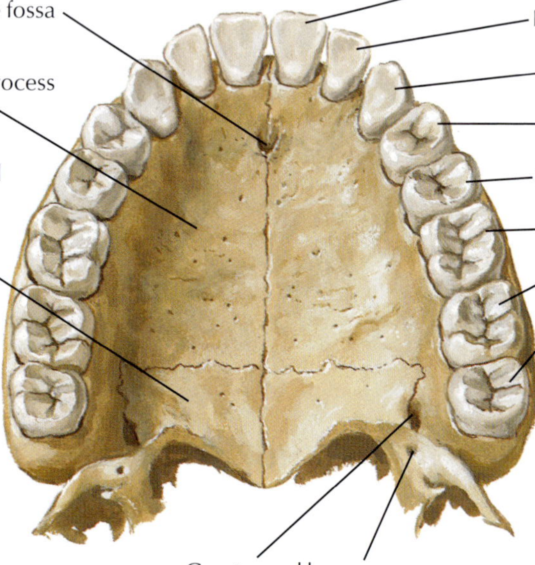

Upper permanent teeth

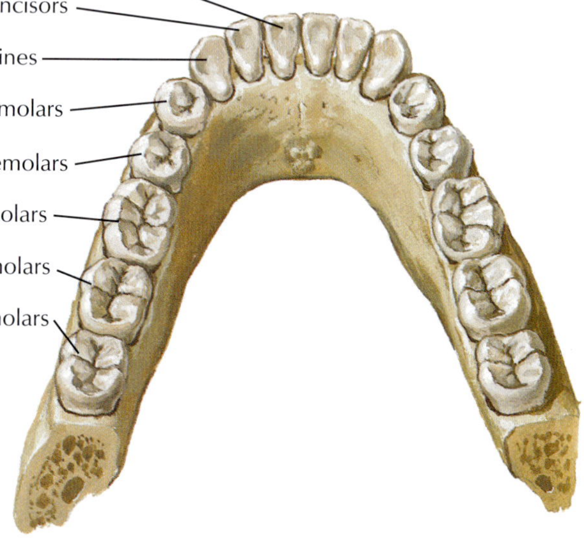

Lower permanent teeth

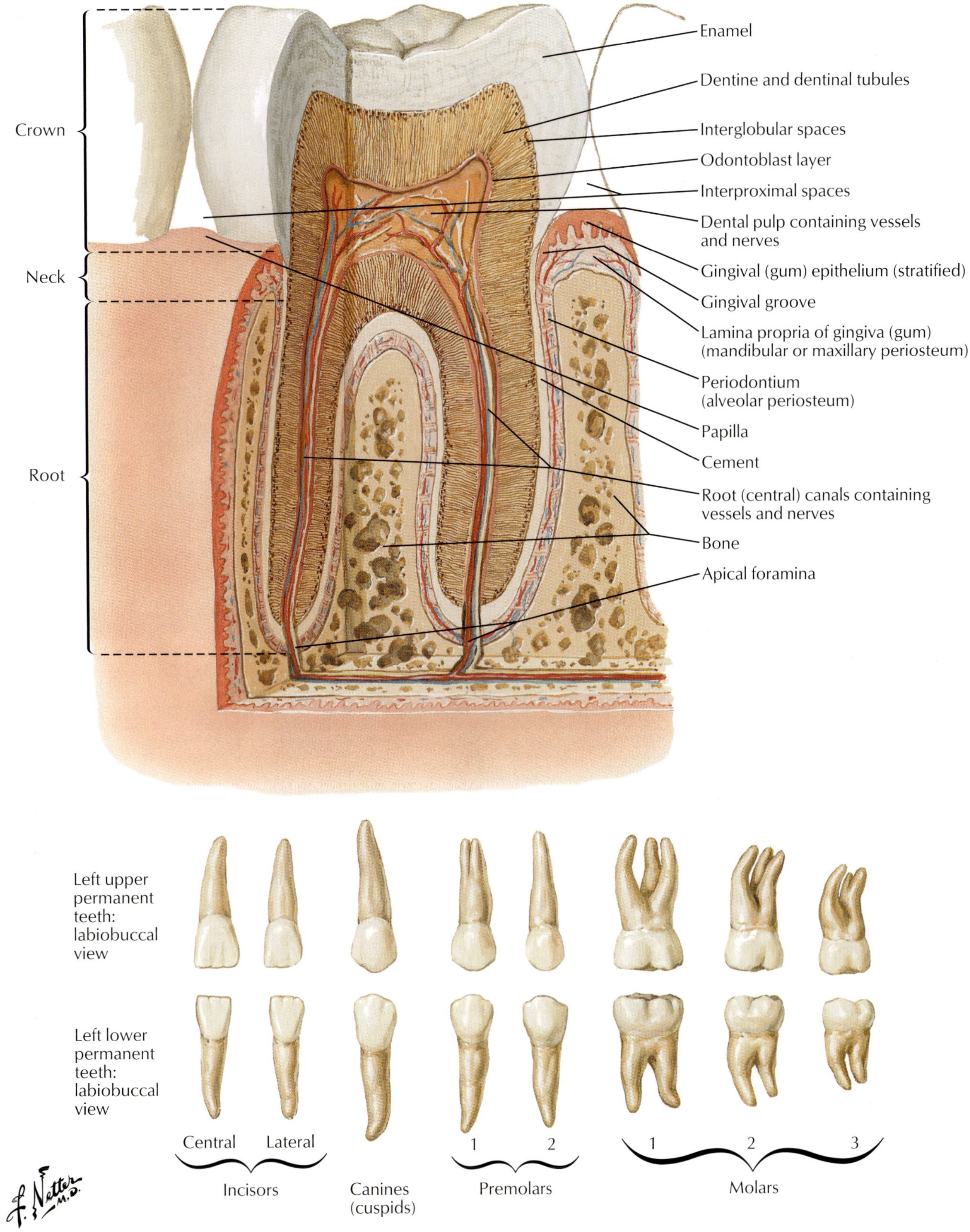
Crown
Neck
Root
Enamel
Dentine and dentinal tubules
Interglobular spaces
Odontoblast layer
Interproximal spaces
Dental pulp containing vessels and nerves
Gingival (gum) epithelium (stratified)
Gingival groove
Lamina propria of gingiva (gum) (mandibular or maxillary periosteum)
Periodontium (alveolar periosteum)
Papilla
Cement
Root (central) canals containing vessels and nerves
Bone
Apical foramina
Left upper permanent teeth: labiobuccal view
Left lower permanent teeth: labiobuccal view
Central
Lateral
Incisors
Canines (cuspids)
1
2
Premolars
1
2
3
Molars
F. Netter M.D.

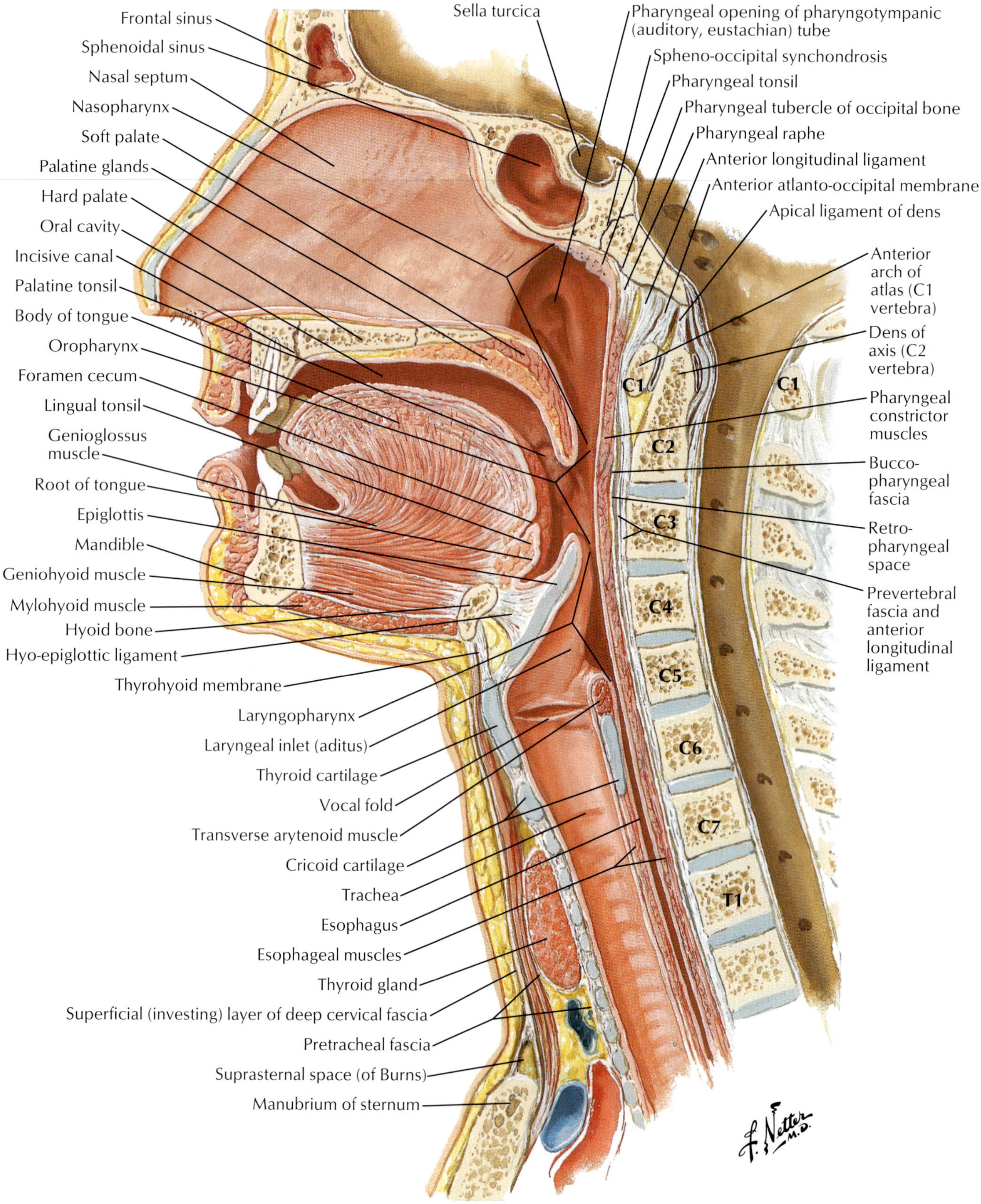
Frontal sinus
Sphenoidal sinus
Nasal septum
Nasopharynx
Soft palate
Palatine glands
Hard palate
Oral cavity
Incisive canal
Palatine tonsil
Body of tongue
Oropharynx
Foramen cecum
Lingual tonsil
Genioglossus muscle
Root of tongue
Epiglottis
Mandible
Geniohyoid muscle
Mylohyoid muscle
Hyoid bone
Hyo-epiglottic ligament
Thyrohyoid membrane
Laryngopharynx
Laryngeal inlet (aditus)
Thyroid cartilage
Vocal fold
Transverse arytenoid muscle
Cricoid cartilage
Trachea
Esophagus
Esophageal muscles
Thyroid gland
Superficial (investing) layer of deep cervical fascia
Pretracheal fascia
Suprasternal space (of Burns)
Manubrium of sternum
Sella turcica
Pharyngeal opening of pharyngotympanic (auditory, eustachian) tube
Spheno-occipital synchondrosis
Pharyngeal tonsil
Pharyngeal tubercle of occipital bone
Pharyngeal raphe
Anterior longitudinal ligament
Anterior atlanto-occipital membrane
Apical ligament of dens
Anterior arch of atlas (C1 vertebra)
Dens of axis (C2 vertebra)
Pharyngeal constrictor muscles
Bucco-pharyngeal fascia
Retro-pharyngeal space
Prevertebral fascia and anterior longitudinal ligament
C1
C2
C3
C4
C5
C6
C7
T1
C1

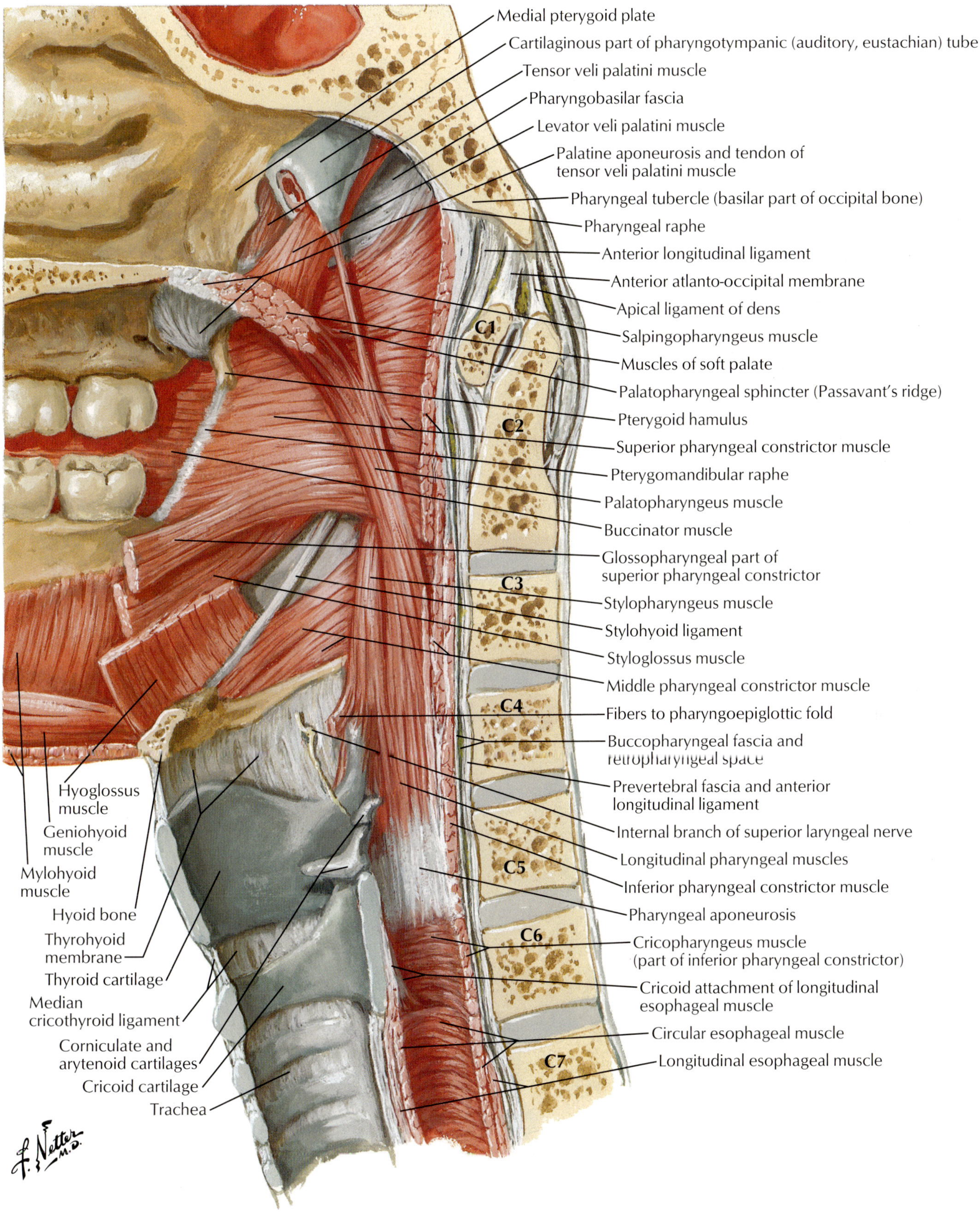
Medial pterygoid plate
Cartilaginous part of pharyngotympanic (auditory, eustachian) tube
Tensor veli palatini muscle
Pharyngobasilar fascia
Levator veli palatini muscle
Palatine aponeurosis and tendon of tensor veli palatini muscle
Pharyngeal tubercle (basilar part of occipital bone)
Pharyngeal raphe
Anterior longitudinal ligament
Anterior atlanto-occipital membrane
Apical ligament of dens
Salpingopharyngeus muscle
Muscles of soft palate
Palatopharyngeal sphincter (Passavant's ridge)
Pterygoid hamulus
Superior pharyngeal constrictor muscle
Pterygomandibular raphe
Palatopharyngeus muscle
Buccinator muscle
Glossopharyngeal part of superior pharyngeal constrictor
Stylopharyngeus muscle
Stylohyoid ligament
Styloglossus muscle
Middle pharyngeal constrictor muscle
Fibers to pharyngoepiglottic fold
Buccopharyngeal fascia and retropharyngeal space
Prevertebral fascia and anterior longitudinal ligament
Internal branch of superior laryngeal nerve
Longitudinal pharyngeal muscles
Inferior pharyngeal constrictor muscle
Pharyngeal aponeurosis
Cricopharyngeus muscle (part of inferior pharyngeal constrictor)
Cricoid attachment of longitudinal esophageal muscle
Circular esophageal muscle
Longitudinal esophageal muscle
C1
C2
C3
C4
C5
C6
C7
Hyoglossus muscle
Geniohyoid muscle
Mylohyoid muscle
Hyoid bone
Thyrohyoid membrane
Thyroid cartilage
Median cricothyroid ligament
Corniculate and arytenoid cartilages
Cricoid cartilage
Trachea
F. Netter M.D.

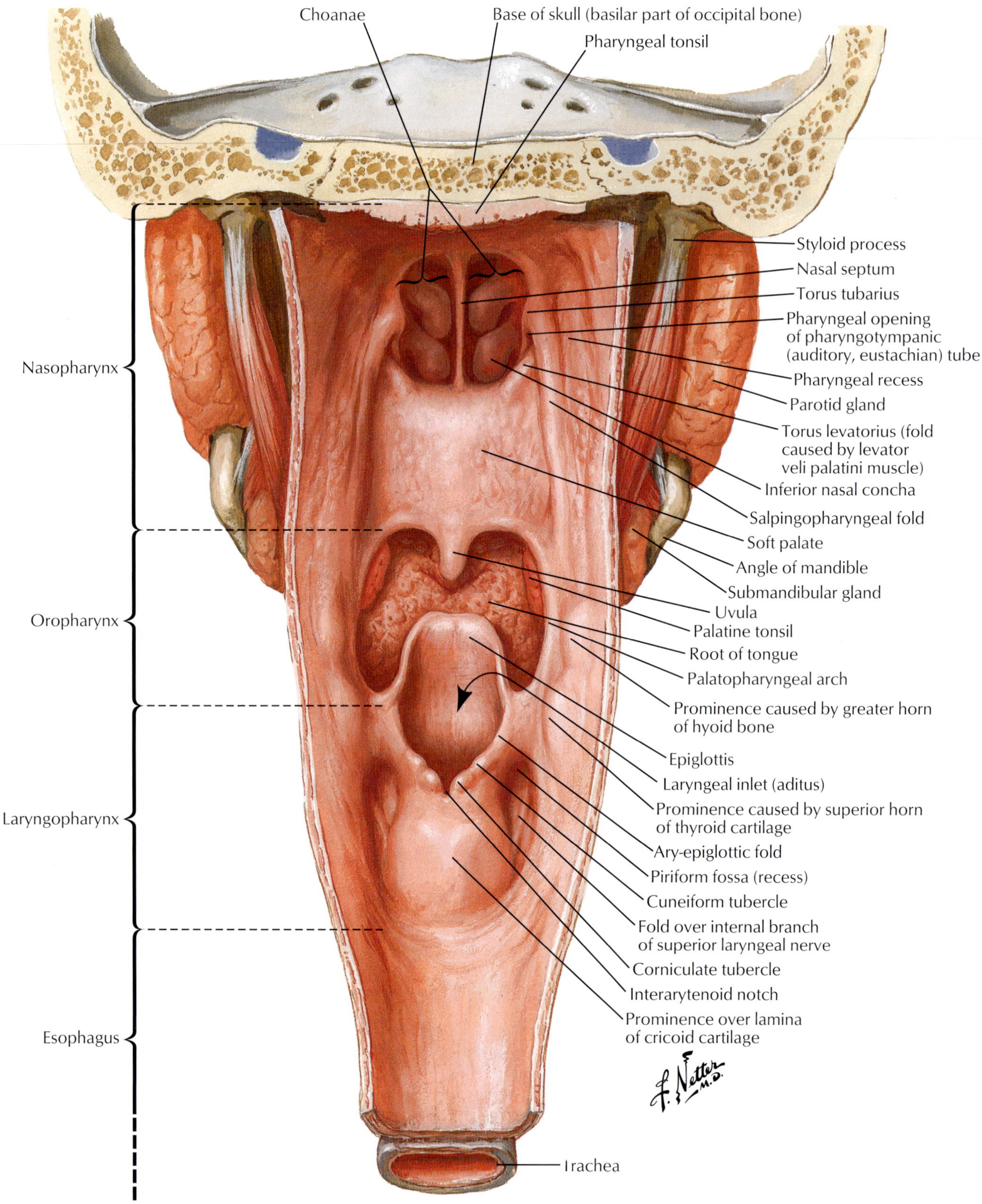
Choanae
Base of skull (basilar part of occipital bone)
Pharyngeal tonsil
Styloid process
Nasal septum
Torus tubarius
Pharyngeal opening of pharyngotympanic (auditory, eustachian) tube
Pharyngeal recess
Parotid gland
Torus levatorius (fold caused by levator veli palatini muscle)
Inferior nasal concha
Salpingopharyngeal fold
Soft palate
Angle of mandible
Submandibular gland
Uvula
Palatine tonsil
Root of tongue
Palatopharyngeal arch
Prominence caused by greater horn of hyoid bone
Epiglottis
Laryngeal inlet (aditus)
Prominence caused by superior horn of thyroid cartilage
Ary-epiglottic fold
Piriform fossa (recess)
Cuneiform tubercle
Fold over internal branch of superior laryngeal nerve
Corniculate tubercle
Interarytenoid notch
Prominence over lamina of cricoid cartilage
Trachea
Nasopharynx
Oropharynx
Laryngopharynx
Esophagus
F. Netter M.D.

Muscles of Pharynx: Partially Opened Posterior View

See also Plate 70

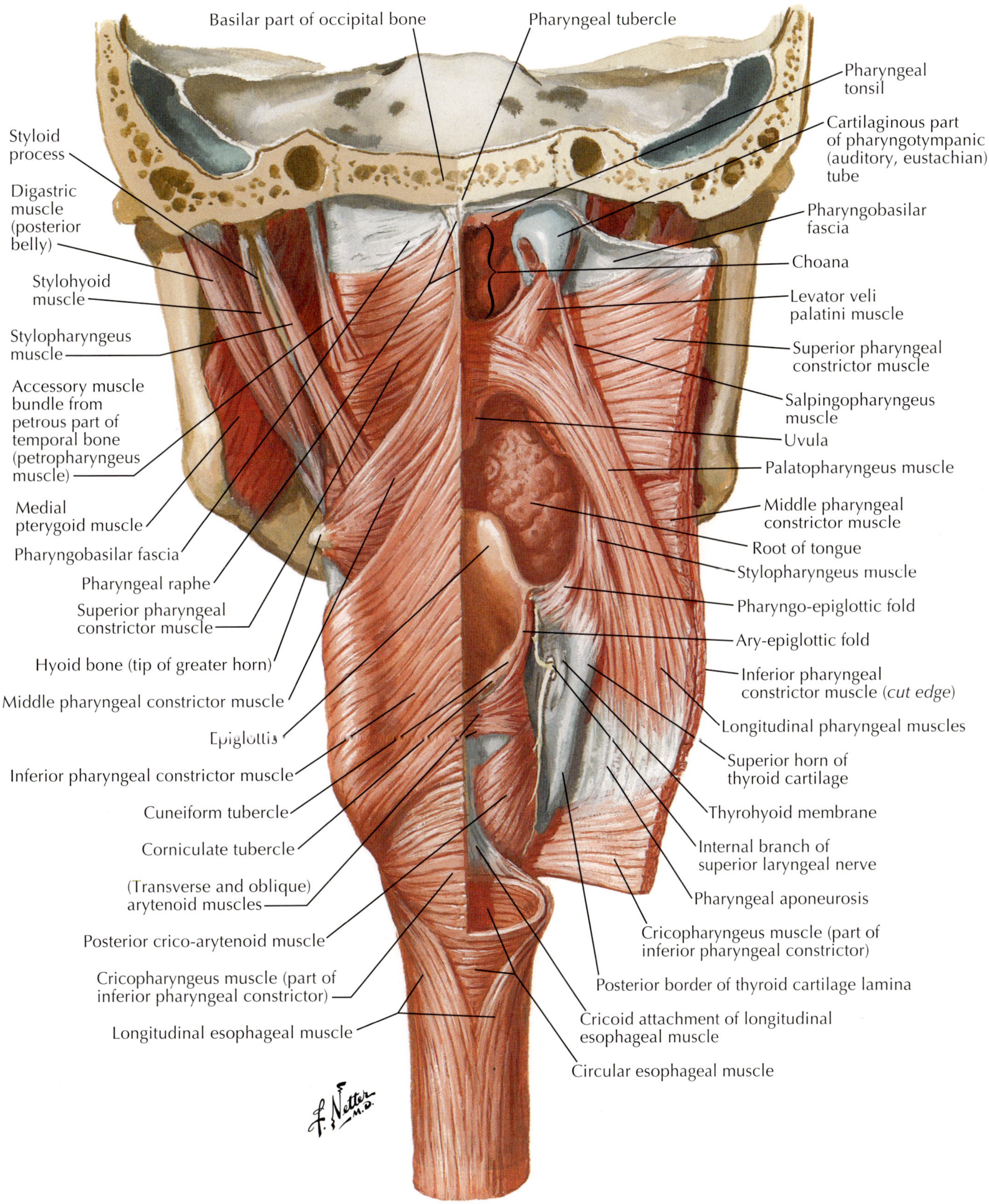

Medial view sagittal section

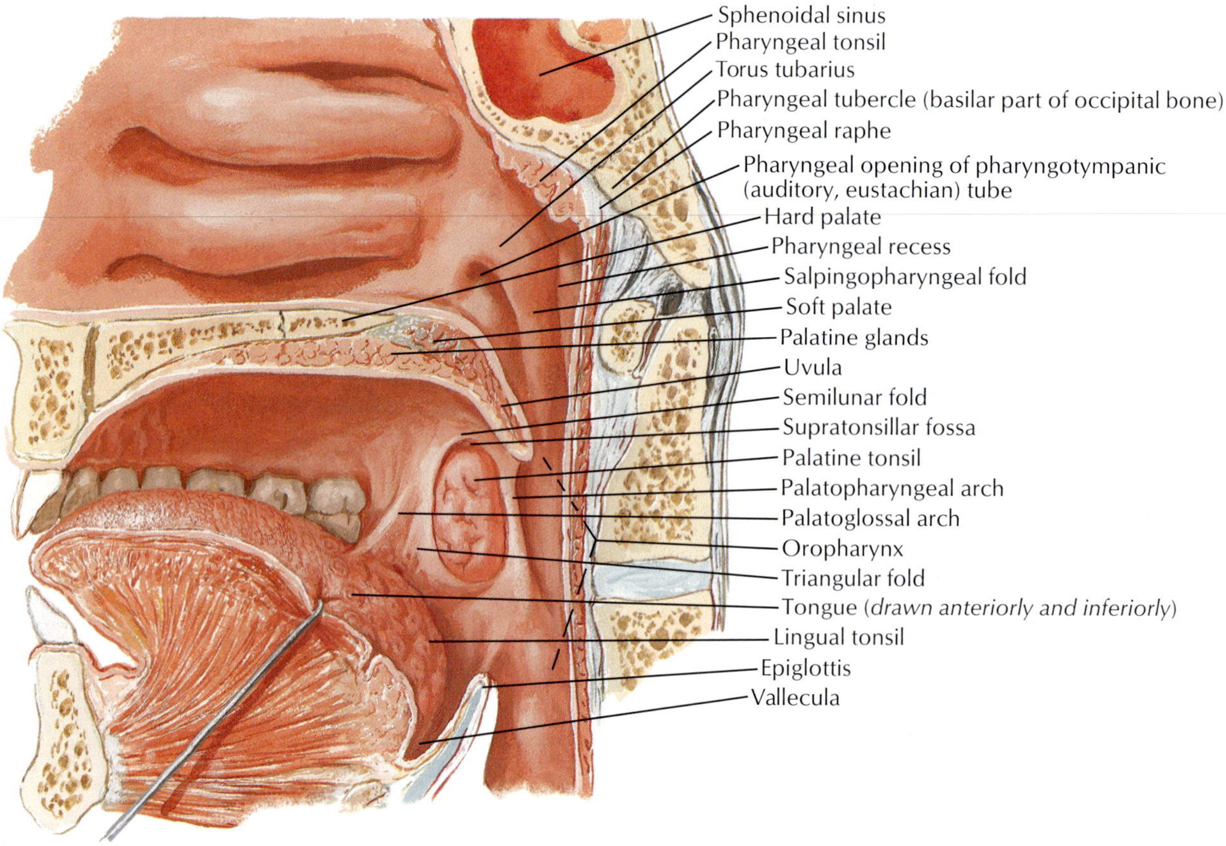

Pharyngeal mucosa removed

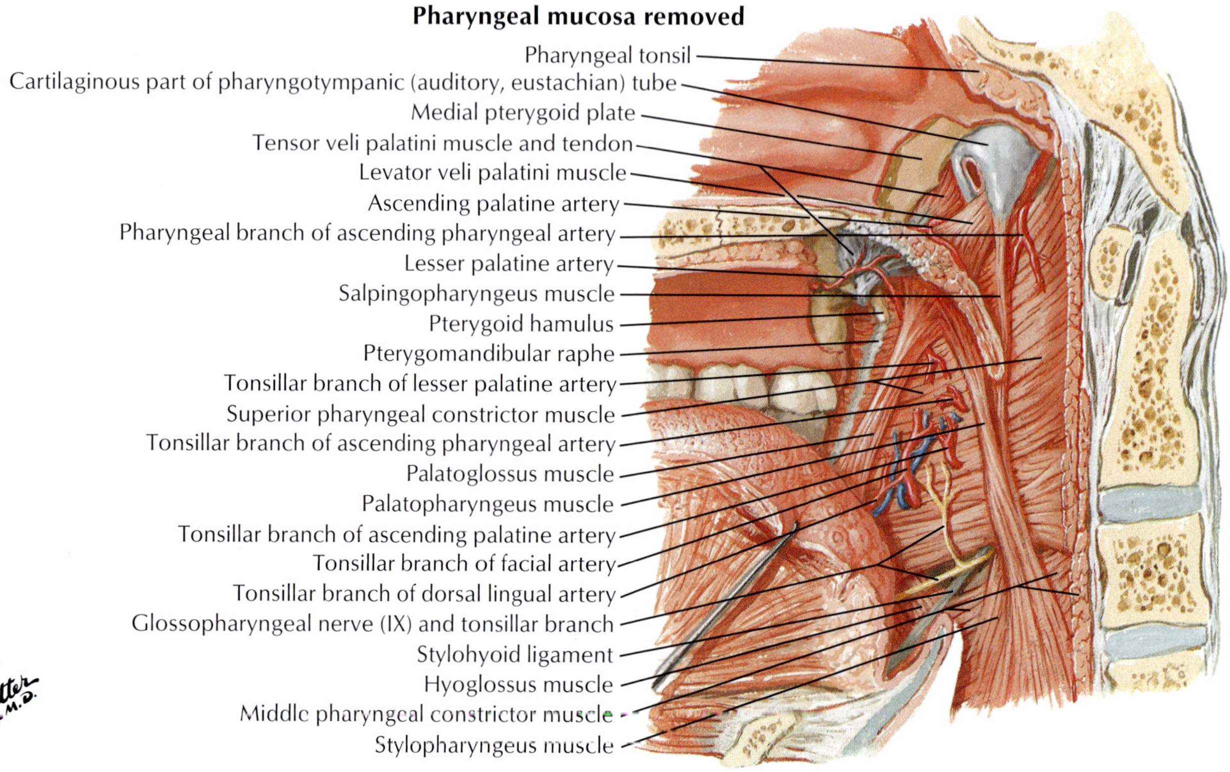

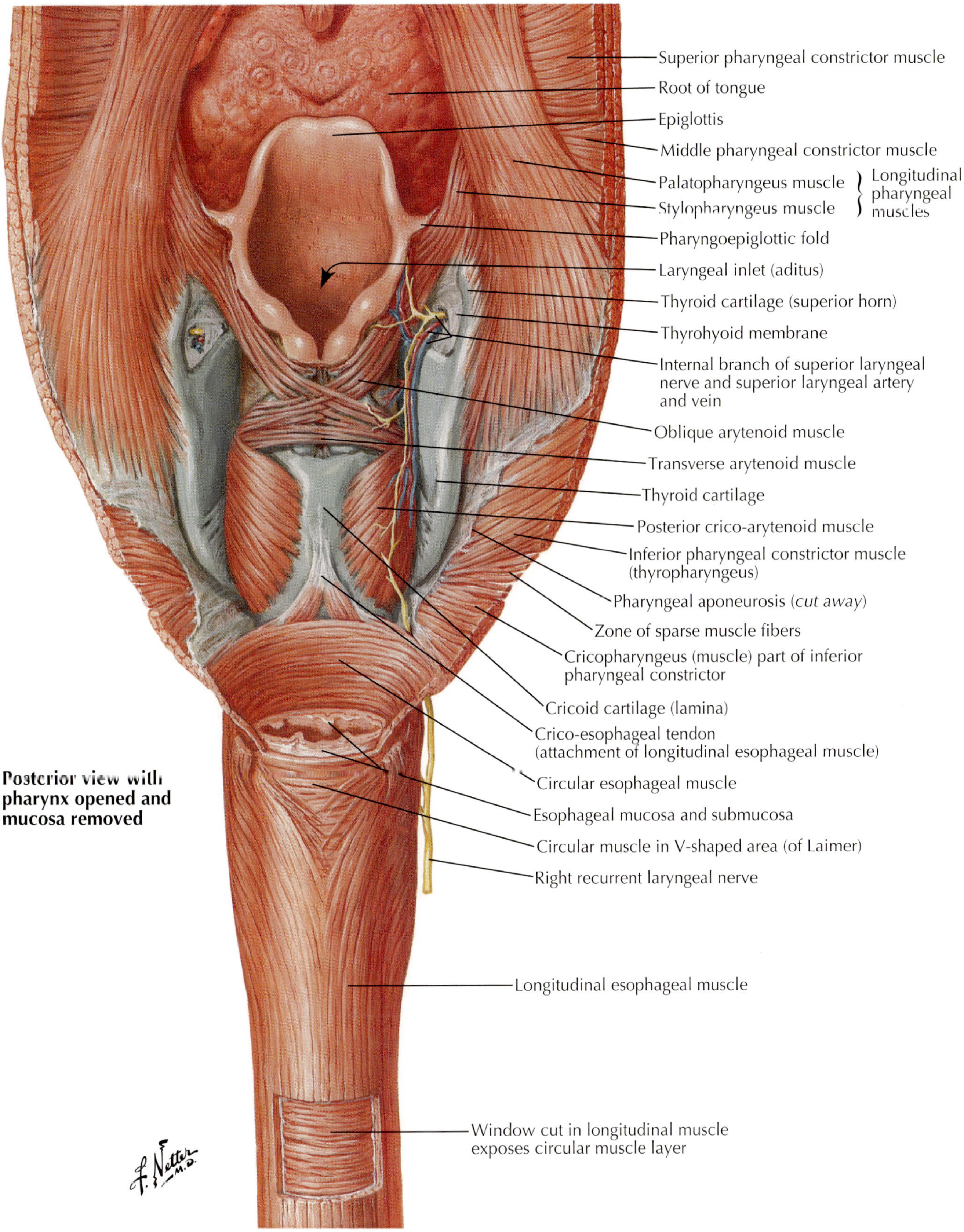

Posterior view with pharynx opened and mucosa removed

Muscles of Pharynx: Lateral View

See also **Plate 67**

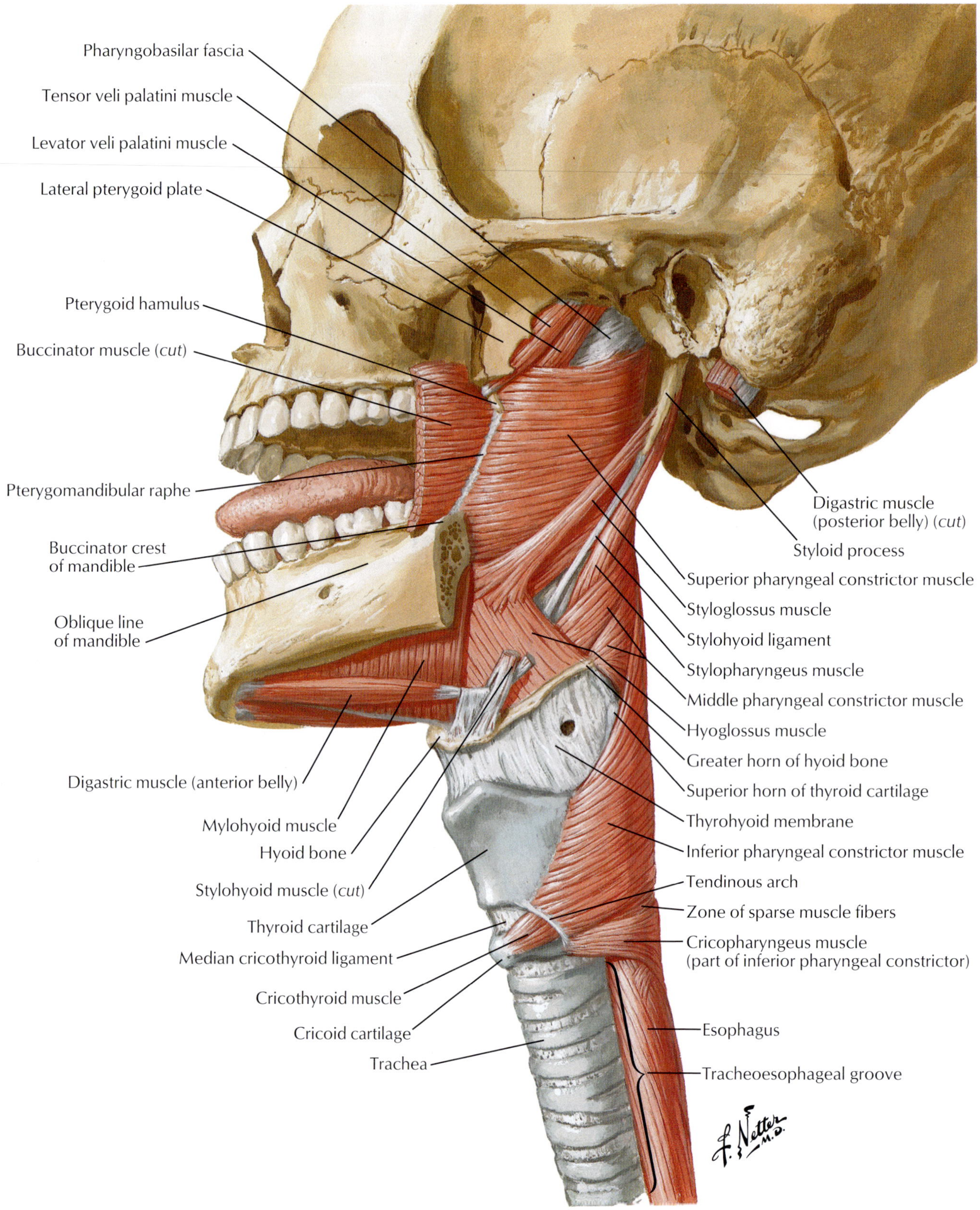

Nerves of Oral and Pharyngeal Regions

See also Plates 50, 123, 126

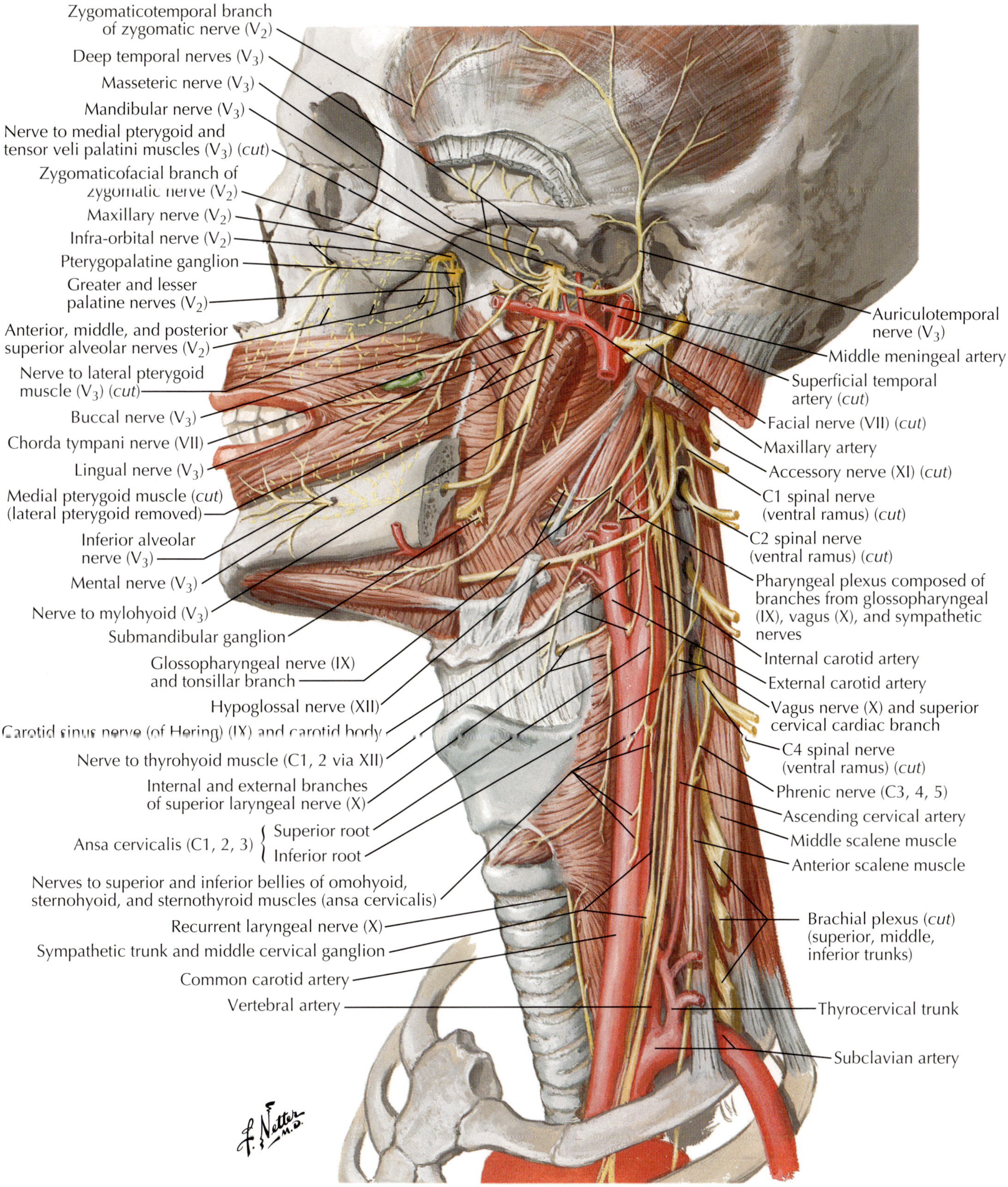

Arteries of Oral and Pharyngeal Regions

See also **Plates 34, 51**

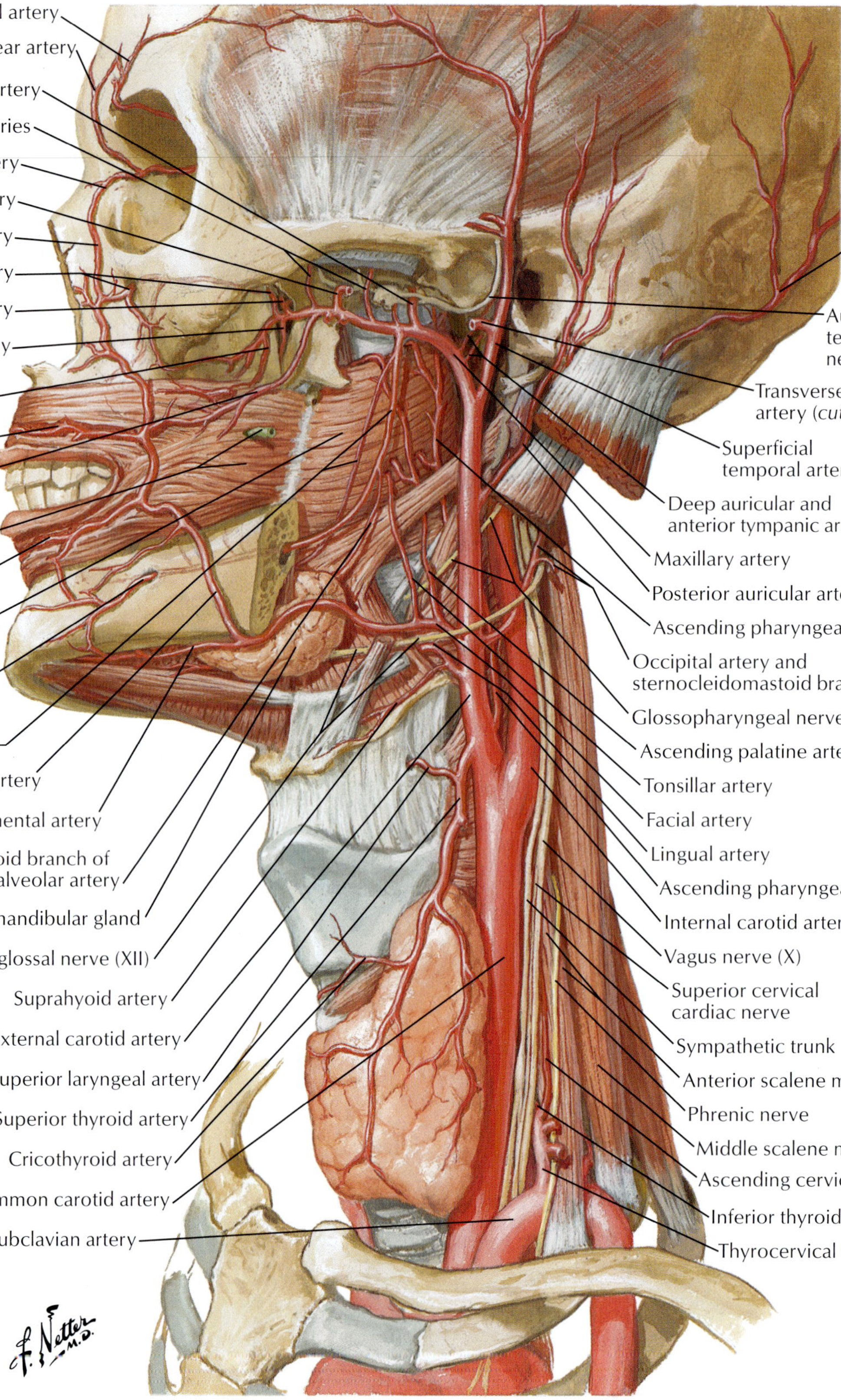

Veins of Oral and Pharyngeal Regions

See also Plate 74

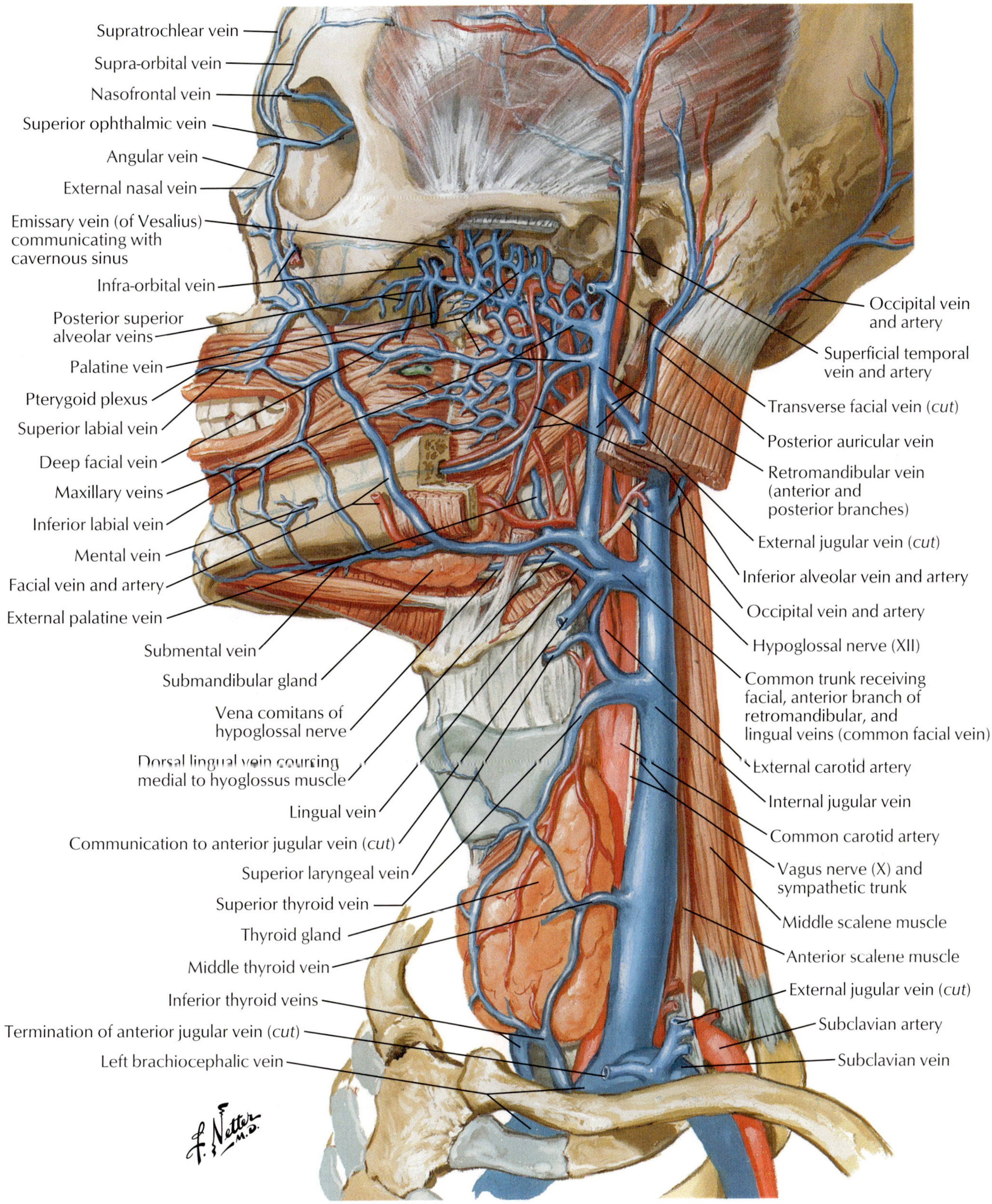

Lymph Vessels and Nodes of Head and Neck

See also **Plates 73, 105**

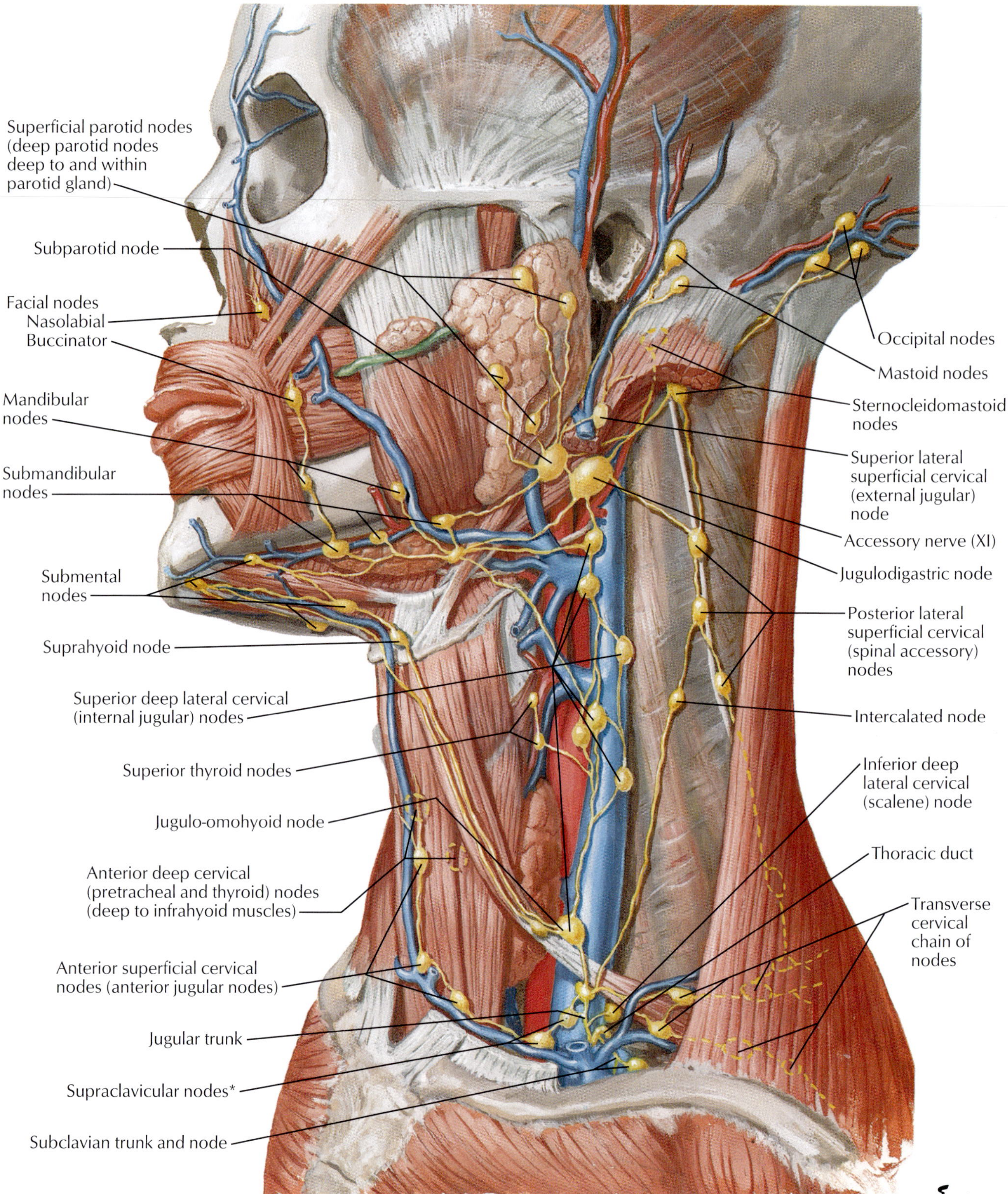

**The supraclavicular group of nodes (also known as the lower deep cervical group), especially on the left, are also sometimes referred to as the signal or sentinel lymph nodes of Virchow or Troisier, especially when sufficiently enlarged and palpable. These nodes (or a single node) are so termed because they may be the first recognized presumptive evidence of malignant disease in the viscera.*

Lymph Vessels and Nodes of Pharynx and Tongue

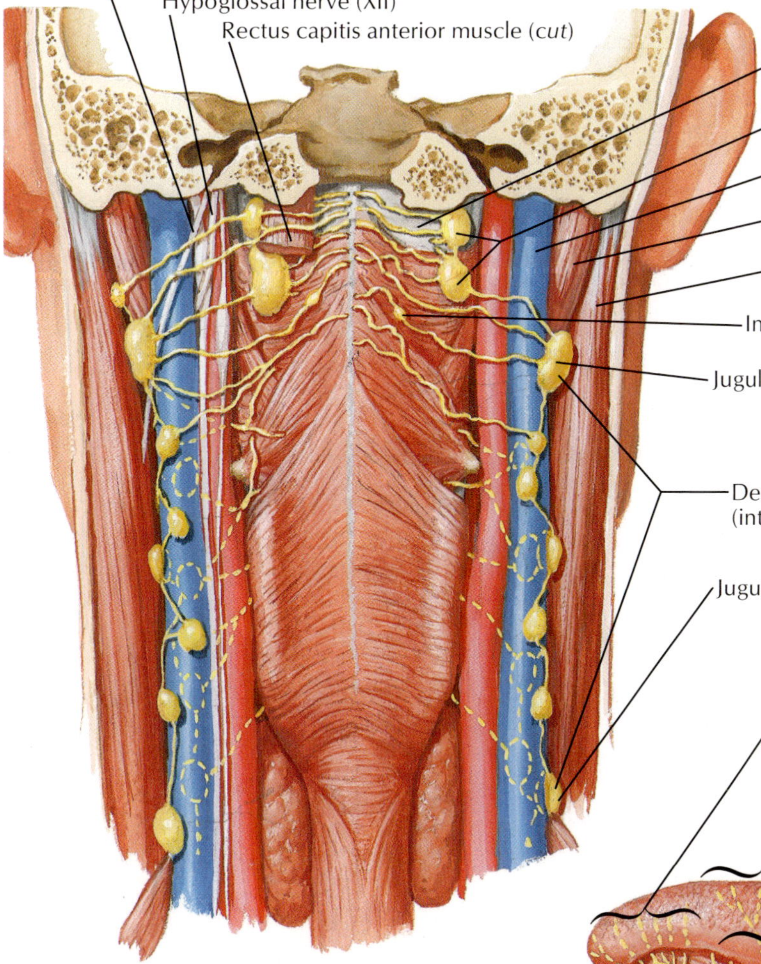

Lymphatic drainage of pharynx: posterior view

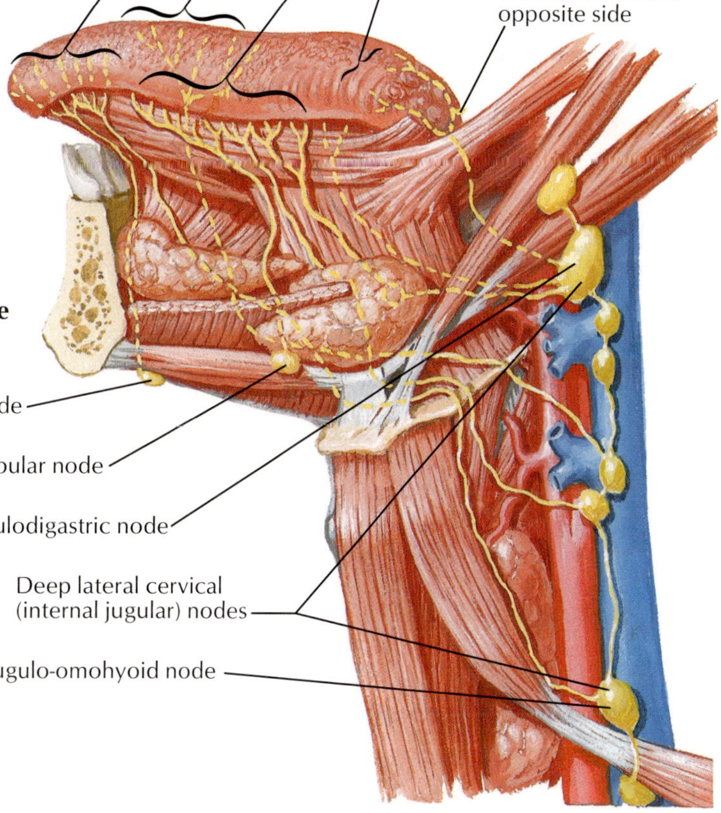

Lymphatic drainage of tongue

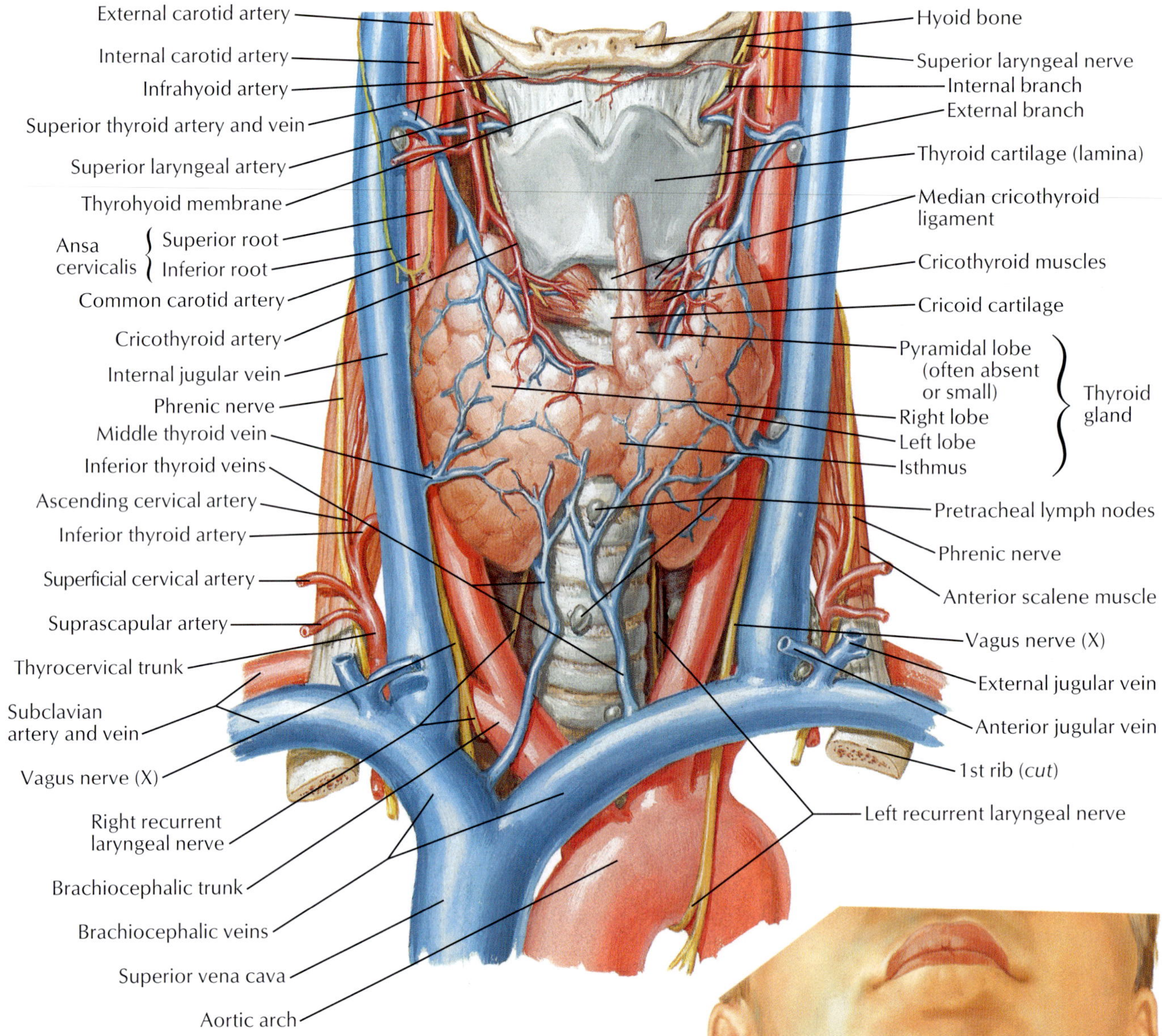
External carotid artery
Internal carotid artery
Infrahyoid artery
Superior thyroid artery and vein
Superior laryngeal artery
Thyrohyoid membrane
Ansa cervicalis
Superior root
Inferior root
Common carotid artery
Cricothyroid artery
Internal jugular vein
Phrenic nerve
Middle thyroid vein
Inferior thyroid veins
Ascending cervical artery
Inferior thyroid artery
Superficial cervical artery
Suprascapular artery
Thyrocervical trunk
Subclavian artery and vein
Vagus nerve (X)
Right recurrent laryngeal nerve
Brachiocephalic trunk
Brachiocephalic veins
Superior vena cava
Aortic arch
Hyoid bone
Superior laryngeal nerve
Internal branch
External branch
Thyroid cartilage (lamina)
Median cricothyroid ligament
Cricothyroid muscles
Cricoid cartilage
Pyramidal lobe (often absent or small)
Right lobe
Left lobe
Isthmus
Thyroid gland
Pretracheal lymph nodes
Phrenic nerve
Anterior scalene muscle
Vagus nerve (X)
External jugular vein
Anterior jugular vein
1st rib (*cut*)
Left recurrent laryngeal nerve

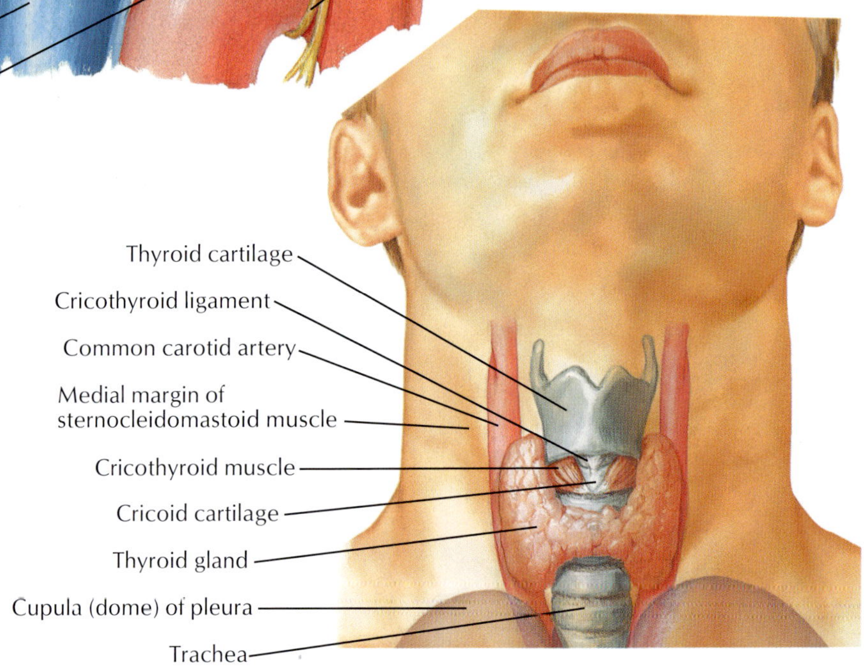
Thyroid cartilage
Cricothyroid ligament
Common carotid artery
Medial margin of sternocleidomastoid muscle
Cricothyroid muscle
Cricoid cartilage
Thyroid gland
Cupula (dome) of pleura
Trachea

Thyroid Gland and Pharynx: Posterior View

See also Plate 78

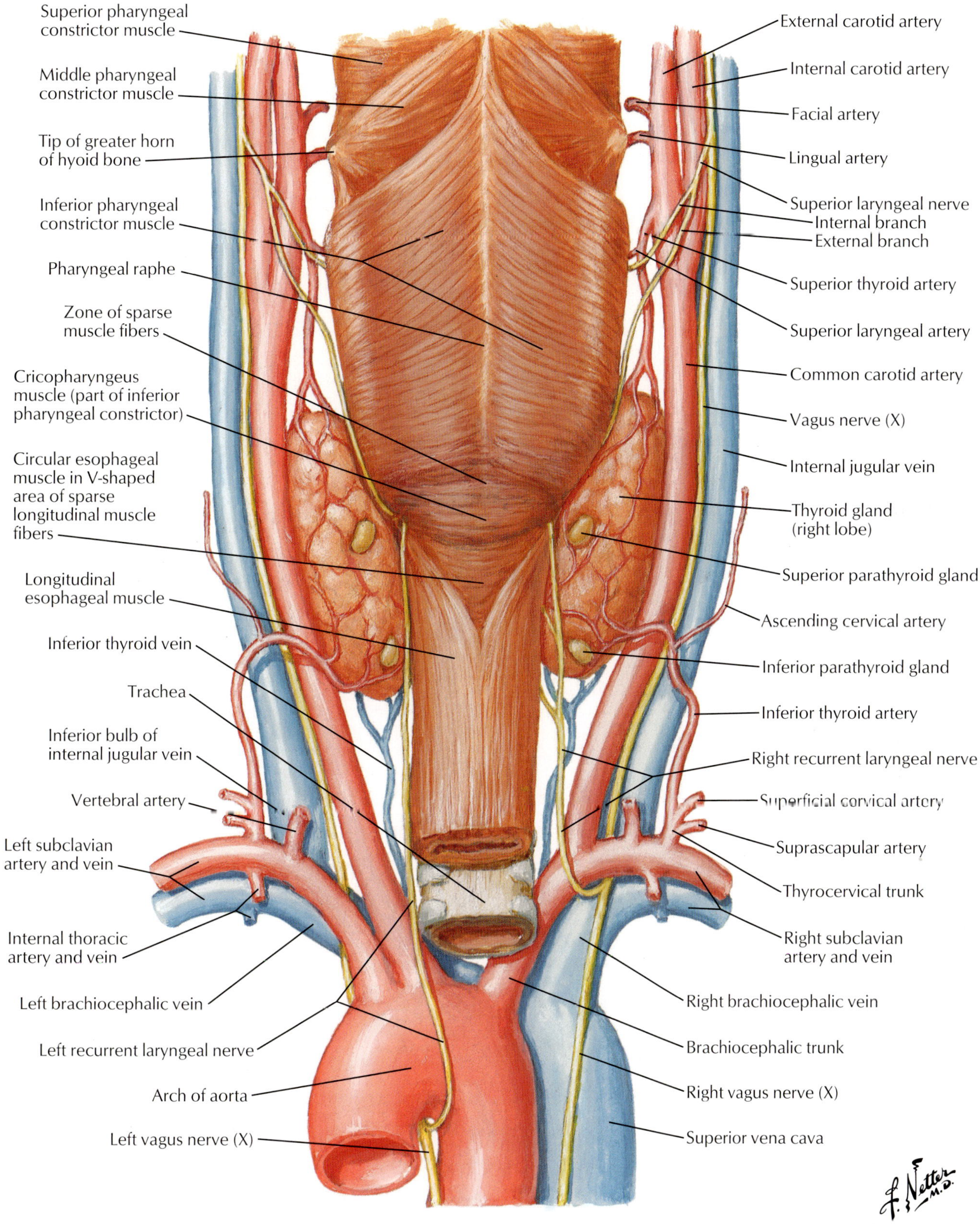

See also Plates 69, 77, 82

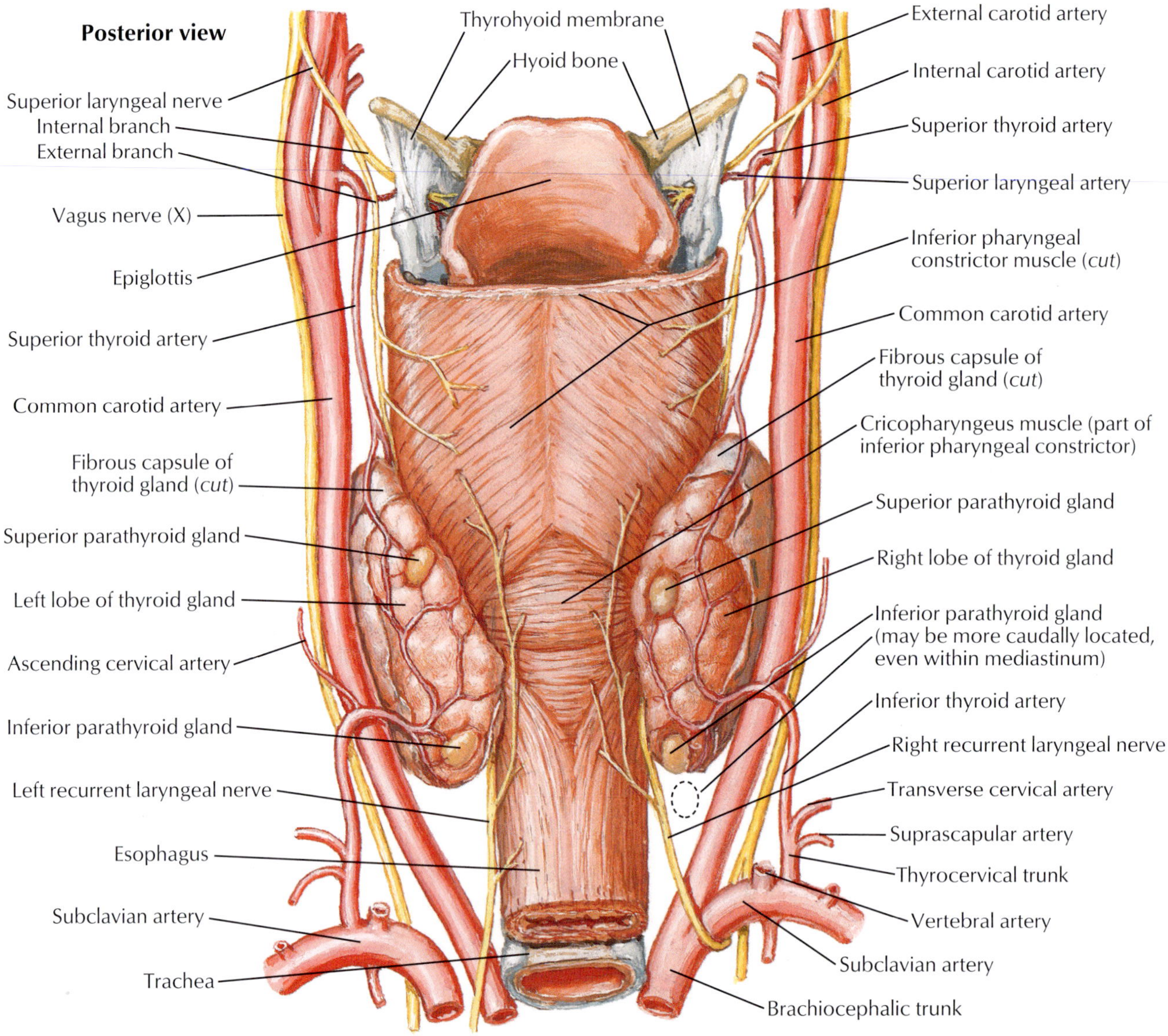

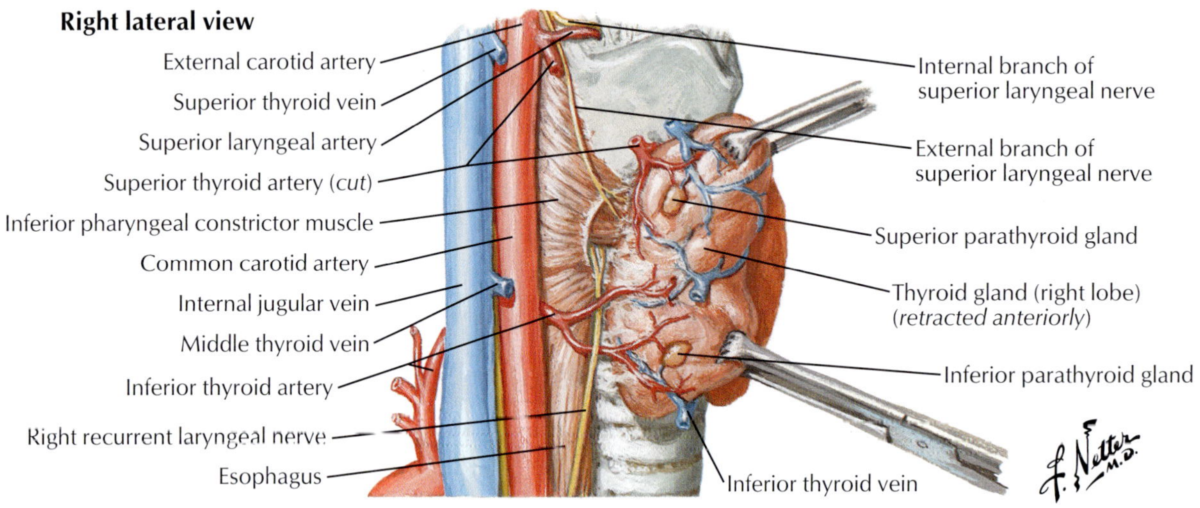

Cartilages of Larynx

See also Plates 80, 81, 82

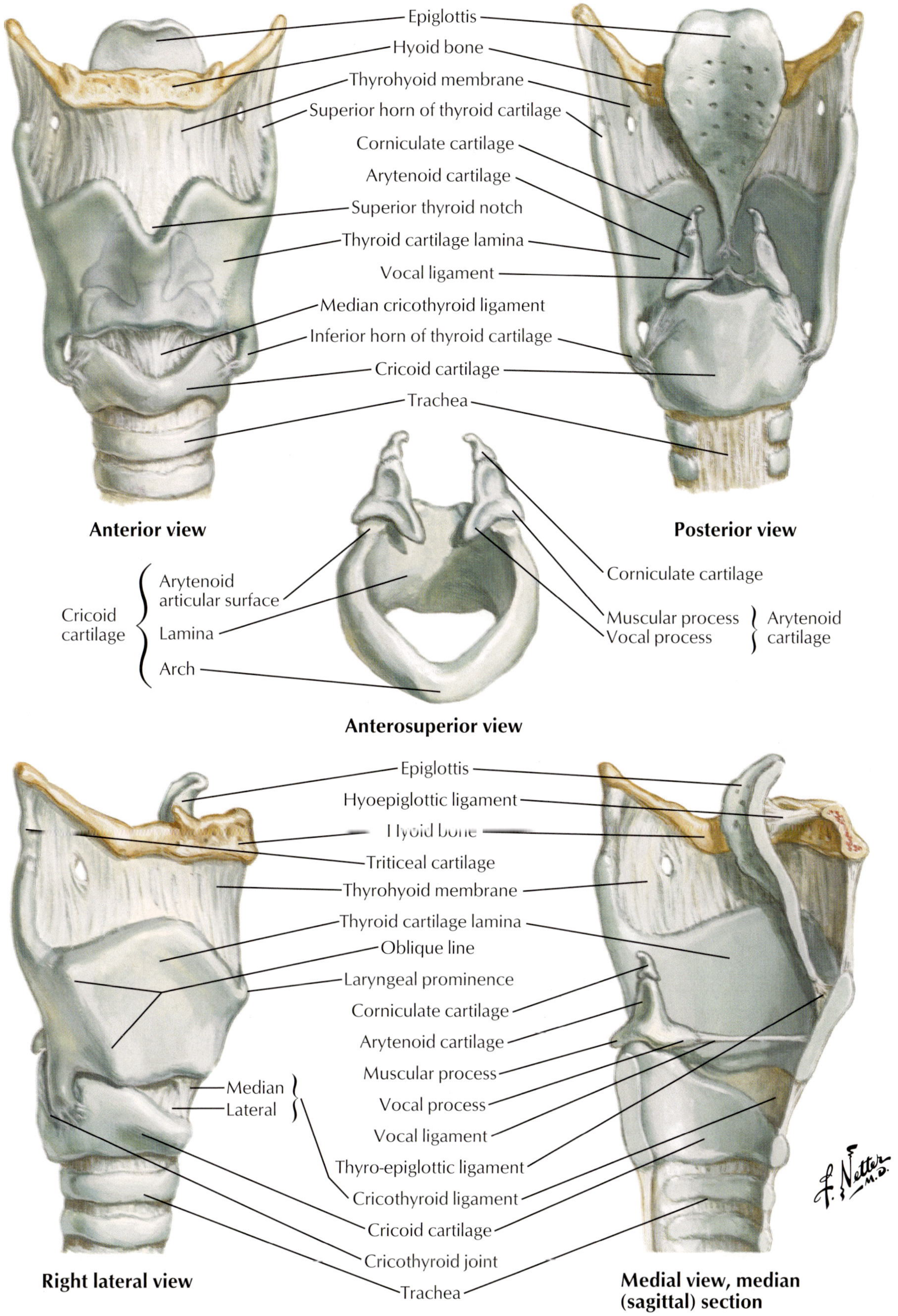

Intrinsic Muscles of Larynx

See also Plates 79, 81, 82

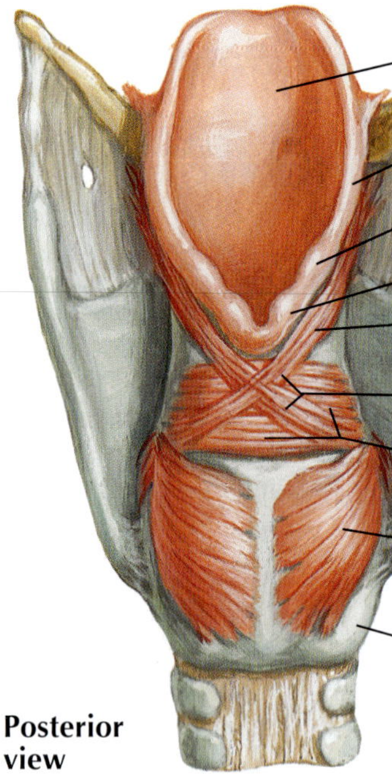

Posterior view

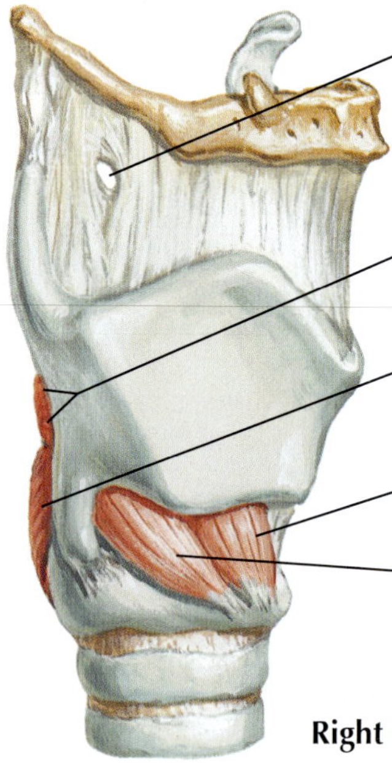

Right lateral view

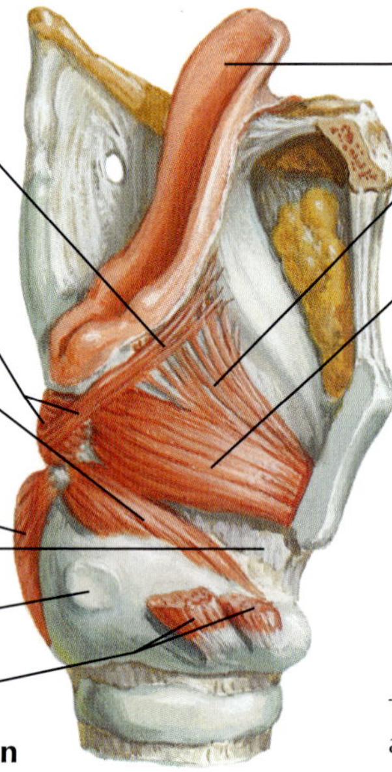

Lateral dissection

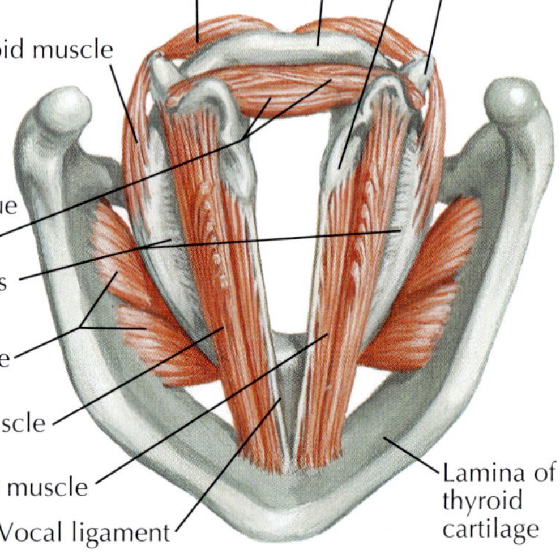

Superior view

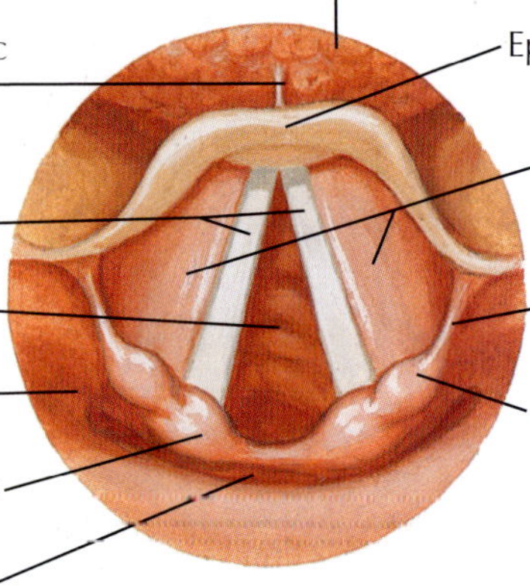

Normal larynx: inspiration

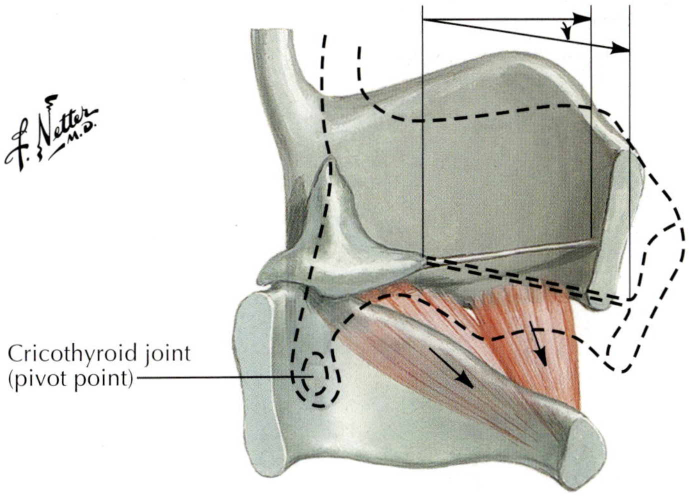

Action of cricothyroid muscles

Lengthening (increasing tension) of vocal ligaments

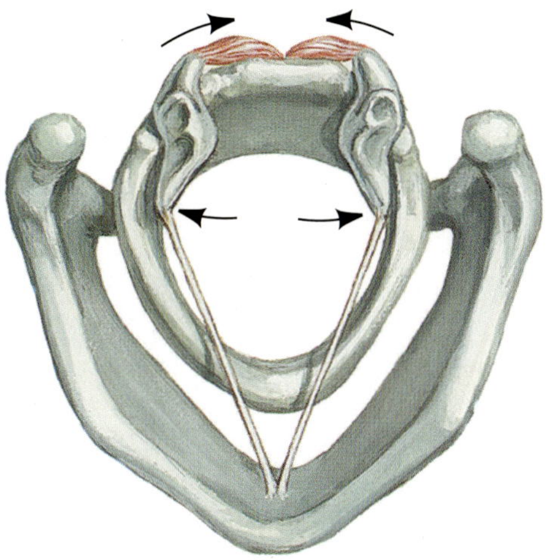

Action of posterior crico-arytenoid muscles

Abduction of vocal ligaments

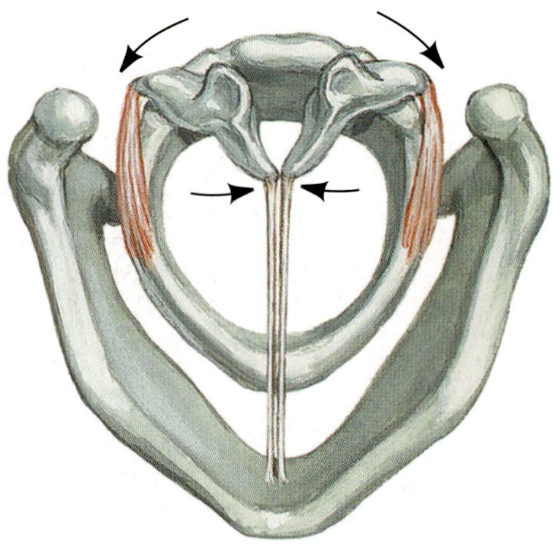

Action of lateral crico-arytenoid muscles

Adduction of vocal ligaments

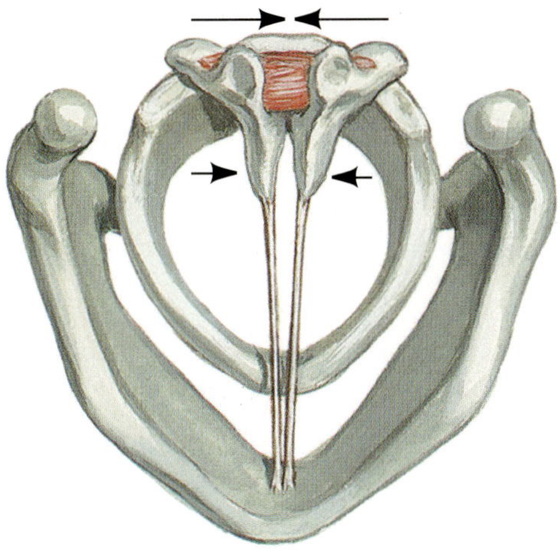

Action of transverse and oblique arytenoid muscles

Adduction of vocal ligaments

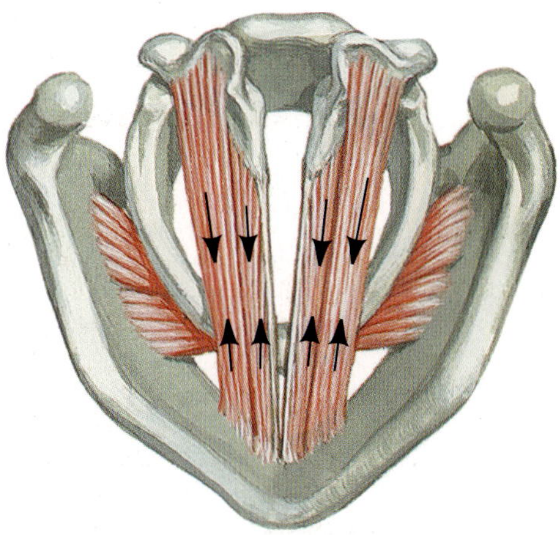

Action of vocalis and thyro-arytenoid muscles

Shortening (relaxation) of vocal ligaments

Nerves of Larynx

See also Plates 79, 80, 81

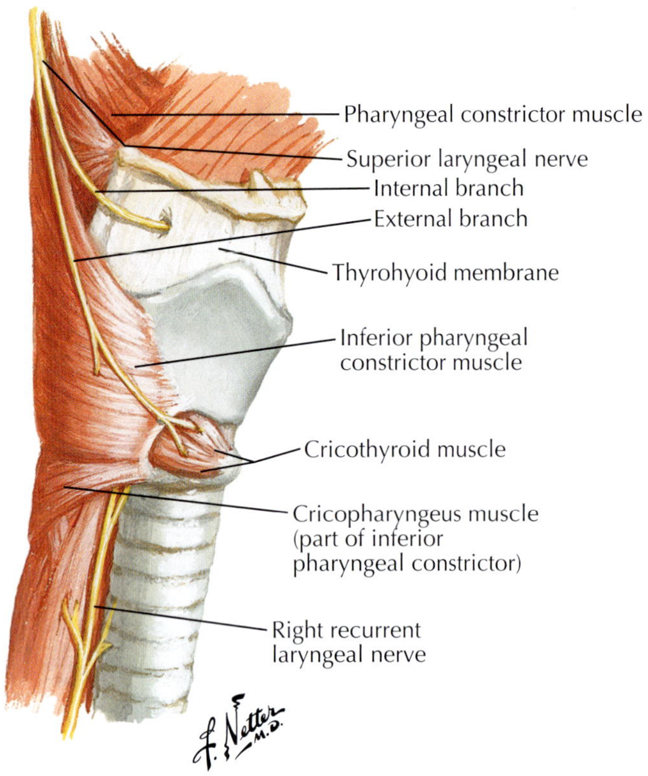

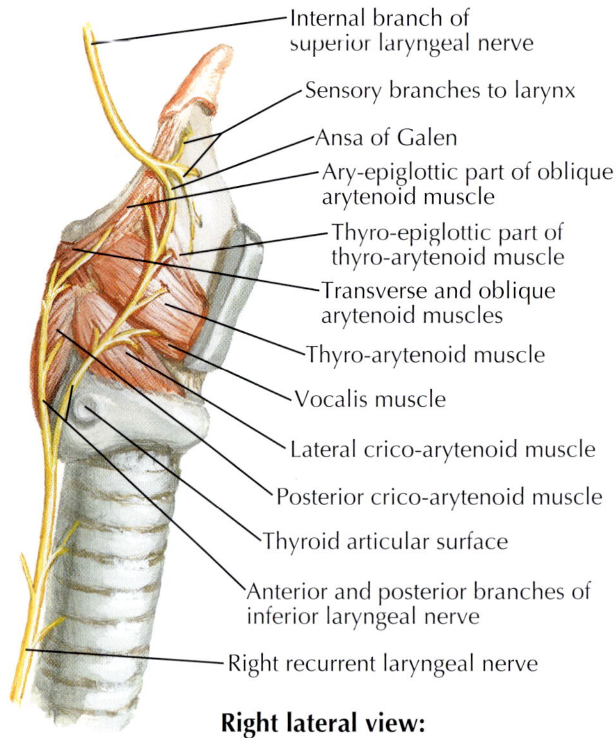

Right lateral view: thyroid cartilage lamina removed

Coronal section through larynx

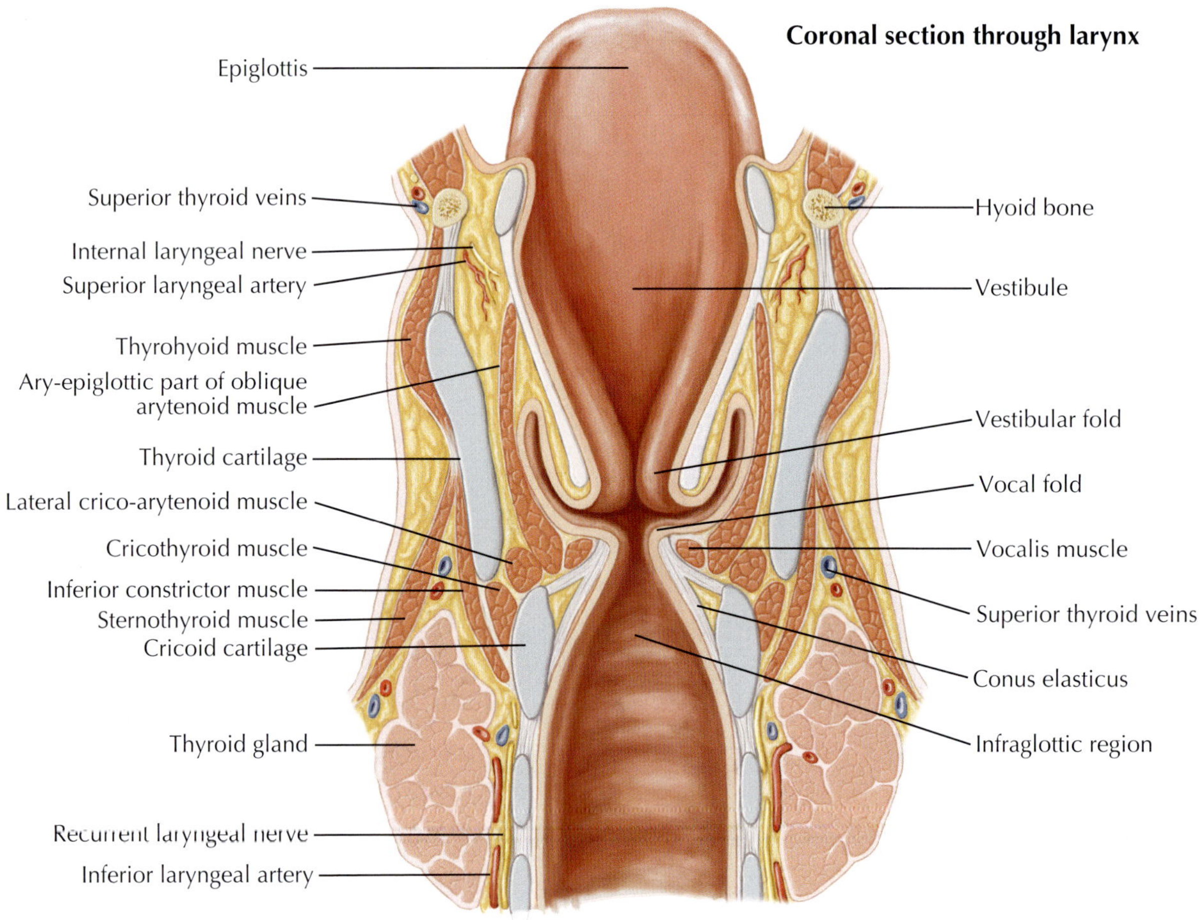

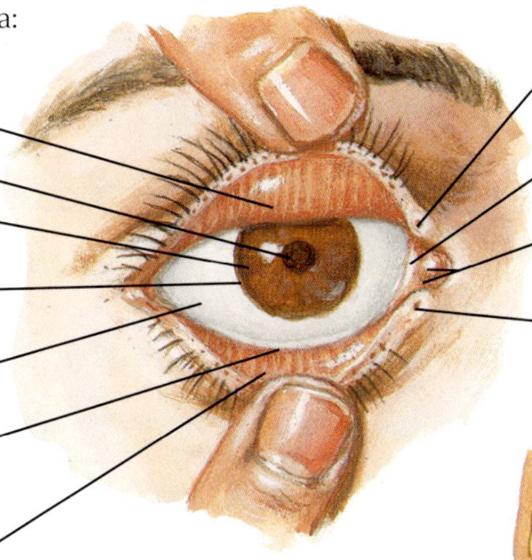
Superior palpebral conjunctiva: tarsal (meibomian) glands shining through
Seen through cornea
Pupil
Iris
Corneoscleral junction (corneal limbus)
Bulbar conjunctiva over sclera
Inferior conjunctival fornix
Inferior palpebral conjunctiva: tarsal glands shining through
Superior lacrimal papilla and punctum
Plica semilunaris
Lacrimal caruncle in lacrimal lake (lacus lacrimalis)
Inferior lacrimal papilla and punctum

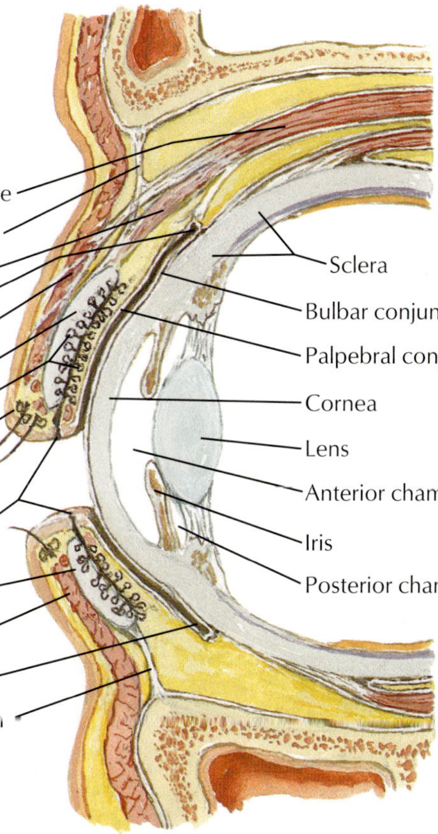
Levator palpebrae superioris muscle
Orbital septum
Superior tarsal (Müller's) muscle (smooth)
Superior conjunctival fornix
Orbicularis oculi muscle (palpebral part)
Superior tarsus
Tarsal (meibomian) glands
Sebaceous glands
Eyelashes (cilia)
Openings of tarsal glands
Inferior tarsus
Orbicularis oculi muscle (palpebral part)
Inferior conjunctival fornix
Orbital septum
Sclera
Bulbar conjunctiva
Palpebral conjunctiva
Cornea
Lens
Anterior chamber
Iris
Posterior chamber
F. Netter M.D.

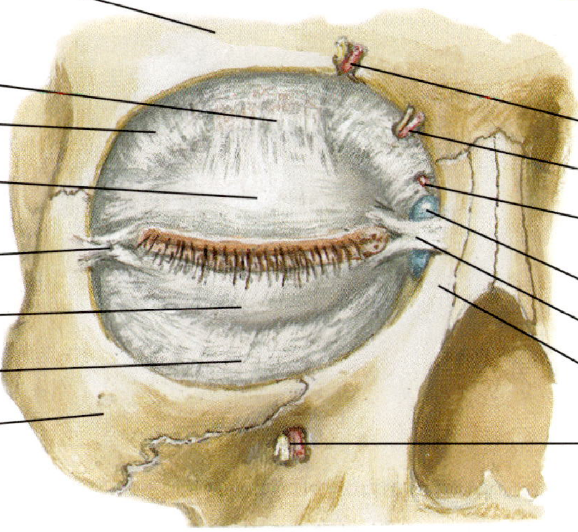
Frontal bone
Insertion of levator palpebrae superioris muscle
Orbital septum
Superior tarsus
Lateral palpebral ligament and overlying raphe
Inferior tarsus
Orbital septum
Zygomatic bone
Supra-orbital artery and nerve
Supratrochlear artery and nerve
Dorsal nasal artery and infratrochlear nerve
Lacrimal sac
Medial palpebral ligament
Maxilla (frontal process)
Infra-orbital artery and nerve

See also Plate 134

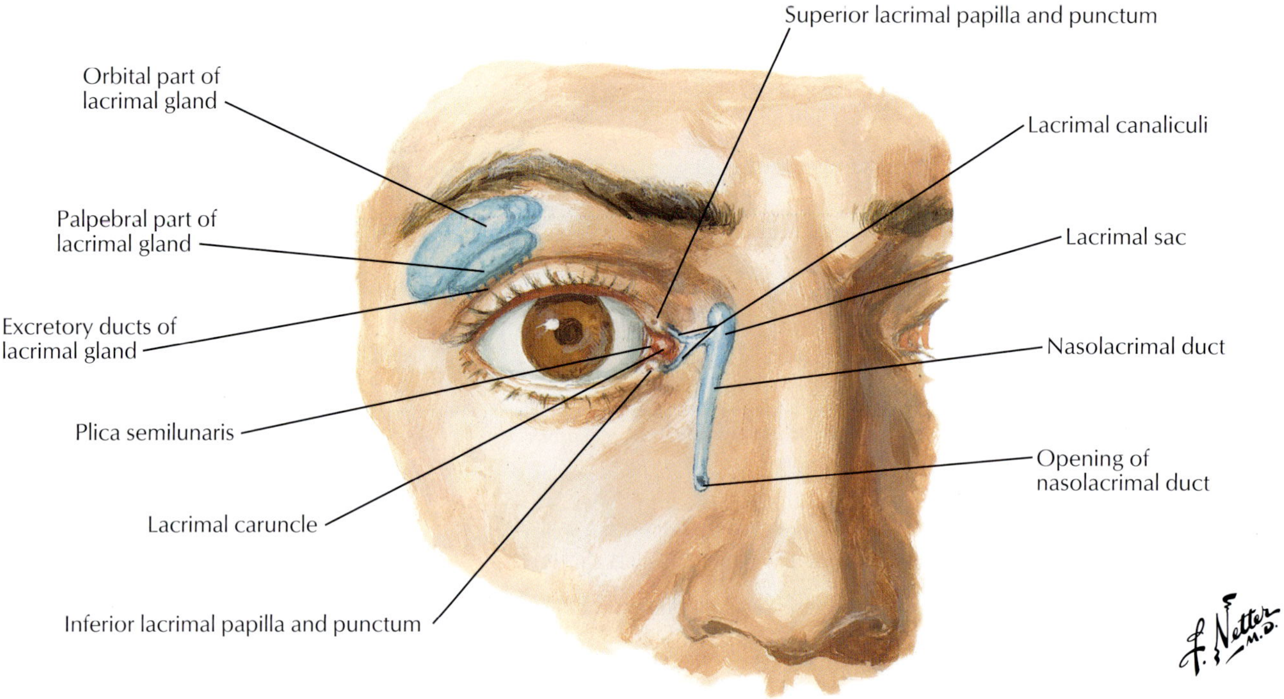

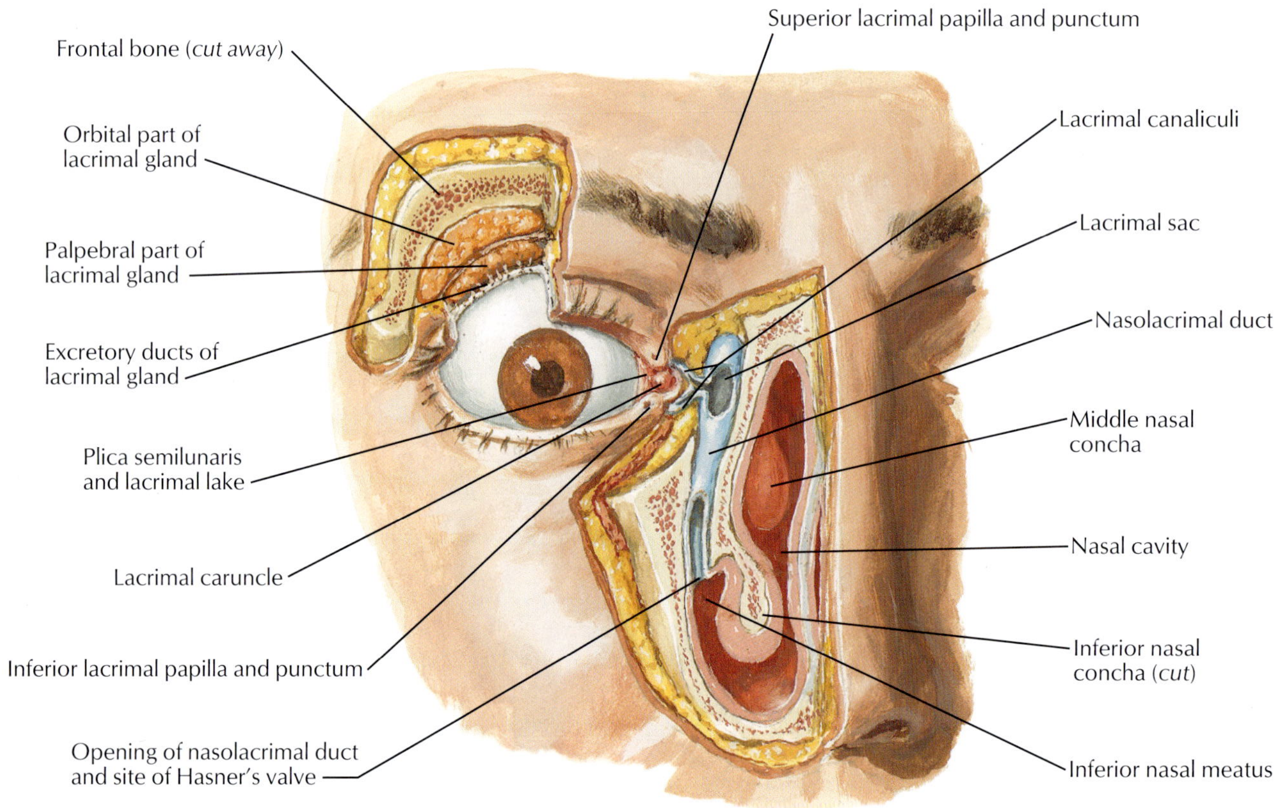

Horizontal section

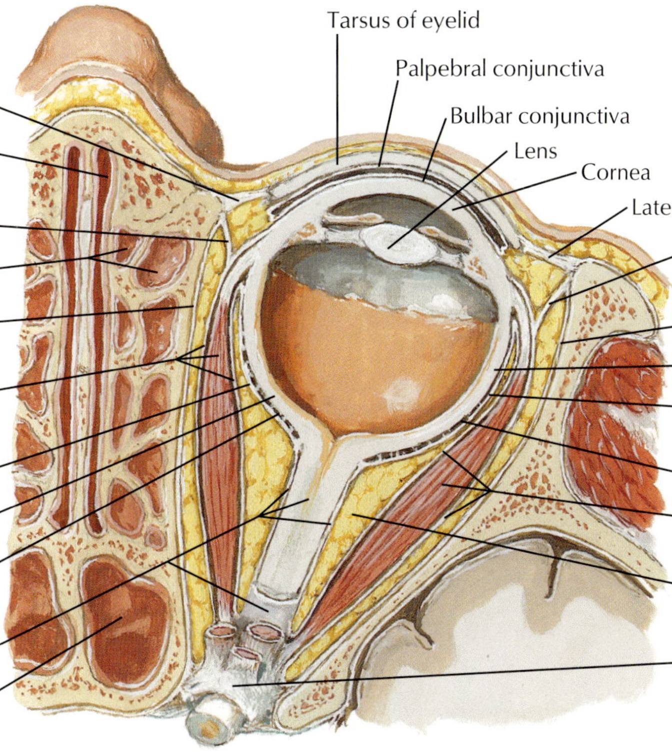

Frontal section

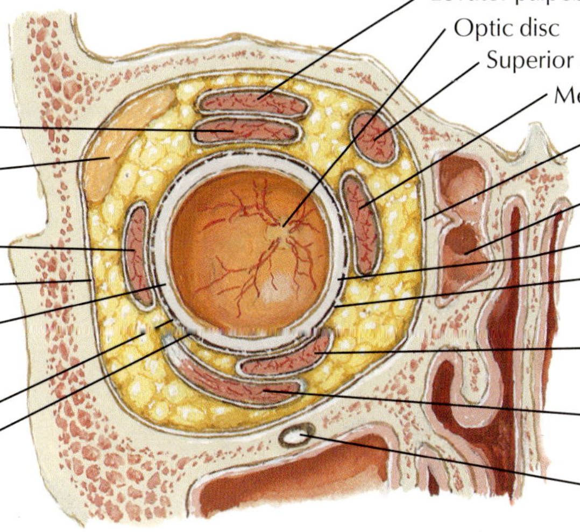

Muscle attachments and nerves and vessels entering orbit

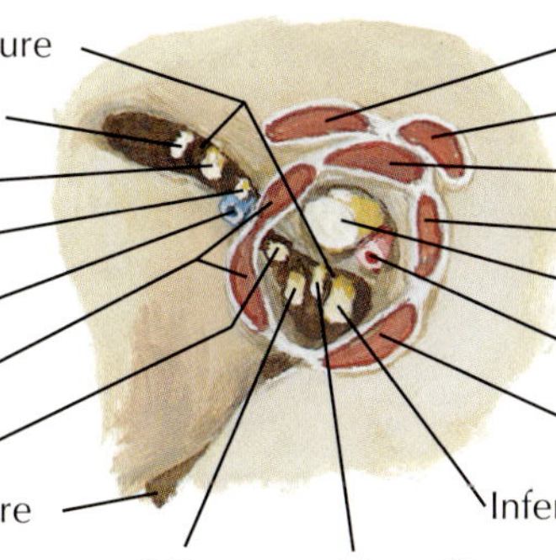

Extrinsic Eye Muscles

Right lateral view

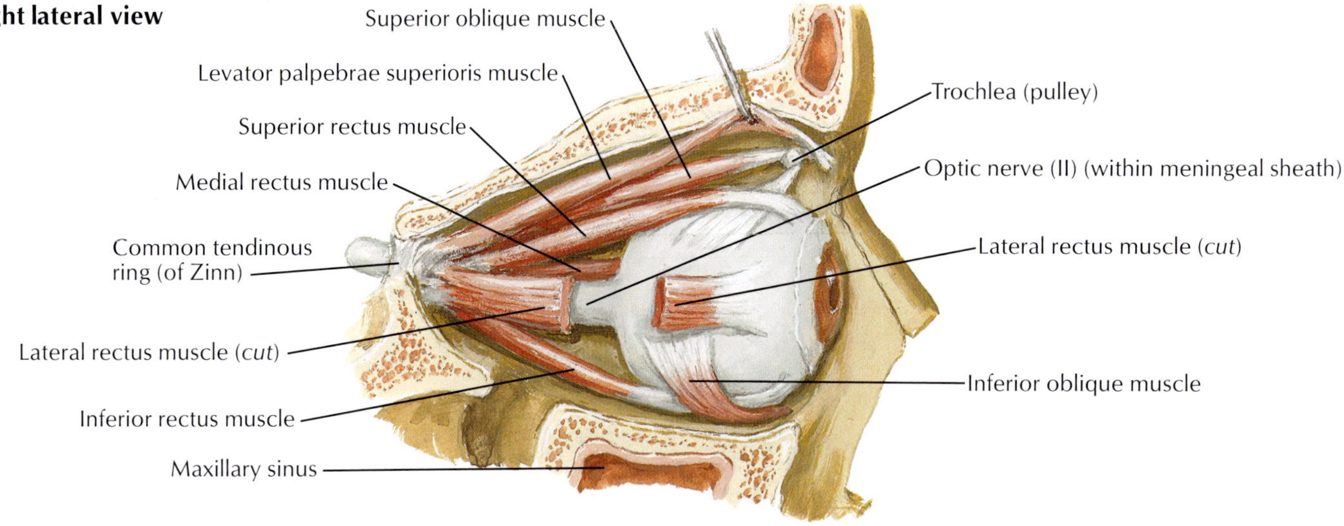

Superior view

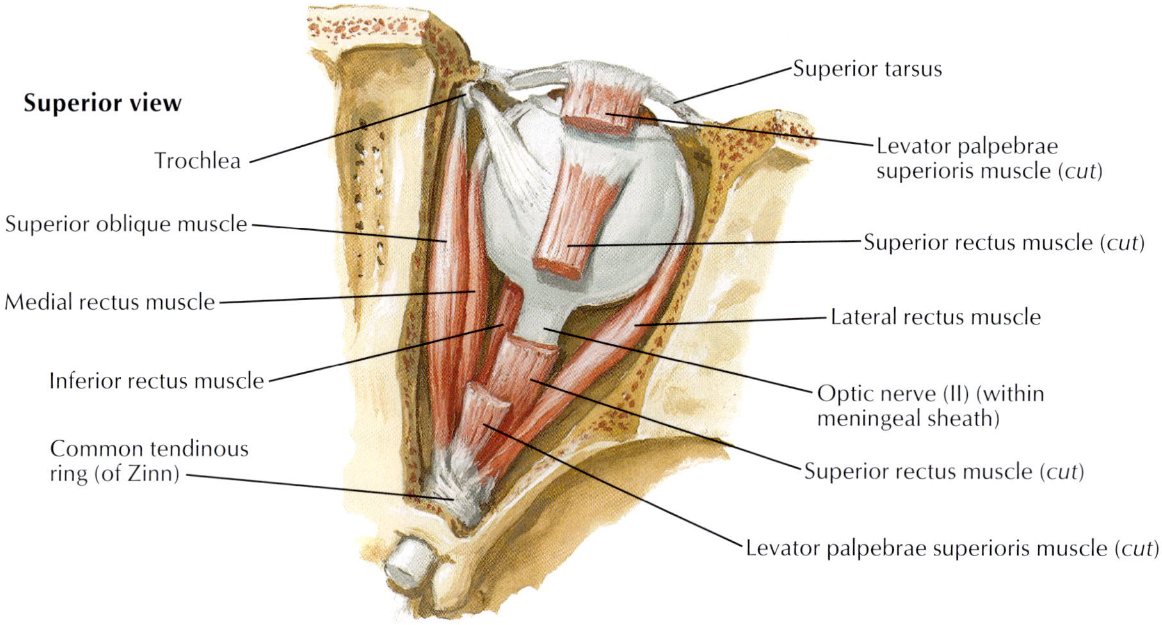

Innervation of extrinsic eye muscles: anterior view

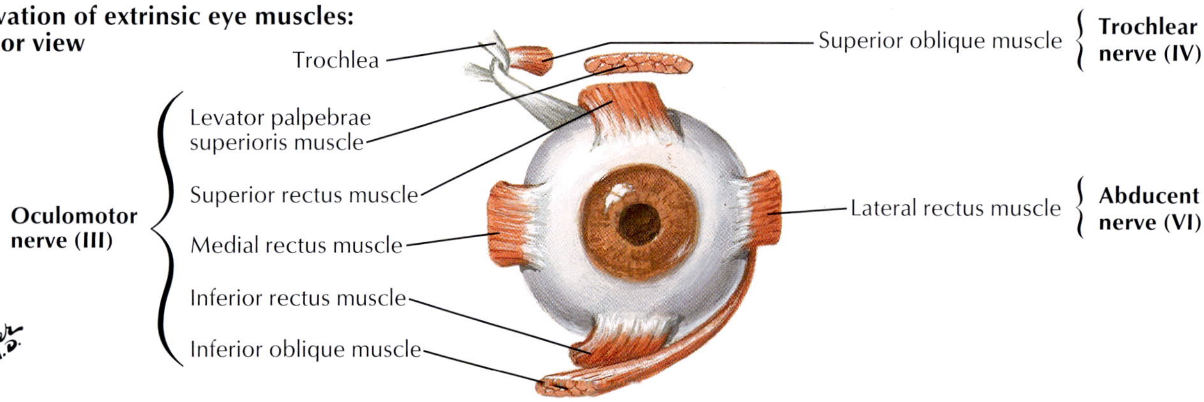

Arteries and Veins of Orbit and Eyelids

See also Plates 3, 105

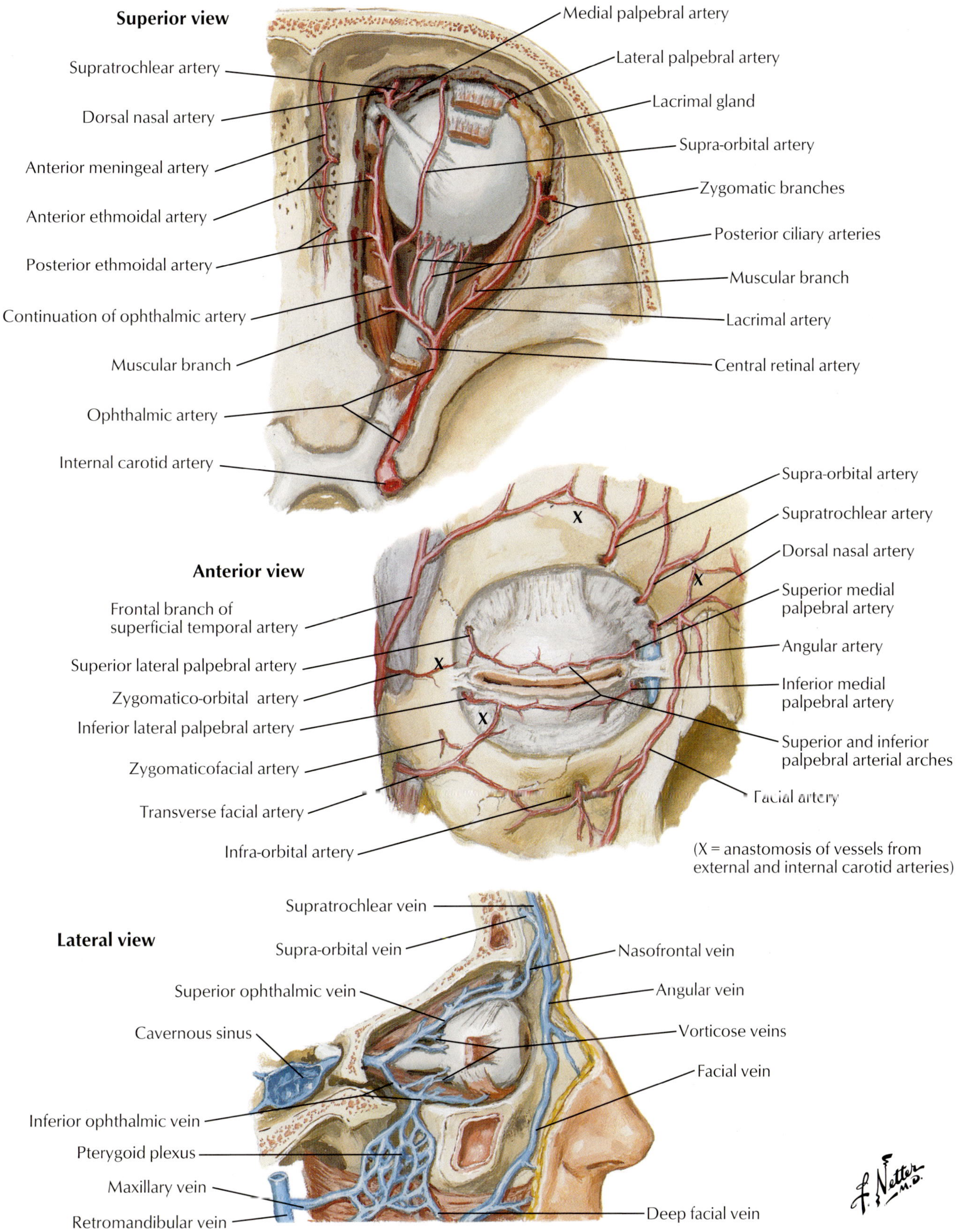

Nerves of Orbit

See also **Plates 52, 122, 123**

Superior view

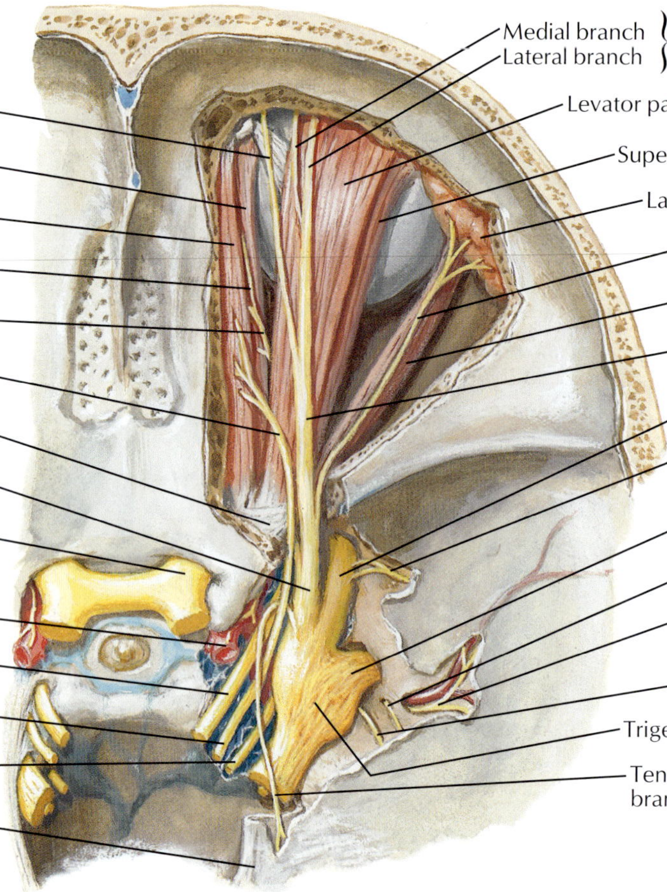

Superior view:
levator palpebrae superioris, superior rectus, and superior oblique muscles partially cut away

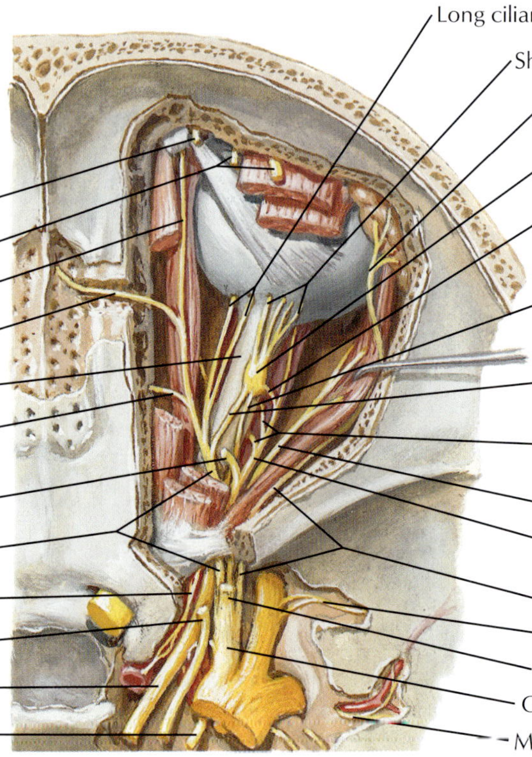

Horizontal section

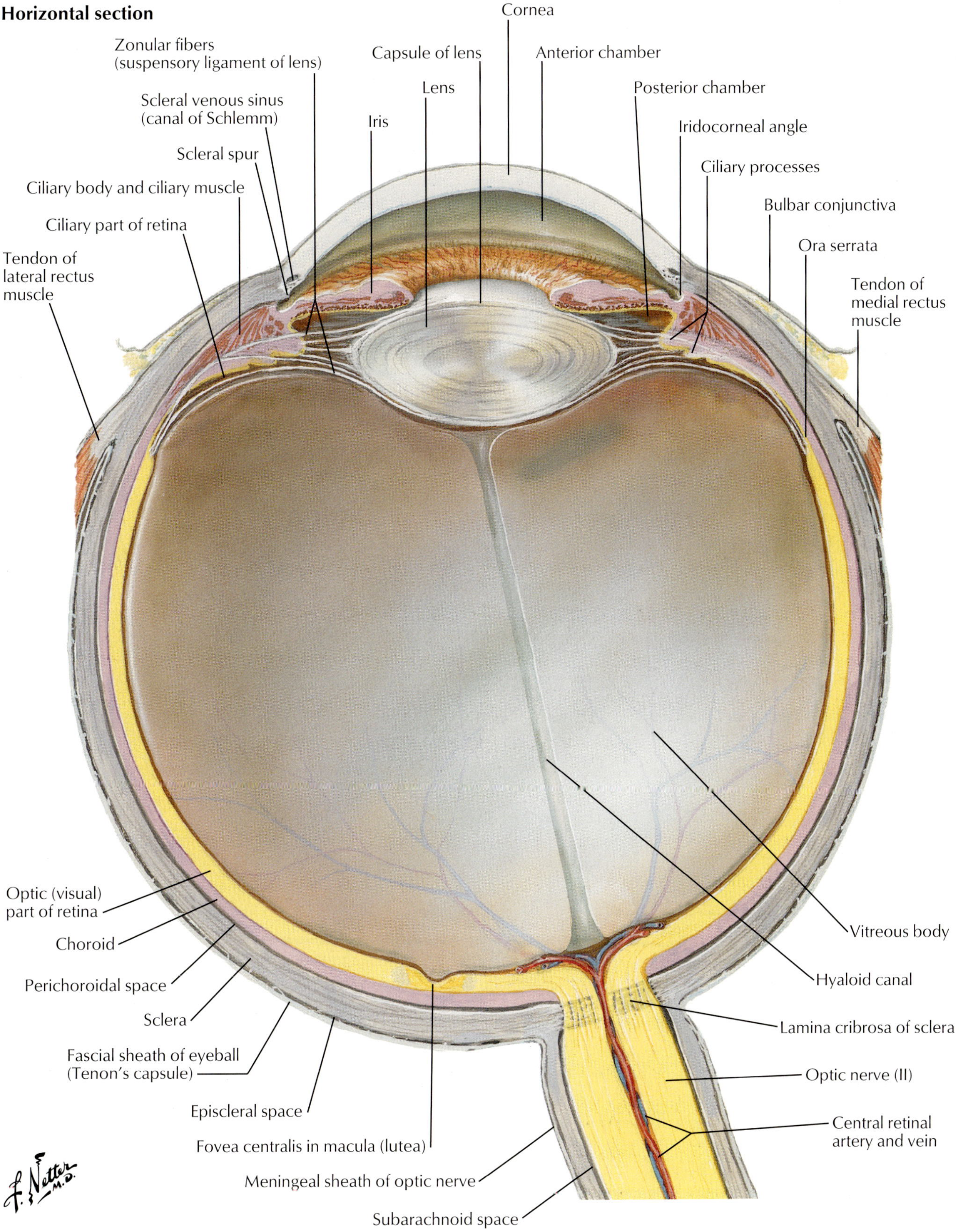

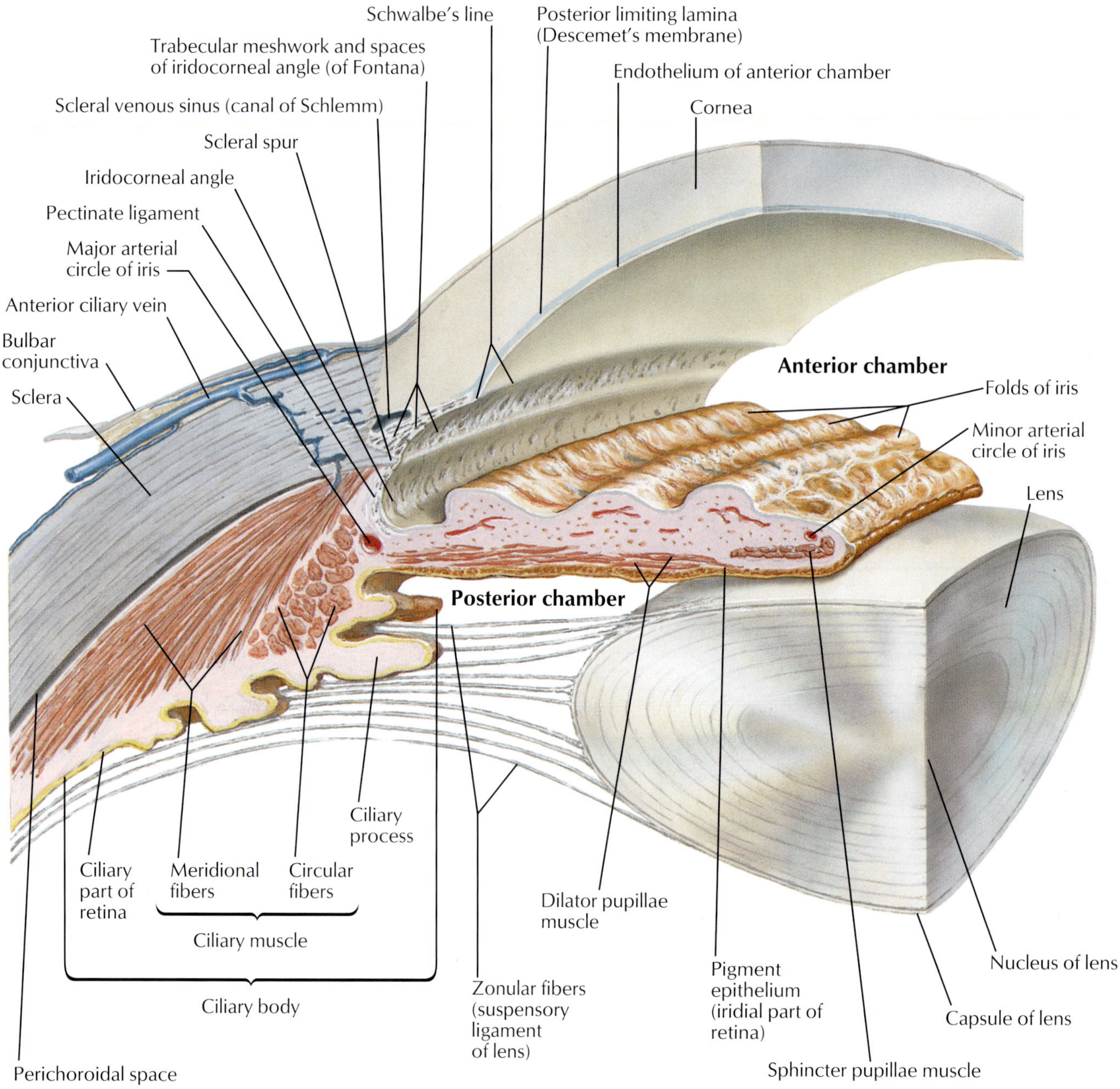

Note: For clarity, only single plane of zonular fibers shown; actually, fibers surround entire circumference of lens.

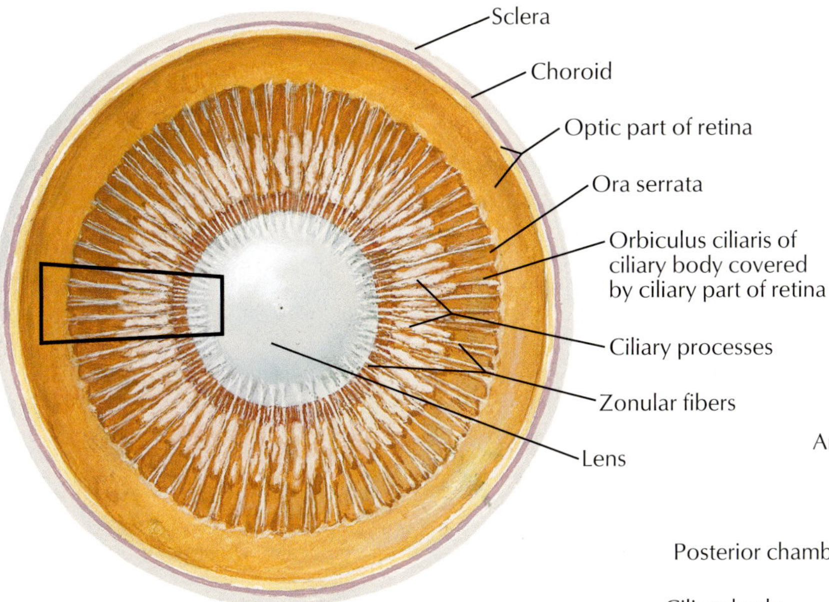

Eyeball sectioned in coronal plane: anterior segment viewed from behind

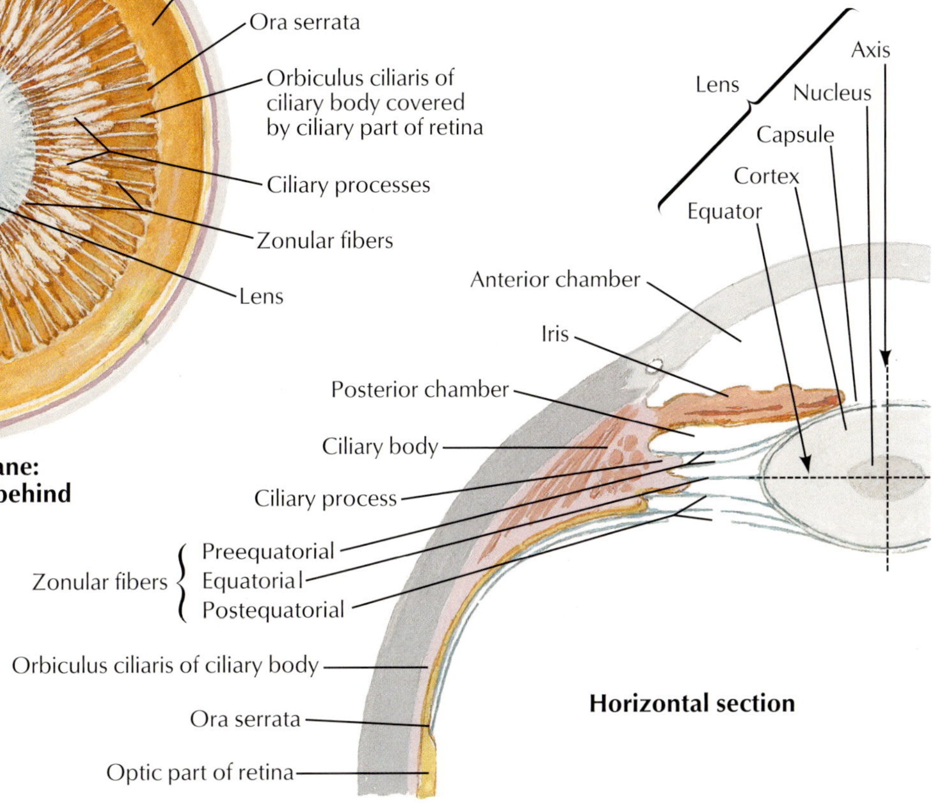

Horizontal section

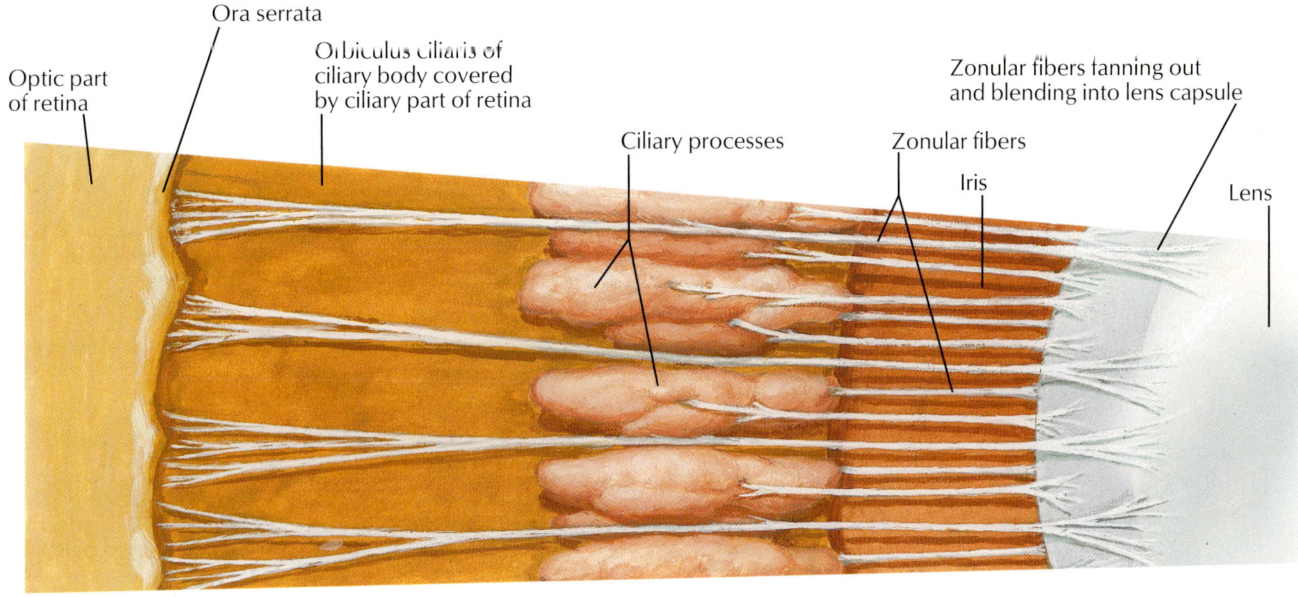

Enlargement of segment outlined in top illustration (semischematic)

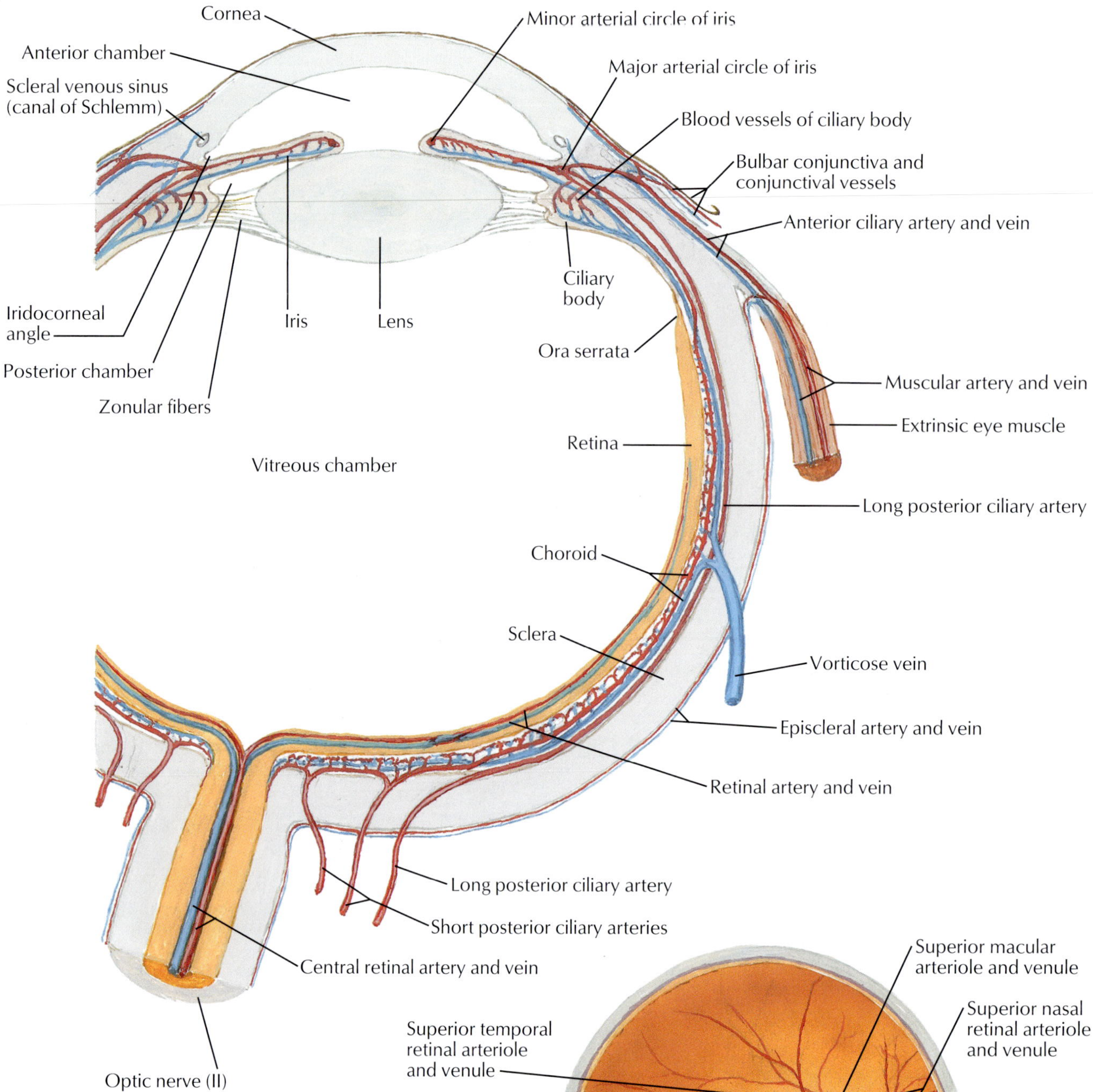

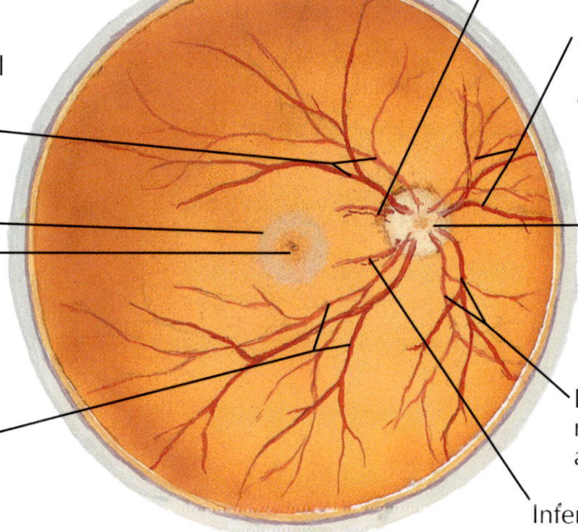

Right retinal vessels: funduscopic view

Vascular arrangements within the choroid (vascular tunic) of the eyeball

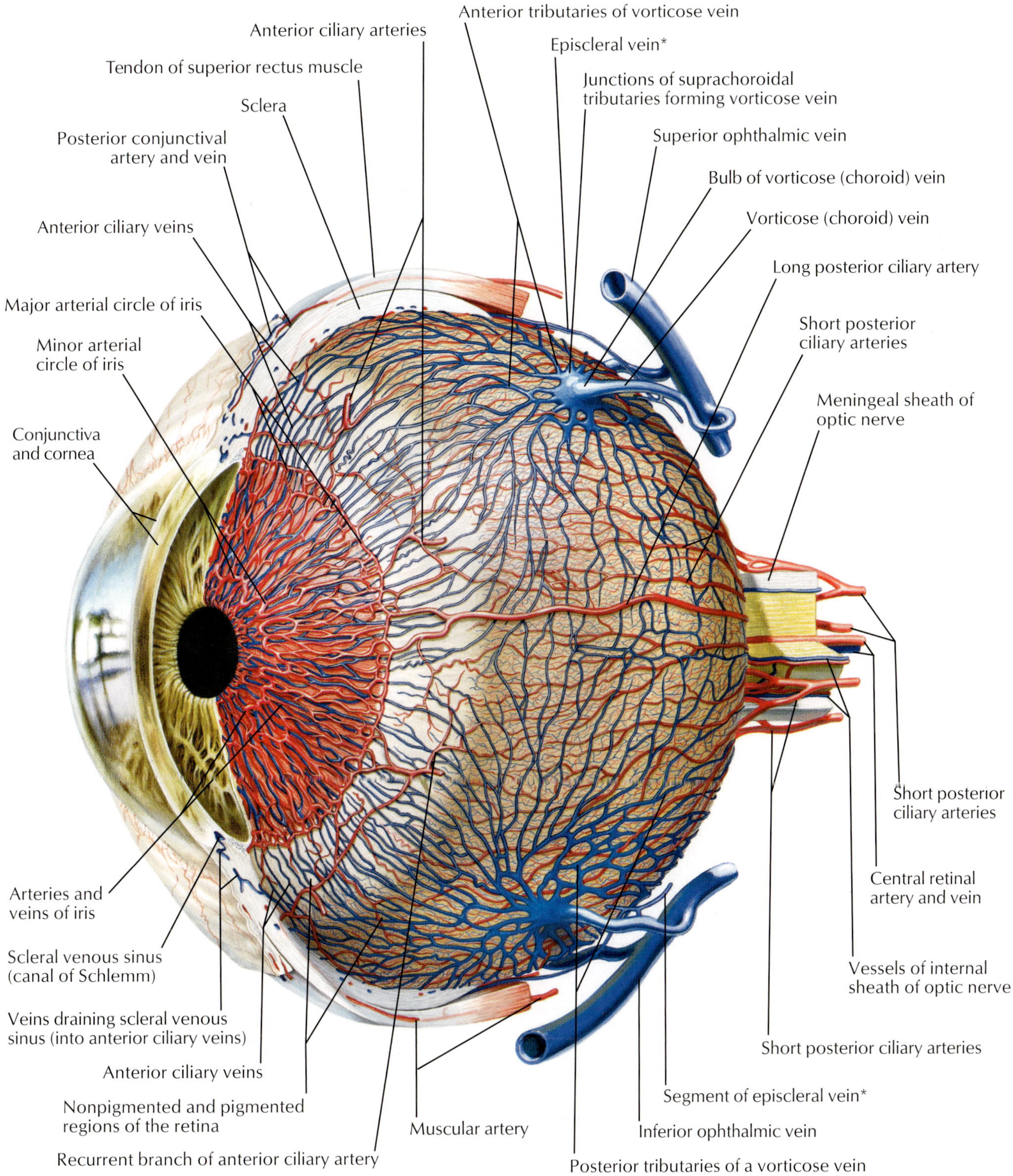

*The episcleral veins are shown here anastomosing with the vorticose veins, which they do; however, they also drain into the anterior ciliary veins.

Pathway of Sound Reception

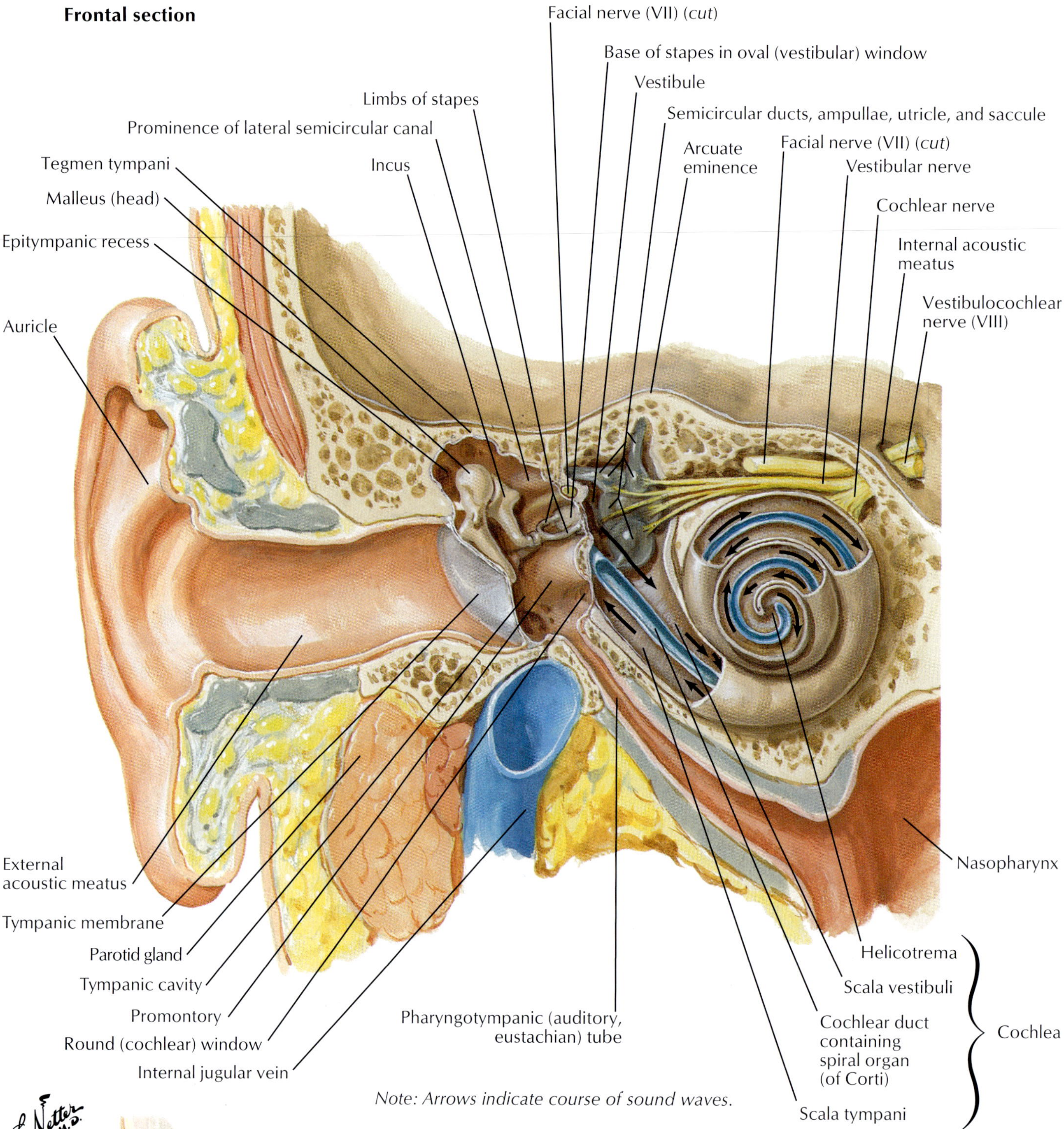

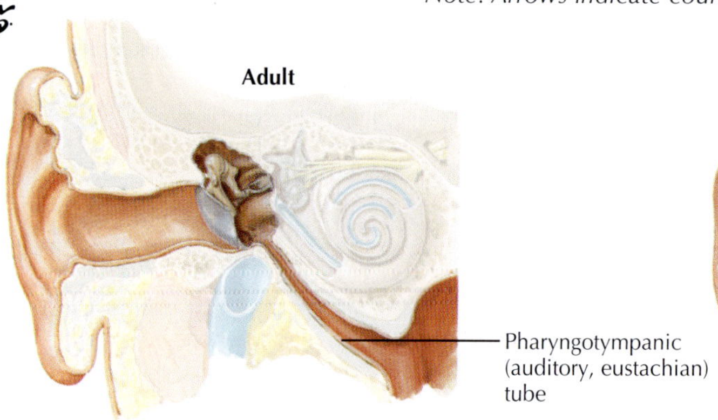

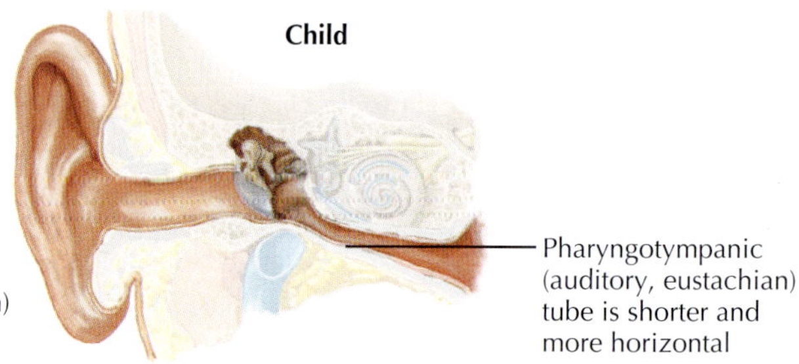

Right auricle (pinna)

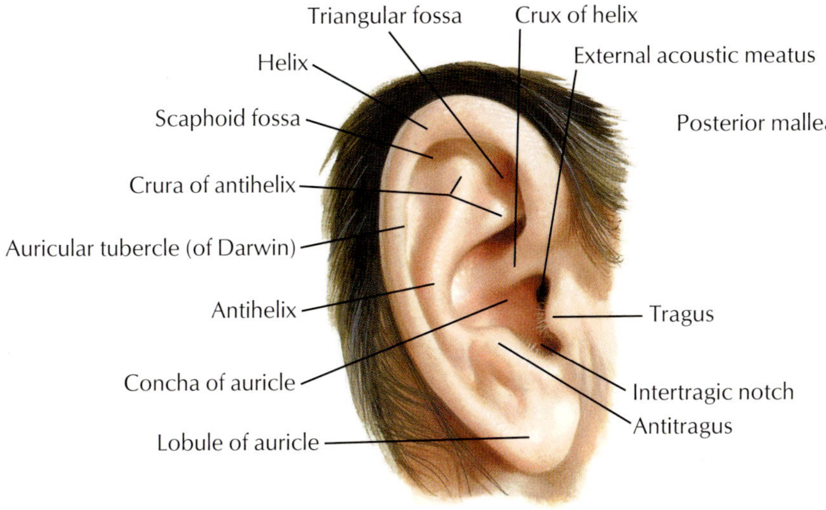

Otoscopic view of right tympanic membrane

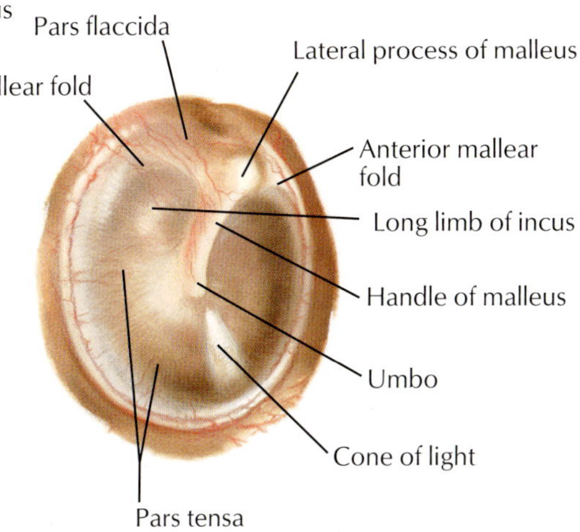

Coronal oblique section of external acoustic meatus and middle ear (tympanic cavity)

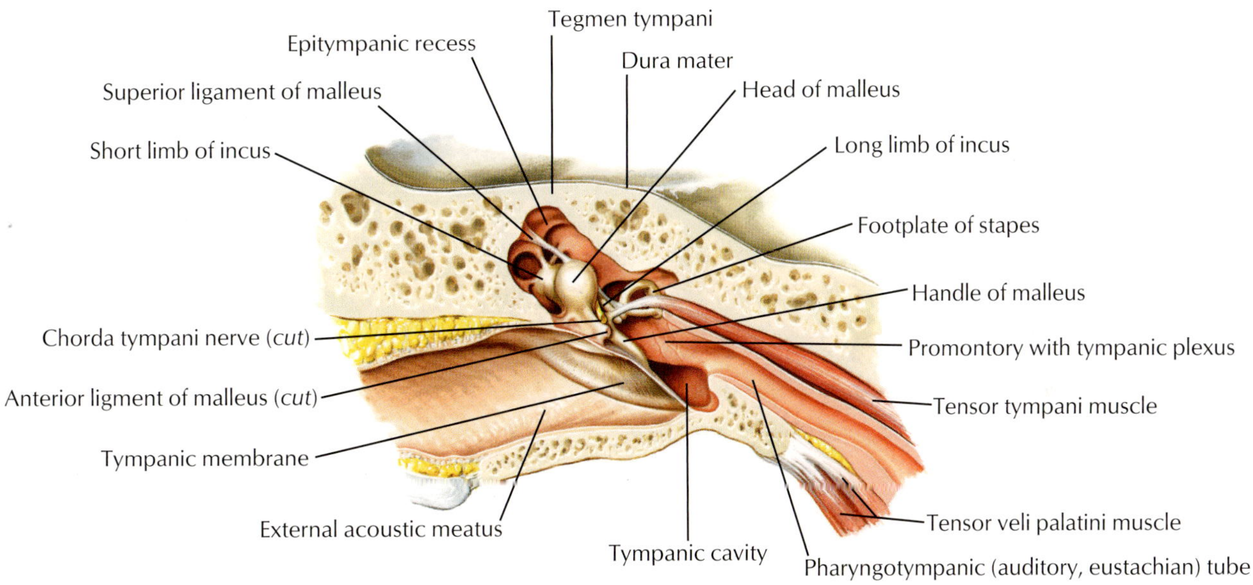

Right tympanic cavity after removal of tympanic membrane (lateral view)

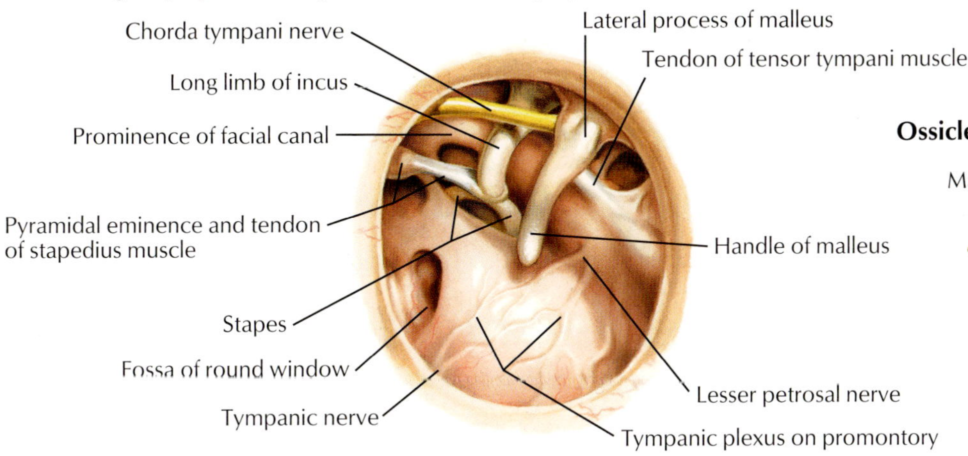

Ossicles articulated: medial view

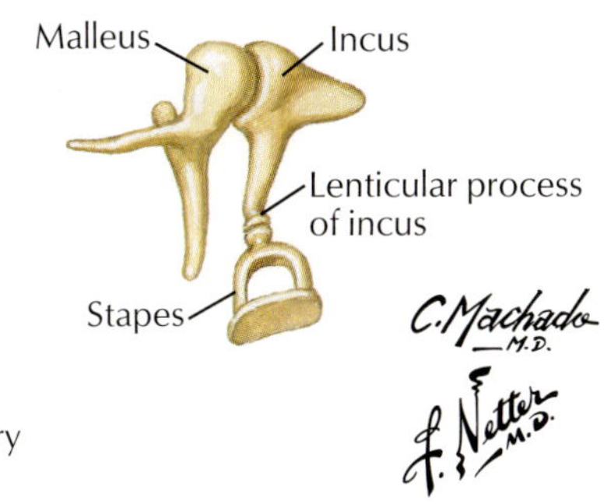

Tympanic Cavity

See also **Plates 50, 124, 136**

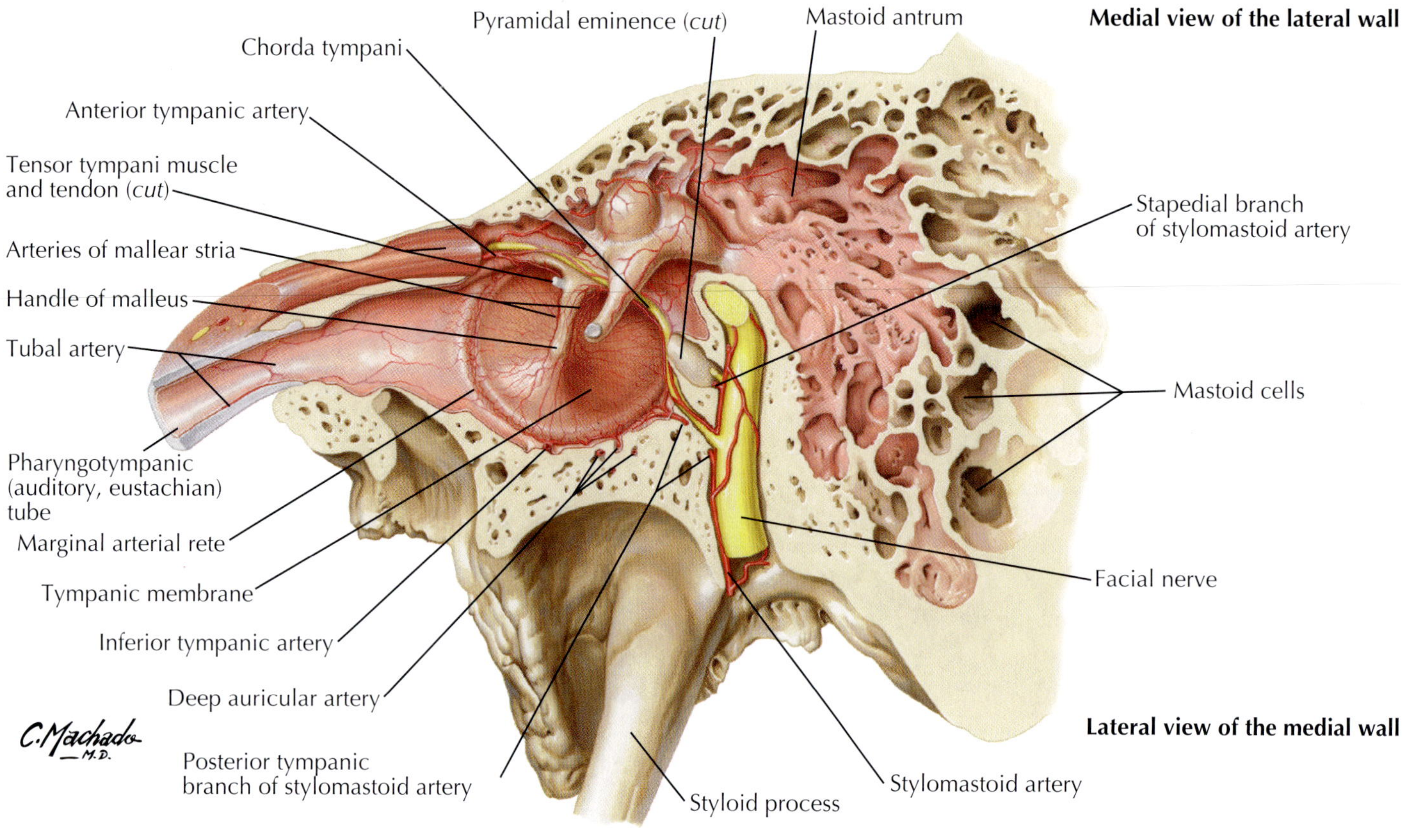

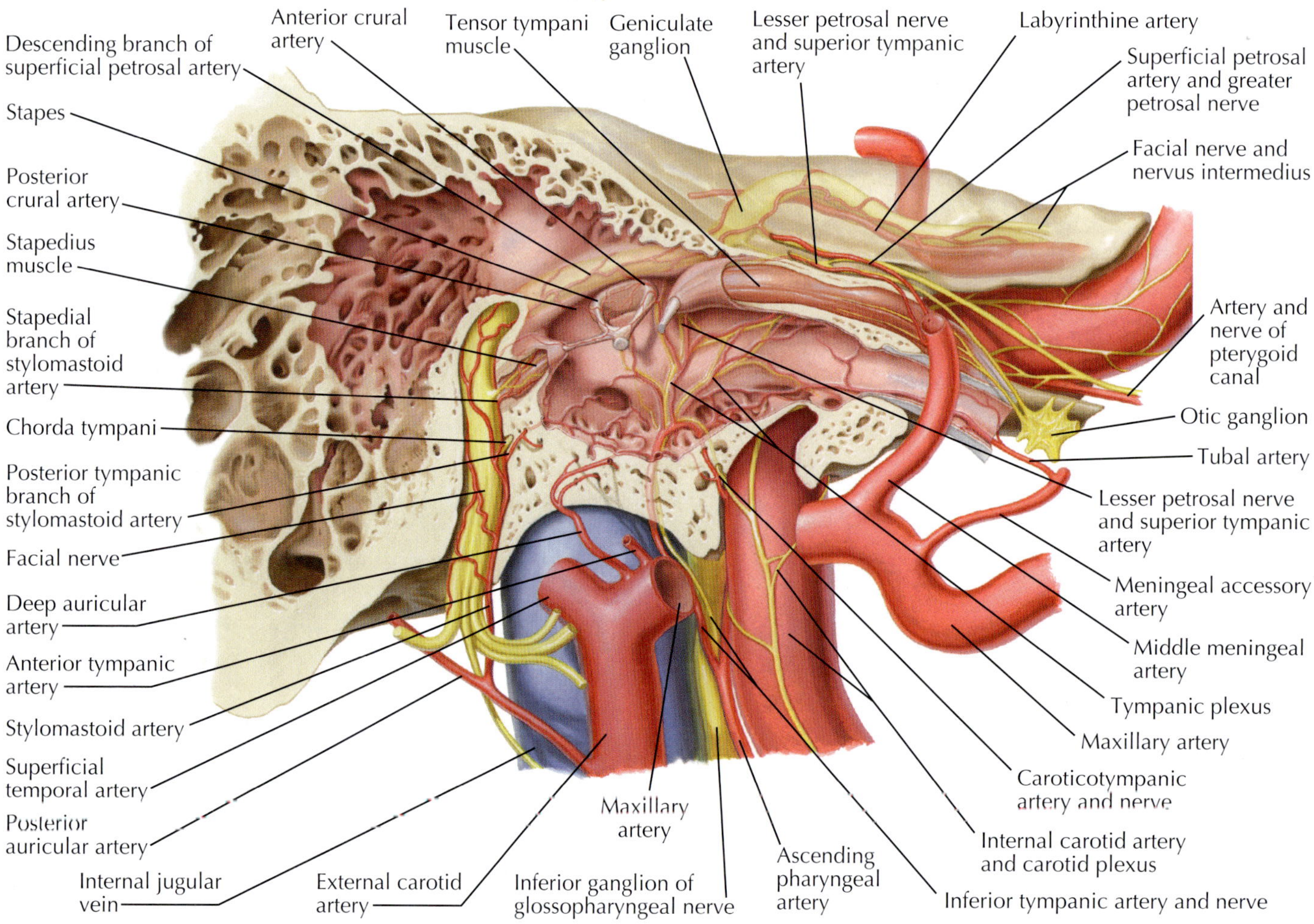

Bony and Membranous Labyrinths

Right bony labyrinth (otic capsule), anterolateral view: surrounding cancellous bone removed

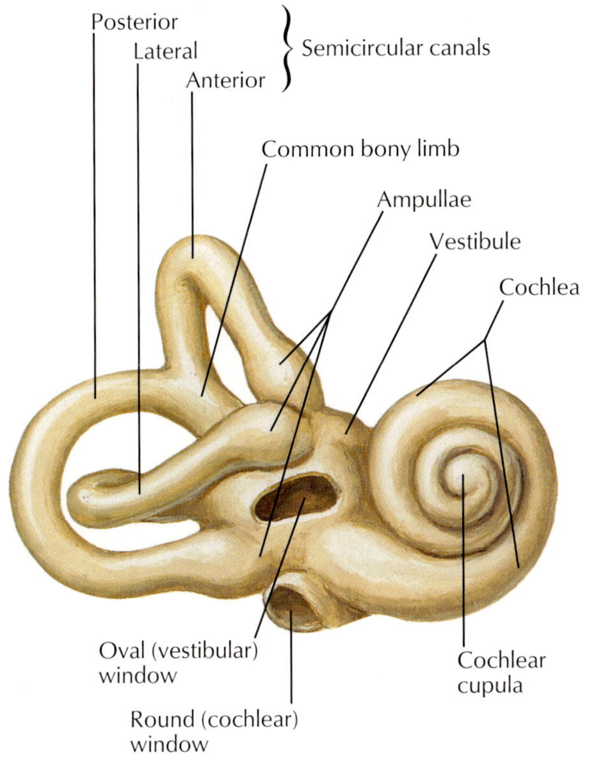

Dissected right bony labyrinth (otic capsule): membranous labyrinth removed

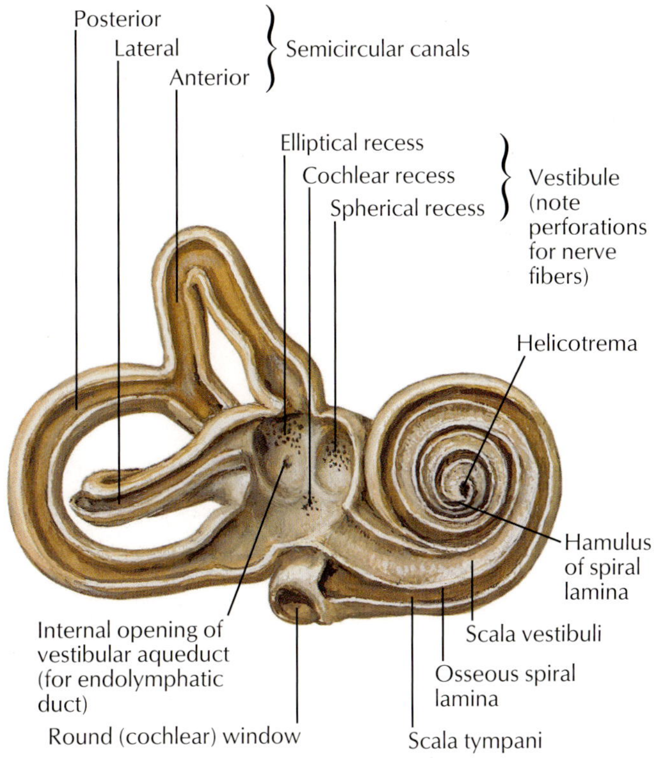

Right membranous labyrinth with nerves: medial view

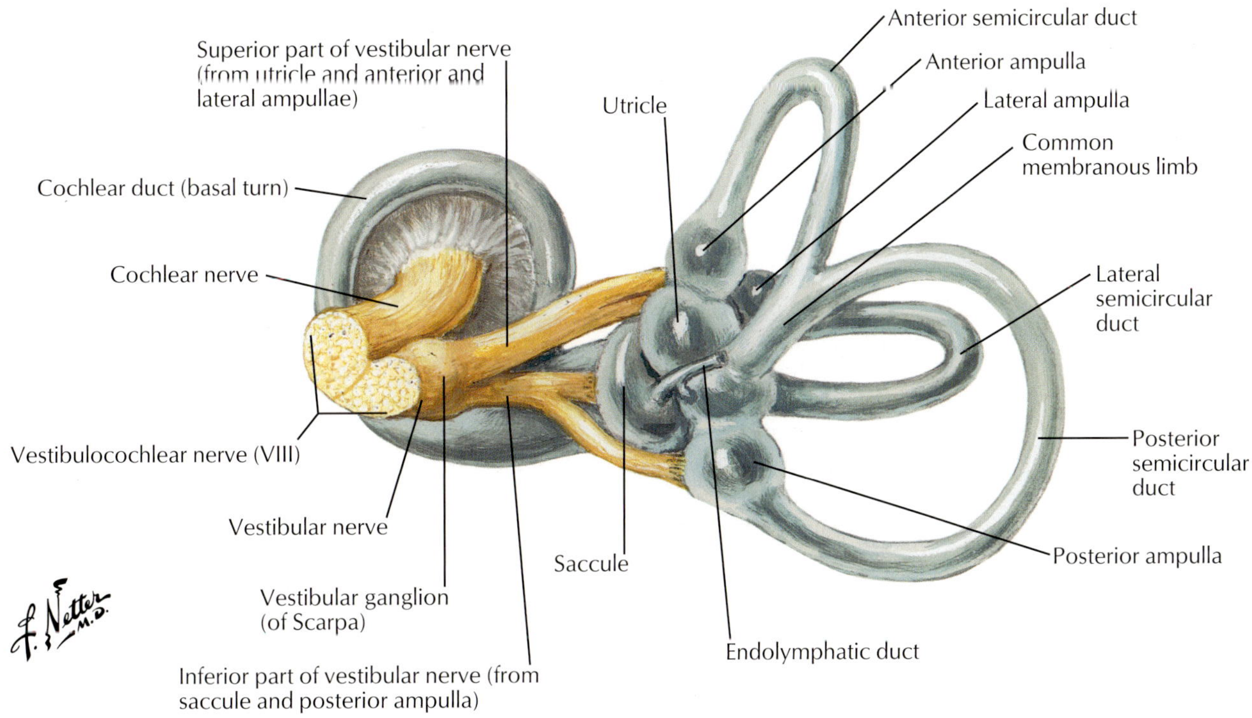

Bony and membranous labyrinths: schema

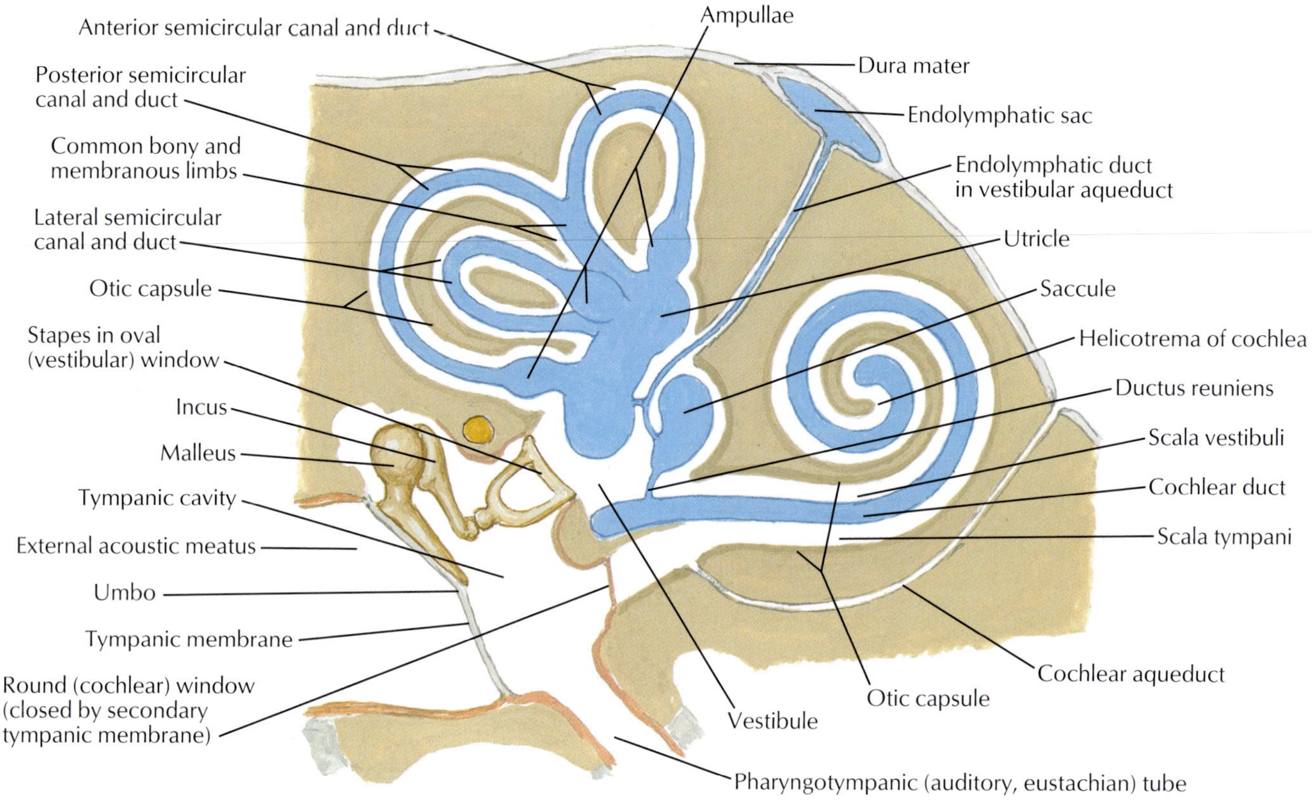

Section through turn of cochlea

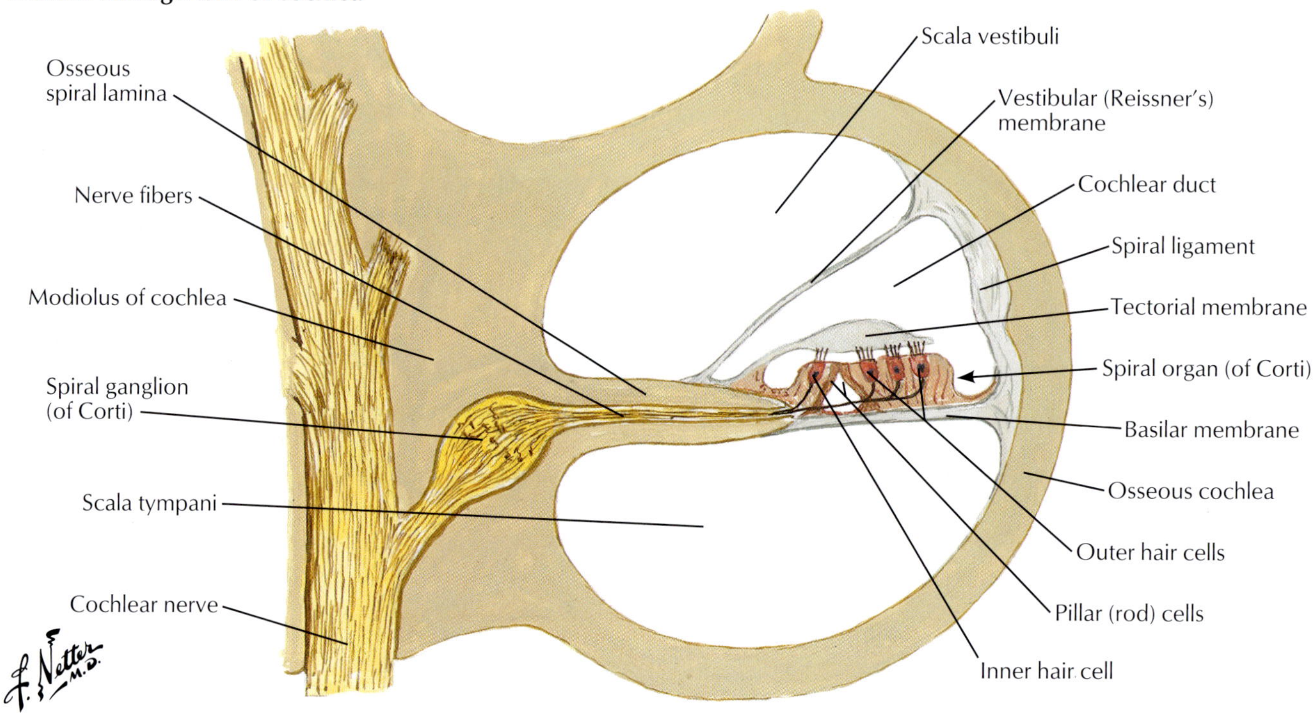

Orientation of Labyrinths in Skull

Superior projection of right bony labyrinth on floor of skull

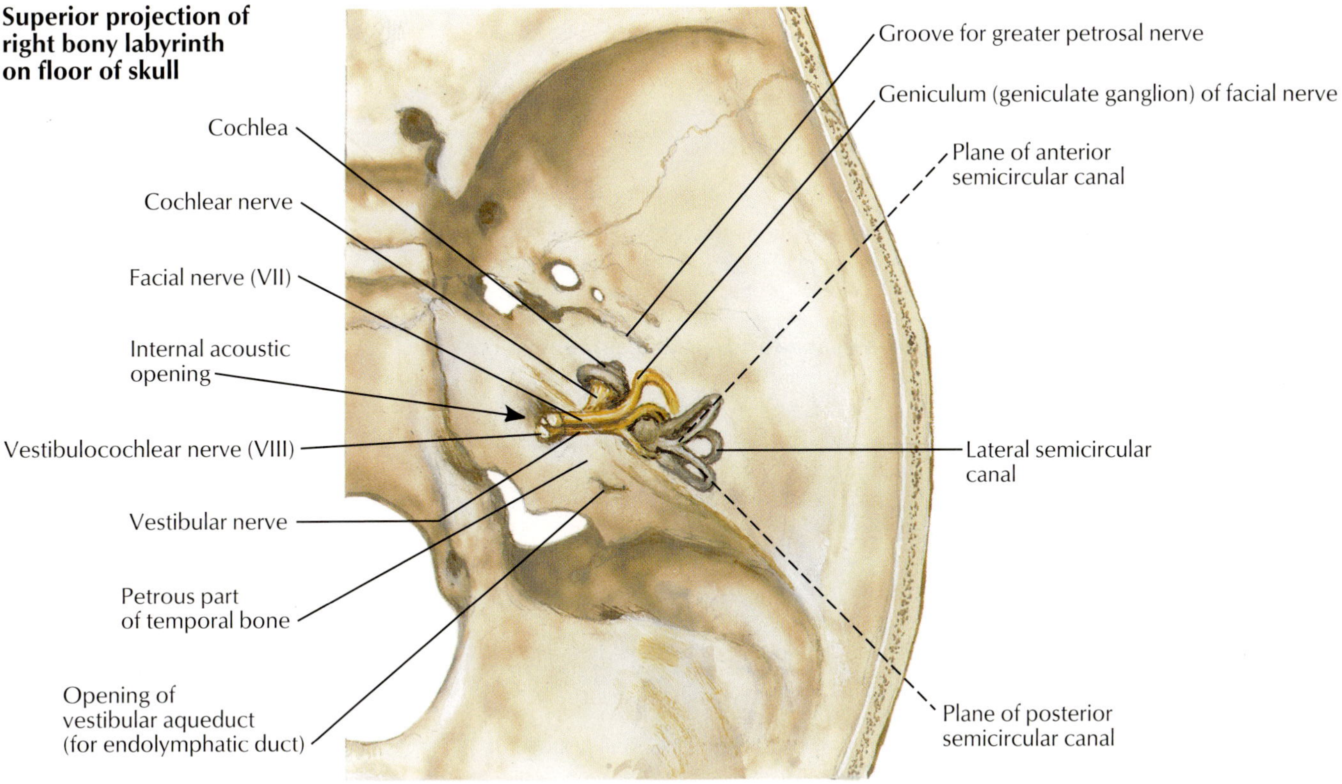

Lateral projection of right membranous labyrinth

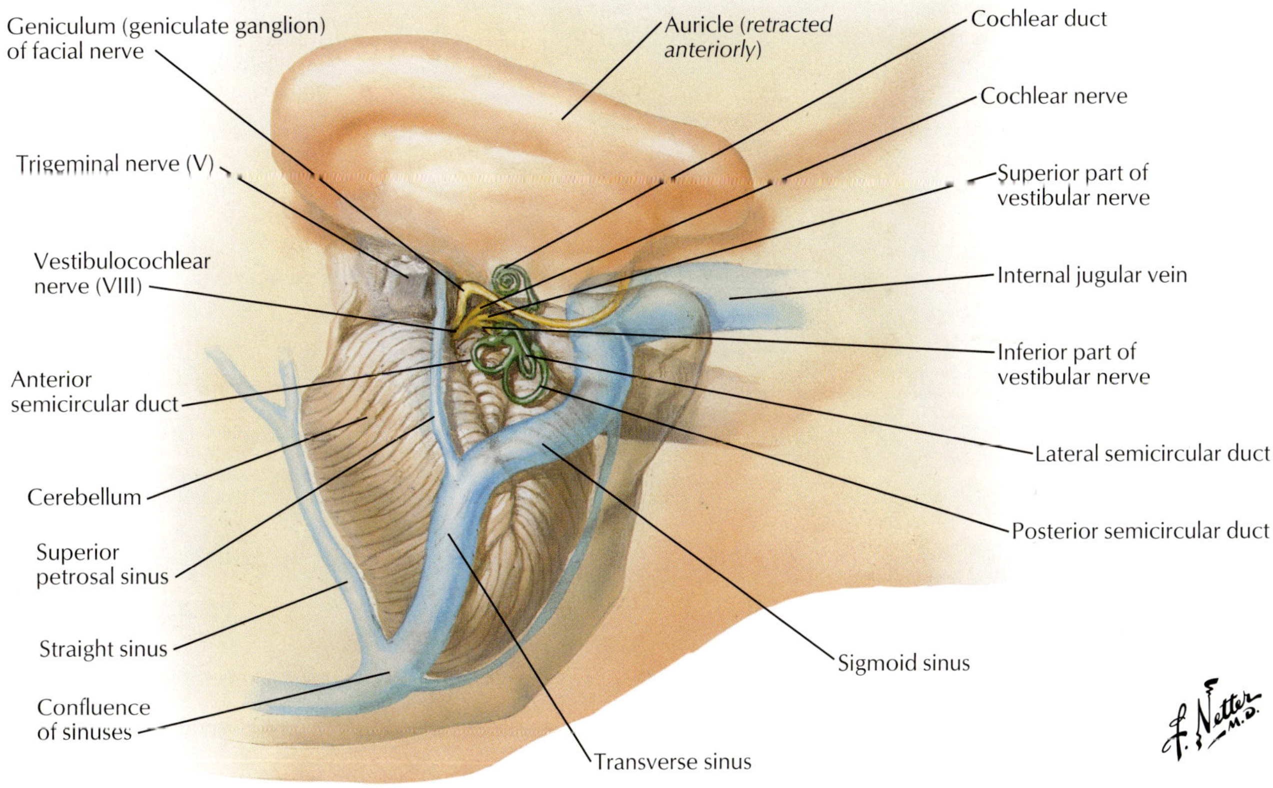

Pharyngotympanic (Auditory, Eustachian) Tube

See also Plate 49

Cartilaginous part of pharyngotympanic (auditory, eustachian) tube at base of skull: inferior view

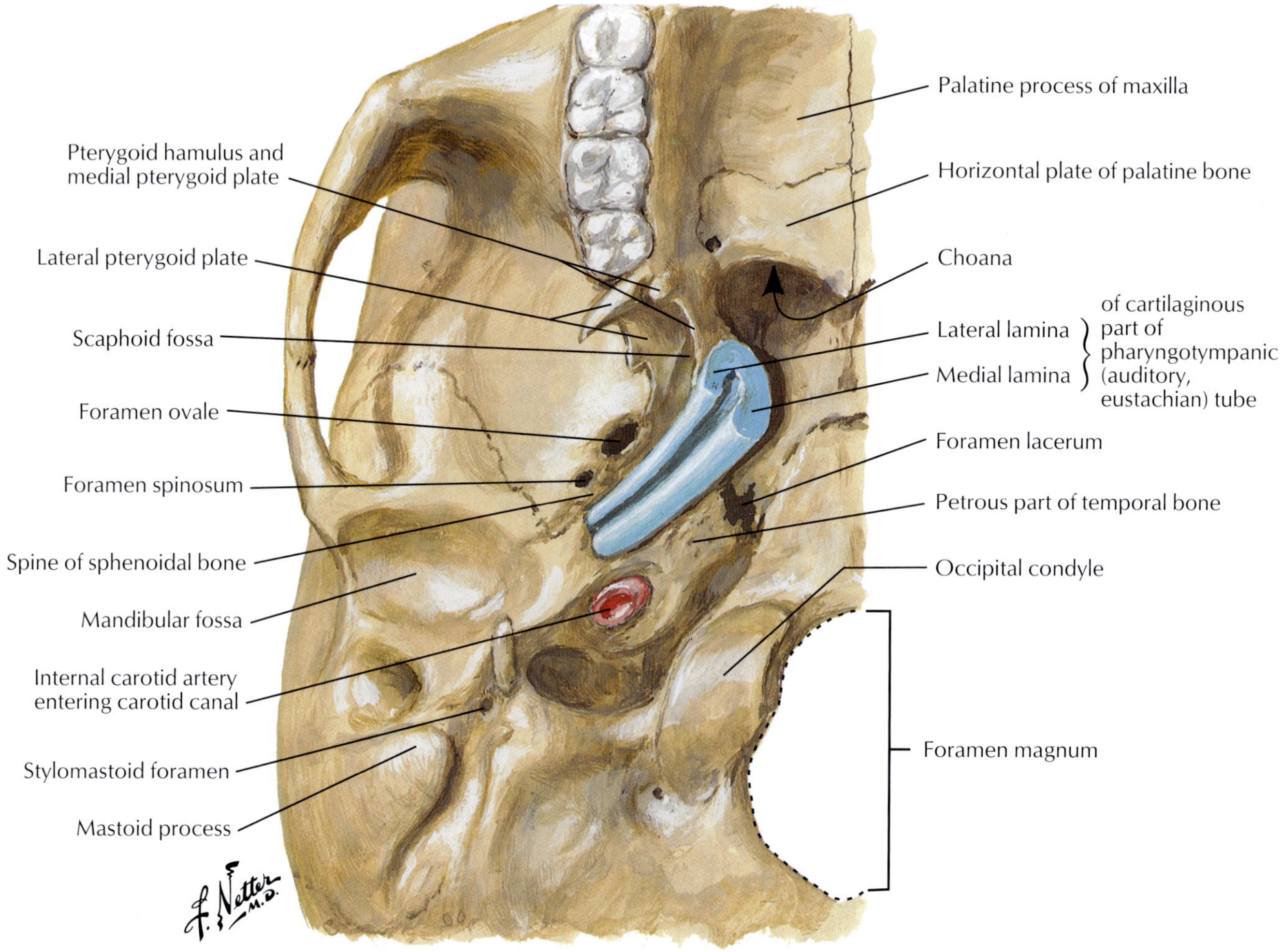

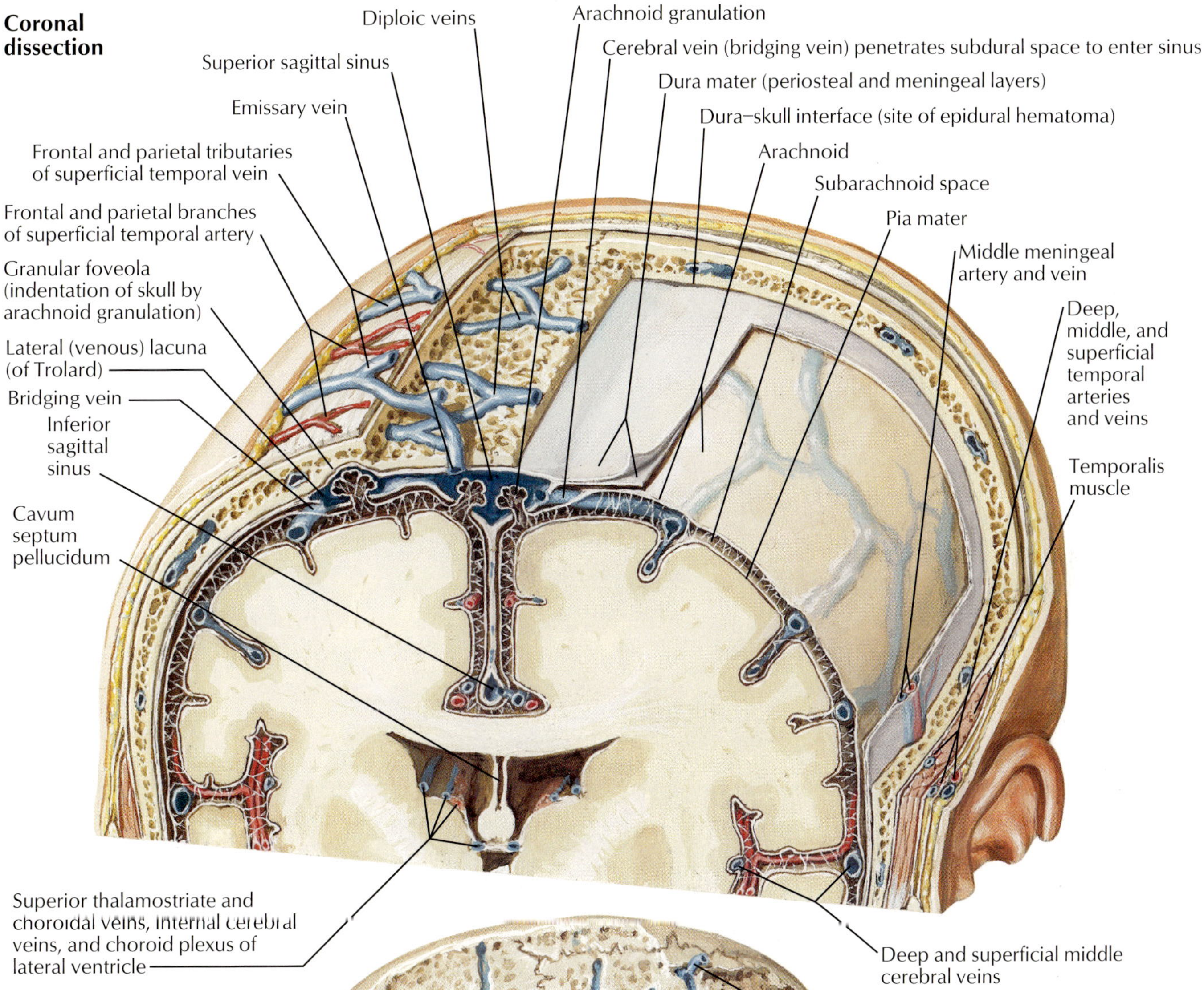
Coronal dissection
Diploic veins
Arachnoid granulation
Superior sagittal sinus
Cerebral vein (bridging vein) penetrates subdural space to enter sinus
Dura mater (periosteal and meningeal layers)
Emissary vein
Dura–skull interface (site of epidural hematoma)
Frontal and parietal tributaries of superficial temporal vein
Arachnoid
Subarachnoid space
Frontal and parietal branches of superficial temporal artery
Pia mater
Granular foveola (indentation of skull by arachnoid granulation)
Middle meningeal artery and vein
Deep, middle, and superficial temporal arteries and veins
Lateral (venous) lacuna (of Trolard)
Bridging vein
Inferior sagittal sinus
Temporalis muscle
Cavum septum pellucidum
Superior thalamostriate and choroidal veins, internal cerebral veins, and choroid plexus of lateral ventricle
Deep and superficial middle cerebral veins

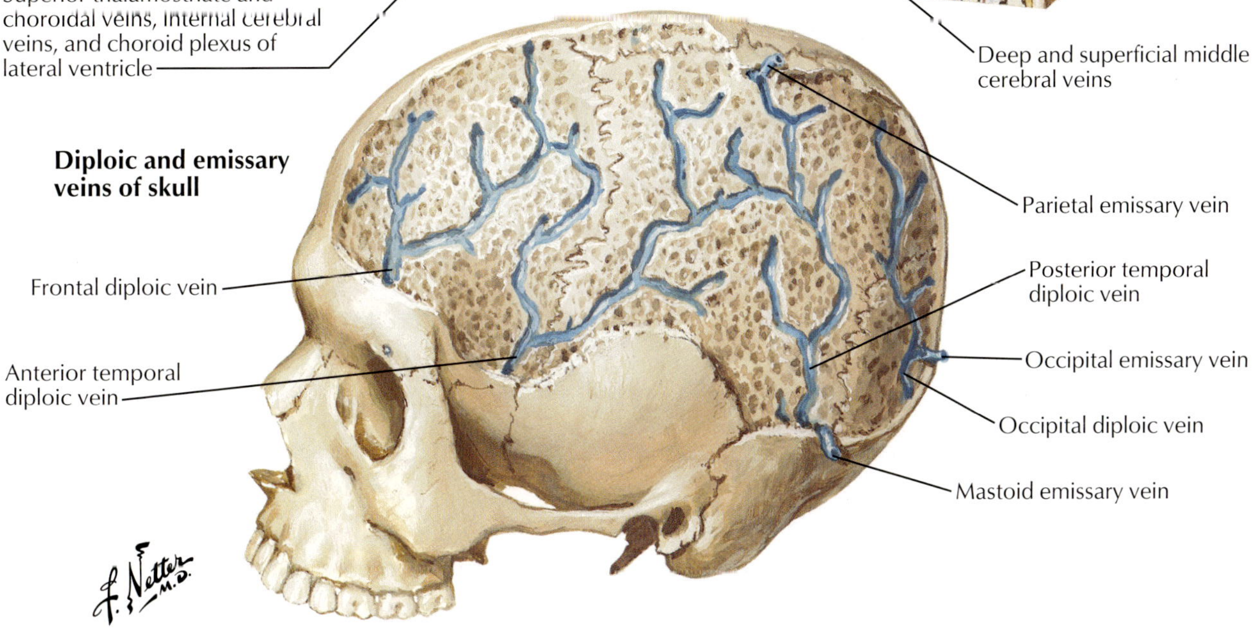
Diploic and emissary veins of skull
Parietal emissary vein
Frontal diploic vein
Posterior temporal diploic vein
Anterior temporal diploic vein
Occipital emissary vein
Occipital diploic vein
Mastoid emissary vein
F. Netter M.D.

Meningeal Arteries

See also Plates 9, 51, 137

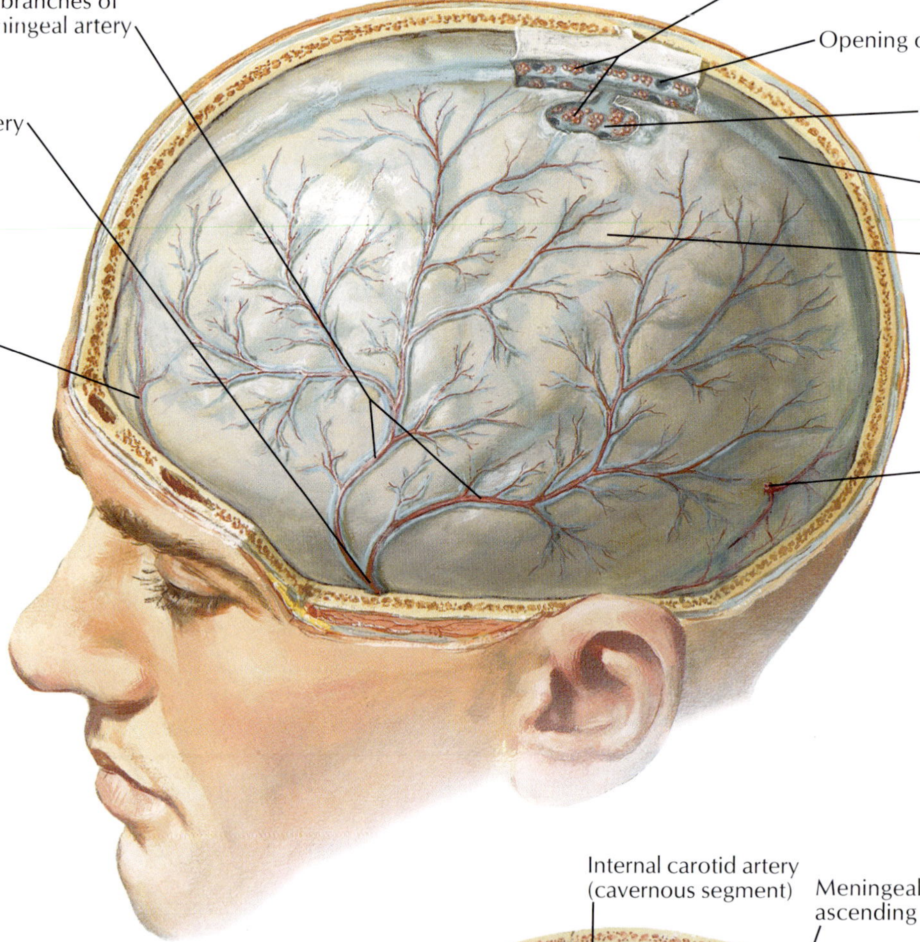

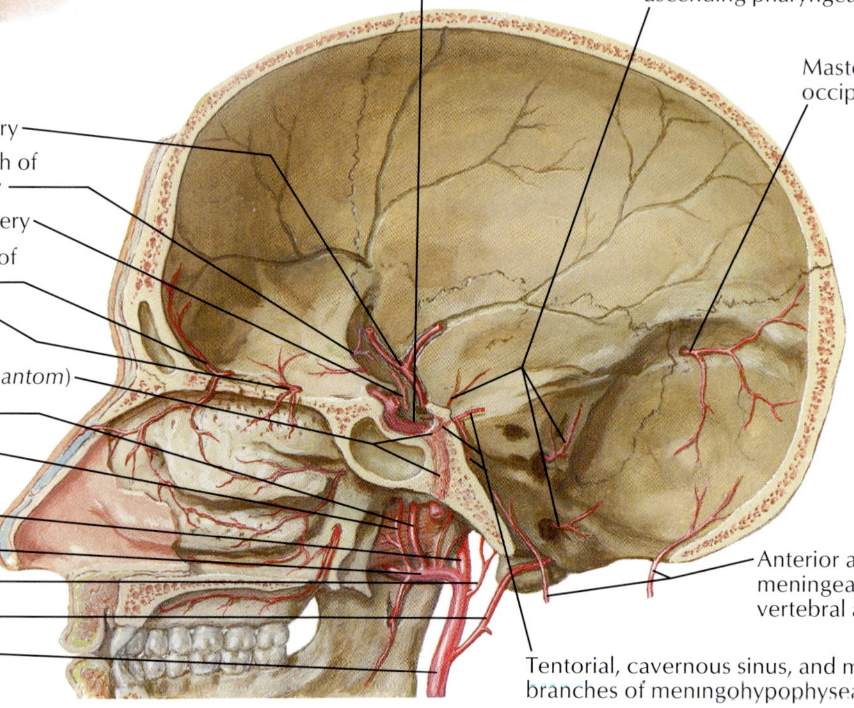

Meninges and Superficial Cerebral Veins

For deep veins of brain see Plate 146

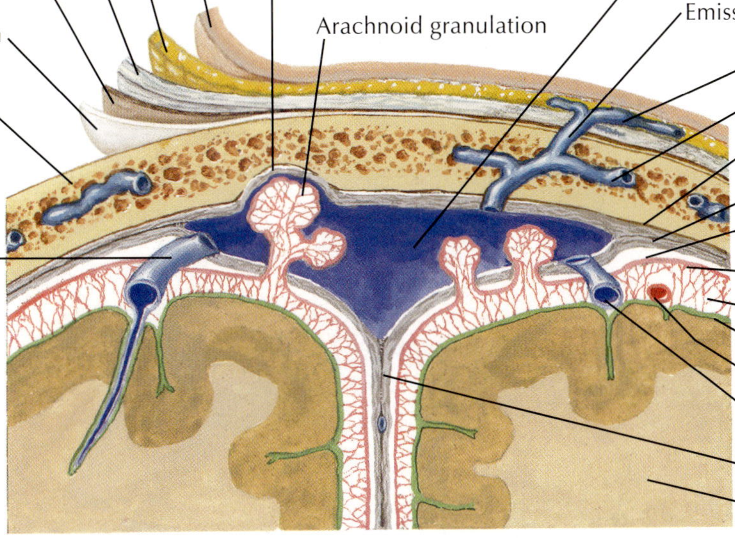

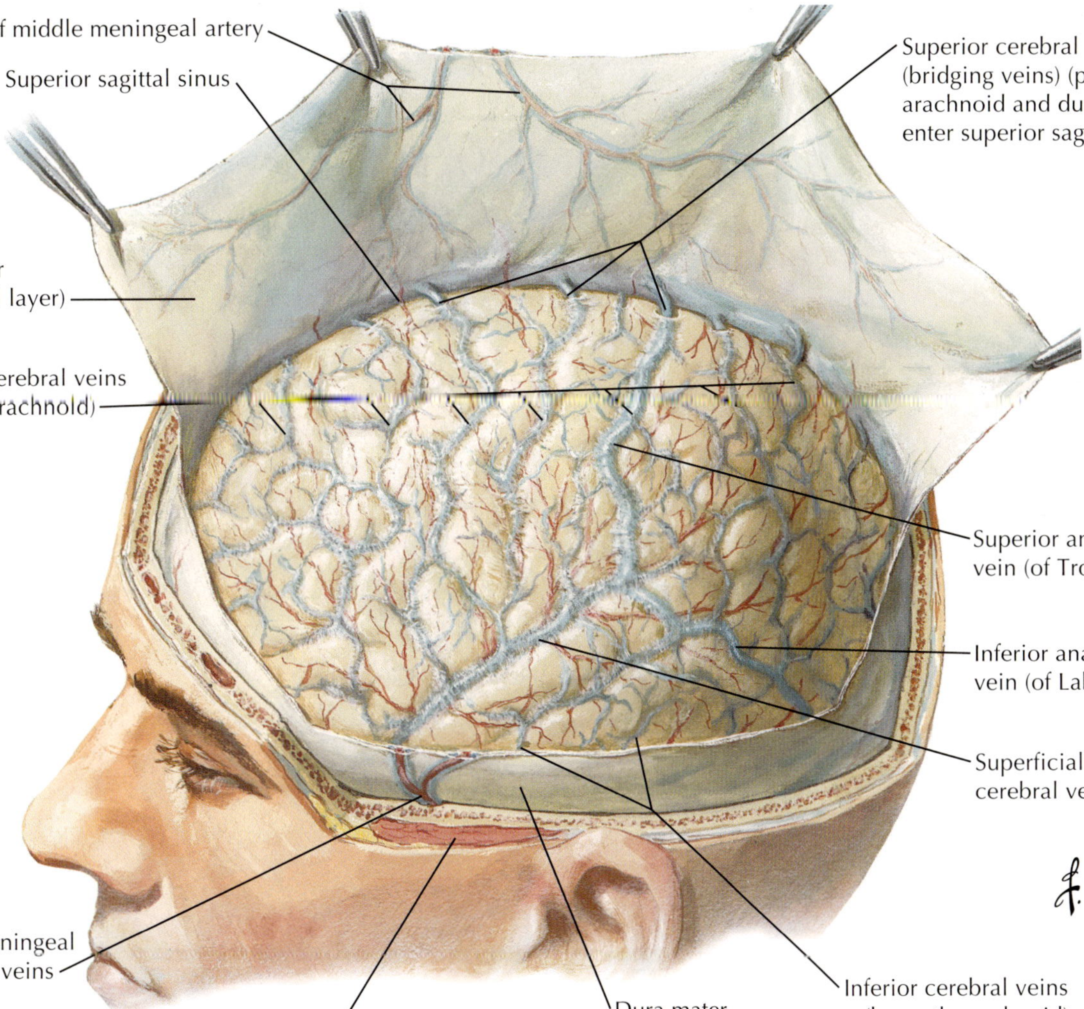

Sagittal section

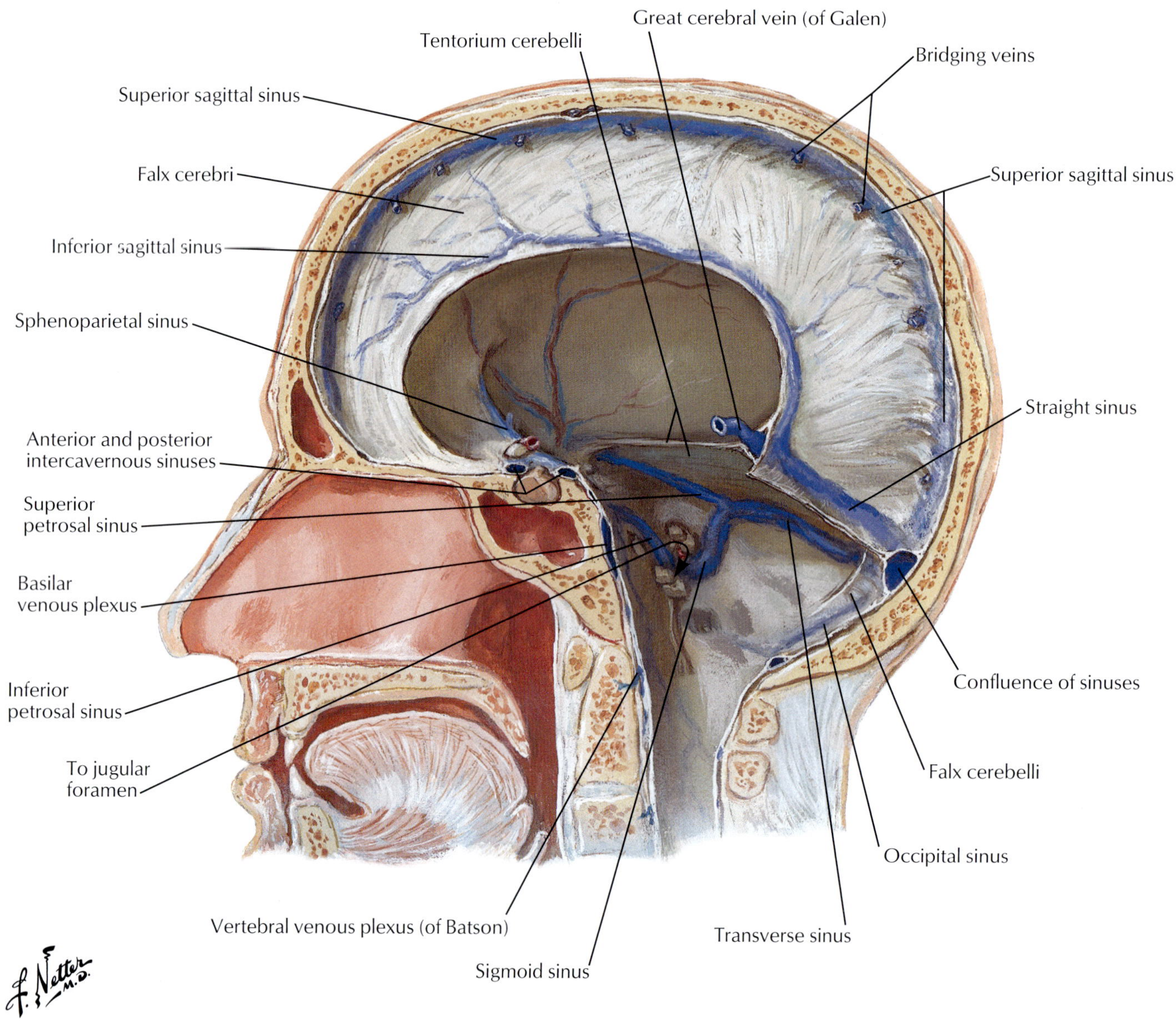

Skull sectioned horizontally: superior view

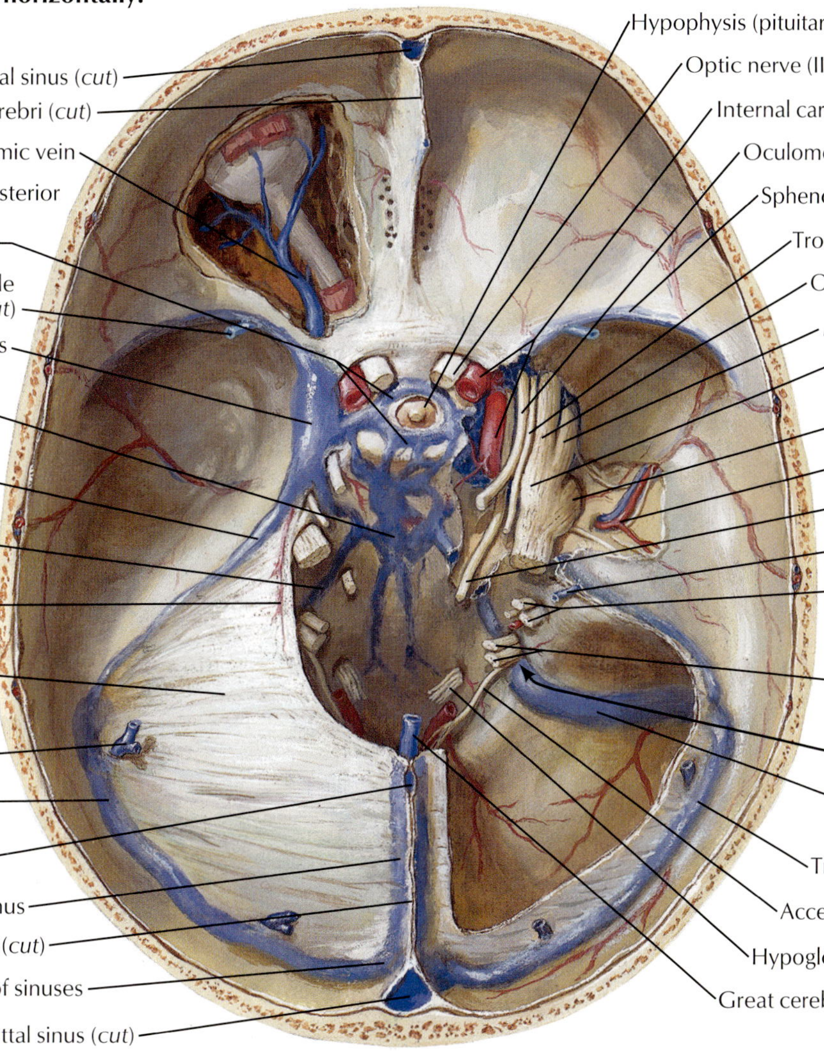

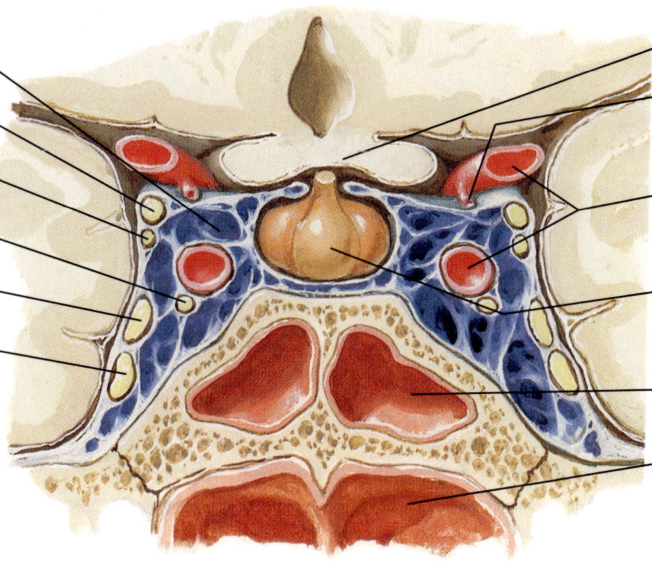

Coronal section through cavernous sinus: posterior view

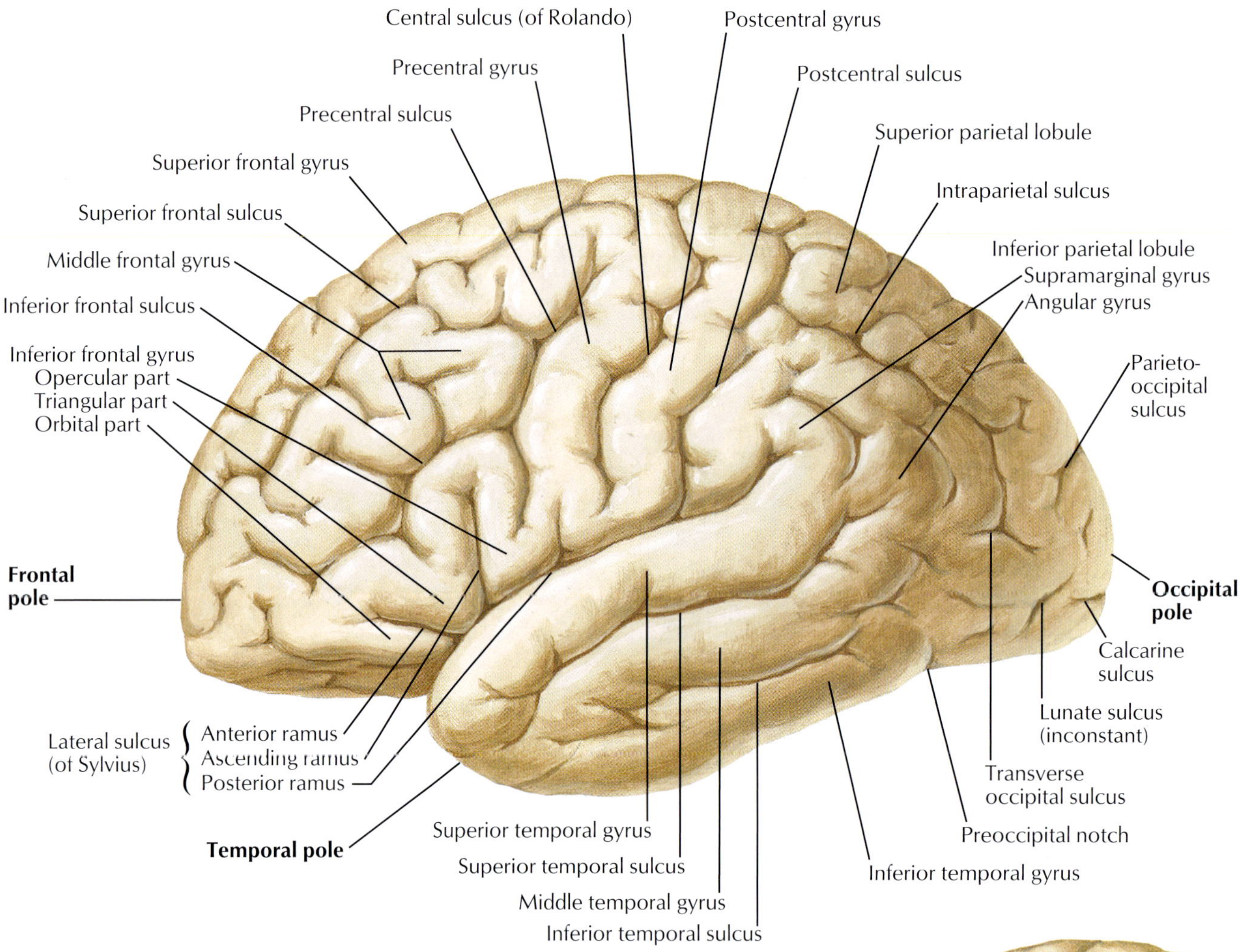
Central sulcus (of Rolando)
Postcentral gyrus
Precentral gyrus
Postcentral sulcus
Precentral sulcus
Superior parietal lobule
Superior frontal gyrus
Intraparietal sulcus
Superior frontal sulcus
Inferior parietal lobule
Supramarginal gyrus
Angular gyrus
Middle frontal gyrus
Inferior frontal sulcus
Inferior frontal gyrus
Opercular part
Triangular part
Orbital part
Parieto-occipital sulcus
Frontal pole
Occipital pole
Calcarine sulcus
Lunate sulcus (inconstant)
Lateral sulcus (of Sylvius)
Anterior ramus
Ascending ramus
Posterior ramus
Transverse occipital sulcus
Temporal pole
Superior temporal gyrus
Preoccipital notch
Superior temporal sulcus
Inferior temporal gyrus
Middle temporal gyrus
Inferior temporal sulcus

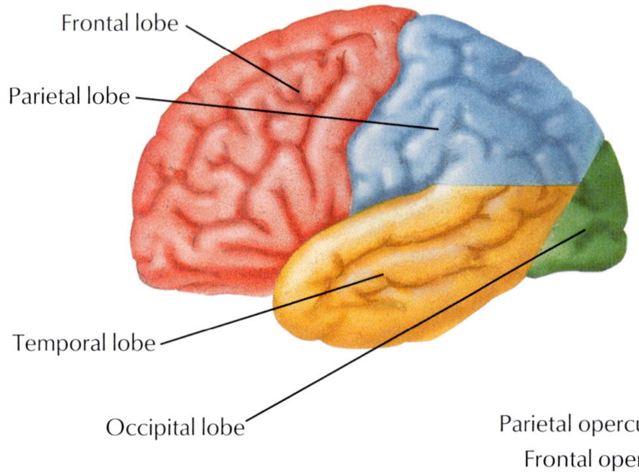
Frontal lobe
Parietal lobe
Temporal lobe
Occipital lobe

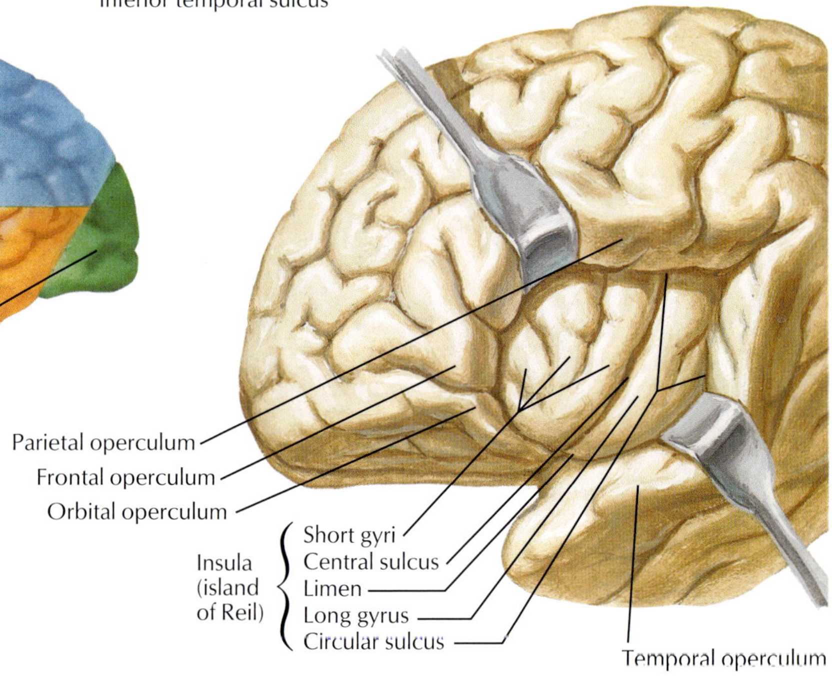
Parietal operculum
Frontal operculum
Orbital operculum
Insula (island of Reil)
Short gyri
Central sulcus
Limen
Long gyrus
Circular sulcus
Temporal operculum

See also Plate 148

Sagittal section of brain in situ

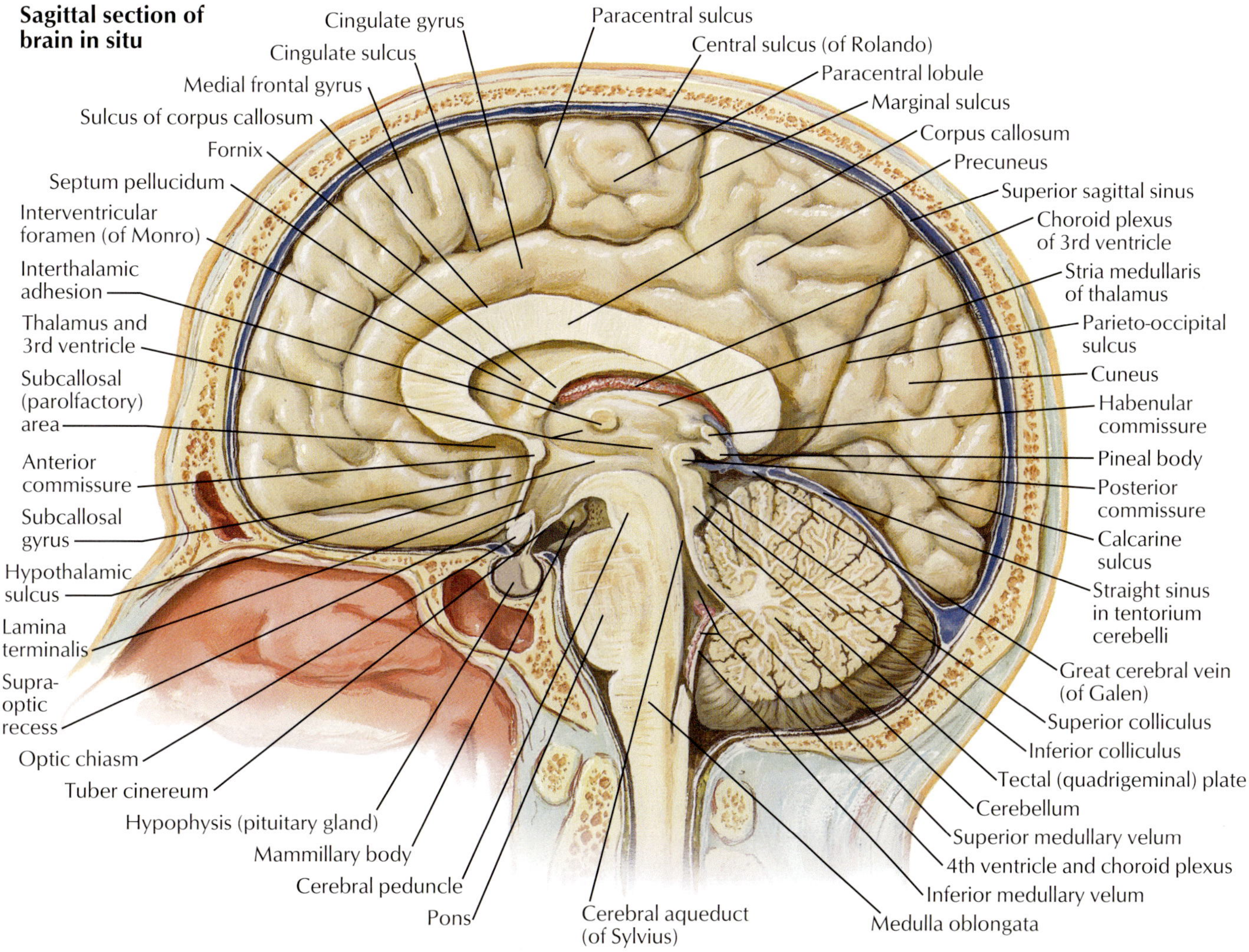

Medial surface of cerebral hemisphere: brainstem excised

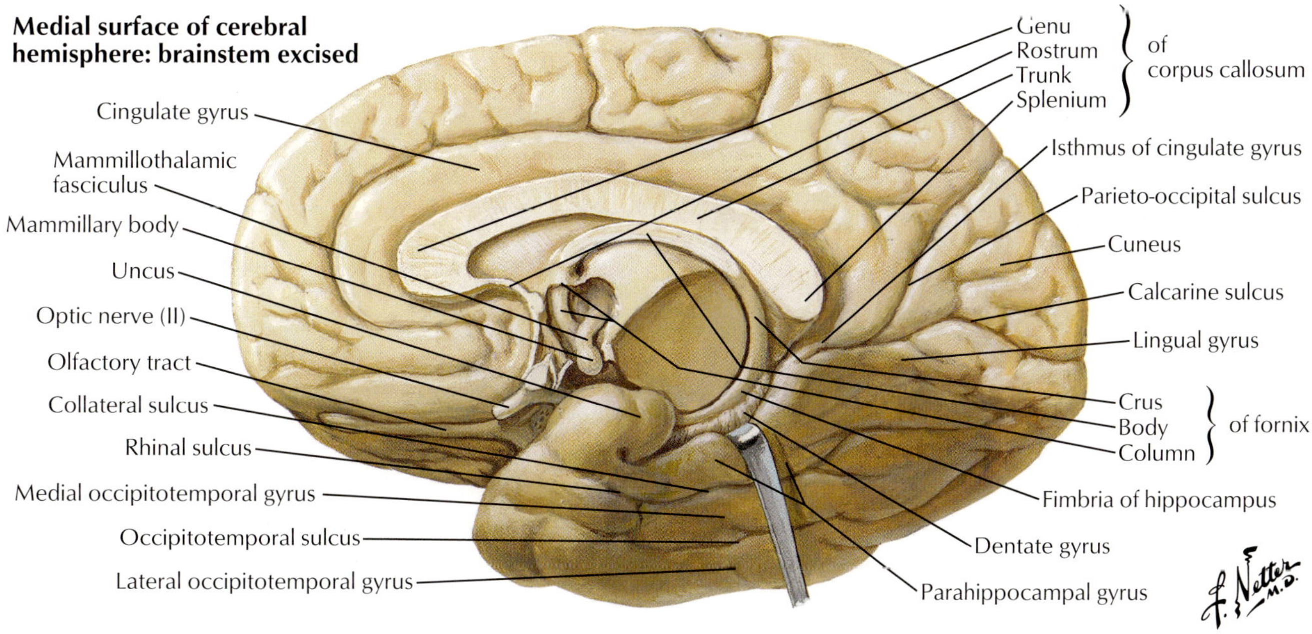

Cerebrum: Inferior View

See also Plate 148

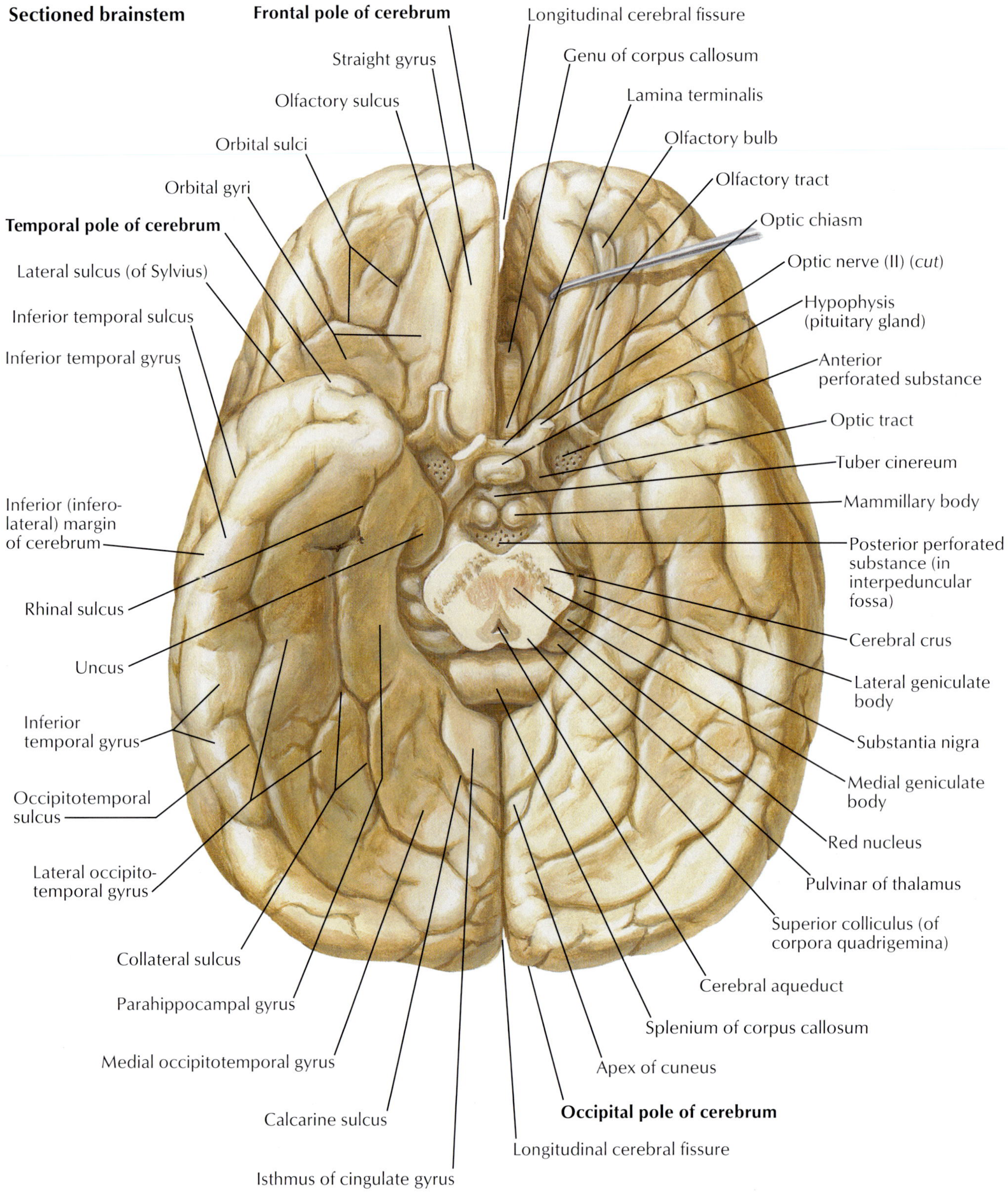

Left lateral phantom view

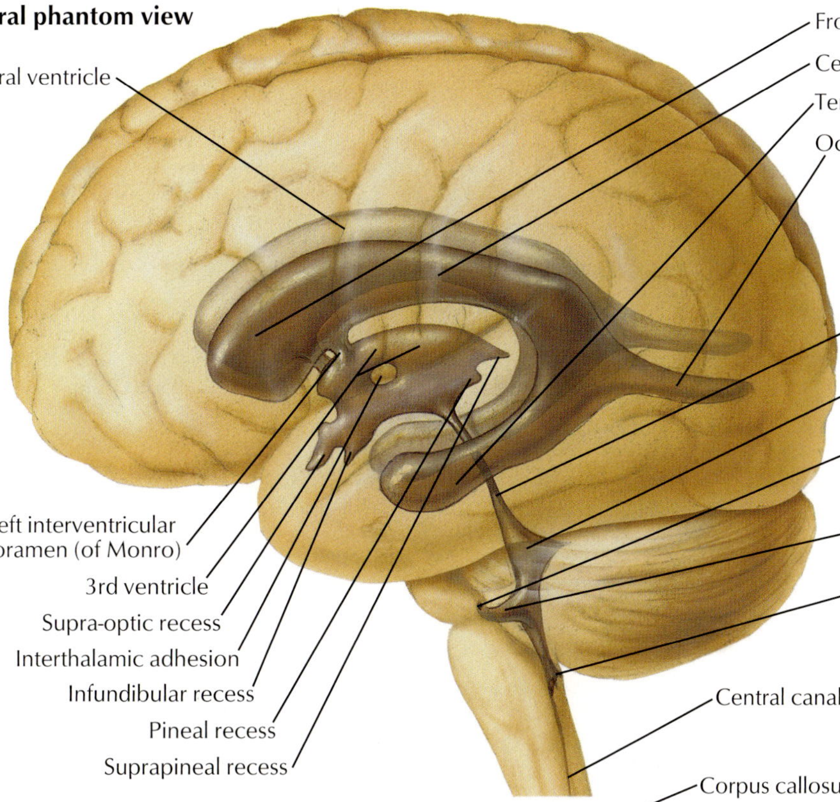

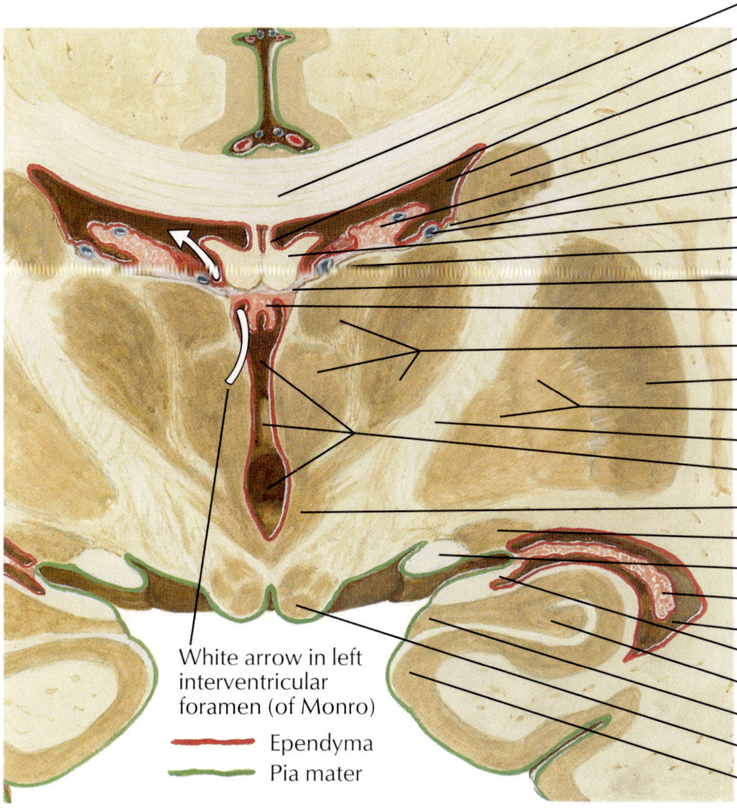

Coronal section of brain: posterior view

Circulation of Cerebrospinal Fluid

See also **Plates 109, 147**

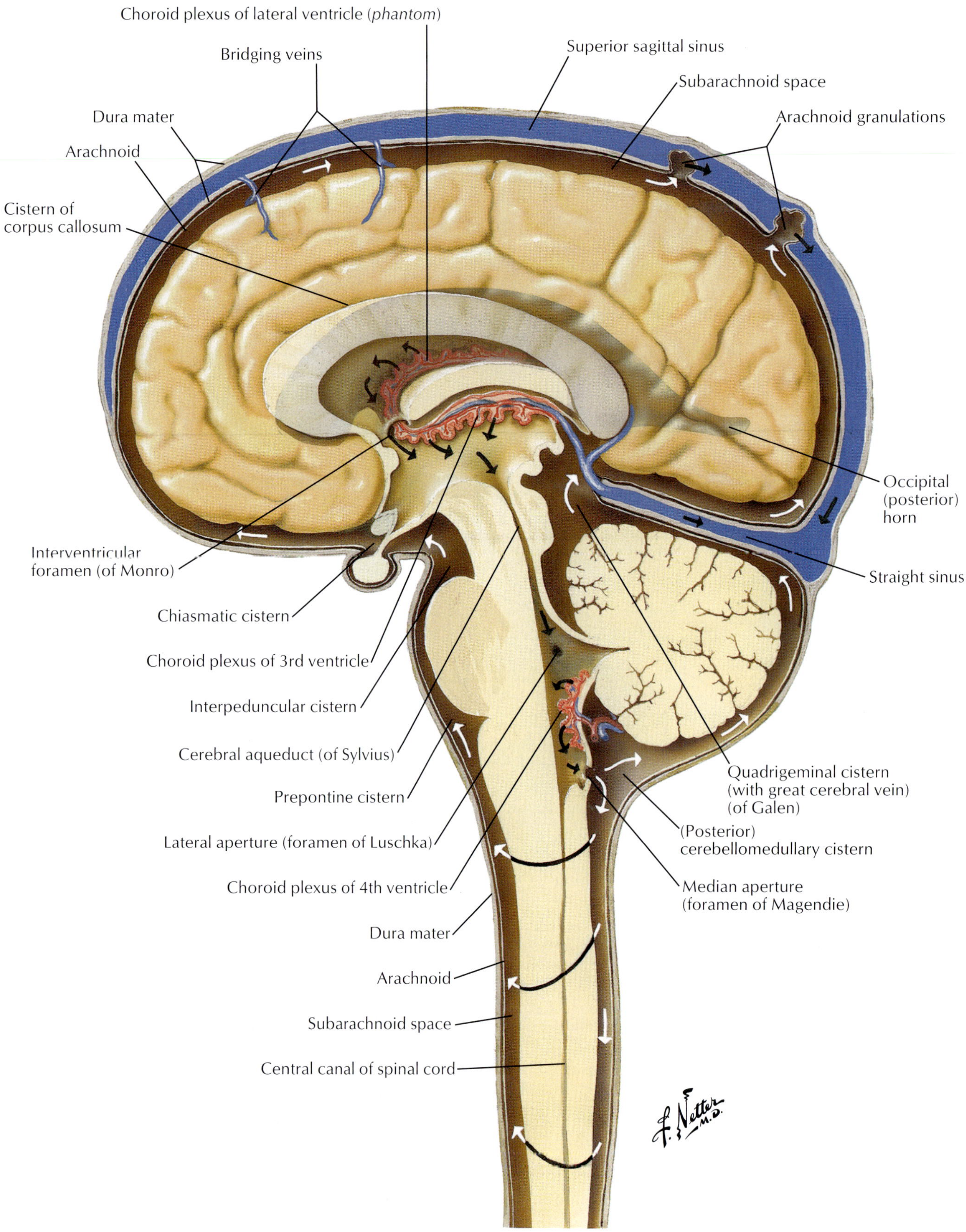

Horizontal sections through cerebrum

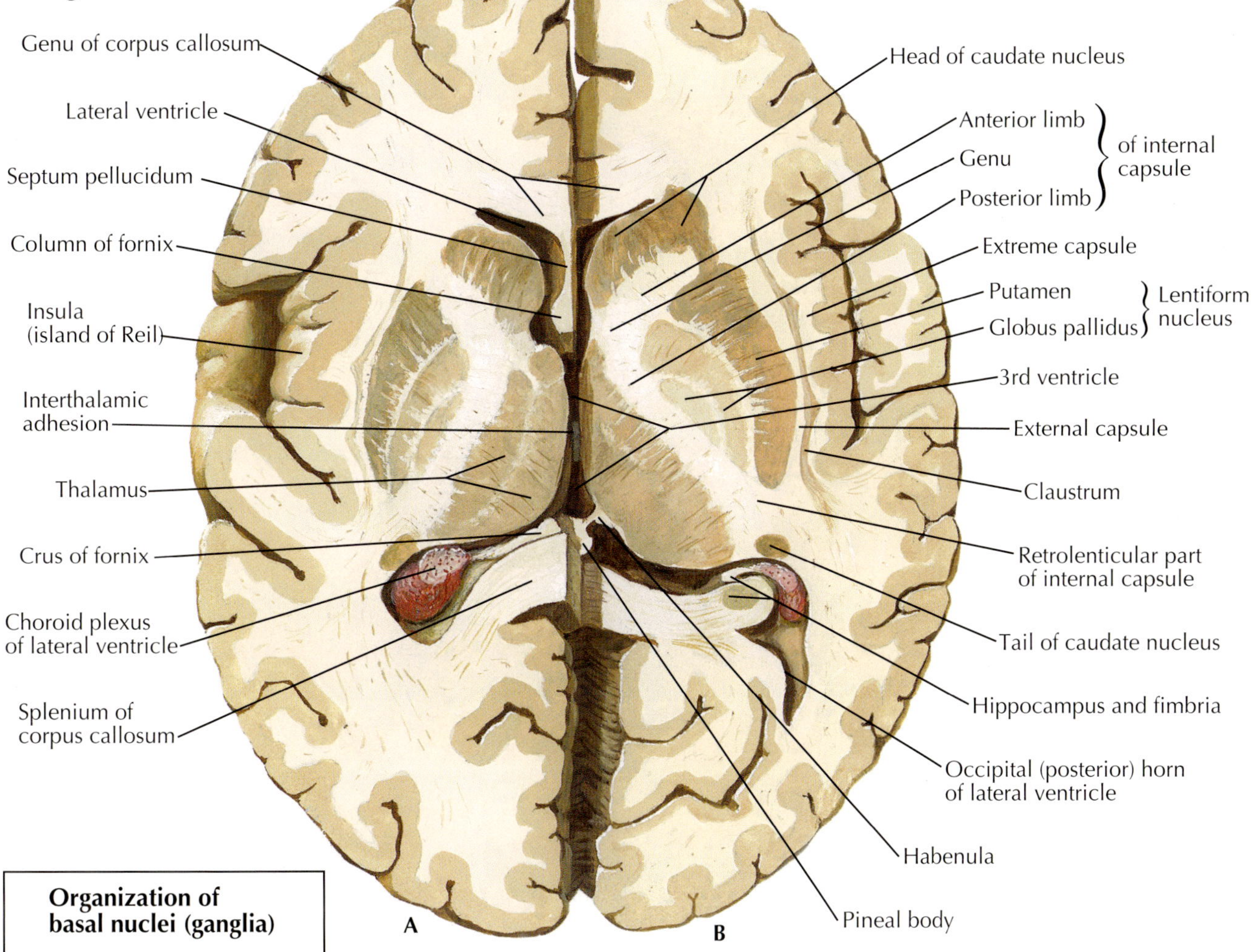

Organization of basal nuclei (ganglia)

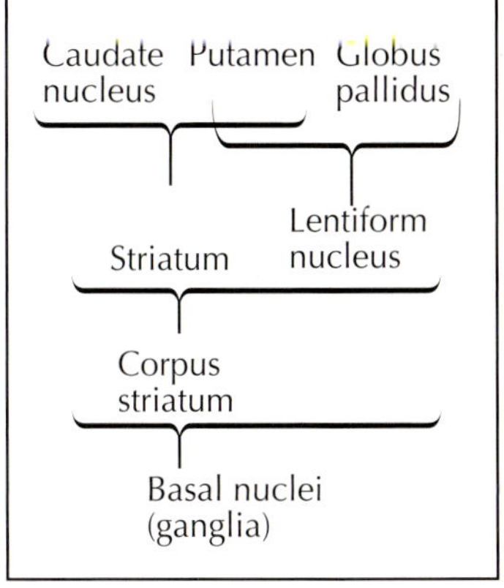

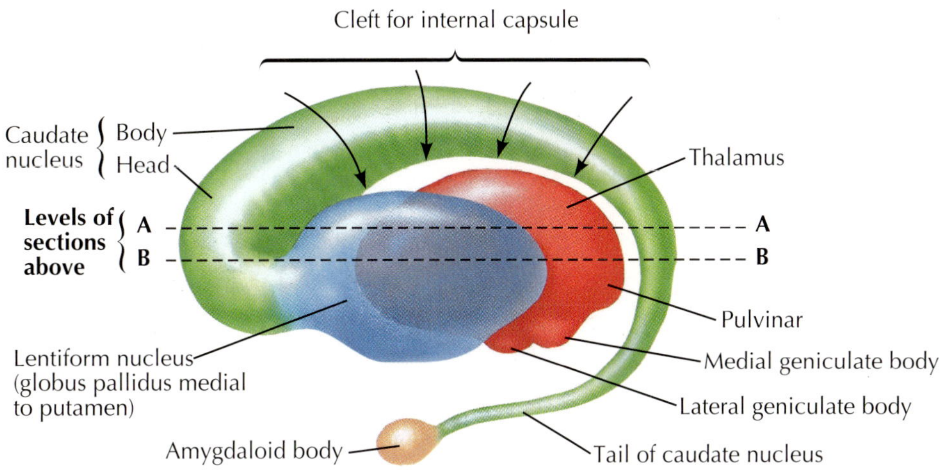

Interrelationship of thalamus, lentiform nucleus, caudate nucleus, and amygdaloid body (schema): left lateral view

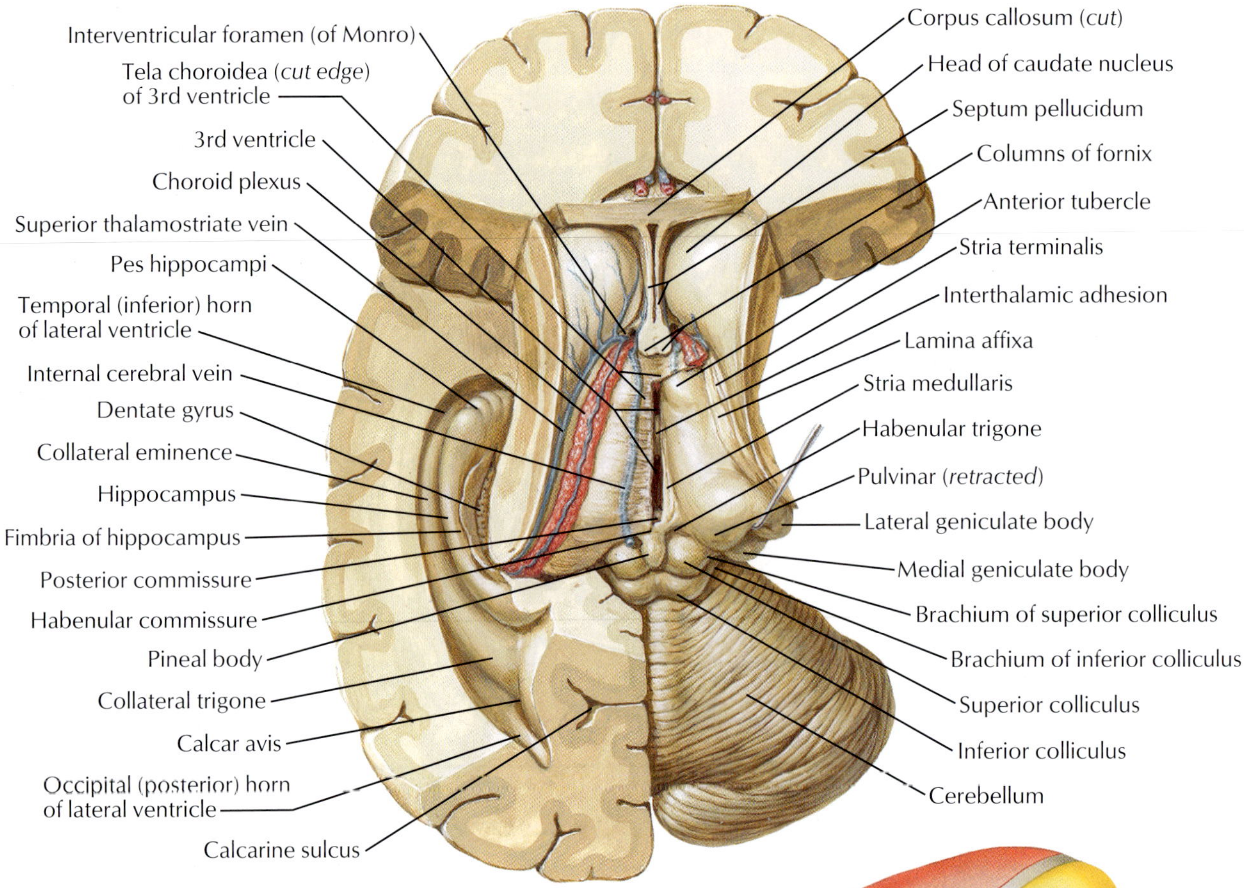

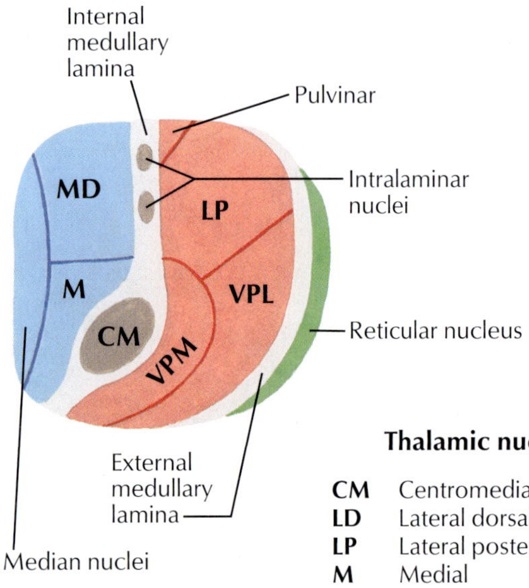

Schematic section through thalamus
(at level of broken line shown in figure at right)

Thalamic nuclei

CM Centromedian
LD Lateral dorsal
LP Lateral posterior
M Medial
MD Medial dorsal
VA Ventral anterior
VI Ventral intermedial
VL Ventral lateral
VP Ventral posterior
VPL Ventral posterolateral
VPM Ventral posteromedial

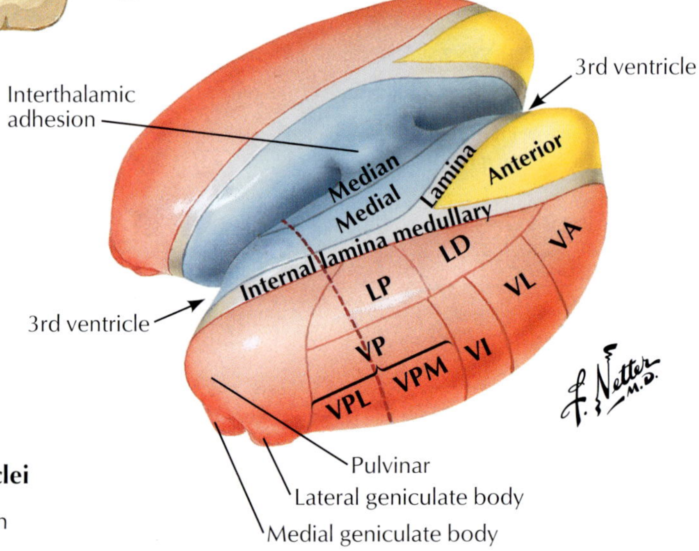

Schematic representation of thalamus
(external medullary lamina and reticular nuclei removed)

Lateral nuclei
Medial nuclei
Anterior nuclei

Superior dissection

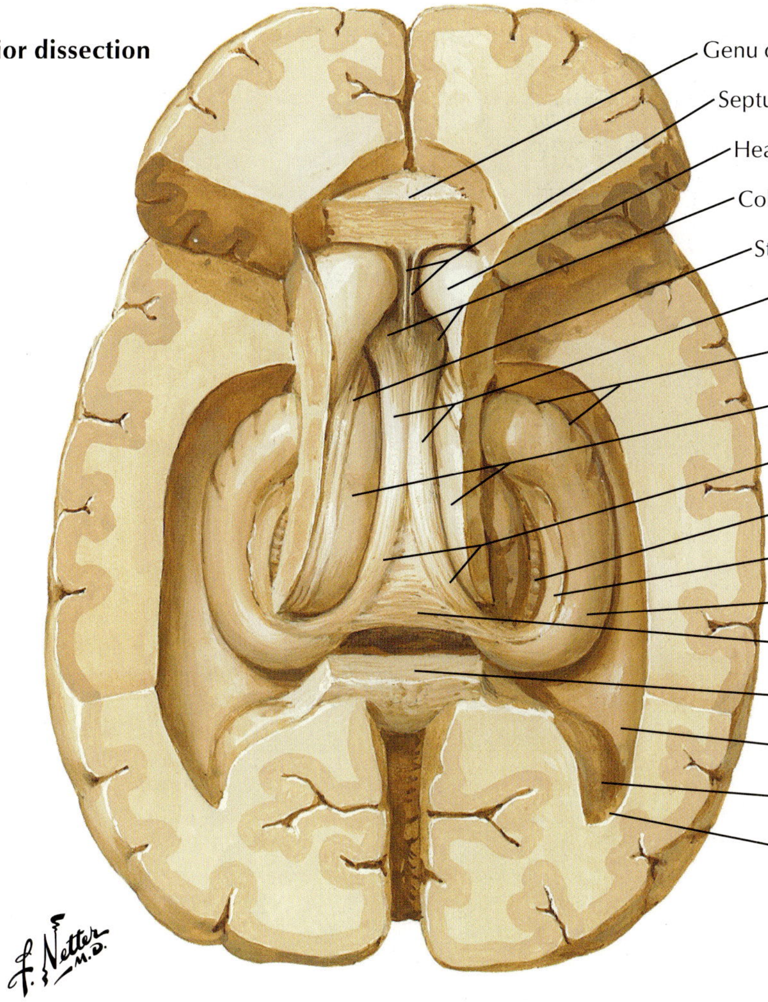

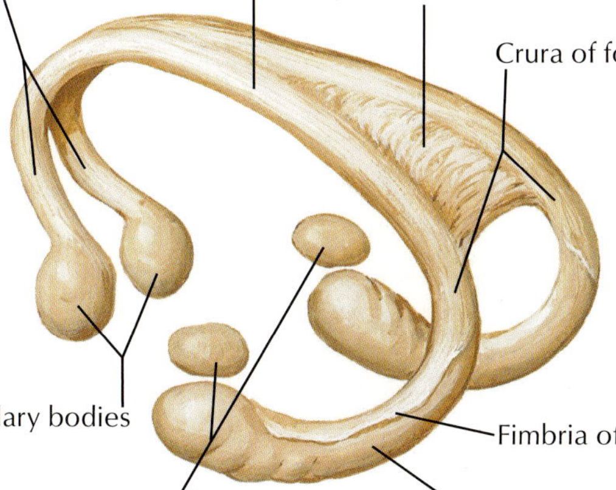

Fornix: schema

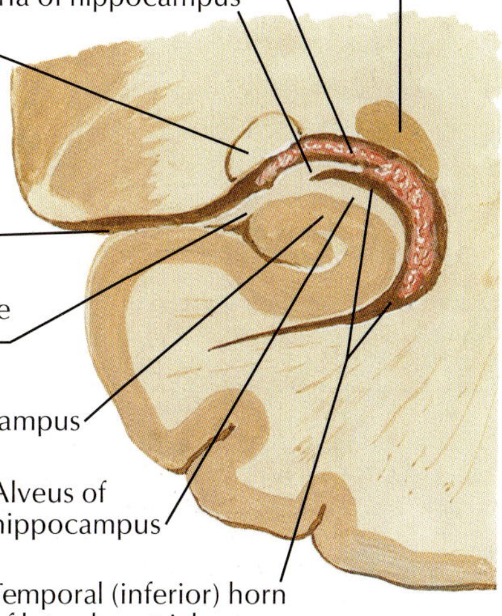

Coronal section: posterior view

Cerebellum

See also Plate 116

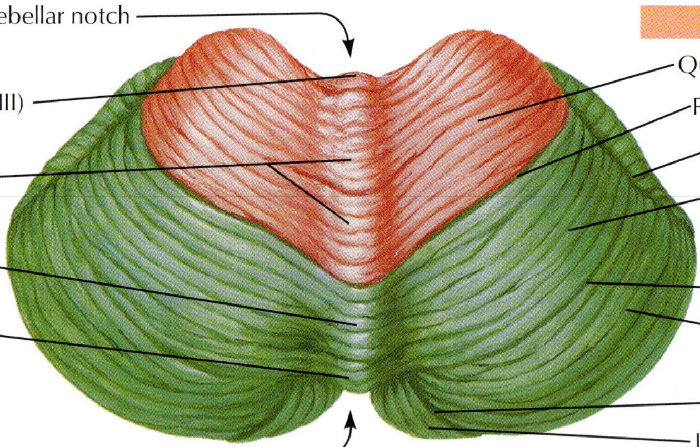

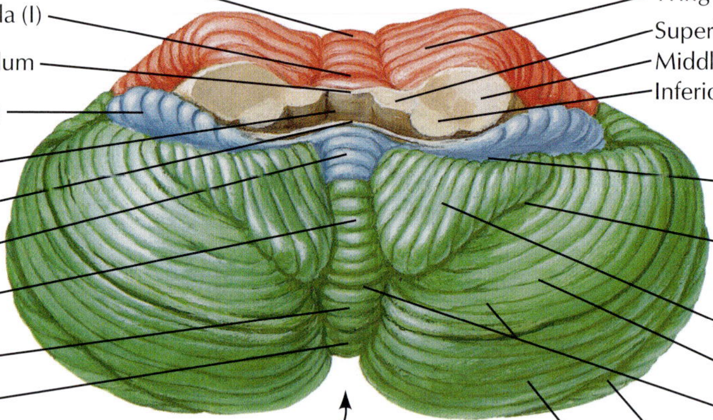

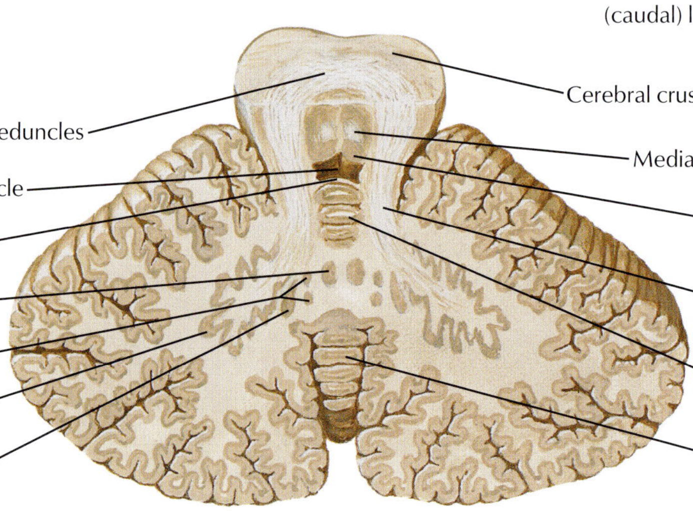

Section in plane of superior cerebellar peduncle

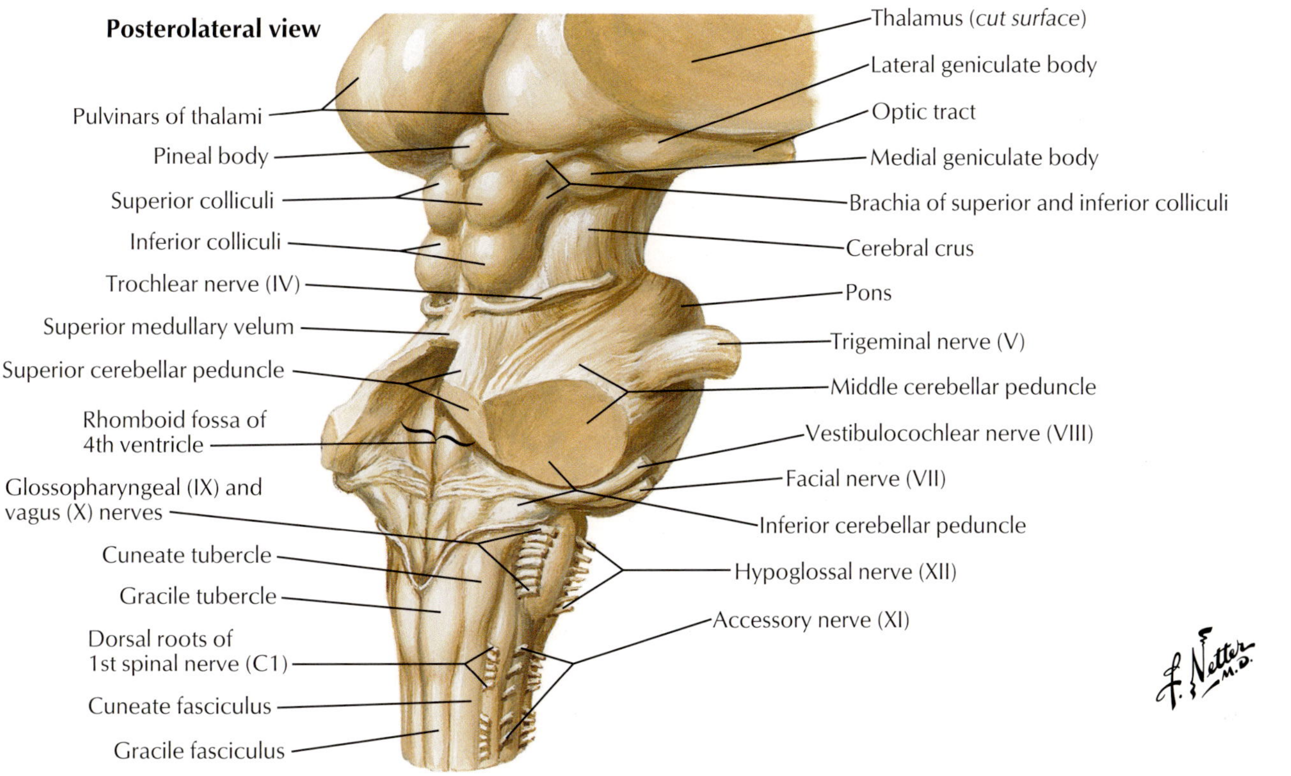
Posterolateral view
Thalamus (*cut surface*)
Lateral geniculate body
Optic tract
Medial geniculate body
Brachia of superior and inferior colliculi
Cerebral crus
Pons
Trigeminal nerve (V)
Middle cerebellar peduncle
Vestibulocochlear nerve (VIII)
Facial nerve (VII)
Inferior cerebellar peduncle
Hypoglossal nerve (XII)
Accessory nerve (XI)
Pulvinars of thalami
Pineal body
Superior colliculi
Inferior colliculi
Trochlear nerve (IV)
Superior medullary velum
Superior cerebellar peduncle
Rhomboid fossa of
4th ventricle
Glossopharyngeal (IX) and
vagus (X) nerves
Cuneate tubercle
Gracile tubercle
Dorsal roots of
1st spinal nerve (C1)
Cuneate fasciculus
Gracile fasciculus
F. Netter M.D.

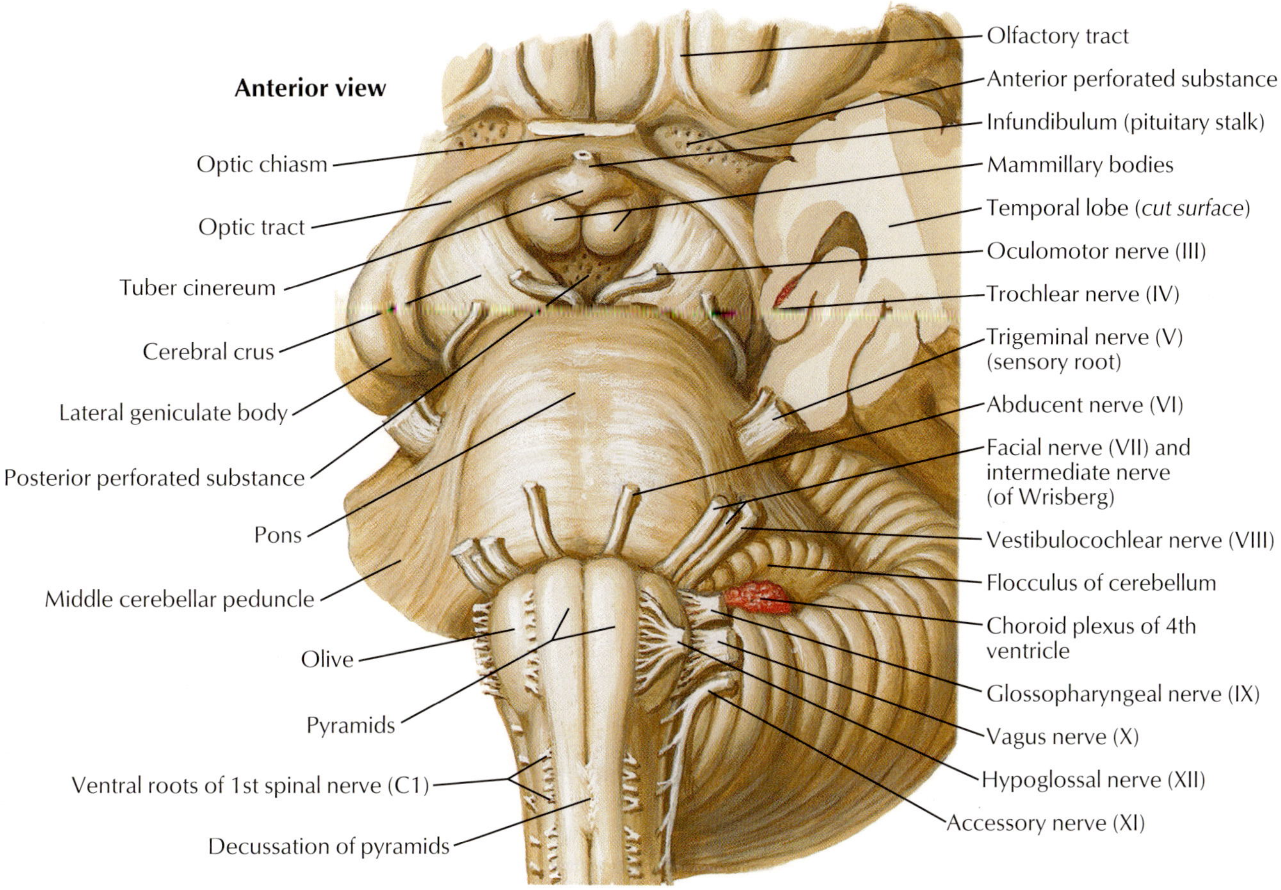
Anterior view
Olfactory tract
Anterior perforated substance
Infundibulum (pituitary stalk)
Mammillary bodies
Temporal lobe (*cut surface*)
Oculomotor nerve (III)
Trochlear nerve (IV)
Trigeminal nerve (V)
(sensory root)
Abducent nerve (VI)
Facial nerve (VII) and
intermediate nerve
(of Wrisberg)
Vestibulocochlear nerve (VIII)
Flocculus of cerebellum
Choroid plexus of 4th
ventricle
Glossopharyngeal nerve (IX)
Vagus nerve (X)
Hypoglossal nerve (XII)
Accessory nerve (XI)
Optic chiasm
Optic tract
Tuber cinereum
Cerebral crus
Lateral geniculate body
Posterior perforated substance
Pons
Middle cerebellar peduncle
Olive
Pyramids
Ventral roots of 1st spinal nerve (C1)
Decussation of pyramids

Fourth Ventricle and Cerebellum

See also Plate 114

Posterior view

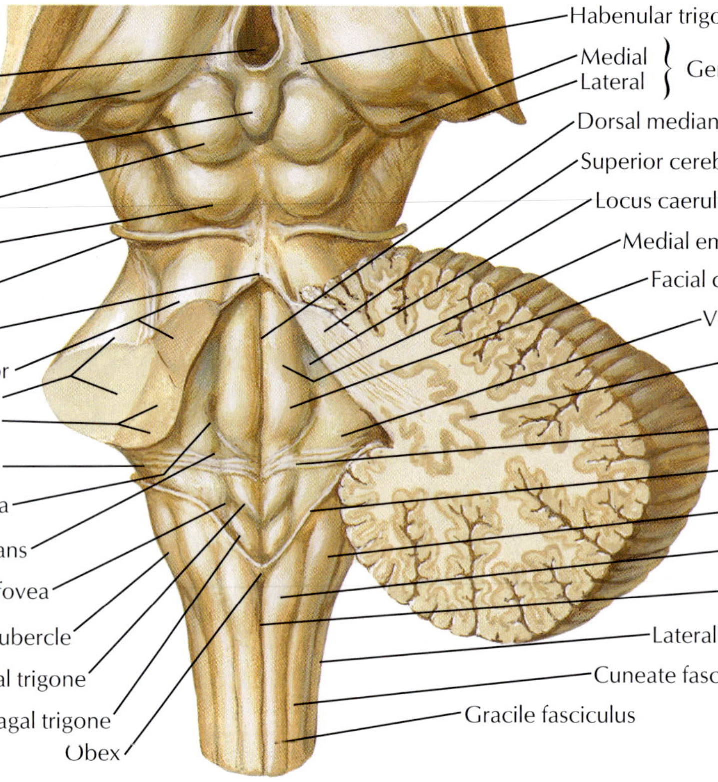

Median sagittal section

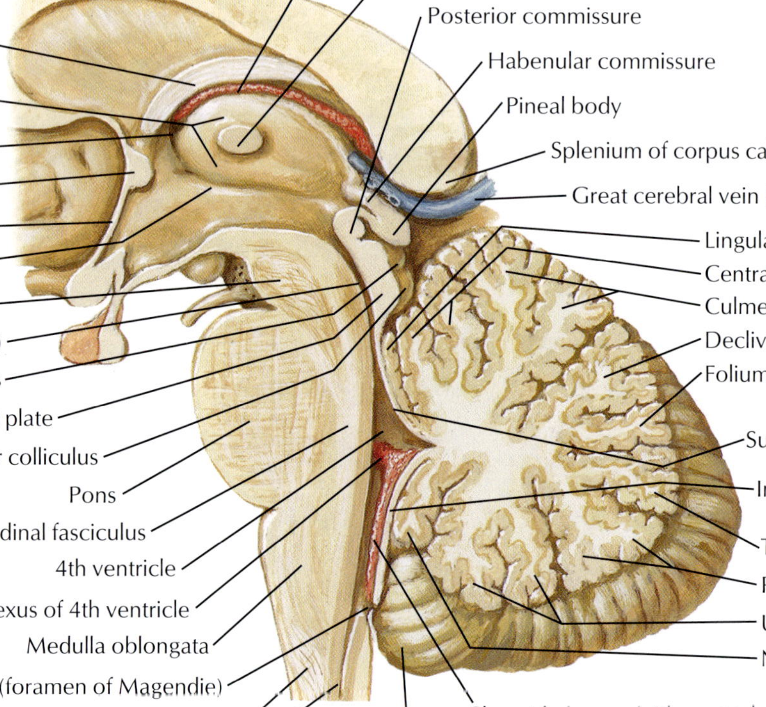

Cranial Nerve Nuclei in Brainstem: Schema

Posterior phantom view

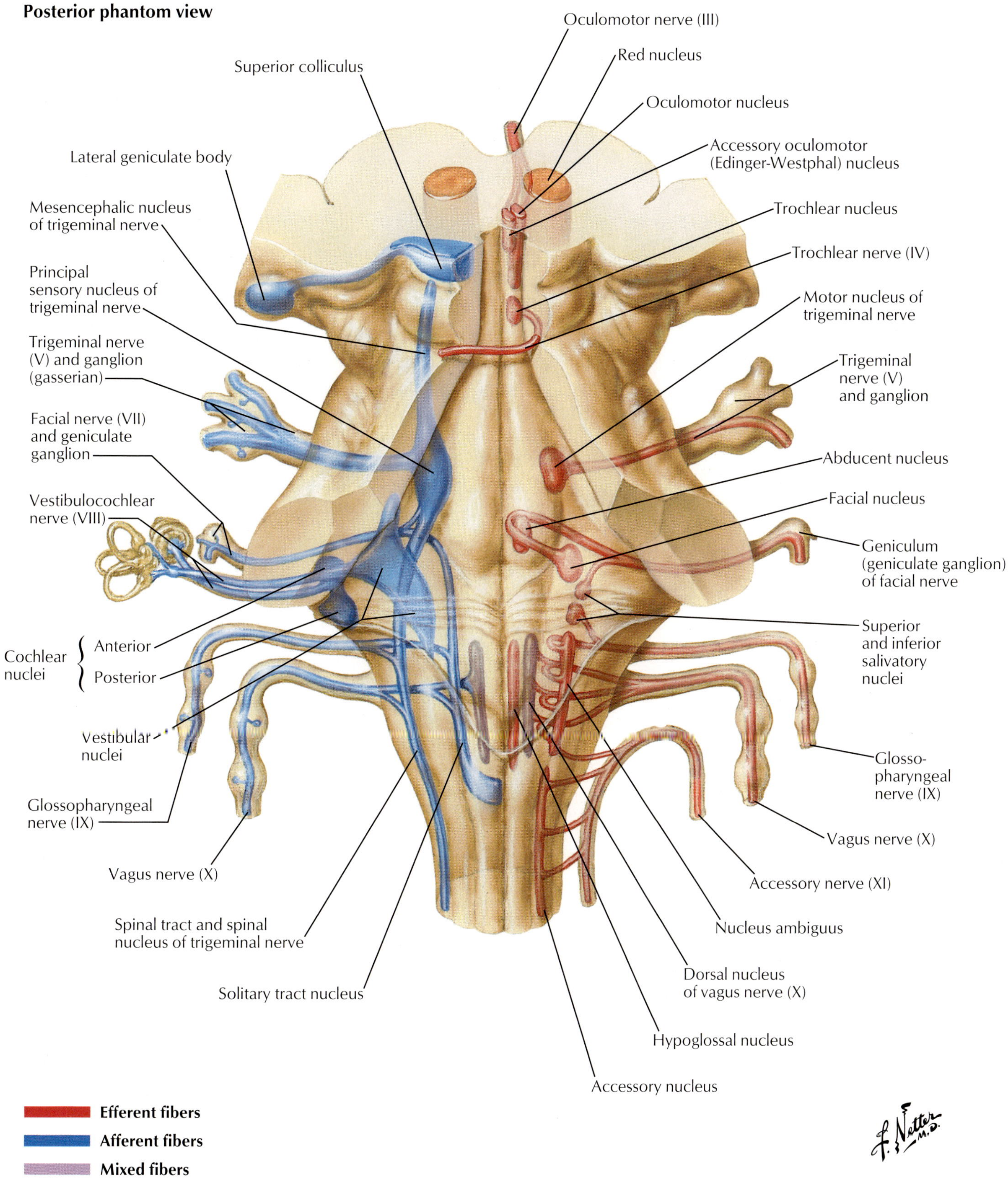

Medial dissection

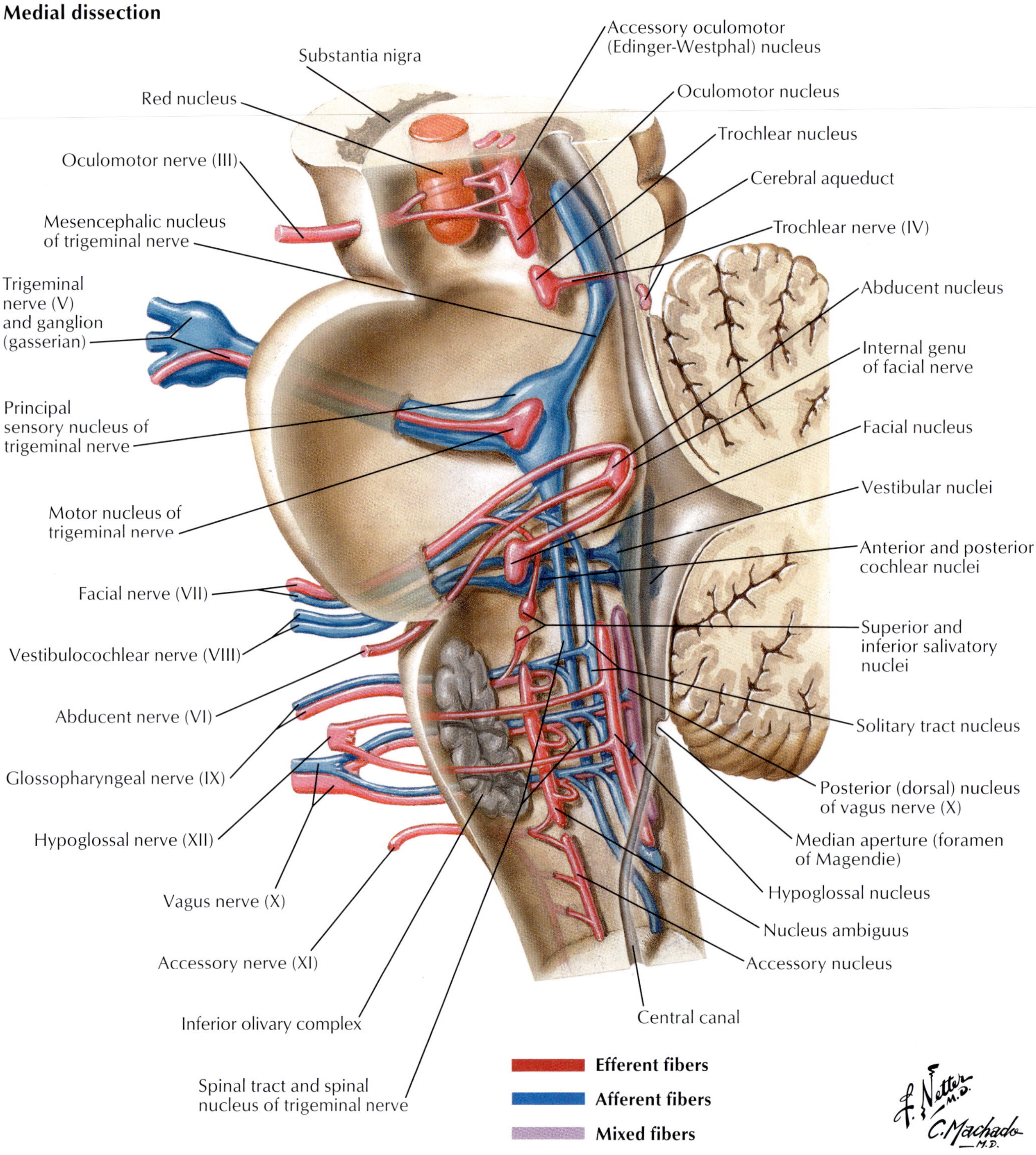

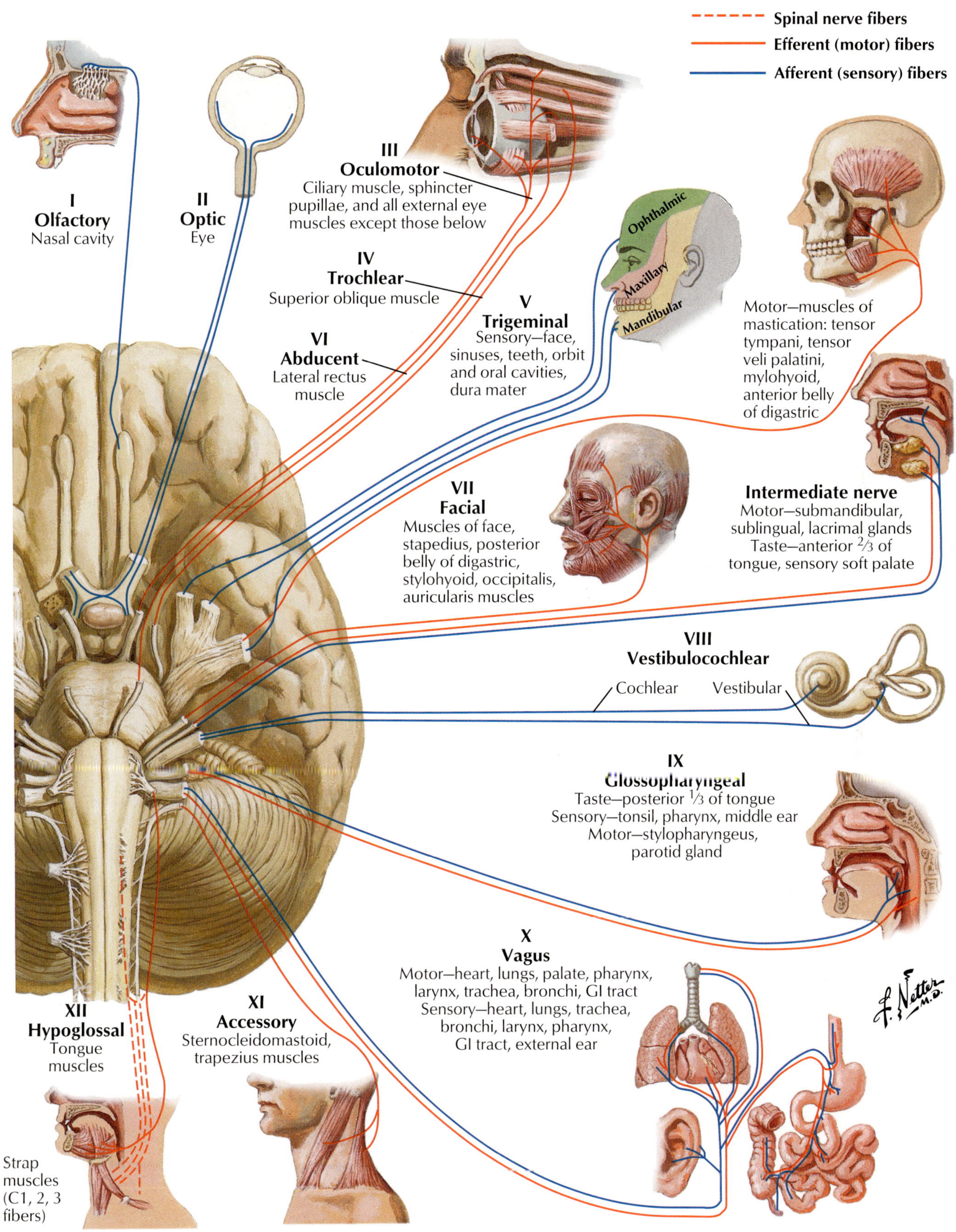
Spinal nerve fibers
Efferent (motor) fibers
Afferent (sensory) fibers
I
Olfactory
Nasal cavity
II
Optic
Eye
III
Oculomotor
Ciliary muscle, sphincter pupillae, and all external eye muscles except those below
IV
Trochlear
Superior oblique muscle
VI
Abducent
Lateral rectus muscle
V
Trigeminal
Sensory—face, sinuses, teeth, orbit and oral cavities, dura mater
Ophthalmic
Maxillary
Mandibular
Motor—muscles of mastication: tensor tympani, tensor veli palatini, mylohyoid, anterior belly of digastric
VII
Facial
Muscles of face, stapedius, posterior belly of digastric, stylohyoid, occipitalis, auricularis muscles
Intermediate nerve
Motor—submandibular, sublingual, lacrimal glands
Taste—anterior 2/3 of tongue, sensory soft palate
VIII
Vestibulocochlear
Cochlear
Vestibular
IX
Glossopharyngeal
Taste—posterior 1/3 of tongue
Sensory—tonsil, pharynx, middle ear
Motor—stylopharyngeus, parotid gland
X
Vagus
Motor—heart, lungs, palate, pharynx, larynx, trachea, bronchi, GI tract
Sensory—heart, lungs, trachea, bronchi, larynx, pharynx, GI tract, external ear
XI
Accessory
Sternocleidomastoid, trapezius muscles
XII
Hypoglossal
Tongue muscles
Strap muscles (C1, 2, 3 fibers)
F. Netter M.D.

Olfactory Nerve (I): Schema

See also Plate 39

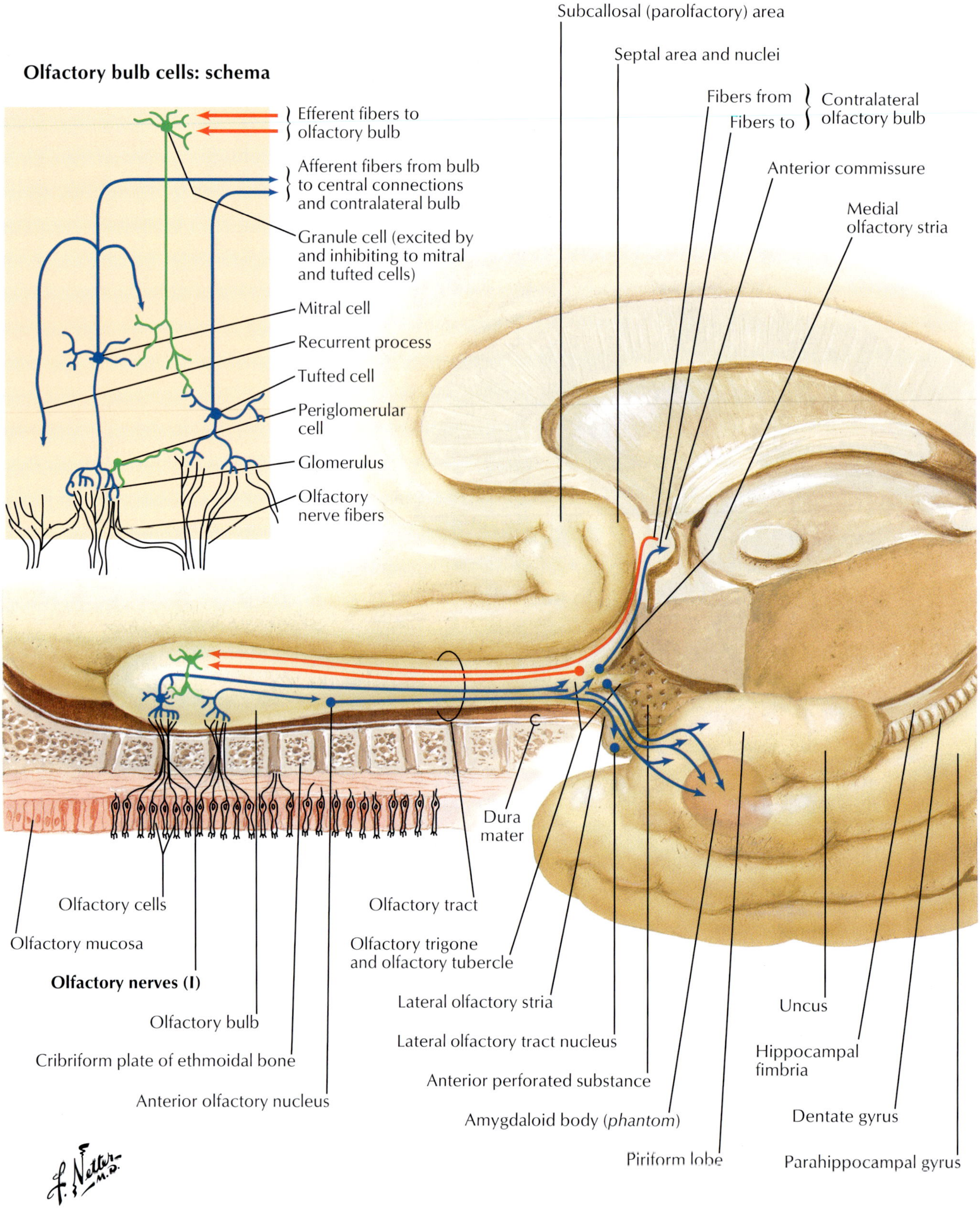

Optic Nerve (II) (Visual Pathway): Schema

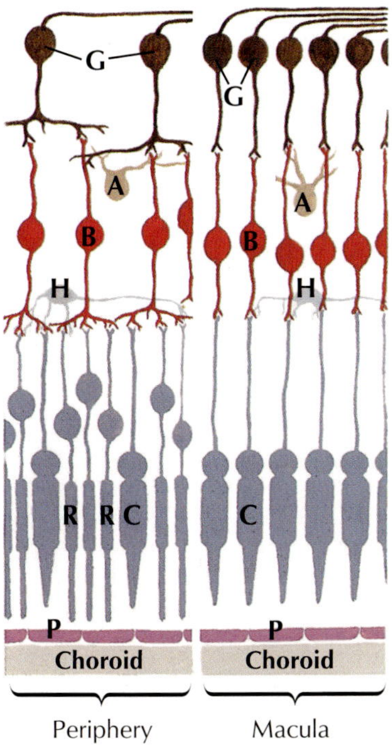

Structure of retina: schema

A Amacrine cells
B Bipolar cells
C Cones
G Ganglion cells
H Horizontal cells
P Pigment cells
R Rods

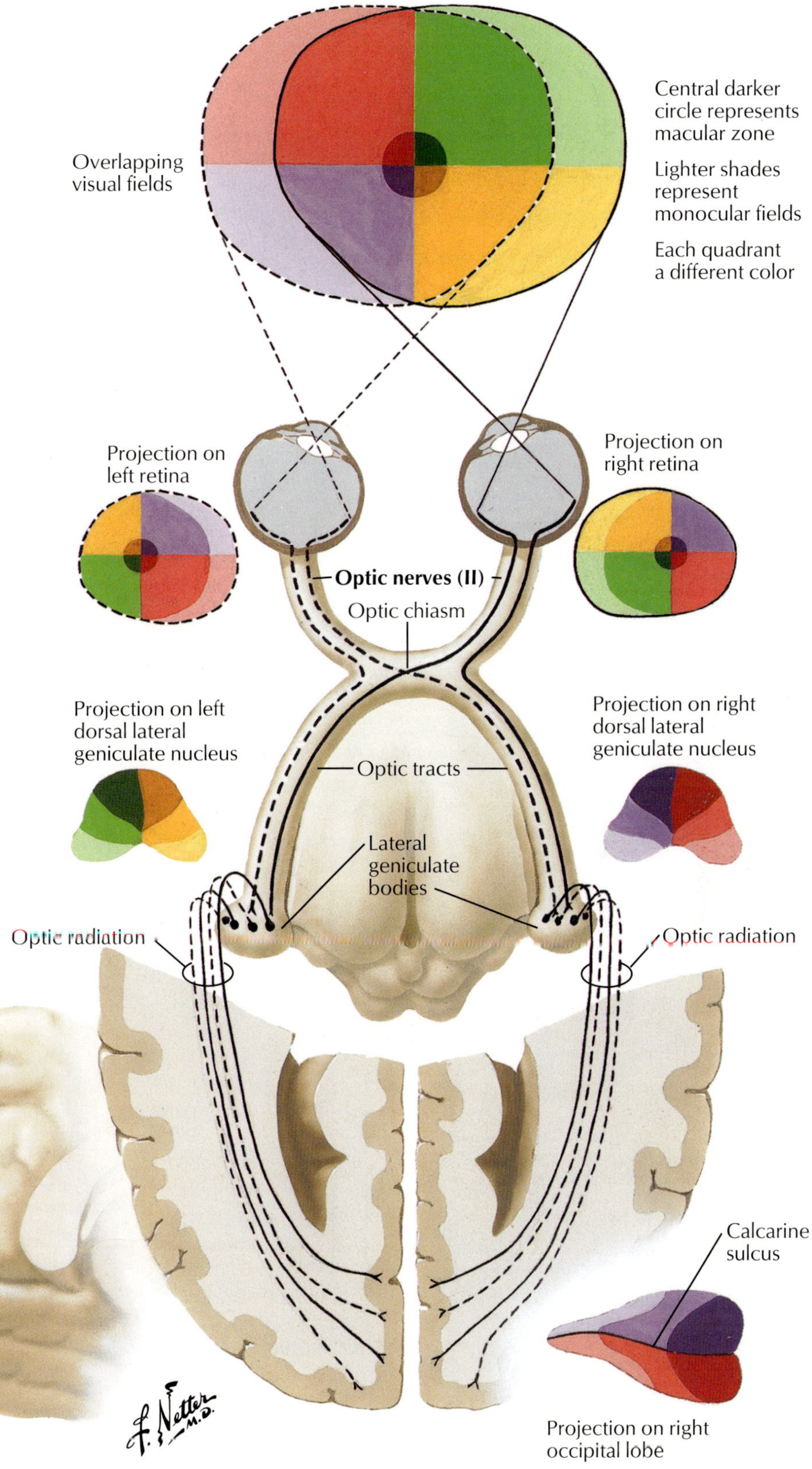

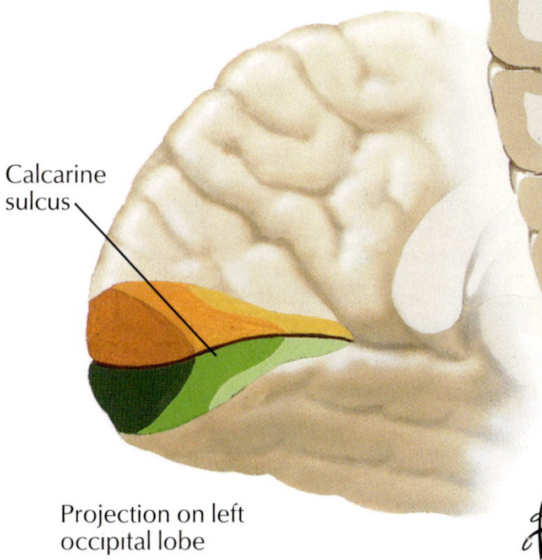

Oculomotor (III), Trochlear (IV), and Abducent (VI) Nerves: Schema

See also Plates 88, 133

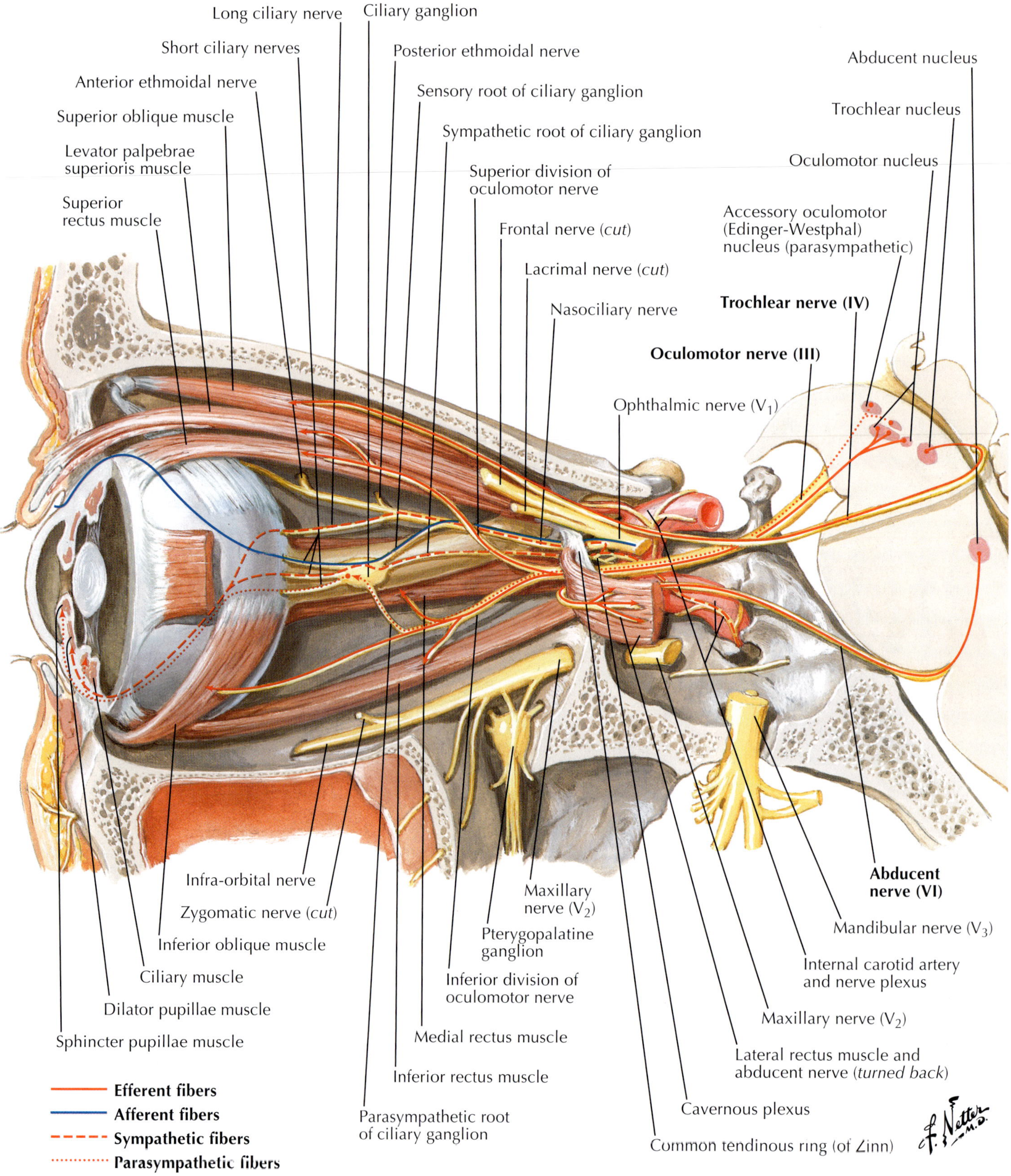

Trigeminal Nerve (V): Schema

See also Plates 2, 50, 52

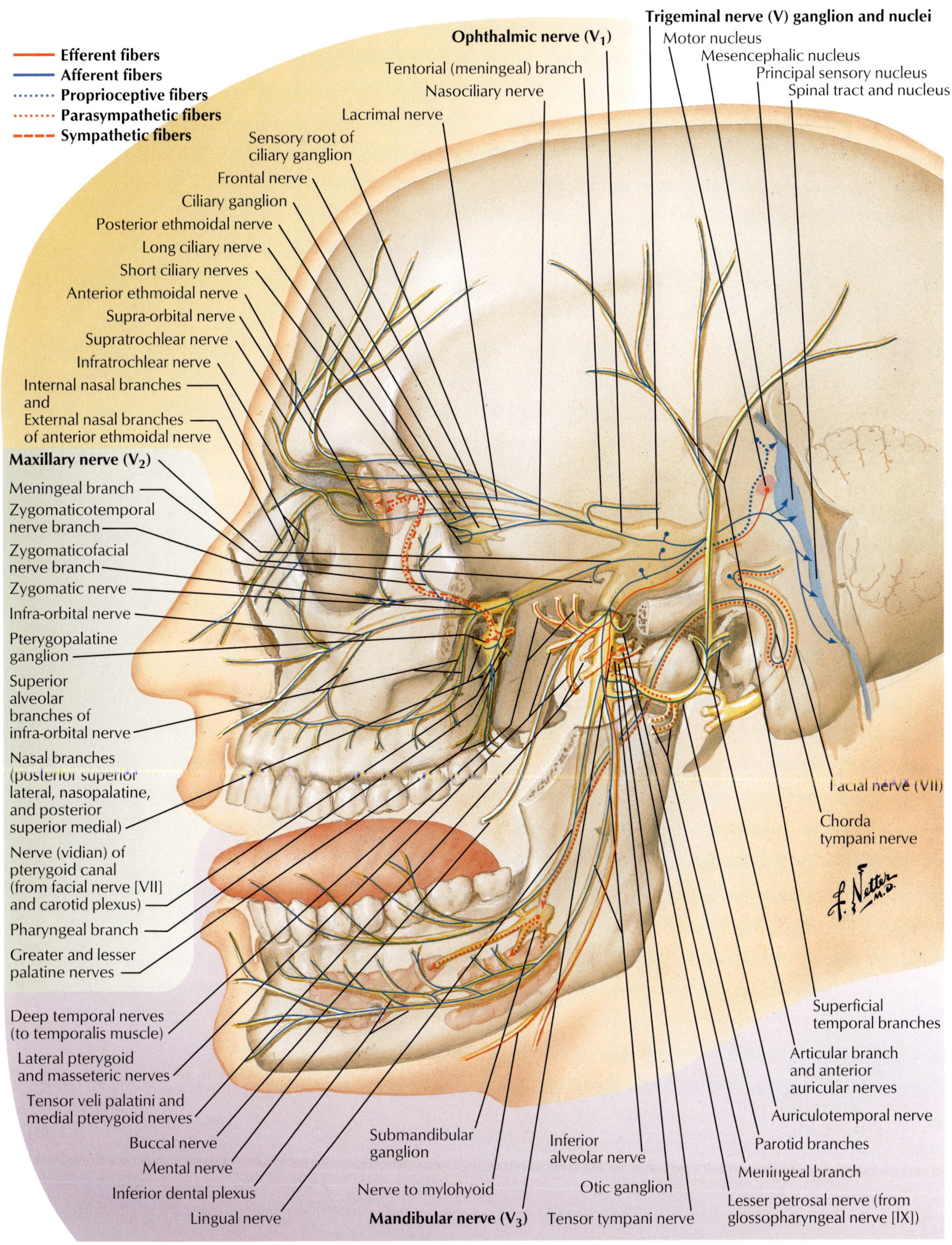

Facial Nerve (VII): Schema

See also Plate 24

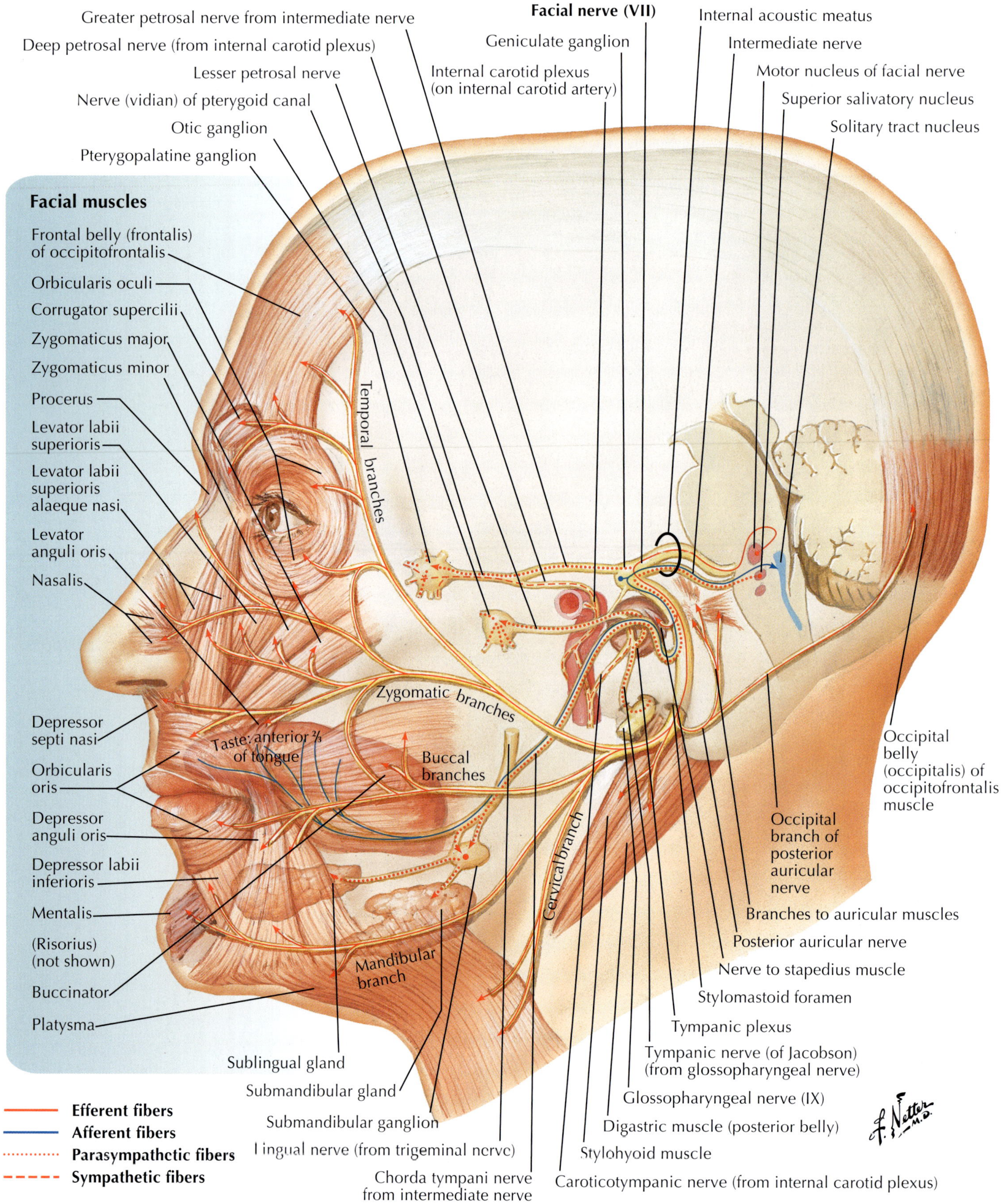

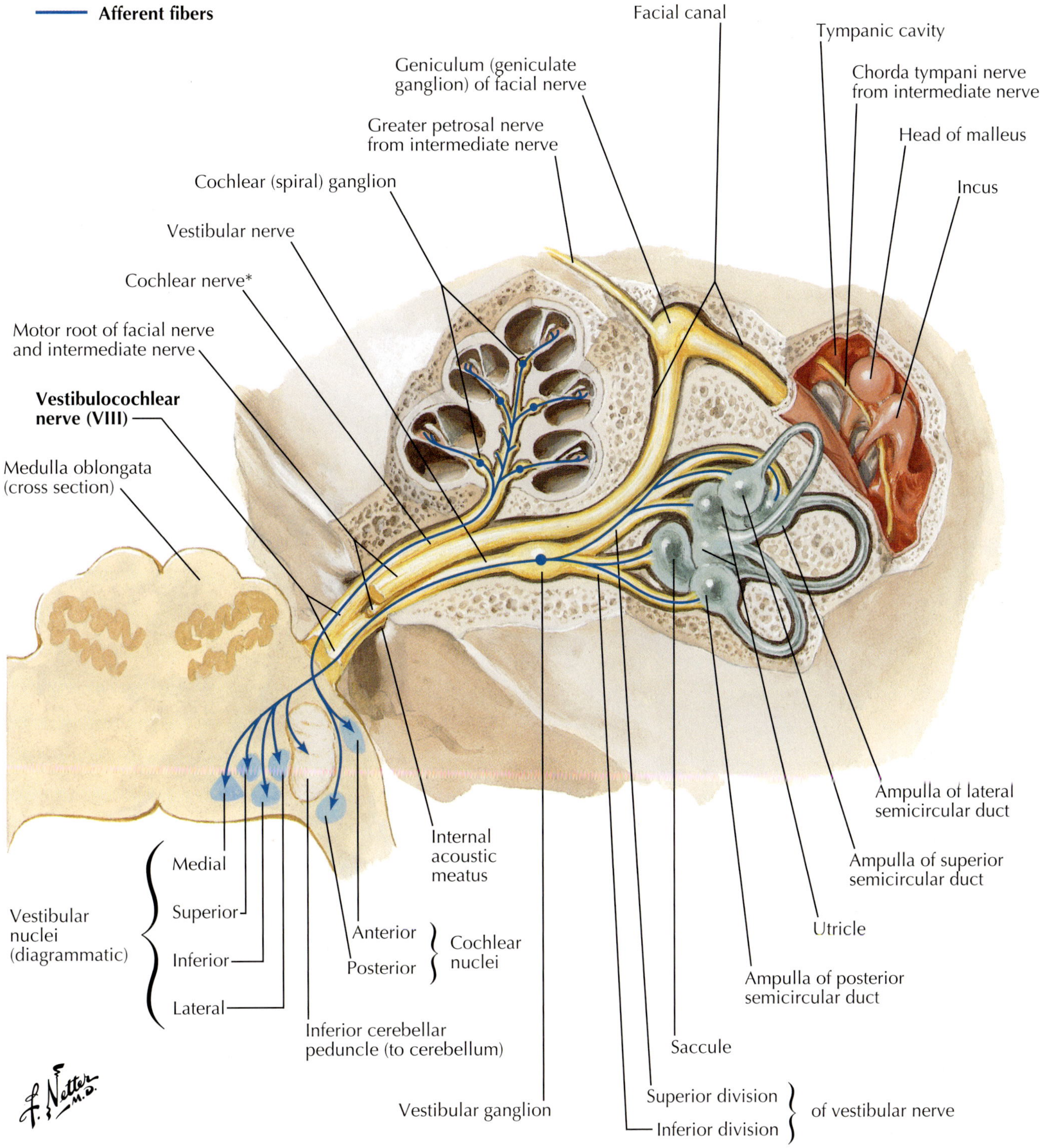

*Note: The cochlear nerve also contains efferent fibers to the sensory epithelium. These fibers are derived from the vestibular nerve while in the internal auditory meatus.

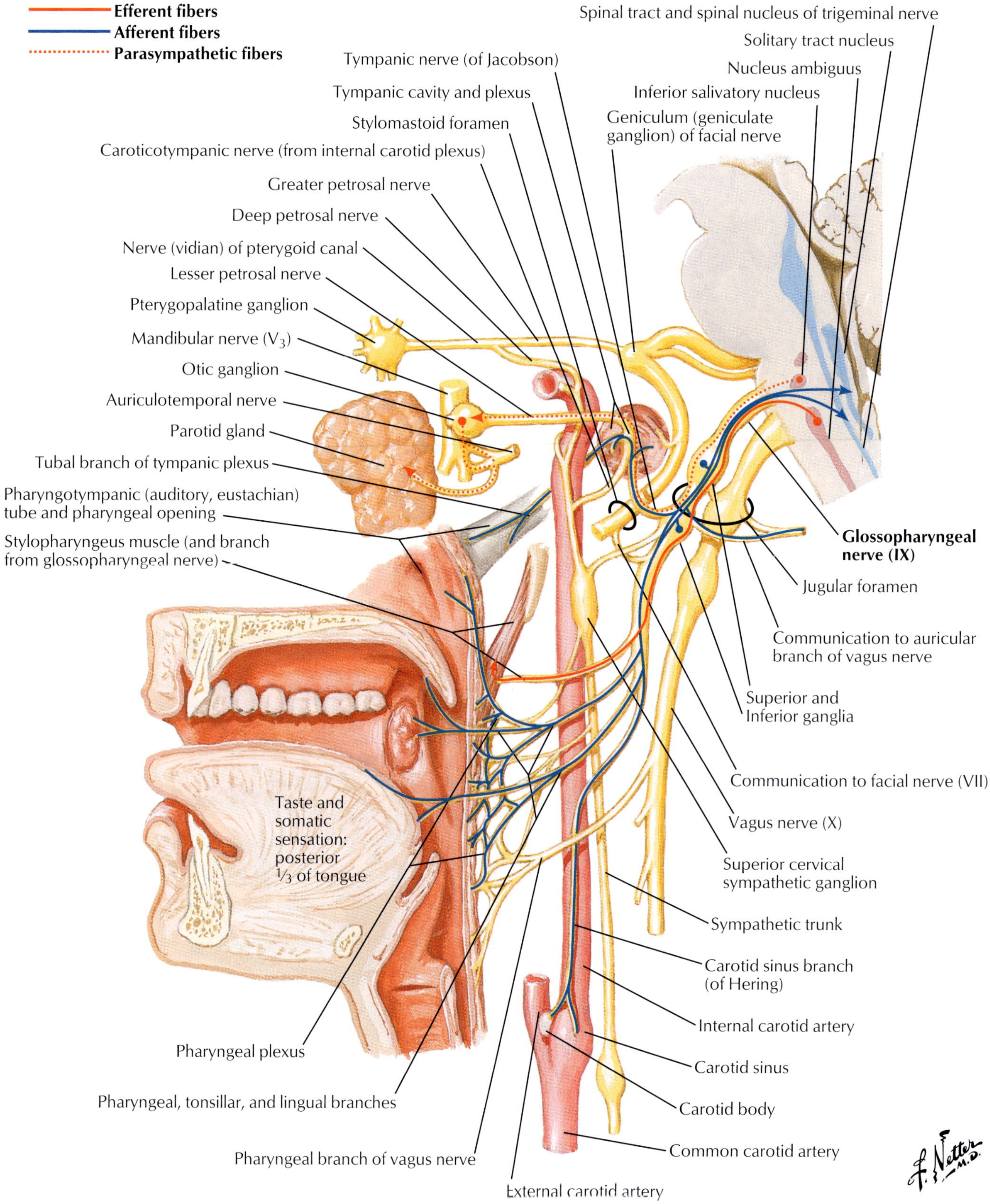
Efferent fibers
Afferent fibers
Parasympathetic fibers
Spinal tract and spinal nucleus of trigeminal nerve
Solitary tract nucleus
Nucleus ambiguus
Inferior salivatory nucleus
Geniculum (geniculate ganglion) of facial nerve
Tympanic nerve (of Jacobson)
Tympanic cavity and plexus
Stylomastoid foramen
Caroticotympanic nerve (from internal carotid plexus)
Greater petrosal nerve
Deep petrosal nerve
Nerve (vidian) of pterygoid canal
Lesser petrosal nerve
Pterygopalatine ganglion
Mandibular nerve (V_3)
Otic ganglion
Auriculotemporal nerve
Parotid gland
Tubal branch of tympanic plexus
Pharyngotympanic (auditory, eustachian) tube and pharyngeal opening
Stylopharyngeus muscle (and branch from glossopharyngeal nerve)
Glossopharyngeal nerve (IX)
Jugular foramen
Communication to auricular branch of vagus nerve
Superior and Inferior ganglia
Communication to facial nerve (VII)
Vagus nerve (X)
Superior cervical sympathetic ganglion
Taste and somatic sensation: posterior ⅓ of tongue
Sympathetic trunk
Carotid sinus branch (of Hering)
Internal carotid artery
Carotid sinus
Carotid body
Common carotid artery
Pharyngeal plexus
Pharyngeal, tonsillar, and lingual branches
Pharyngeal branch of vagus nerve
External carotid artery

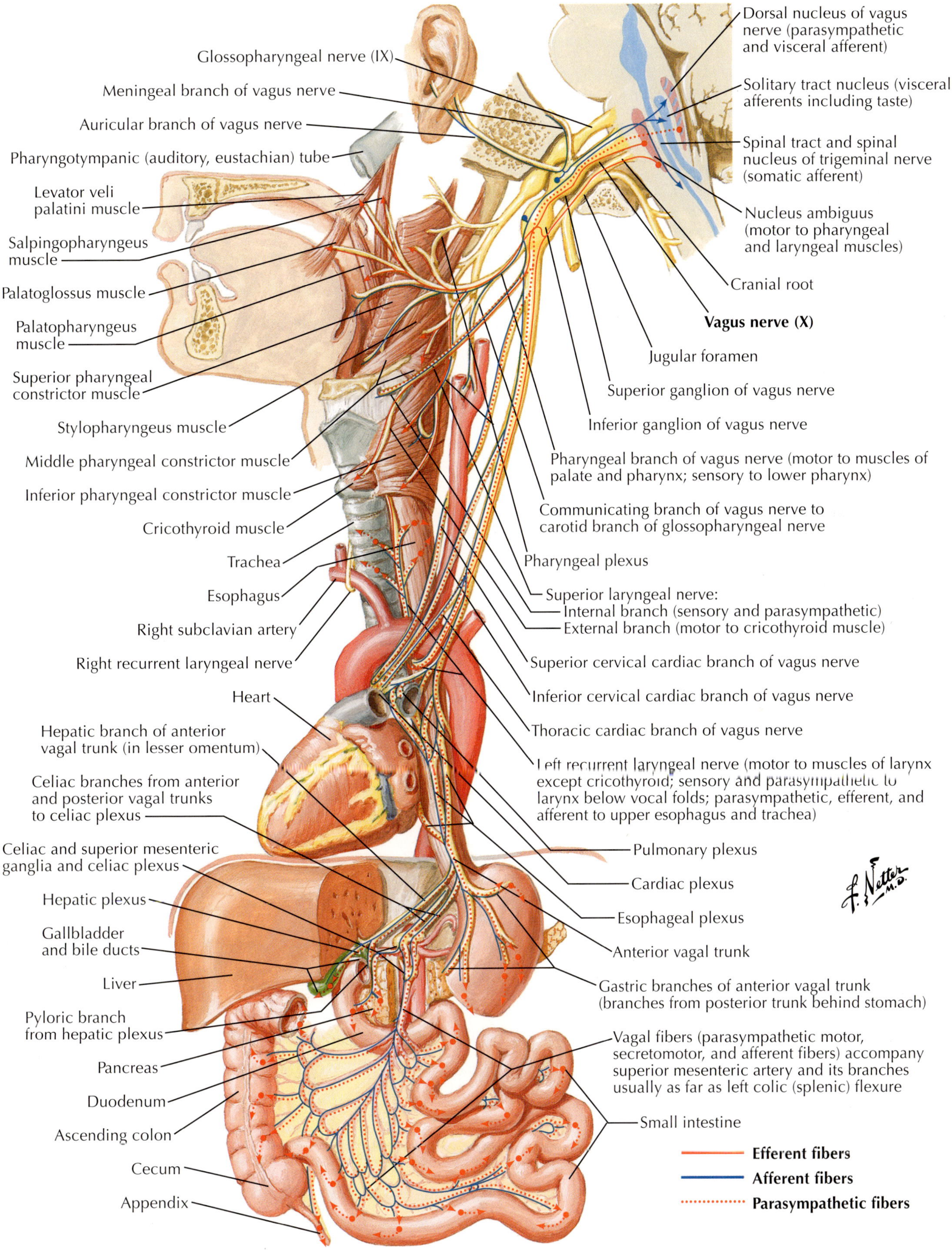
Glossopharyngeal nerve (IX)
Meningeal branch of vagus nerve
Auricular branch of vagus nerve
Pharyngotympanic (auditory, eustachian) tube
Levator veli palatini muscle
Salpingopharyngeus muscle
Palatoglossus muscle
Palatopharyngeus muscle
Superior pharyngeal constrictor muscle
Stylopharyngeus muscle
Middle pharyngeal constrictor muscle
Inferior pharyngeal constrictor muscle
Cricothyroid muscle
Trachea
Esophagus
Right subclavian artery
Right recurrent laryngeal nerve
Heart
Hepatic branch of anterior vagal trunk (in lesser omentum)
Celiac branches from anterior and posterior vagal trunks to celiac plexus
Celiac and superior mesenteric ganglia and celiac plexus
Hepatic plexus
Gallbladder and bile ducts
Liver
Pyloric branch from hepatic plexus
Pancreas
Duodenum
Ascending colon
Cecum
Appendix
Dorsal nucleus of vagus nerve (parasympathetic and visceral afferent)
Solitary tract nucleus (visceral afferents including taste)
Spinal tract and spinal nucleus of trigeminal nerve (somatic afferent)
Nucleus ambiguus (motor to pharyngeal and laryngeal muscles)
Cranial root
Vagus nerve (X)
Jugular foramen
Superior ganglion of vagus nerve
Inferior ganglion of vagus nerve
Pharyngeal branch of vagus nerve (motor to muscles of palate and pharynx; sensory to lower pharynx)
Communicating branch of vagus nerve to carotid branch of glossopharyngeal nerve
Pharyngeal plexus
Superior laryngeal nerve:
Internal branch (sensory and parasympathetic)
External branch (motor to cricothyroid muscle)
Superior cervical cardiac branch of vagus nerve
Inferior cervical cardiac branch of vagus nerve
Thoracic cardiac branch of vagus nerve
Left recurrent laryngeal nerve (motor to muscles of larynx except cricothyroid; sensory and parasympathetic to larynx below vocal folds; parasympathetic, efferent, and afferent to upper esophagus and trachea)
Pulmonary plexus
Cardiac plexus
Esophageal plexus
Anterior vagal trunk
Gastric branches of anterior vagal trunk (branches from posterior trunk behind stomach)
Vagal fibers (parasympathetic motor, secretomotor, and afferent fibers) accompany superior mesenteric artery and its branches usually as far as left colic (splenic) flexure
Small intestine
Efferent fibers
Afferent fibers
Parasympathetic fibers
F. Netter M.D.

Accessory Nerve (XI): Schema

See also Plate 32

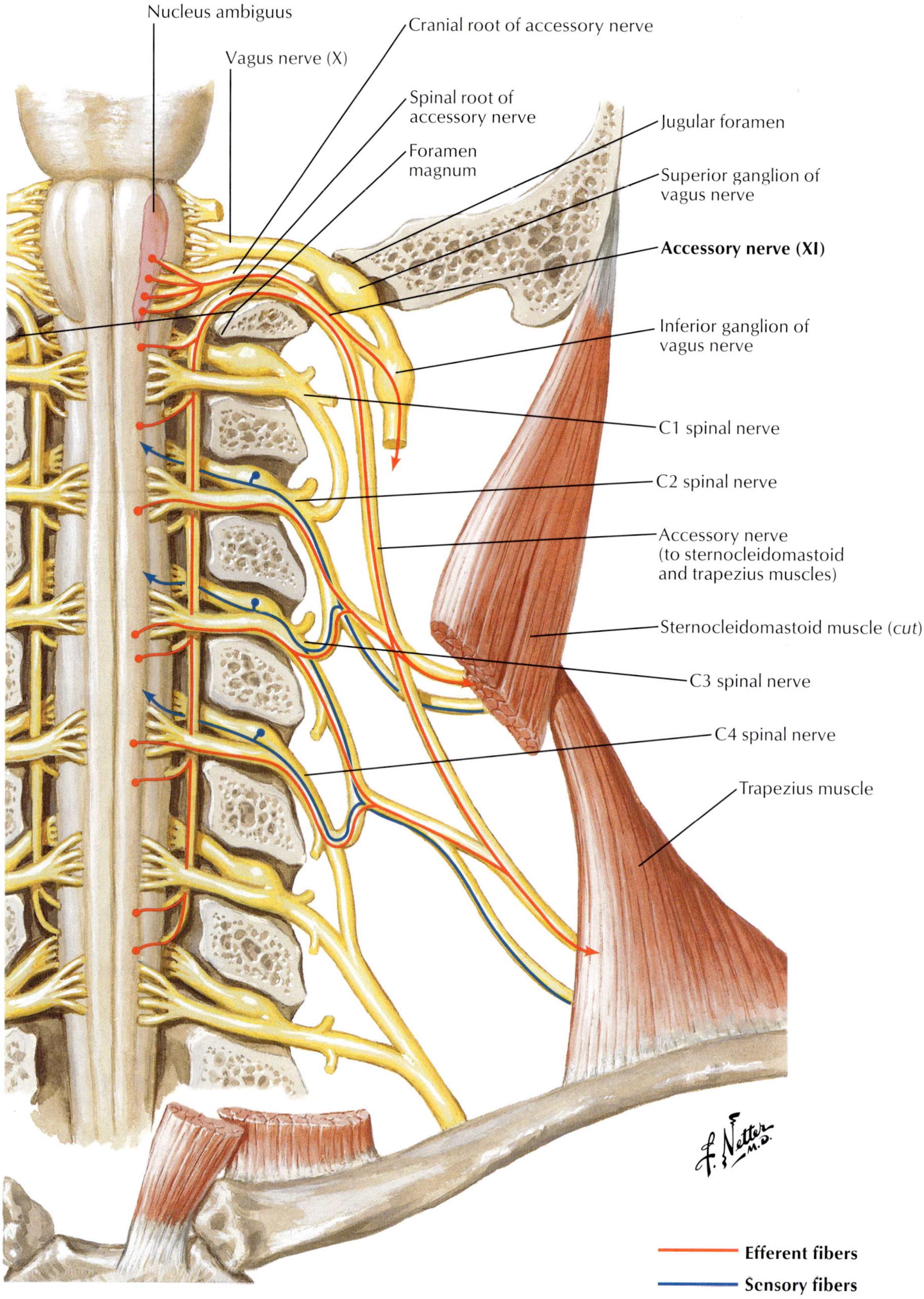

Hypoglossal Nerve (XII): Schema

See also Plate 32

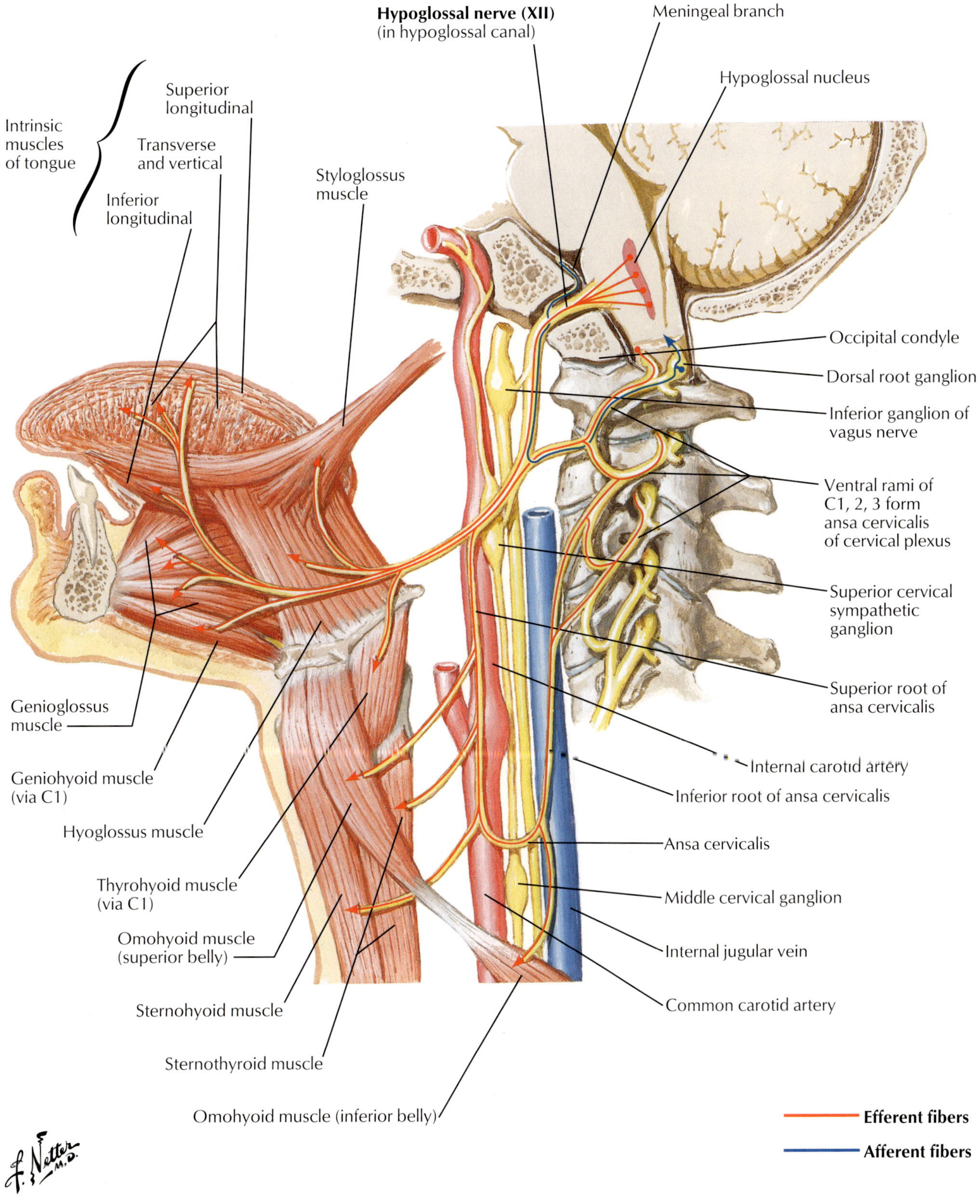

See also Plates 32, 33

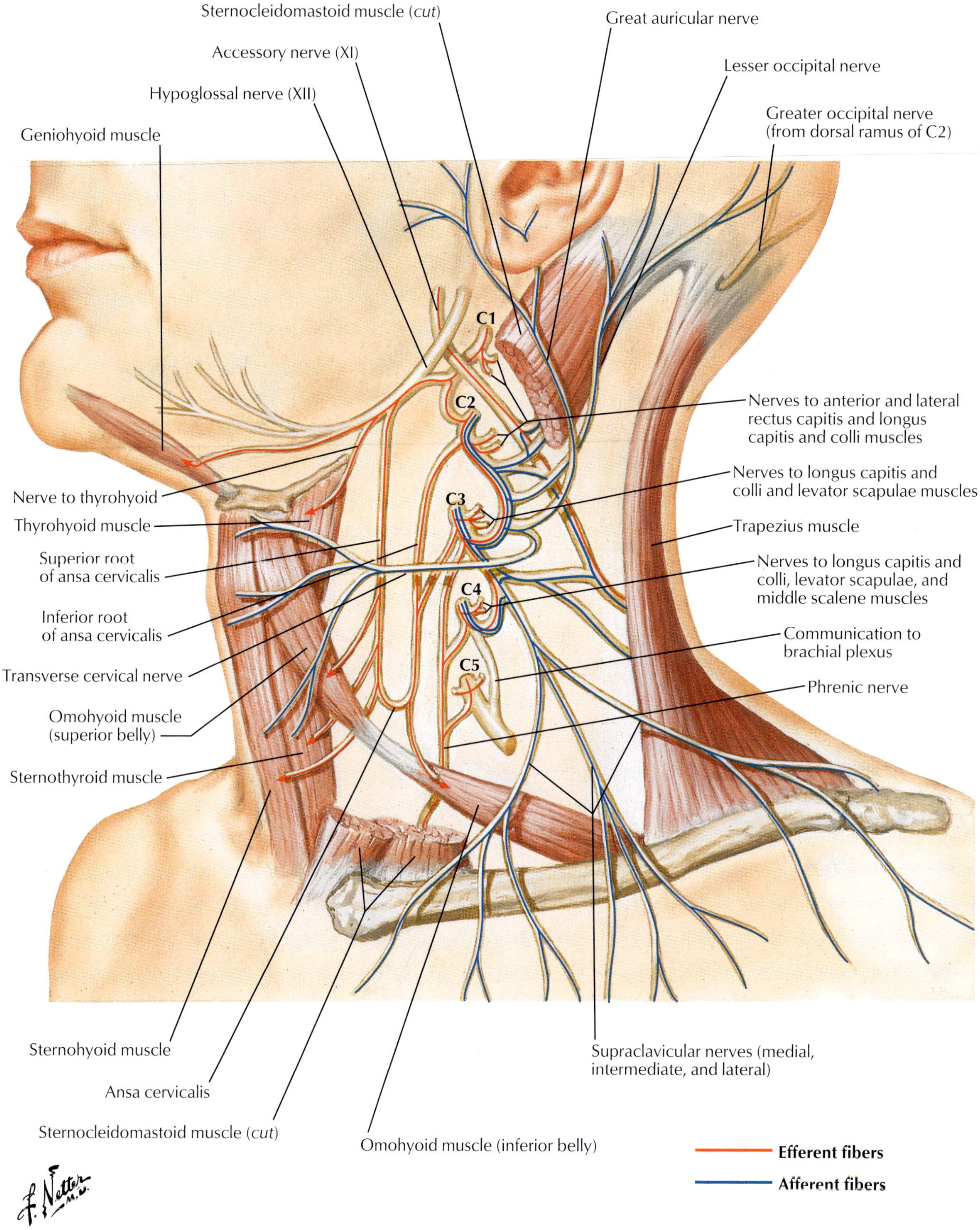

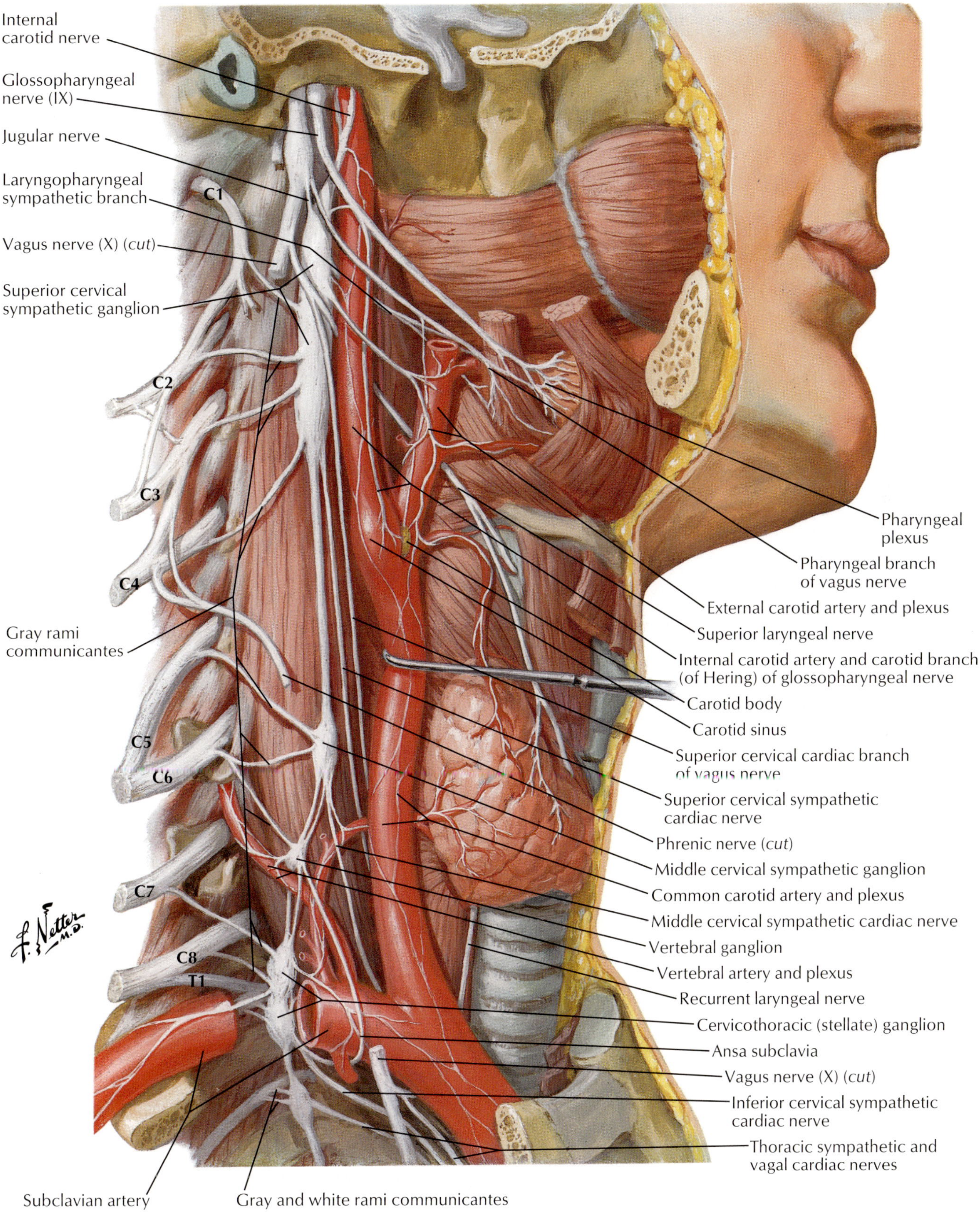
Internal carotid nerve
Glossopharyngeal nerve (IX)
Jugular nerve
Laryngopharyngeal sympathetic branch
C1
Vagus nerve (X) (cut)
Superior cervical sympathetic ganglion
C2
C3
C4
Gray rami communicantes
C5
C6
C7
C8
T1
Subclavian artery
Gray and white rami communicantes
Pharyngeal plexus
Pharyngeal branch of vagus nerve
External carotid artery and plexus
Superior laryngeal nerve
Internal carotid artery and carotid branch (of Hering) of glossopharyngeal nerve
Carotid body
Carotid sinus
Superior cervical cardiac branch of vagus nerve
Superior cervical sympathetic cardiac nerve
Phrenic nerve (cut)
Middle cervical sympathetic ganglion
Common carotid artery and plexus
Middle cervical sympathetic cardiac nerve
Vertebral ganglion
Vertebral artery and plexus
Recurrent laryngeal nerve
Cervicothoracic (stellate) ganglion
Ansa subclavia
Vagus nerve (X) (cut)
Inferior cervical sympathetic cardiac nerve
Thoracic sympathetic and vagal cardiac nerves
F. Netter M.D.

Autonomic Nerves in Head

See also **Plates 53, 123, 134**

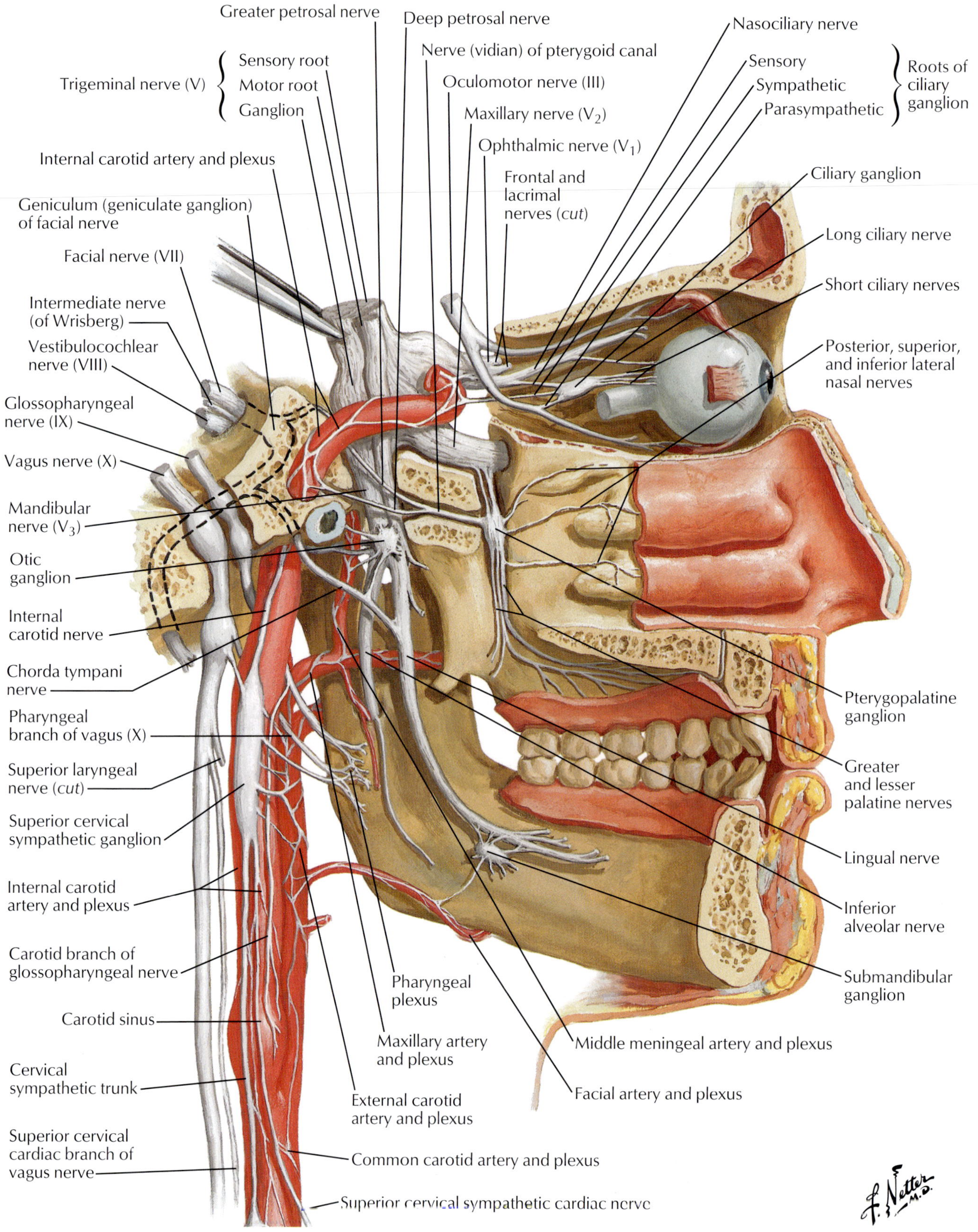

Ciliary Ganglion: Schema

See also Plate 53

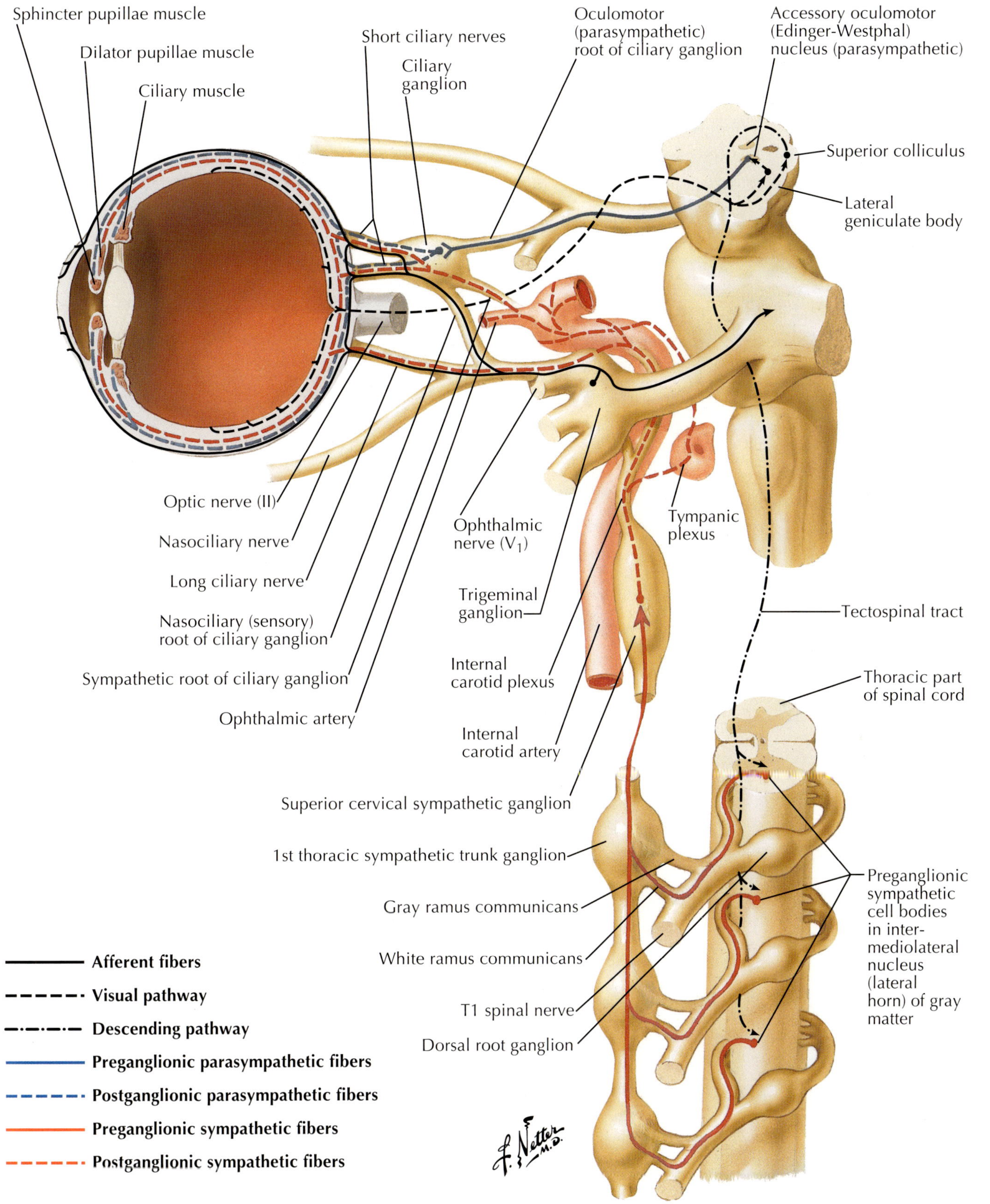

Pterygopalatine and Submandibular Ganglia: Schema

See also Plate 84

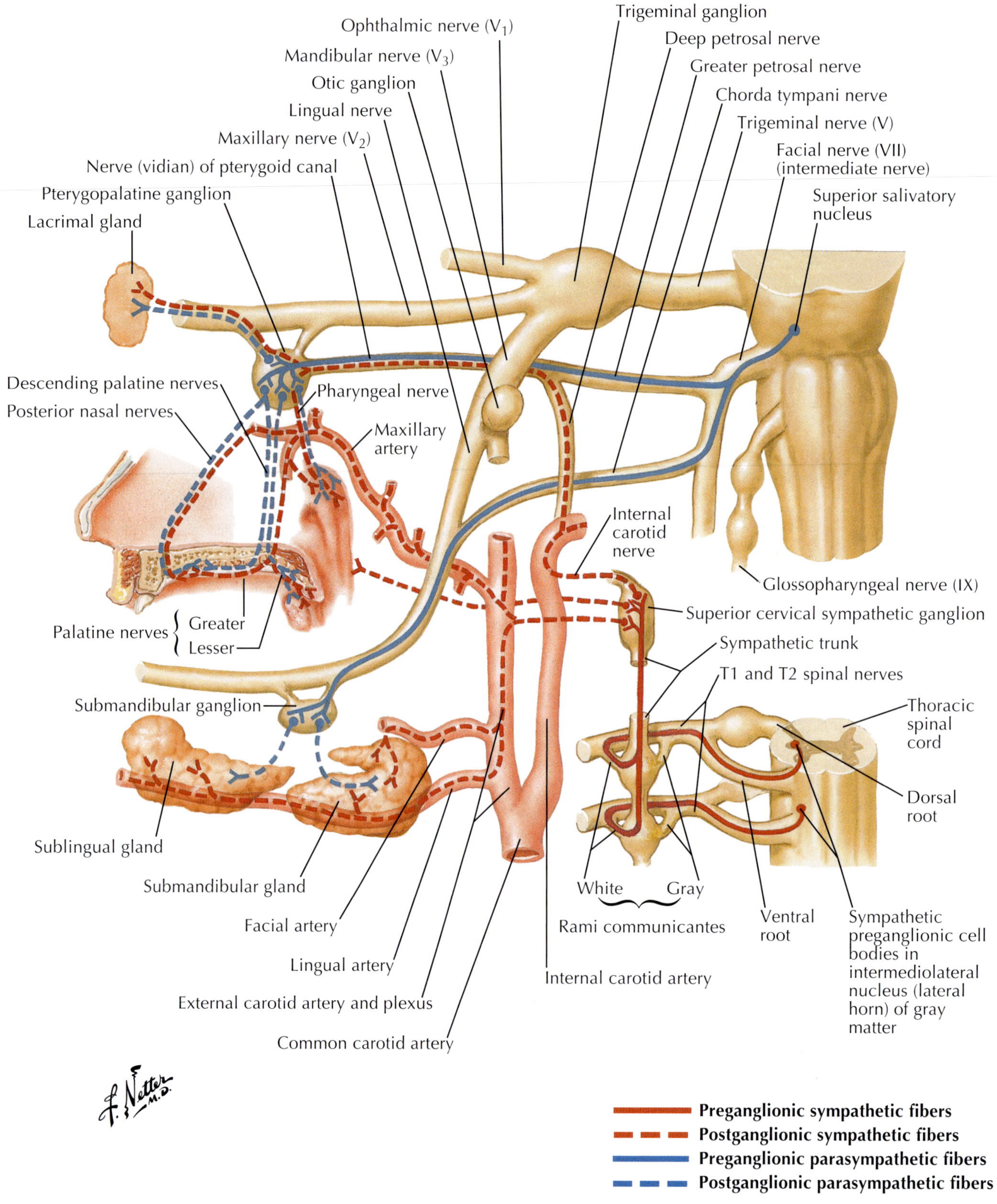

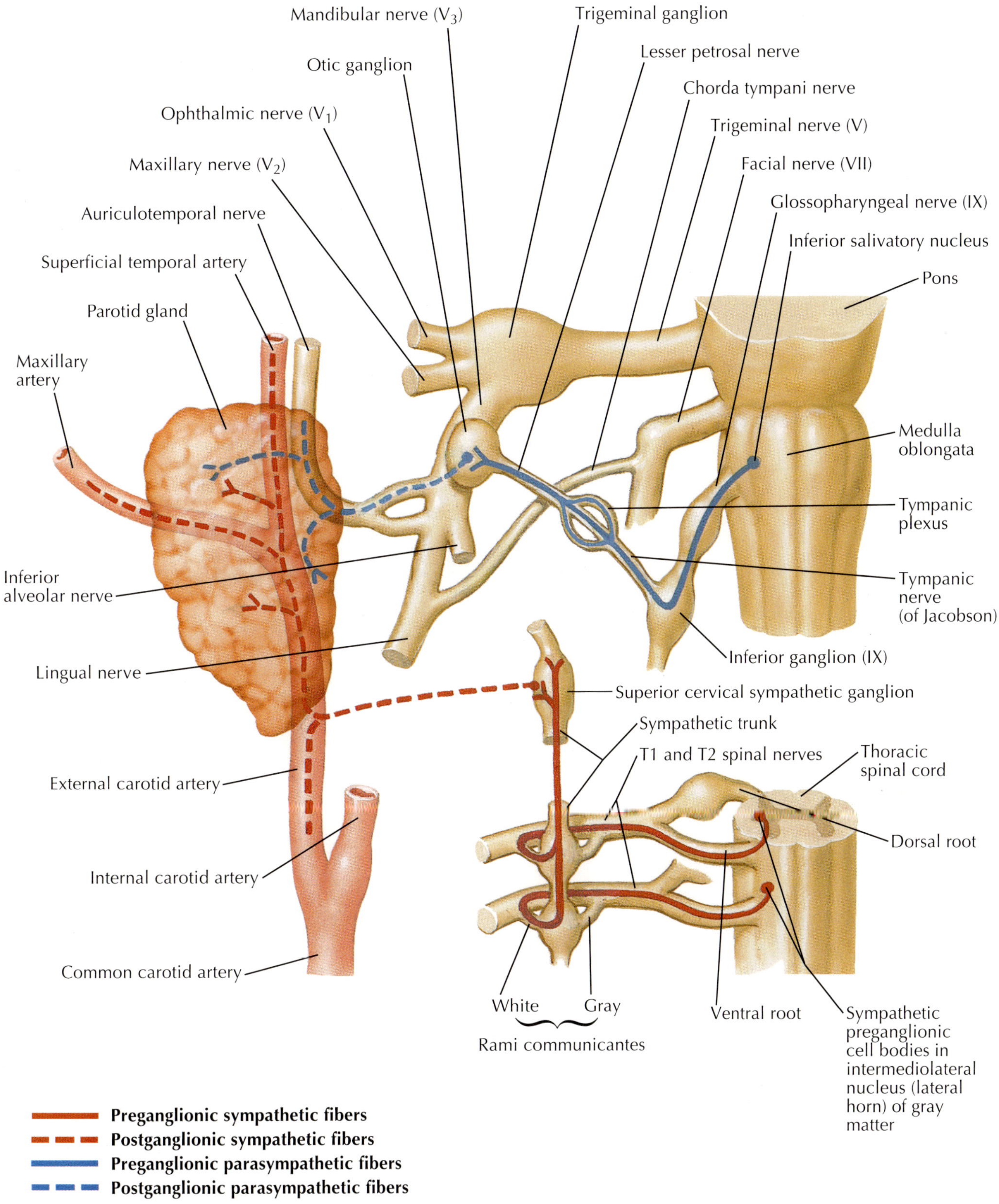
Mandibular nerve (V_3)
Trigeminal ganglion
Lesser petrosal nerve
Otic ganglion
Chorda tympani nerve
Ophthalmic nerve (V_1)
Trigeminal nerve (V)
Maxillary nerve (V_2)
Facial nerve (VII)
Auriculotemporal nerve
Glossopharyngeal nerve (IX)
Inferior salivatory nucleus
Superficial temporal artery
Pons
Parotid gland
Maxillary artery
Medulla oblongata
Tympanic plexus
Inferior alveolar nerve
Tympanic nerve (of Jacobson)
Inferior ganglion (IX)
Lingual nerve
Superior cervical sympathetic ganglion
Sympathetic trunk
T1 and T2 spinal nerves
Thoracic spinal cord
External carotid artery
Dorsal root
Internal carotid artery
Common carotid artery
White
Gray
Rami communicantes
Ventral root
Sympathetic preganglionic cell bodies in intermediolateral nucleus (lateral horn) of gray matter
Preganglionic sympathetic fibers
Postganglionic sympathetic fibers
Preganglionic parasympathetic fibers
Postganglionic parasympathetic fibers
F. Netter M.D.

Taste Pathways: Schema

See also Plates 124, 126, 127

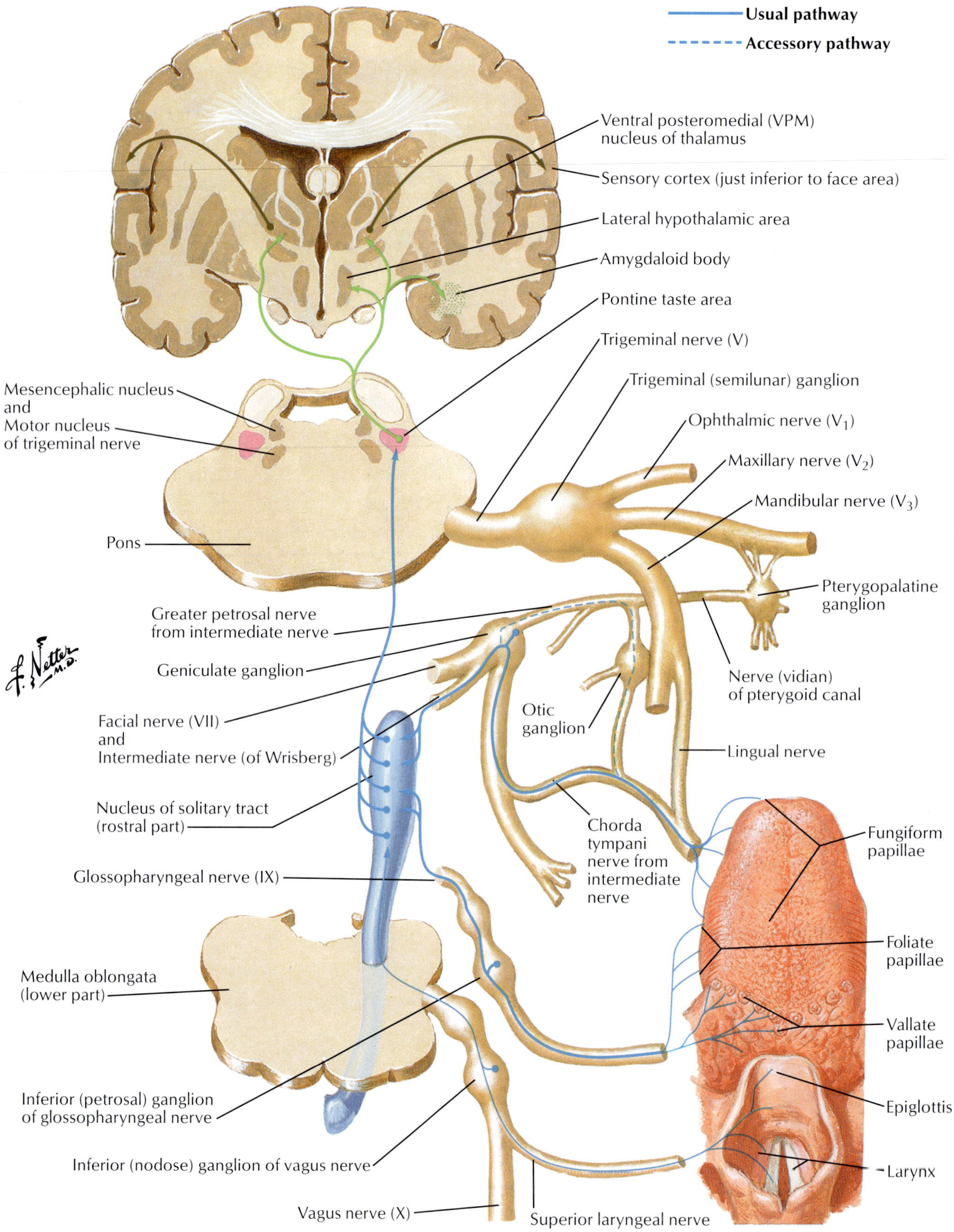

Arteries to Brain and Meninges

See also Plate 34

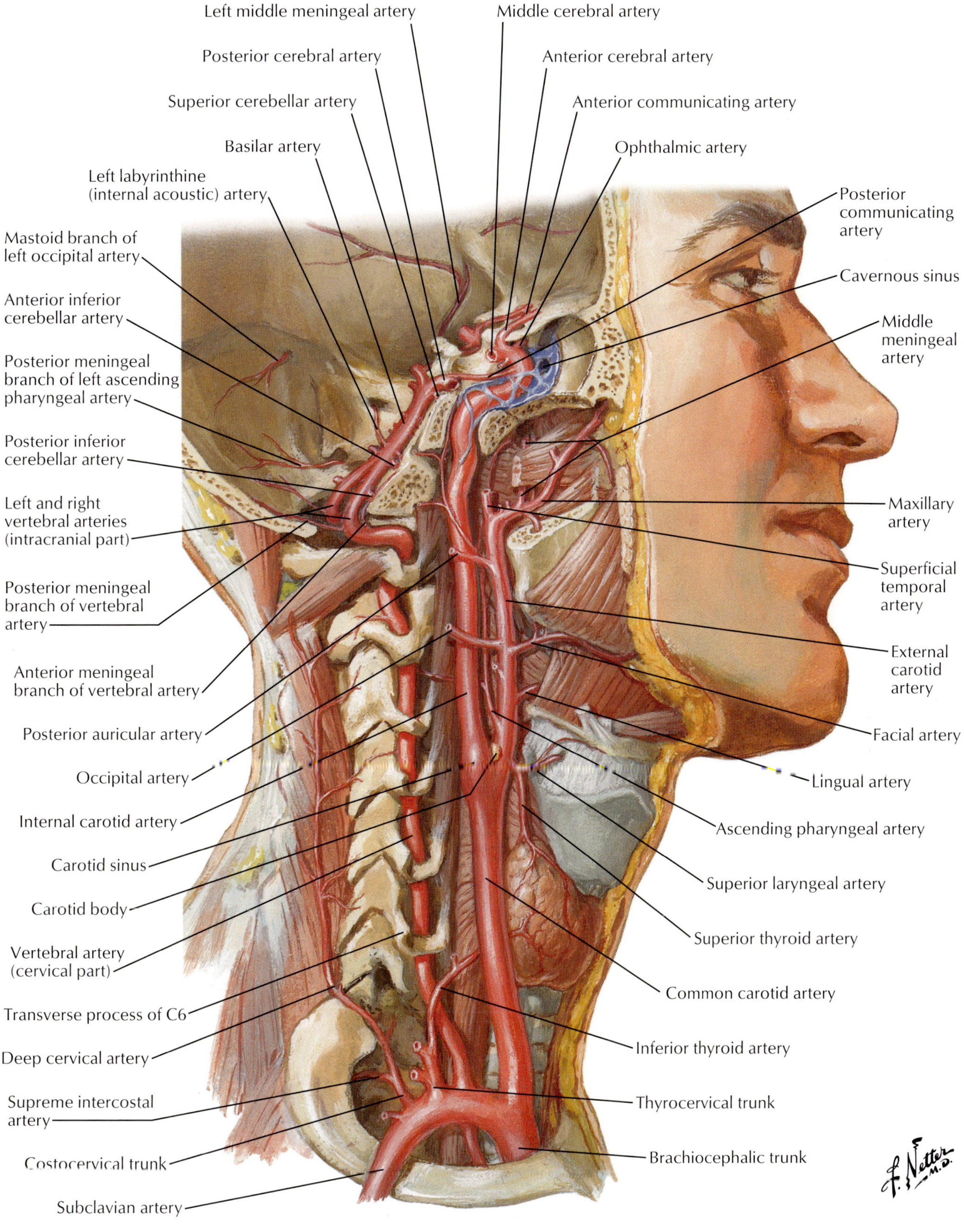

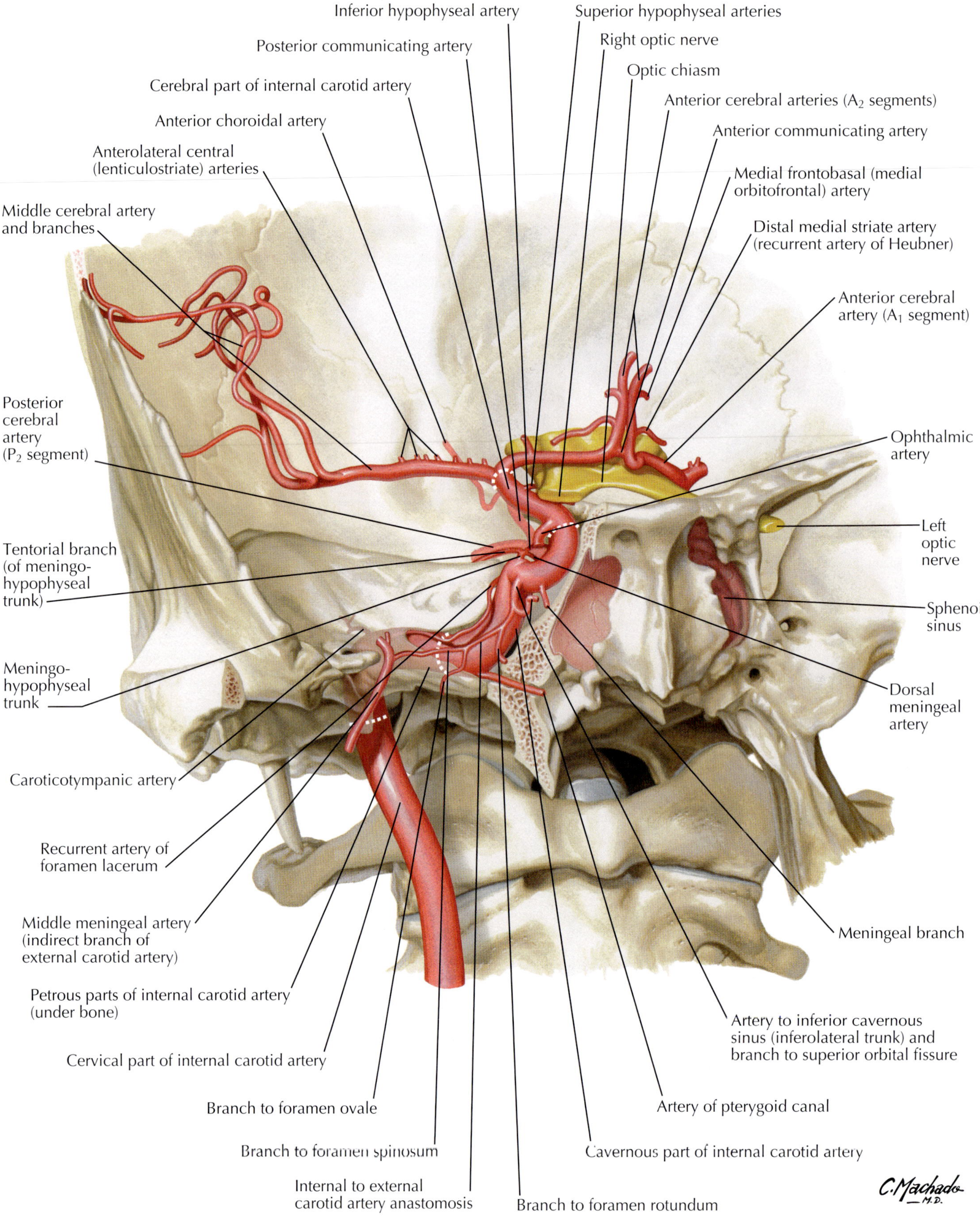

Inferior hypophyseal artery
Superior hypophyseal arteries
Posterior communicating artery
Right optic nerve
Cerebral part of internal carotid artery
Optic chiasm
Anterior cerebral arteries (A_2 segments)
Anterior choroidal artery
Anterior communicating artery
Anterolateral central (lenticulostriate) arteries
Medial frontobasal (medial orbitofrontal) artery
Middle cerebral artery and branches
Distal medial striate artery (recurrent artery of Heubner)
Anterior cerebral artery (A_1 segment)
Posterior cerebral artery (P_2 segment)
Ophthalmic artery
Left optic nerve
Tentorial branch (of meningo-hypophyseal trunk)
Sphenoidal sinus
Meningo-hypophyseal trunk
Dorsal meningeal artery
Caroticotympanic artery
Recurrent artery of foramen lacerum
Middle meningeal artery (indirect branch of external carotid artery)
Meningeal branch
Petrous parts of internal carotid artery (under bone)
Artery to inferior cavernous sinus (inferolateral trunk) and branch to superior orbital fissure
Cervical part of internal carotid artery
Branch to foramen ovale
Artery of pterygoid canal
Branch to foramen spinosum
Cavernous part of internal carotid artery
Internal to external carotid artery anastomosis
Branch to foramen rotundum
C. Machado M.D.

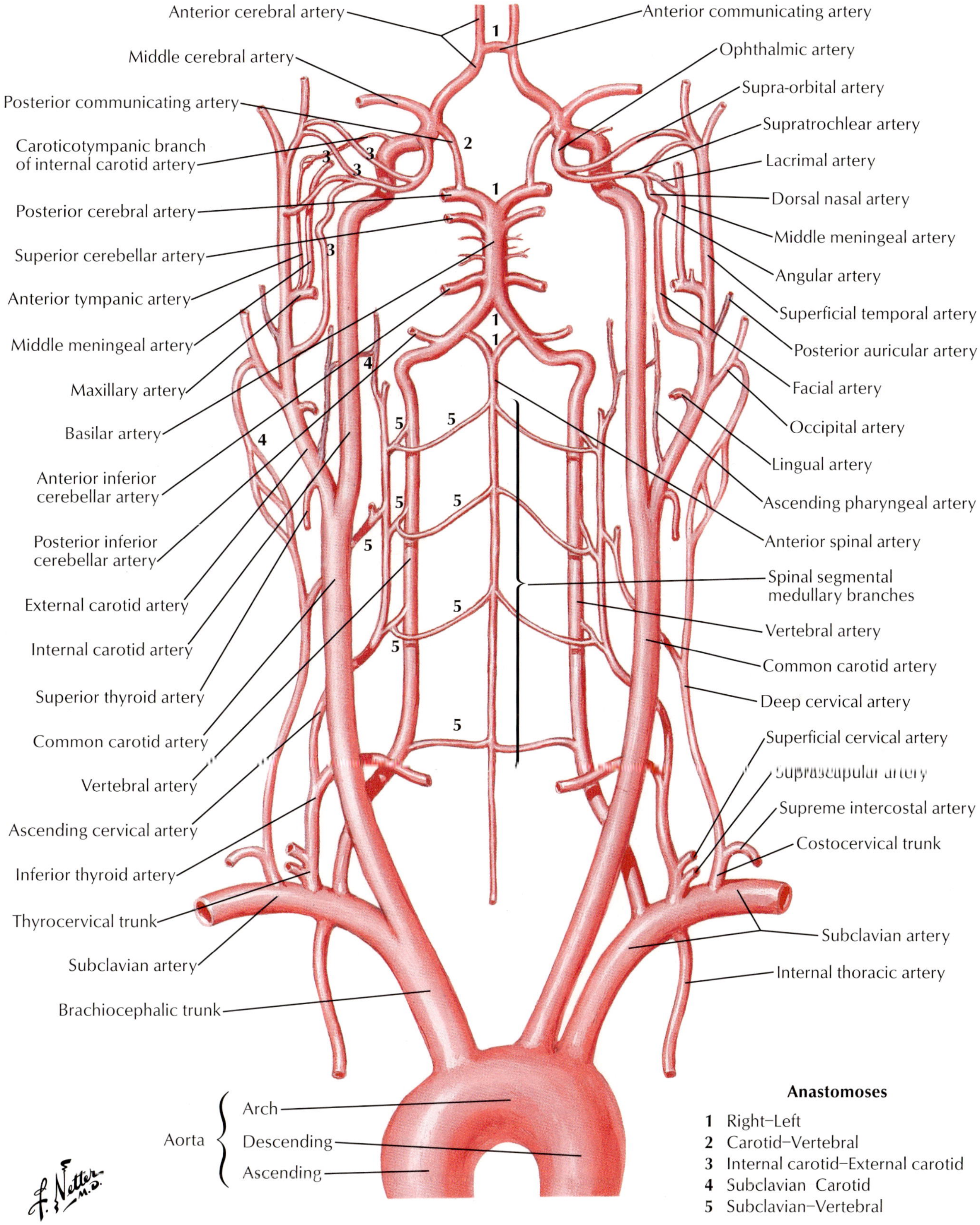
Anterior cerebral artery
Middle cerebral artery
Posterior communicating artery
Caroticotympanic branch of internal carotid artery
Posterior cerebral artery
Superior cerebellar artery
Anterior tympanic artery
Middle meningeal artery
Maxillary artery
Basilar artery
Anterior inferior cerebellar artery
Posterior inferior cerebellar artery
External carotid artery
Internal carotid artery
Superior thyroid artery
Common carotid artery
Vertebral artery
Ascending cervical artery
Inferior thyroid artery
Thyrocervical trunk
Subclavian artery
Brachiocephalic trunk
Anterior communicating artery
Ophthalmic artery
Supra-orbital artery
Supratrochlear artery
Lacrimal artery
Dorsal nasal artery
Middle meningeal artery
Angular artery
Superficial temporal artery
Posterior auricular artery
Facial artery
Occipital artery
Lingual artery
Ascending pharyngeal artery
Anterior spinal artery
Spinal segmental medullary branches
Vertebral artery
Common carotid artery
Deep cervical artery
Superficial cervical artery
Suprascapular artery
Supreme intercostal artery
Costocervical trunk
Subclavian artery
Internal thoracic artery
Aorta
Arch
Descending
Ascending
1
2
3
4
5
Anastomoses
1 Right–Left
2 Carotid–Vertebral
3 Internal carotid–External carotid
4 Subclavian Carotid
5 Subclavian–Vertebral
F. Netter M.D.

Arteries of Brain: Inferior Views

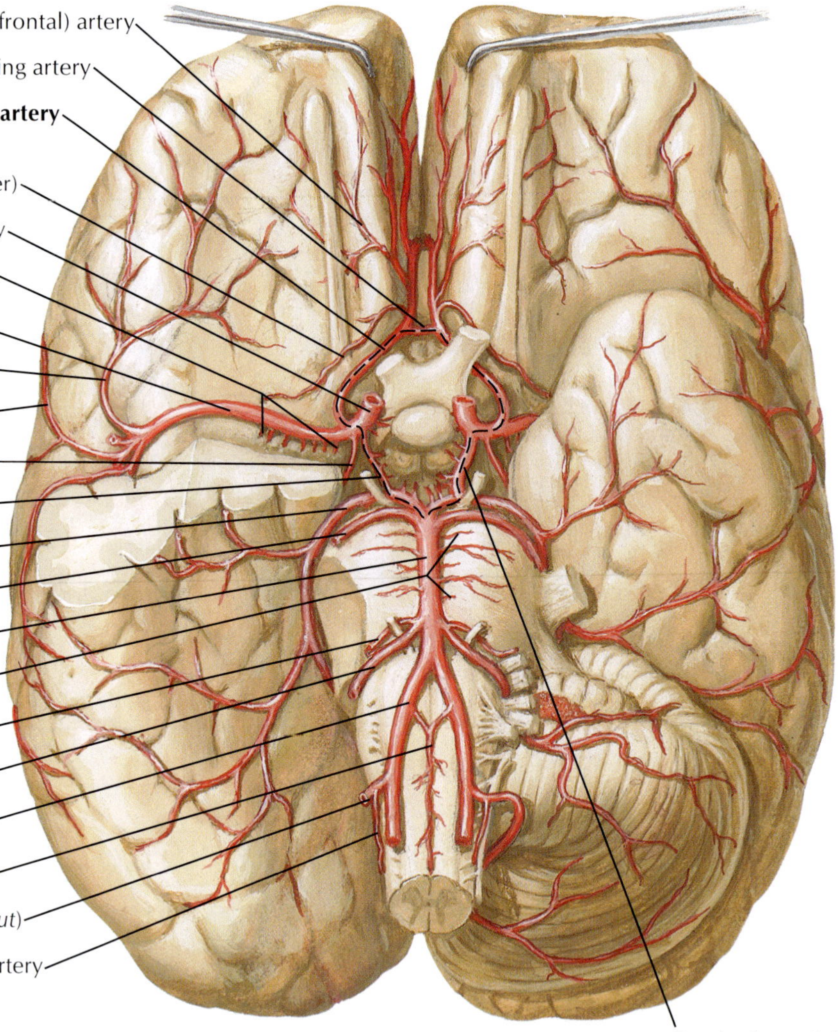

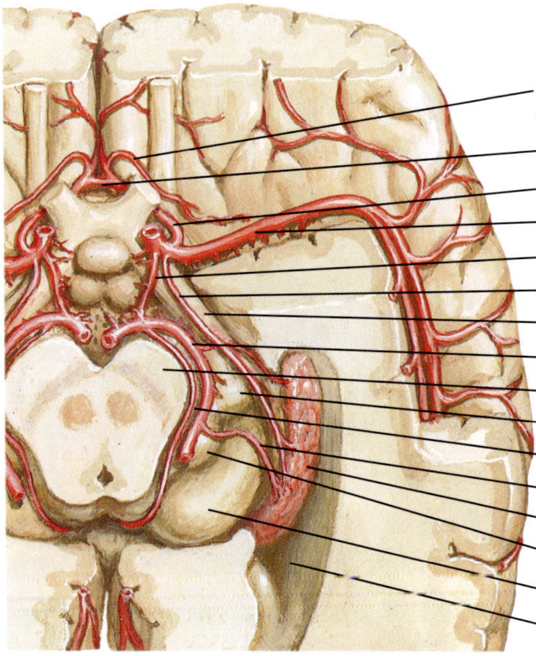

For hypophyseal arteries see Plate 149

Vessels dissected out: inferior view

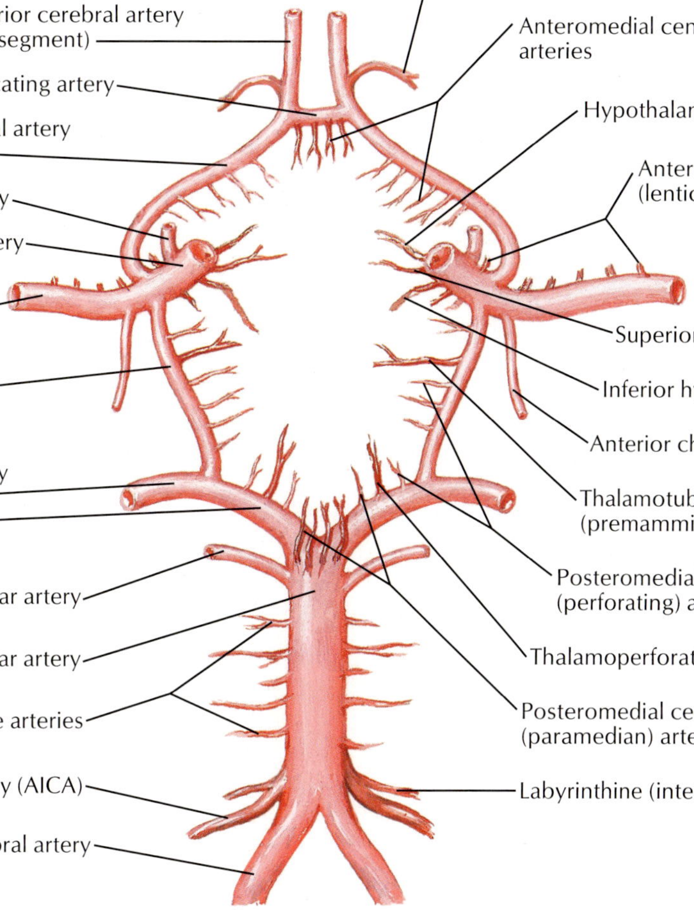

Vessels in situ: inferior view

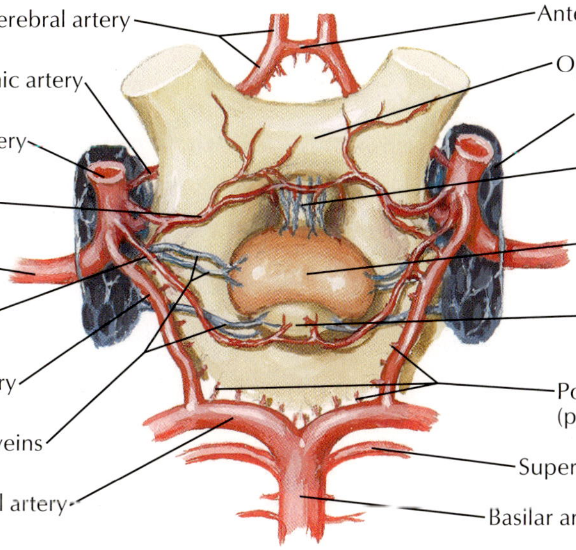

Arteries of Brain: Frontal View and Section

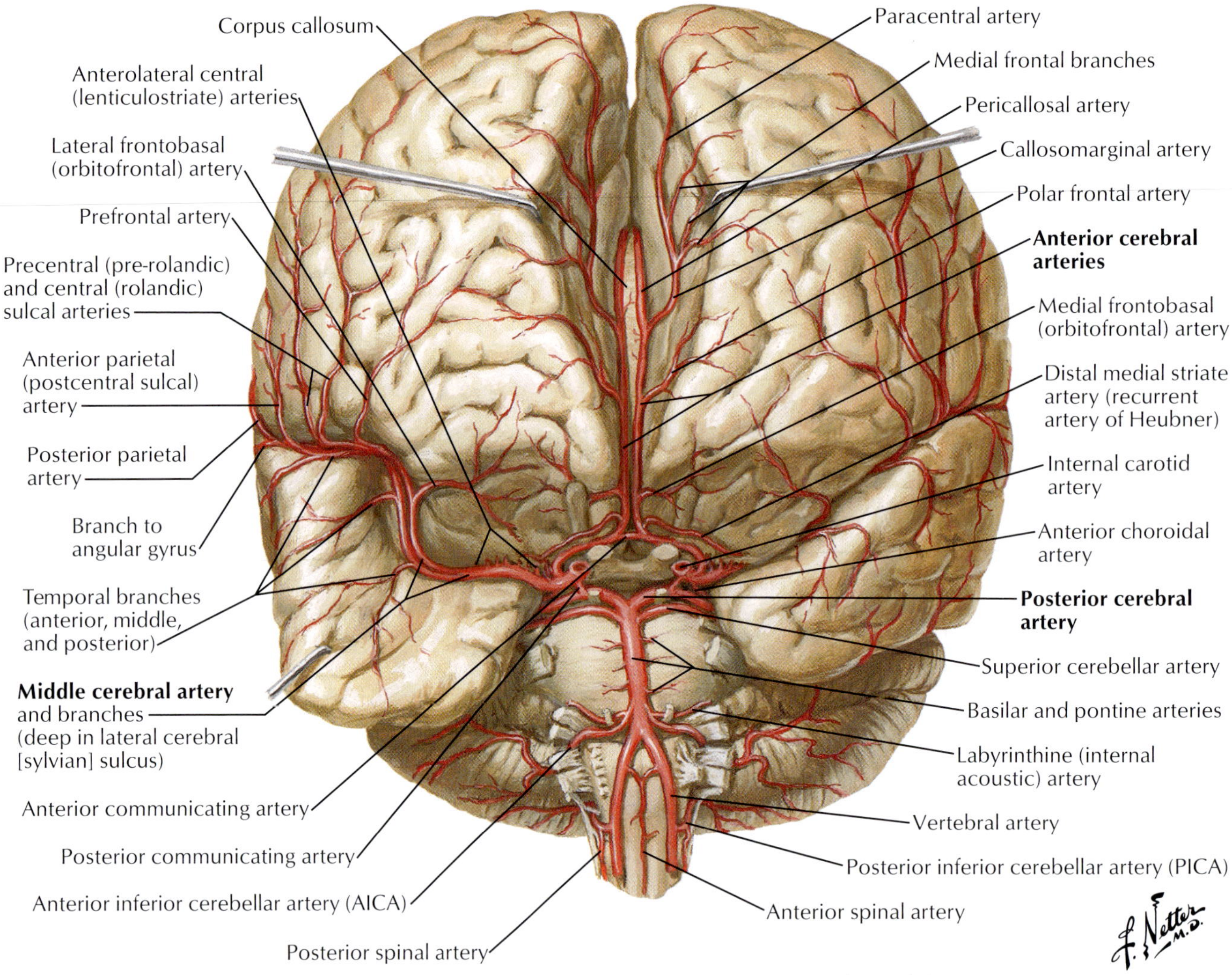

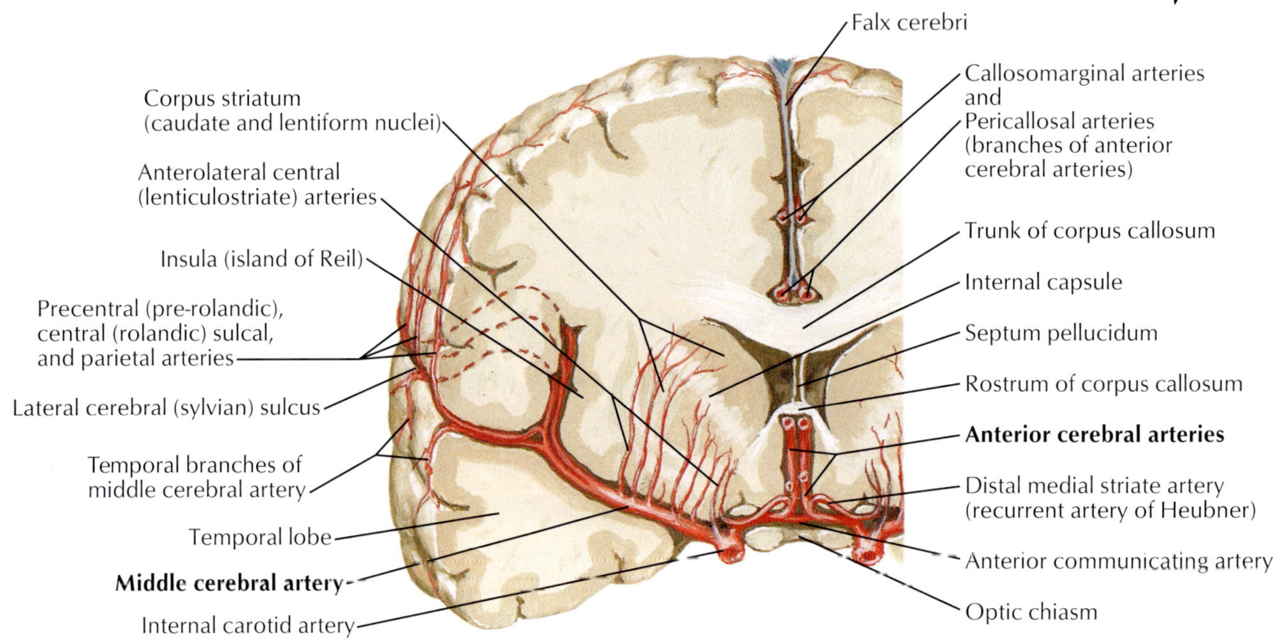

Arteries of Brain: Lateral and Medial Views

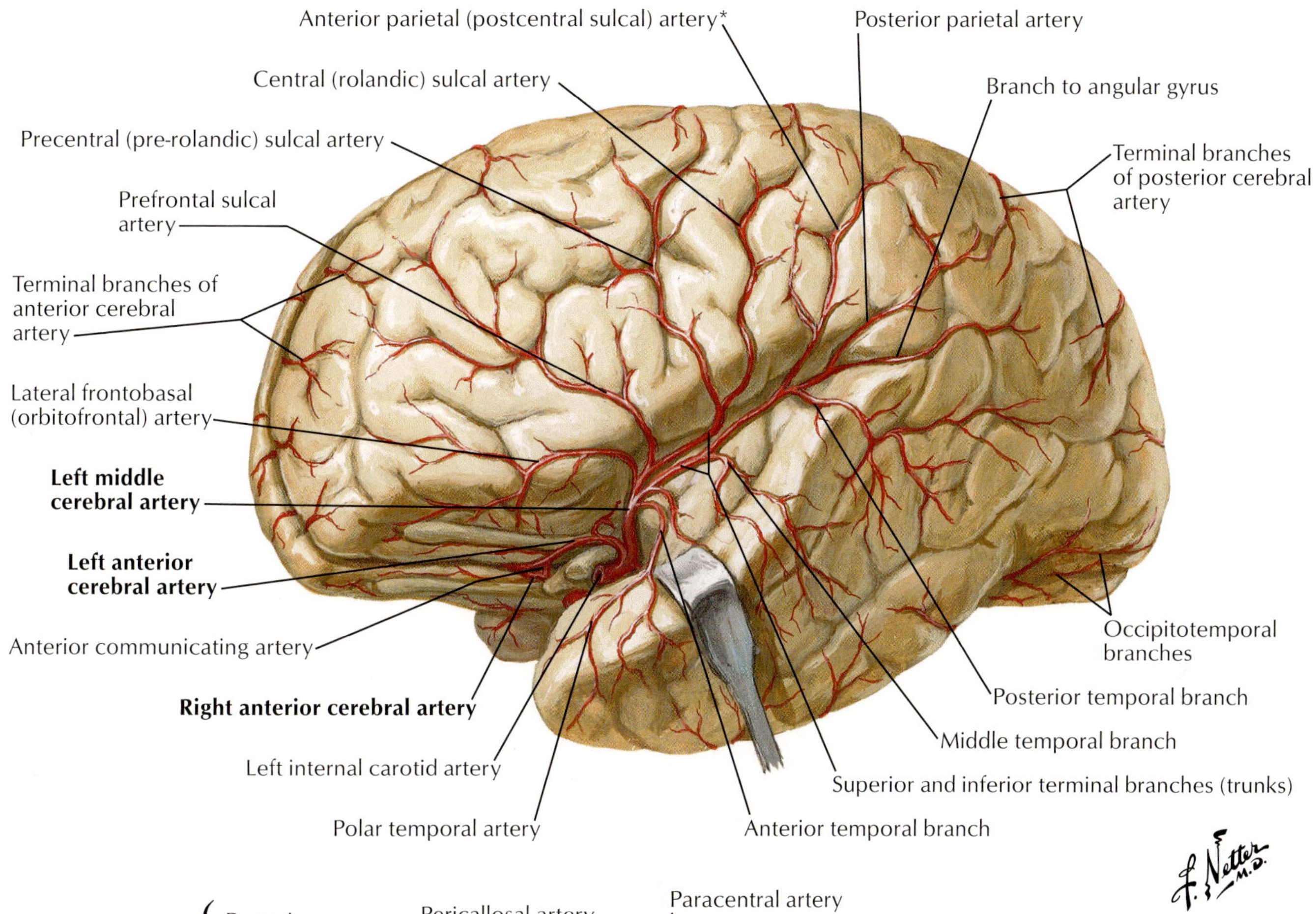

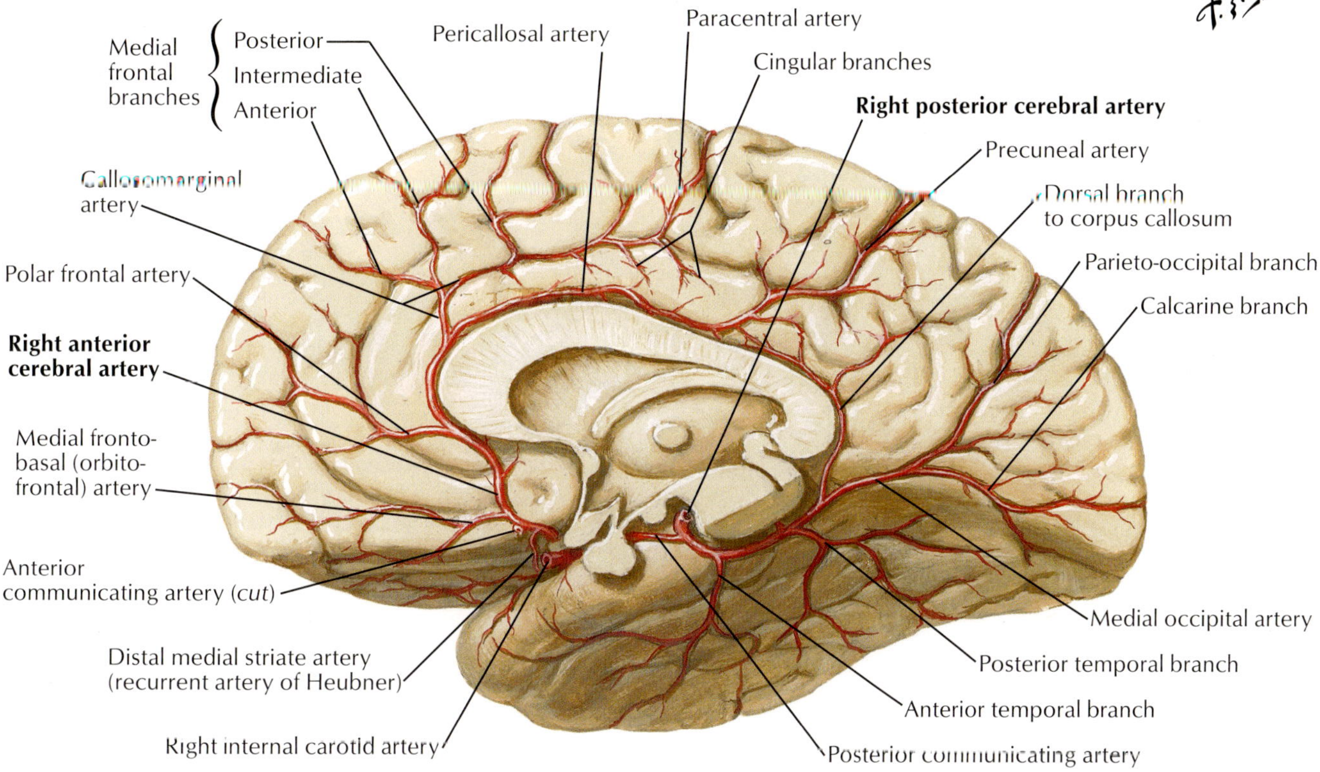

Note: Anterior parietal (postcentral sulcal) artery also occurs as separate anterior parietal and postcentral sulcal arteries.

Arteries of Posterior Cranial Fossa

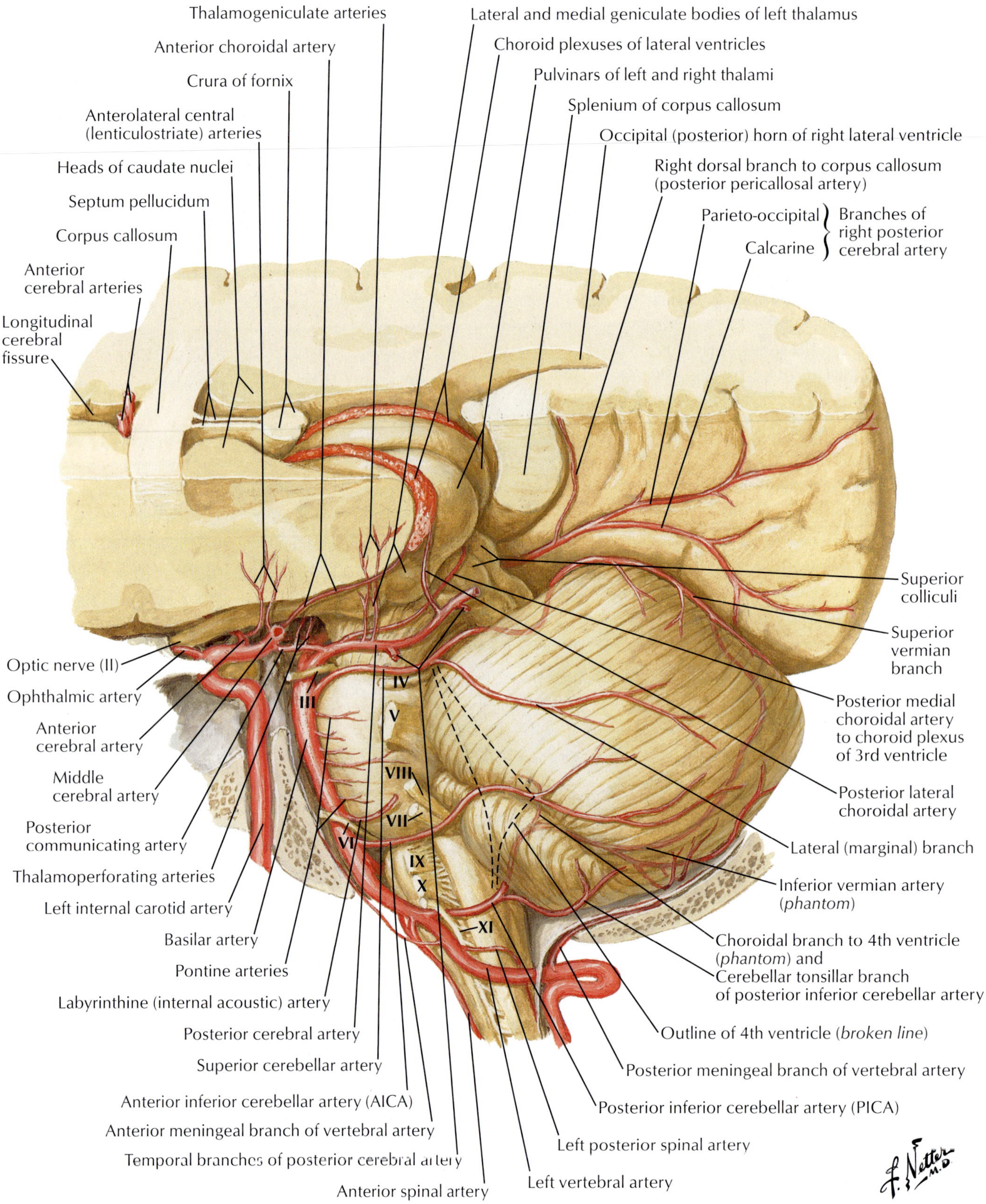

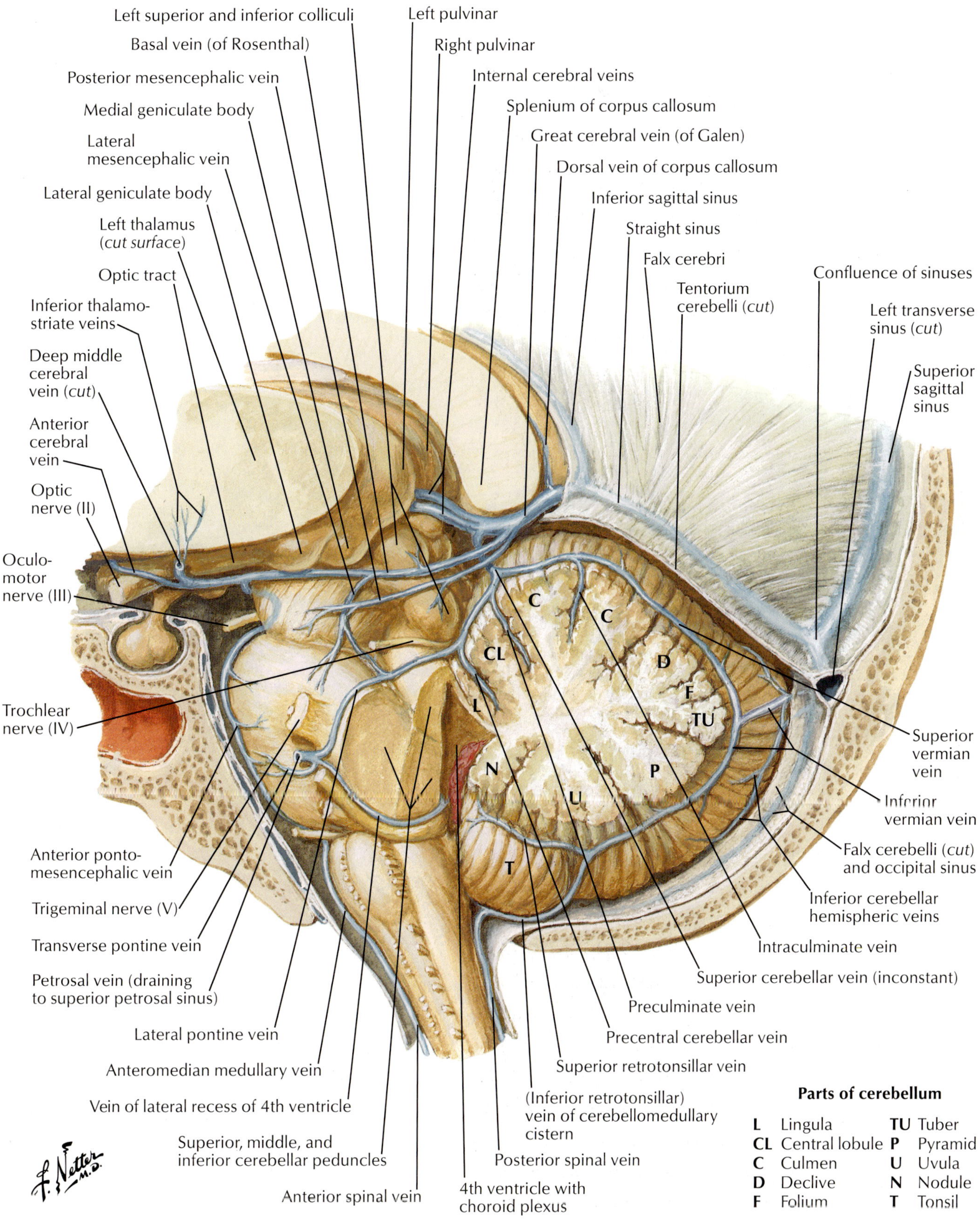

Parts of cerebellum

L	Lingula	**TU**	Tuber
CL	Central lobule	**P**	Pyramid
C	Culmen	**U**	Uvula
D	Declive	**N**	Nodule
F	Folium	**T**	Tonsil

For superficial veins of brain see **Plate 103**

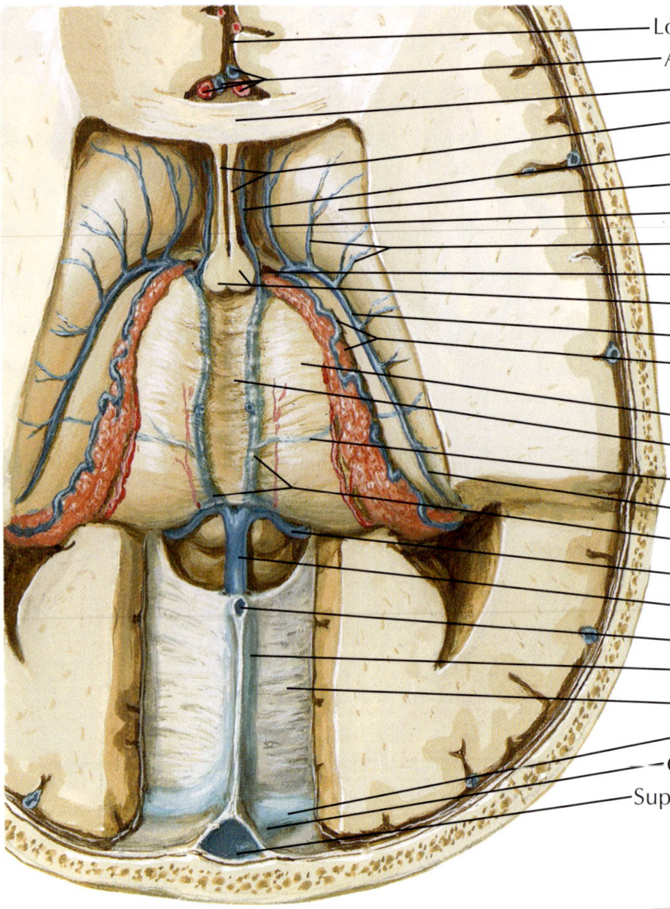

Dissection: superior view

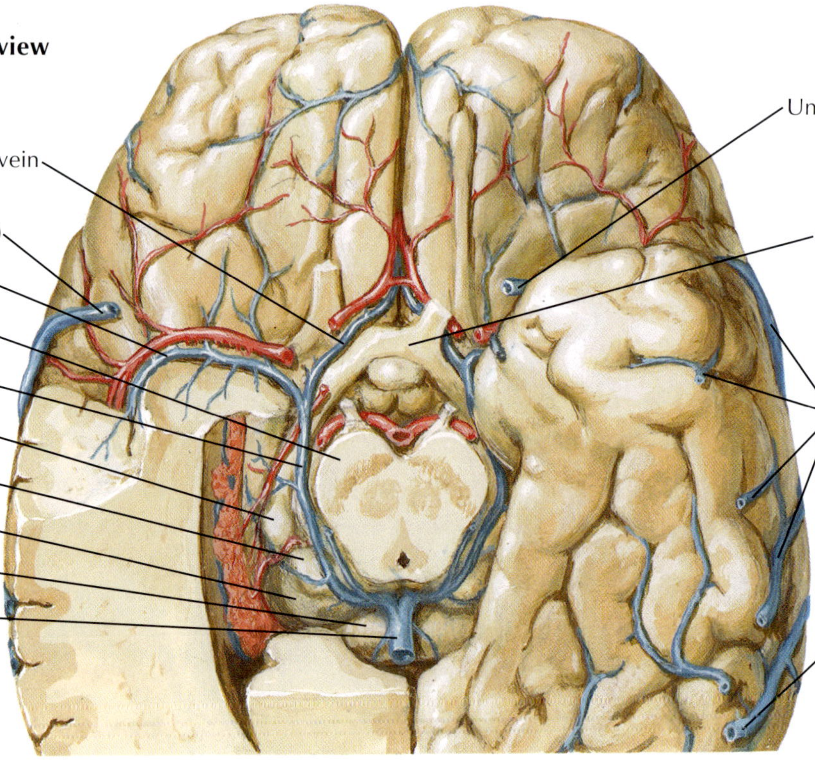

Dissection: inferior view

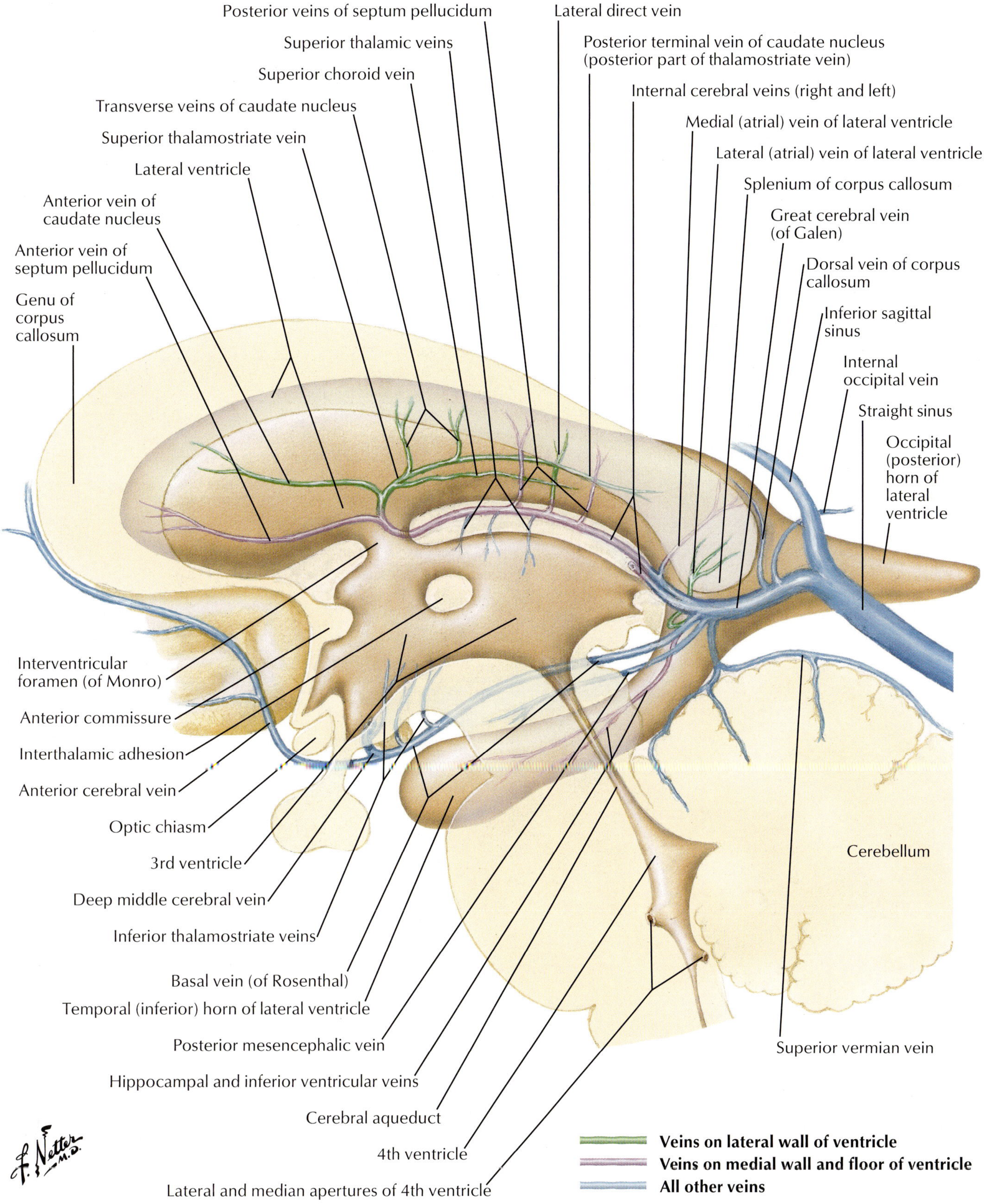
Posterior veins of septum pellucidum
Superior thalamic veins
Superior choroid vein
Transverse veins of caudate nucleus
Superior thalamostriate vein
Lateral ventricle
Anterior vein of caudate nucleus
Anterior vein of septum pellucidum
Genu of corpus callosum
Lateral direct vein
Posterior terminal vein of caudate nucleus (posterior part of thalamostriate vein)
Internal cerebral veins (right and left)
Medial (atrial) vein of lateral ventricle
Lateral (atrial) vein of lateral ventricle
Splenium of corpus callosum
Great cerebral vein (of Galen)
Dorsal vein of corpus callosum
Inferior sagittal sinus
Internal occipital vein
Straight sinus
Occipital (posterior) horn of lateral ventricle
Interventricular foramen (of Monro)
Anterior commissure
Interthalamic adhesion
Anterior cerebral vein
Optic chiasm
3rd ventricle
Deep middle cerebral vein
Inferior thalamostriate veins
Basal vein (of Rosenthal)
Temporal (inferior) horn of lateral ventricle
Posterior mesencephalic vein
Hippocampal and inferior ventricular veins
Cerebral aqueduct
4th ventricle
Lateral and median apertures of 4th ventricle
Cerebellum
Superior vermian vein
F. Netter M.D.
Veins on lateral wall of ventricle
Veins on medial wall and floor of ventricle
All other veins

See also Plates 107, 108

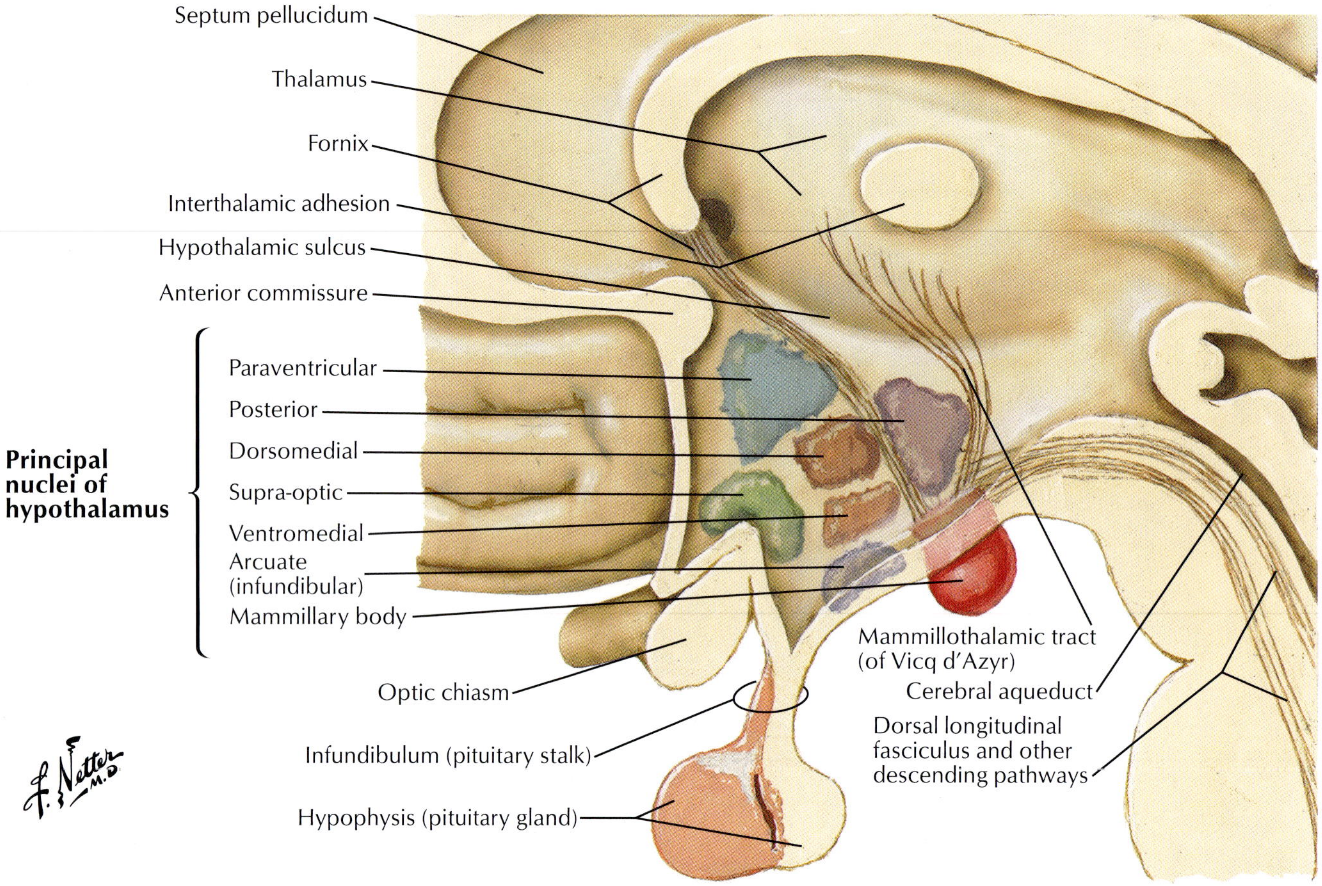

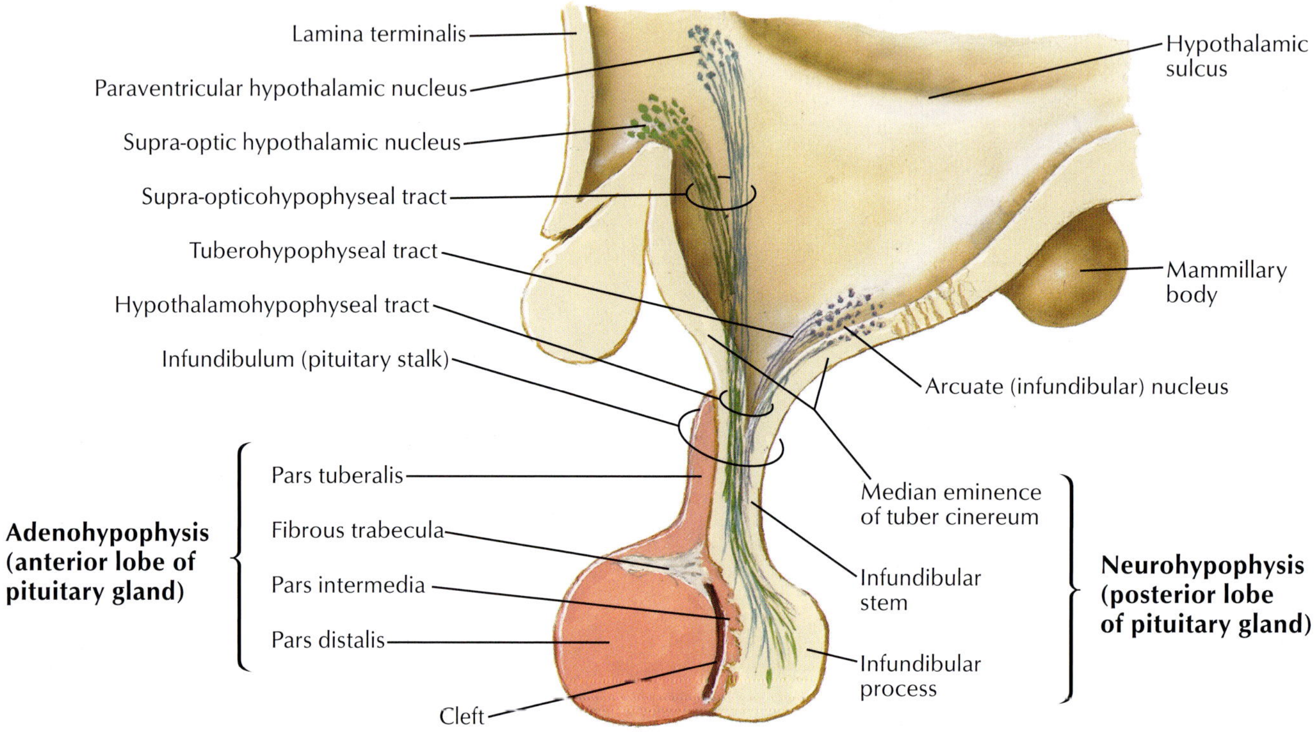

Arteries and Veins of Hypothalamus and Hypophysis

See also Plate 141

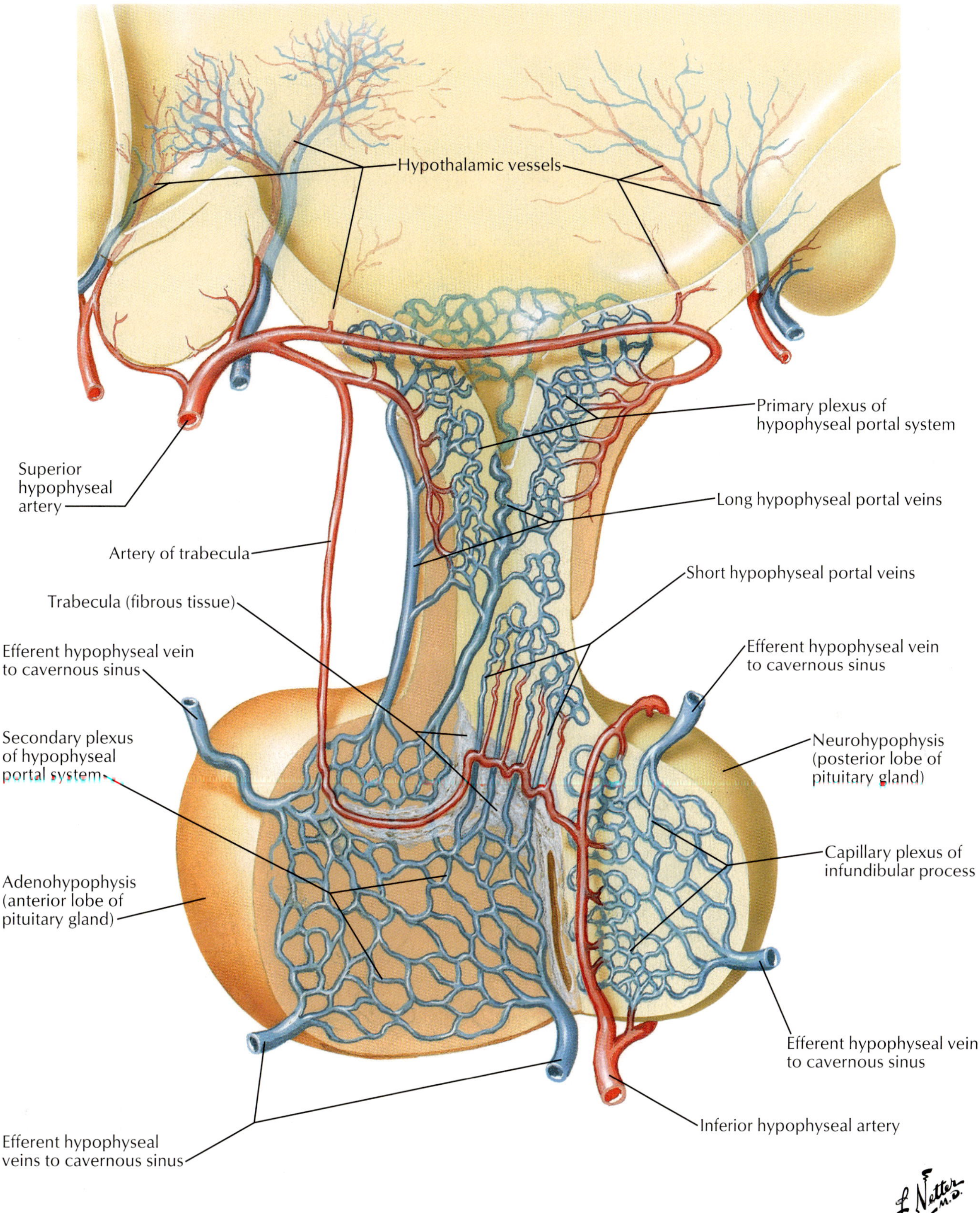

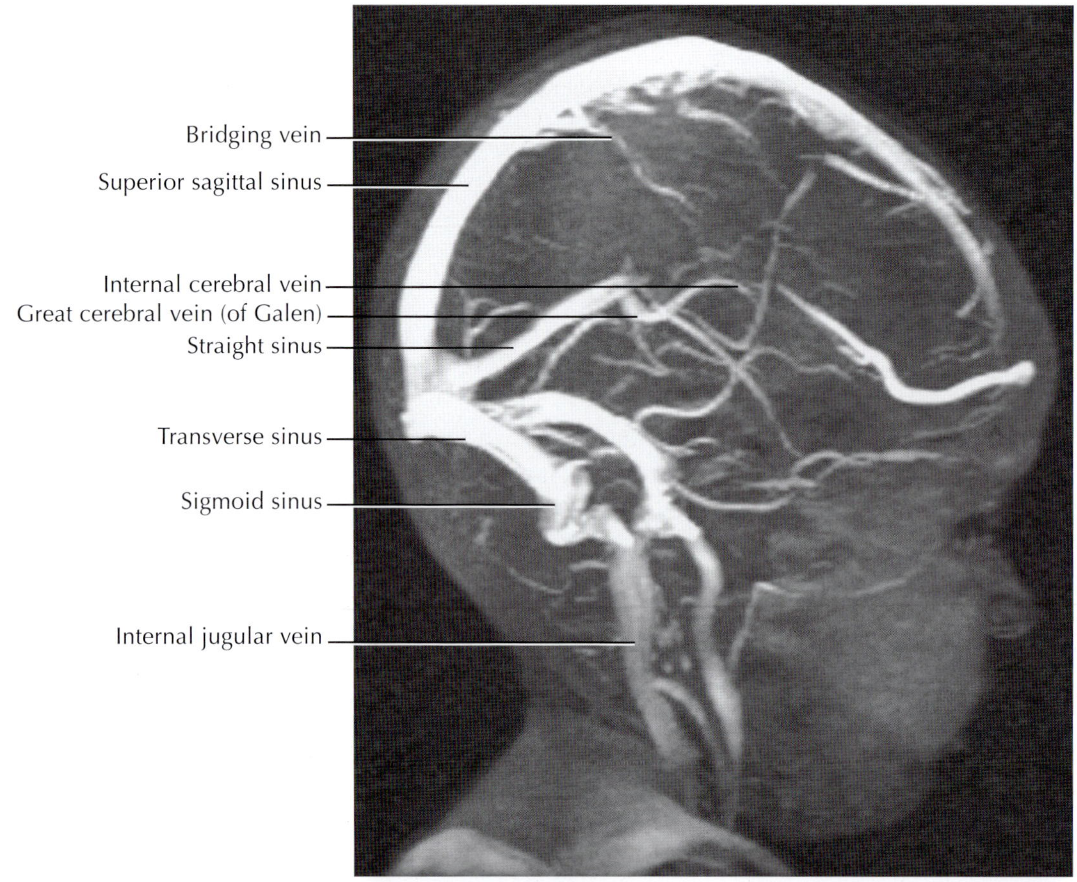
Bridging vein
Superior sagittal sinus
Internal cerebral vein
Great cerebral vein (of Galen)
Straight sinus
Transverse sinus
Sigmoid sinus
Internal jugular vein

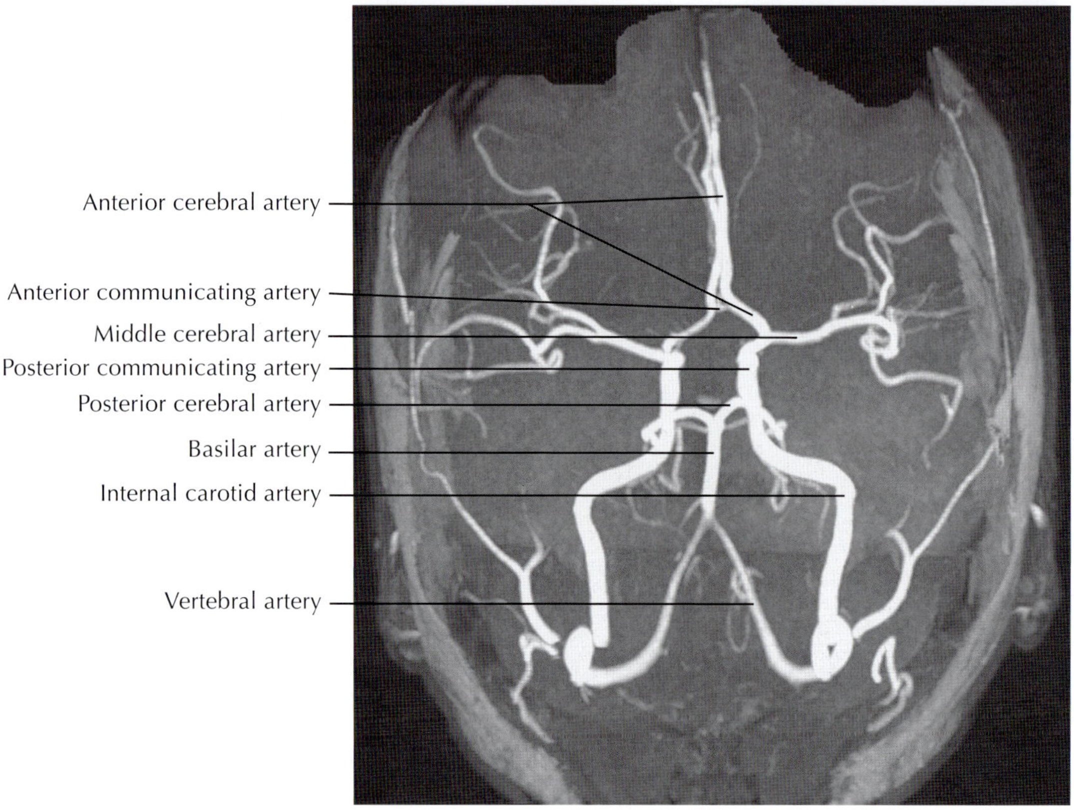
Anterior cerebral artery
Anterior communicating artery
Middle cerebral artery
Posterior communicating artery
Posterior cerebral artery
Basilar artery
Internal carotid artery
Vertebral artery

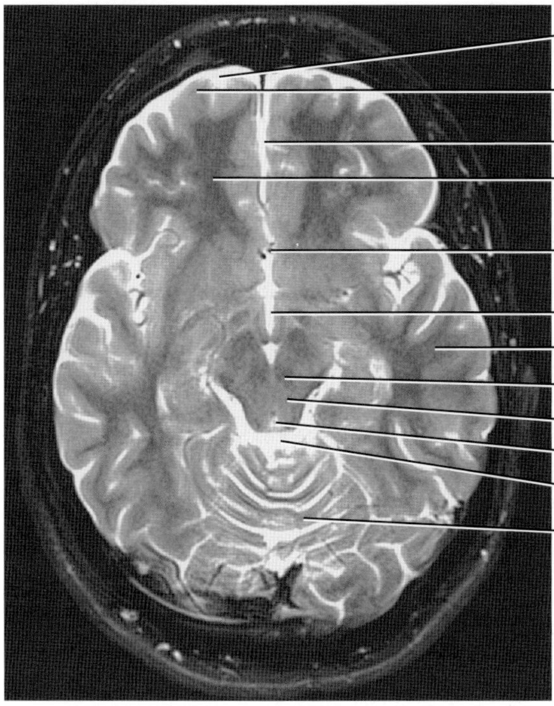
Subarachnoid space
Gray matter
Longitudinal fissure
White matter
Anterior cerebral artery
Third ventricle
Temporal lobe
Red nucleus
Midbrain
Cerebral aqueduct
Quadrigeminal cistern
Cerebellum

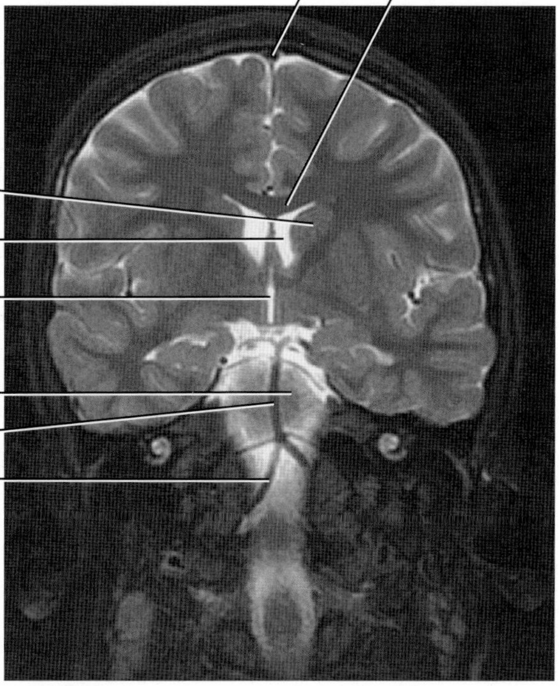
Superior sagittal sinus
Corpus callosum
Head of caudate
Lateral ventricle
Third ventricle
Pons
Basilar artery
Vertebral artery

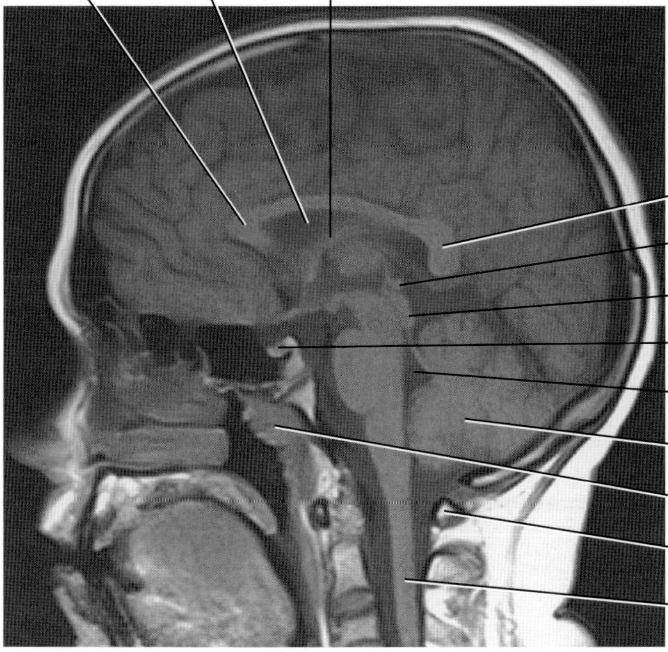
Genu of corpus callosum
Lateral ventricle
Fornix
Splenium of corpus callosum
Pineal gland
Tectum
Pituitary gland
Fourth ventricle
Cerebellum
Pharyngeal tonsil
Posterior arch of atlas
Spinal cord

MUSCLE	PROXIMAL ATTACHMENT (ORIGIN)	DISTAL ATTACHMENT (INSERTION)	INNERVATION	MAIN ACTIONS	BLOOD SUPPLY	MUSCLE GROUP
Auricularis anterior	Temporal fascia, epicranial aponeurosis	Anterior part of medial surface of helix of ear	Posterior auricular and temporal branches of facial nerve	Elevates and draws ear forward	Auricular branch of posterior auricular artery, parietal branch of superficial temporal artery	External ear
Auricularis posterior	Base of mastoid process	Lower part of cranial surface of auricle	Posterior auricular and temporal branches of facial nerve	Retracts and elevates ear	Auricular branch of posterior auricular artery, parietal branch of superficial temporal artery	External ear
Auricularis superior	Temporal fascia, epicranial aponeurosis	Upper part of medial surface of auricle	Posterior auricular and temporal branches of facial nerve	Retracts and elevates ear	Auricular branch of posterior auricular artery, parietal branch of superficial temporal artery	External ear
Buccinator	Posterior portion of alveolar process of maxilla and mandible opposite sockets of molar teeth, anterior border of pterygomandibular raphe	Angle of mouth	Buccal branches of facial nerve	Compresses cheeks, expels air between lips, aids in mastication	Muscular branches of facial artery, buccal branch of maxillary artery	Facial expression
Ciliary	Corneoscleral junction	Ciliary body	Parasympathetic fibers via short ciliary nerves (CN III)	Constricts ciliary body and lens rounds up (accommodation)	Ophthalmic artery	Intrinsic eye
Corrugator supercilii	Medial part of supra-orbital margin	Skin of medial half of eyebrow	Zygomatic and temporal branches of facial nerve	Draws eyebrows downward and medially, produces wrinkles in frowning	Zygomatic and anterior branches of superficial temporal artery	Facial expression
Cricothyroid	Anterior cricoid cartilage	Inferior border of thyroid cartilage and its inferior horn	External branch of superior laryngeal nerve	Lengthens and tenses vocal ligaments	Superior and inferior thyroid arteries	Laryngeal
Depressor anguli oris	Continuous with platysma on oblique line of mandible	Angle of mouth into orbicularis and skin	Mandibular and buccal branches of facial nerve	Depresses angle of mouth	Inferior labial branch of facial artery	Facial expression
Depressor labii inferioris	Lateral surface of mandible between symphysis and mental foramen deep to depressor anguli oris	Skin to lower lip, mingling with orbicularis oris, medial fibers joining those of opposite side	Mandibular and buccal branches of facial nerve	Depresses lower lip and draws it lateralward	Inferior labial branch of facial artery	Facial expression
Depressor septi nasi	Incisive fossa of maxilla	Septum and posterior part of ala of nose	Zygomatic and buccal branches of facial nerve	Narrows nostril, draws septum downward	Superior labial branch of facial artery	Facial expression
Digastric	*Anterior belly:* digastric fossa of mandible *Posterior belly*: mastoid notch of temporal bone	Intermediate tendon attached to body of hyoid	*Anterior belly:* nerve to mylohyoid *Posterior belly:* facial nerve	Raises hyoid bone and base of tongue, steadies hyoid bone, opens mouth by lowering mandible	*Anterior belly*: branches of submental artery *Posterior belly:* muscular branches of posterior auricular artery, muscular branches of occipital artery	Suprahyoid
Dilator pupillae	Radial fibers in iris	Blends with sphincter pupillae fibers	Sympathetic fibers from SCG	Dilates pupil	Ophthalmic artery	Intrinsic eye
Frontal belly of occipitofrontalis	Epicranial aponeurosis at level of coronal suture	Skin of frontal region, epicranial aponeurosis	Temporal branches of facial nerve	Wrinkles forehead skin, raises eyebrows	Frontal branch of superficial temporal artery	Facial expression

Variations in spinal nerve contributions to the innervation of muscles, their arterial supply, their attachments, and their actions are common themes in human anatomy. Therefore, expect differences between texts and realize that anatomical variation is normal.

MUSCLE	PROXIMAL ATTACHMENT (ORIGIN)	DISTAL ATTACHMENT (INSERTION)	INNERVATION	MAIN ACTIONS	BLOOD SUPPLY	MUSCLE GROUP
Genioglossus	Mental spine of mandible	Dorsum of tongue, hyoid bone	Hypoglossal nerve (CN XII)	Depresses and protrudes tongue	Sublingual and submental arteries	Extrinsic tongue
Geniohyoid	Inferior genial tubercle on back of symphysis of mandible	Anterior surface of body of hyoid bone	Branch of C1 through hypoglossal nerve (CN XII)	Elevates hyoid bone and depresses mandible	Sublingual branch of lingual artery	Suprahyoid
Hyoglossus	Body and greater horn of hyoid bone	Lateral and inferior aspect of tongue	Hypoglossal nerve (CN XII)	Depresses and retracts tongue	Sublingual and submental arteries	Extrinsic tongue
Inferior longitudinal muscle of tongue	Under surface of tongue between genioglossus and hyoglossus	Tip of tongue blending with styloglossus	Hypoglossal nerve (CN XII)	Shortens tongue, turns tip and sides downward	Deep lingual branch of lingual artery, branches from facial artery	Intrinsic tongue
Inferior oblique	Anterior floor of orbit lateral to nasolacrimal canal	Lateral sclera deep to lateral rectus	Oculomotor nerve (CN III), inferior division	Abducts, elevates, and laterally rotates eyeball	Ophthalmic artery	Extra-ocular
Inferior pharyngeal constrictor	Oblique line of thyroid cartilage and cricoid cartilage	Median raphe of pharynx	Vagus nerve via pharyngeal plexus	Constricts wall of pharynx during swallowing	Ascending pharyngeal artery, branches of superior thyroid artery	Circular pharyngeal
Inferior rectus	Common tendinous ring	Inferior aspect of eyeball, posterior to corneoscleral junction	Oculomotor nerve (CN III), inferior division	Depresses, adducts, and laterally rotates eyeball	Ophthalmic artery	Extra-ocular
Lateral crico-arytenoid	Arch of cricoid cartilage	Muscular process of arytenoid cartilage	Recurrent laryngeal nerve	Adducts vocal folds	Superior and inferior thyroid arteries	Laryngeal
Lateral pterygoid	*Superior head:* infratemporal surface of greater wing of sphenoid *Inferior head:* lateral pterygoid plate	Pterygoid fovea, capsule of temporomandibular joint, articular disc	Mandibular nerve (CN V_3), muscular branches from anterior division	*Bilaterally:* protrude mandible *Unilaterally and alternately:* produces side-to-side grinding	Muscular branches of maxillary artery	Mastication
Lateral rectus	Common tendinous ring	Lateral aspect of eyeball, posterior to corneoscleral junction	Abducent nerve (CN VI)	Abducts eyeball	Ophthalmic artery	Extra-ocular
Levator anguli oris	Canine fossa of maxilla immediately below infra-orbital foramen and under cover of zygomatic head of levator labii superioris	Angle of mouth; fibers intermingle with orbicularis oris, depressor anguli oris, zygomaticus	Zygomatic and buccal branches of facial nerve	Elevates angle of mouth	Superior labial branch of facial artery	Facial expression
Levator labii superioris alaeque nasi	*Angular head:* upper part of frontal process of maxilla *Infra-orbital head:* orbit above infra-orbital foramen *Zygomatic head:* malar surface of zygomatic bone	*Angular head:* into greater alar cartilage, skin of nose, lateral upper lip *Infra-orbital head:* into muscular substance of upper lip between angular head and caninus *Zygomatic head:* into skin of nasolabial groove and upper lip	Zygomatic and buccal branches of facial nerve	*Angular head:* elevates upper lip and dilates nostril *Infra-orbital head:* raises angle of mouth *Zygomatic head:* elevates upper lip laterally	Superior labial branch and angular branches of facial artery	Facial expression

MUSCLE	PROXIMAL ATTACHMENT (ORIGIN)	DISTAL ATTACHMENT (INSERTION)	INNERVATION	MAIN ACTIONS	BLOOD SUPPLY	MUSCLE GROUP
Levator labii superioris	Maxilla above infra-orbital foramen	Skin of upper lip	Zygomatic and buccal branches of facial nerve	Elevates upper lip, dilates nares	Superior labial artery and angular branches of facial artery	Facial expression
Levator palpebrae superioris	Lesser wing of sphenoid, anterior to optic canal	Superior tarsal plate	Oculomotor nerve (CN III), superior division	Raises upper eyelid	Ophthalmic artery	Extra-ocular; eyelid
Levator veli palatini	Temporal bone (petrous portion)	Palatine aponeurosis	Vagus nerve via pharyngeal plexus	Elevates soft palate during swallowing	Ascending palatine artery branch of facial artery, descending palatine artery branch of maxillary artery	Palatal
Longus capitis	Anterior tubercles of transverse processes of C3–C6	Inferior surface of basilar part of occipital bone	Ventral rami of cervical nerves (C1–C4)	Flexes and assists in rotating cervical vertebrae and head	Ascending cervical branch of inferior thyroid artery, ascending pharyngeal artery, muscular branches of vertebral artery	Prevertebral
Longus colli	*Vertical portion:* C5–T3 vertebrae *Inferior oblique portion:* T1–T3 vertebrae *Superior oblique portion*: anterior tubercles of transverse processes of C3–C5 vertebrae	*Vertical portion:* into C2–C4 vertebrae *Inferior oblique portion* on anterior tubercles of transverse processes of C5–C6 vertebrae *Superior oblique portion:* tubercle of anterior arch of atlas	Ventral primary rami of cervical nerves (C2–C8)	*Bilaterally*: flex and assist in rotating cervical vertebrae and head *Unilaterally:* flexes vertebral column laterally	Prevertebral branches of ascending pharyngeal artery, muscular branches of ascending cervical and vertebral arteries	Prevertebral
Masseter	Zygomatic arch	Ramus of mandible, coronoid process	Mandibular nerve (CN V_3), via masseteric nerve	Elevates and protrudes mandible; deep fibers retrude it	Transverse facial artery; masseteric branch of maxillary and facial arteries	Mastication
Medial pterygoid	Medial surface of lateral plate of pterygoid, pyramidal process of palatine bone, maxillary tuberosity	Medial surface of ramus and angle of mandible inferior to mandibular foramen	Mandibular nerve (V_3), nerve to medial pterygoid	*Bilaterally:* protrude and elevate mandible *Unilaterally and alternately:* produces side-to-side movements	Facial and maxillary arteries	Mastication
Medial rectus	Common tendinous ring	Medial aspect of eyeball, posterior to corneoscleral junction	Oculomotor nerve (CN III), inferior division	Adducts eyeball	Ophthalmic artery	Extra-ocular
Mentalis	Incisive fossa of mandible	Skin of chin	Mandibular branch of facial nerve	Raises and protrudes lower lip	Inferior labial branch of facial artery	Facial expression
Middle pharyngeal constrictor	Stylohyoid ligament and horns of hyoid bone	Median raphe of pharynx	Vagus nerve via pharyngeal plexus	Constricts wall of pharynx during swallowing	Ascending pharyngeal artery, ascending palatine and tonsillar branches of facial artery, dorsal lingual branches of lingual artery	Circular pharyngeal
Mylohyoid	Mylohyoid line of mandible	Median raphe and body of hyoid bone	Nerve to mylohyoid nerve (branch of trigeminal nerve)	Elevates hyoid bone, base of tongue, floor of mouth; depresses mandible	Sublingual branch of lingual artery, submental branch of facial artery	Suprahyoid

MUSCLE	PROXIMAL ATTACHMENT (ORIGIN)	DISTAL ATTACHMENT (INSERTION)	INNERVATION	MAIN ACTIONS	BLOOD SUPPLY	MUSCLE GROUP
Nasalis	Canine eminence above and lateral to incisive fossa of maxilla	Aponeurosis on nasal cartilages	Zygomatic and buccal branches of facial nerve	Draws ala of nose toward septum, compresses nostrils; alar part opens nostrils	Superior labial, septal, and lateral nasal branches of facial artery	Facial expression
Occipital belly (occipitalis) of epicranius	Lateral 2/3 of superior nuchal line and mastoid process	Skin of occipital region, epicranial aponeurosis	Posterior auricular branches of facial nerve	Moves scalp backward	Occipital branch of posterior auricular artery, descending branch of occipital artery	Facial expression
Omohyoid	*Inferior belly:* from upper border of scapula and suprascapular ligament, ending in tendon under sternocleidomastoid muscle *Superior belly:* from this tendon	*Inferior belly:* to intermediate tendon *Superior belly:* to body of hyoid bone	Ansa cervicalis	Steadies hyoid bone and depresses hyoid	Hyoid branch of lingual artery, sternocleidomastoid branch of superior thyroid artery	Infrahyoid
Orbicularis oculi	Medial orbital margin, palpebral ligament, lacrimal bone	Skin around orbit, palpebral ligament, upper and lower eyelids	Facial nerve (CN VII)	Closes eyelids	Facial and superficial temporal arteries	Facial expression
Orbicularis oris	Maxilla above incisor teeth	Skin around lips	Zygomatic, buccal, and mandibular branches of facial nerve	Compression, contraction, and protrusion of lips	Inferior and superior labial branches of facial artery	Facial expression
Palatoglossus	Palatine aponeurosis of soft palate	Lateral aspect of tongue	Vagus nerve via pharyngeal plexus	Elevates posterior tongue, depresses palate	Ascending pharyngeal arteries, palatine branches of facial and maxillary arteries	Palatal
Palatopharyngeus	Hard palate, superior palatine aponeurosis	Lateral pharyngeal wall	Vagus nerve via pharyngeal plexus	Tenses soft palate; pulls walls of pharynx superiorly, anteriorly, and medially during swallowing	Ascending palatine artery branch of facial artery, descending palatine artery branch of maxillary artery	Longitudinal pharyngeal
Platysma	Skin below clavicle, upper thorax	Mandible, oral muscles	Facial nerve	Tenses skin of neck	Submental and suprascapular arteries	Facial expression
Posterior crico-arytenoid	Posterior surface of lamina of cricoid cartilage	Muscular process of arytenoid cartilage	Recurrent laryngeal nerve	Abducts vocal folds	Superior and inferior thyroid arteries	Laryngeal
Procerus	Fascia covering lower parts of nasal bone and upper part of lateral nasal cartilage	Skin between and above eyebrow	Temporal and zygomatic branches of facial nerve	Draws down medial angle of eyebrows, produces transverse wrinkles over bridge of nose	Angular and lateral nasal branches of facial artery	Facial expression
Rectus capitis anterior	Lateral mass of atlas	Base of occipital bone in front of foramen magnum	Ventral rami of cervical nerves (C1–C2)	Flexes head	Muscular branches of vertebral artery, ascending pharyngeal artery	Prevertebral
Rectus capitis lateralis	Upper surface of transverse process of atlas	Inferior surface of jugular process of occipital bone	Ventral rami of cervical nerves (C1–C2)	Flexes head laterally to same side	Muscular branches of vertebral artery, occipital artery, ascending pharyngeal artery	Prevertebral
Risorius	Fascia over masseter superficial to platysma	Skin at angle of mouth	Zygomatic and buccal branches of facial nerve	Retracts angle of mouth	Superior labial branch of facial artery	Facial expression
Salpingopharyngeus	Pharyngotympanic (auditory, eustachian) tube	Side of pharyngeal wall	Vagus nerve via pharyngeal plexus	Elevates pharynx and larynx during swallowing and speaking	Pharyngeal branch of ascending pharyngeal artery	Longitudinal pharyngeal

MUSCLE	PROXIMAL ATTACHMENT (ORIGIN)	DISTAL ATTACHMENT (INSERTION)	INNERVATION	MAIN ACTIONS	BLOOD SUPPLY	MUSCLE GROUP
Scalene (anterior)	Anterior tubercles of transverse processes of C3–C6	Scalene tubercle on 1st rib	Anterior rami of cervical nerves (C5–C8)	Elevates 1st rib, bends neck	Ascending cervical branch of inferior thyroid artery	Prevertebral
Scalene (medius)	Posterior tubercles of transverse processes of C2–C7	Upper surface of 1st rib (behind subclavian groove)	Anterior rami of cervical nerves (C3–C7)	Elevates 1st rib, bends neck	Muscular branches of ascending cervical artery	Prevertebral
Scalene (posterior)	Posterior tubercles of transverse processes of C4–C6	Outer surface of 2nd rib (behind attachment of serratus anterior)	Anterior rami of lower four cervical nerves	Elevates 2nd rib, bends neck	Muscular branches of ascending cervical division of inferior thyroid artery, superficial branch of transverse cervical artery	Prevertebral
Sphincter pupillae	Circular smooth muscle of iris that passes around pupil	Blends with dilator pupillae fibers	Parasympathetic fibers via oculomotor nerve (CN III)	Constricts pupil	Ophthalmic artery	Intrinsic eye
Stapedius	Pyramidal eminence of temporal bone	Stapes	Facial nerve	Pulls stapes posteriorly to lessen oscillation of tympanic membrane	Posterior auricular, anterior tympanic, and middle meningeal arteries	Middle ear
Sternocleidomastoid	*Sternal head:* anterior surface of manubrium *Clavicular head:* upper surface of medial 1/3 of clavicle	Lateral surface of mastoid process; lateral half of superior nuchal line of occipital bone	Accessory nerve (CN XI)	*Bilaterally:* flex head, raise thorax *Unilaterally:* turns face toward opposite side	Sternocleidomastoid branch of superior thyroid and occipital arteries, muscular branch of suprascapular artery, occipital branch of posterior auricular artery	Neck
Sternohyoid	Posterior surface of manubrium sterni, posterior sternoclavicular ligament, medial end of clavicle	Medial part of lower border of body of hyoid bone	Ansa cervicalis	Depresses larynx and hyoid bone, steadies hyoid bone	Sternocleidomastoid and hyoid branches of superior thyroid artery, hyoid branch of lingual artery	Infrahyoid
Sternothyroid	Posterior surface of manubrium sterni below and deep to origin of sternohyoid, edge of first costal cartilage	Oblique line on lamina of thyroid cartilage	Ansa cervicalis	Depresses larynx and thyroid cartilage	Cricothyroid branch of superior thyroid artery	Infrahyoid
Styloglossus	Styloid process and stylohyoid ligament	Lateral and inferior aspect of tongue	Hypoglossal nerve (CN XII)	Retracts tongue and draws it up for swallowing	Sublingual artery	Extrinsic tongue
Stylohyoid	Posterior border of styloid process	Body of hyoid bone at junction with greater horn	Facial nerve	Elevates hyoid bone and base of tongue	Muscular branches of facial artery, muscular branches of occipital artery	Suprahyoid
Stylopharyngeus	Medial aspect of styloid process	Pharyngeal wall	Glossopharyngeal nerve (CN IX)	Elevates pharynx and larynx during swallowing and speaking	Ascending pharyngeal artery, ascending palatine and tonsillar branches of facial artery, dorsal branches of lingual artery	Longitudinal pharyngeal
Subclavius	Upper border of 1st rib and its cartilage	Inferior surface of middle third of clavicle	Nerve to subclavius	Anchors and depresses clavicle	Clavicular branch of thoraco-acromial artery	Neck
Superior longitudinal muscle of tongue	Submucous fibers at back of tongue	Tip of tongue; unites with muscle of opposite side	Hypoglossal nerve (CN XII)	Shortens tongue, turns tip and sides upward	Deep lingual branch of lingual artery, branches from facial artery	Intrinsic tongue
Superior oblique	Body of sphenoid (above optic foramen), medial to origin of superior rectus	Passes through trochlea, attaches to superior sclera between superior and lateral recti	Trochlear nerve (CN IV)	Abducts, depresses, and medially rotates eyeball	Ophthalmic artery	Extra-ocular

MUSCLE	PROXIMAL ATTACHMENT (ORIGIN)	DISTAL ATTACHMENT (INSERTION)	INNERVATION	MAIN ACTIONS	BLOOD SUPPLY	MUSCLE GROUP
Superior pharyngeal constrictor	Hamulus, pterygomandibular raphe, mylohyoid line of mandible	Median raphe of pharynx	Vagus nerve via pharyngeal plexus	Constricts wall of pharynx during swallowing	Ascending pharyngeal artery, ascending palatine and tonsillar branches of facial artery, dorsal branches of lingual artery	Circular pharyngeal
Superior rectus	Common tendinous ring	Superior aspect of eyeball, posterior to the corneoscleral junction	Oculomotor nerve (CN III), superior division	Elevates, adducts, and medially rotates eyeball	Ophthalmic artery	Extra-ocular
Temporalis	Floor of temporal fossa, deep temporal fascia	Coronoid process and ramus of mandible	Mandibular nerve (CN V_3),deep temporal nerves	Elevates mandible; posterior fibers retrude mandible	Superficial temporal and maxillary arteries, middle, anterior, and posterior deep temporal arteries	Mastication
Tensor tympani	Cartilage of pharyngotympanic (auditory, eustachian) tube	Handle of malleus	Mandibular branch of trigeminal nerve (CN V_3)	Tenses tympanic membrane by drawing it medially	Superior tympanic branch of middle meningeal division of maxillary artery	Middle ear
Tensor veli palatini	Scaphoid fossa of medial pterygoid plate, spine of sphenoid, pharyngotympanic (auditory, eustachian) tube	Palatine aponeurosis	Mandibular nerve	Tenses soft palate, opens pharyngotympanic (auditory, eustachian) tube during swallowing and yawning	Ascending palatine artery branch of facial artery, descending palatine artery branch of maxillary artery	Palatal
Thyro-arytenoid	Posterior aspect of thyroid cartilage	Muscular process of arytenoid cartilage	Recurrent laryngeal nerve	Shortens and relaxes vocal cords, sphincter of vestibule	Superior and inferior thyroid arteries	Laryngeal
Thyrohyoid	Oblique line on lamina of thyroid cartilage	Lower border of body and greater horn of hyoid bone	Thyrohyoid branch of C1 nerve via hypoglossal nerve (CN XII)	Depresses larynx and hyoid bone, elevates thyroid cartilage	Hyoid branch of superior thyroid artery	Infrahyoid
Transverse and oblique arytenoid	Arytenoid cartilage	Opposite arytenoid cartilage	Recurrent laryngeal nerve	Closes intercartilaginous portion of rima glottides	Superior and inferior thyroid arteries	Laryngeal
Transverse (tongue)	Median fibrous septum of tongue	Dorsum and sides of tongue	Hypoglossal nerve (CN XII)	Narrows and elongates tongue	Deep lingual branch of lingual artery, branches from facial artery	Intrinsic tongue
Uvular muscle	Nasal spine, palatine aponeurosis	Mucosa of uvula	Vagus nerve via pharyngeal plexus	Shortens, elevates, and retracts uvula	Ascending palatine artery branch of facial artery, descending palatine artery branch of maxillary artery	Palatal
Vertical (tongue)	Mucous membrane on dorsum of forepart of tongue	Fibers extend from dorsum to undersurface of tongue	Hypoglossal nerve (CN XII)	Flattens and broadens tongue	Deep lingual branch of lingual artery, branches from facial artery	Intrinsic tongue
Vocalis	Vocal process of arytenoid cartilage	Vocal ligament	Recurrent laryngeal nerve	Tenses anterior vocal ligament, relaxes posterior vocal ligament	Superior and inferior thyroid arteries	Laryngeal
Zygomaticus major	Zygomatic arch	Angle of mouth	Zygomatic and buccal branches of facial nerve	Draws angle of mouth backward and upward	Superior labial branch of facial artery	Facial expression
Zygomaticus minor	Zygomatic arch	Angle of mouth, upper lip	Zygomatic and buccal branches of facial nerve	Elevates upper lip	Superior labial branch of facial artery	Facial expression

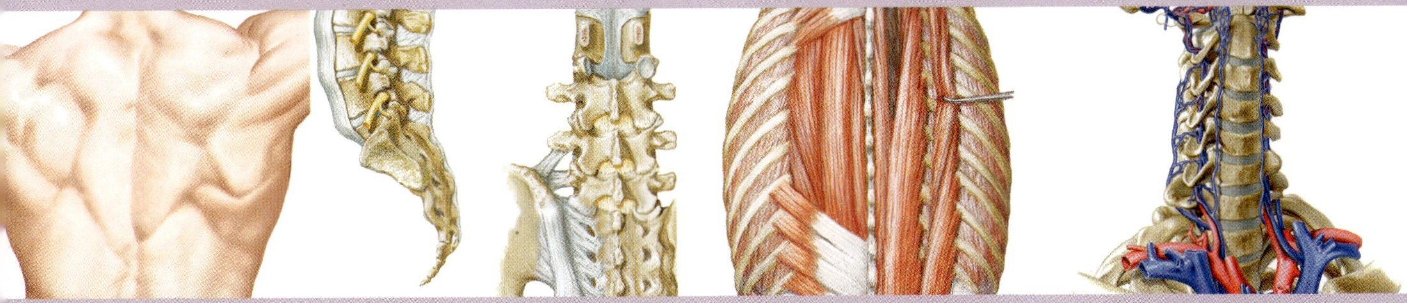

2 BACK AND SPINAL CORD

Topographic Anatomy
Plate 152

152 Back: Surface Anatomy

Bones and Ligaments
Plates 153–159

153 Vertebral Column
154 Thoracic Vertebrae
155 Lumbar Vertebrae
156 Vertebrae: Radiology
157 Sacrum and Coccyx
158 Vertebral Ligaments: Lumbosacral Region
159 Vertebral Ligaments: Lumbar Region

Spinal Cord
Plates 160–170

160 Spinal Cord and Ventral Rami in Situ
161 Relation of Spinal Nerve Roots to Vertebrae
162 Dermatomes
163 Sympathetic Nervous System: Schema
164 Parasympathetic Nervous System: Schema
165 Spinal Membranes and Nerve Roots
166 Spinal Nerve Origin: Cross Sections
167 Arteries of Spinal Cord: Schema
168 Arteries of Spinal Cord: Intrinsic Distribution
169 Veins of Spinal Cord and Vertebral Column
170 Veins of Vertebral Column: Vertebral Veins

Muscles and Nerves

Plates 171–175

171 Muscles of Back: Superficial Layers
172 Muscles of Back: Intermediate Layers
173 Muscles of Back: Deep Layers
174 Nerves of Back
175 Suboccipital Triangle

Cross-Sectional Anatomy

Plates 176–177

176 Lumbar Region of Back: Cross Section
177 Typical Thoracic Spinal Nerve: Cross Section

Muscle Tables

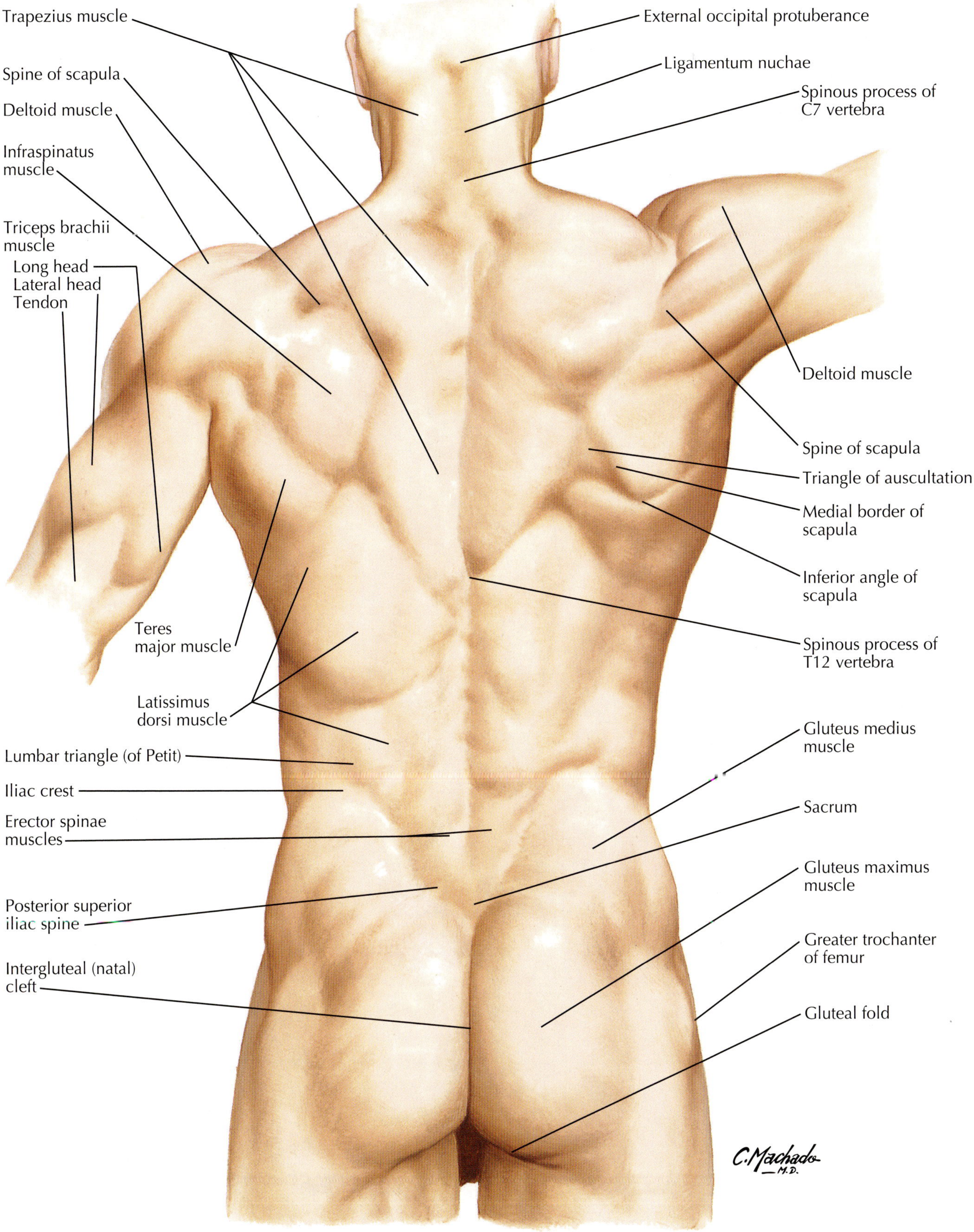
Trapezius muscle
Spine of scapula
Deltoid muscle
Infraspinatus muscle
Triceps brachii muscle
Long head
Lateral head
Tendon
Teres major muscle
Latissimus dorsi muscle
Lumbar triangle (of Petit)
Iliac crest
Erector spinae muscles
Posterior superior iliac spine
Intergluteal (natal) cleft
External occipital protuberance
Ligamentum nuchae
Spinous process of C7 vertebra
Deltoid muscle
Spine of scapula
Triangle of auscultation
Medial border of scapula
Inferior angle of scapula
Spinous process of T12 vertebra
Gluteus medius muscle
Sacrum
Gluteus maximus muscle
Greater trochanter of femur
Gluteal fold
C. Machado M.D.

Vertebral Column

See also Plates 21, 183, 243

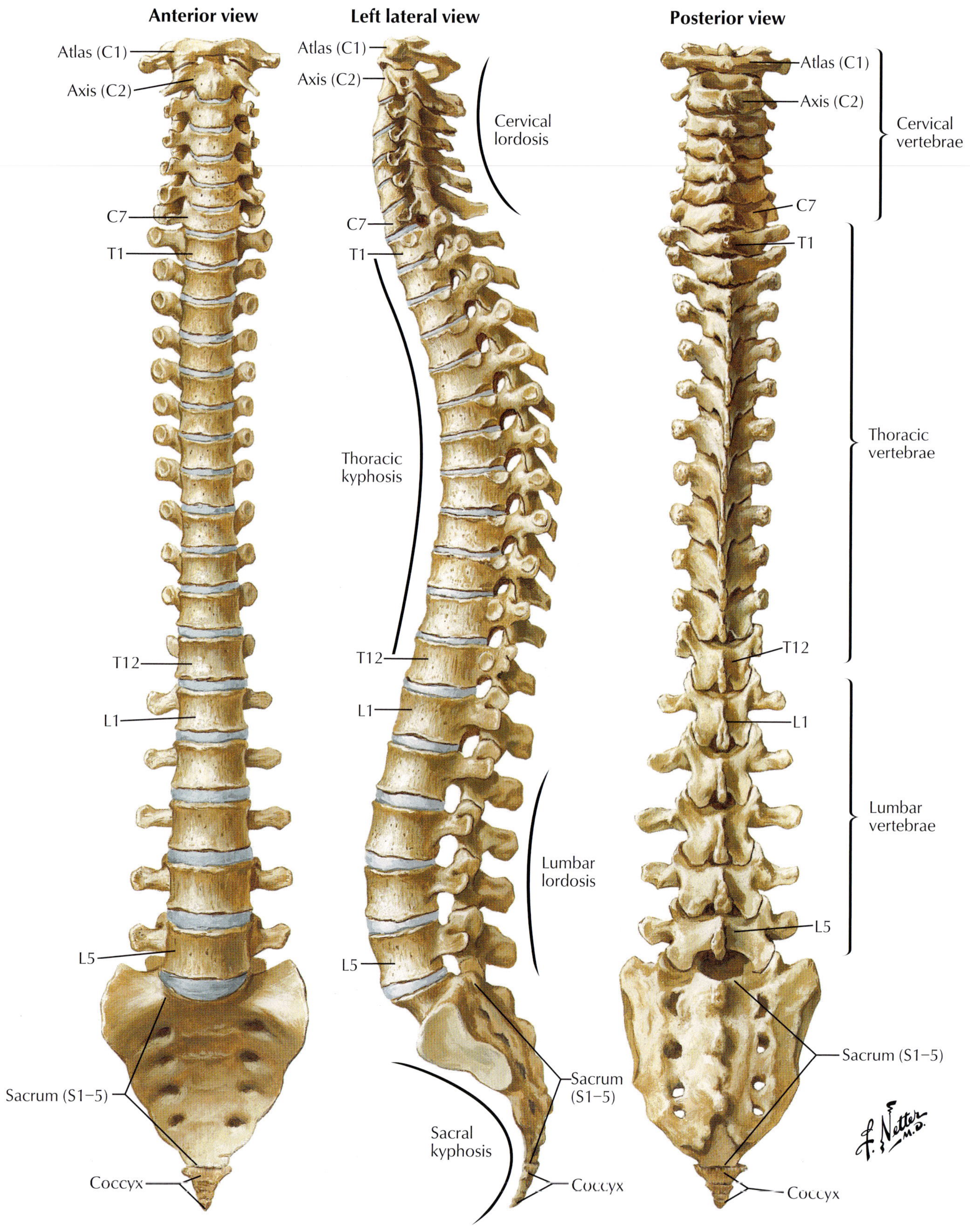

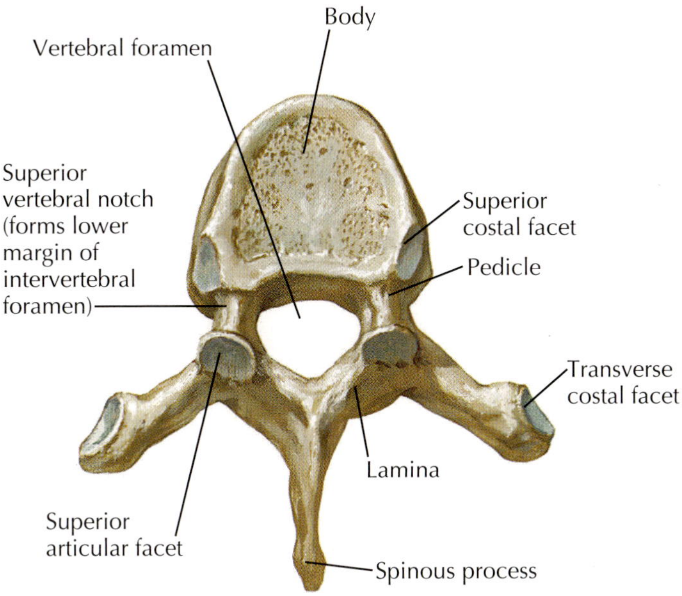

T6 vertebra: superior view

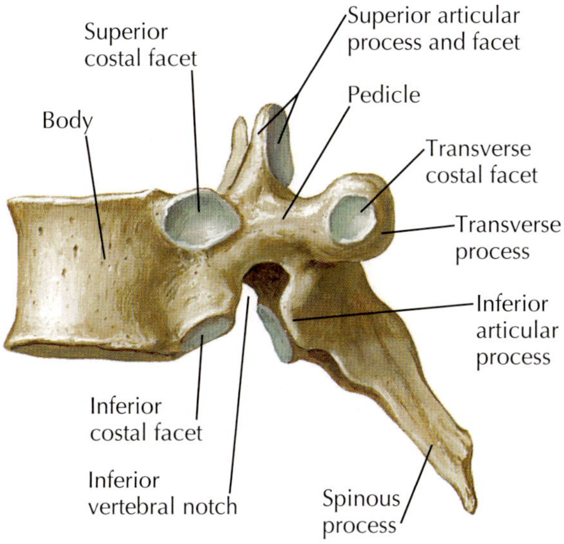

T6 vertebra: lateral view

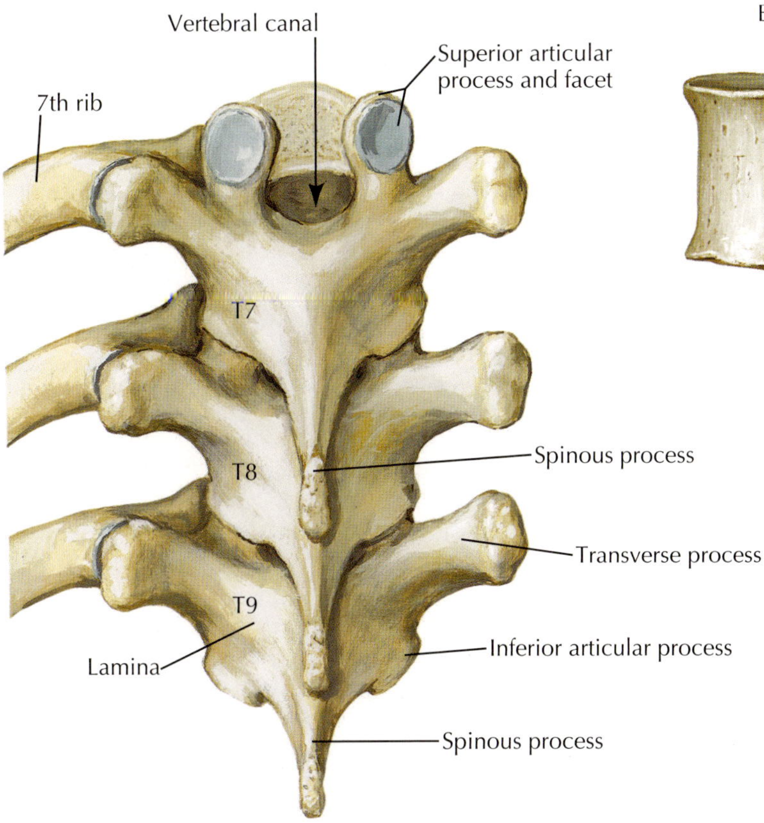

T7, T8, and T9 vertebrae: posterior view

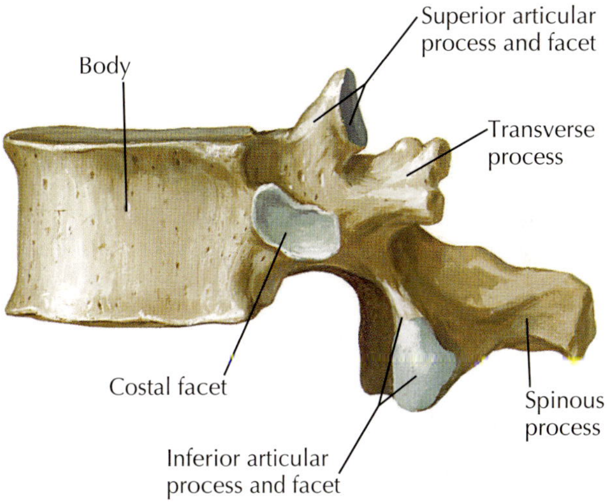

T12 vertebra: lateral view

Lumbar Vertebrae

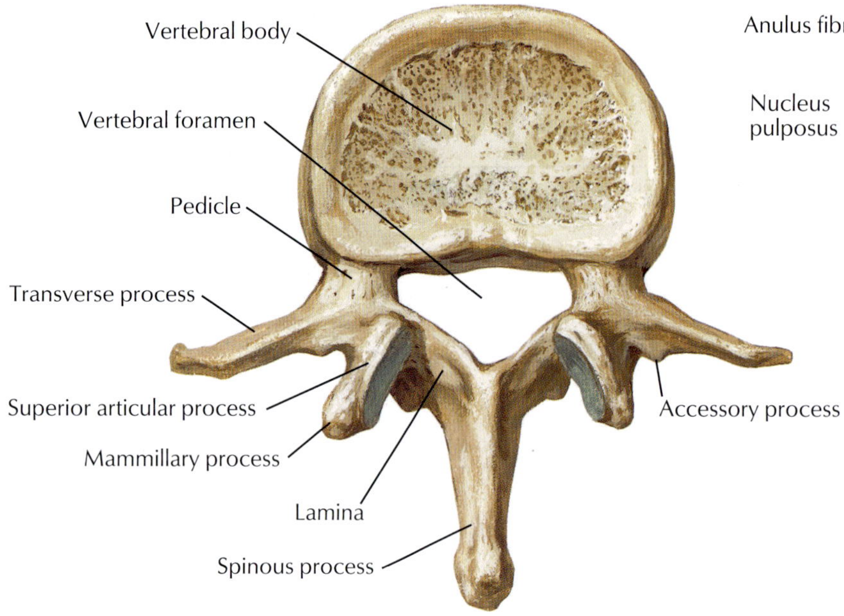

L2 vertebra: superior view

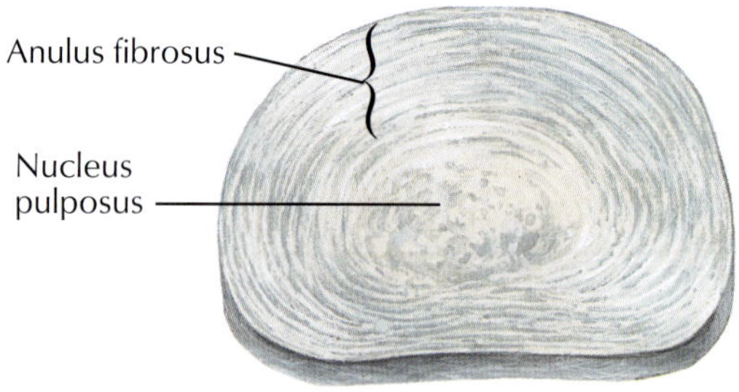

Intervertebral disc

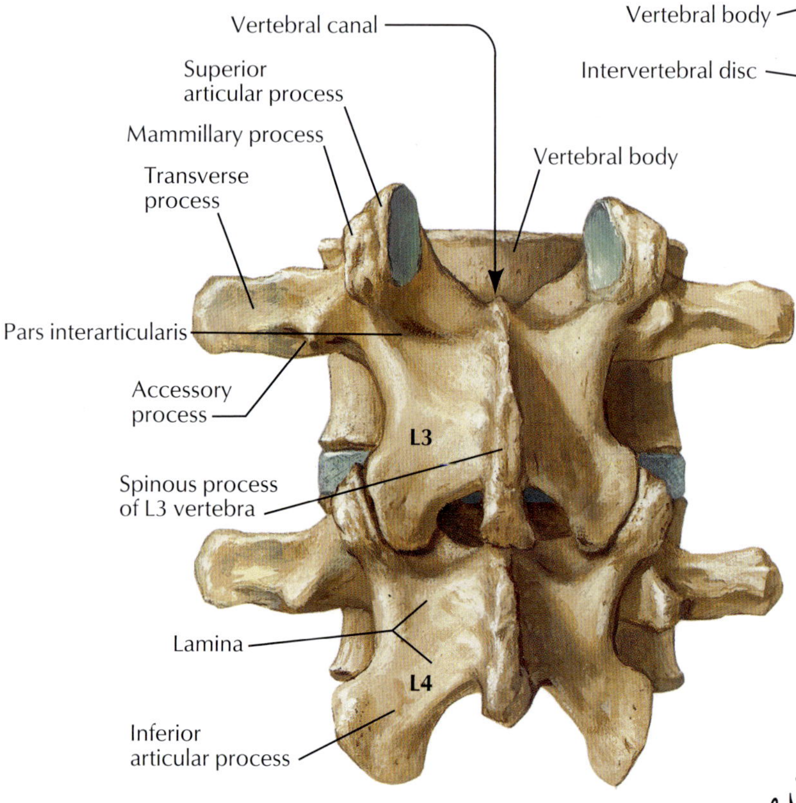

L3 and L4 vertebrae: posterior view

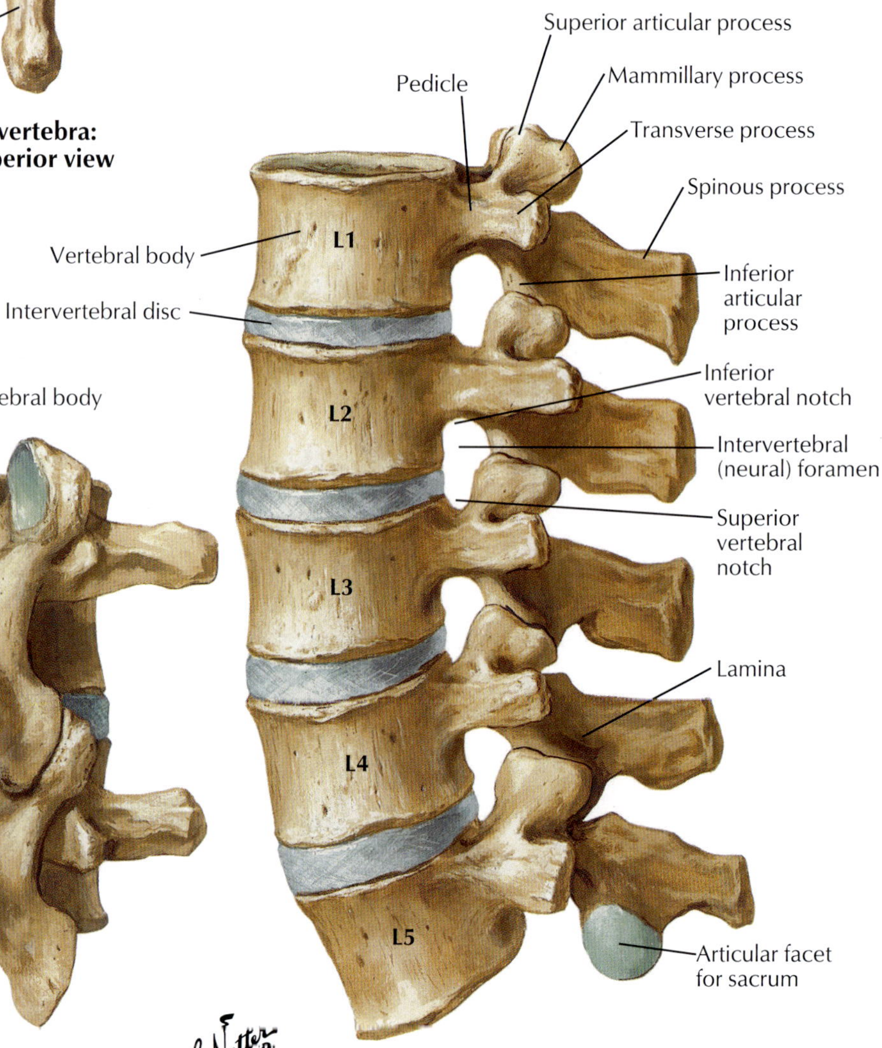

Lumbar vertebrae, articulated: left lateral view

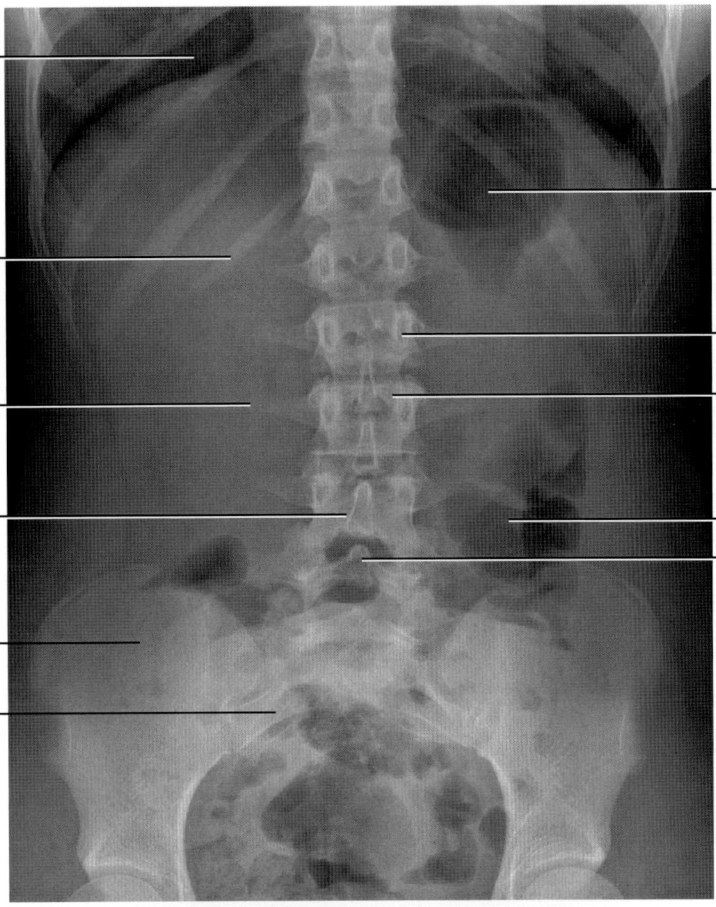
Lung
12th rib
Transverse process L3
Lamina L4
Ilium
Sacrum
Air in stomach
Pedicle L2
Inferior articular process L2
Air in colon
Spinous process

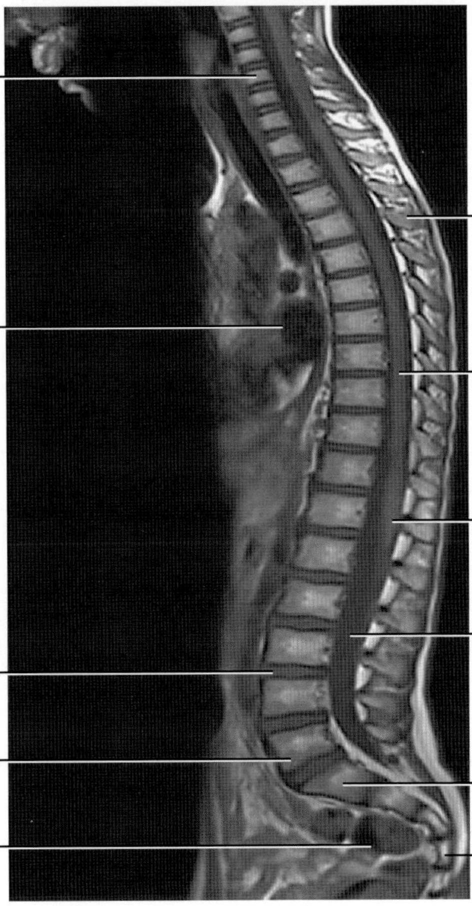
Body of cervical vertebra
Heart
L3/L4 intervertebral disc
Body L5
Rectum
Spinous process of thoracic vertebra
Spinal cord
Conus medullaris
Lumbar cistern
S1 vertebra
Coccyx

Sacrum and Coccyx

See also **Plates 330, 334**

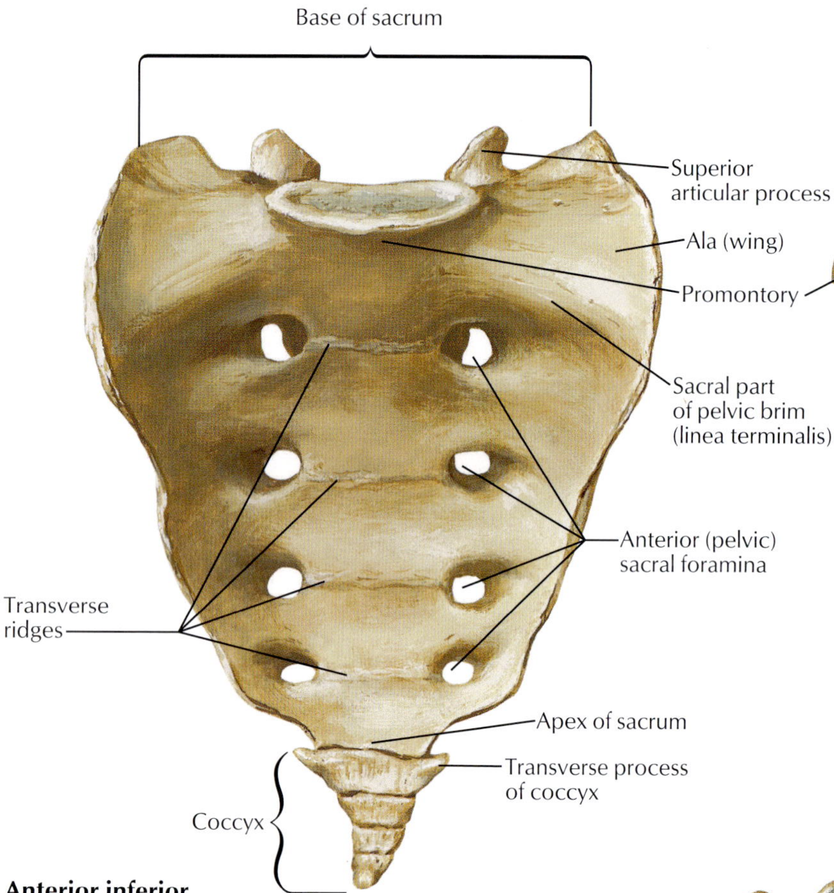

Anterior inferior view

Pelvic surface

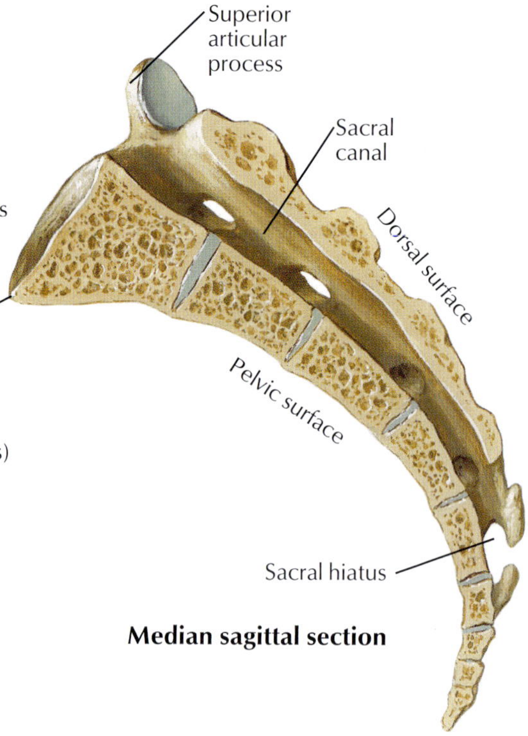

Median sagittal section

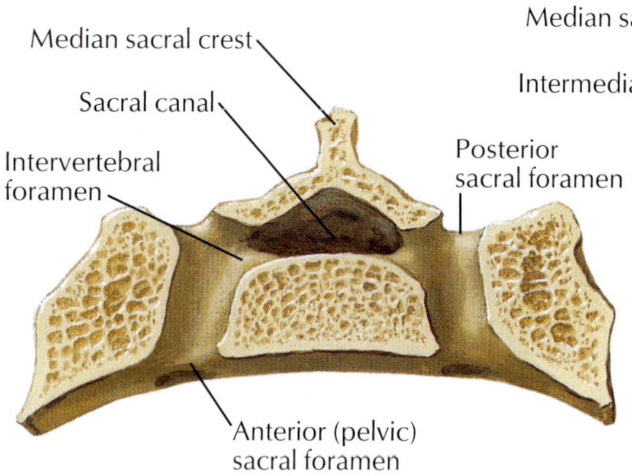

Transverse section through S2 foramina

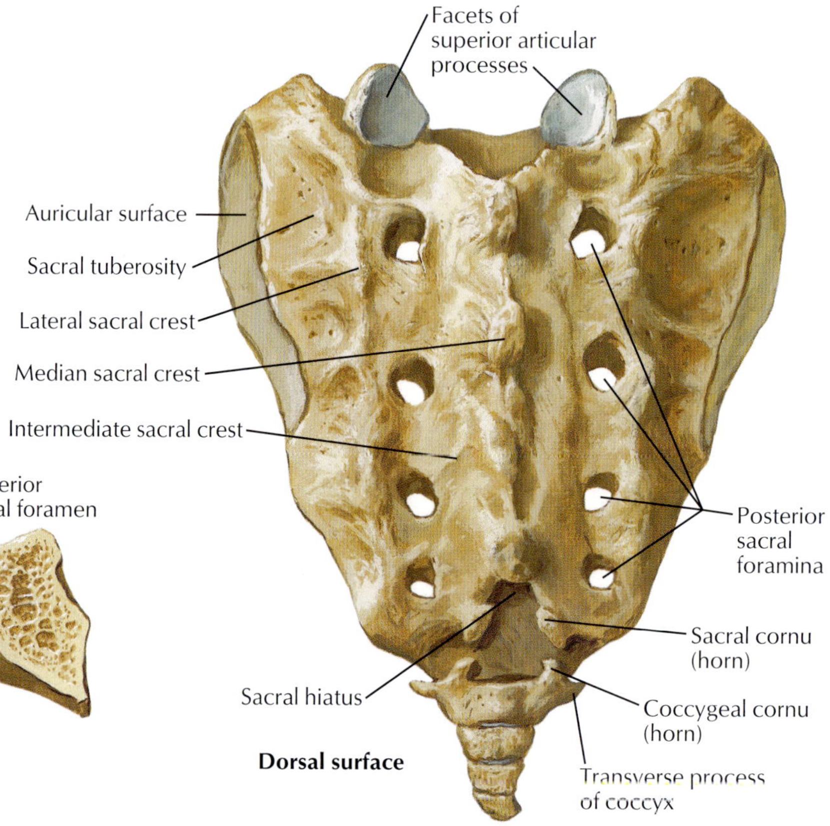

Dorsal surface

Posterior superior view

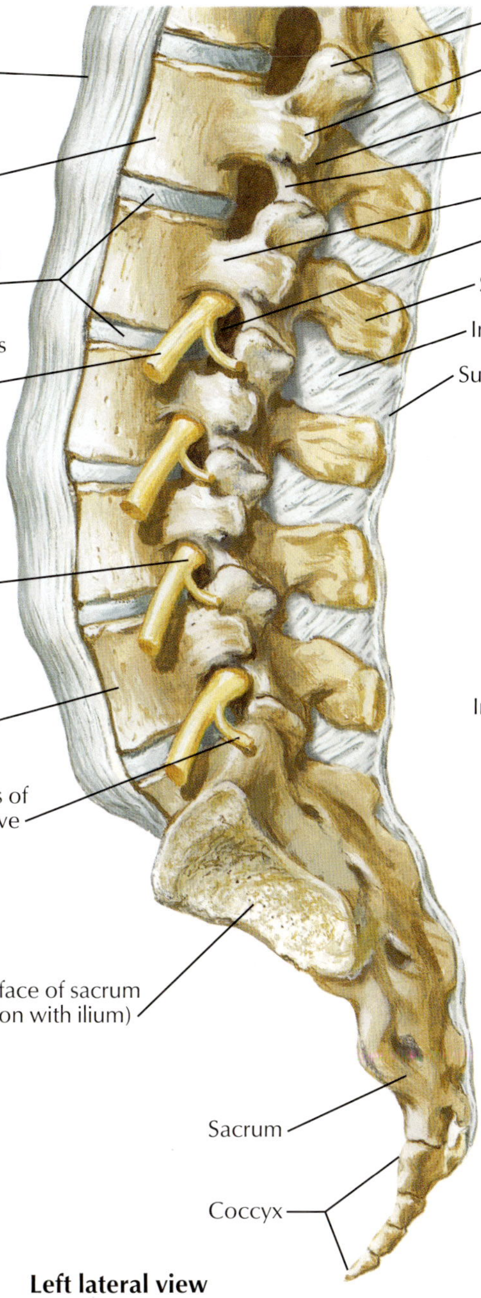

Left lateral view

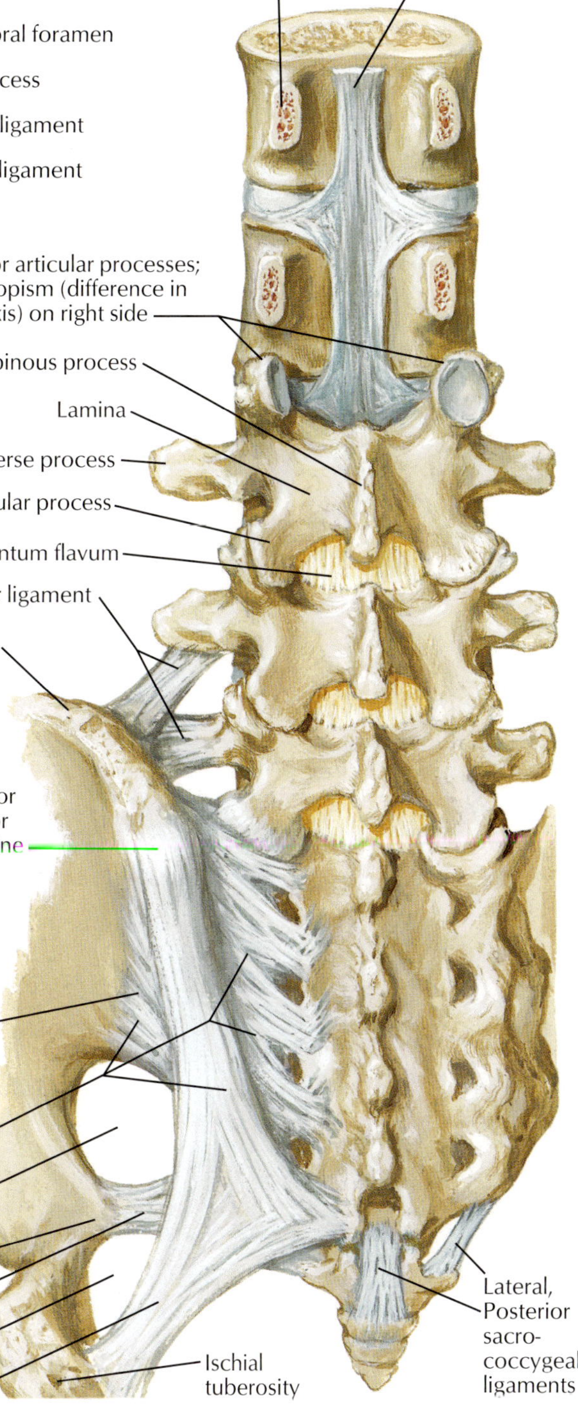

Posterior view

Vertebral Ligaments: Lumbar Region

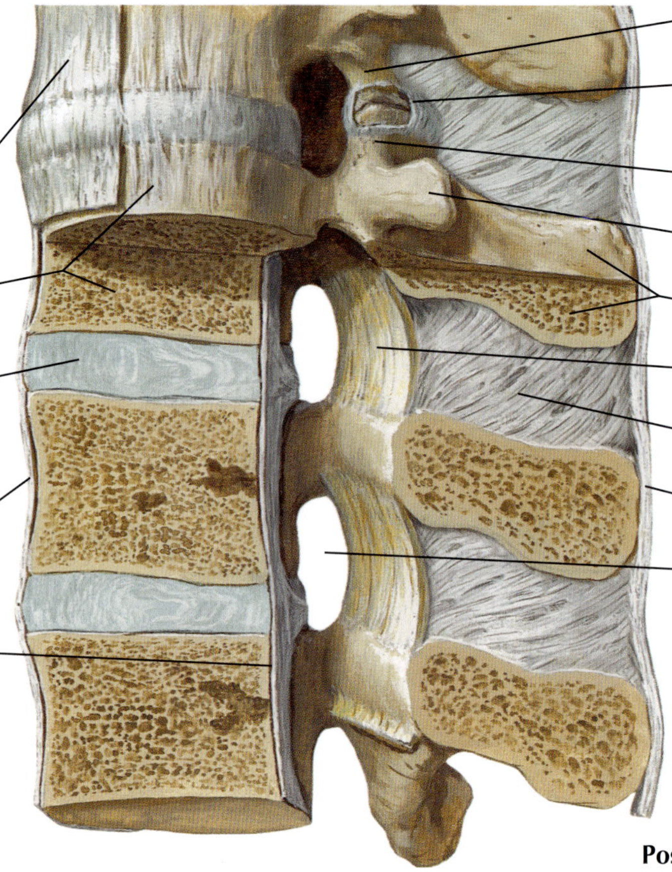

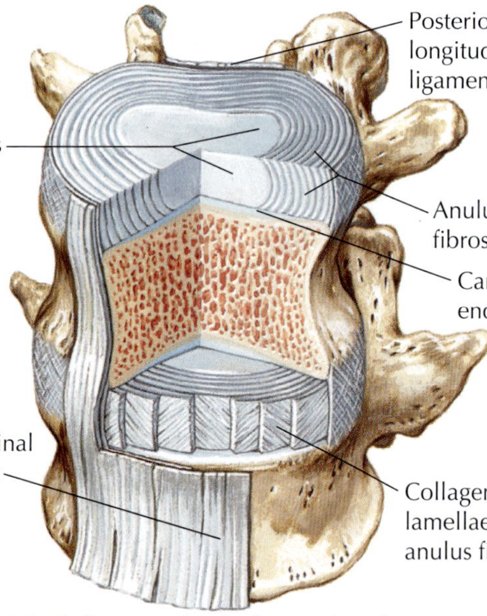

Intervertebral disc composed of central nuclear zone of collagen and hydrated proteoglycans surrounded by concentric lamellae of collagen fibers

Posterior vertebral arches: anterior view

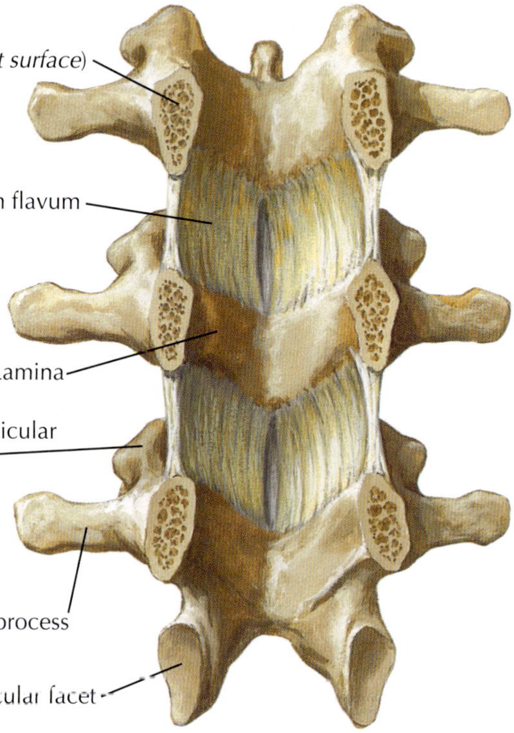

F. Netter M.D. C. Machado M.D.

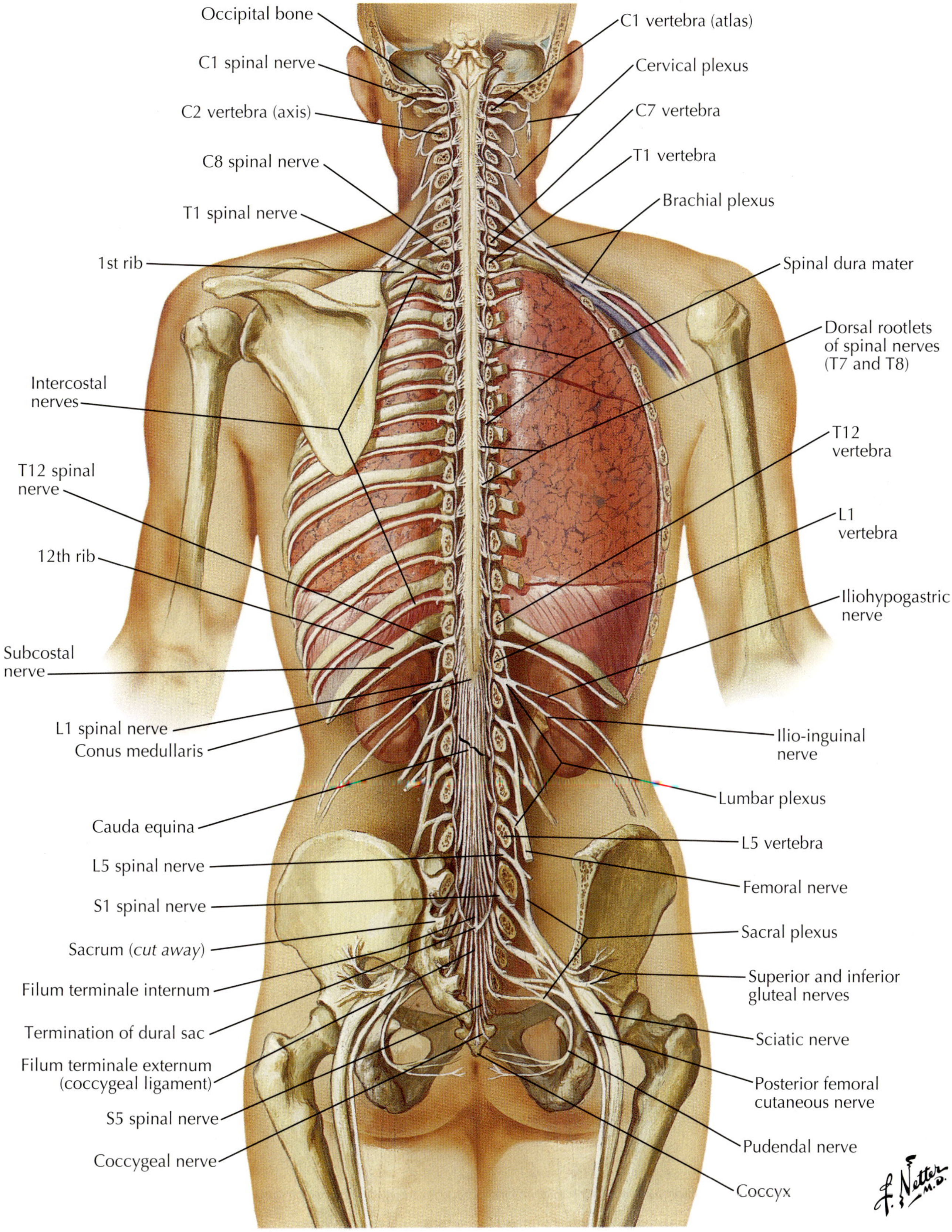
Occipital bone
C1 spinal nerve
C2 vertebra (axis)
C8 spinal nerve
T1 spinal nerve
1st rib
Intercostal nerves
T12 spinal nerve
12th rib
Subcostal nerve
L1 spinal nerve
Conus medullaris
Cauda equina
L5 spinal nerve
S1 spinal nerve
Sacrum (cut away)
Filum terminale internum
Termination of dural sac
Filum terminale externum (coccygeal ligament)
S5 spinal nerve
Coccygeal nerve
C1 vertebra (atlas)
Cervical plexus
C7 vertebra
T1 vertebra
Brachial plexus
Spinal dura mater
Dorsal rootlets of spinal nerves (T7 and T8)
T12 vertebra
L1 vertebra
Iliohypogastric nerve
Ilio-inguinal nerve
Lumbar plexus
L5 vertebra
Femoral nerve
Sacral plexus
Superior and inferior gluteal nerves
Sciatic nerve
Posterior femoral cutaneous nerve
Pudendal nerve
Coccyx
F. Netter M.D.

Relation of Spinal Nerve Roots to Vertebrae

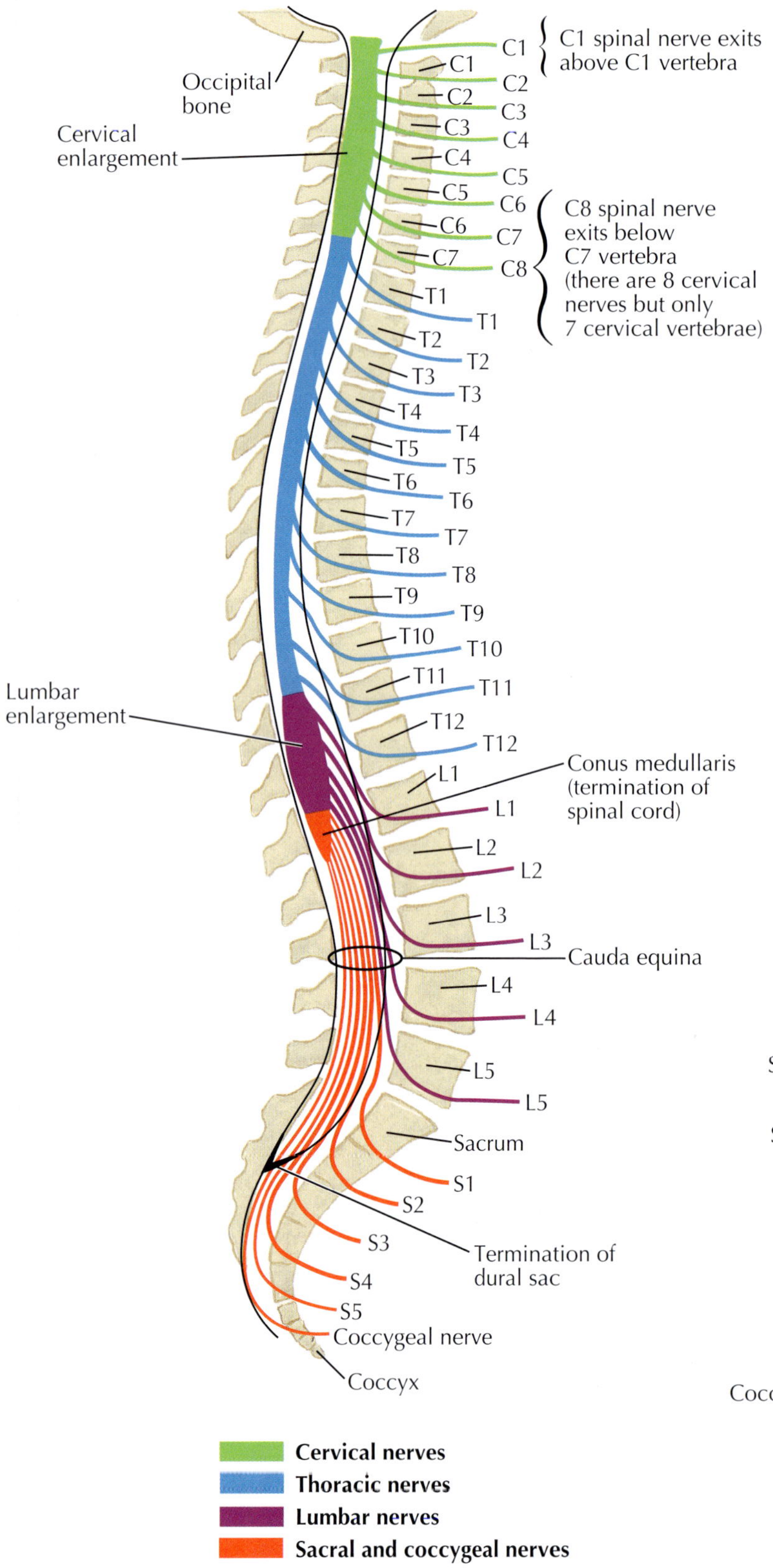

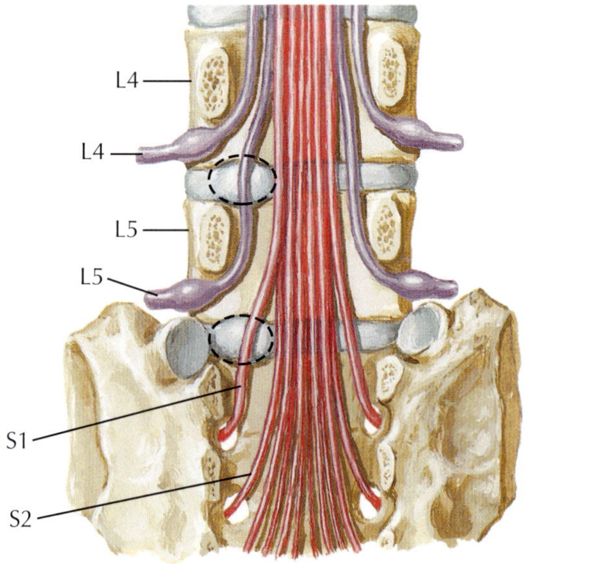

Lumbar disc protrusion (*dashed ovals*) does not usually affect nerve exiting above disc. Lateral protrusion at disc level L4–5 affects L5 spinal nerve, not L4 spinal nerve. Protrusion at disc level L5–S1 affects S1 spinal nerve, not L5 spinal nerve.

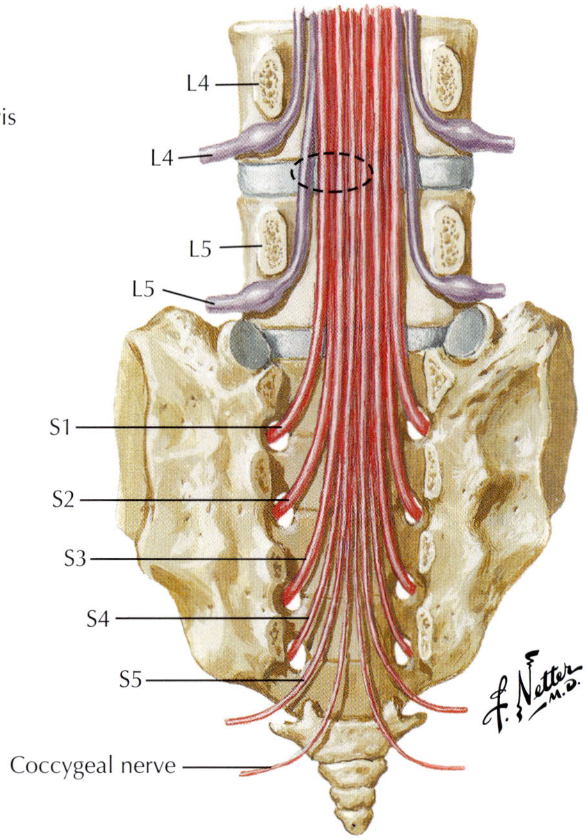

Medial protrusion at disc level L4–5 (*dashed oval*) rarely affects L4 spinal nerve but may affect L5 spinal nerve and sometimes S1–4 spinal nerves.

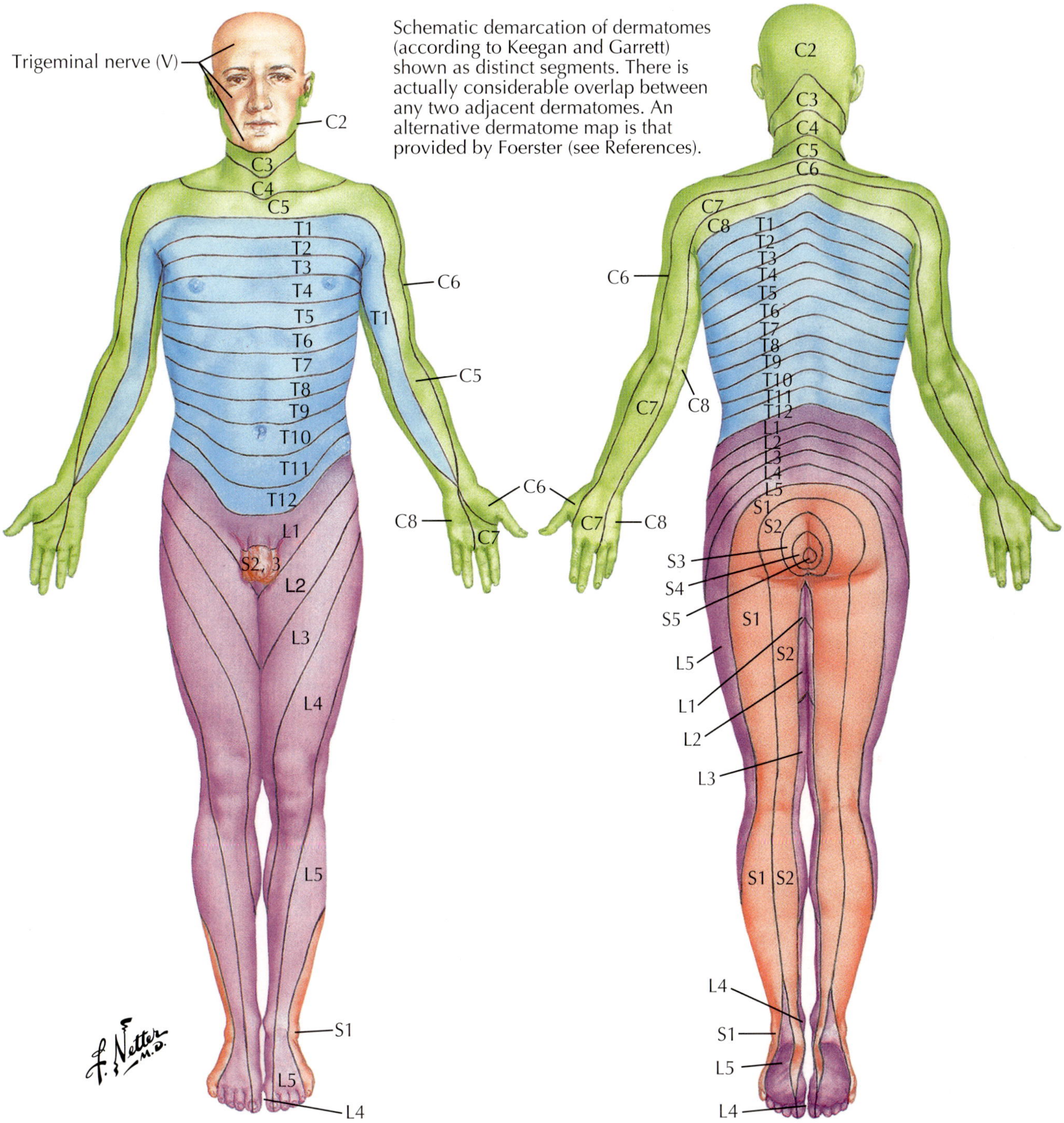

Schematic demarcation of dermatomes (according to Keegan and Garrett) shown as distinct segments. There is actually considerable overlap between any two adjacent dermatomes. An alternative dermatome map is that provided by Foerster (see References).

Levels of principal dermatomes

C5	Clavicles
C5, 6	Lateral sides of upper limbs
C8, T1	Medial sides of upper limbs
C6	Digit I (thumb)
C6, 7, 8	Hand
C8	Digits IV and V (ring and little fingers)
T4	Level of nipples
T10	Level of umbilicus
L1	Inguinal region
L1, 2, 3, 4	Anterior and inner surfaces of lower limbs
L4, 5, S1	Foot
L4	Medial side digit I (great toe)
L5, S1, 2	Lateral and posterior surfaces of lower limbs
S1	Lateral margin of foot and digit V (little toe)
S2, 3, 4	Perineum

Sympathetic Nervous System: Schema

See also **Plates 206, 317, 319**

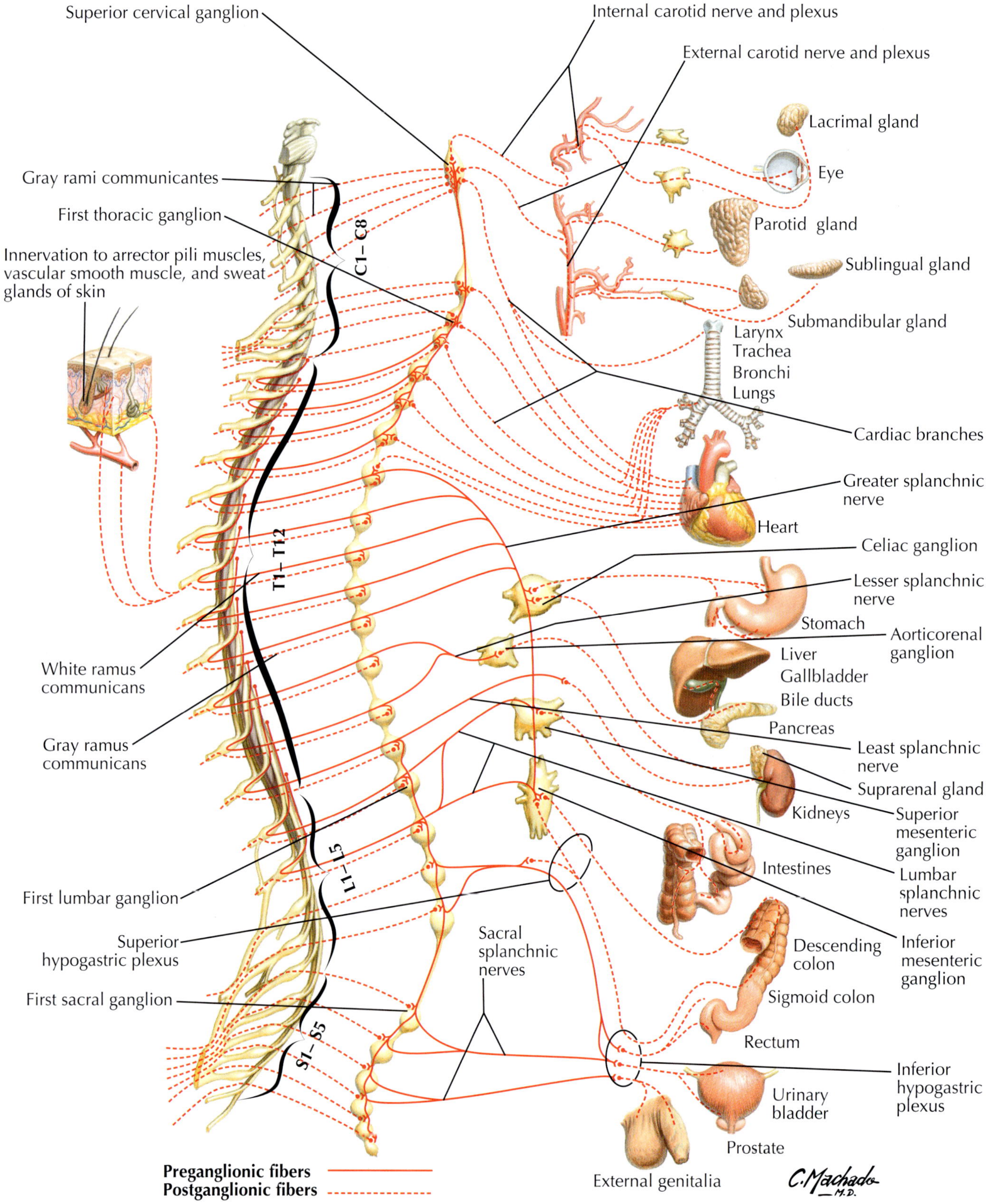

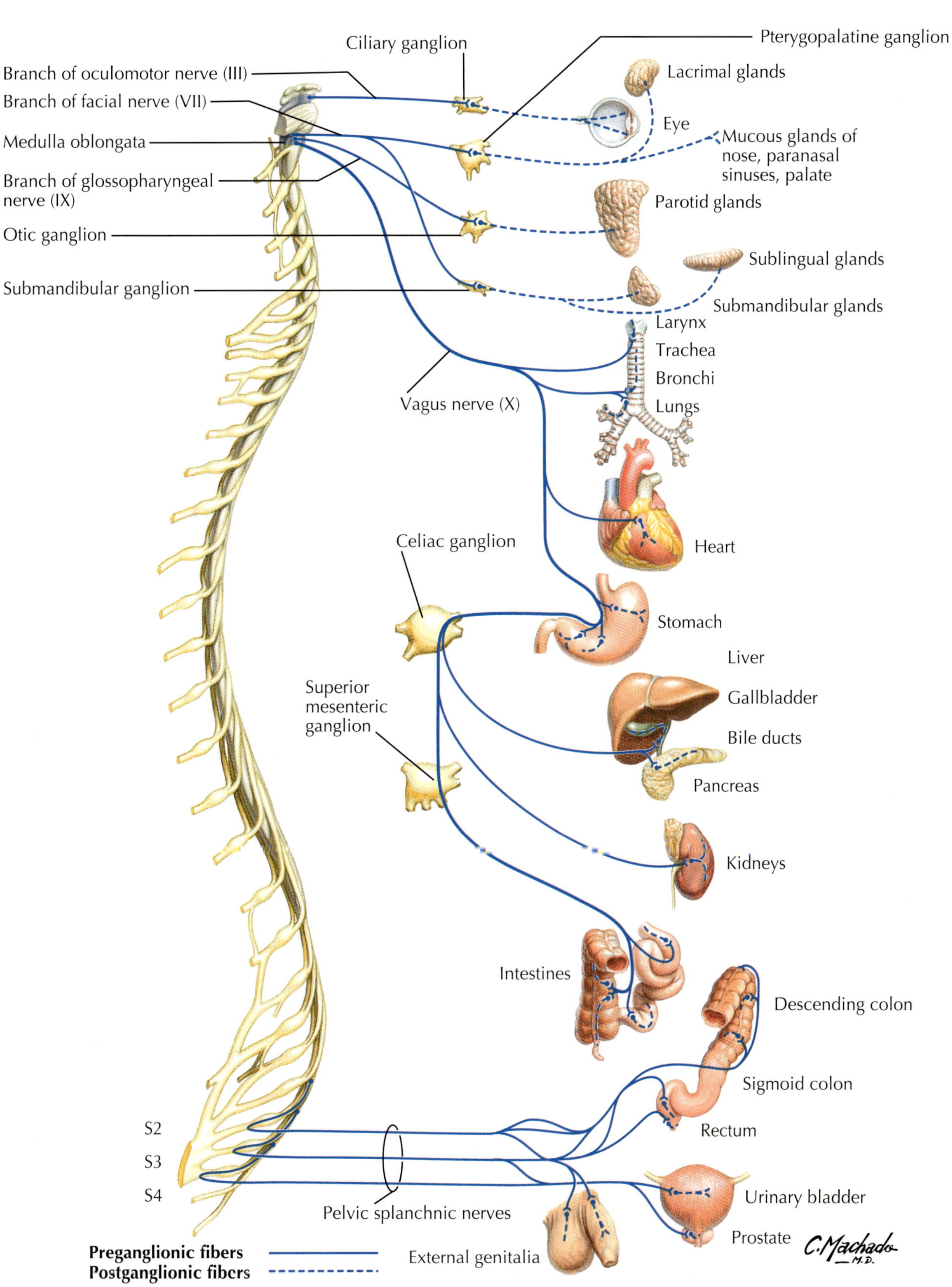
Ciliary ganglion
Pterygopalatine ganglion
Branch of oculomotor nerve (III)
Branch of facial nerve (VII)
Medulla oblongata
Branch of glossopharyngeal nerve (IX)
Otic ganglion
Submandibular ganglion
Lacrimal glands
Eye
Mucous glands of nose, paranasal sinuses, palate
Parotid glands
Sublingual glands
Submandibular glands
Larynx
Trachea
Bronchi
Lungs
Vagus nerve (X)
Heart
Celiac ganglion
Stomach
Liver
Gallbladder
Bile ducts
Superior mesenteric ganglion
Pancreas
Kidneys
Intestines
Descending colon
Sigmoid colon
Rectum
S2
S3
S4
Urinary bladder
Prostate
Pelvic splanchnic nerves
External genitalia
Preganglionic fibers
Postganglionic fibers
C.Machado M.D.

Spinal Membranes and Nerve Roots

Posterior view

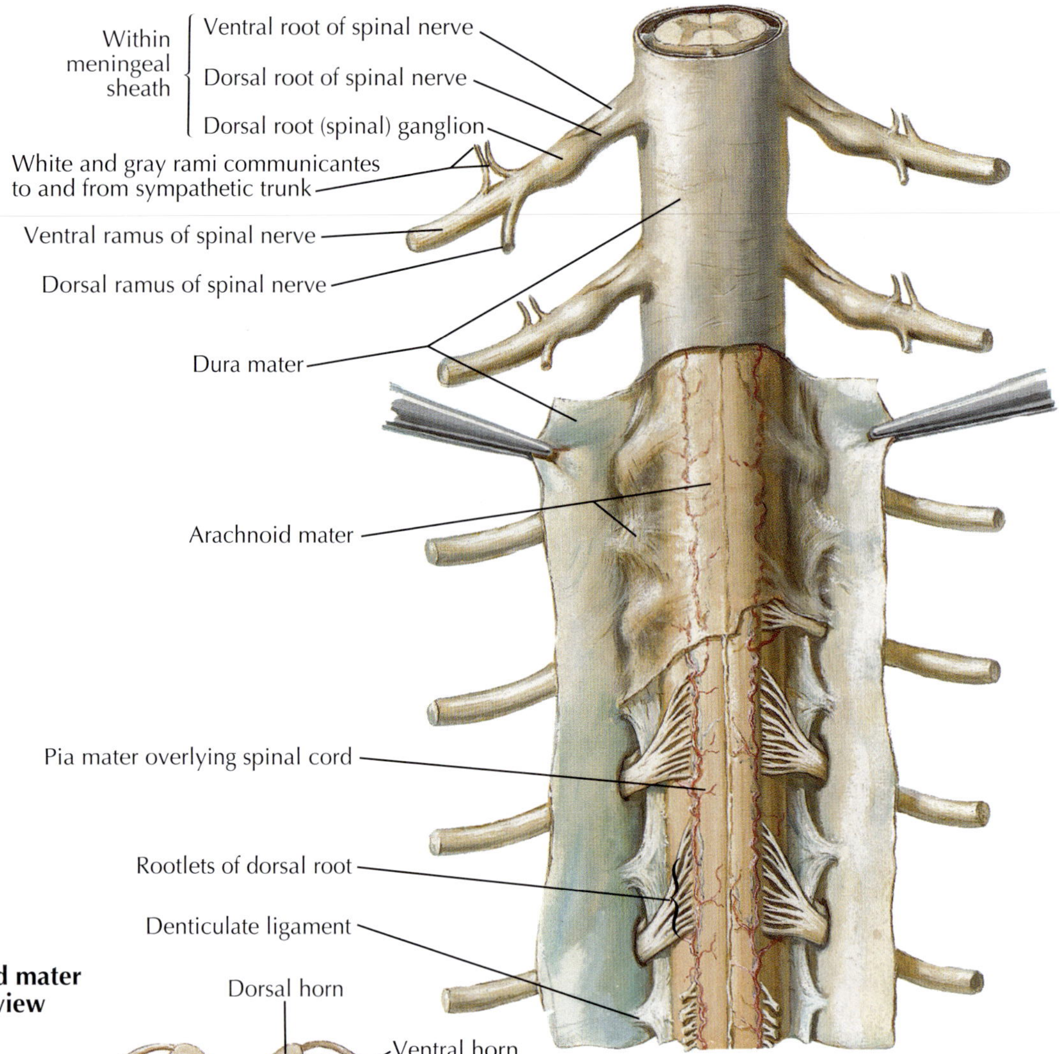

Dura and arachnoid mater removed: anterior view *(greatly magnified)*

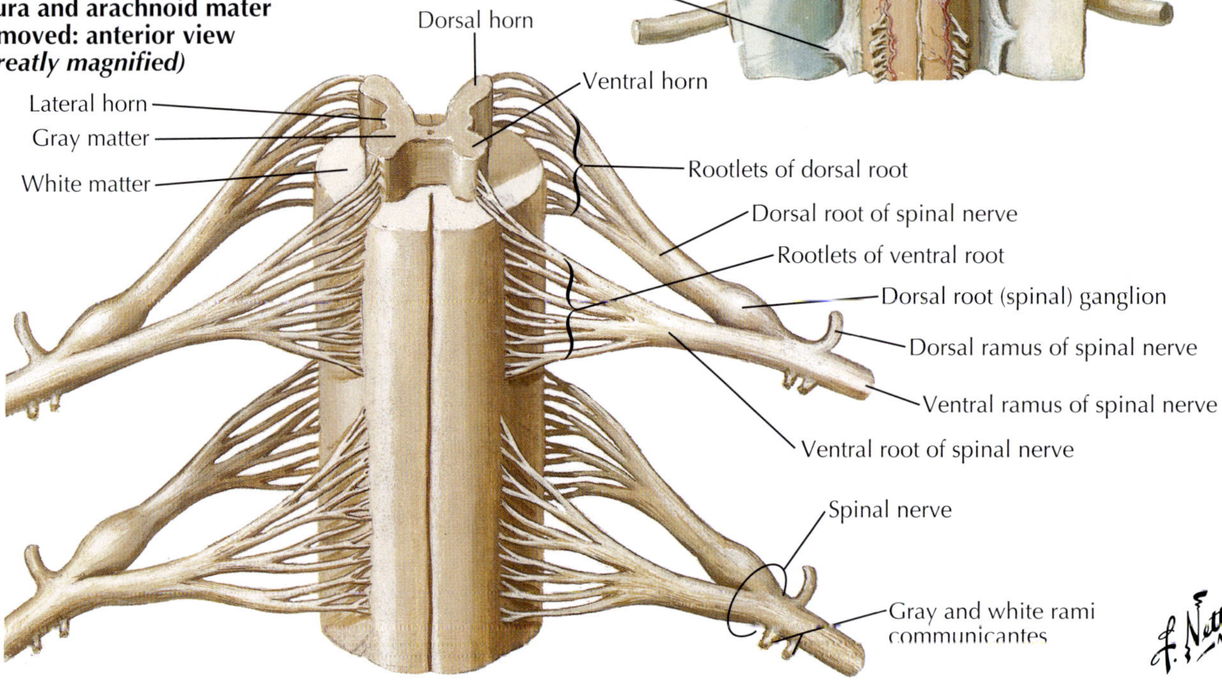

Section through thoracic vertebra

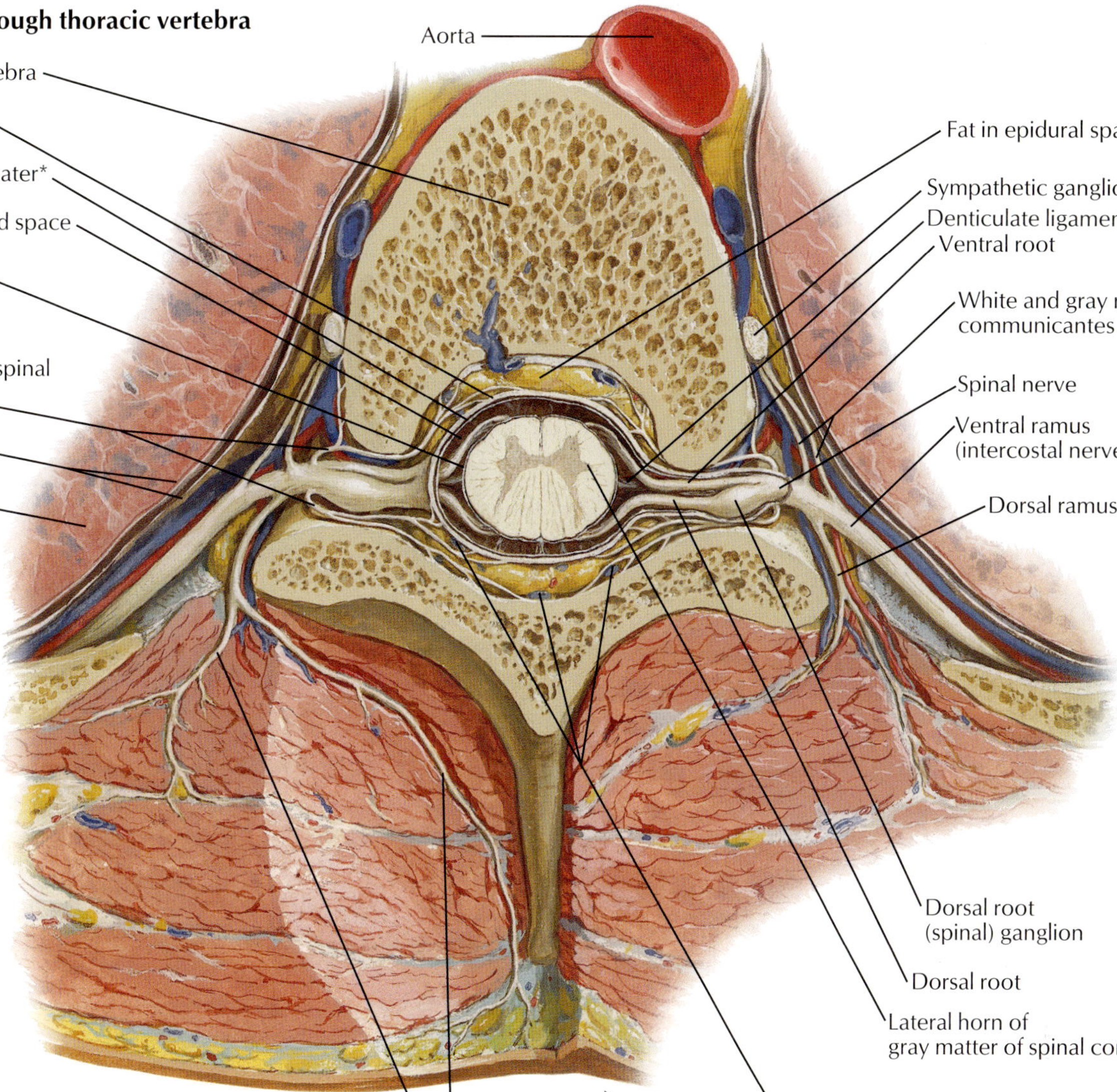

Section through lumbar vertebra

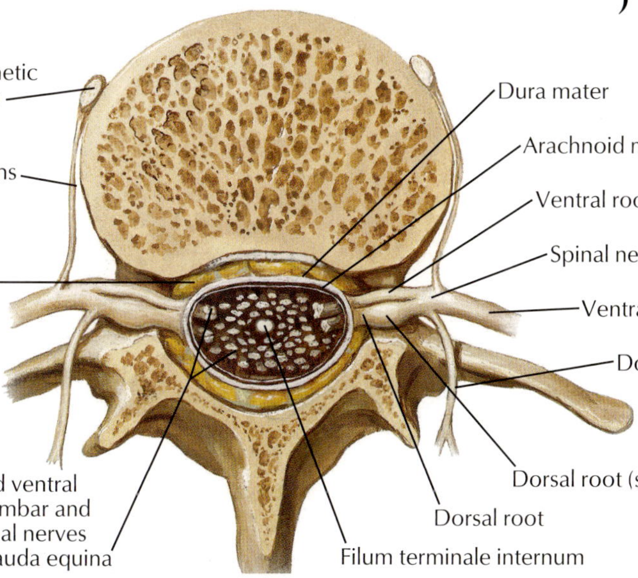

*Leptomeninges

Arteries of Spinal Cord: Schema

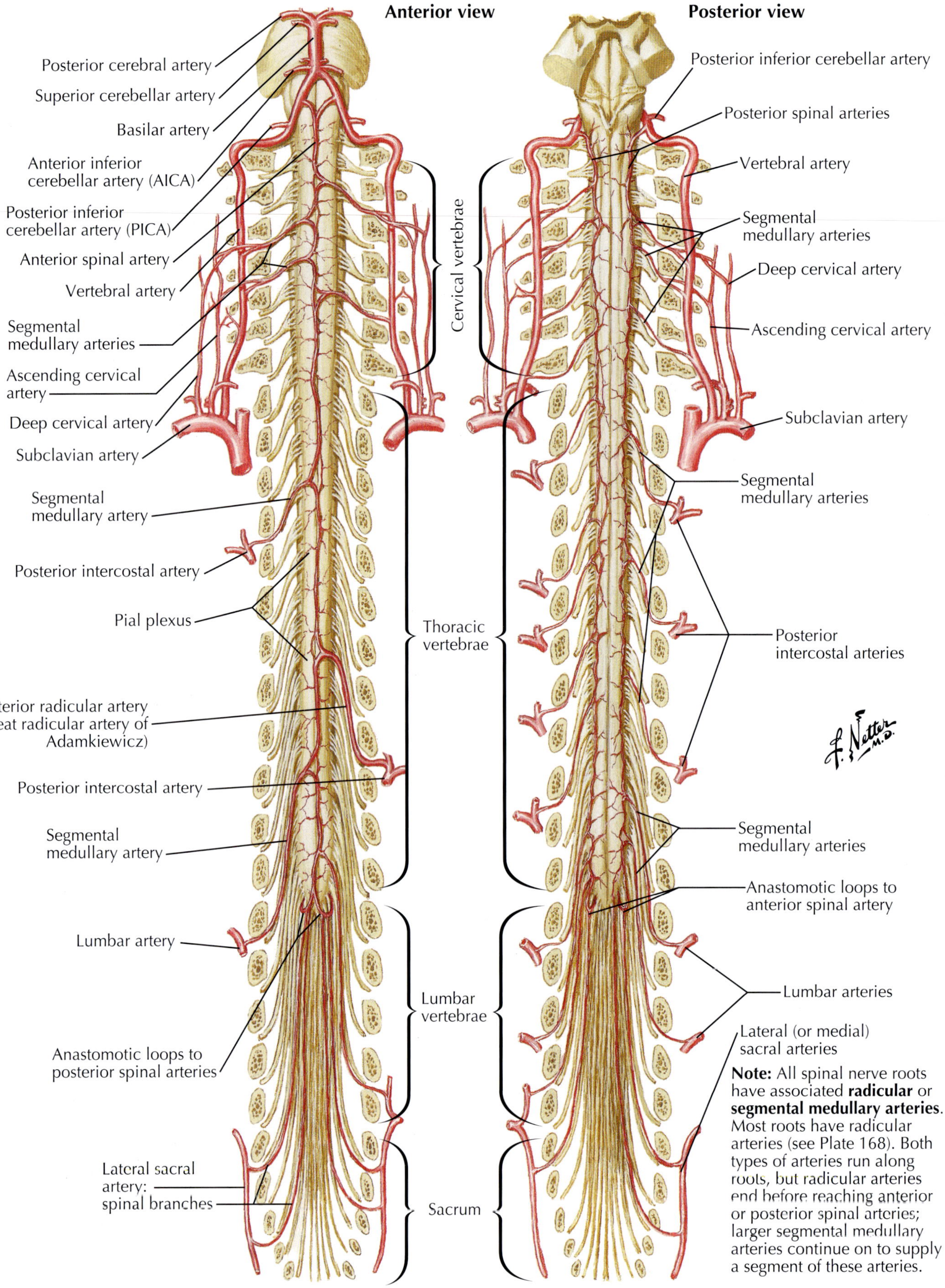

Note: All spinal nerve roots have associated **radicular** or **segmental medullary arteries**. Most roots have radicular arteries (see Plate 168). Both types of arteries run along roots, but radicular arteries end before reaching anterior or posterior spinal arteries; larger segmental medullary arteries continue on to supply a segment of these arteries.

Arteries of Spinal Cord: Intrinsic Distribution

See also Plate 188

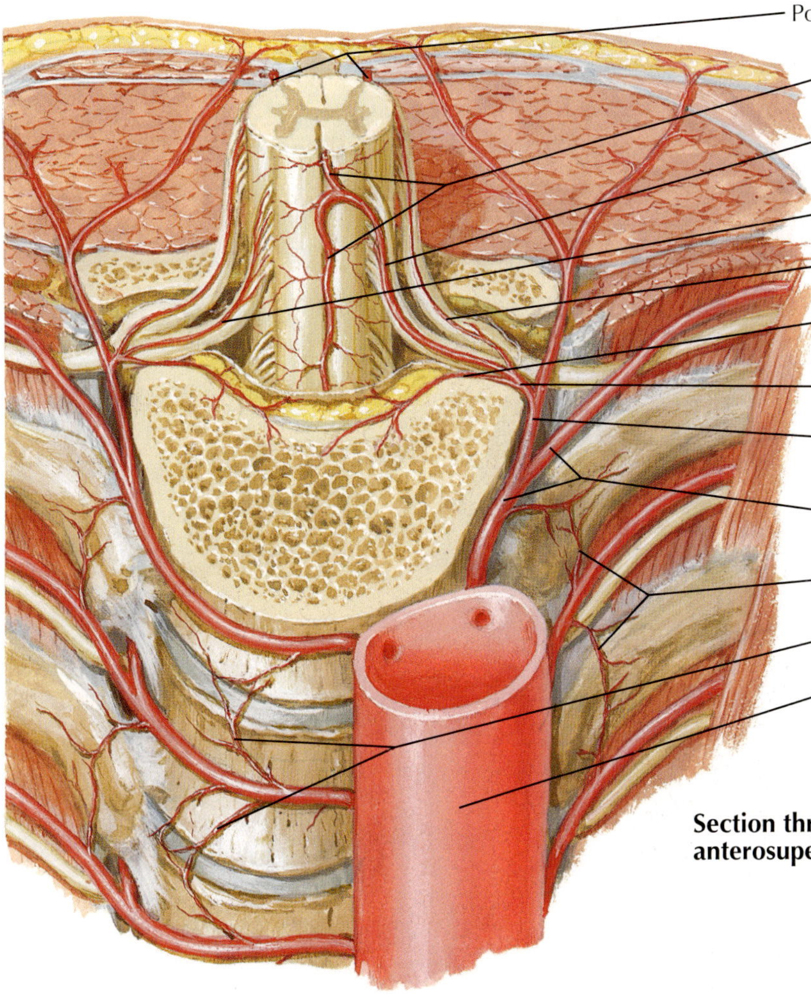

Section through thoracic level: anterosuperior view

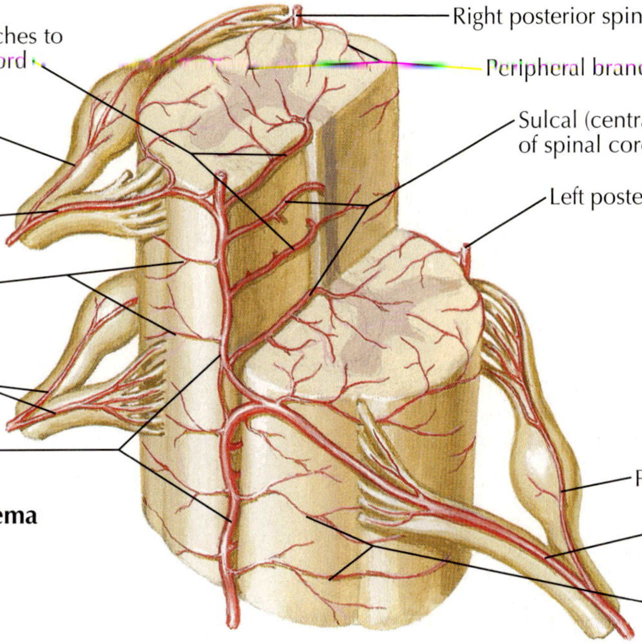

Arterial distribution: schema

Veins of Spinal Cord and Vertebral Column

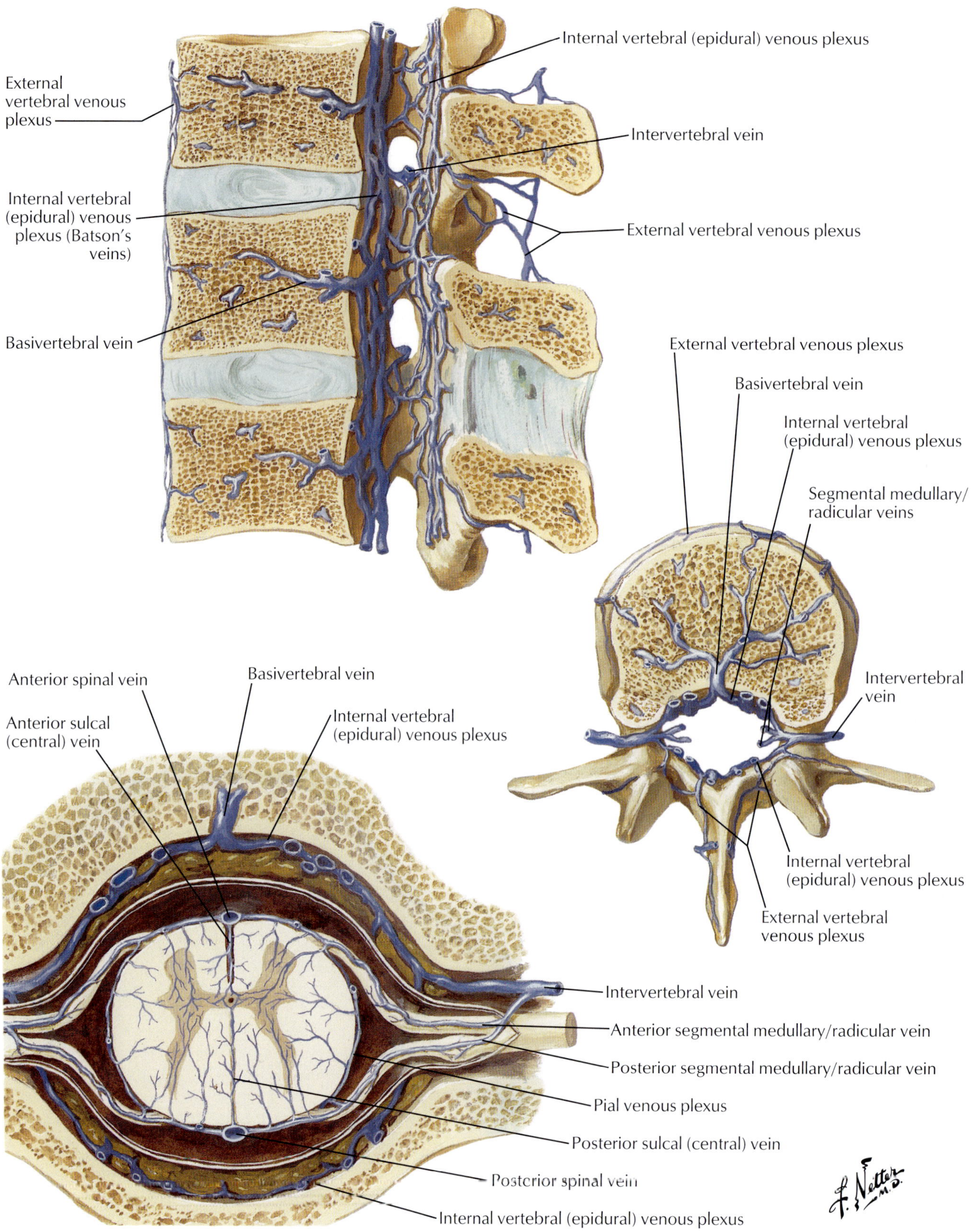

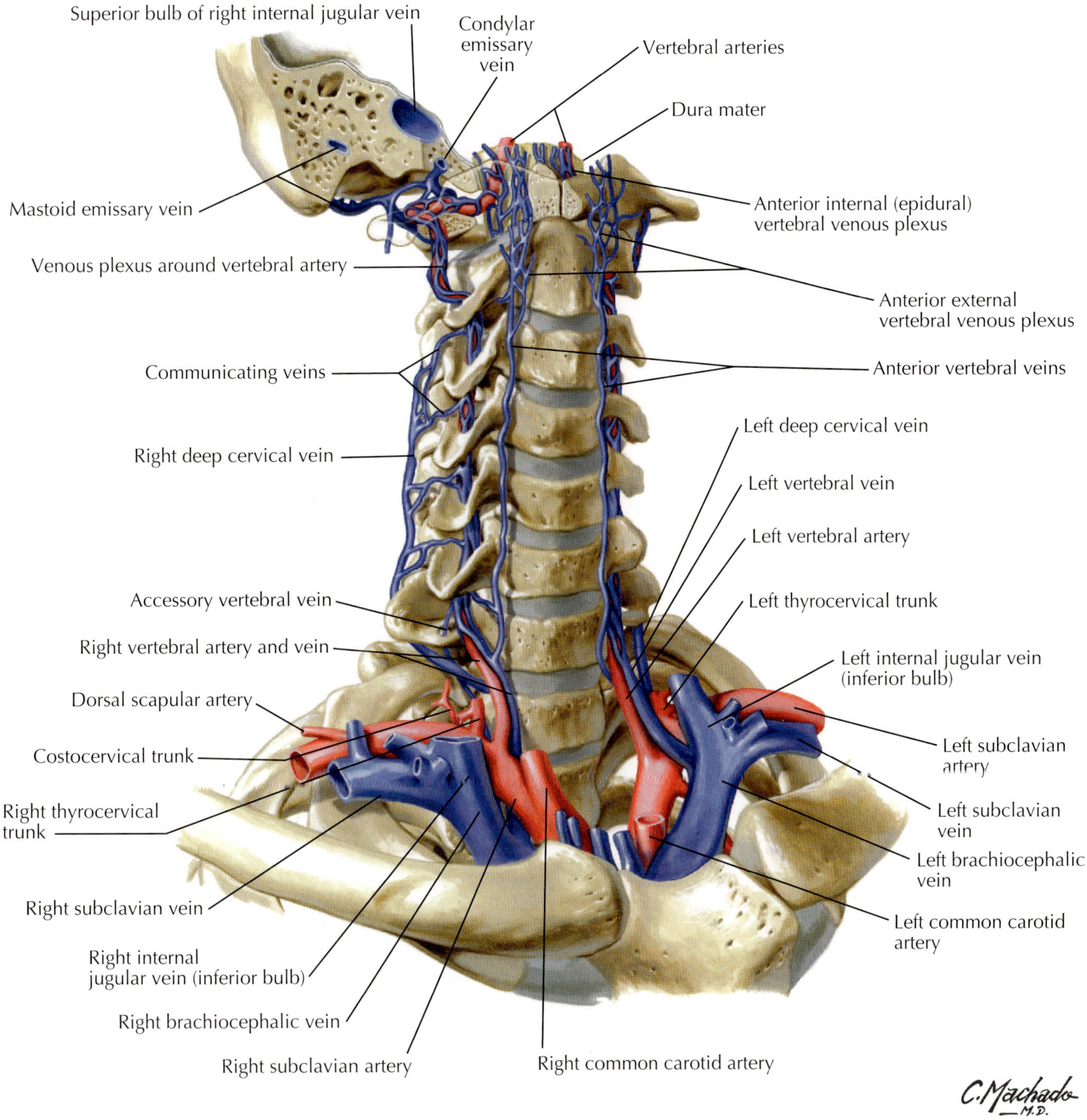

Superior bulb of right internal jugular vein
Condylar emissary vein
Vertebral arteries
Dura mater
Mastoid emissary vein
Anterior internal (epidural) vertebral venous plexus
Venous plexus around vertebral artery
Anterior external vertebral venous plexus
Communicating veins
Anterior vertebral veins
Left deep cervical vein
Right deep cervical vein
Left vertebral vein
Left vertebral artery
Accessory vertebral vein
Left thyrocervical trunk
Right vertebral artery and vein
Left internal jugular vein (inferior bulb)
Dorsal scapular artery
Costocervical trunk
Left subclavian artery
Right thyrocervical trunk
Left subclavian vein
Left brachiocephalic vein
Right subclavian vein
Left common carotid artery
Right internal jugular vein (inferior bulb)
Right brachiocephalic vein
Right subclavian artery
Right common carotid artery
C. Machado M.D.

See also Plates 29, 250

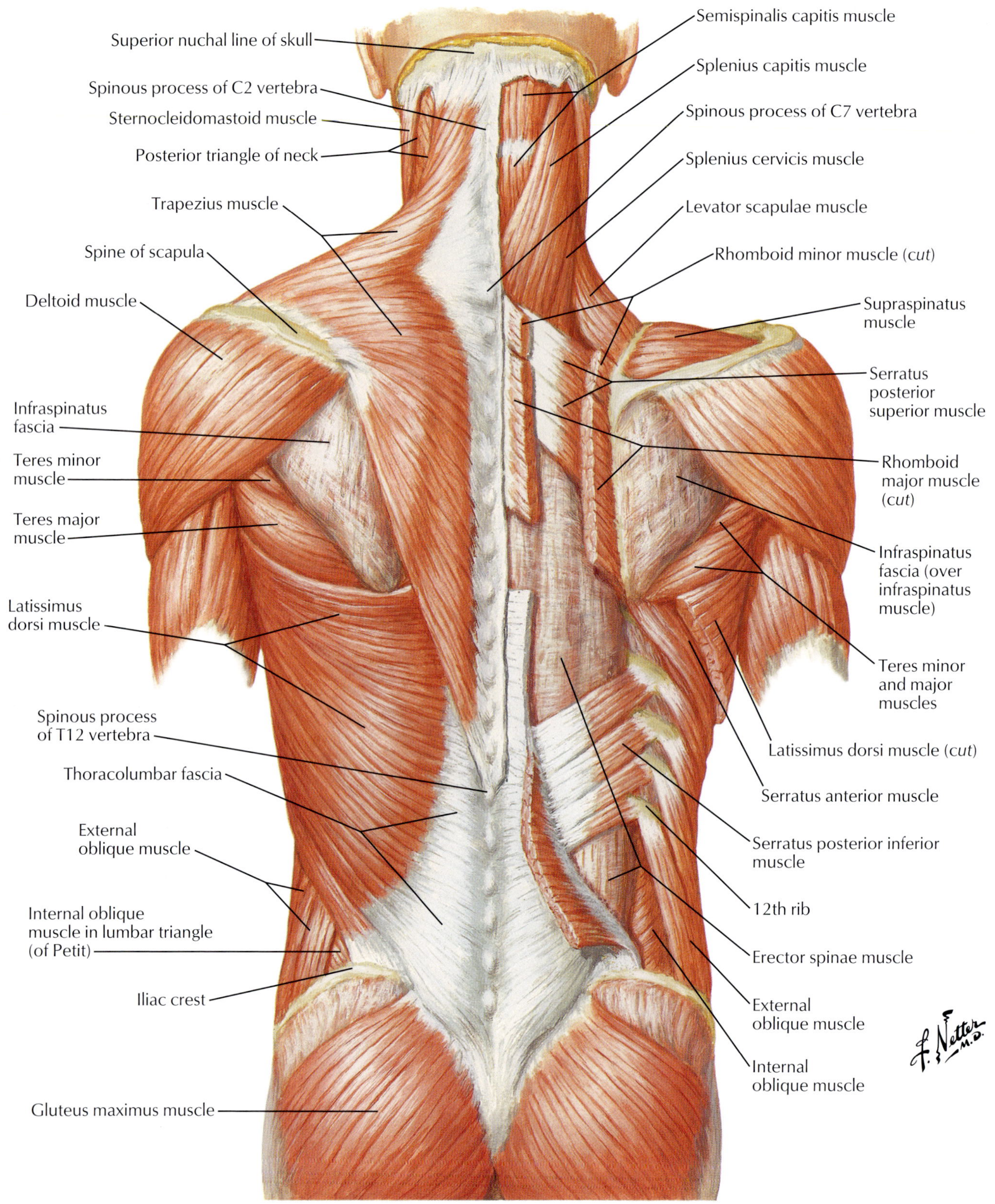

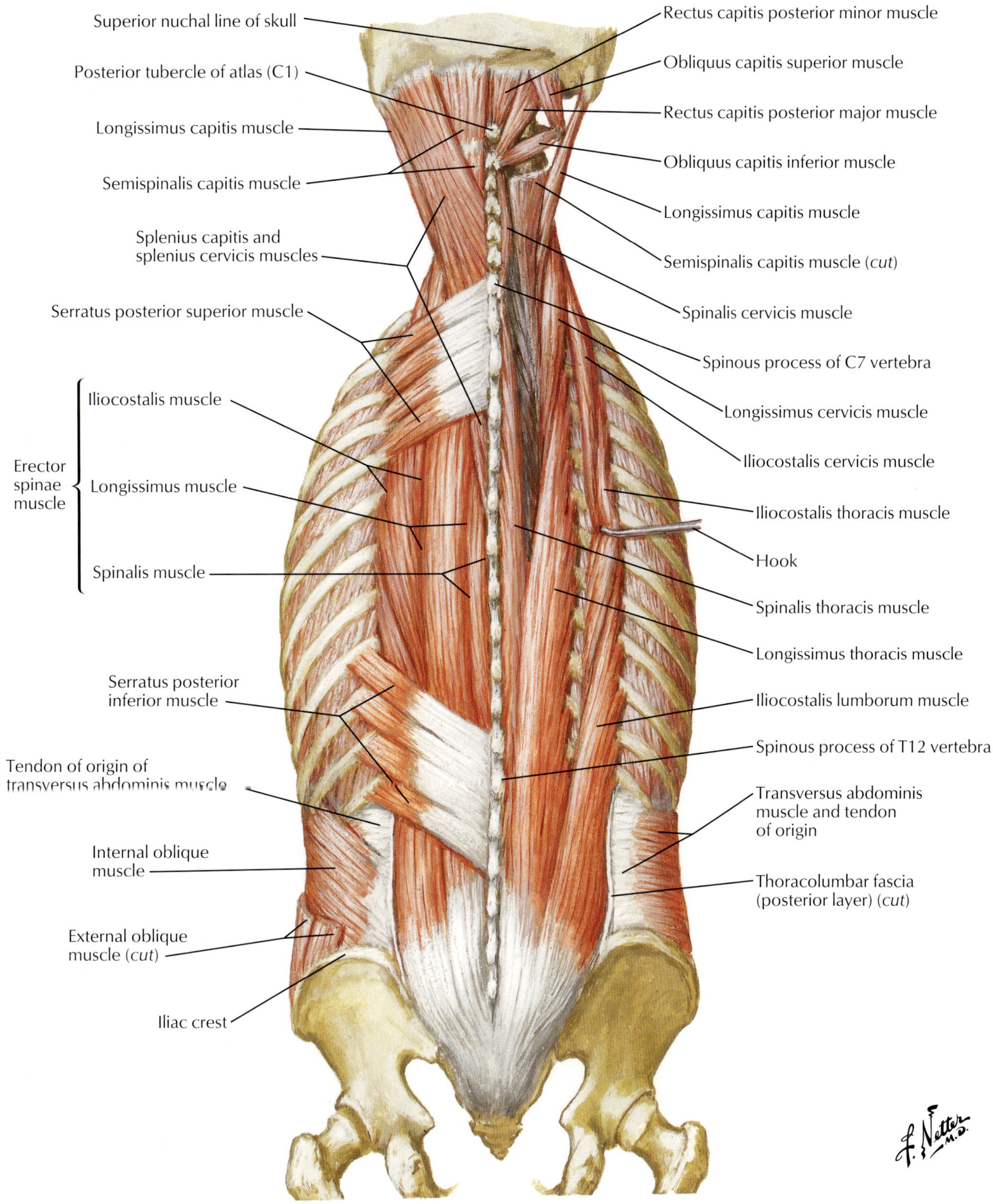
Superior nuchal line of skull
Posterior tubercle of atlas (C1)
Longissimus capitis muscle
Semispinalis capitis muscle
Splenius capitis and splenius cervicis muscles
Serratus posterior superior muscle
Iliocostalis muscle
Erector spinae muscle
Longissimus muscle
Spinalis muscle
Serratus posterior inferior muscle
Tendon of origin of transversus abdominis muscle
Internal oblique muscle
External oblique muscle (cut)
Iliac crest
Rectus capitis posterior minor muscle
Obliquus capitis superior muscle
Rectus capitis posterior major muscle
Obliquus capitis inferior muscle
Longissimus capitis muscle
Semispinalis capitis muscle (cut)
Spinalis cervicis muscle
Spinous process of C7 vertebra
Longissimus cervicis muscle
Iliocostalis cervicis muscle
Iliocostalis thoracis muscle
Hook
Spinalis thoracis muscle
Longissimus thoracis muscle
Iliocostalis lumborum muscle
Spinous process of T12 vertebra
Transversus abdominis muscle and tendon of origin
Thoracolumbar fascia (posterior layer) (cut)
F. Netter M.D.

Muscles of Back: Deep Layers

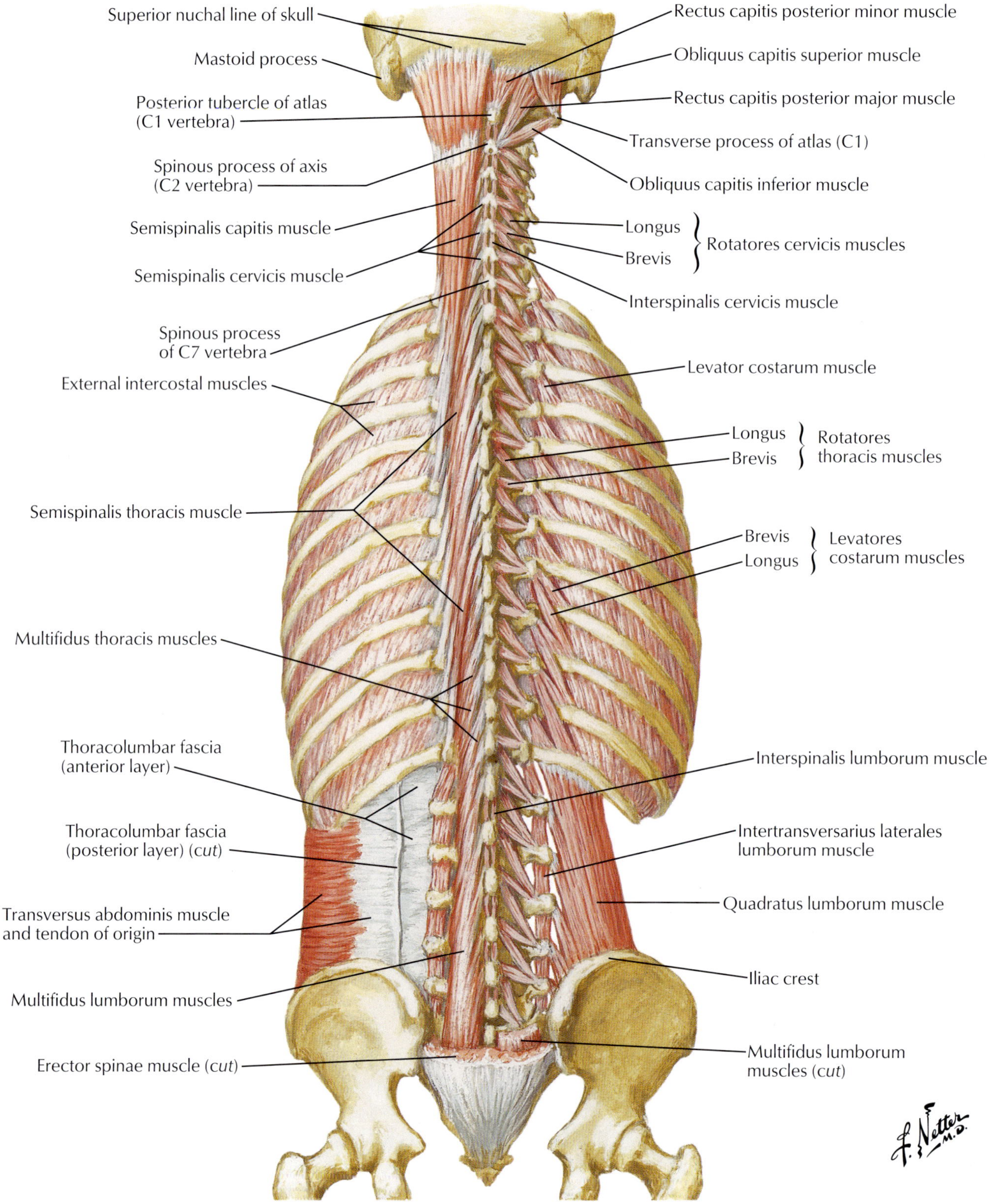

See also Plates 409, 481

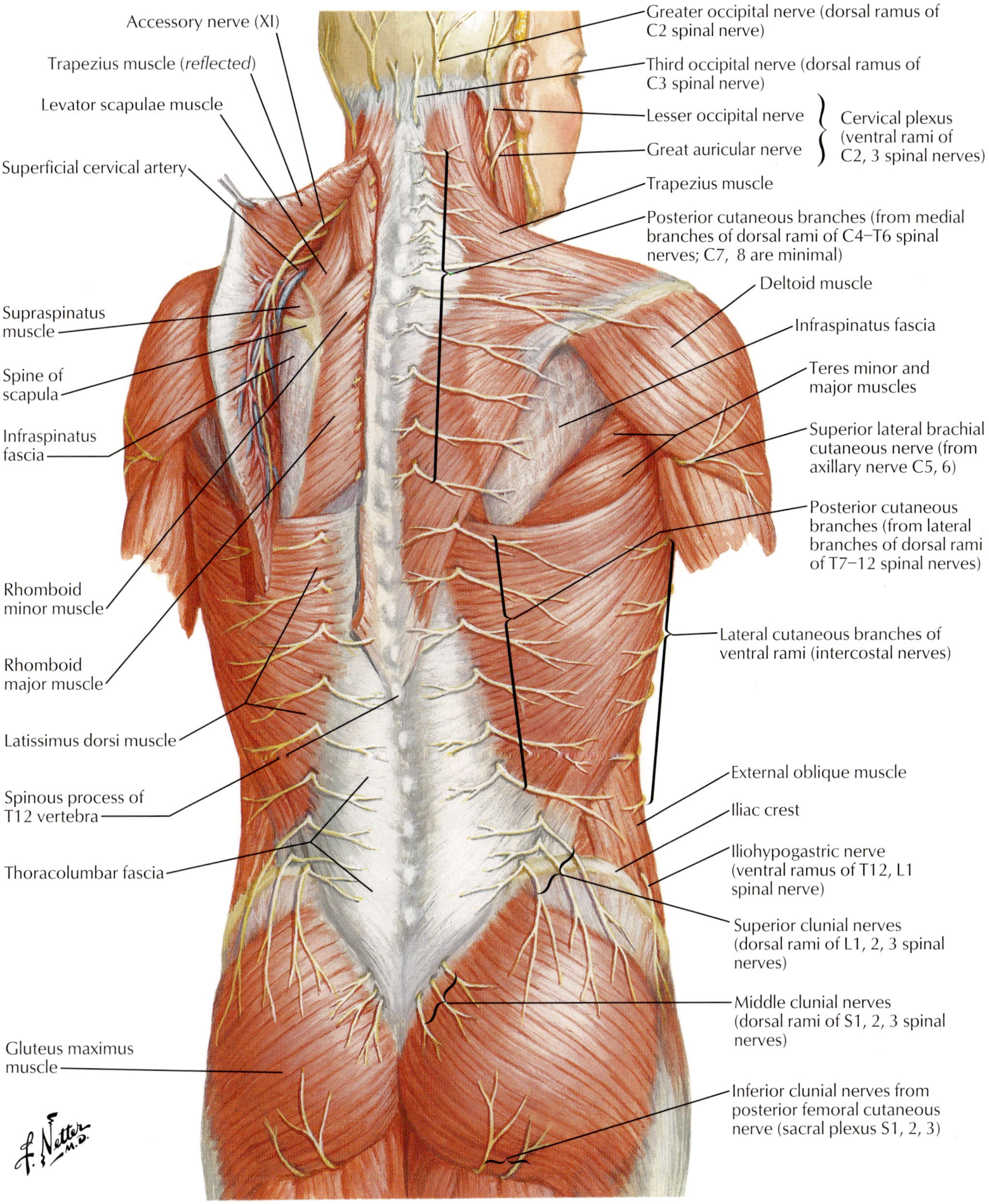

Suboccipital Triangle

See also **Plates 29, 32**

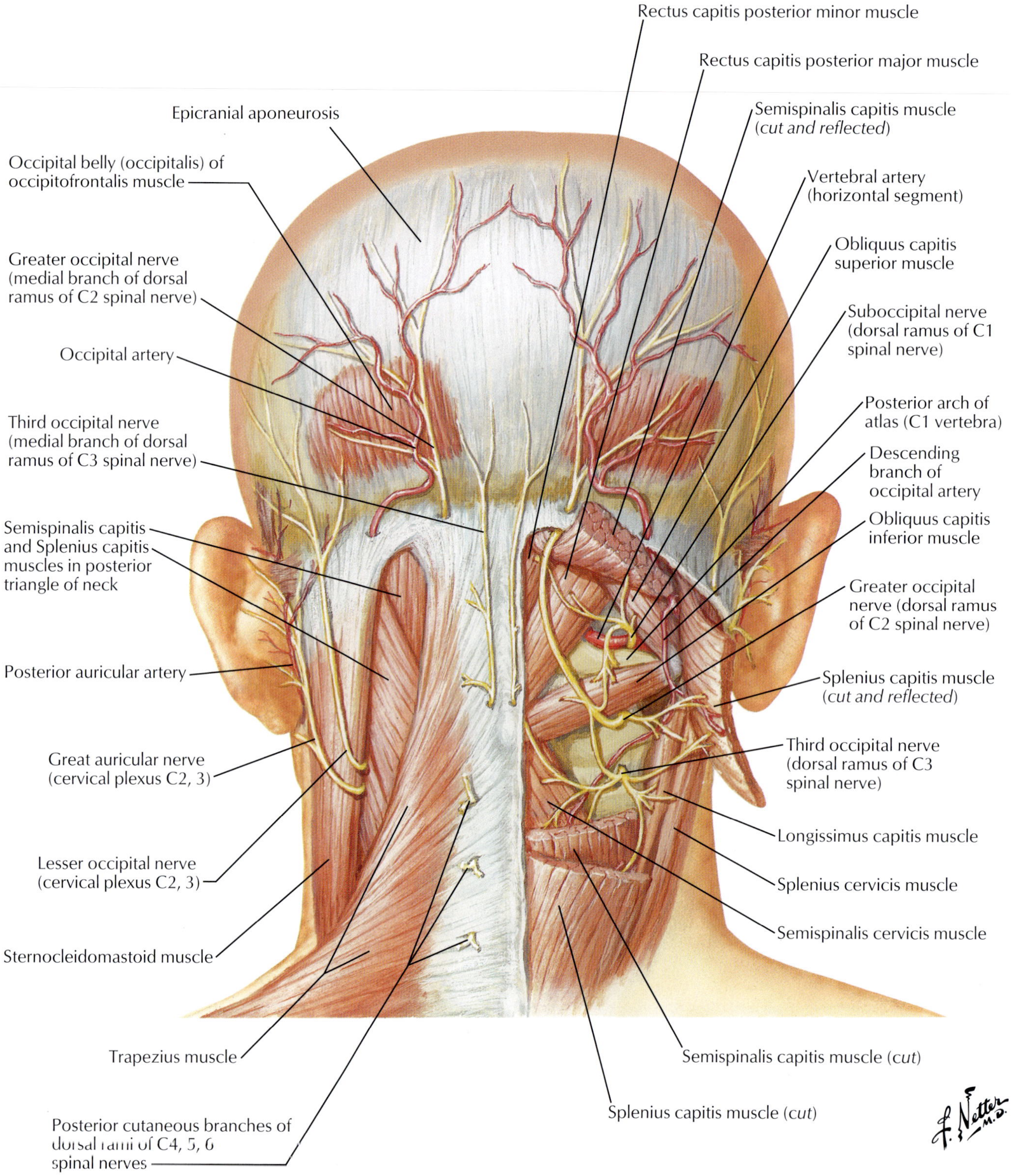

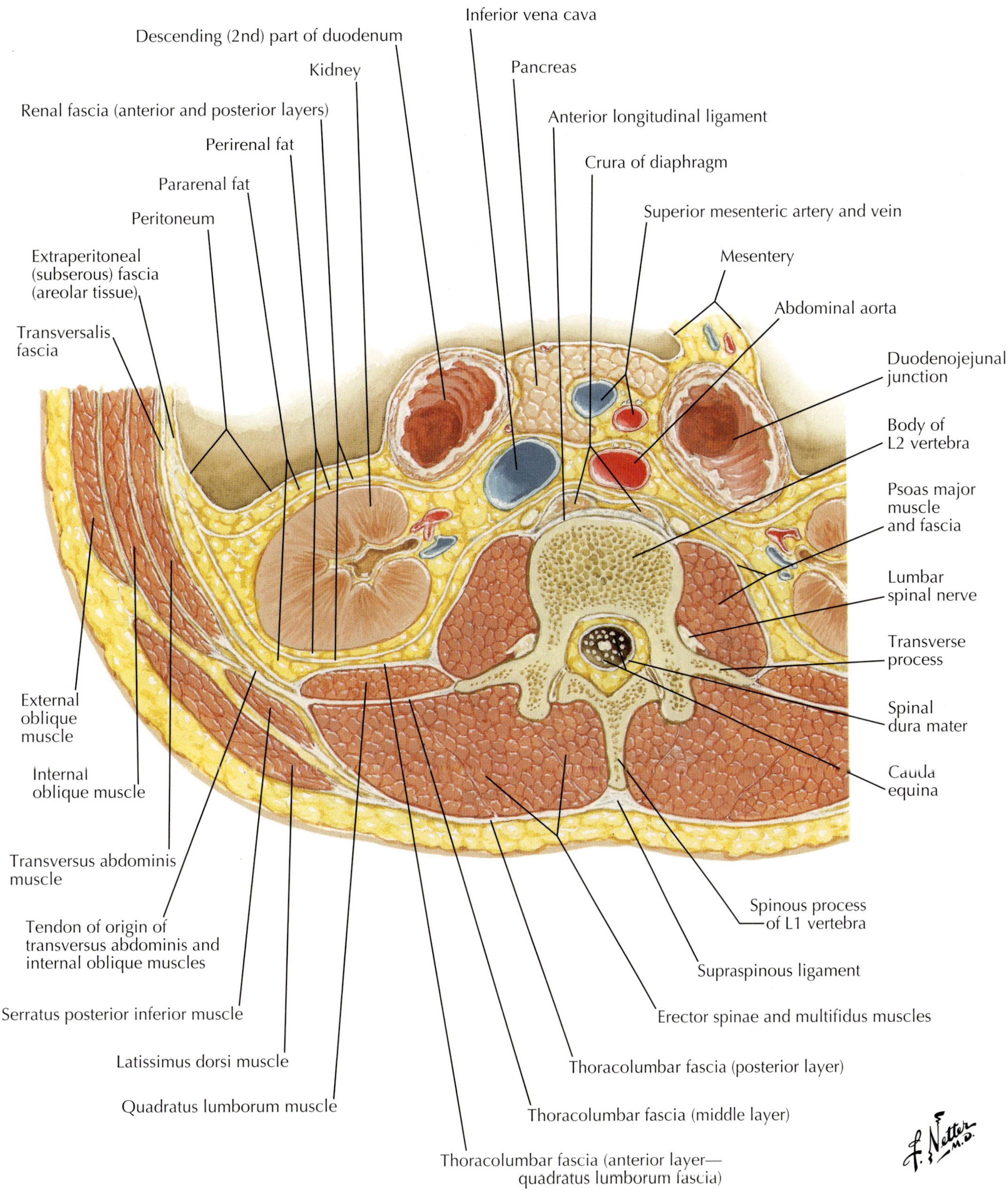
Inferior vena cava
Descending (2nd) part of duodenum
Kidney
Pancreas
Renal fascia (anterior and posterior layers)
Anterior longitudinal ligament
Perirenal fat
Crura of diaphragm
Pararenal fat
Superior mesenteric artery and vein
Peritoneum
Mesentery
Extraperitoneal (subserous) fascia (areolar tissue)
Abdominal aorta
Transversalis fascia
Duodenojejunal junction
Body of L2 vertebra
Psoas major muscle and fascia
Lumbar spinal nerve
Transverse process
External oblique muscle
Spinal dura mater
Internal oblique muscle
Cauda equina
Transversus abdominis muscle
Spinous process of L1 vertebra
Tendon of origin of transversus abdominis and internal oblique muscles
Supraspinous ligament
Serratus posterior inferior muscle
Erector spinae and multifidus muscles
Latissimus dorsi muscle
Thoracolumbar fascia (posterior layer)
Quadratus lumborum muscle
Thoracolumbar fascia (middle layer)
Thoracolumbar fascia (anterior layer—quadratus lumborum fascia)
F. Netter M.D.

Typical Thoracic Spinal Nerve: Cross Section

See also Plate 254

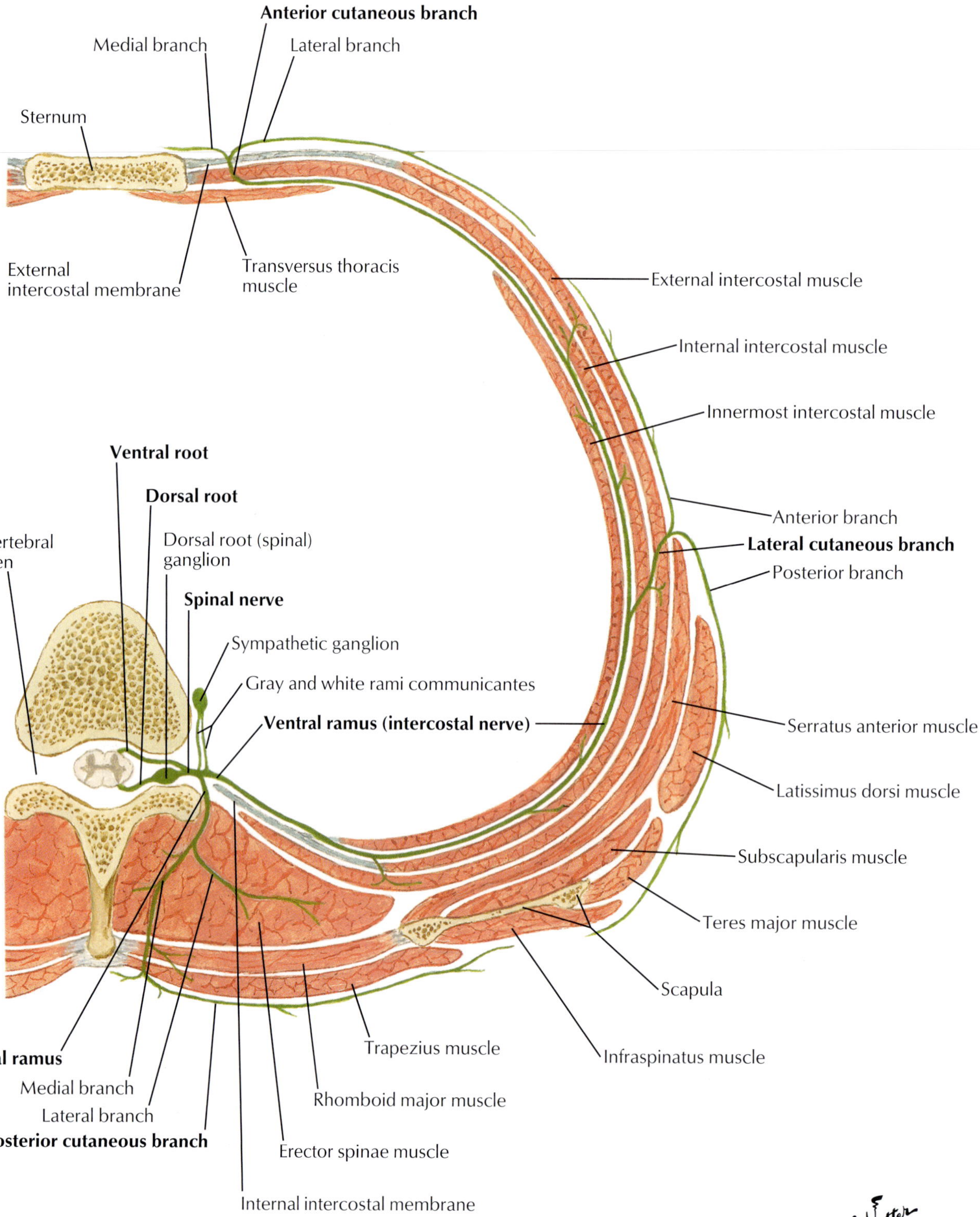

***Note:** In lower thoracic region, lateral branch of dorsal ramus is longer, motor, and cutaneous; medial branch is shorter and motor only.*

MUSCLE	PROXIMAL ATTACHMENT (ORIGIN)	DISTAL ATTACHMENT (INSERTION)	INNERVATION	MAIN ACTIONS	BLOOD SUPPLY	MUSCLE GROUP
Erector spinae	Posterior sacrum, iliac crest, sacrospinous ligament, supraspinous ligament, spinous processes of lower lumbar and sacral vertebrae	*Iliocostalis:* angles of lower ribs, cervical transverse processes *Longissimus:* between tubercles and angles of ribs, transverse processes of thoracic and cervical vertebrae, mastoid process *Spinalis:* spinous processes of upper thoracic and midcervical vertebrae	Dorsal rami of each region	Extends and laterally bends vertebral column and head	*Cervical portions:* occipital, deep cervical, and vertebral arteries *Thoracic portions:* dorsal branches of posterior intercostal, subcostal, and lumbar arteries *Sacral portions:* dorsal branches of lateral sacral arteries	Sacrospinalis
Interspinales (cervical, thoracic, lumbar)	Spinous process	Adjacent spinous process	Dorsal rami of spinal nerves	Aid in extension of vertebral column	*Cervical portions:* occipital, deep cervical, and vertebral arteries *Thoracic portions:* dorsal branches of posterior intercostal arteries *Lumbar portions:* dorsal branches of lumbar arteries	Segmental
Intertransversarii (cervical, thoracic, lumbar)	Extend between adjacent transverse processes of vertebrae	Extend between adjacent transverse processes of vertebrae	Dorsal rami of spinal nerves	Assist in lateral flexion of vertebral column	*Cervical portions:* occipital, deep cervical, and vertebral arteries *Thoracic portions:* dorsal branches of posterior intercostal, subcostal, and lumbar arteries *Lumbar portions:* dorsal branches of lateral lumbar arteries	Segmental
Latissimus dorsi	Spinous processes of T7–L5, thoracolumbar fascia, iliac crest, and last three ribs	Humerus (intertubercular sulcus)	Thoracodorsal nerve	Extends, adducts, and medially rotates humerus	Thoracodorsal artery, dorsal perforating branches of 9th, 10th, and 11th posterior intercostal, subcostal, and first three lumbar arteries	Superficial back
Levator scapulae	Posterior tubercles of transverse processes of C1–C4	Medial border of scapula from superior angle to spine	Ventral rami of C3–C4 and dorsal scapular nerve	Elevates scapula medially, inferiorly rotates glenoid cavity	Dorsal scapular artery, transverse cervical artery, ascending cervical artery	Superficial back
Multifidus	Sacrum, ilium, transverse processes of T1–T12, and articular processes of C4–C7	Spinous processes of vertebrae above, spanning two to four segments	Dorsal rami of each region	Stabilizes spine	*Cervical portions:* occipital, deep cervical, and vertebral arteries *Thoracic portions:* dorsal branches of posterior intercostal, subcostal, and lumbar arteries *Sacral portions:* dorsal branches of lateral sacral arteries	Transversospinalis
Obliquus capitis inferior	Spine of axis	Transverse process of atlas	Suboccipital nerve	Rotates atlas to turn face to same side	Vertebral artery, descending branch of occipital artery	Suboccipital
Obliquus capitis superior	Transverse process of atlas	Occipital bone	Suboccipital nerve	Extends and bends head laterally	Vertebral artery, descending branch of occipital artery	Suboccipital
Rectus capitis posterior major	Spine of axis	Inferior nuchal line	Suboccipital nerve	Extends and rotates head to same side	Vertebral artery, descending branch of occipital artery	Suboccipital

Variations in spinal nerve contributions to the innervation of muscles, their arterial supply, their attachments, and their actions are common themes in human anatomy. Therefore, expect differences between texts and realize that anatomical variation is normal.

MUSCLE	PROXIMAL ATTACHMENT (ORIGIN)	DISTAL ATTACHMENT (INSERTION)	INNERVATION	MAIN ACTIONS	BLOOD SUPPLY	MUSCLE GROUP
Rectus capitis posterior minor	Tubercle of posterior arch of atlas	Median inferior nuchal line	Suboccipital nerve	Extends head	Vertebral artery, descending branch of occipital artery	Suboccipital
Rhomboid major	Spinous processes of T2–T5 vertebrae	Medial border of scapula below base of spine of scapula	Dorsal scapular nerve	Fixes scapula to thoracic wall and retracts and rotates it to depress glenoid cavity	Dorsal scapular artery *OR* deep branch of transverse cervical artery, dorsal perforating branches of the upper five or six posterior intercostal arteries	Superficial back
Rhomboid minor	Ligamentum nuchae, spines of C7 and T1 vertebrae	Medial border of scapula at spine of scapula	Dorsal scapular nerve	Fixes scapula to thoracic wall and retracts and rotates it to depress glenoid cavity	Dorsal scapular artery *OR* deep branch of transverse cervical artery, dorsal perforating branches of the upper five or six posterior intercostal arteries	Superficial back
Rotatores	Transverse processes of cervical, thoracic, and lumbar regions	Lamina and transverse process of spine above, spanning one or two segments	Dorsal rami of spinal nerves	Stabilizes, extends, and rotates spine	Dorsal branches of segmental arteries	Transversospinalis
Semispinalis	Transverse processes of C4–T12	Spinous processes of cervical and thoracic regions	Dorsal rami of spinal nerves	Extends head, neck, and thorax and rotates them to opposite side	*Cervical portions:* occipital, deep cervical, and vertebral arteries *Thoracic portions:* dorsal branches of posterior intercostal arteries	Transversospinalis
Serratus posterior inferior	Spinous processes of T11–L2	Inferior aspect of ribs 9–12	Ventral rami of lower thoracic nerves	Depresses ribs	Posterior intercostal arteries	Intermediate back
Serratus posterior superior	Ligamentum nuchae, spinous processes of C7–T3	Superior aspect of ribs 2–4	Ventral rami of upper thoracic nerves	Elevates ribs	Posterior intercostal arteries	Intermediate back
Splenius capitis	Nuchal ligament, spinous process of C7–T3	Mastoid process of temporal bone, lateral third of superior nuchal line	Dorsal rami of middle cervical nerves	*Bilaterally:* extend head *Unilaterally:* laterally bends (flexes) and rotates face to same side	Descending branch of occipital artery, deep cervical artery	Spinotransverse
Splenius cervicis	Spinous process of T3–T6	Transverse processes (C1–C3)	Dorsal rami of lower cervical nerves	*Bilaterally:* extend neck *Unilaterally:* laterally bends (flexes) and rotates neck toward same side	Descending branch of occipital artery, deep cervical artery	Spinotransverse
Trapezius	Superior nuchal line, external occipital protuberance, nuchal ligament, spinous processes of C7–T12	Lateral third of clavicle, acromion, spine of scapula	Accessory nerve (CN XI)	Elevates, retracts, and rotates scapula; lower fibers depress scapula	Transverse cervical artery, dorsal perforating branches of posterior intercostal arteries	Superficial back

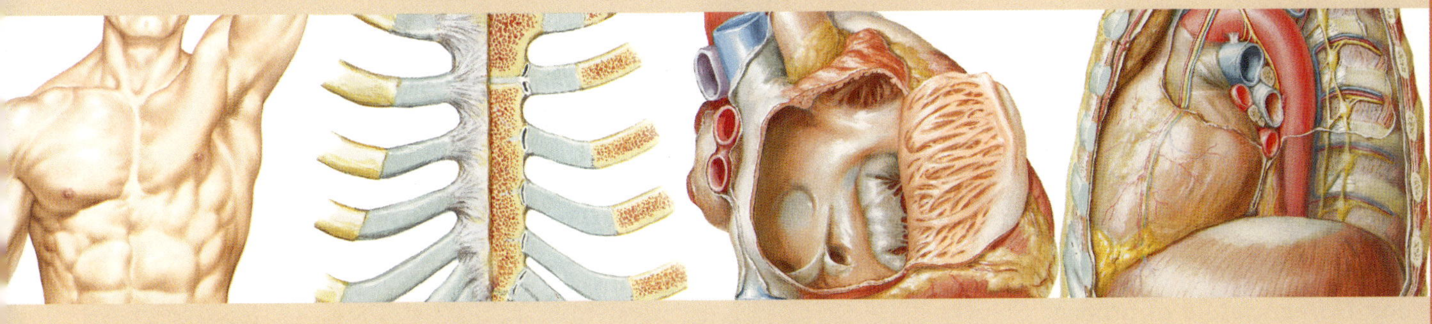

3 THORAX

Topographic Anatomy
Plate 178

178 Thorax: Surface Anatomy

Mammary Gland
Plates 179–182

179 Mammary Gland

180 Arteries of Mammary Gland

181 Lymph Vessels and Nodes of Mammary Gland

182 Lymphatic Drainage of Breast

Body Wall
Plates 183–192

183 Bony Framework of Thorax

184 Ribs and Associated Joints

185 Anterior Thoracic Wall

186 Anterior Thoracic Wall (continued)

187 Anterior Thoracic Wall: Internal View

188 Intercostal Nerves and Arteries

189 Veins of Internal Thoracic Wall

190 Phrenic Nerve

191 Diaphragm: Thoracic Surface

192 Diaphragm: Abdominal Surface

Lungs
Plates 193–207

193 Topography of Lungs: Anterior View

194 Topography of Lungs: Posterior View

195 Lungs in Situ: Anterior View
196 Lungs: Medial Views
197 Bronchopulmonary Segments
198 Bronchopulmonary Segments (continued)
199 Trachea and Major Bronchi
200 Nomenclature of Bronchi: Schema
201 Intrapulmonary Airways: Schema
202 Intrapulmonary Blood Circulation: Schema
203 Great Vessels of Superior Mediastinum
204 Bronchial Arteries and Veins
205 Lymph Vessels and Nodes of Lung
206 Autonomic Nerves in Thorax
207 Innervation of Tracheobronchial Tree: Schema

Heart

Plates 208–226

208 Heart in Situ
209 Heart: Anterior Exposure
210 Radiology and Auscultation of Heart
211 Heart: Base and Diaphragmatic Surface
212 Pericardial Sac
213 Mediastinum: Cross Section
214 Thorax: Coronal Section of Heart, Ascending Aorta
215 Coronary Arteries and Cardiac Veins
216 Coronary Arteries: Imaging
217 Right Atrium and Ventricle
218 Left Atrium and Ventricle
219 Valves and Fibrous Skeleton of Heart
220 Valves and Fibrous Skeleton of Heart (continued)
221 Atria, Ventricles, and Interventricular Septum
222 Conducting System of Heart
223 Nerves of Heart
224 Innervation of Heart: Schema
225 Innervation of Blood Vessels: Schema
226 Prenatal and Postnatal Circulation

Mediastinum

Plates 227–236

227 Mediastinum: Right Lateral View
228 Mediastinum: Left Lateral View
229 Esophagus in Situ
230 Topography and Constrictions of Esophagus
231 Musculature of Esophagus
232 Esophagogastric Junction
233 Arteries of Esophagus
234 Veins of Esophagus
235 Lymph Vessels and Nodes of Esophagus
236 Nerves of Esophagus

Regional Scans

Plate 237

237 Chest Scans: Axial CT Images

Cross-Sectional Anatomy

Plates 238–241

238 Cross Section of Thorax at T3 Level
239 Cross Section of Thorax at T3-4 Disc Level
240 Cross Section of Thorax at T4-5 Disc Level
241 Cross Section of Thorax at T7 Level

Muscle Table

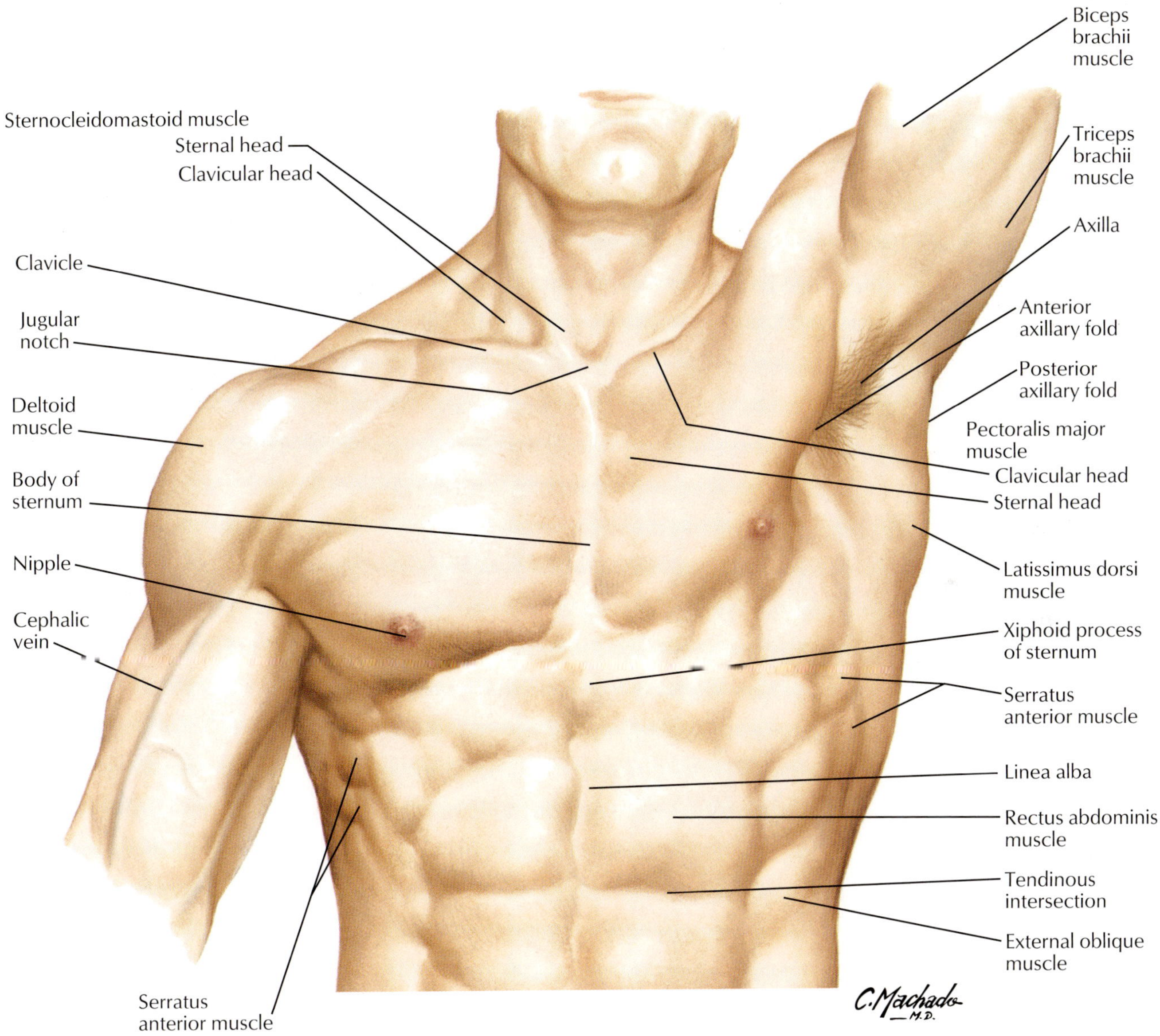
Sternocleidomastoid muscle
Sternal head
Clavicular head
Clavicle
Jugular notch
Deltoid muscle
Body of sternum
Nipple
Cephalic vein
Serratus anterior muscle
Biceps brachii muscle
Triceps brachii muscle
Axilla
Anterior axillary fold
Posterior axillary fold
Pectoralis major muscle
Clavicular head
Sternal head
Latissimus dorsi muscle
Xiphoid process of sternum
Serratus anterior muscle
Linea alba
Rectus abdominis muscle
Tendinous intersection
External oblique muscle
C. Machado M.D.

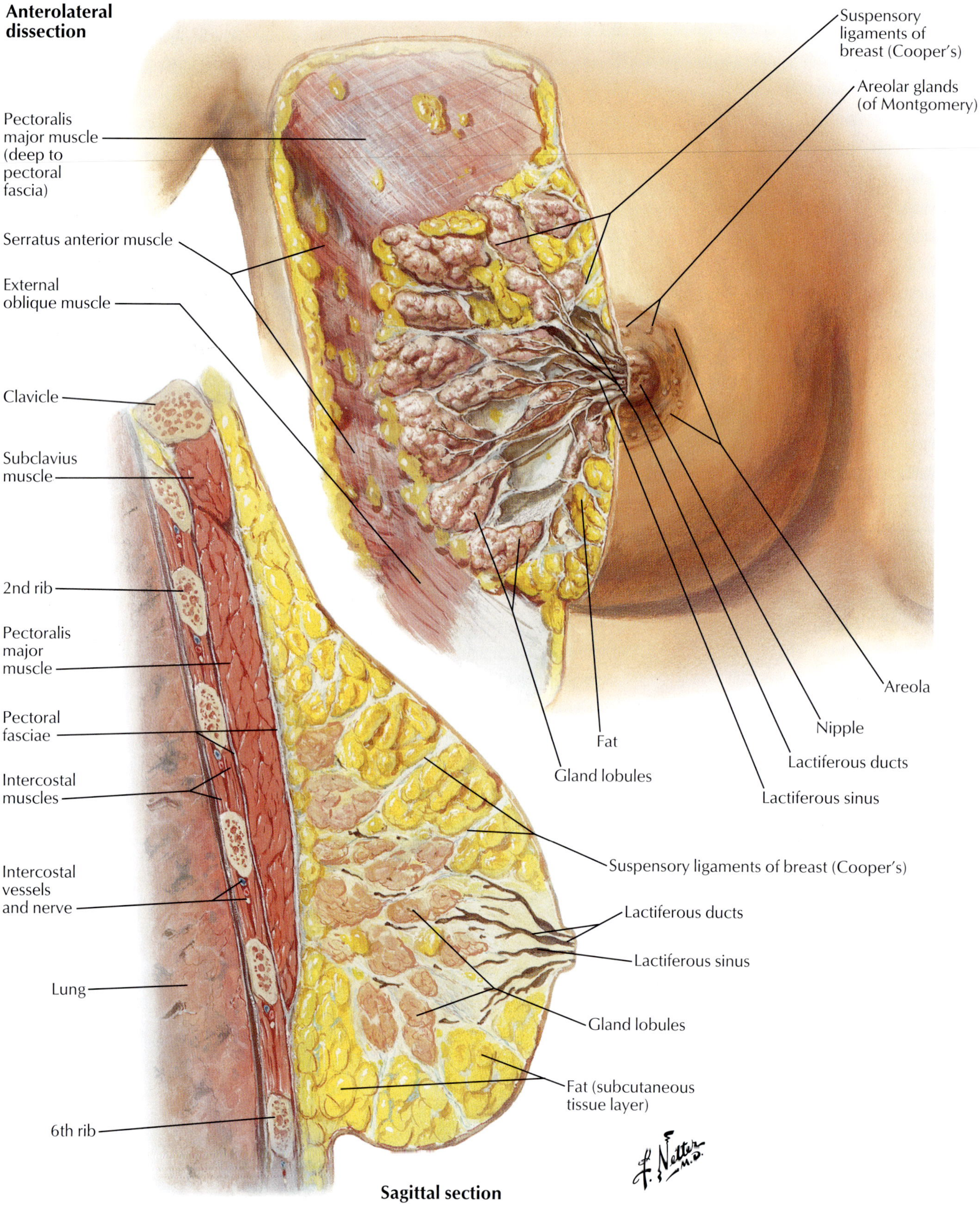

Anterolateral dissection
Pectoralis major muscle (deep to pectoral fascia)
Serratus anterior muscle
External oblique muscle
Suspensory ligaments of breast (Cooper's)
Areolar glands (of Montgomery)
Areola
Nipple
Lactiferous ducts
Lactiferous sinus
Fat
Gland lobules
Clavicle
Subclavius muscle
2nd rib
Pectoralis major muscle
Pectoral fasciae
Intercostal muscles
Intercostal vessels and nerve
Lung
6th rib
Suspensory ligaments of breast (Cooper's)
Lactiferous ducts
Lactiferous sinus
Gland lobules
Fat (subcutaneous tissue layer)
Sagittal section

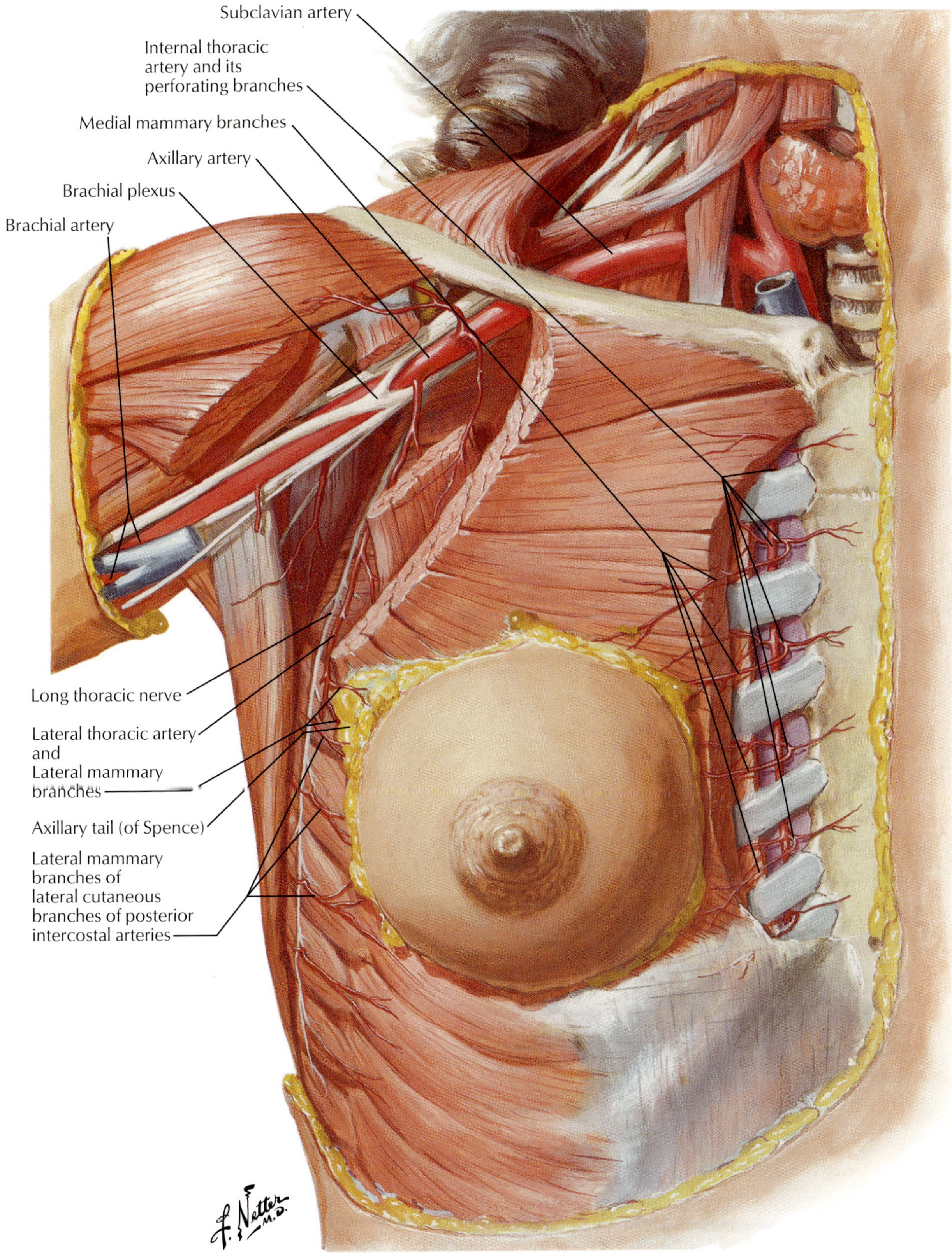
Subclavian artery
Internal thoracic artery and its perforating branches
Medial mammary branches
Axillary artery
Brachial plexus
Brachial artery
Long thoracic nerve
Lateral thoracic artery and Lateral mammary branches
Axillary tail (of Spence)
Lateral mammary branches of lateral cutaneous branches of posterior intercostal arteries
F. Netter M.D.

Lymph Vessels and Nodes of Mammary Gland

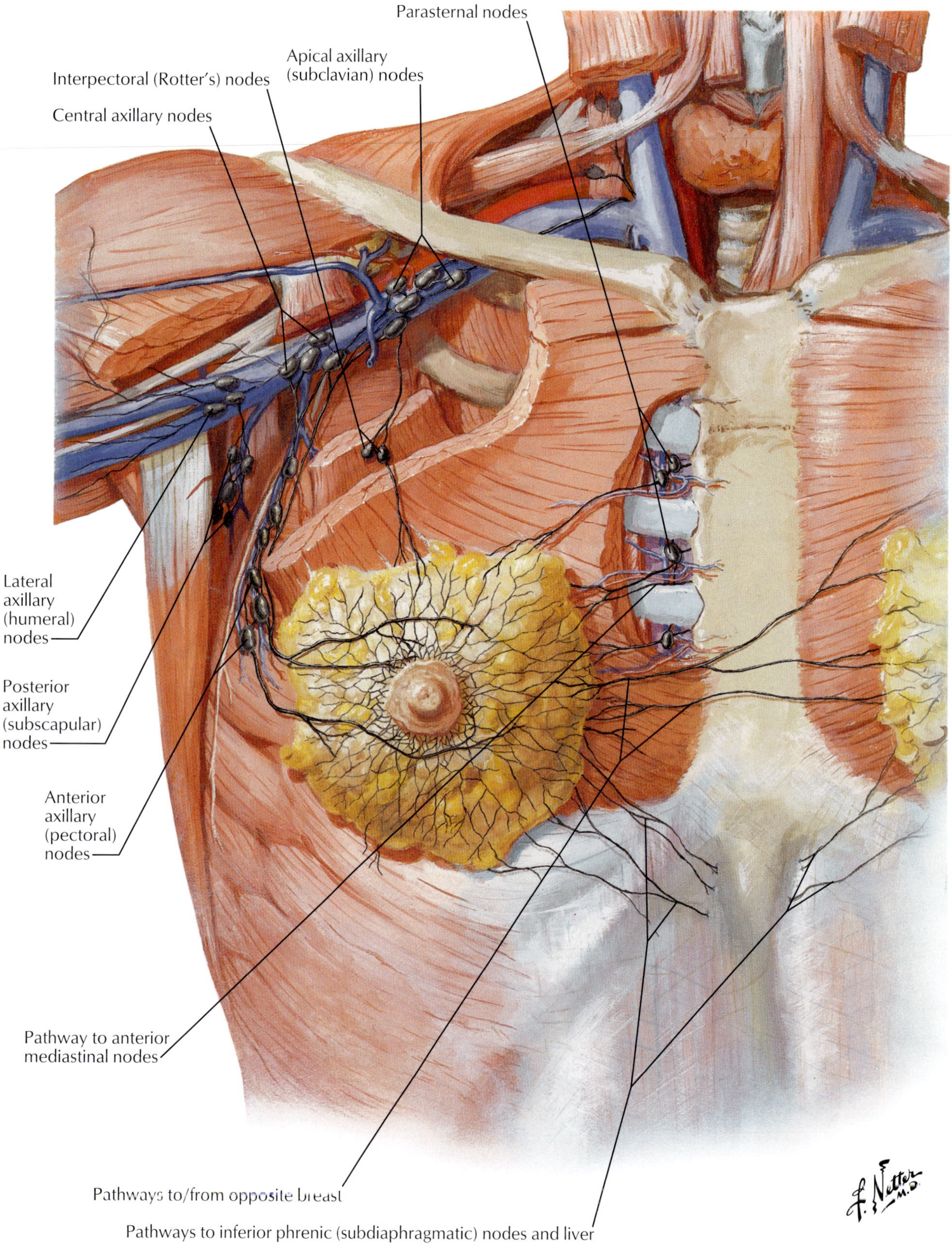

See also Plate 181

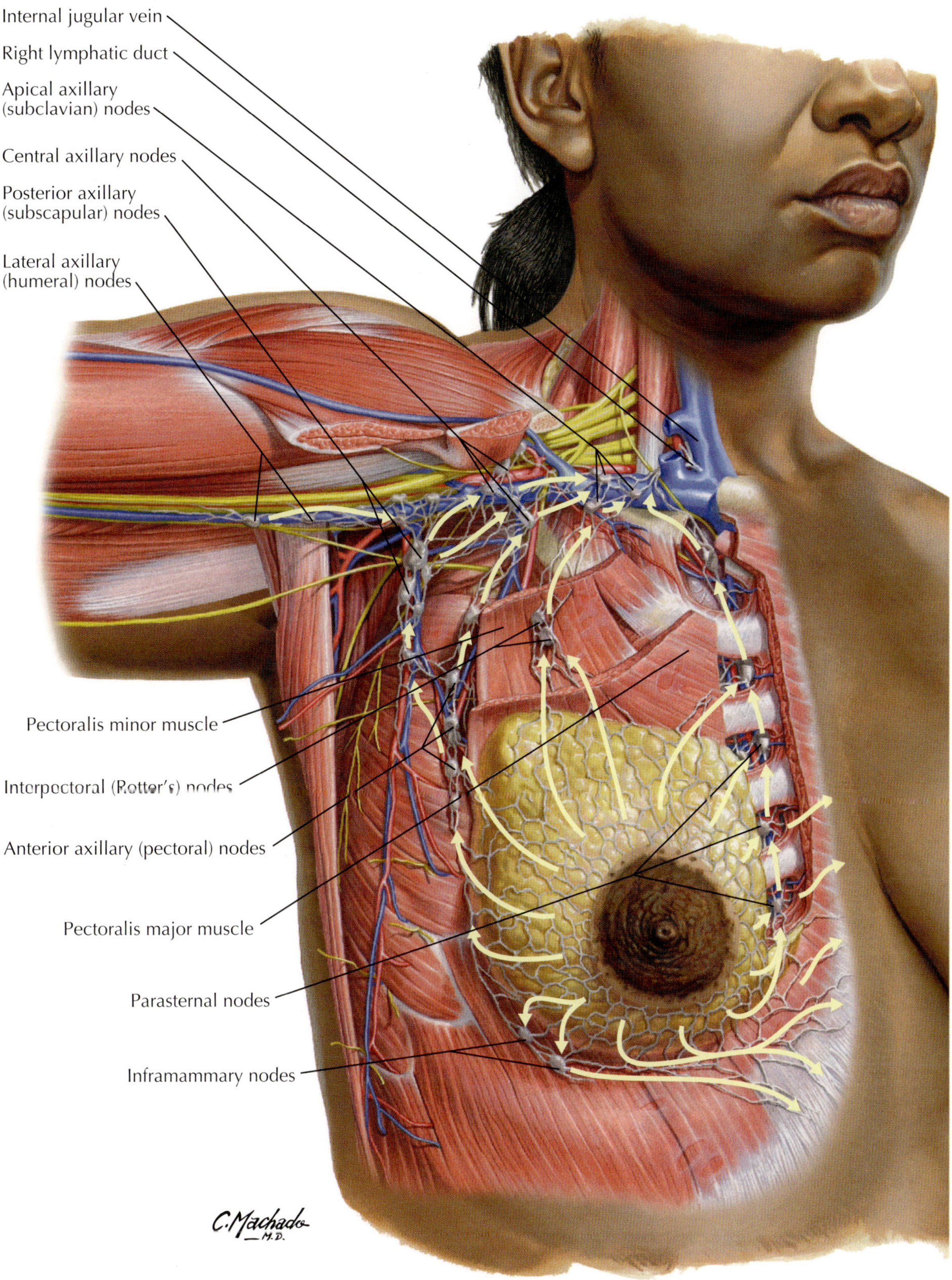

Anterior view

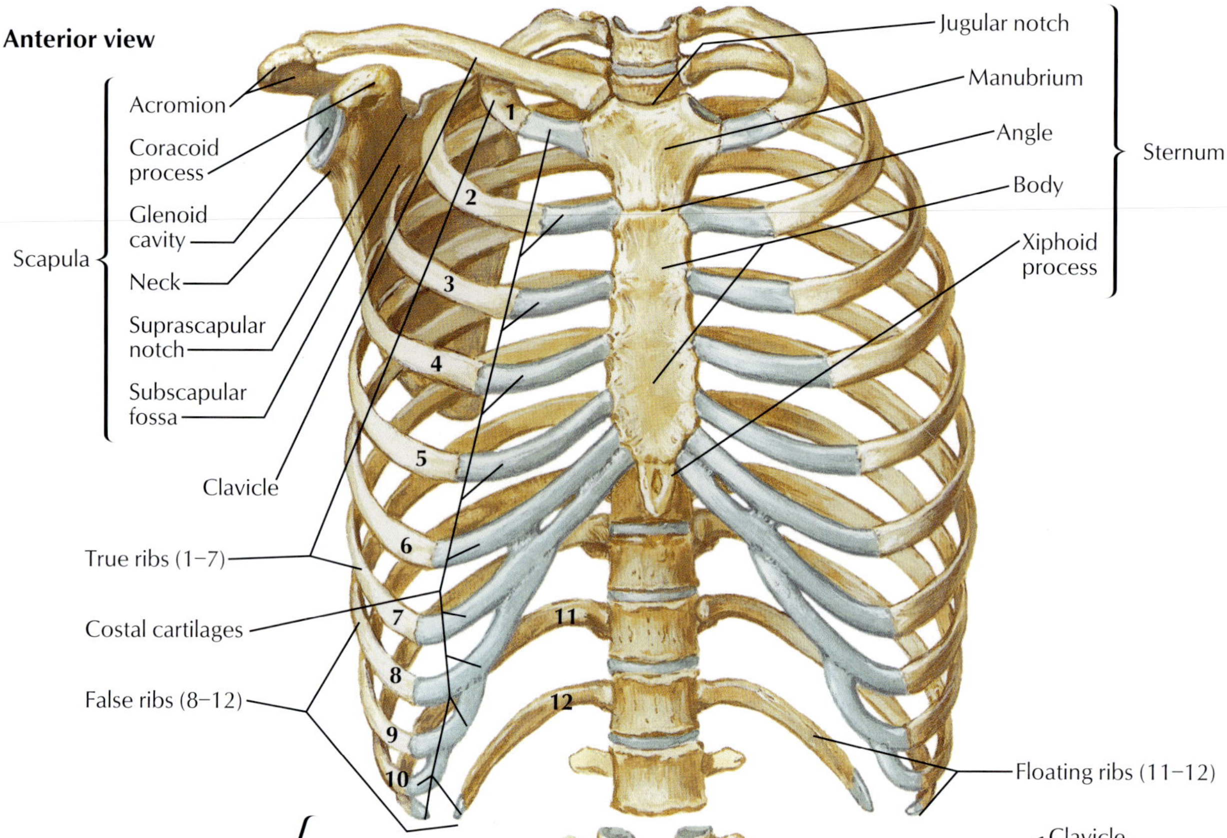

Posterior view

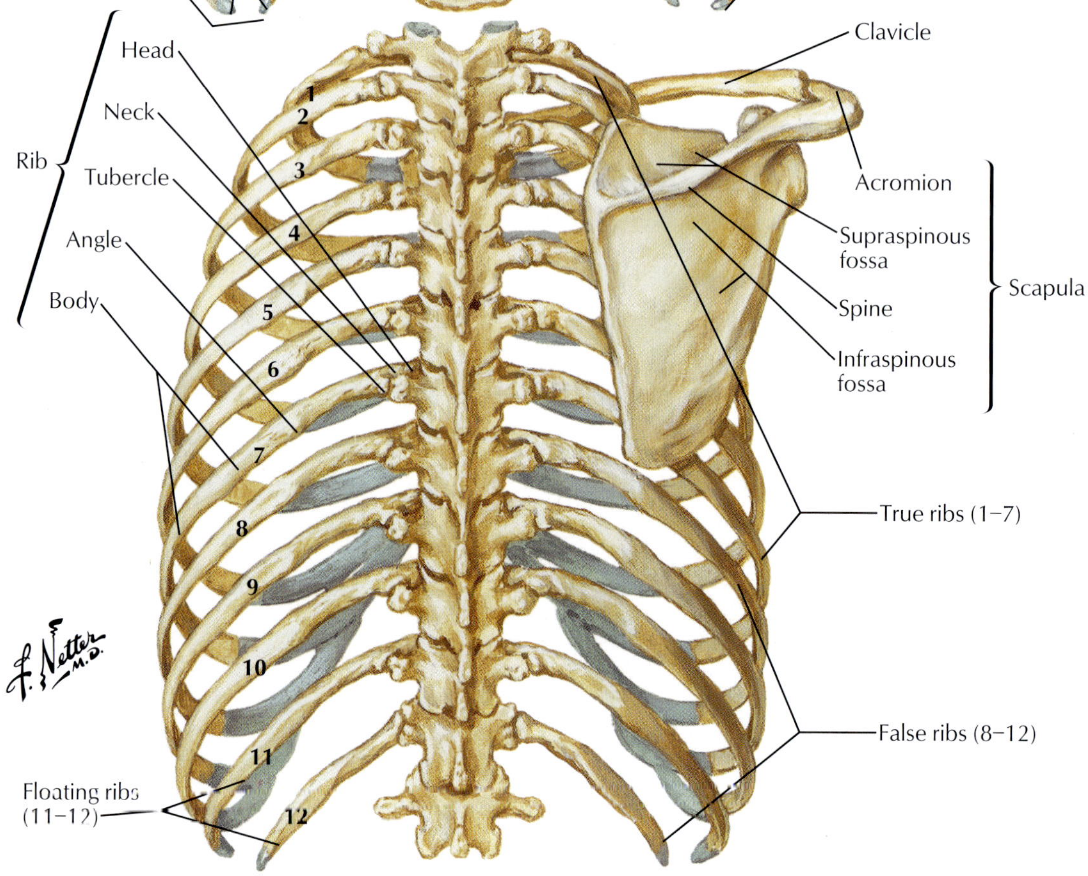

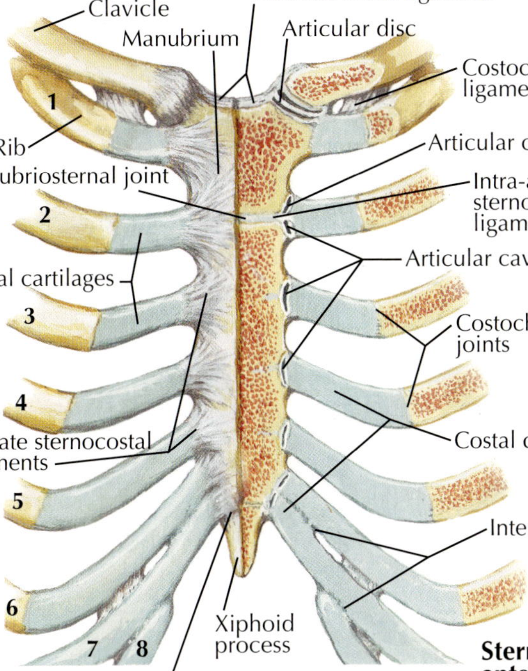

Sternocostal articulations: anterior view

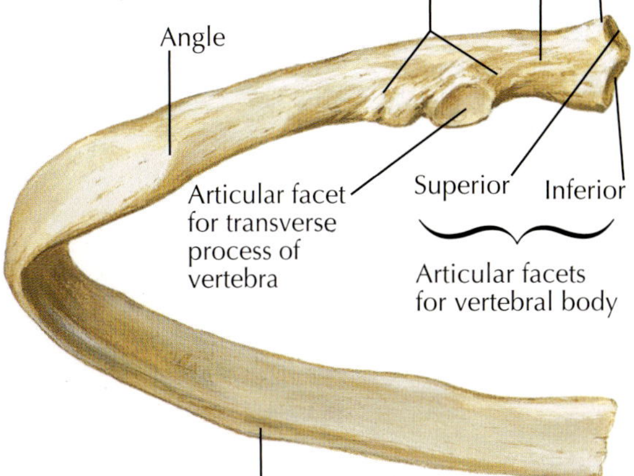

6th rib: posterior view

Note: The head of a typical rib articulates with the superior costal facet of the thoracic vertebra of the same number (by its inferior articular facet), the inferior costal facet of the vertebra above (by its superior articular facet), and the intervertebral disc between the two vertebrae. The costal tubercle articulates with the transverse process of the vertebra of the same number.

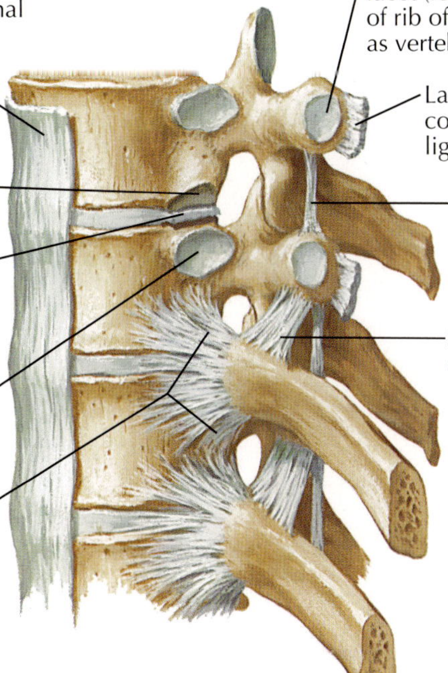

Left anterolateral view

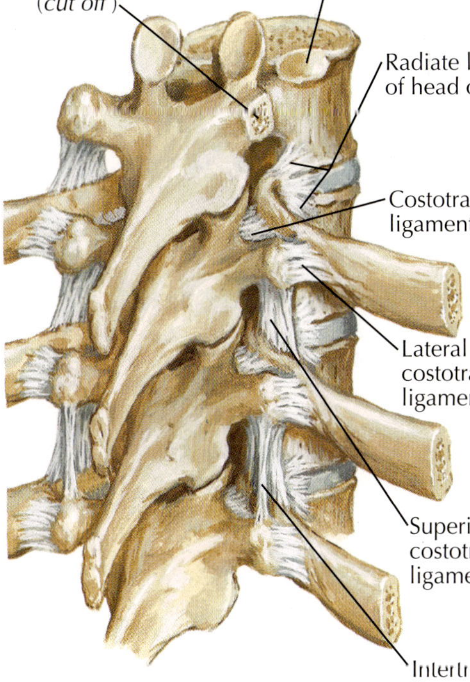

Right posterolateral view

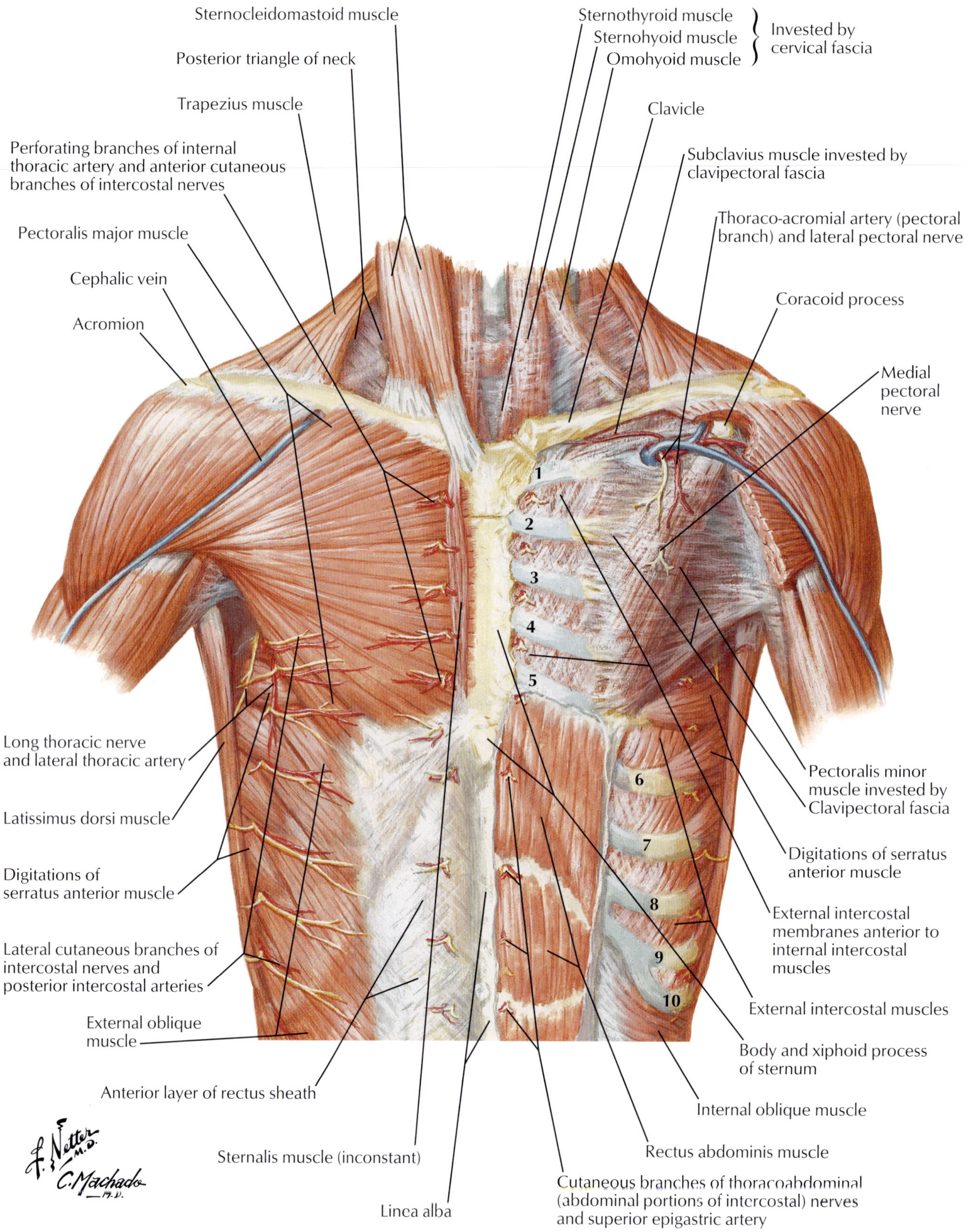
Sternocleidomastoid muscle
Posterior triangle of neck
Trapezius muscle
Perforating branches of internal thoracic artery and anterior cutaneous branches of intercostal nerves
Pectoralis major muscle
Cephalic vein
Acromion
Sternothyroid muscle
Sternohyoid muscle
Omohyoid muscle
Invested by cervical fascia
Clavicle
Subclavius muscle invested by clavipectoral fascia
Thoraco-acromial artery (pectoral branch) and lateral pectoral nerve
Coracoid process
Medial pectoral nerve
1
2
3
4
5
6
7
8
9
10
Long thoracic nerve and lateral thoracic artery
Latissimus dorsi muscle
Digitations of serratus anterior muscle
Lateral cutaneous branches of intercostal nerves and posterior intercostal arteries
External oblique muscle
Anterior layer of rectus sheath
Sternalis muscle (inconstant)
Linea alba
Pectoralis minor muscle invested by Clavipectoral fascia
Digitations of serratus anterior muscle
External intercostal membranes anterior to internal intercostal muscles
External intercostal muscles
Body and xiphoid process of sternum
Internal oblique muscle
Rectus abdominis muscle
Cutaneous branches of thoracoabdominal (abdominal portions of intercostal) nerves and superior epigastric artery
F. Netter M.D.
C. Machado M.D.

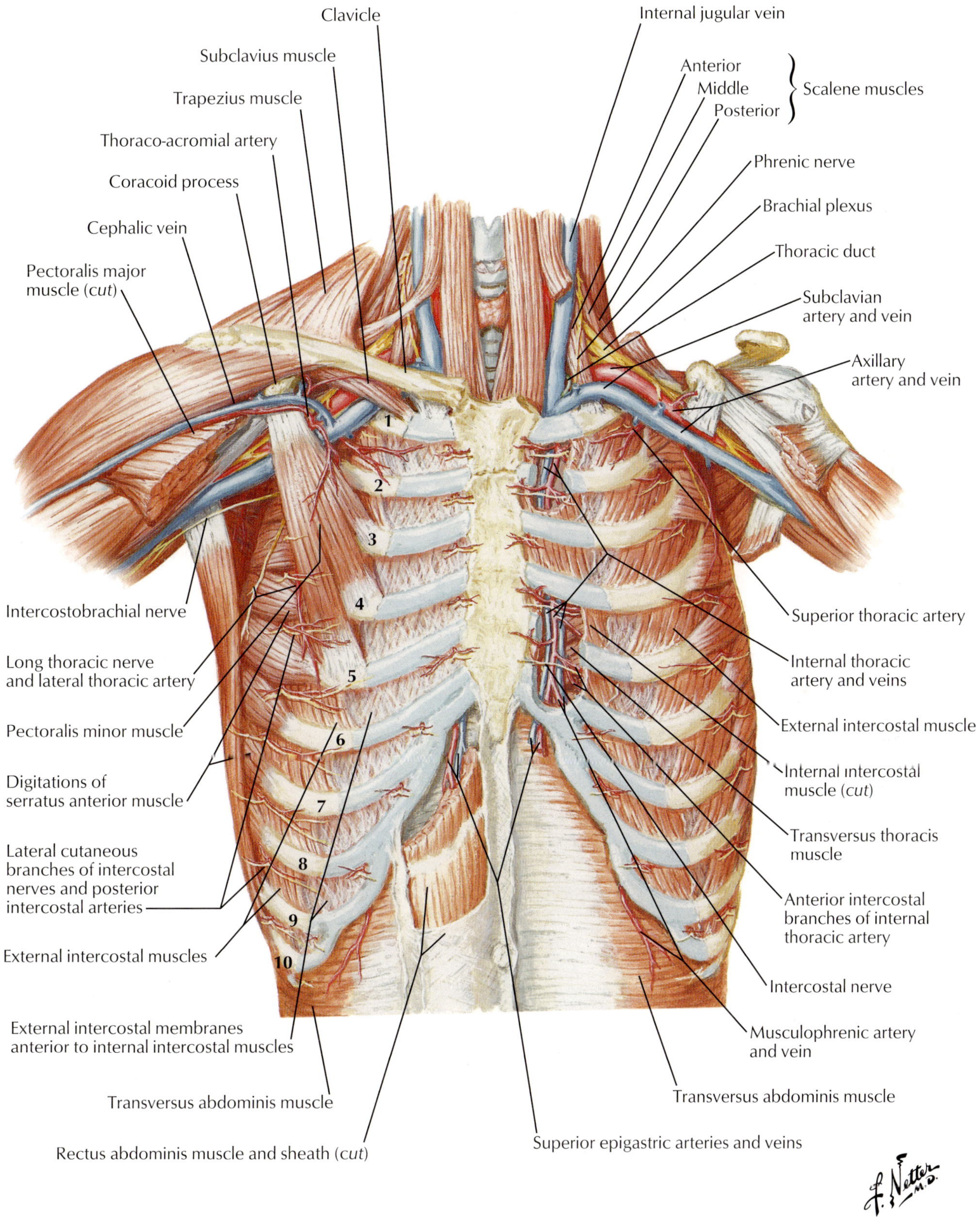
Clavicle
Subclavius muscle
Trapezius muscle
Thoraco-acromial artery
Coracoid process
Cephalic vein
Pectoralis major muscle (cut)
Intercostobrachial nerve
Long thoracic nerve and lateral thoracic artery
Pectoralis minor muscle
Digitations of serratus anterior muscle
Lateral cutaneous branches of intercostal nerves and posterior intercostal arteries
External intercostal muscles
External intercostal membranes anterior to internal intercostal muscles
Transversus abdominis muscle
Rectus abdominis muscle and sheath (cut)
Internal jugular vein
Anterior
Middle
Posterior
Scalene muscles
Phrenic nerve
Brachial plexus
Thoracic duct
Subclavian artery and vein
Axillary artery and vein
Superior thoracic artery
Internal thoracic artery and veins
External intercostal muscle
Internal intercostal muscle (cut)
Transversus thoracis muscle
Anterior intercostal branches of internal thoracic artery
Intercostal nerve
Musculophrenic artery and vein
Transversus abdominis muscle
Superior epigastric arteries and veins
1
2
3
4
5
6
7
8
9
10
F. Netter M.D.

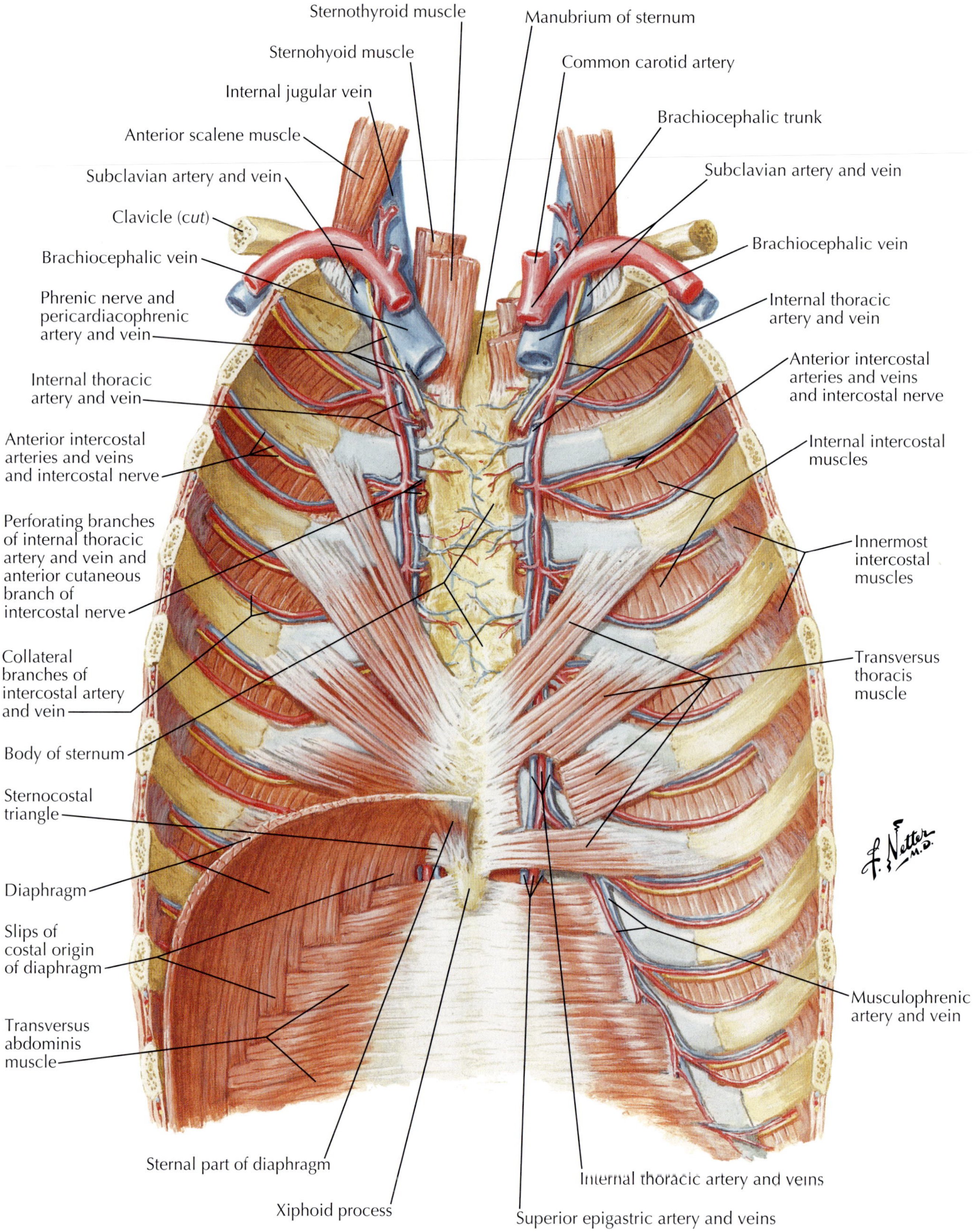
Sternothyroid muscle
Manubrium of sternum
Sternohyoid muscle
Common carotid artery
Internal jugular vein
Brachiocephalic trunk
Anterior scalene muscle
Subclavian artery and vein
Subclavian artery and vein
Clavicle (cut)
Brachiocephalic vein
Brachiocephalic vein
Phrenic nerve and pericardiacophrenic artery and vein
Internal thoracic artery and vein
Internal thoracic artery and vein
Anterior intercostal arteries and veins and intercostal nerve
Anterior intercostal arteries and veins and intercostal nerve
Internal intercostal muscles
Perforating branches of internal thoracic artery and vein and anterior cutaneous branch of intercostal nerve
Innermost intercostal muscles
Collateral branches of intercostal artery and vein
Transversus thoracis muscle
Body of sternum
Sternocostal triangle
Diaphragm
Slips of costal origin of diaphragm
Musculophrenic artery and vein
Transversus abdominis muscle
Sternal part of diaphragm
Internal thoracic artery and veins
Xiphoid process
Superior epigastric artery and veins

Intercostal Nerves and Arteries

See also Plates 254, 262

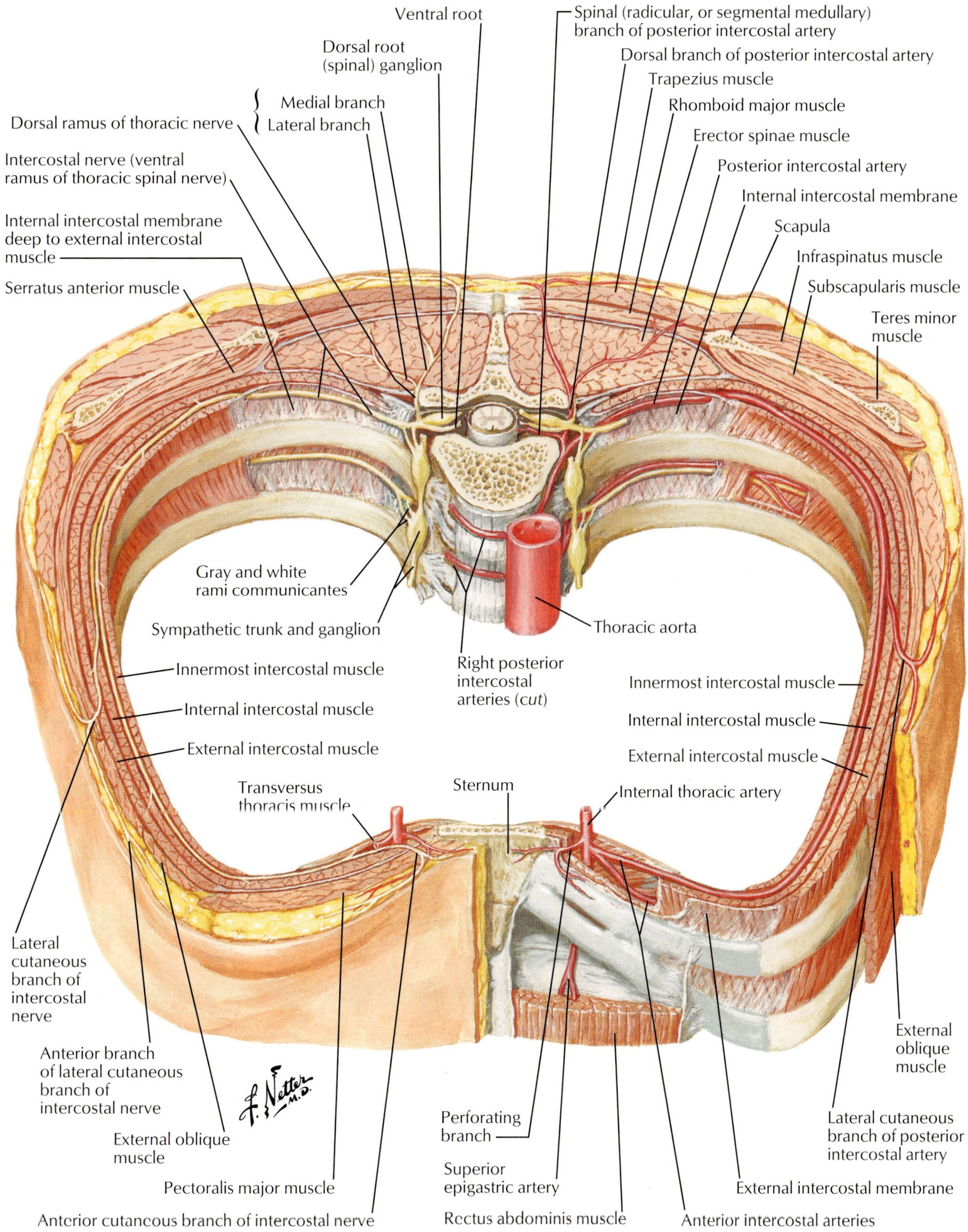

Veins of Internal Thoracic Wall

See also **Plates 187, 227, 252**

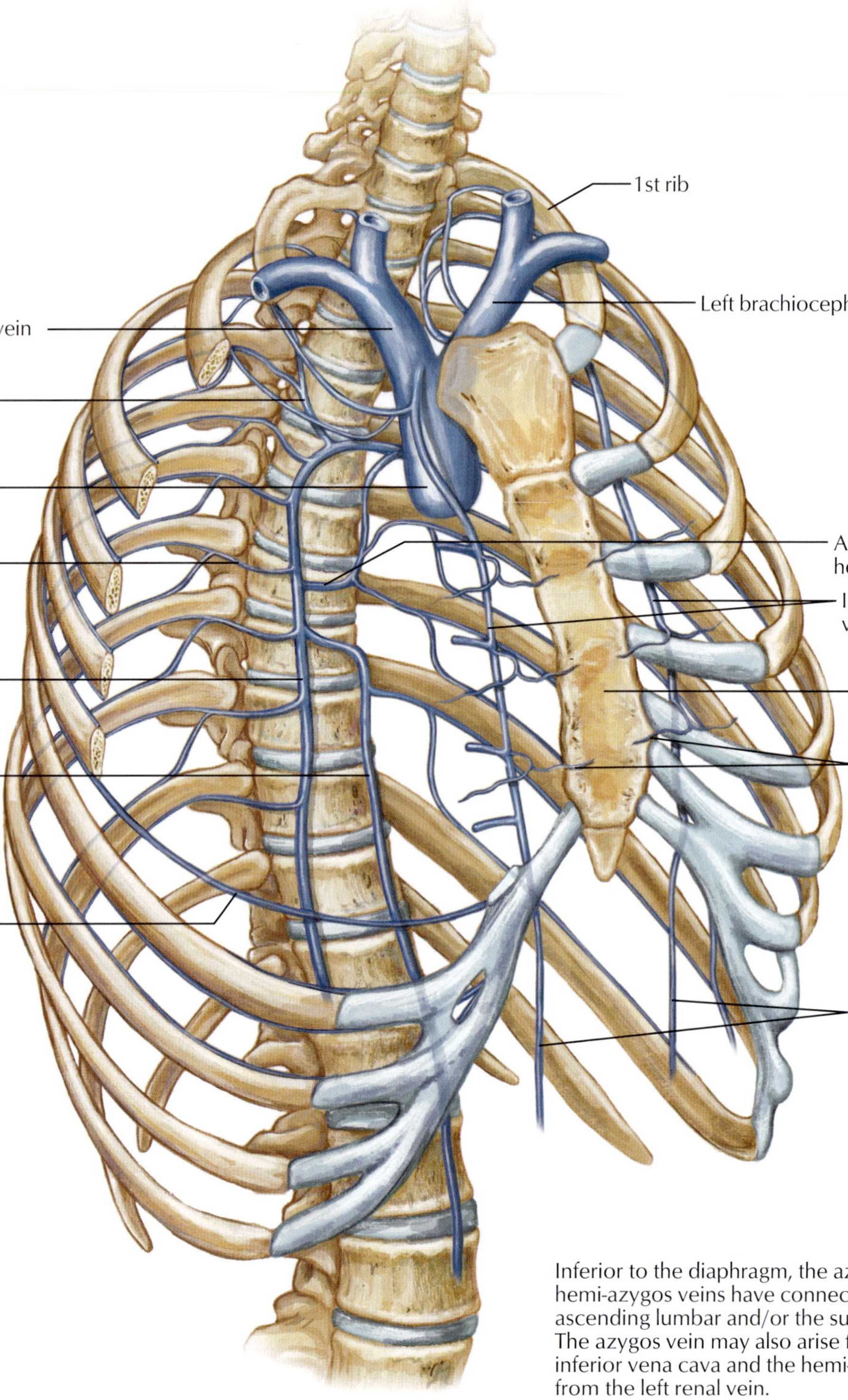

Inferior to the diaphragm, the azygos and hemi-azygos veins have connections with the ascending lumbar and/or the subcostal veins. The azygos vein may also arise from the inferior vena cava and the hemi-azygos vein from the left renal vein.

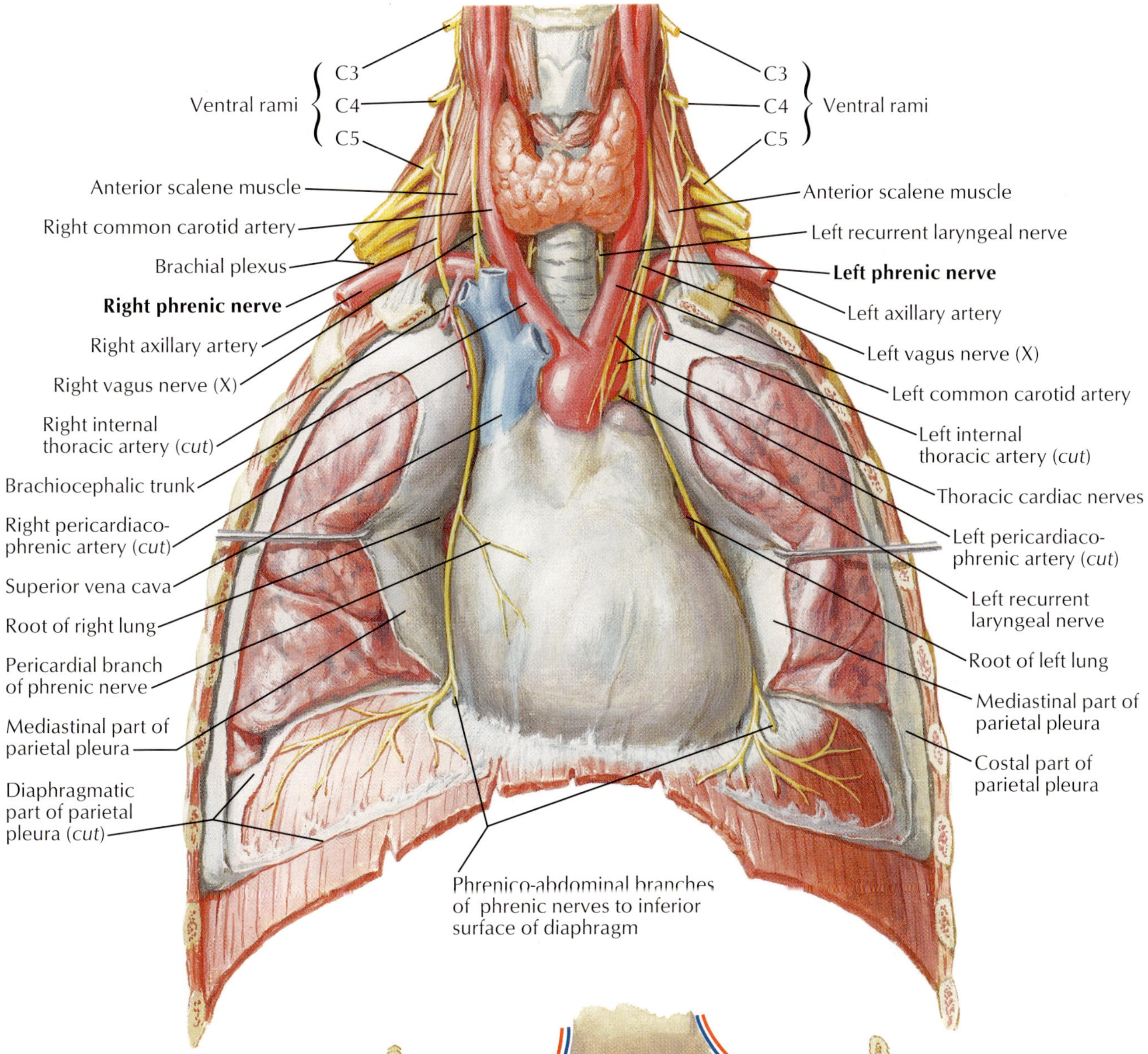
Ventral rami
C3
C4
C5
C3
C4
C5
Ventral rami
Anterior scalene muscle
Right common carotid artery
Brachial plexus
Right phrenic nerve
Right axillary artery
Right vagus nerve (X)
Right internal thoracic artery (*cut*)
Brachiocephalic trunk
Right pericardiacophrenic artery (*cut*)
Superior vena cava
Root of right lung
Pericardial branch of phrenic nerve
Mediastinal part of parietal pleura
Diaphragmatic part of parietal pleura (*cut*)
Anterior scalene muscle
Left recurrent laryngeal nerve
Left phrenic nerve
Left axillary artery
Left vagus nerve (X)
Left common carotid artery
Left internal thoracic artery (*cut*)
Thoracic cardiac nerves
Left pericardiacophrenic artery (*cut*)
Left recurrent laryngeal nerve
Root of left lung
Mediastinal part of parietal pleura
Costal part of parietal pleura
Phrenico-abdominal branches of phrenic nerves to inferior surface of diaphragm

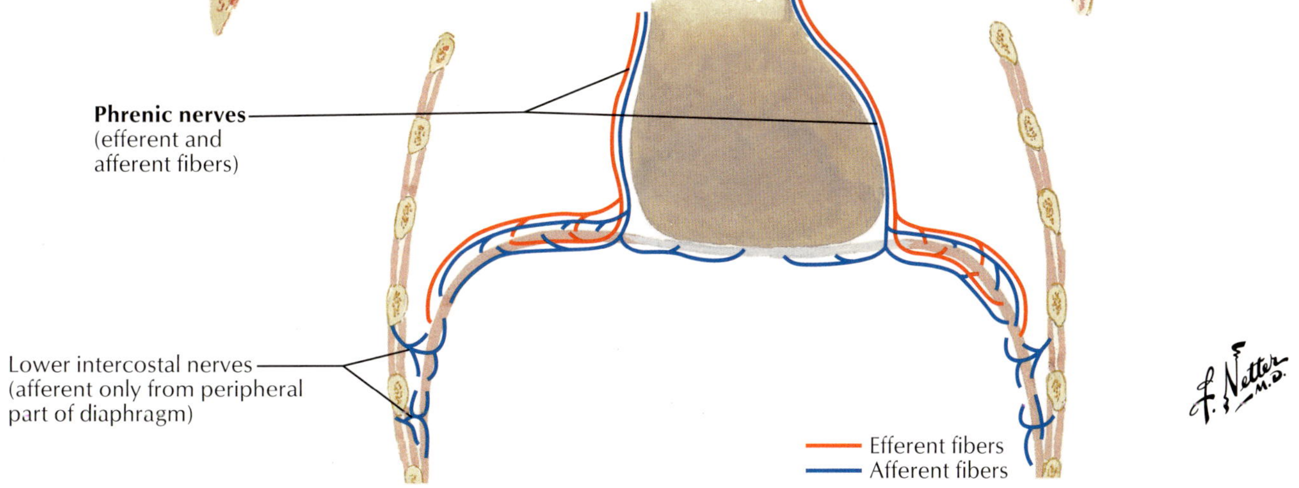
Phrenic nerves (efferent and afferent fibers)
Lower intercostal nerves (afferent only from peripheral part of diaphragm)
Efferent fibers
Afferent fibers
F. Netter M.D.

Diaphragm: Thoracic Surface

See also Plate 229

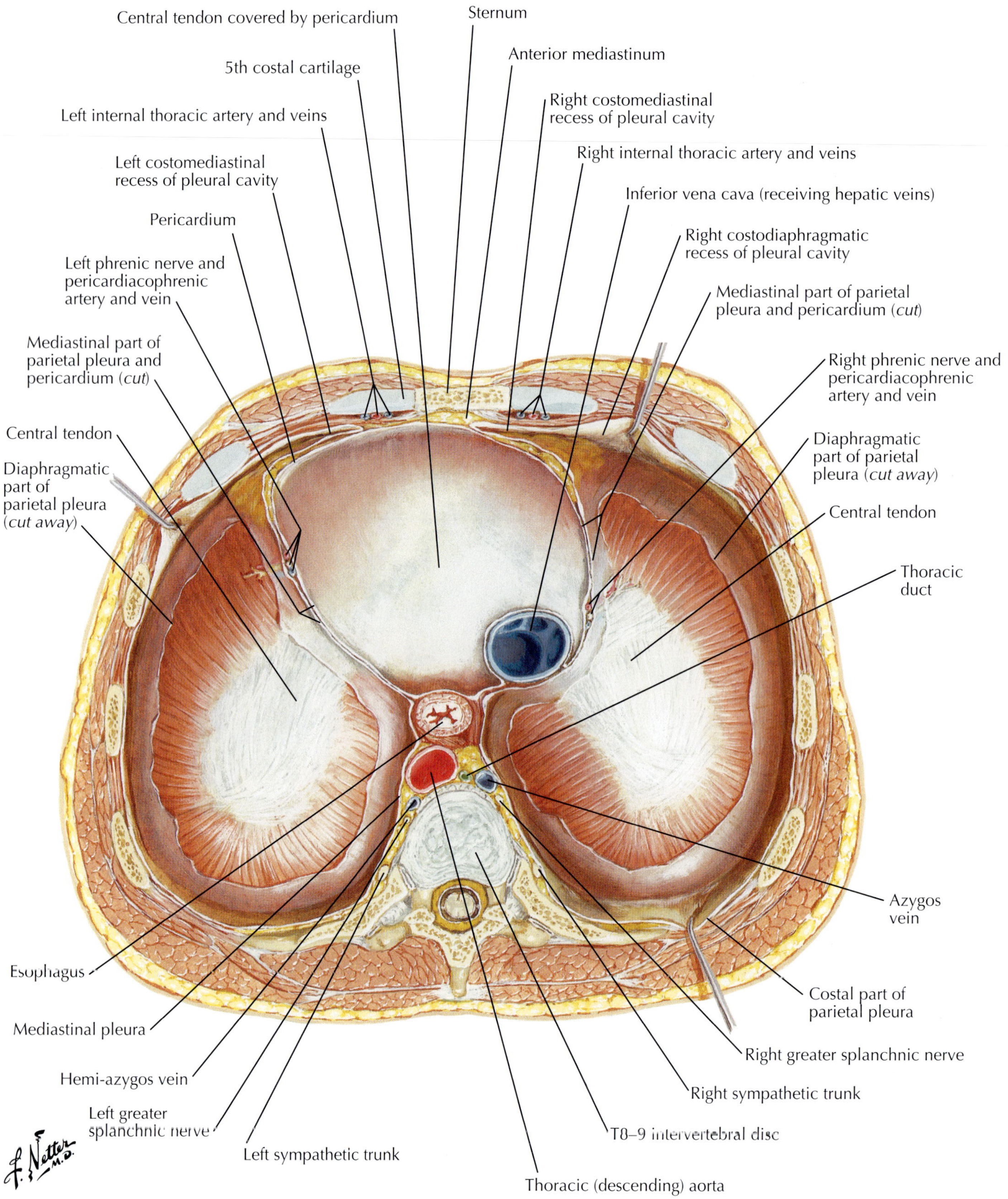

Diaphragm: Abdominal Surface

See also Plates 258, 259

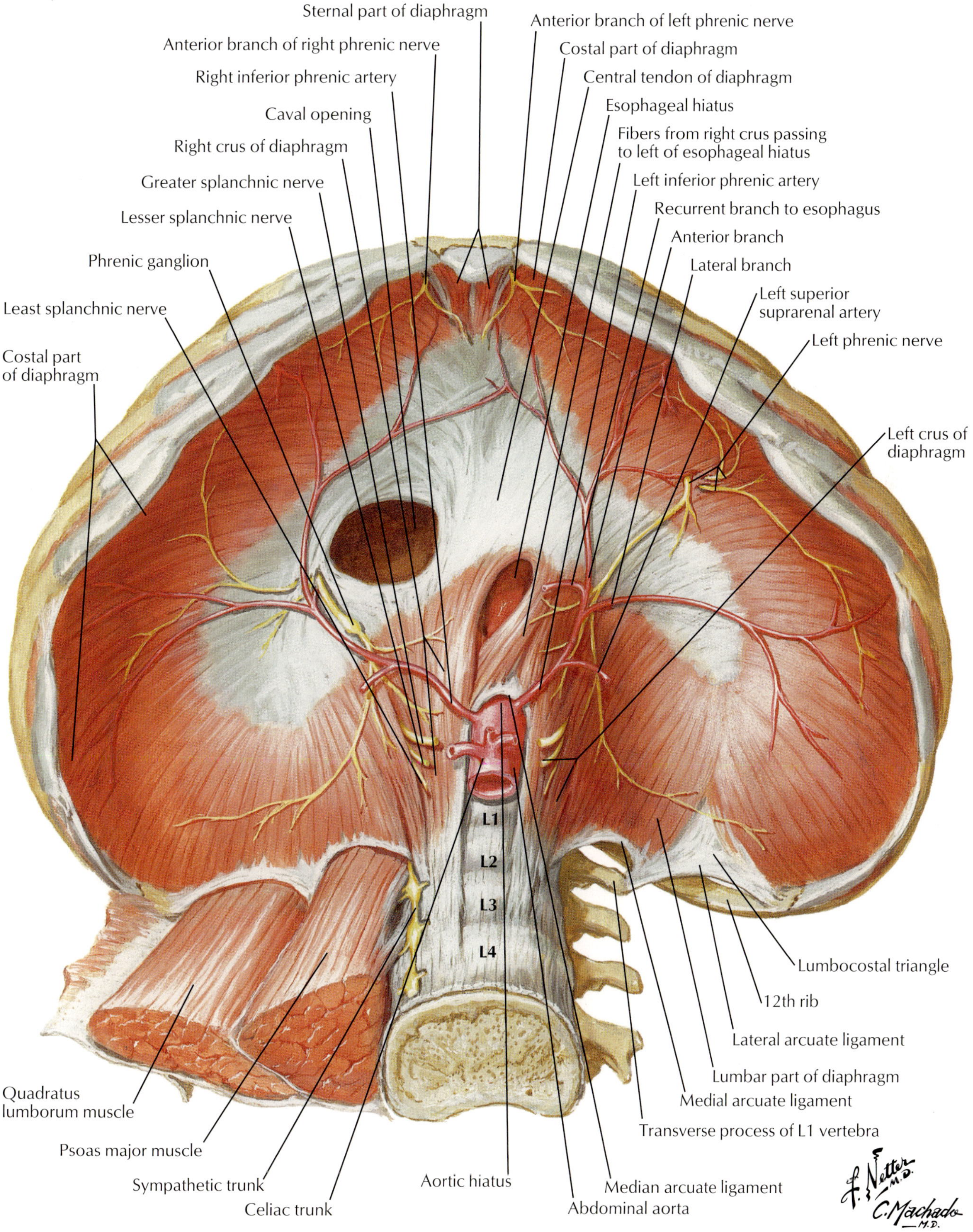

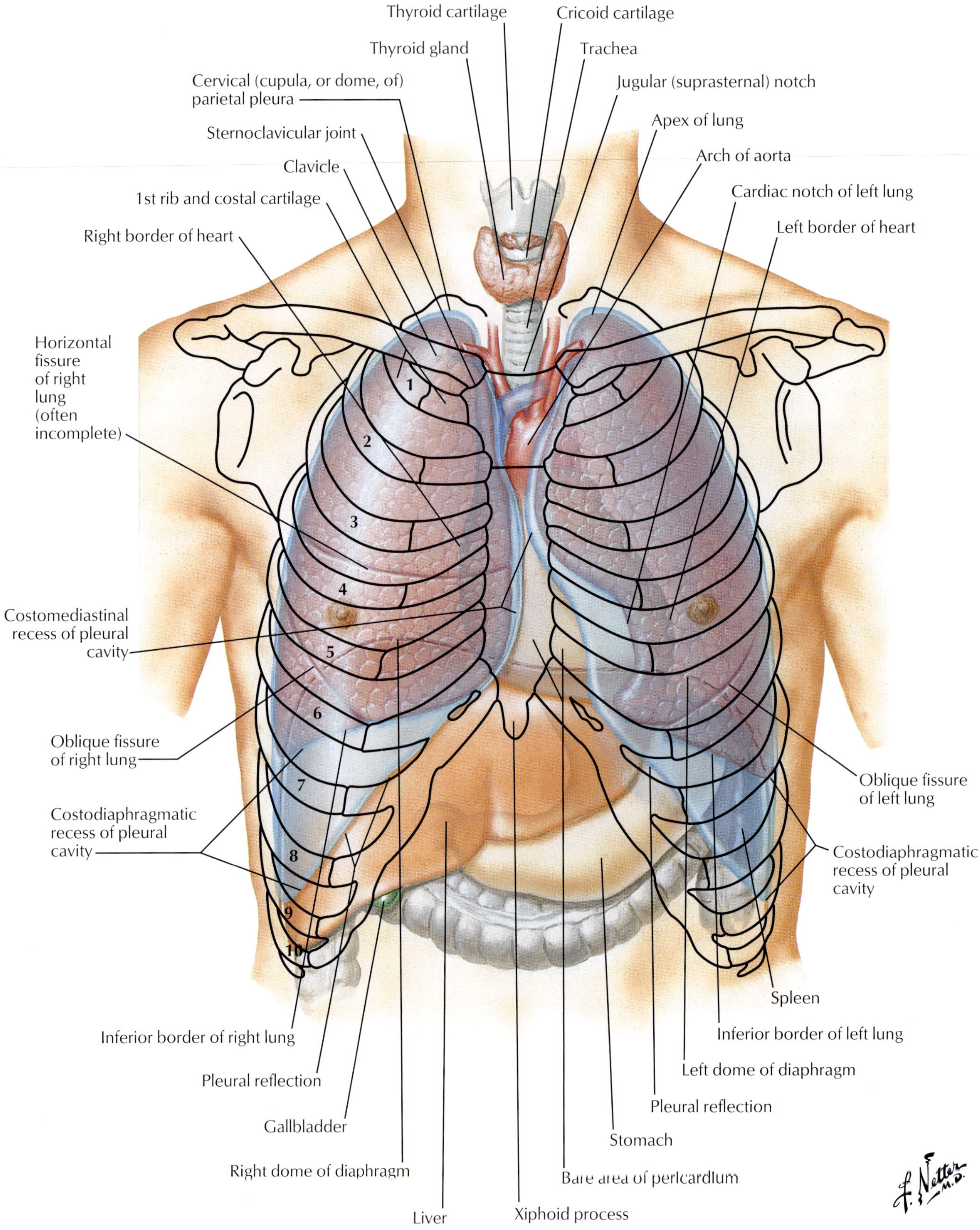
Thyroid cartilage
Cricoid cartilage
Thyroid gland
Trachea
Cervical (cupula, or dome, of) parietal pleura
Jugular (suprasternal) notch
Sternoclavicular joint
Apex of lung
Arch of aorta
Clavicle
1st rib and costal cartilage
Cardiac notch of left lung
Right border of heart
Left border of heart
Horizontal fissure of right lung (often incomplete)
1
2
3
4
5
6
7
8
9
10
Costomediastinal recess of pleural cavity
Oblique fissure of right lung
Oblique fissure of left lung
Costodiaphragmatic recess of pleural cavity
Costodiaphragmatic recess of pleural cavity
Spleen
Inferior border of right lung
Inferior border of left lung
Left dome of diaphragm
Pleural reflection
Pleural reflection
Gallbladder
Stomach
Right dome of diaphragm
Bare area of pericardium
Liver
Xiphoid process

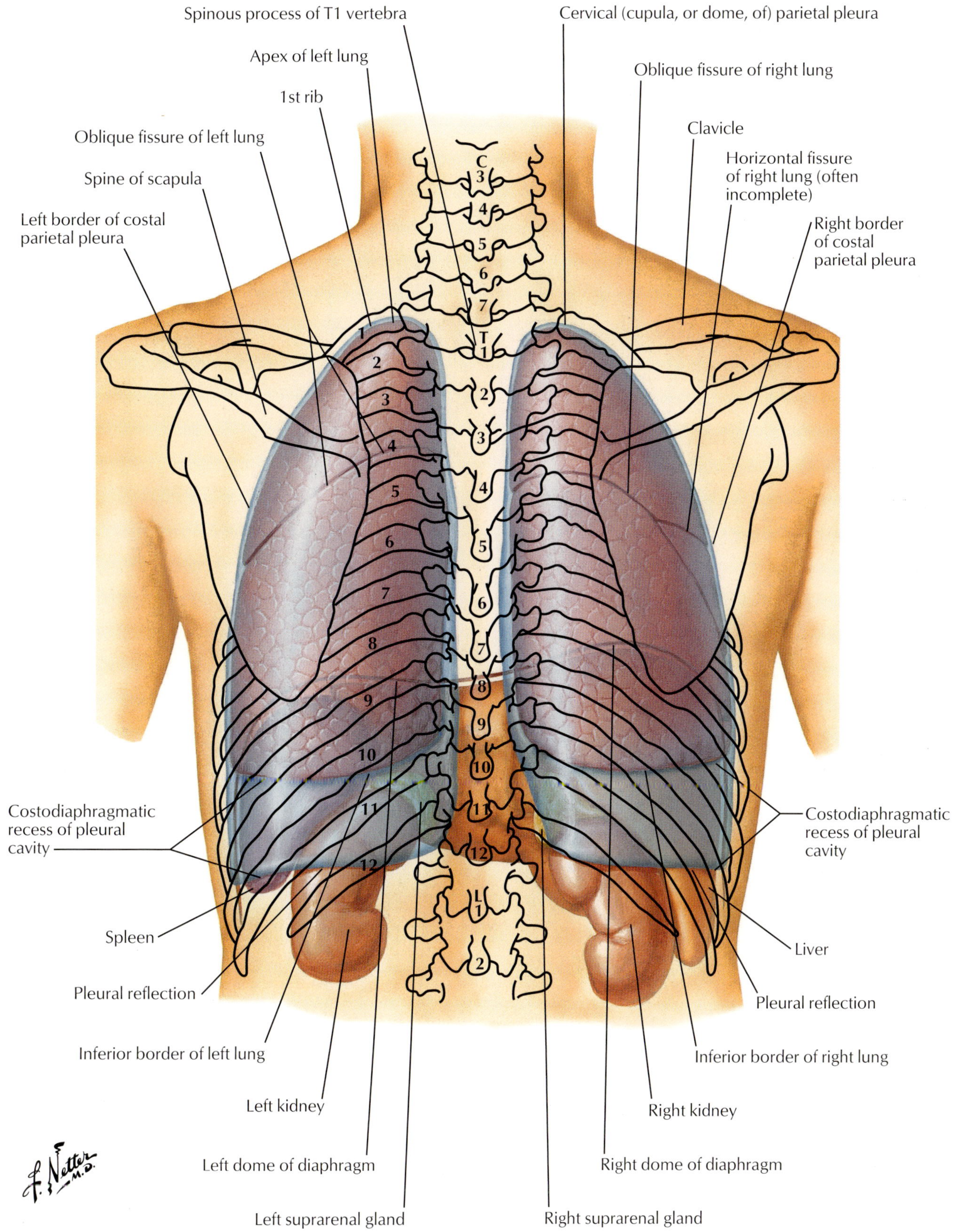

Spinous process of T1 vertebra
Cervical (cupula, or dome, of) parietal pleura
Apex of left lung
Oblique fissure of right lung
1st rib
Oblique fissure of left lung
Clavicle
Horizontal fissure of right lung (often incomplete)
Spine of scapula
Left border of costal parietal pleura
Right border of costal parietal pleura
Costodiaphragmatic recess of pleural cavity
Costodiaphragmatic recess of pleural cavity
Spleen
Liver
Pleural reflection
Pleural reflection
Inferior border of left lung
Inferior border of right lung
Left kidney
Right kidney
Left dome of diaphragm
Right dome of diaphragm
Left suprarenal gland
Right suprarenal gland
F. Netter M.D.

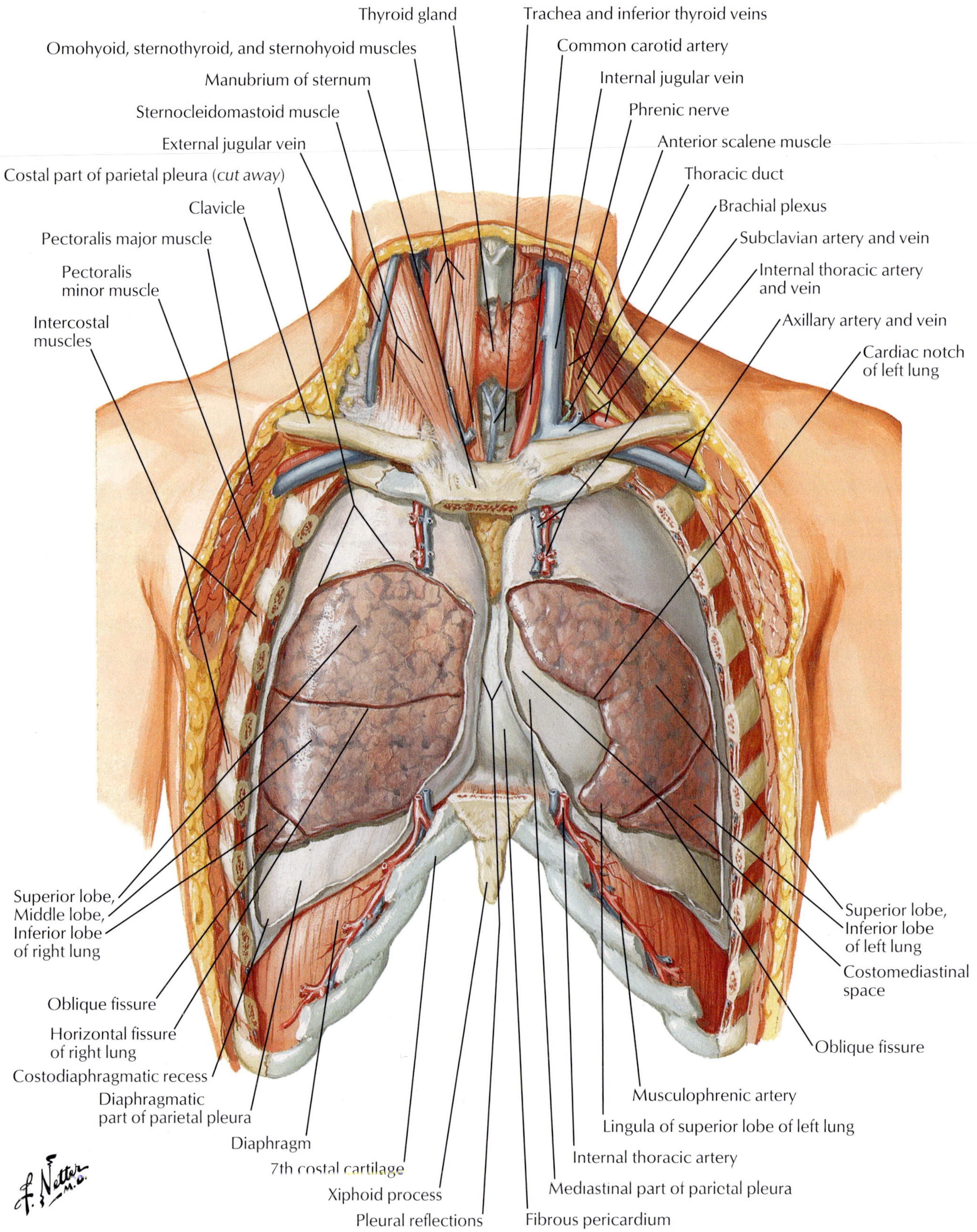
Thyroid gland
Trachea and inferior thyroid veins
Omohyoid, sternothyroid, and sternohyoid muscles
Common carotid artery
Manubrium of sternum
Internal jugular vein
Sternocleidomastoid muscle
Phrenic nerve
External jugular vein
Anterior scalene muscle
Costal part of parietal pleura (*cut away*)
Thoracic duct
Clavicle
Brachial plexus
Pectoralis major muscle
Subclavian artery and vein
Pectoralis minor muscle
Internal thoracic artery and vein
Intercostal muscles
Axillary artery and vein
Cardiac notch of left lung
Superior lobe, Middle lobe, Inferior lobe of right lung
Superior lobe, Inferior lobe of left lung
Costomediastinal space
Oblique fissure
Horizontal fissure of right lung
Oblique fissure
Costodiaphragmatic recess
Diaphragmatic part of parietal pleura
Musculophrenic artery
Lingula of superior lobe of left lung
Diaphragm
Internal thoracic artery
7th costal cartilage
Mediastinal part of parietal pleura
Xiphoid process
Pleural reflections
Fibrous pericardium
F. Netter M.D.

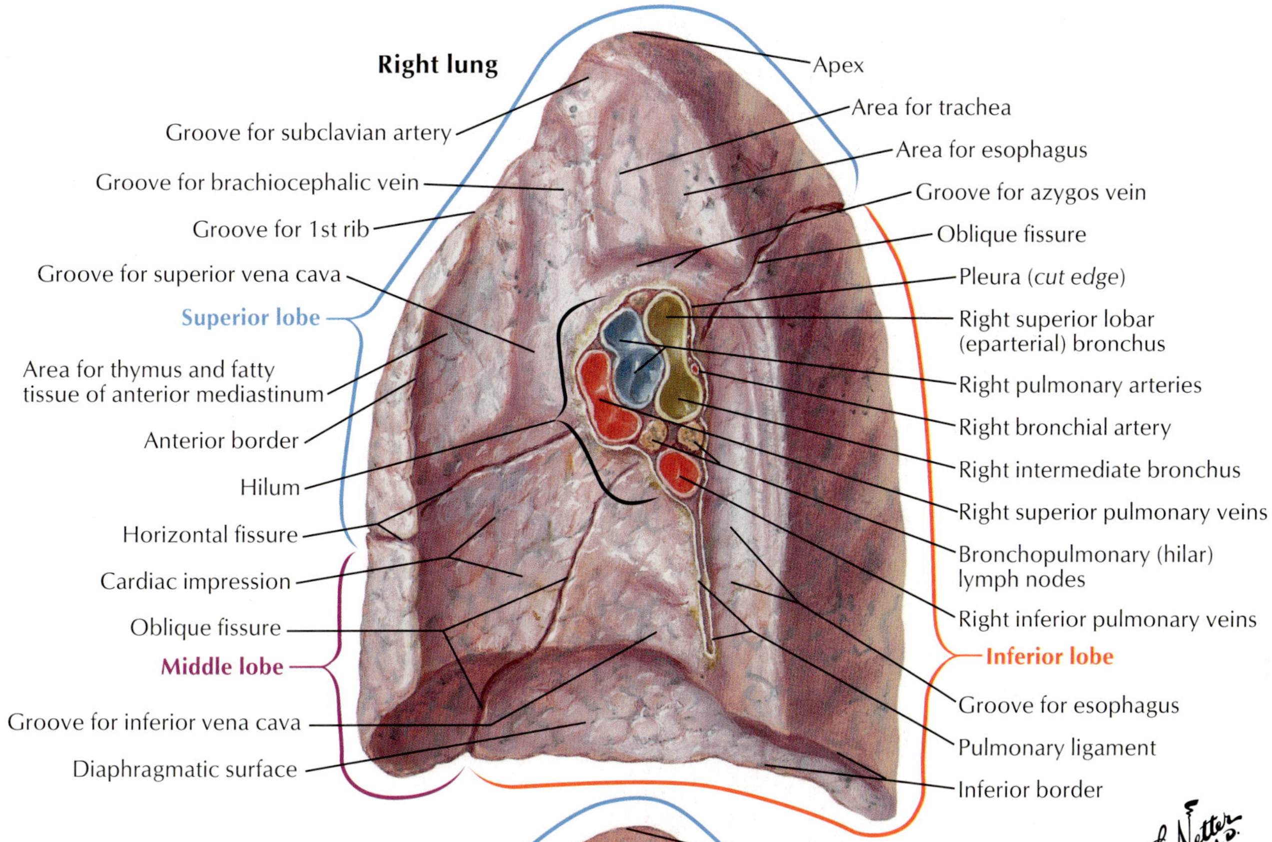
Right lung
Apex
Area for trachea
Area for esophagus
Groove for azygos vein
Oblique fissure
Pleura (cut edge)
Right superior lobar (eparterial) bronchus
Right pulmonary arteries
Right bronchial artery
Right intermediate bronchus
Right superior pulmonary veins
Bronchopulmonary (hilar) lymph nodes
Right inferior pulmonary veins
Inferior lobe
Groove for esophagus
Pulmonary ligament
Inferior border
Groove for subclavian artery
Groove for brachiocephalic vein
Groove for 1st rib
Groove for superior vena cava
Superior lobe
Area for thymus and fatty tissue of anterior mediastinum
Anterior border
Hilum
Horizontal fissure
Cardiac impression
Oblique fissure
Middle lobe
Groove for inferior vena cava
Diaphragmatic surface

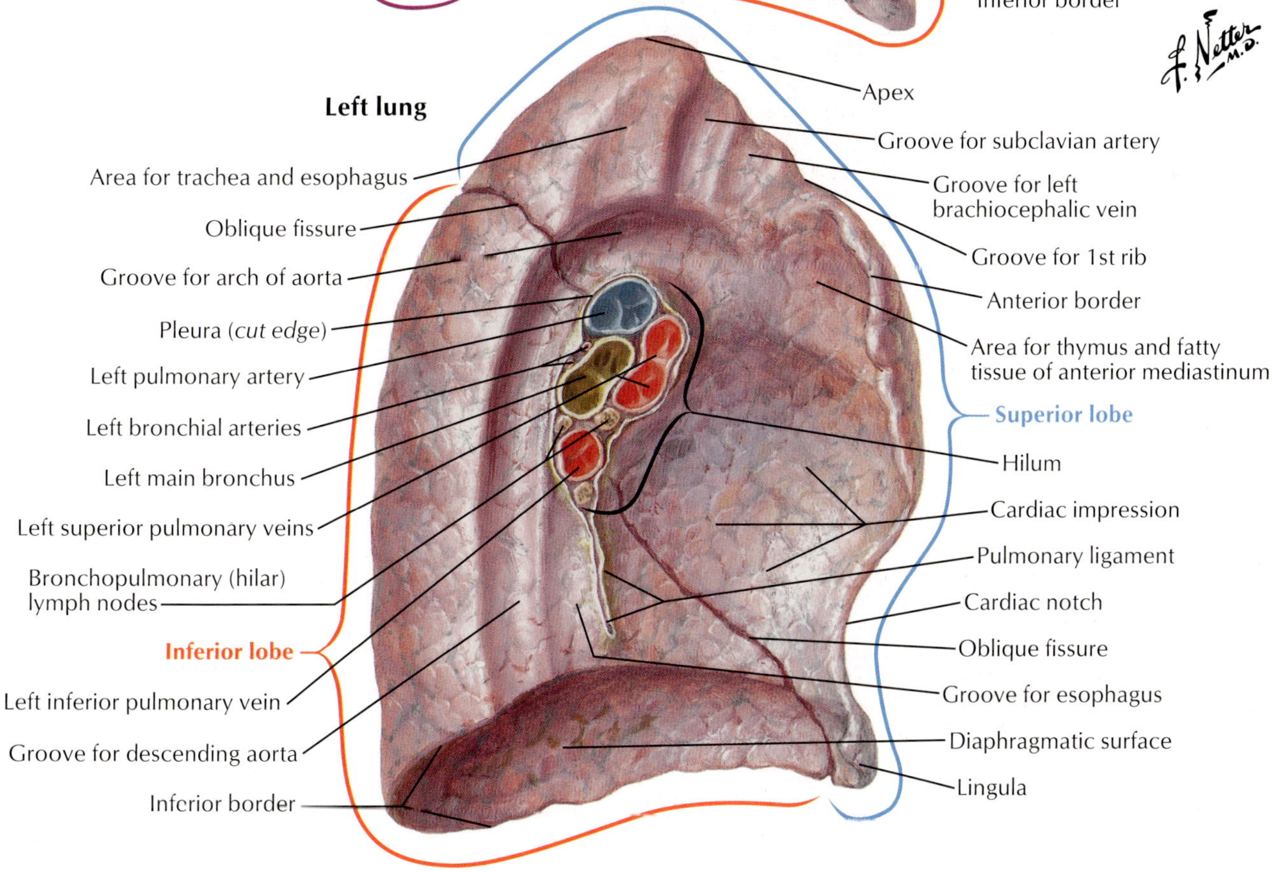
Left lung
Apex
Groove for subclavian artery
Groove for left brachiocephalic vein
Groove for 1st rib
Anterior border
Area for thymus and fatty tissue of anterior mediastinum
Superior lobe
Hilum
Cardiac impression
Pulmonary ligament
Cardiac notch
Oblique fissure
Groove for esophagus
Diaphragmatic surface
Lingula
Area for trachea and esophagus
Oblique fissure
Groove for arch of aorta
Pleura (cut edge)
Left pulmonary artery
Left bronchial arteries
Left main bronchus
Left superior pulmonary veins
Bronchopulmonary (hilar) lymph nodes
Inferior lobe
Left inferior pulmonary vein
Groove for descending aorta
Inferior border

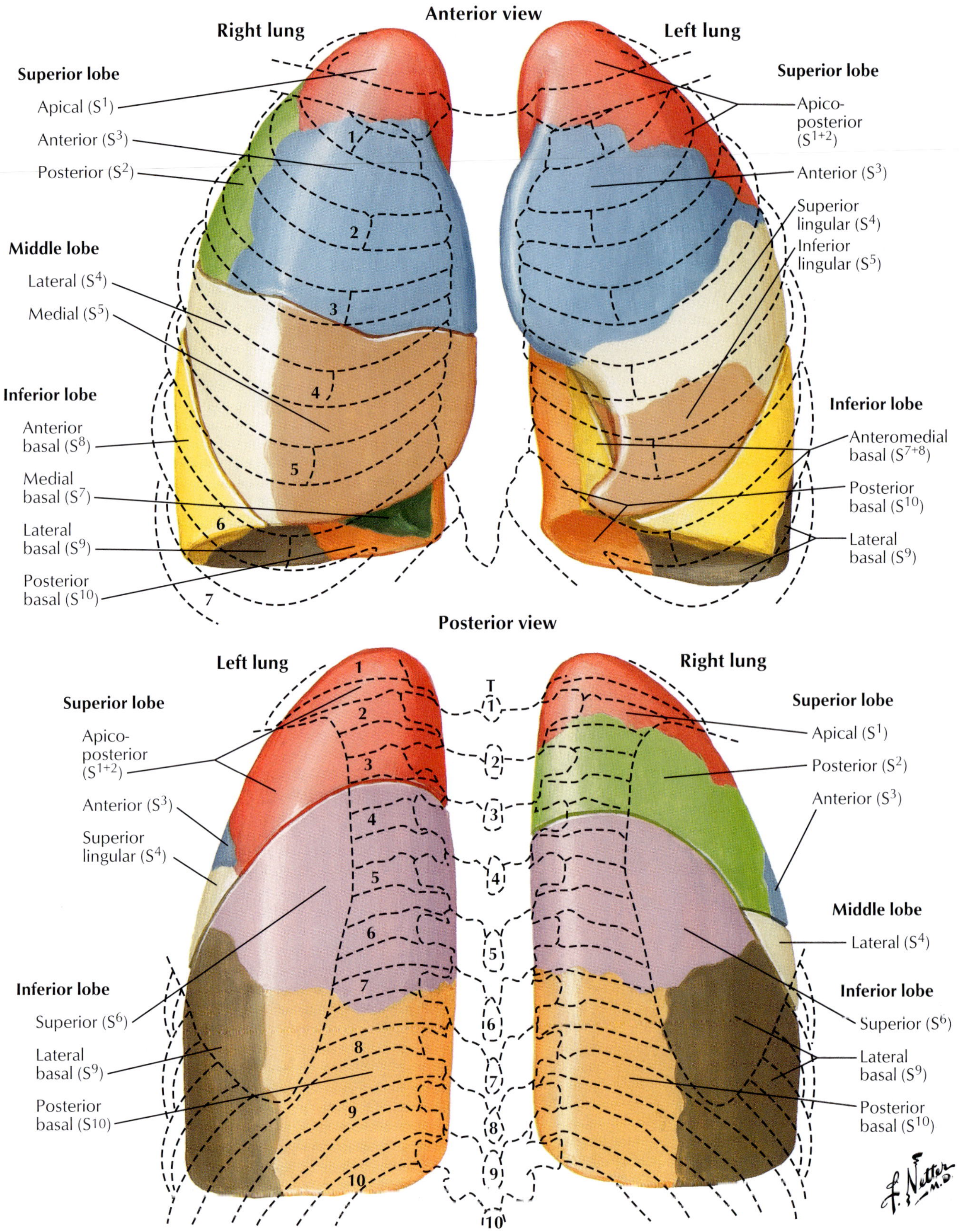
Anterior view
Right lung
Superior lobe
Apical (S^1)
Anterior (S^3)
Posterior (S^2)
Middle lobe
Lateral (S^4)
Medial (S^5)
Inferior lobe
Anterior basal (S^8)
Medial basal (S^7)
Lateral basal (S^9)
Posterior basal (S^{10})
Left lung
Superior lobe
Apico-posterior (S^{1+2})
Anterior (S^3)
Superior lingular (S^4)
Inferior lingular (S^5)
Inferior lobe
Anteromedial basal (S^{7+8})
Posterior basal (S^{10})
Lateral basal (S^9)
Posterior view
Left lung
Superior lobe
Apico-posterior (S^{1+2})
Anterior (S^3)
Superior lingular (S^4)
Inferior lobe
Superior (S^6)
Lateral basal (S^9)
Posterior basal (S^{10})
Right lung
Superior lobe
Apical (S^1)
Posterior (S^2)
Anterior (S^3)
Middle lobe
Lateral (S^4)
Inferior lobe
Superior (S^6)
Lateral basal (S^9)
Posterior basal (S^{10})
T

Lateral views

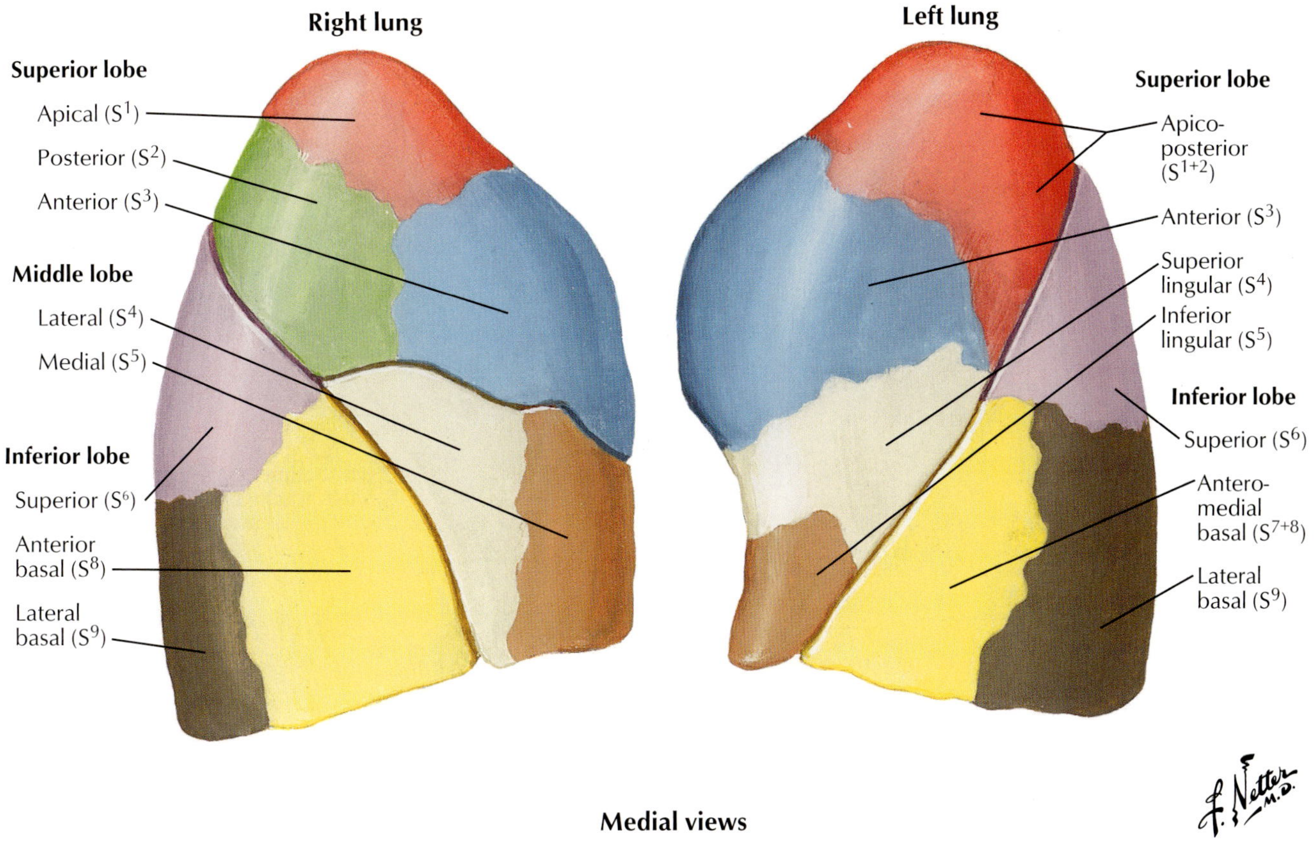

Medial views

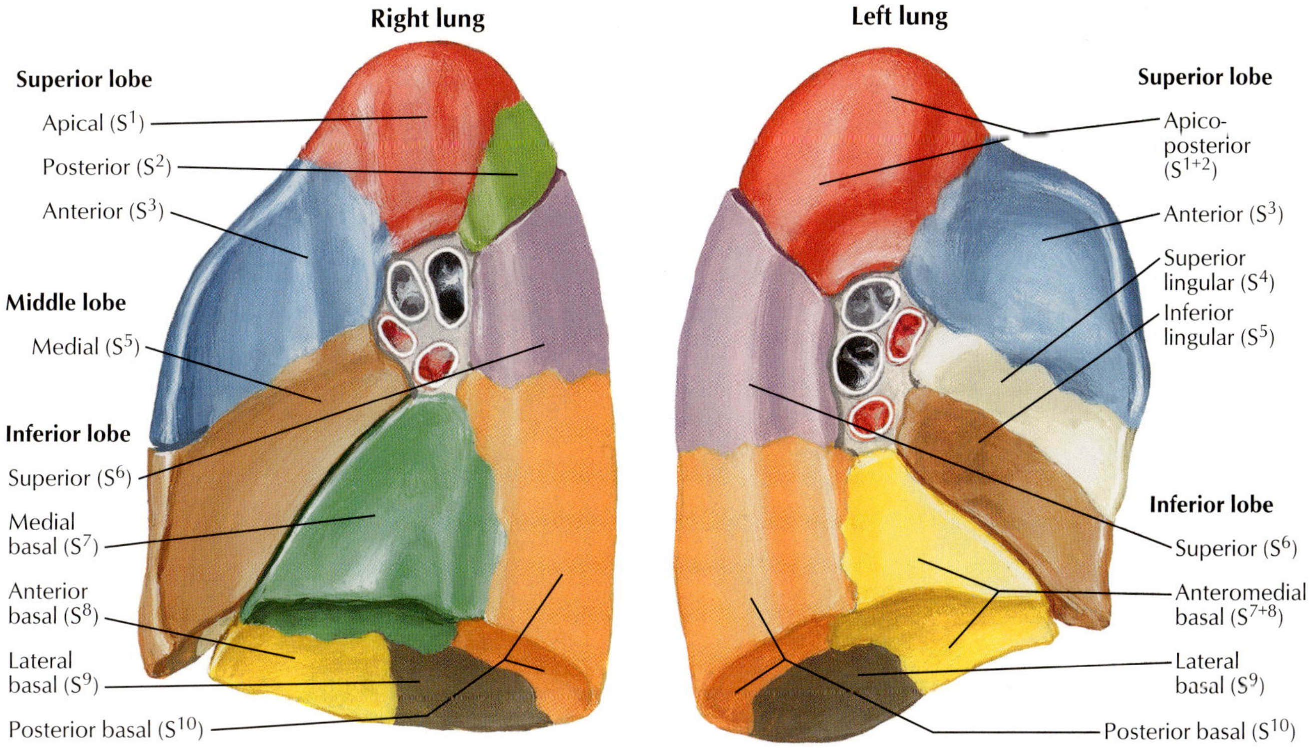

Trachea and Major Bronchi

See also **Plates 70, 204, 207**

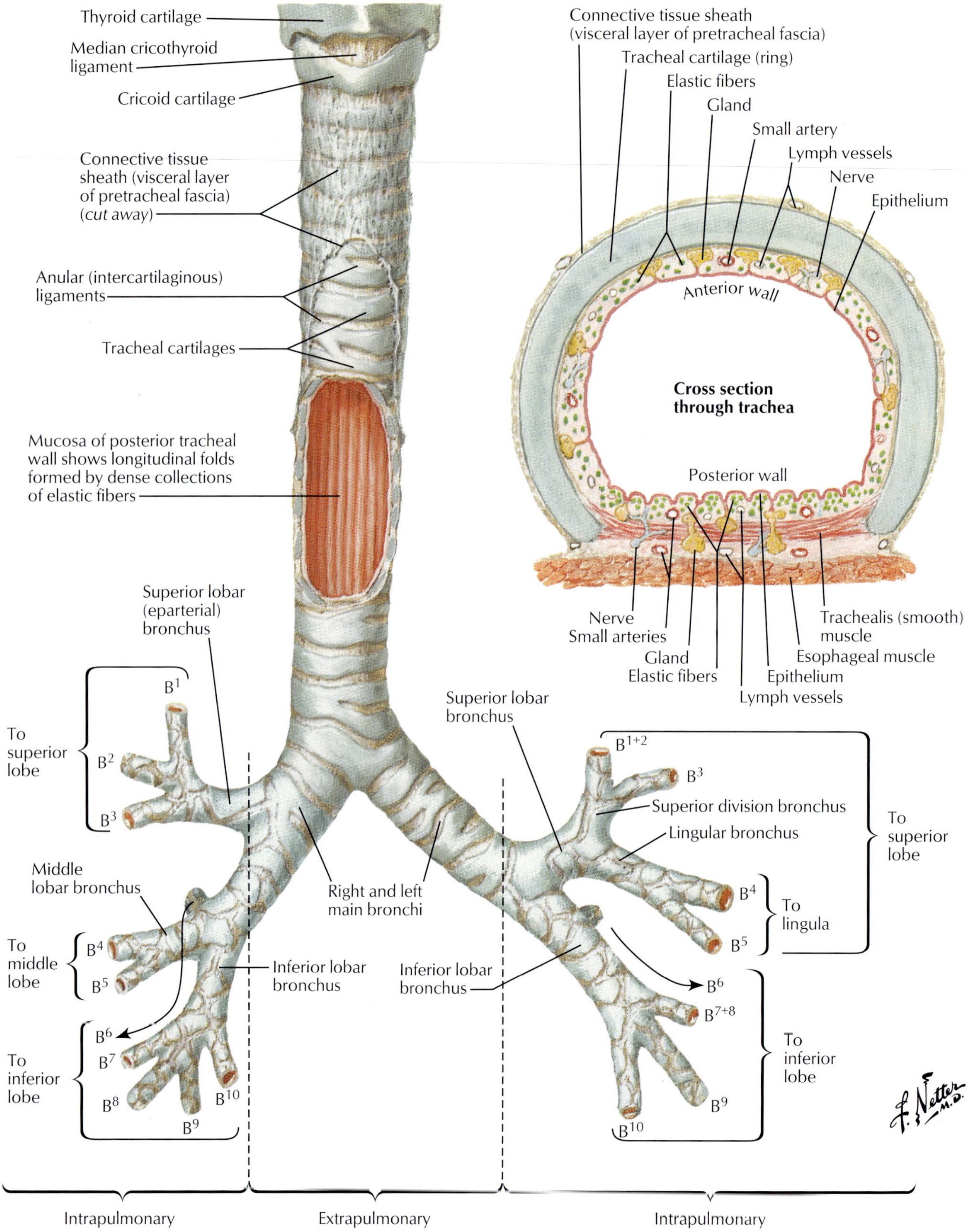

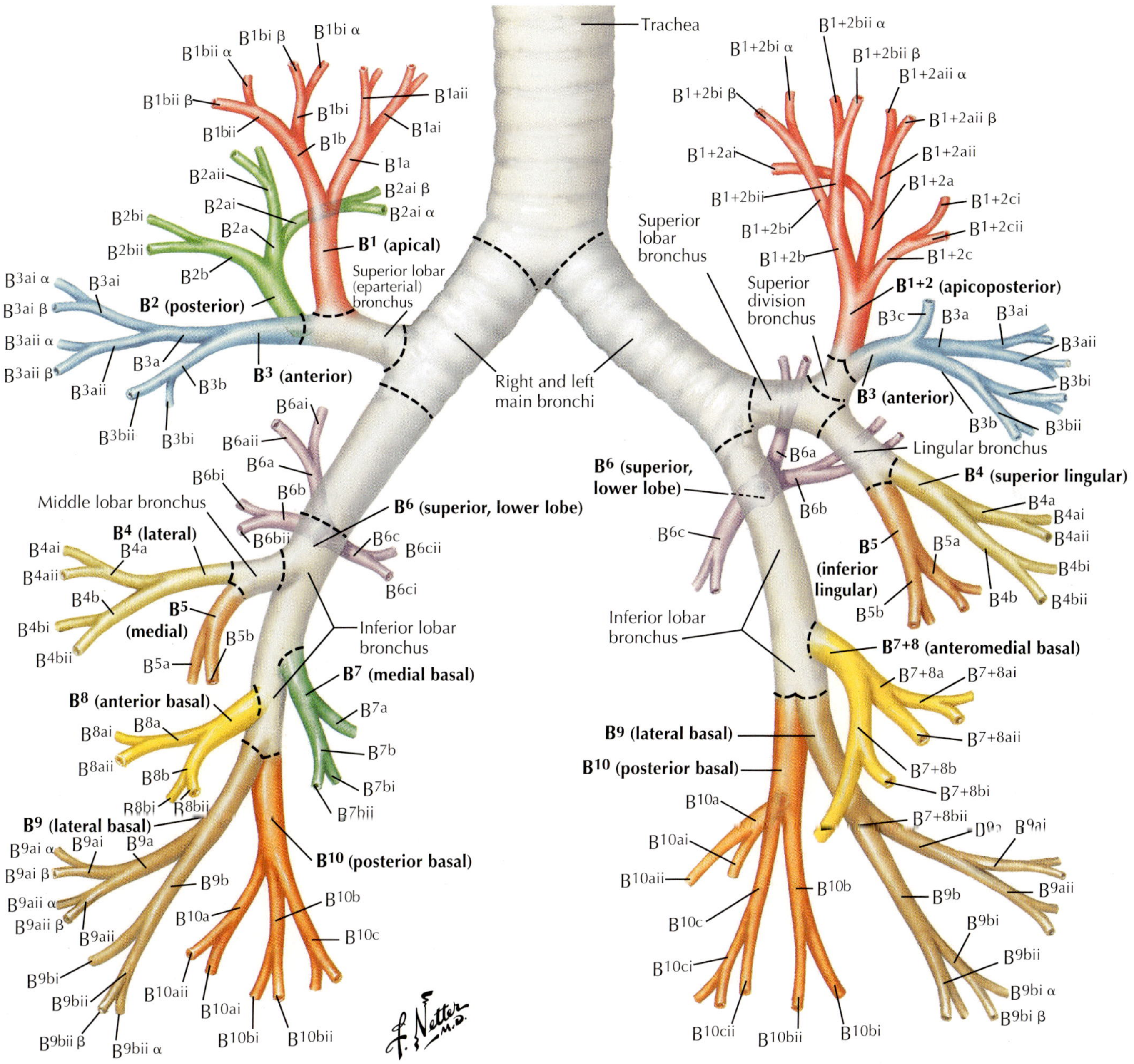

Nomenclature in common usage for bronchopulmonary segments (Plates 197 and 198) is that of Jackson and Huber, and segmental bronchi are named accordingly. Ikeda proposed nomenclature (as demonstrated here) for bronchial subdivisions as far as the 6th generation. For simplification on this illustration, only some bronchial subdivisions are labeled as far as the 5th or 6th generation. Segmental bronchi (B) are numbered from 1 to 10 in each lung, corresponding to pulmonary segments. In the left lung, B^1 and B^2 are combined as are B^7 and B^8. Subsegmental, or 4th order, bronchi are indicated by the addition of lowercase letters a, b, or c when an additional branch is present. Fifth order bronchi are designated by Roman numerals i (anterior) or ii (posterior) and 6th order bronchi by Greek letters α or β. Several texts use alternate numbers (as proposed by Boyden) for segmental bronchi.

Variations of the standard bronchial pattern shown here are common, especially in peripheral airways.

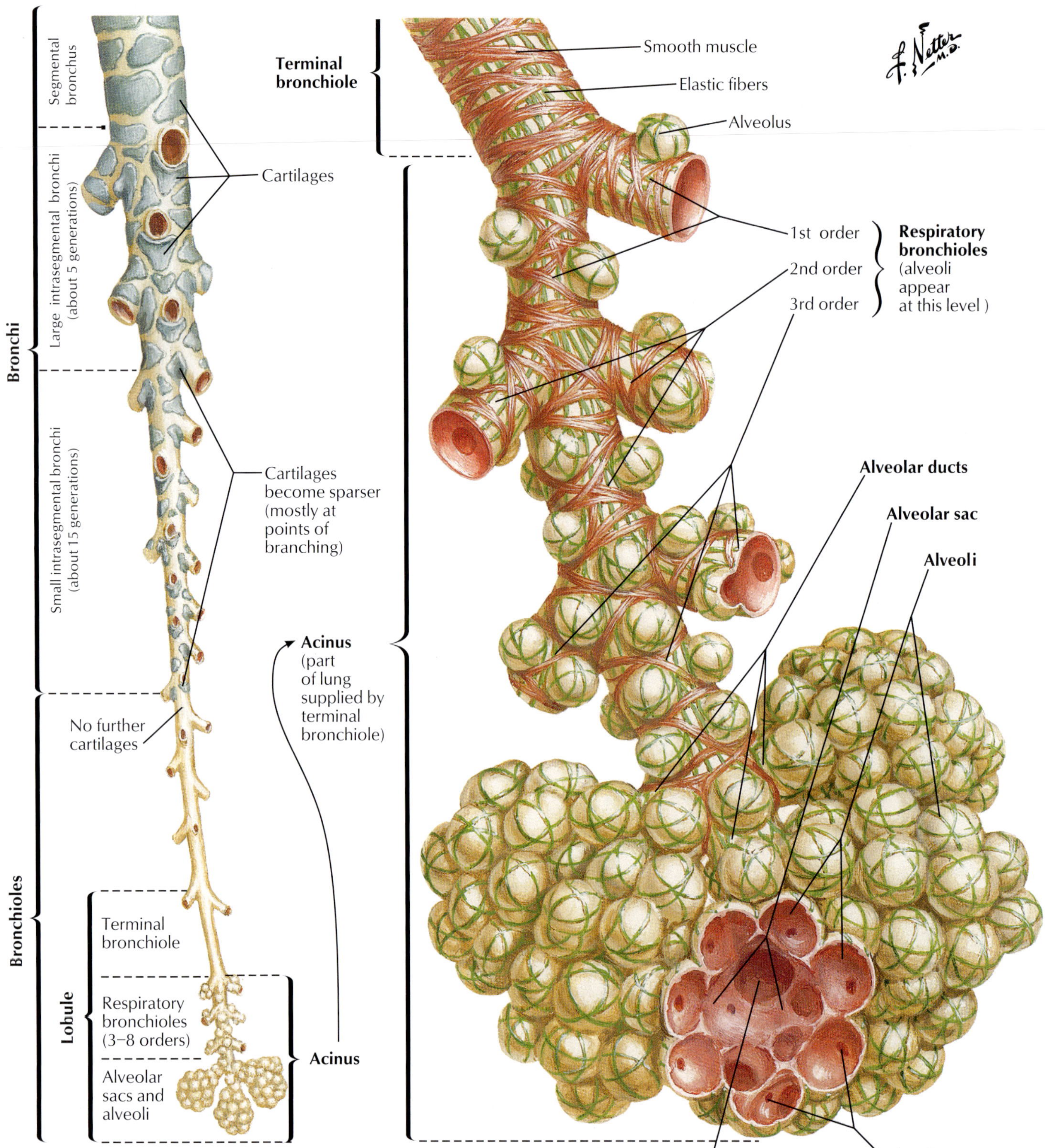

Subdivisions of intrapulmonary airways

Structure of intrapulmonary airways

Intrapulmonary Blood Circulation: Schema

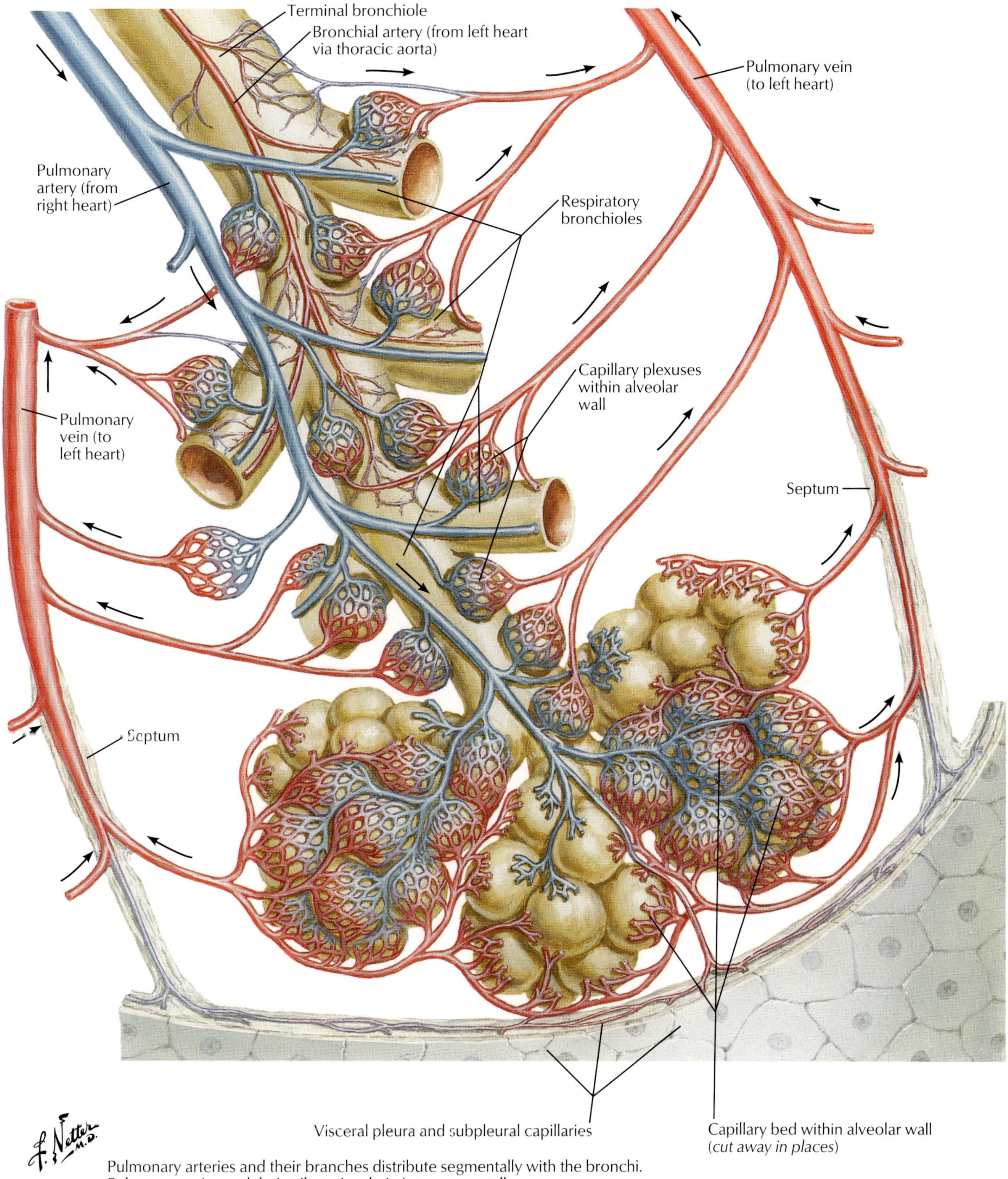

Pulmonary arteries and their branches distribute segmentally with the bronchi. Pulmonary veins and their tributaries drain intersegmentally.

Great Vessels of Superior Mediastinum

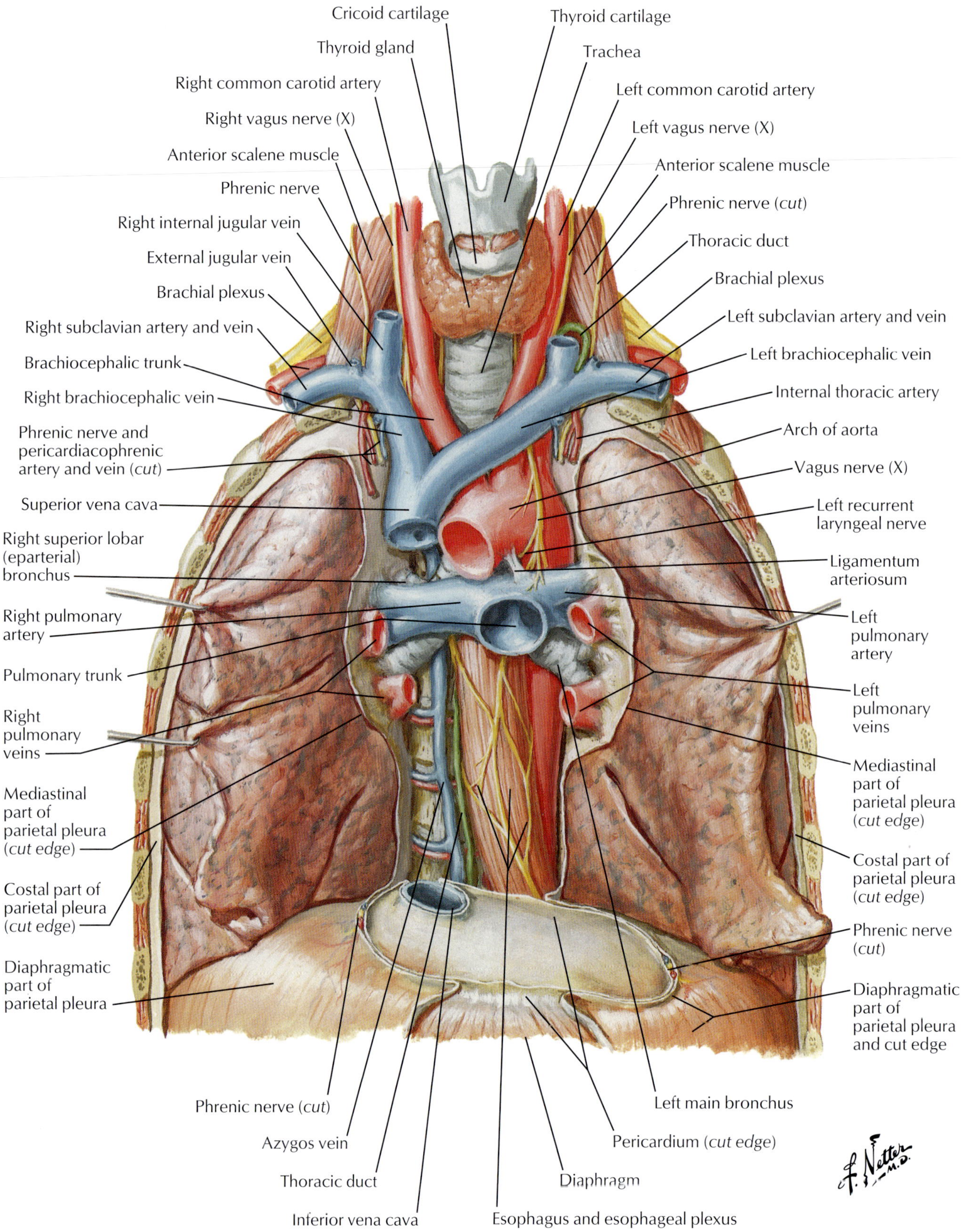

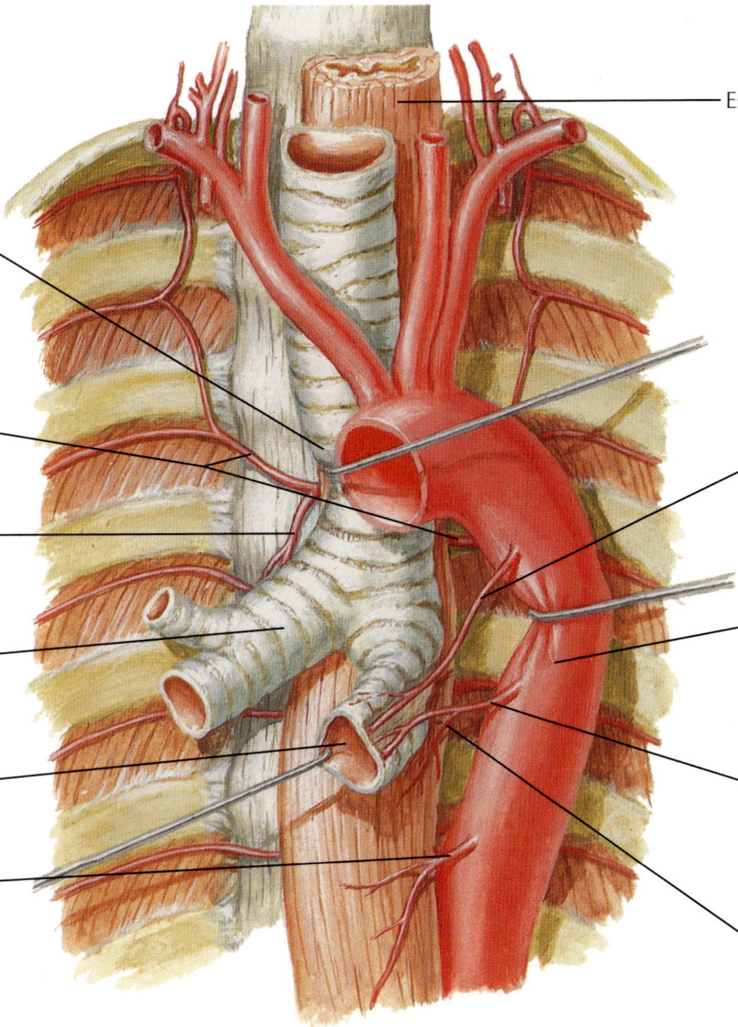
Esophagus
Trachea (*pulled to left by hook*)
3rd right posterior intercostal artery
Right bronchial artery
Right main bronchus
Left main bronchus (*pulled to right by hook*)
Esophageal artery
Superior left bronchial artery
Aorta (*pulled aside by hook*)
Inferior left bronchial artery
Esophageal branch of bronchial artery

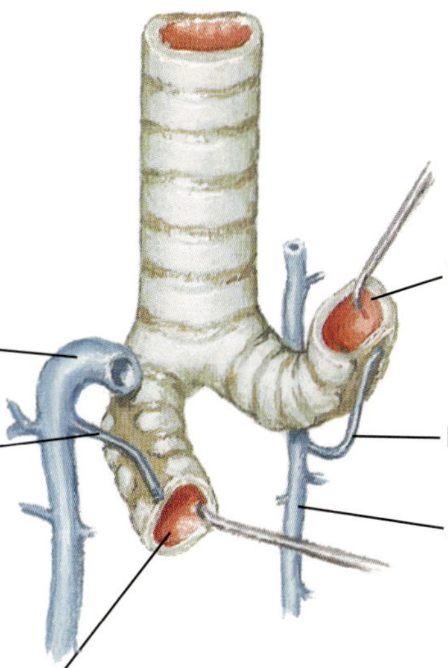
Azygos vein
Right bronchial vein
Right main bronchus (*pulled to left and rotated by hook*)
Left main bronchus (*turned up by hook*)
Left bronchial vein
Accessory hemiazygos vein

Lymph Vessels and Nodes of Lung

See also Plates 74, 235

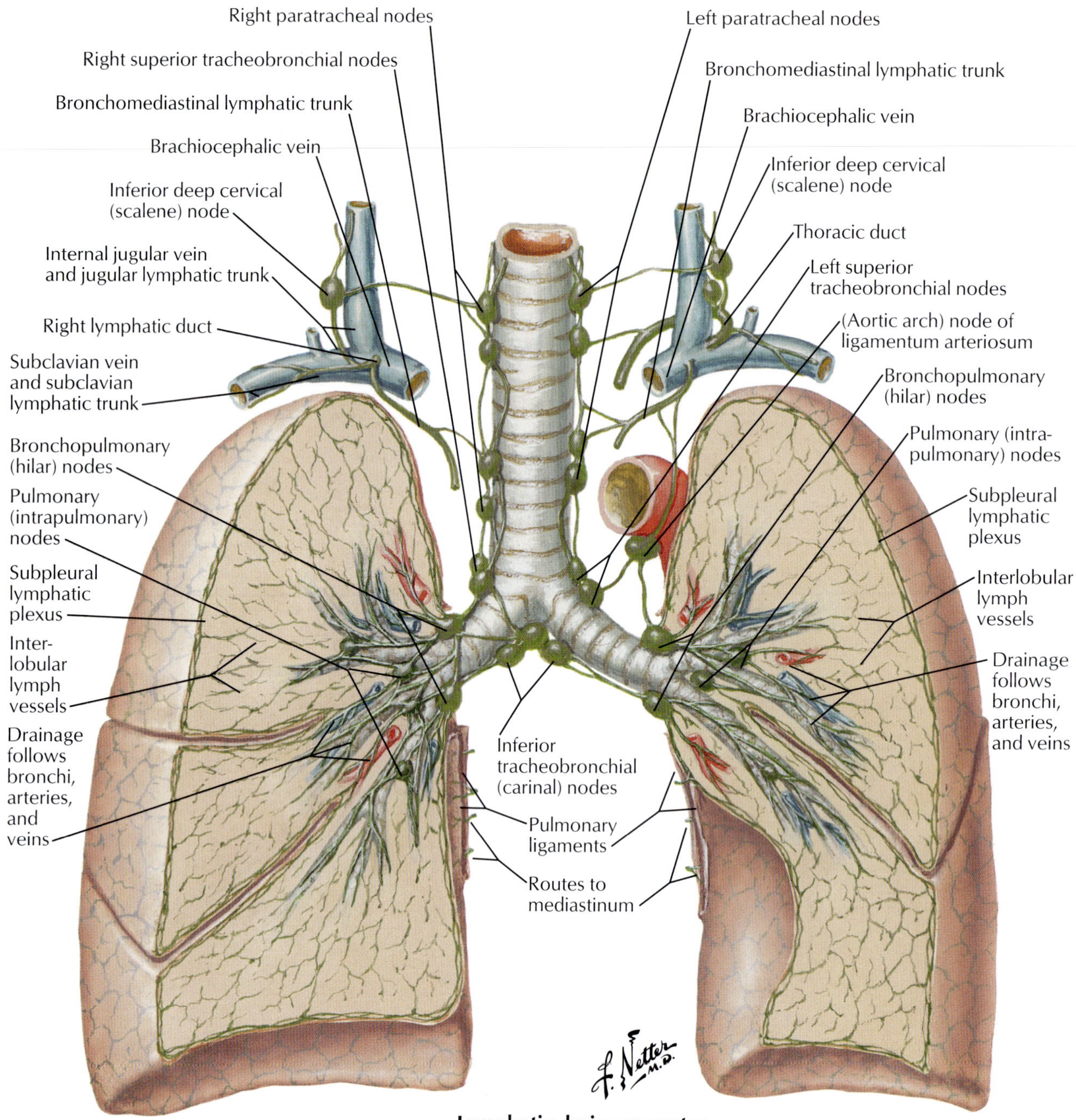

Lymphatic drainage routes

Right lung: All lobes drain to pulmonary and bronchopulmonary (hilar) nodes, then to inferior tracheobronchial (carinal) nodes, right superior tracheobronchial nodes, and right paratracheal nodes on the way to the brachiocephalic vein via the bronchomediastinal lymphatic trunk and/or inferior deep cervical (scalene) node.

Left lung: The superior lobe drains to pulmonary and bronchopulmonary (hilar) nodes, inferior tracheobronchial (carinal) nodes, left superior tracheobronchial nodes, left paratracheal nodes and/or (aortic arch) node of ligamentum arteriosum, then to the brachiocephalic vein via the left bronchomediastinal trunk and thoracic duct. The left inferior lobe also drains to the pulmonary and bronchopulmonary (hilar) nodes and to inferior tracheobronchial (carinal) nodes, but then mostly to right superior tracheobronchial nodes, where it follows the same route as lymph from the right lung.

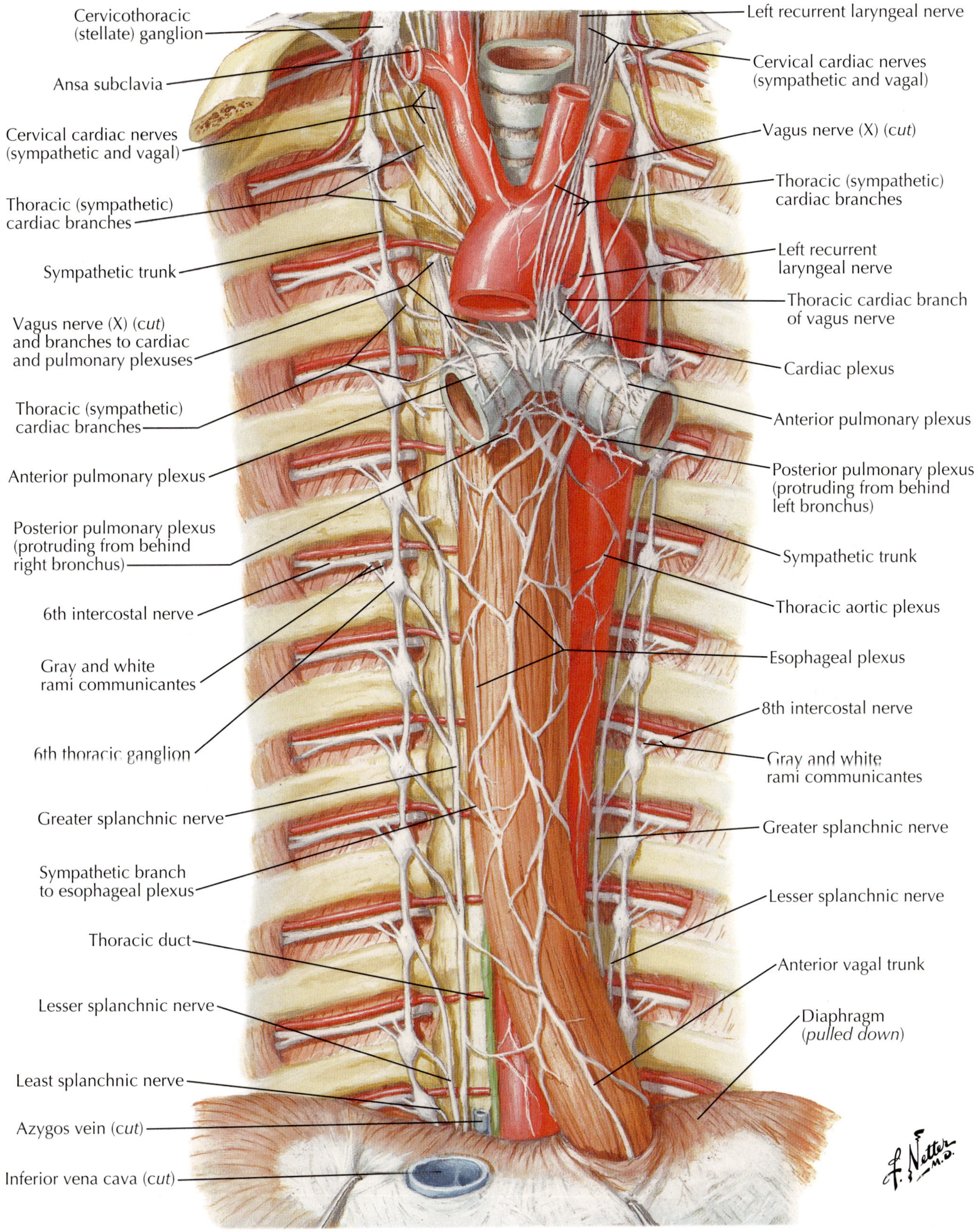
Cervicothoracic (stellate) ganglion
Ansa subclavia
Cervical cardiac nerves (sympathetic and vagal)
Thoracic (sympathetic) cardiac branches
Sympathetic trunk
Vagus nerve (X) (cut) and branches to cardiac and pulmonary plexuses
Thoracic (sympathetic) cardiac branches
Anterior pulmonary plexus
Posterior pulmonary plexus (protruding from behind right bronchus)
6th intercostal nerve
Gray and white rami communicantes
6th thoracic ganglion
Greater splanchnic nerve
Sympathetic branch to esophageal plexus
Thoracic duct
Lesser splanchnic nerve
Least splanchnic nerve
Azygos vein (cut)
Inferior vena cava (cut)
Left recurrent laryngeal nerve
Cervical cardiac nerves (sympathetic and vagal)
Vagus nerve (X) (cut)
Thoracic (sympathetic) cardiac branches
Left recurrent laryngeal nerve
Thoracic cardiac branch of vagus nerve
Cardiac plexus
Anterior pulmonary plexus
Posterior pulmonary plexus (protruding from behind left bronchus)
Sympathetic trunk
Thoracic aortic plexus
Esophageal plexus
8th intercostal nerve
Gray and white rami communicantes
Greater splanchnic nerve
Lesser splanchnic nerve
Anterior vagal trunk
Diaphragm (pulled down)
F. Netter M.D.

Innervation of Tracheobronchial Tree: Schema

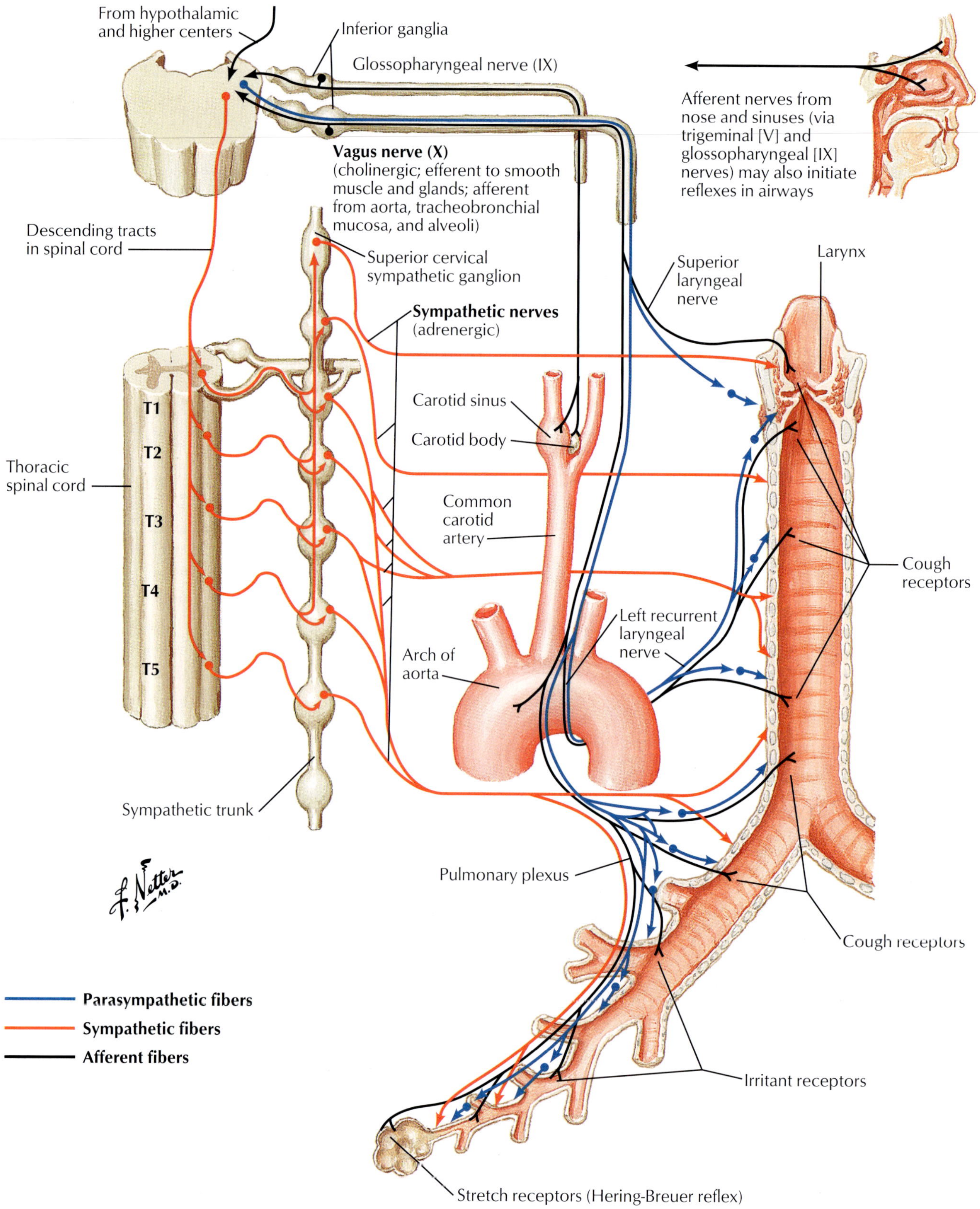

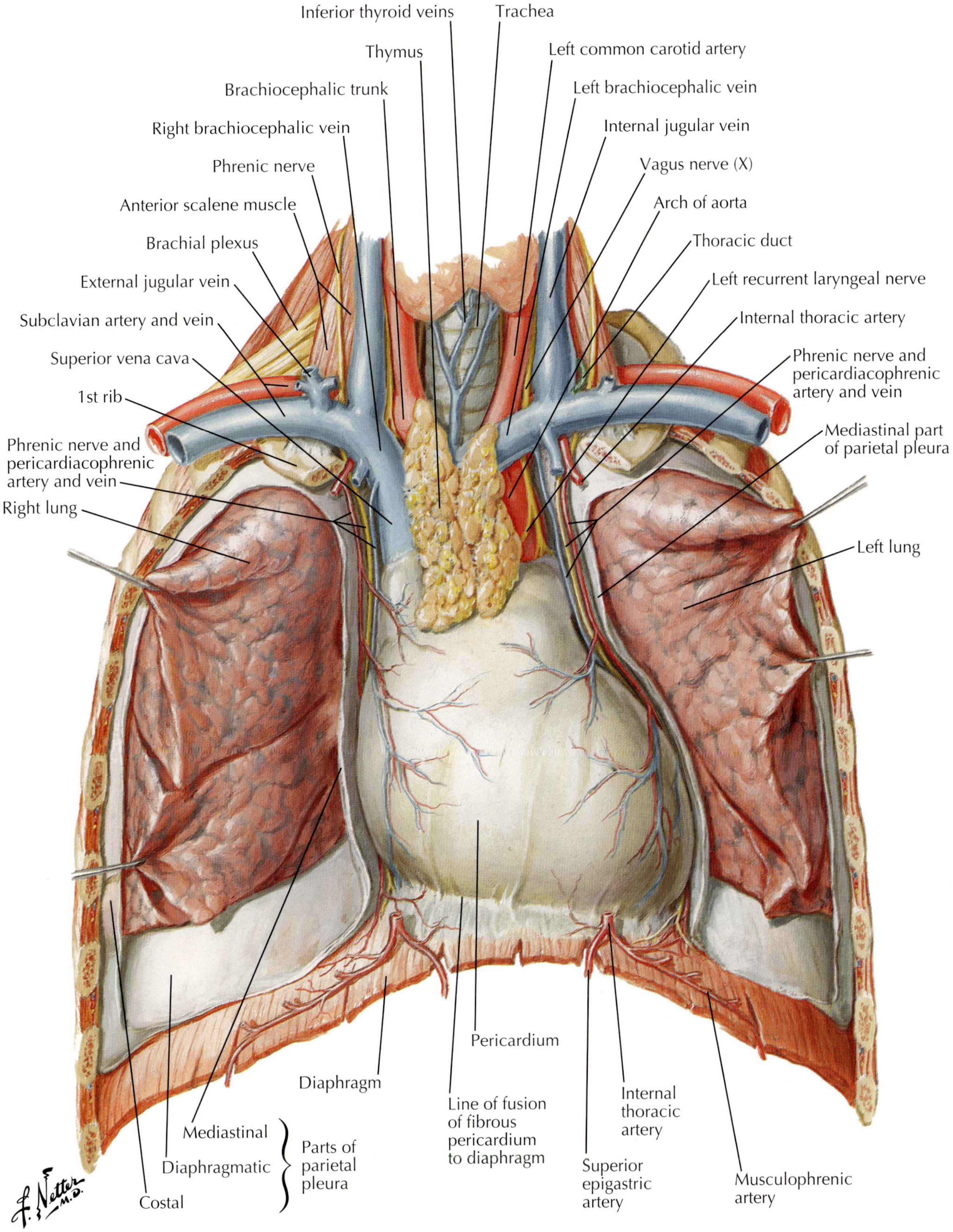
Inferior thyroid veins
Trachea
Thymus
Left common carotid artery
Brachiocephalic trunk
Left brachiocephalic vein
Right brachiocephalic vein
Internal jugular vein
Phrenic nerve
Vagus nerve (X)
Anterior scalene muscle
Arch of aorta
Brachial plexus
Thoracic duct
External jugular vein
Left recurrent laryngeal nerve
Subclavian artery and vein
Internal thoracic artery
Superior vena cava
Phrenic nerve and pericardiacophrenic artery and vein
1st rib
Mediastinal part of parietal pleura
Phrenic nerve and pericardiacophrenic artery and vein
Right lung
Left lung
Pericardium
Diaphragm
Line of fusion of fibrous pericardium to diaphragm
Internal thoracic artery
Mediastinal
Diaphragmatic
Costal
Parts of parietal pleura
Superior epigastric artery
Musculophrenic artery
F. Netter M.D.

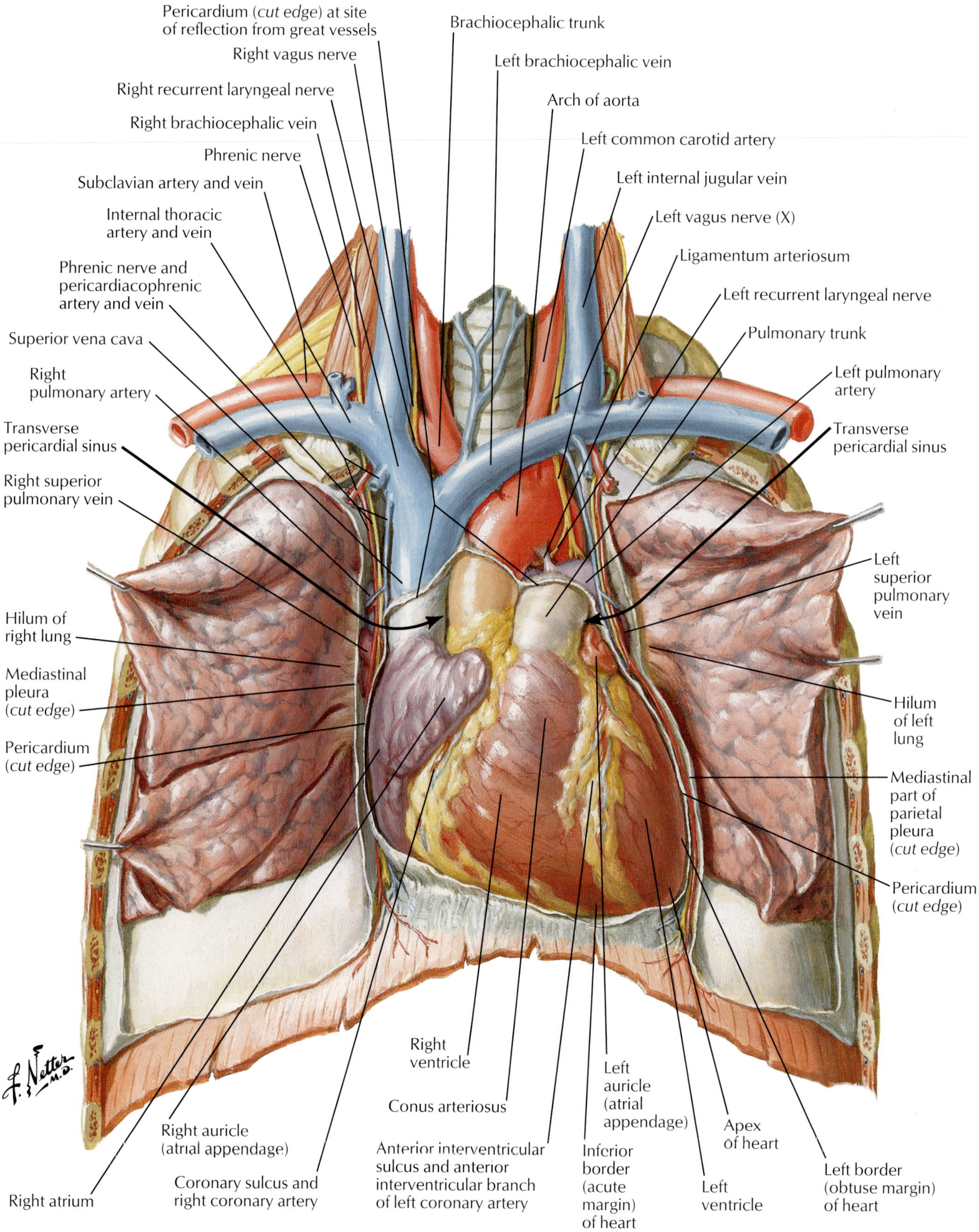

Pericardium (cut edge) at site of reflection from great vessels
Right vagus nerve
Right recurrent laryngeal nerve
Right brachiocephalic vein
Phrenic nerve
Subclavian artery and vein
Internal thoracic artery and vein
Phrenic nerve and pericardiacophrenic artery and vein
Superior vena cava
Right pulmonary artery
Transverse pericardial sinus
Right superior pulmonary vein
Hilum of right lung
Mediastinal pleura (cut edge)
Pericardium (cut edge)
Brachiocephalic trunk
Left brachiocephalic vein
Arch of aorta
Left common carotid artery
Left internal jugular vein
Left vagus nerve (X)
Ligamentum arteriosum
Left recurrent laryngeal nerve
Pulmonary trunk
Left pulmonary artery
Transverse pericardial sinus
Left superior pulmonary vein
Hilum of left lung
Mediastinal part of parietal pleura (cut edge)
Pericardium (cut edge)
Right ventricle
Conus arteriosus
Left auricle (atrial appendage)
Apex of heart
Right auricle (atrial appendage)
Anterior interventricular sulcus and anterior interventricular branch of left coronary artery
Inferior border (acute margin) of heart
Left ventricle
Left border (obtuse margin) of heart
Right atrium
Coronary sulcus and right coronary artery

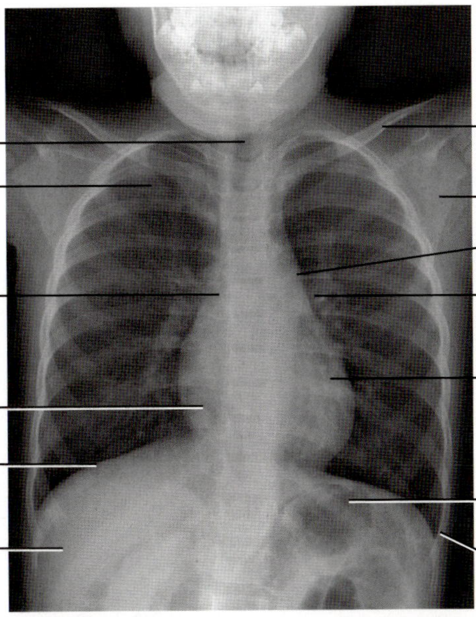

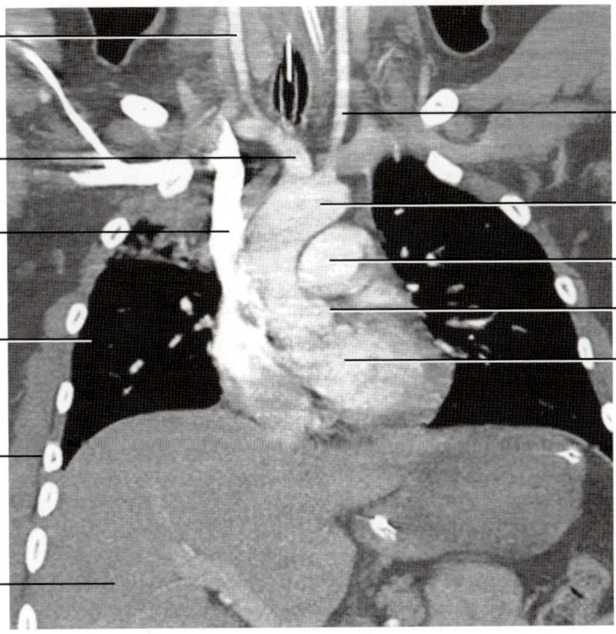

Precordial areas of auscultation

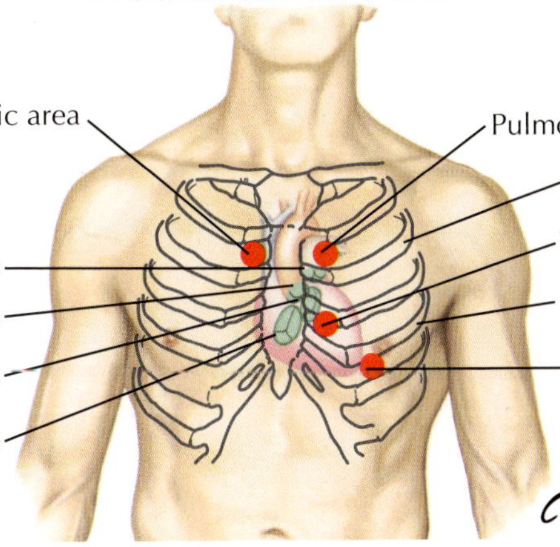

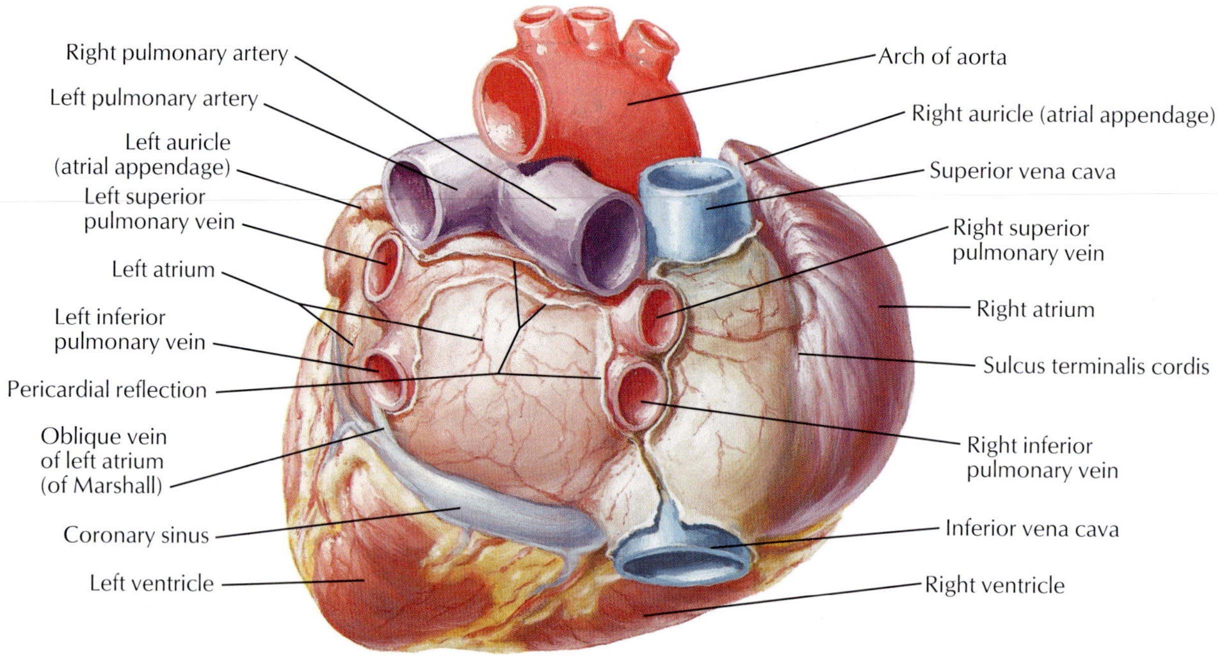

Base of heart: posterior view

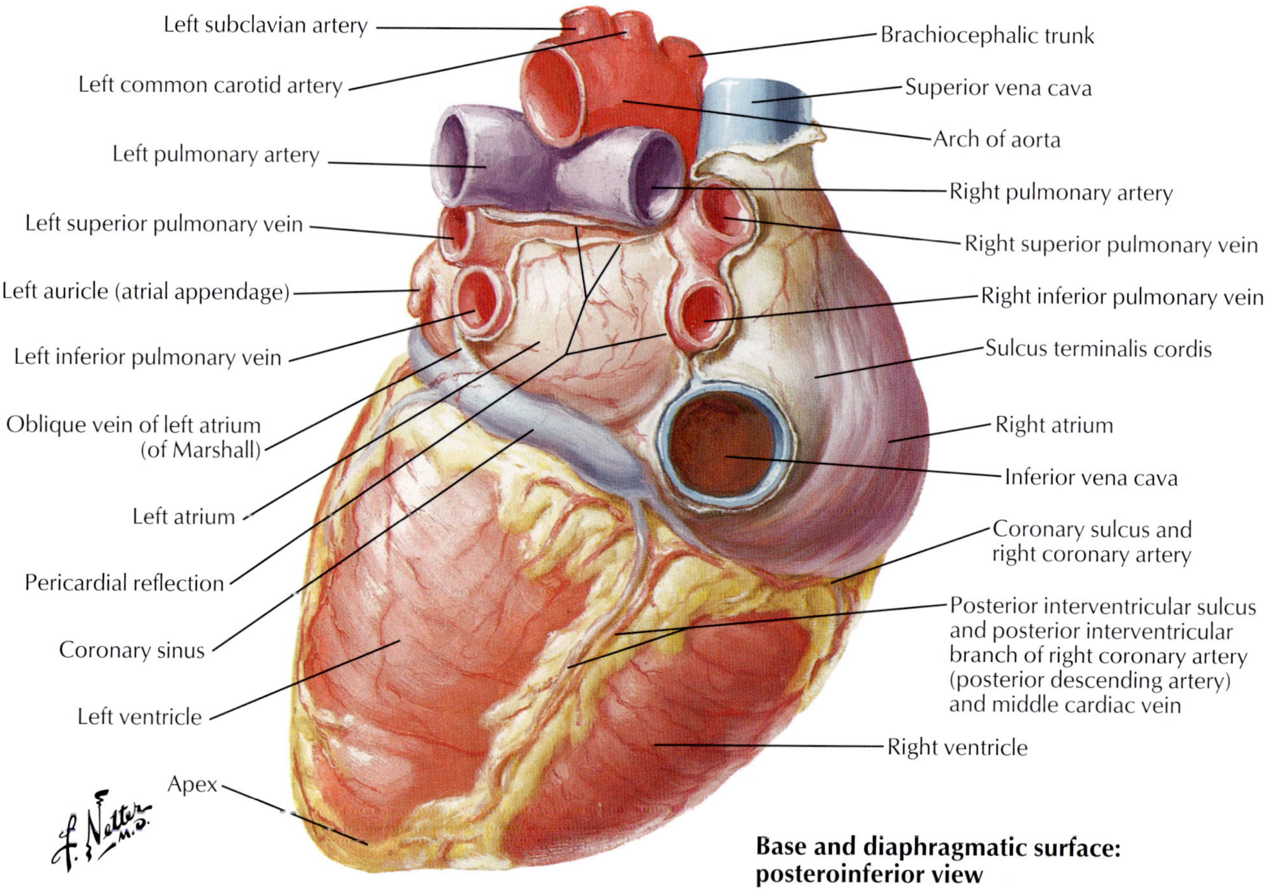

Base and diaphragmatic surface: posteroinferior view

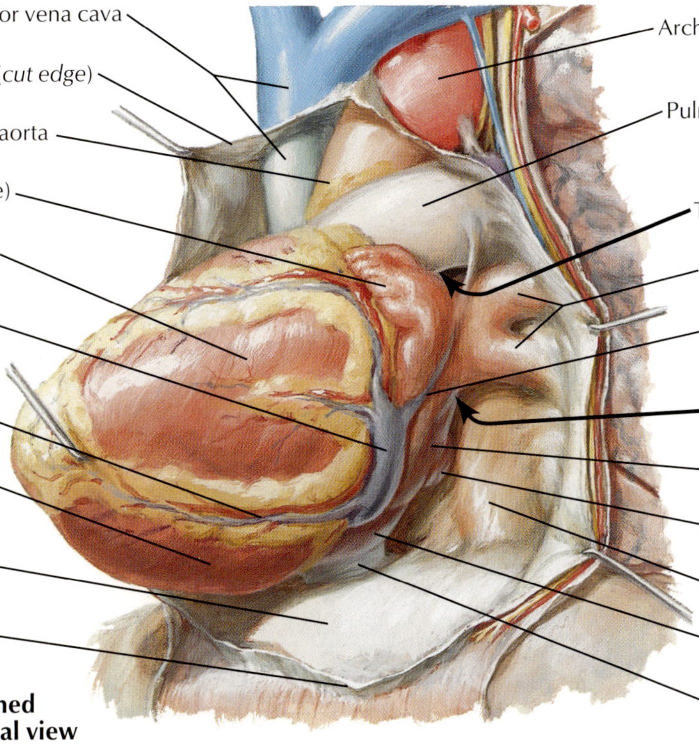

Heart drawn out of opened pericardial sac: left lateral view

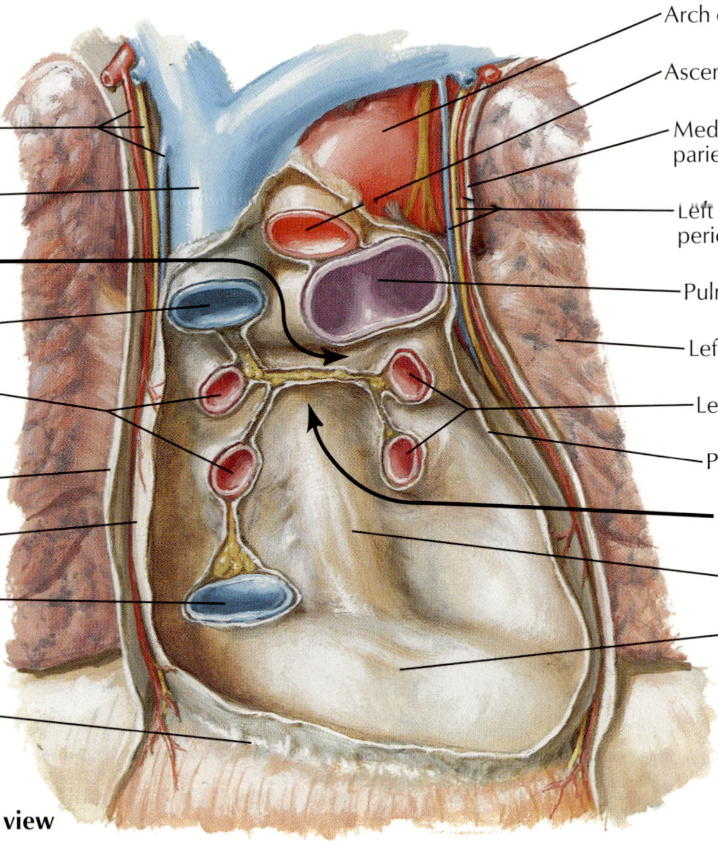

Pericardial sac with heart removed: anterior view

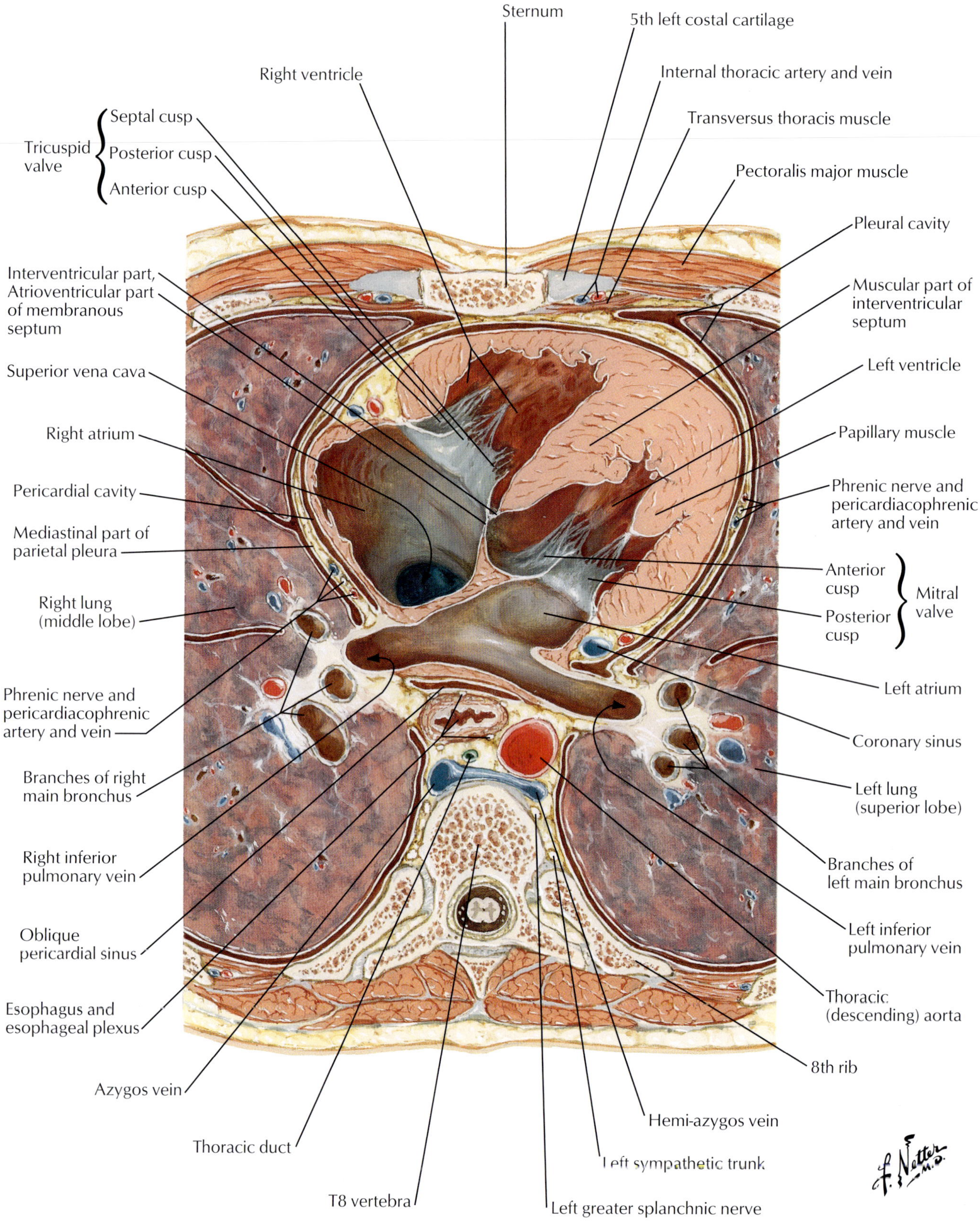
Sternum
5th left costal cartilage
Right ventricle
Internal thoracic artery and vein
Transversus thoracis muscle
Tricuspid valve
Septal cusp
Posterior cusp
Anterior cusp
Pectoralis major muscle
Pleural cavity
Interventricular part, Atrioventricular part of membranous septum
Muscular part of interventricular septum
Left ventricle
Superior vena cava
Right atrium
Papillary muscle
Pericardial cavity
Phrenic nerve and pericardiacophrenic artery and vein
Mediastinal part of parietal pleura
Anterior cusp
Posterior cusp
Mitral valve
Right lung (middle lobe)
Left atrium
Phrenic nerve and pericardiacophrenic artery and vein
Coronary sinus
Branches of right main bronchus
Left lung (superior lobe)
Right inferior pulmonary vein
Branches of left main bronchus
Oblique pericardial sinus
Left inferior pulmonary vein
Esophagus and esophageal plexus
Thoracic (descending) aorta
8th rib
Azygos vein
Hemi-azygos vein
Thoracic duct
Left sympathetic trunk
T8 vertebra
Left greater splanchnic nerve

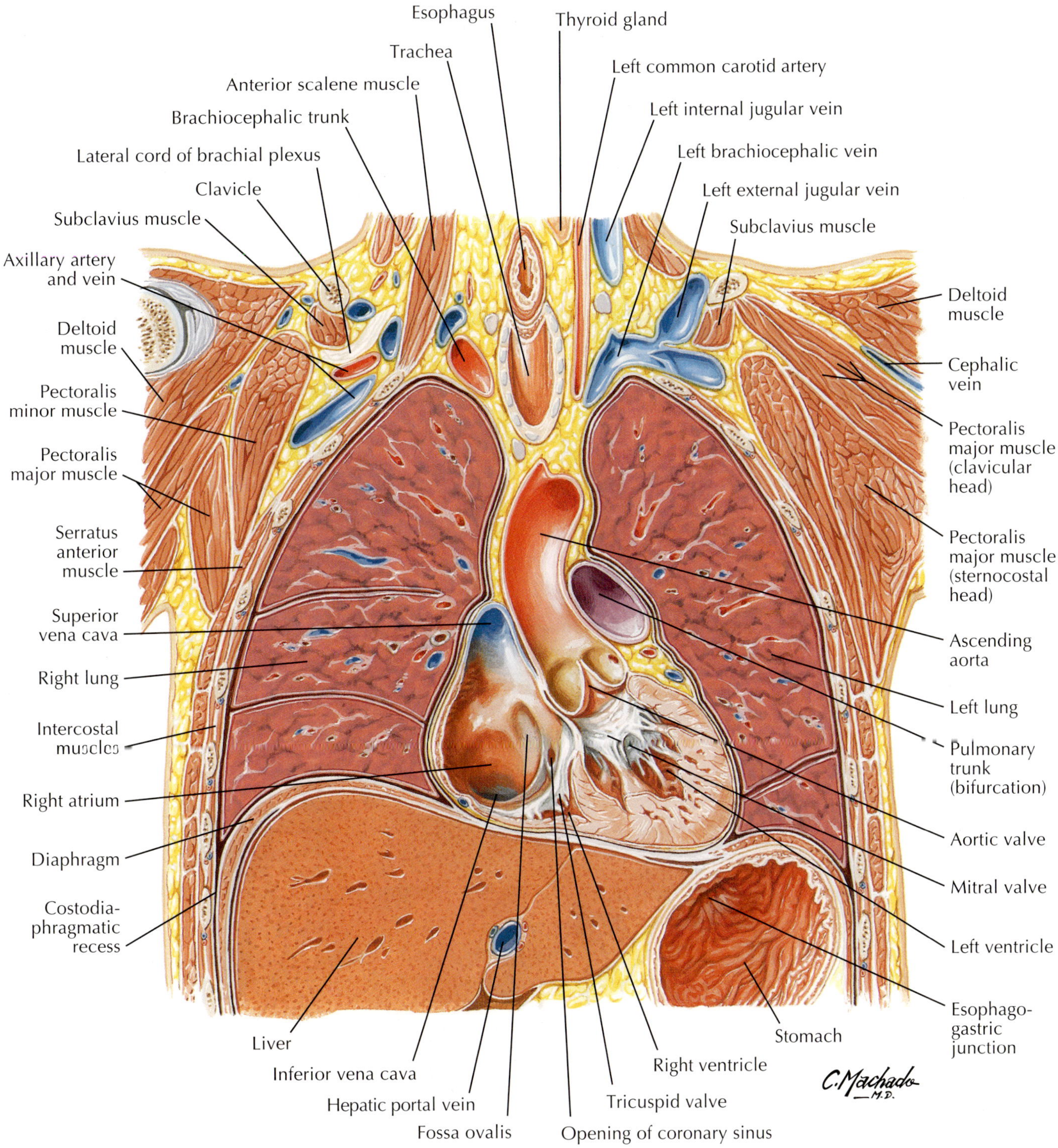
Esophagus
Thyroid gland
Trachea
Left common carotid artery
Anterior scalene muscle
Left internal jugular vein
Brachiocephalic trunk
Left brachiocephalic vein
Lateral cord of brachial plexus
Left external jugular vein
Clavicle
Subclavius muscle
Subclavius muscle
Axillary artery and vein
Deltoid muscle
Deltoid muscle
Cephalic vein
Pectoralis minor muscle
Pectoralis major muscle (clavicular head)
Pectoralis major muscle
Pectoralis major muscle (sternocostal head)
Serratus anterior muscle
Superior vena cava
Ascending aorta
Right lung
Left lung
Intercostal muscles
Pulmonary trunk (bifurcation)
Right atrium
Aortic valve
Diaphragm
Mitral valve
Costodiaphragmatic recess
Left ventricle
Esophagogastric junction
Liver
Stomach
Inferior vena cava
Right ventricle
Hepatic portal vein
Tricuspid valve
Fossa ovalis
Opening of coronary sinus
C. Machado M.D.

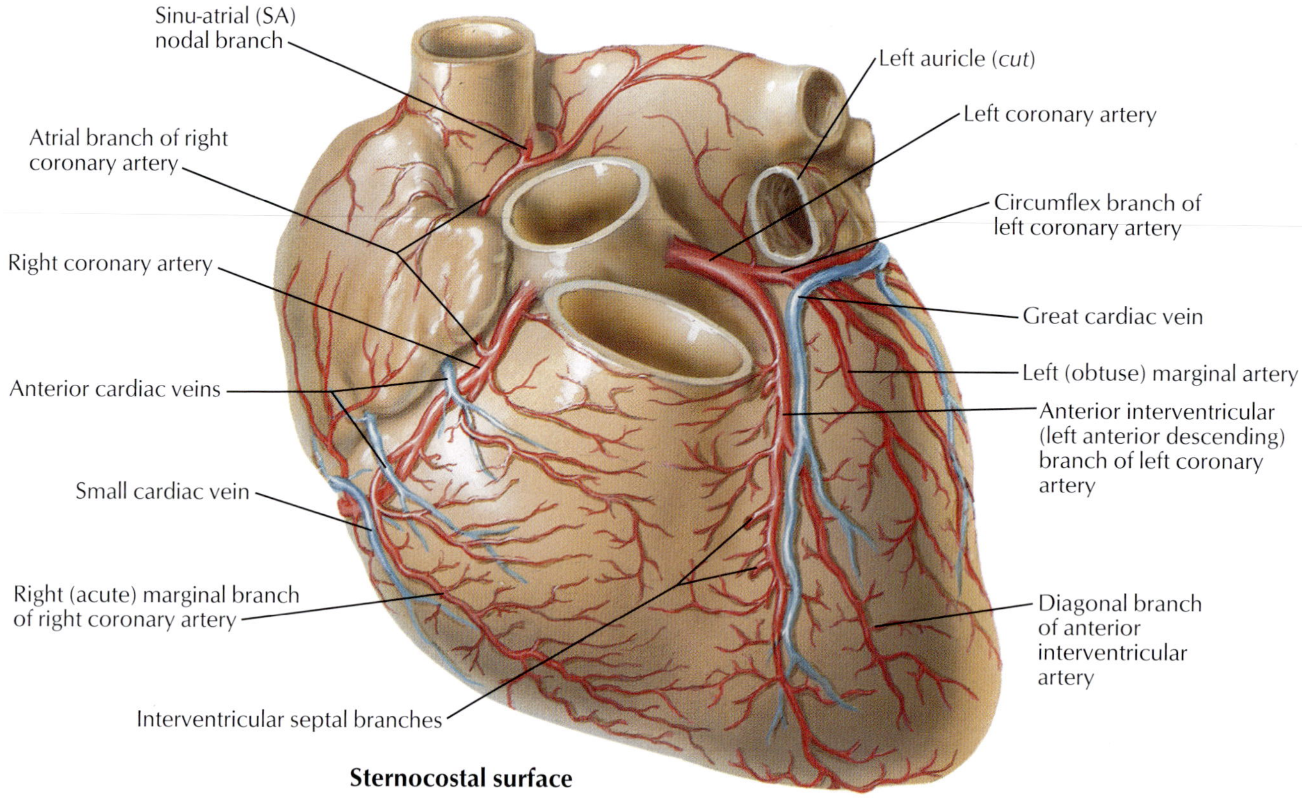

Sternocostal surface

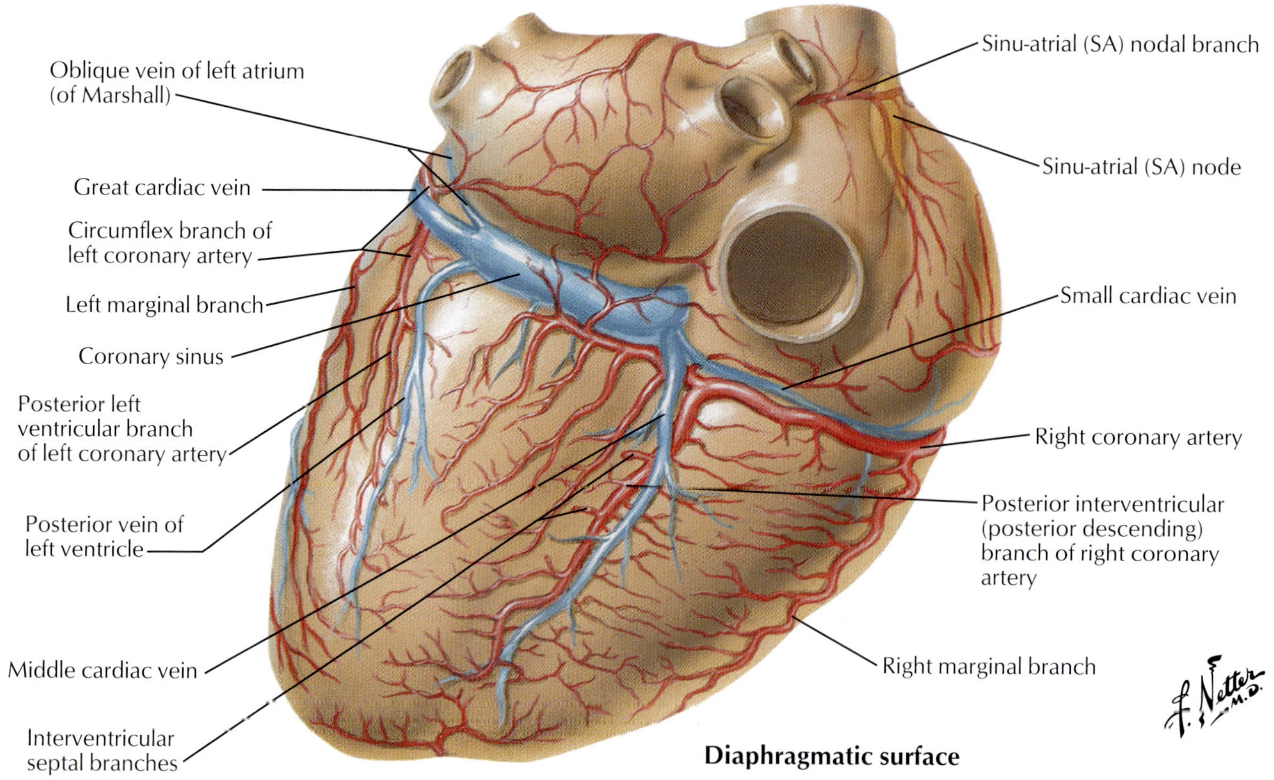

Diaphragmatic surface

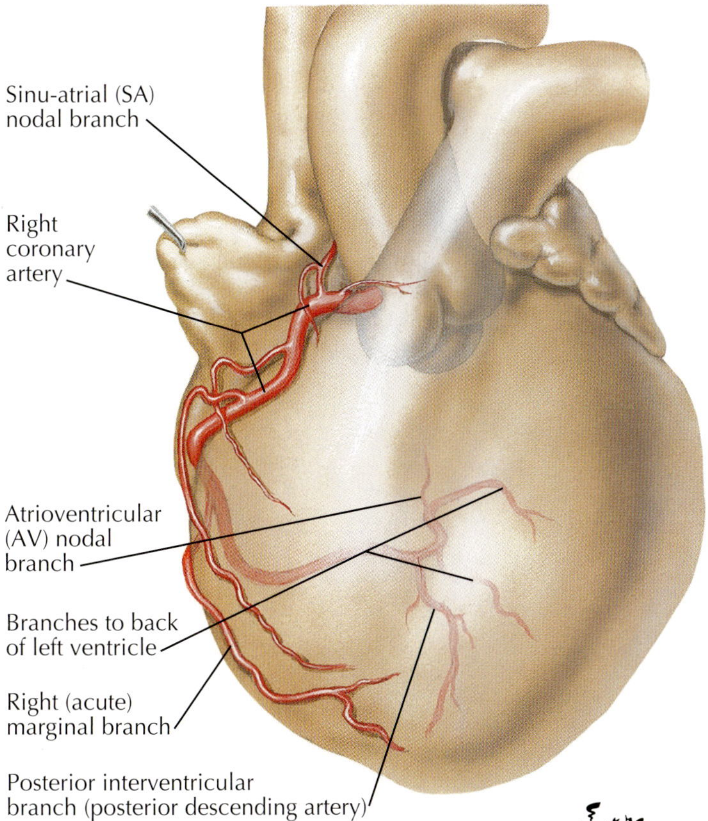
Sinu-atrial (SA) nodal branch
Right coronary artery
Atrioventricular (AV) nodal branch
Branches to back of left ventricle
Right (acute) marginal branch
Posterior interventricular branch (posterior descending artery)

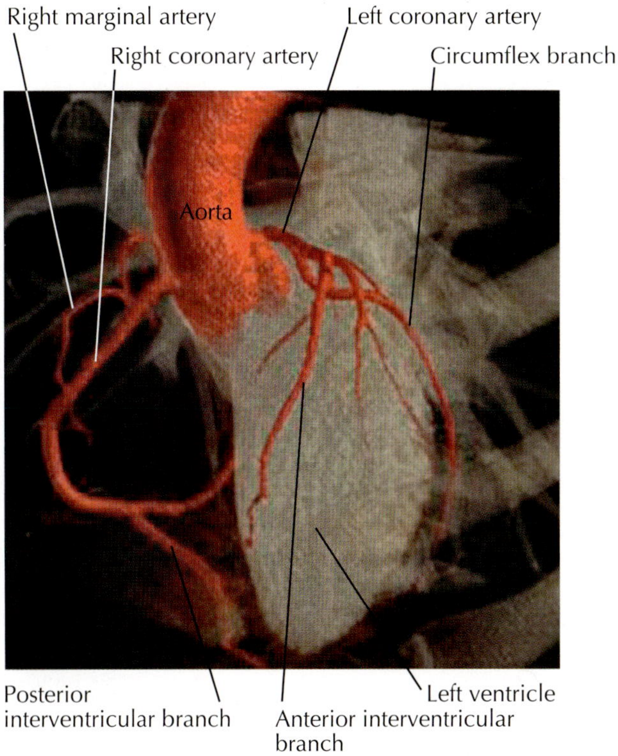
Right marginal artery
Right coronary artery
Left coronary artery
Circumflex branch
Aorta
Posterior interventricular branch
Anterior interventricular branch
Left ventricle

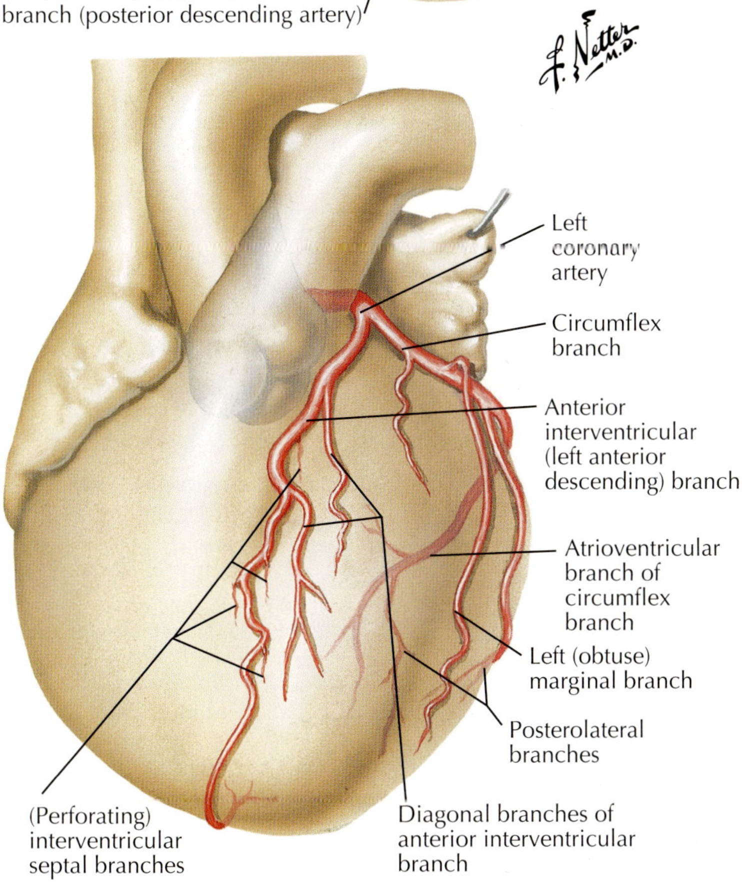
Left coronary artery
Circumflex branch
Anterior interventricular (left anterior descending) branch
Atrioventricular branch of circumflex branch
Left (obtuse) marginal branch
Posterolateral branches
(Perforating) interventricular septal branches
Diagonal branches of anterior interventricular branch

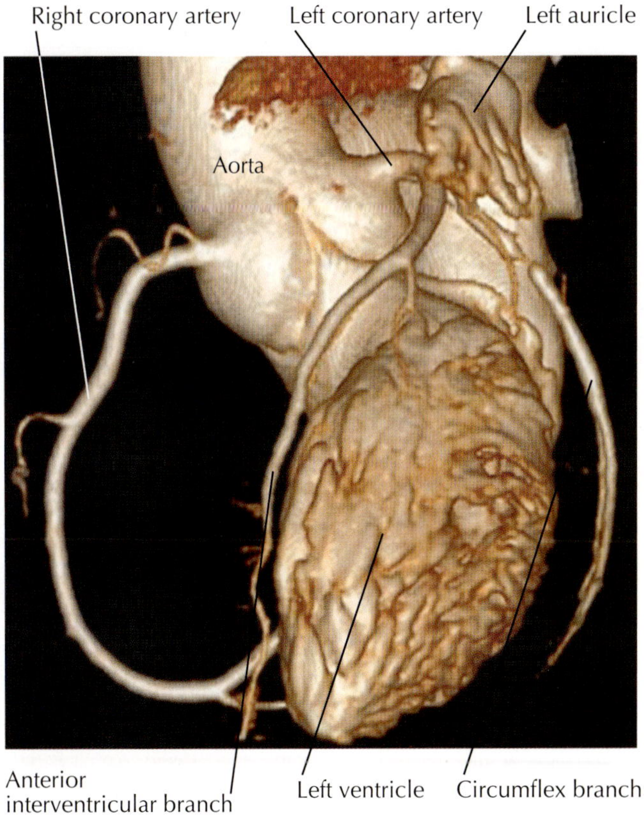
Right coronary artery
Left coronary artery
Left auricle
Aorta
Anterior interventricular branch
Left ventricle
Circumflex branch

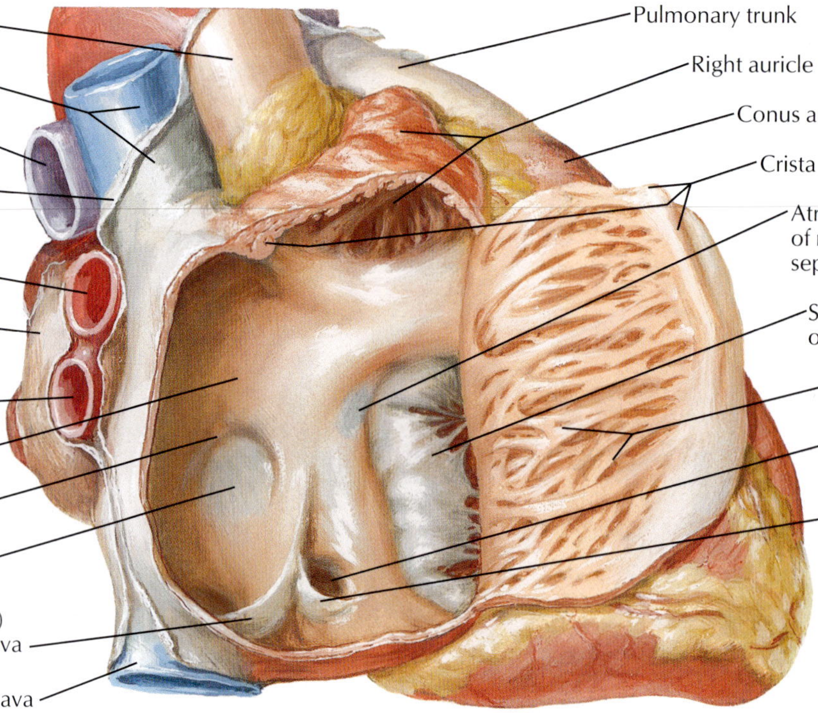

Opened right atrium: right lateral view

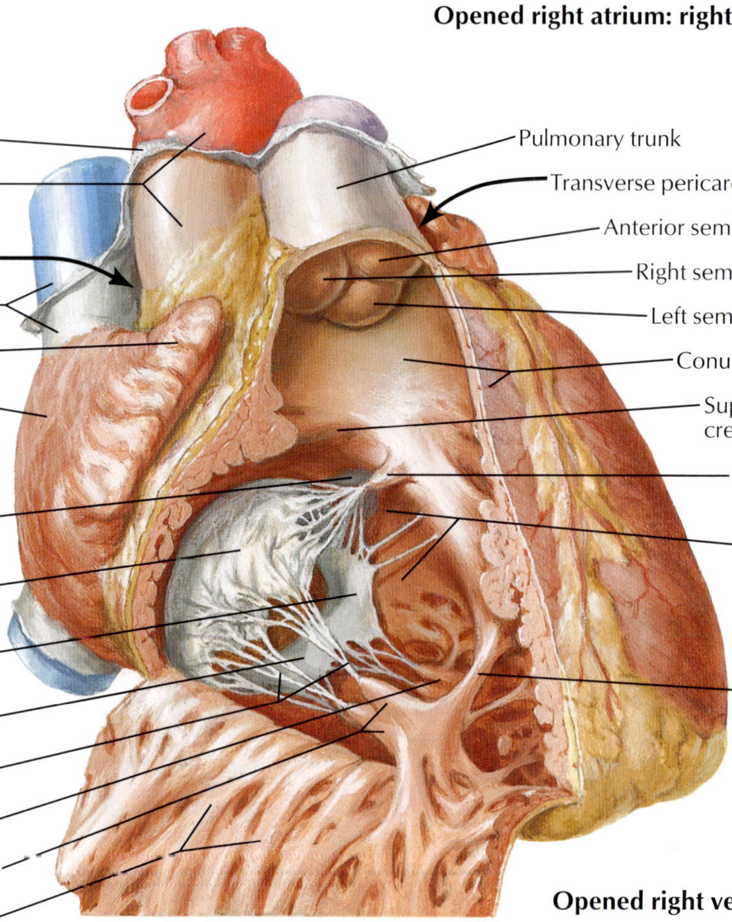

Opened right ventricle: anterior view

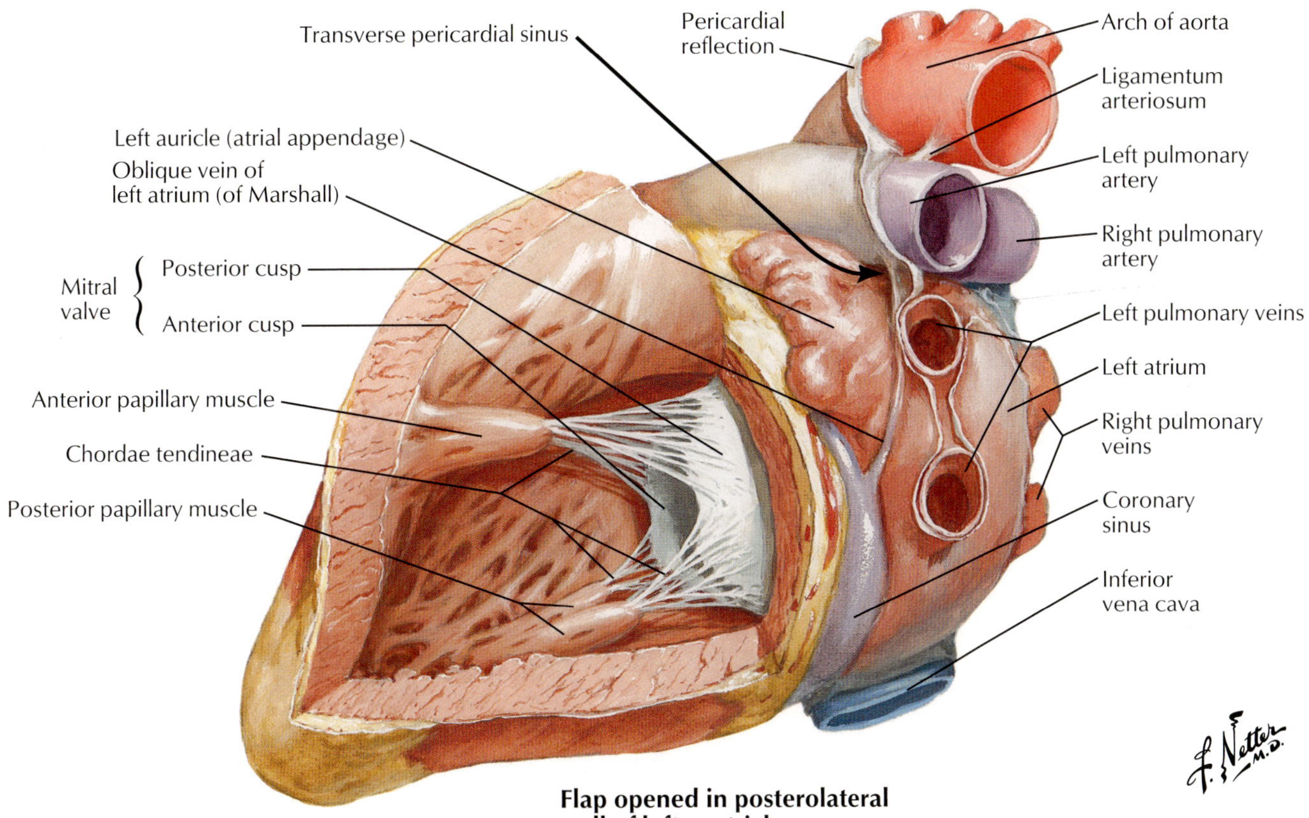

Flap opened in posterolateral wall of left ventricle

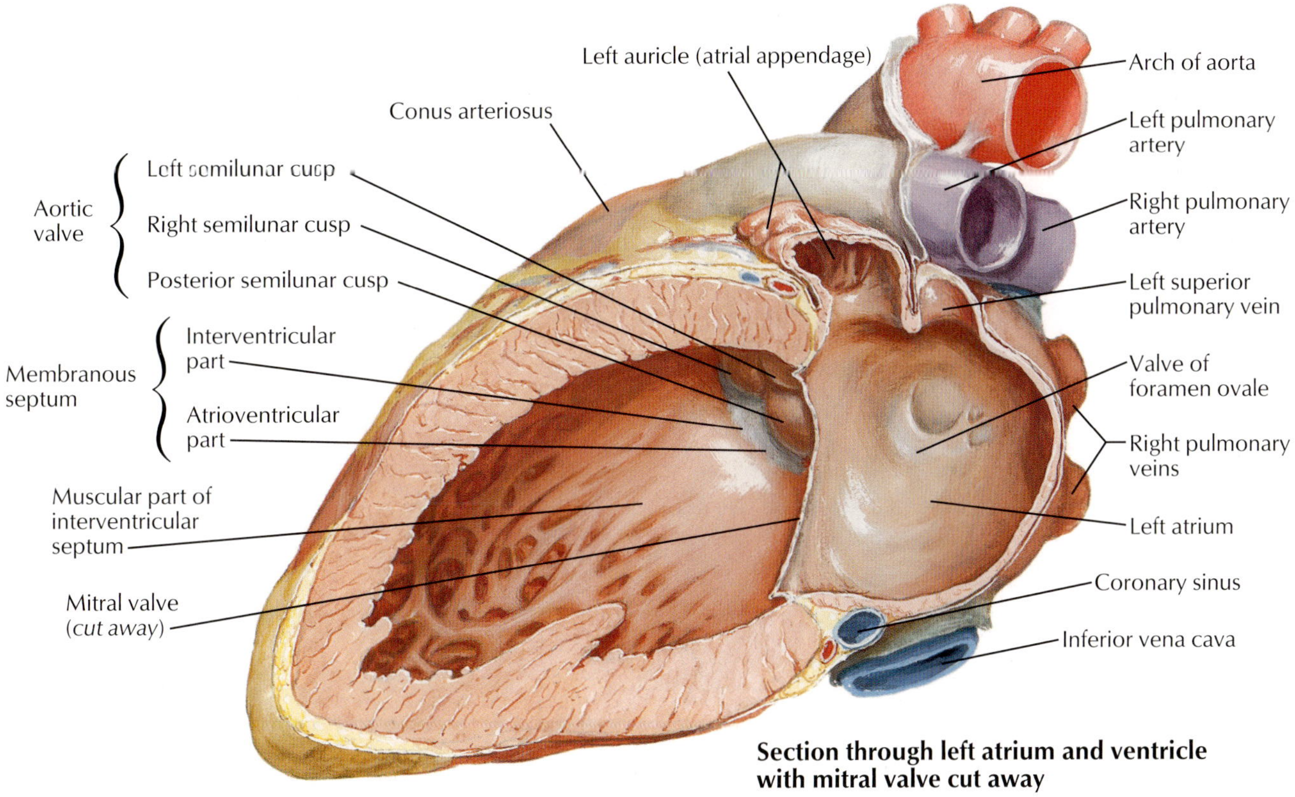

Section through left atrium and ventricle with mitral valve cut away

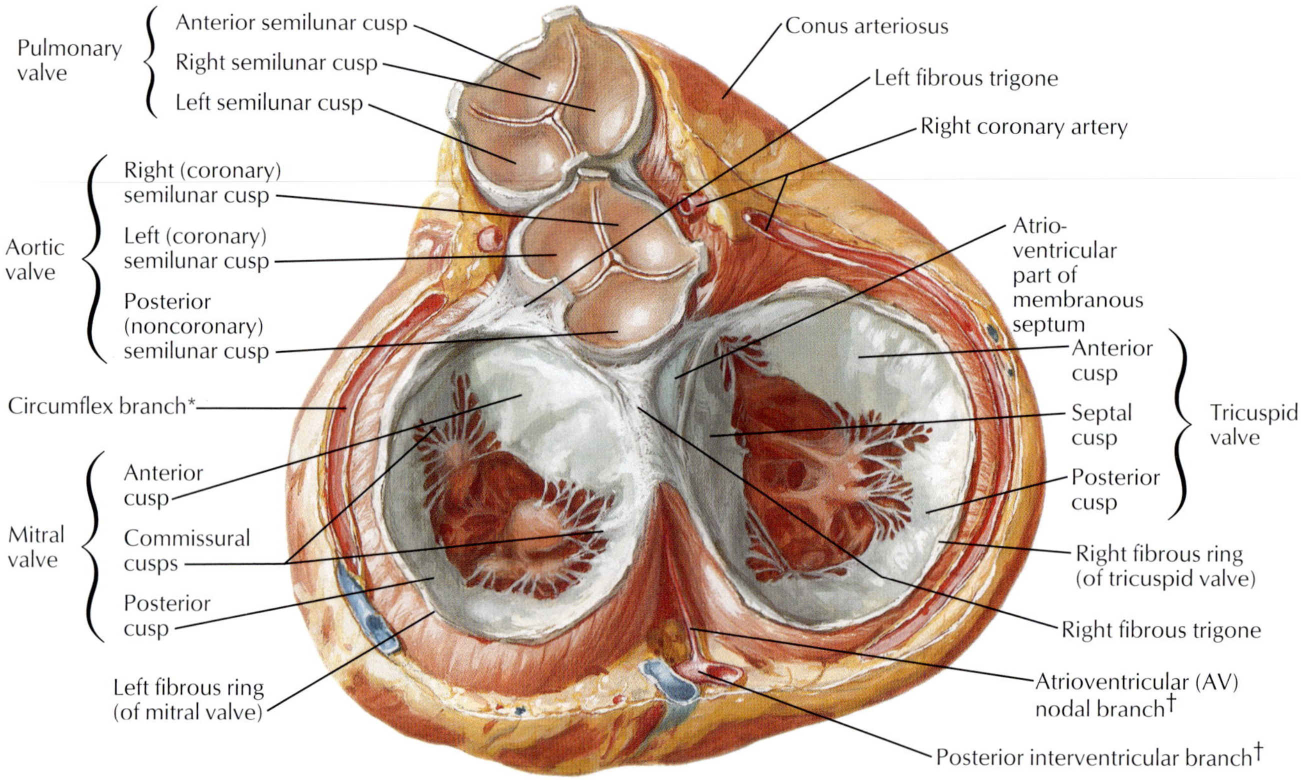

Heart in diastole: viewed from base with atria removed

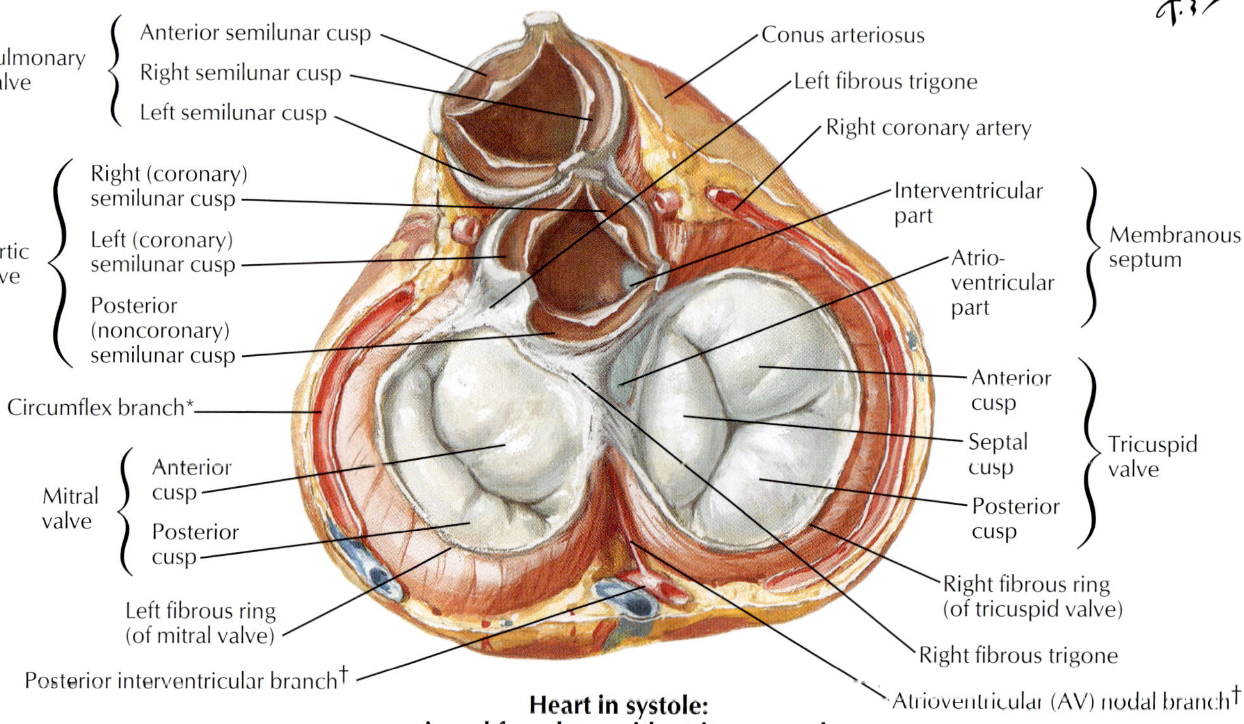

Heart in systole: viewed from base with atria removed

*Of left coronary artery
†Of right coronary artery

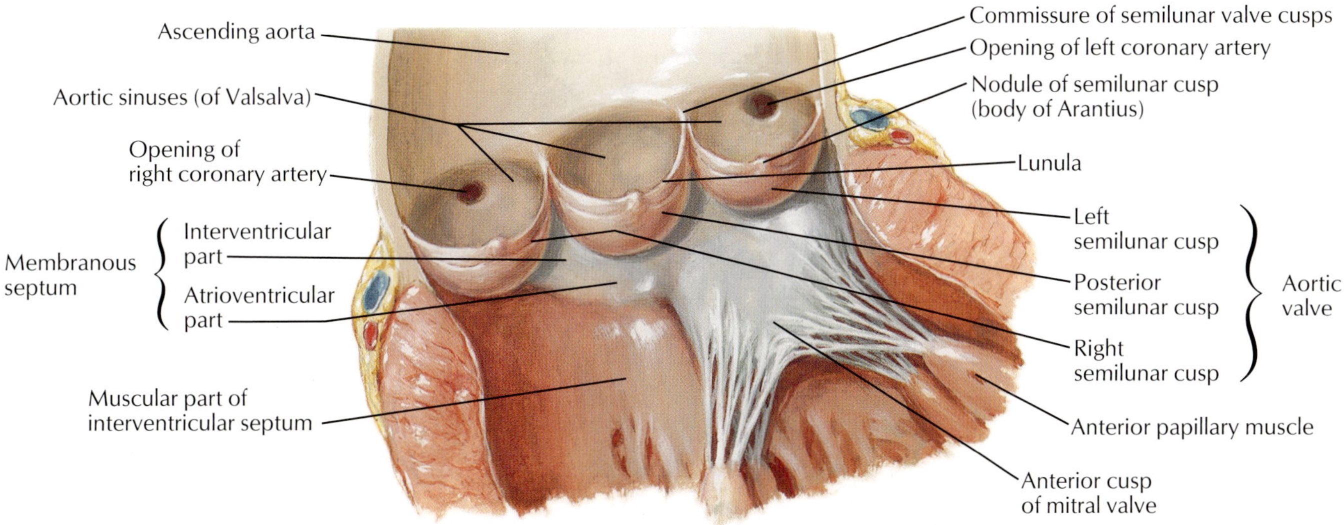

Aortic valve

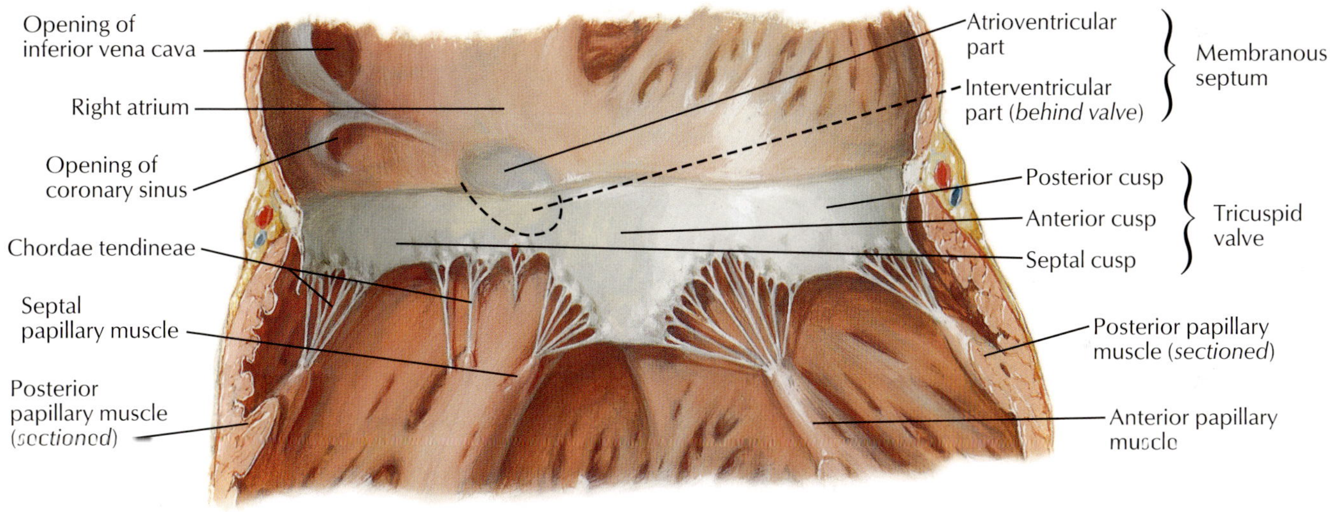

Tricuspid (right atrioventricular) valve

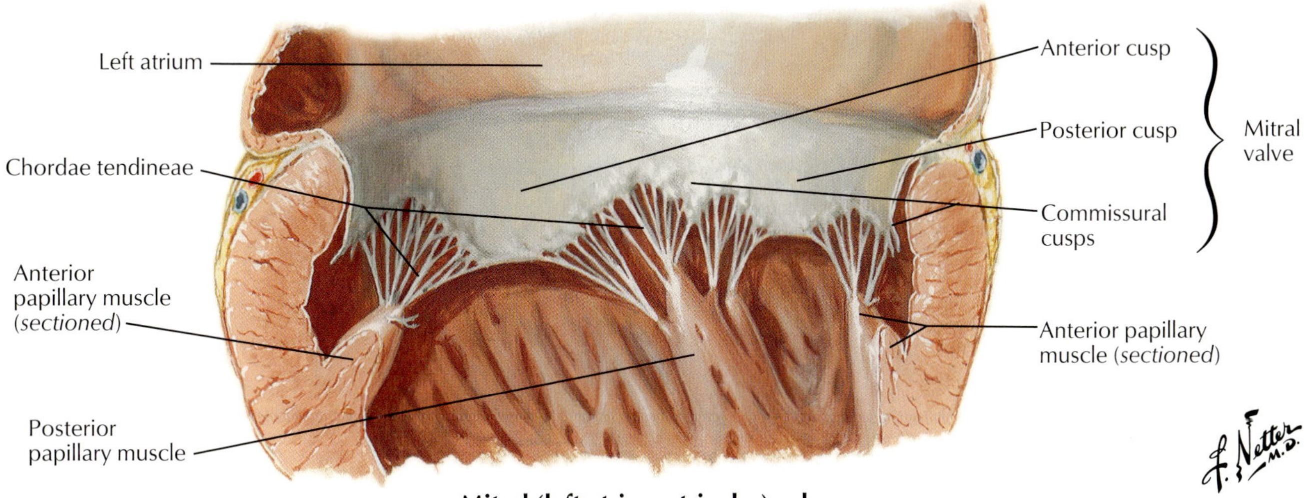

Mitral (left atrioventricular) valve

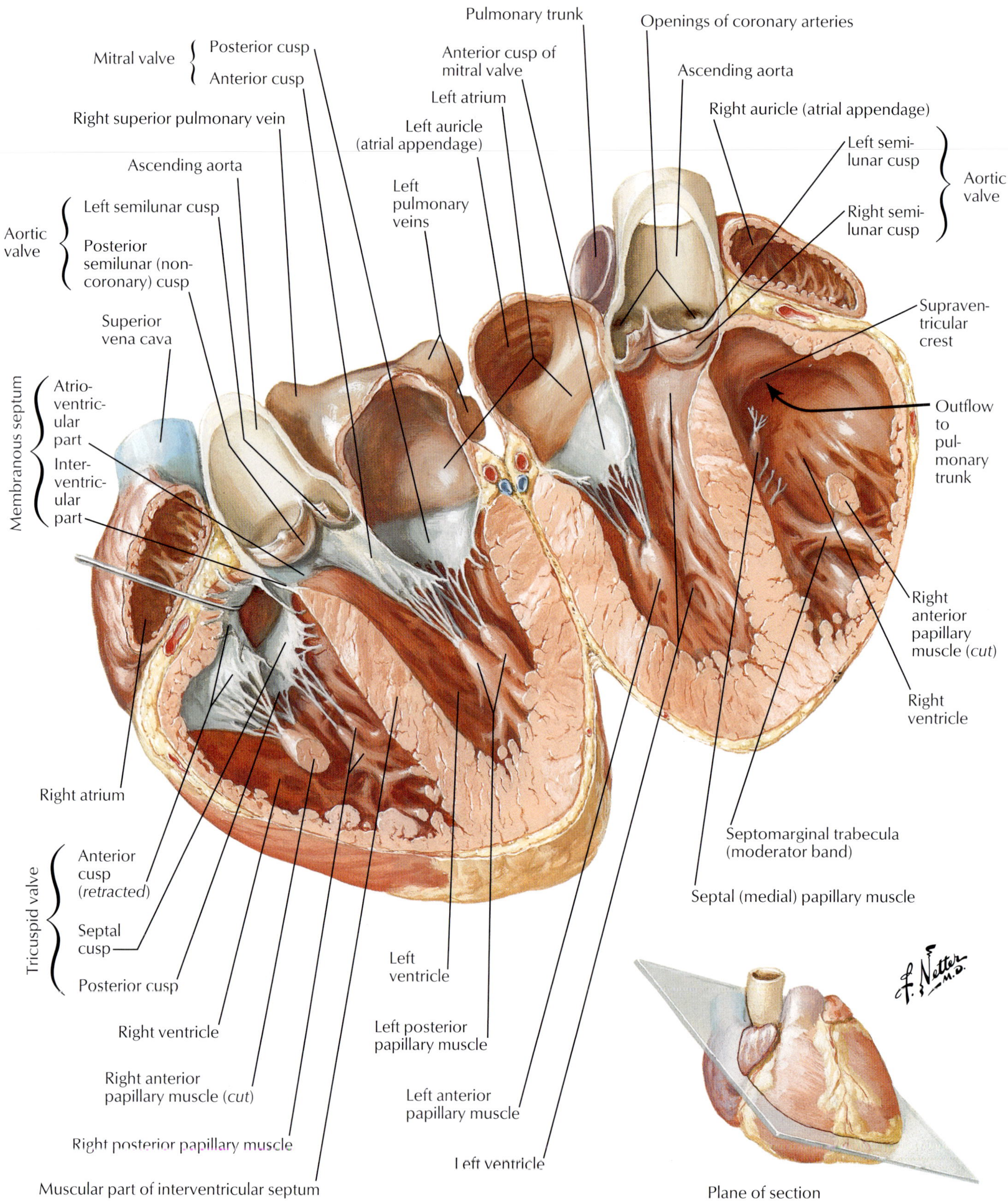
Pulmonary trunk
Openings of coronary arteries
Mitral valve
Posterior cusp
Anterior cusp
Anterior cusp of mitral valve
Ascending aorta
Left atrium
Right superior pulmonary vein
Left auricle (atrial appendage)
Right auricle (atrial appendage)
Ascending aorta
Left semilunar cusp
Right semilunar cusp
Aortic valve
Left pulmonary veins
Aortic valve
Left semilunar cusp
Posterior semilunar (noncoronary) cusp
Superior vena cava
Supraventricular crest
Membranous septum
Atrioventricular part
Interventricular part
Outflow to pulmonary trunk
Right anterior papillary muscle (cut)
Right ventricle
Right atrium
Septomarginal trabecula (moderator band)
Septal (medial) papillary muscle
Tricuspid valve
Anterior cusp (retracted)
Septal cusp
Posterior cusp
Left ventricle
Right ventricle
Left posterior papillary muscle
Right anterior papillary muscle (cut)
Left anterior papillary muscle
Right posterior papillary muscle
Left ventricle
Muscular part of interventricular septum
Plane of section

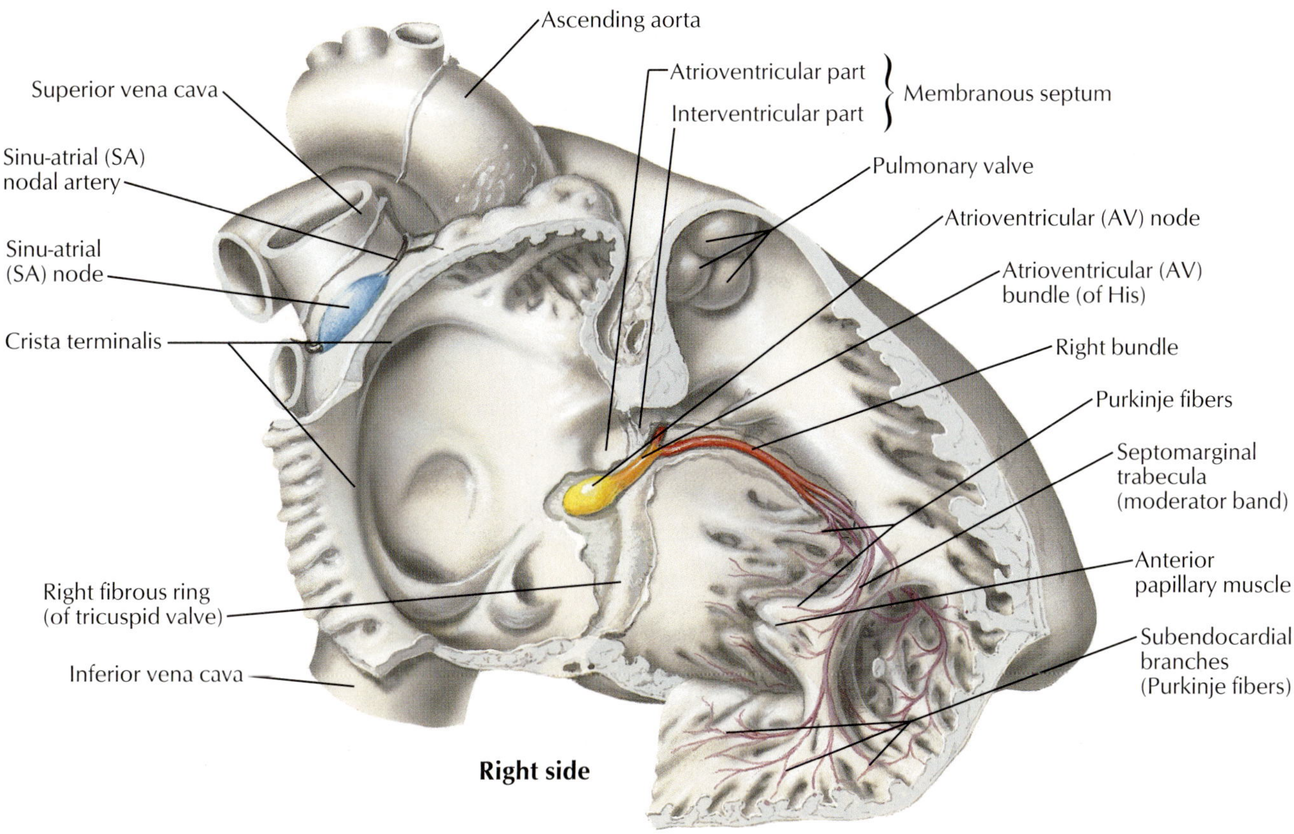

Right side

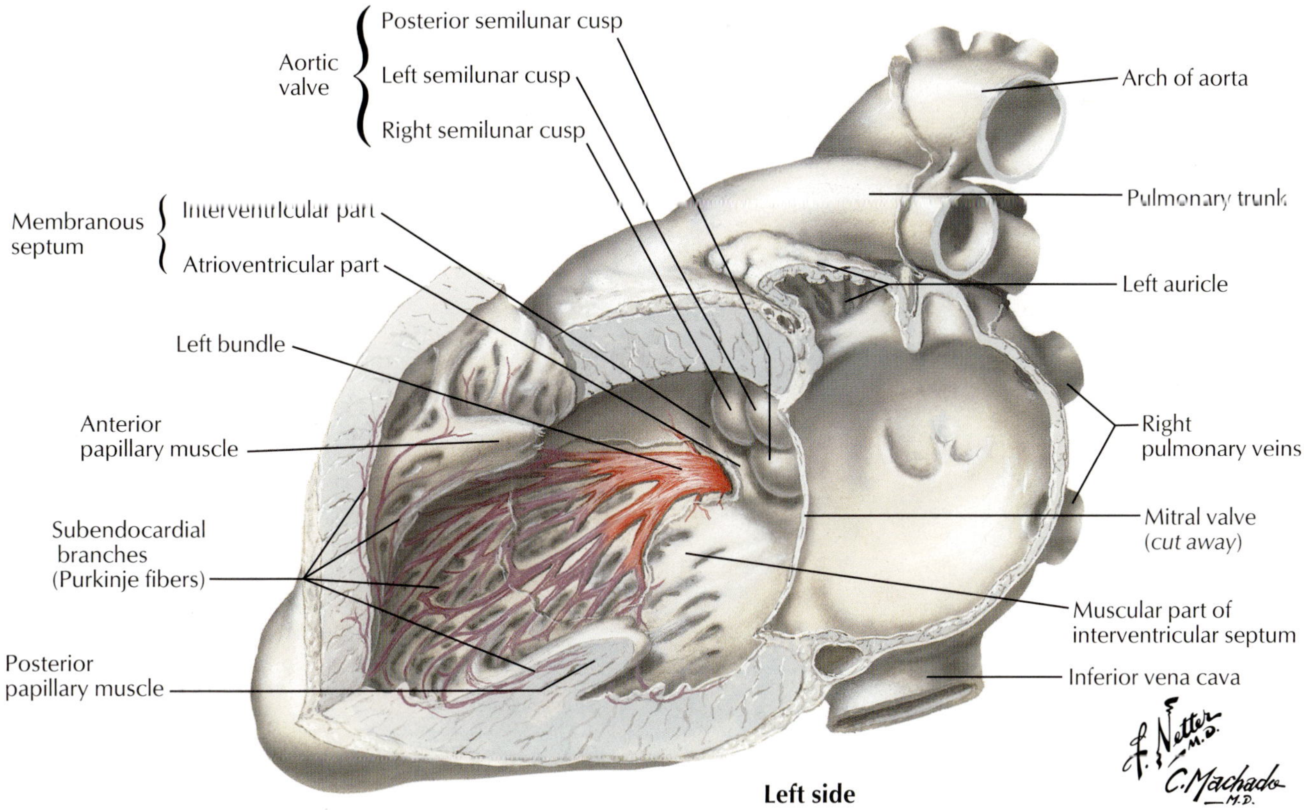

Left side

Nerves of Heart

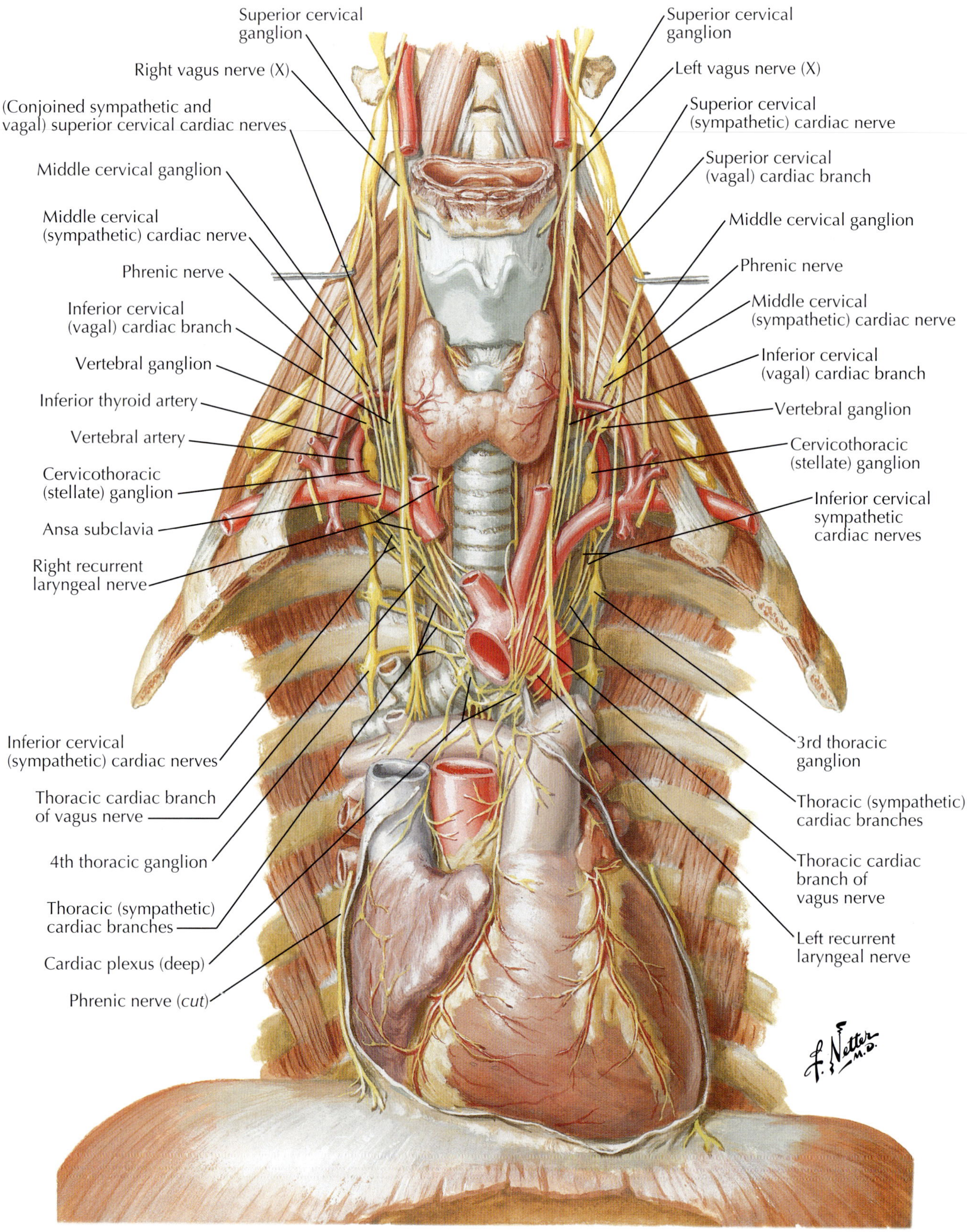

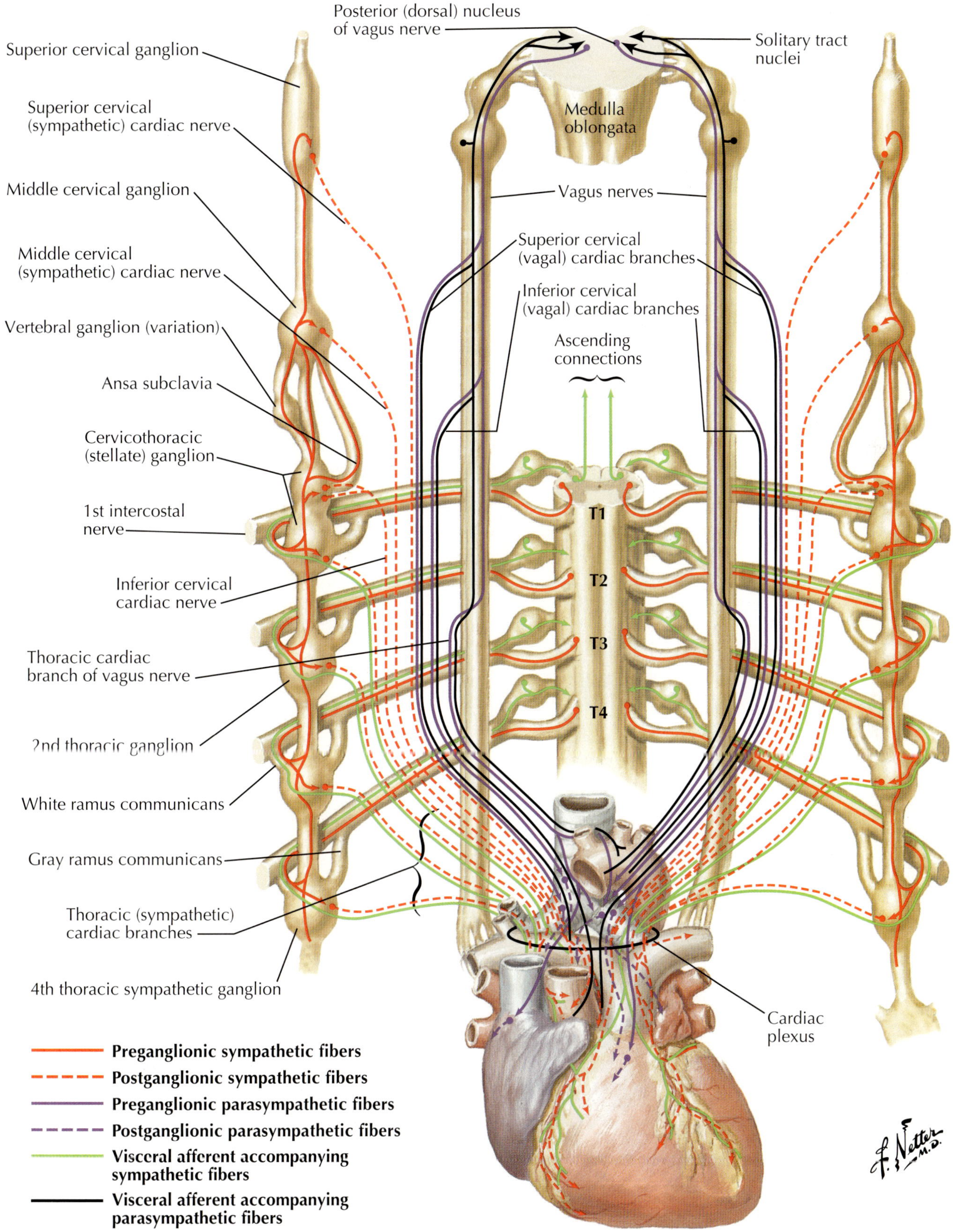
Posterior (dorsal) nucleus of vagus nerve
Solitary tract nuclei
Superior cervical ganglion
Superior cervical (sympathetic) cardiac nerve
Medulla oblongata
Middle cervical ganglion
Vagus nerves
Superior cervical (vagal) cardiac branches
Middle cervical (sympathetic) cardiac nerve
Inferior cervical (vagal) cardiac branches
Vertebral ganglion (variation)
Ascending connections
Ansa subclavia
Cervicothoracic (stellate) ganglion
1st intercostal nerve
T1
Inferior cervical cardiac nerve
T2
T3
Thoracic cardiac branch of vagus nerve
T4
2nd thoracic ganglion
White ramus communicans
Gray ramus communicans
Thoracic (sympathetic) cardiac branches
4th thoracic sympathetic ganglion
Cardiac plexus
Preganglionic sympathetic fibers
Postganglionic sympathetic fibers
Preganglionic parasympathetic fibers
Postganglionic parasympathetic fibers
Visceral afferent accompanying sympathetic fibers
Visceral afferent accompanying parasympathetic fibers
F. Netter M.D.

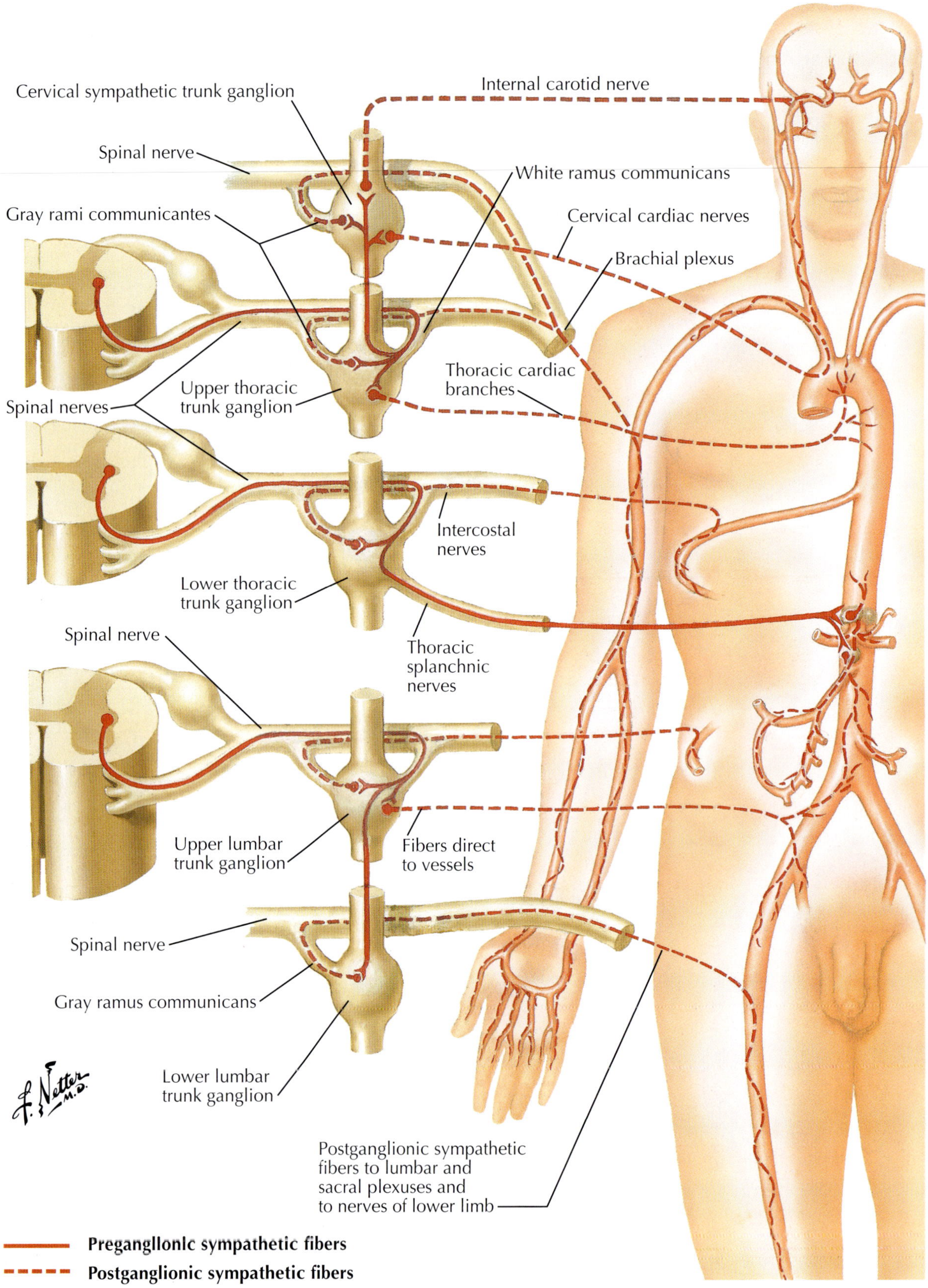

Cervical sympathetic trunk ganglion
Internal carotid nerve
Spinal nerve
White ramus communicans
Gray rami communicantes
Cervical cardiac nerves
Brachial plexus
Thoracic cardiac branches
Spinal nerves
Upper thoracic trunk ganglion
Intercostal nerves
Lower thoracic trunk ganglion
Spinal nerve
Thoracic splanchnic nerves
Upper lumbar trunk ganglion
Fibers direct to vessels
Spinal nerve
Gray ramus communicans
Lower lumbar trunk ganglion
Postganglionic sympathetic fibers to lumbar and sacral plexuses and to nerves of lower limb
Preganglionic sympathetic fibers
Postganglionic sympathetic fibers

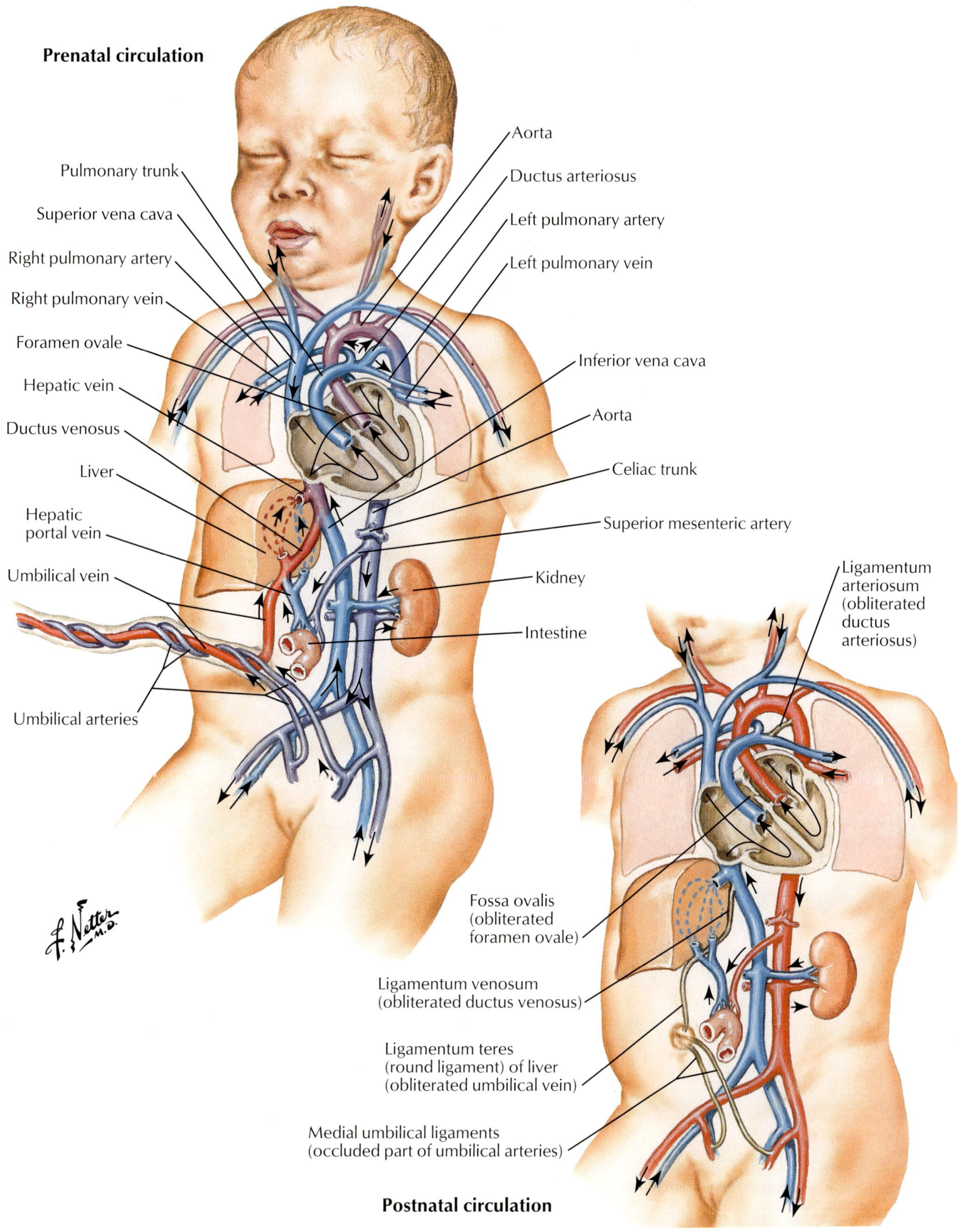
Prenatal circulation
Aorta
Pulmonary trunk
Ductus arteriosus
Superior vena cava
Left pulmonary artery
Right pulmonary artery
Left pulmonary vein
Right pulmonary vein
Foramen ovale
Inferior vena cava
Hepatic vein
Aorta
Ductus venosus
Liver
Celiac trunk
Hepatic portal vein
Superior mesenteric artery
Umbilical vein
Kidney
Intestine
Umbilical arteries
Ligamentum arteriosum (obliterated ductus arteriosus)
Fossa ovalis (obliterated foramen ovale)
Ligamentum venosum (obliterated ductus venosus)
Ligamentum teres (round ligament) of liver (obliterated umbilical vein)
Medial umbilical ligaments (occluded part of umbilical arteries)
Postnatal circulation

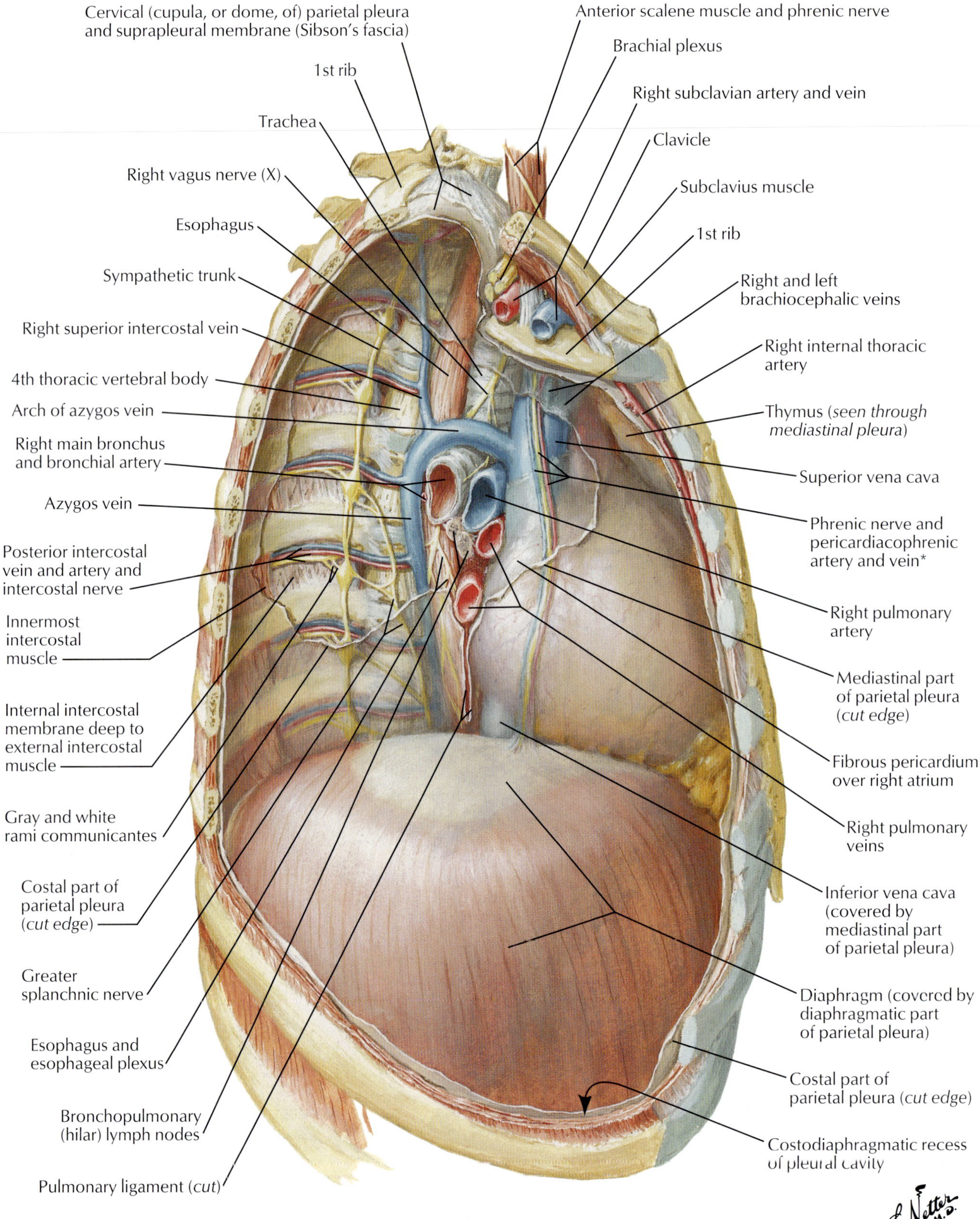

*Nerve and vessels commonly run independently.

Mediastinum: Left Lateral View

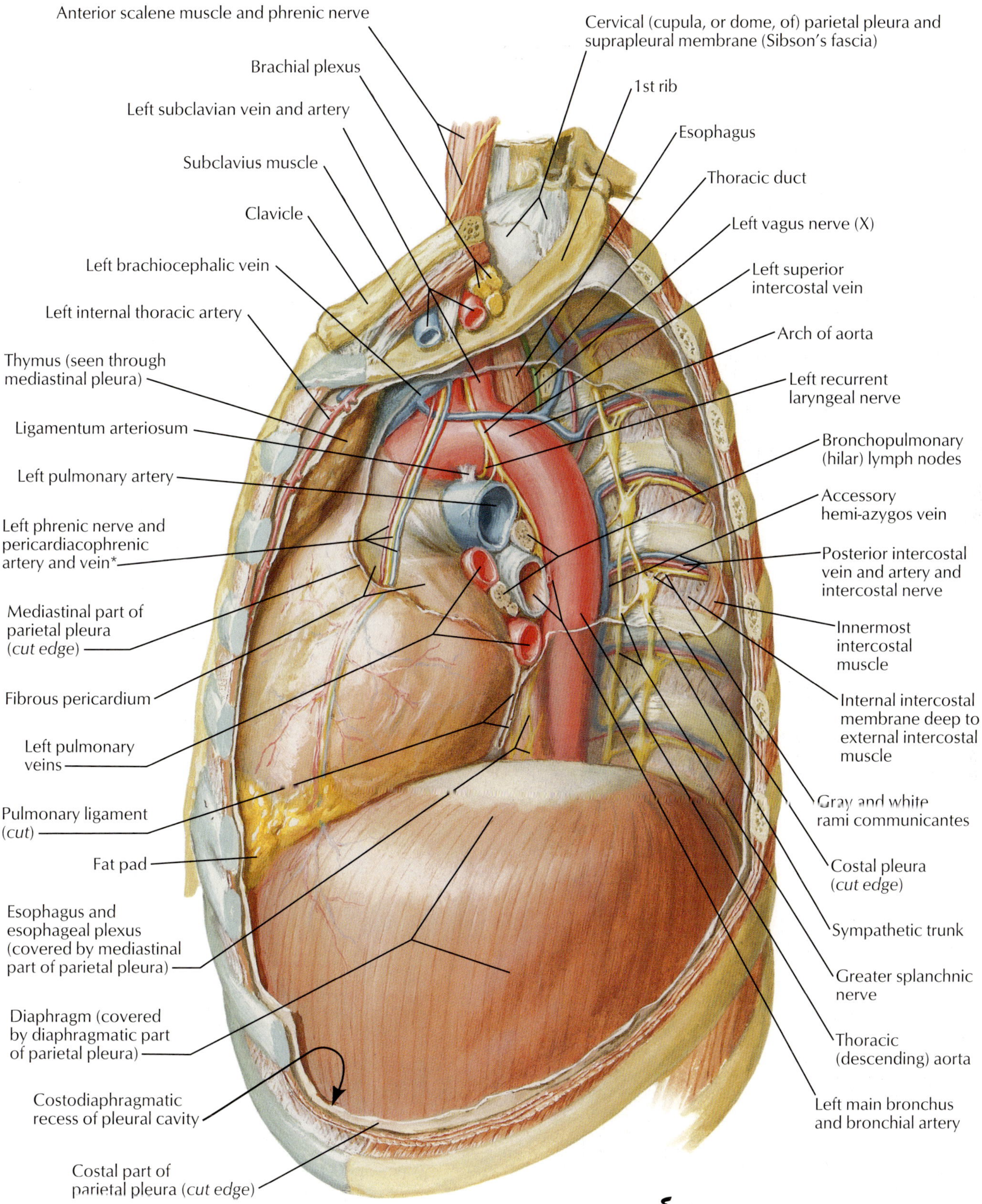

*Nerve and vessels commonly run independently.

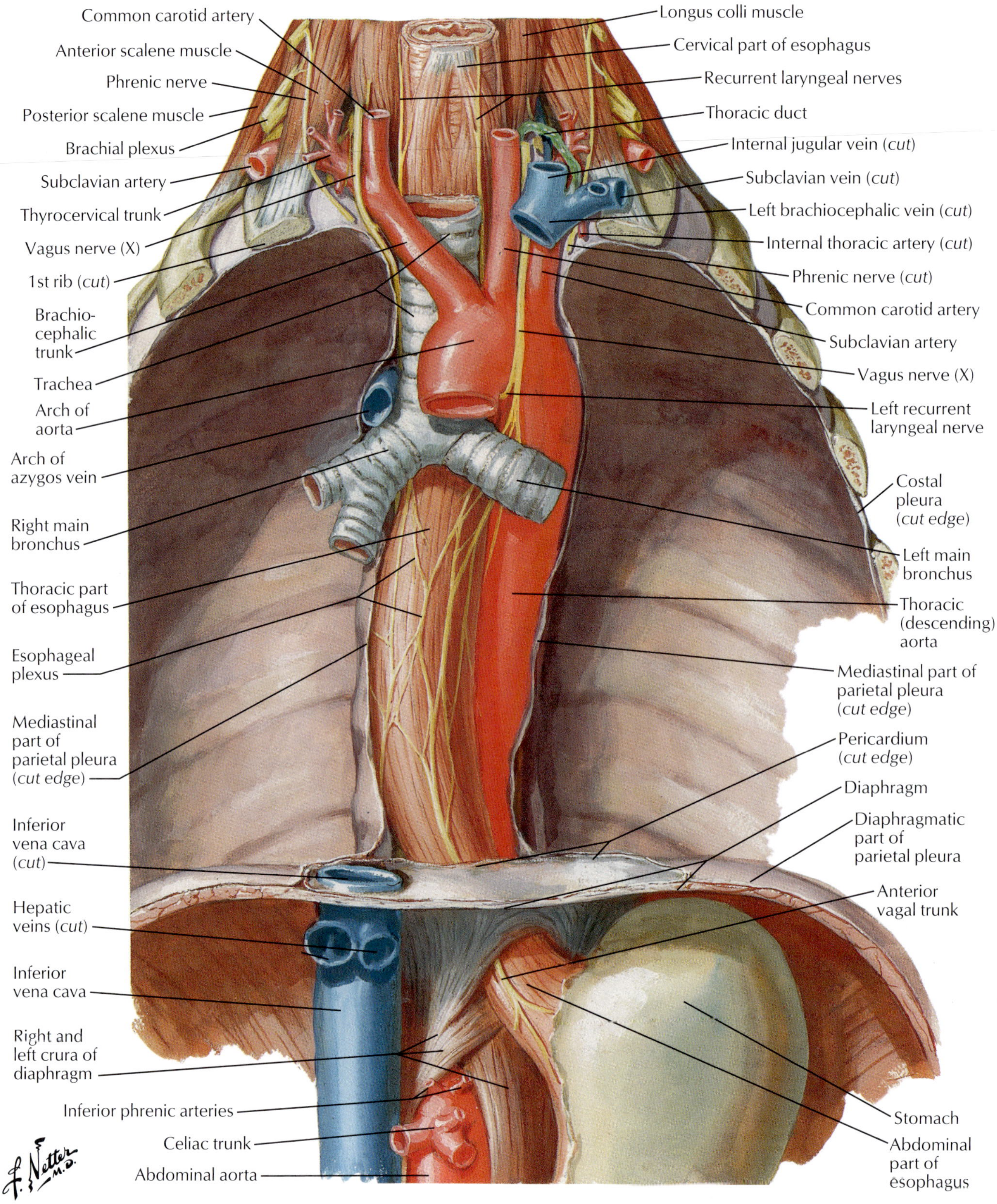
Common carotid artery
Anterior scalene muscle
Phrenic nerve
Posterior scalene muscle
Brachial plexus
Subclavian artery
Thyrocervical trunk
Vagus nerve (X)
1st rib (*cut*)
Brachio-cephalic trunk
Trachea
Arch of aorta
Arch of azygos vein
Right main bronchus
Thoracic part of esophagus
Esophageal plexus
Mediastinal part of parietal pleura (*cut edge*)
Inferior vena cava (*cut*)
Hepatic veins (*cut*)
Inferior vena cava
Right and left crura of diaphragm
Inferior phrenic arteries
Celiac trunk
Abdominal aorta
Longus colli muscle
Cervical part of esophagus
Recurrent laryngeal nerves
Thoracic duct
Internal jugular vein (*cut*)
Subclavian vein (*cut*)
Left brachiocephalic vein (*cut*)
Internal thoracic artery (*cut*)
Phrenic nerve (*cut*)
Common carotid artery
Subclavian artery
Vagus nerve (X)
Left recurrent laryngeal nerve
Costal pleura (*cut edge*)
Left main bronchus
Thoracic (descending) aorta
Mediastinal part of parietal pleura (*cut edge*)
Pericardium (*cut edge*)
Diaphragm
Diaphragmatic part of parietal pleura
Anterior vagal trunk
Stomach
Abdominal part of esophagus

Topography and Constrictions of Esophagus

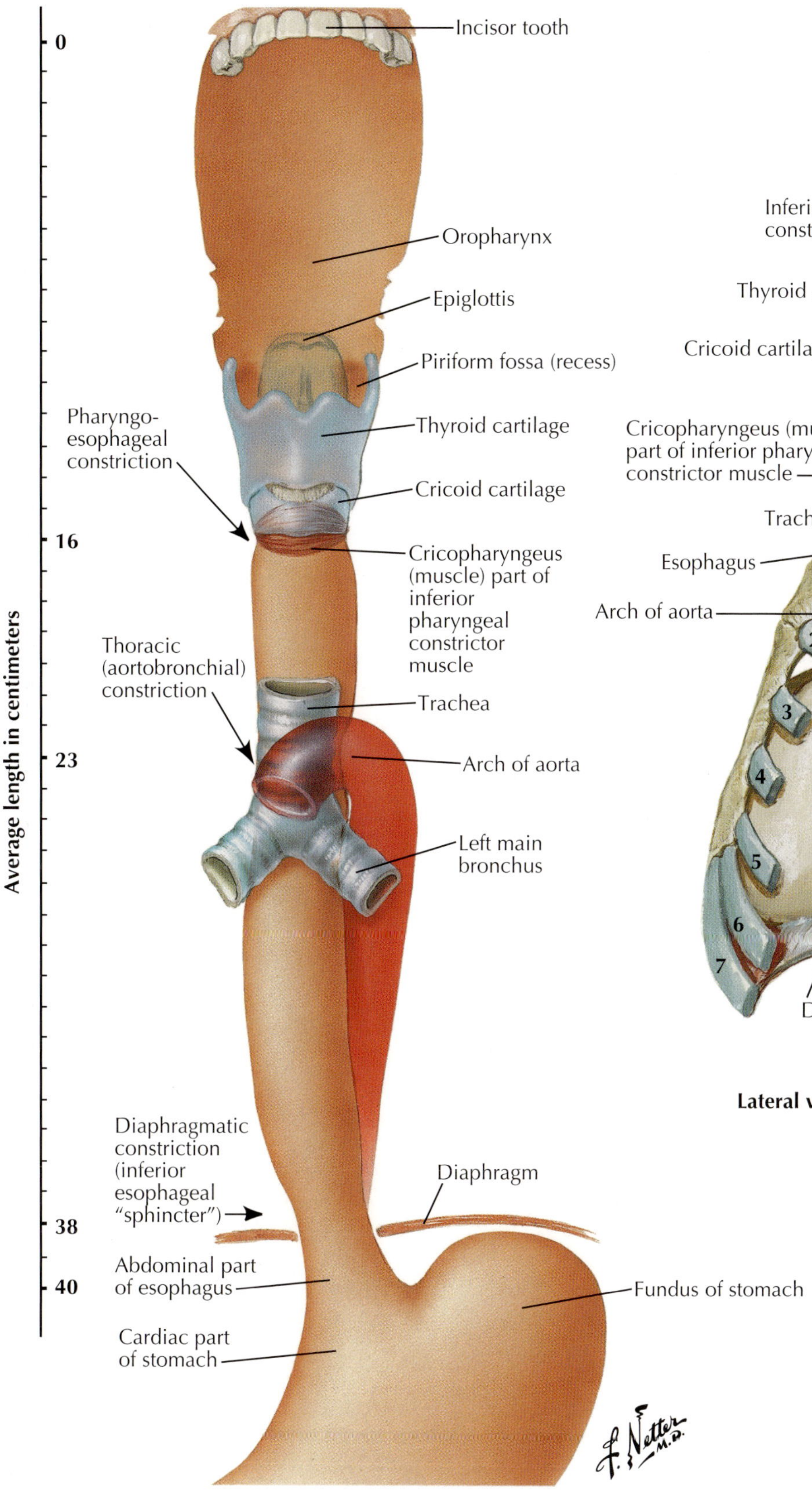

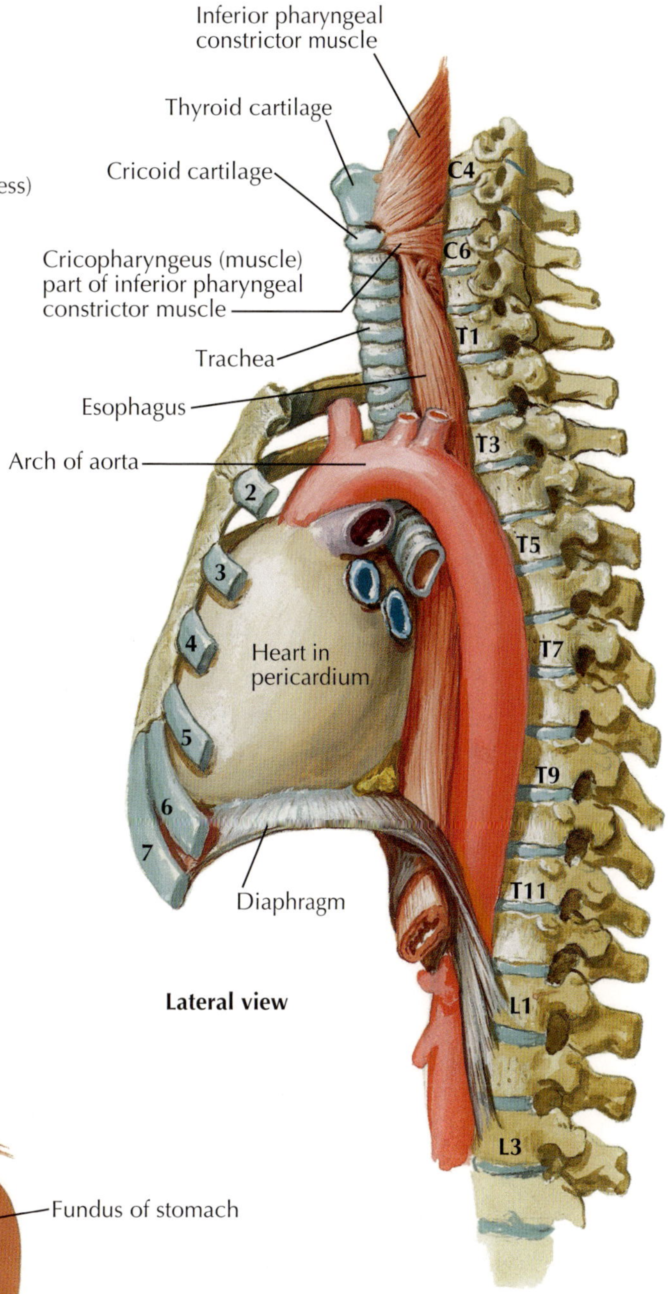

Lateral view

Musculature of Esophagus

See also Plates 67, 70

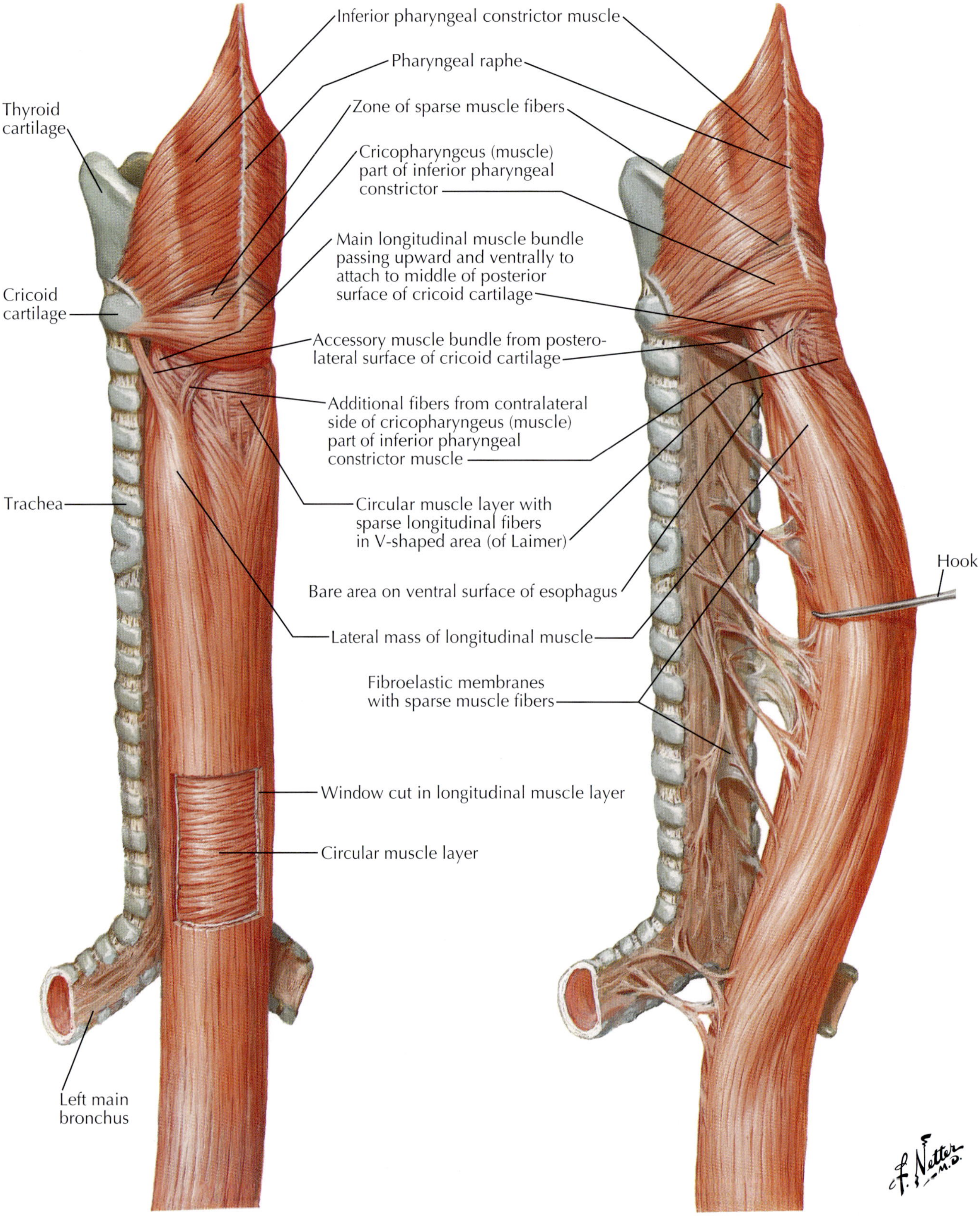

Posterolateral view

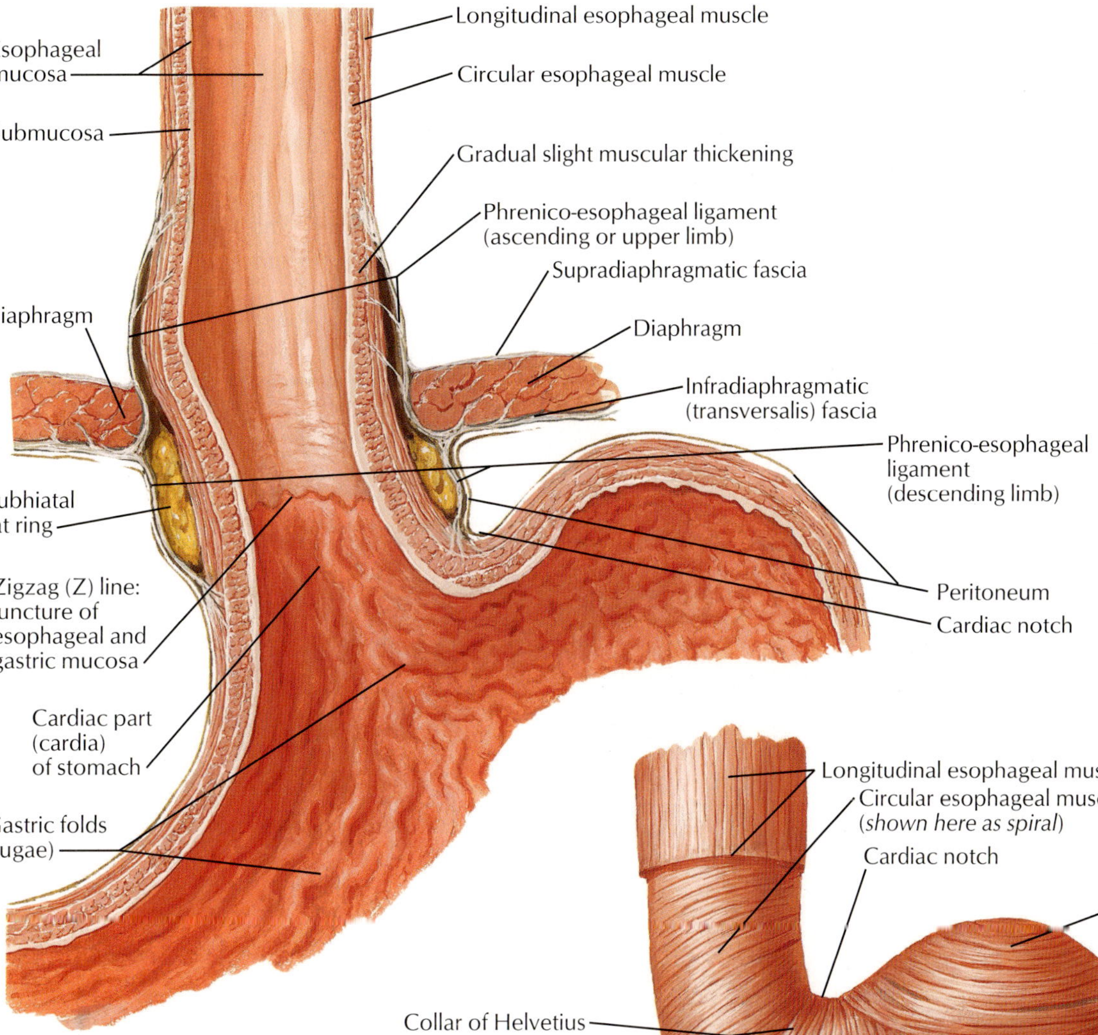
Esophageal mucosa
Submucosa
Diaphragm
Subhiatal fat ring
Zigzag (Z) line: juncture of esophageal and gastric mucosa
Cardiac part (cardia) of stomach
Gastric folds (rugae)
Longitudinal esophageal muscle
Circular esophageal muscle
Gradual slight muscular thickening
Phrenico-esophageal ligament (ascending or upper limb)
Supradiaphragmatic fascia
Diaphragm
Infradiaphragmatic (transversalis) fascia
Phrenico-esophageal ligament (descending limb)
Peritoneum
Cardiac notch

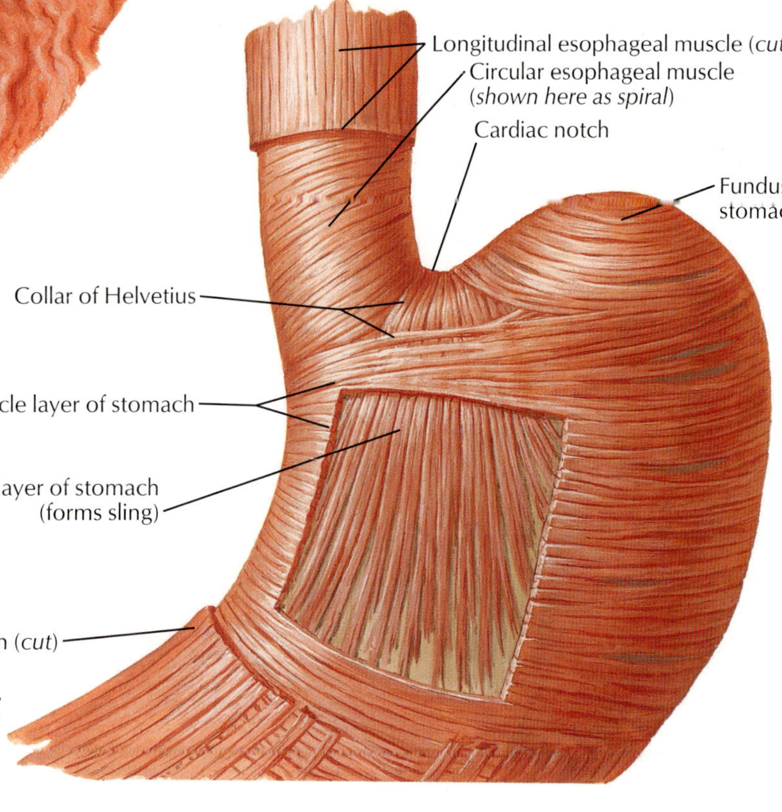
Longitudinal esophageal muscle (*cut*)
Circular esophageal muscle (*shown here as spiral*)
Cardiac notch
Fundus of stomach
Collar of Helvetius
Window cut in middle circular muscle layer of stomach
Innermost oblique muscle layer of stomach (forms sling)
Outer longitudinal muscle layer of stomach (*cut*)
F. Netter M.D.

See also Plates 204, 284

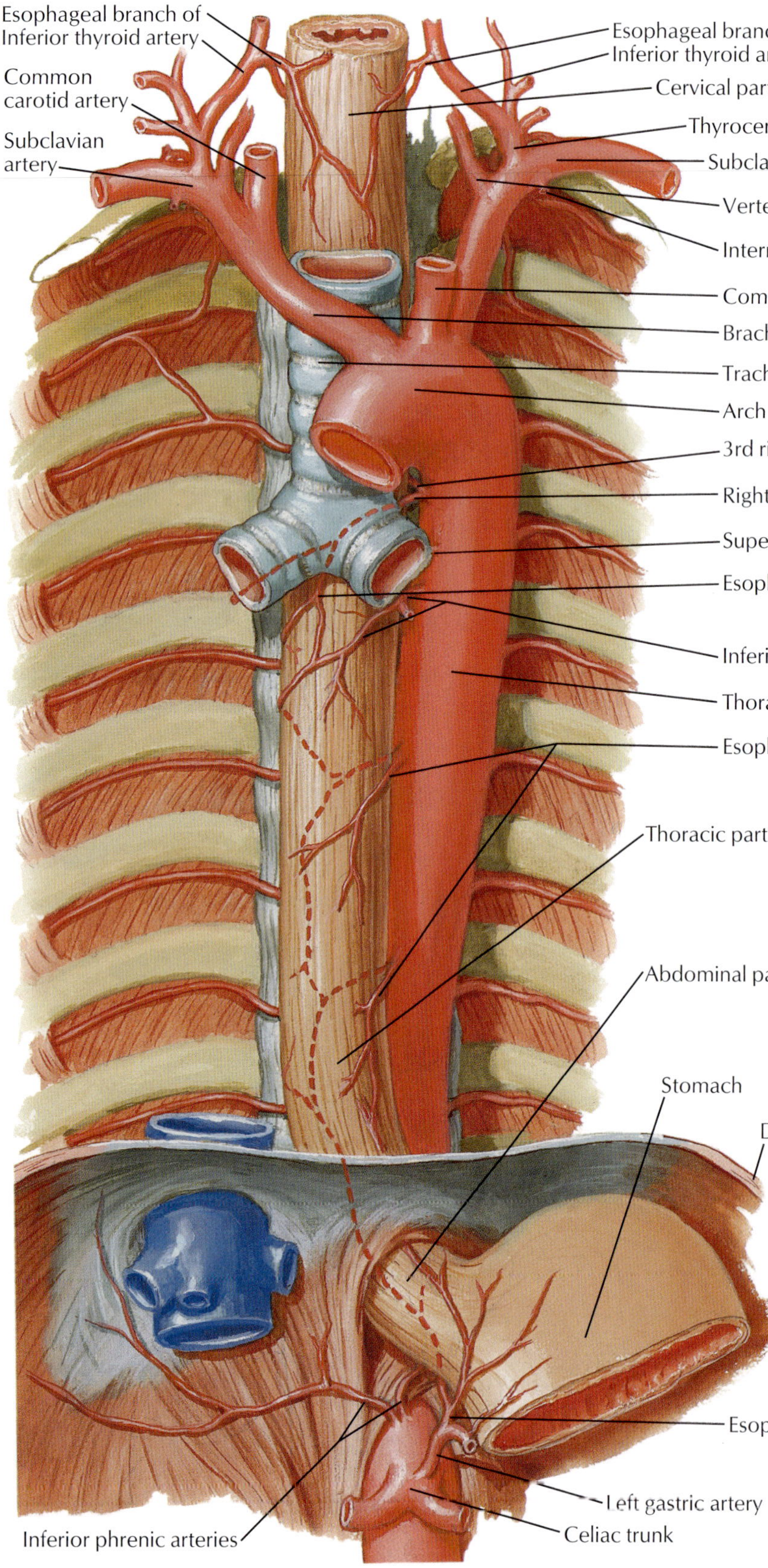

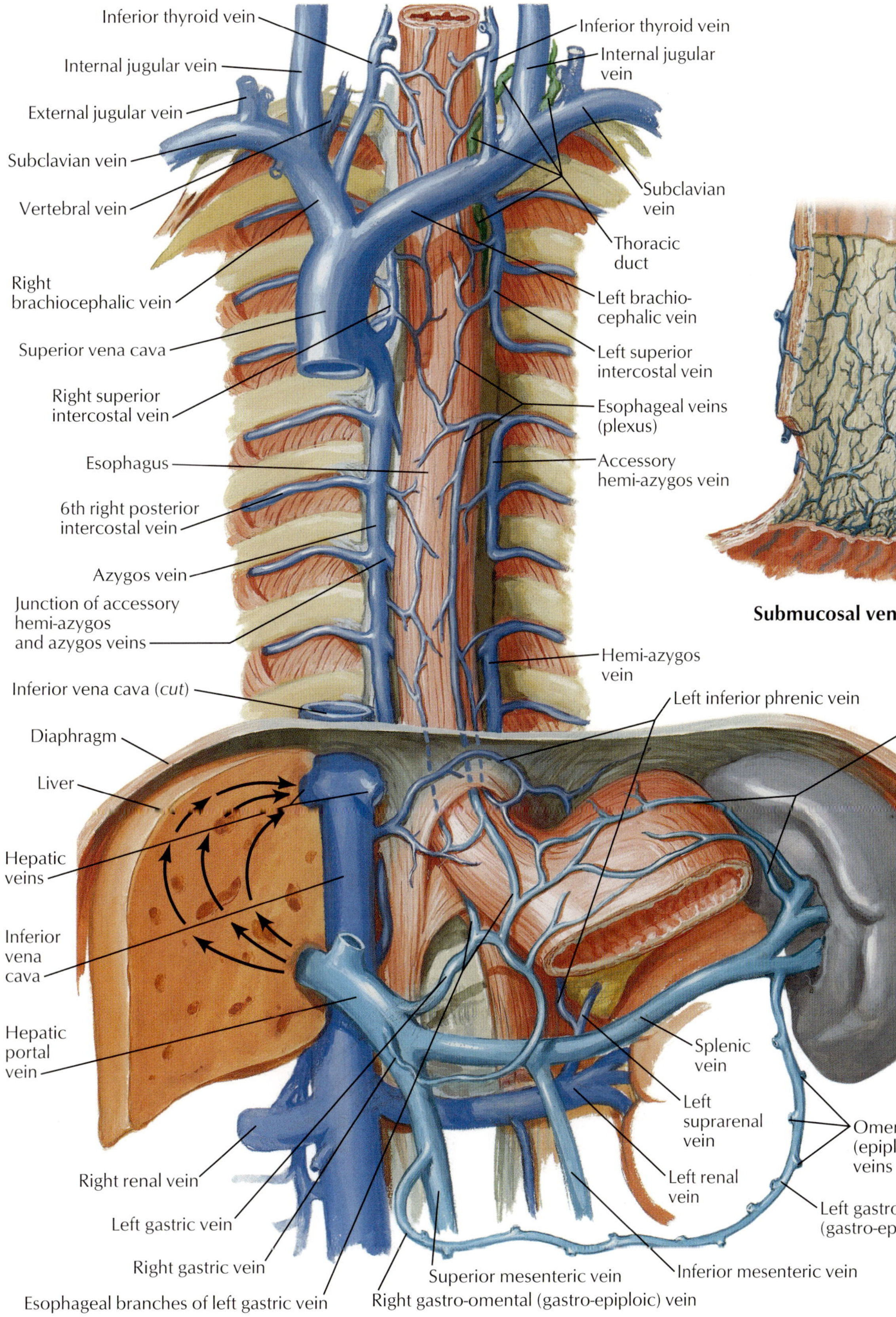

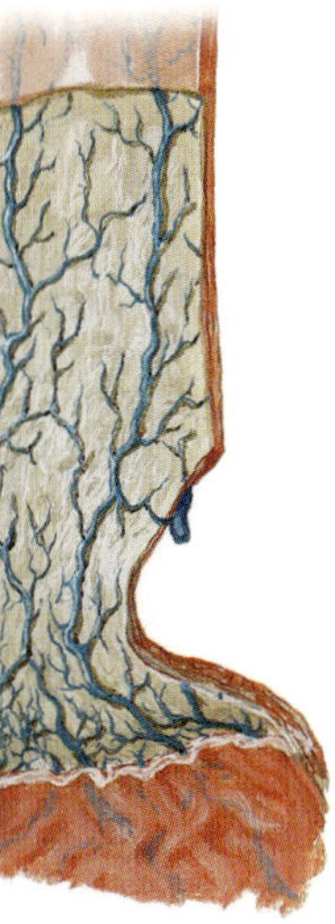

Submucosal venous plexus

Lymph Vessels and Nodes of Esophagus

See also Plates 205, 293

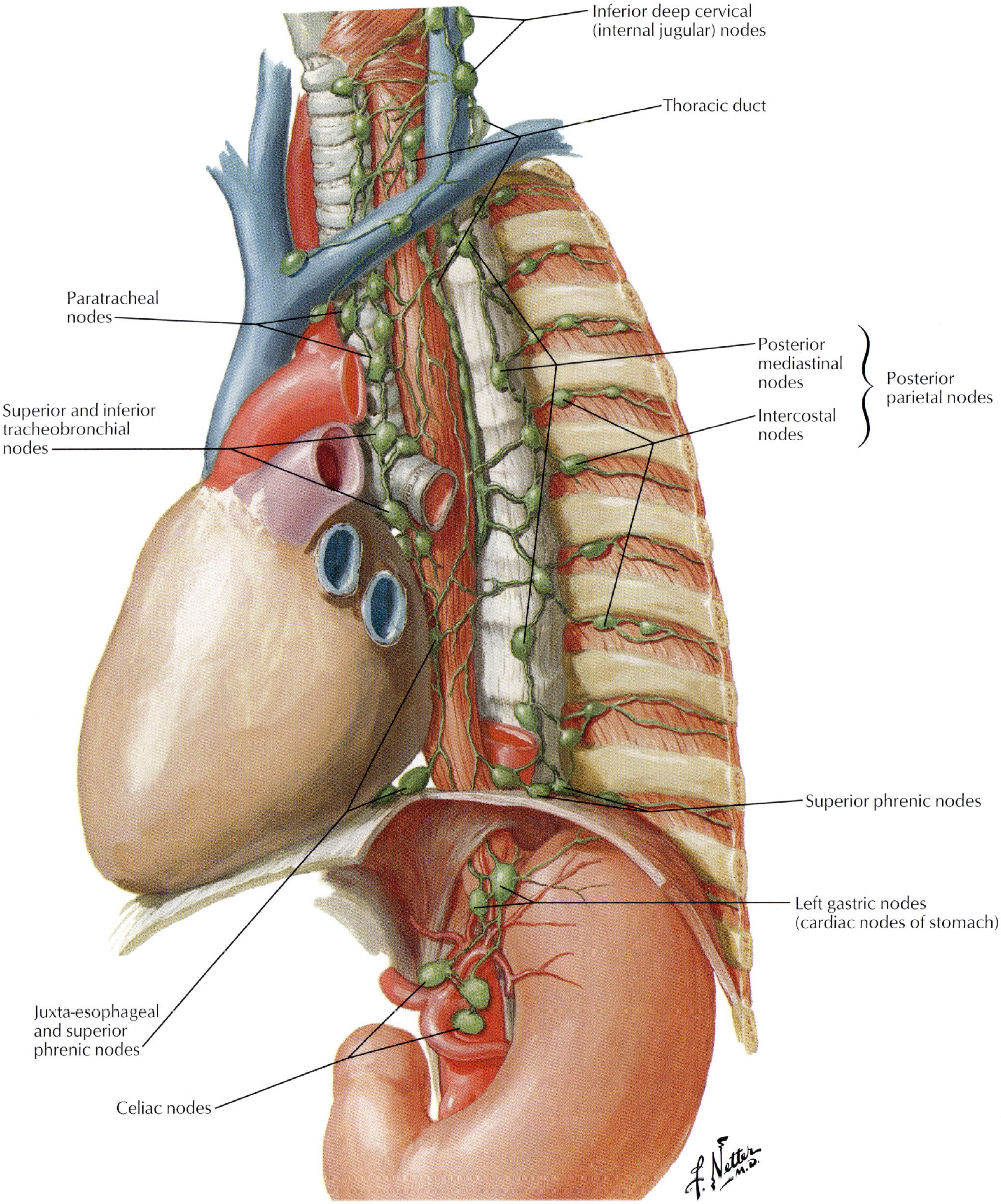

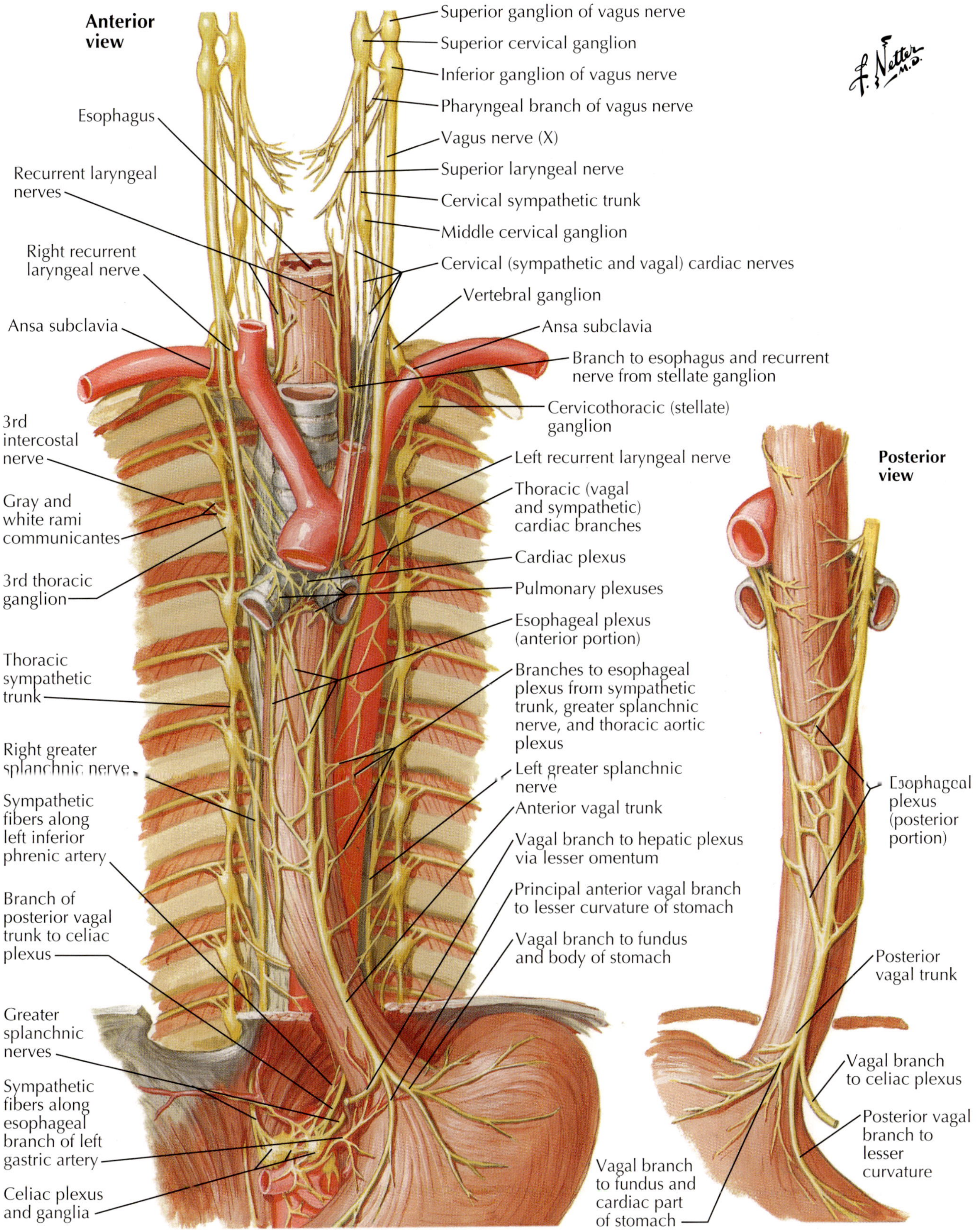
Anterior view
Superior ganglion of vagus nerve
Superior cervical ganglion
Inferior ganglion of vagus nerve
Pharyngeal branch of vagus nerve
Vagus nerve (X)
Superior laryngeal nerve
Cervical sympathetic trunk
Middle cervical ganglion
Cervical (sympathetic and vagal) cardiac nerves
Vertebral ganglion
Ansa subclavia
Branch to esophagus and recurrent nerve from stellate ganglion
Cervicothoracic (stellate) ganglion
Left recurrent laryngeal nerve
Thoracic (vagal and sympathetic) cardiac branches
Cardiac plexus
Pulmonary plexuses
Esophageal plexus (anterior portion)
Branches to esophageal plexus from sympathetic trunk, greater splanchnic nerve, and thoracic aortic plexus
Left greater splanchnic nerve
Anterior vagal trunk
Vagal branch to hepatic plexus via lesser omentum
Principal anterior vagal branch to lesser curvature of stomach
Vagal branch to fundus and body of stomach
Esophagus
Recurrent laryngeal nerves
Right recurrent laryngeal nerve
Ansa subclavia
3rd intercostal nerve
Gray and white rami communicantes
3rd thoracic ganglion
Thoracic sympathetic trunk
Right greater splanchnic nerve
Sympathetic fibers along left inferior phrenic artery
Branch of posterior vagal trunk to celiac plexus
Greater splanchnic nerves
Sympathetic fibers along esophageal branch of left gastric artery
Celiac plexus and ganglia
Vagal branch to fundus and cardiac part of stomach
Posterior view
Esophageal plexus (posterior portion)
Posterior vagal trunk
Vagal branch to celiac plexus
Posterior vagal branch to lesser curvature

Series of chest axial CT images from superior (A) to inferior (C)

A

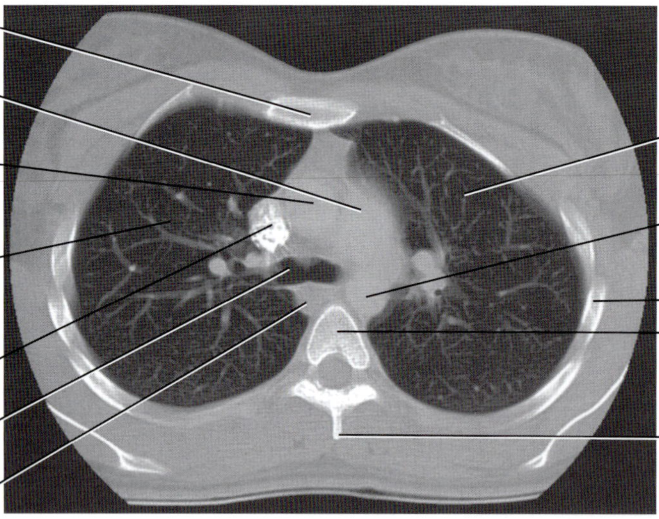

B

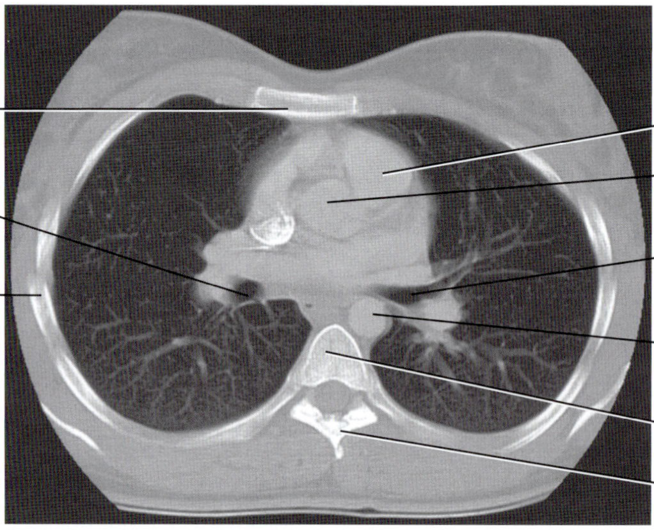

C

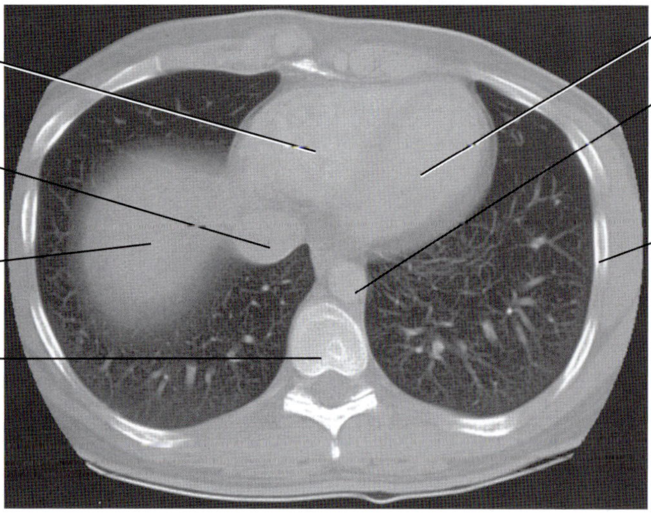

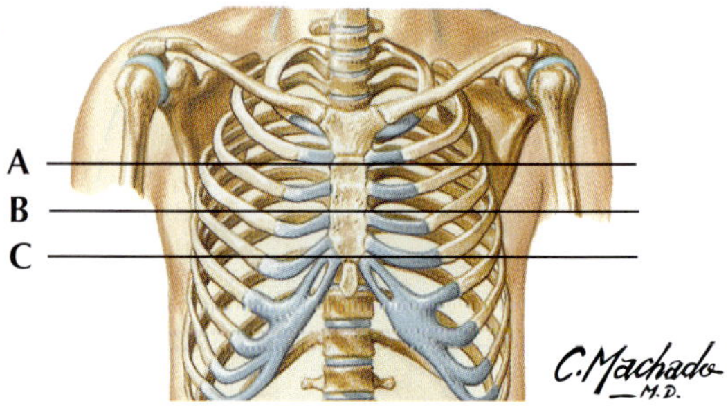

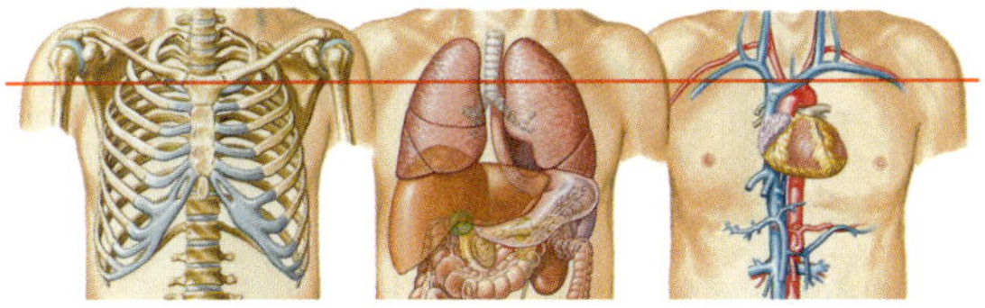

Inferior view

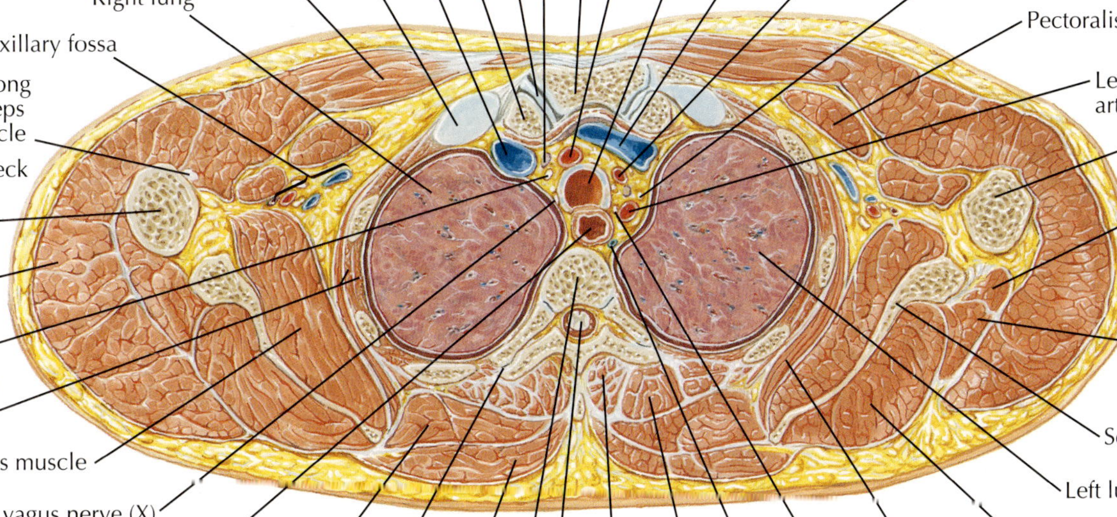

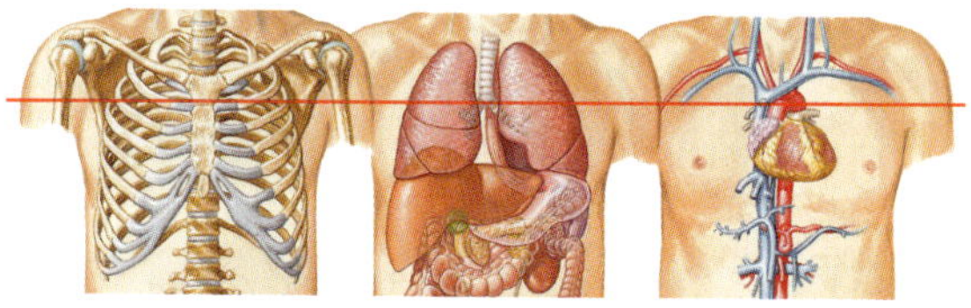

Inferior view

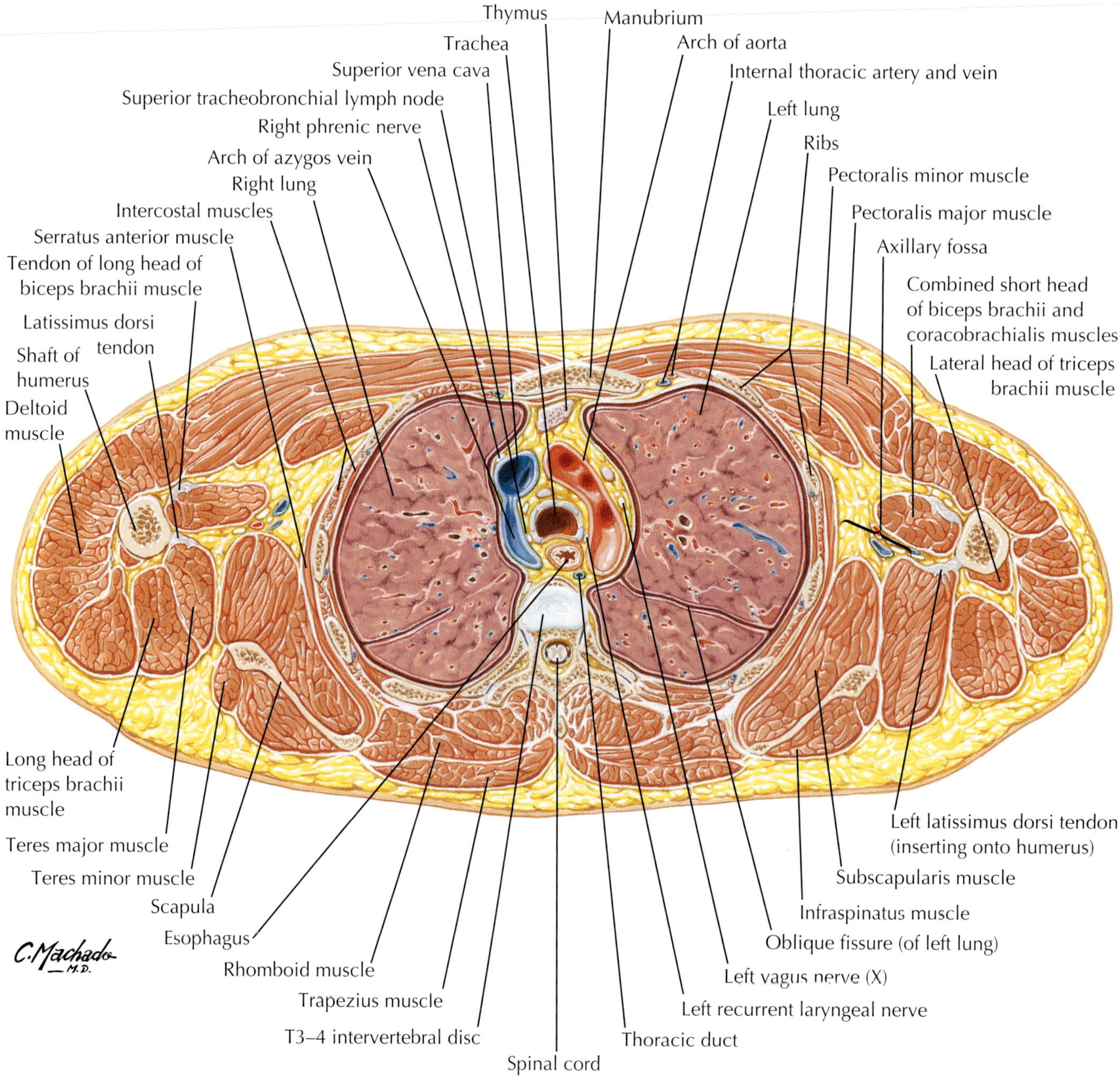

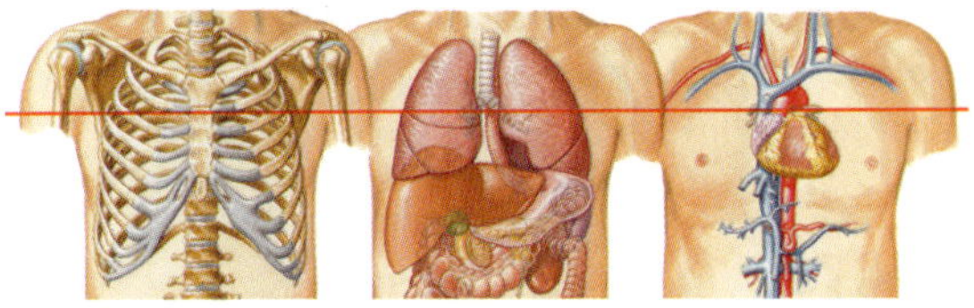

Inferior view

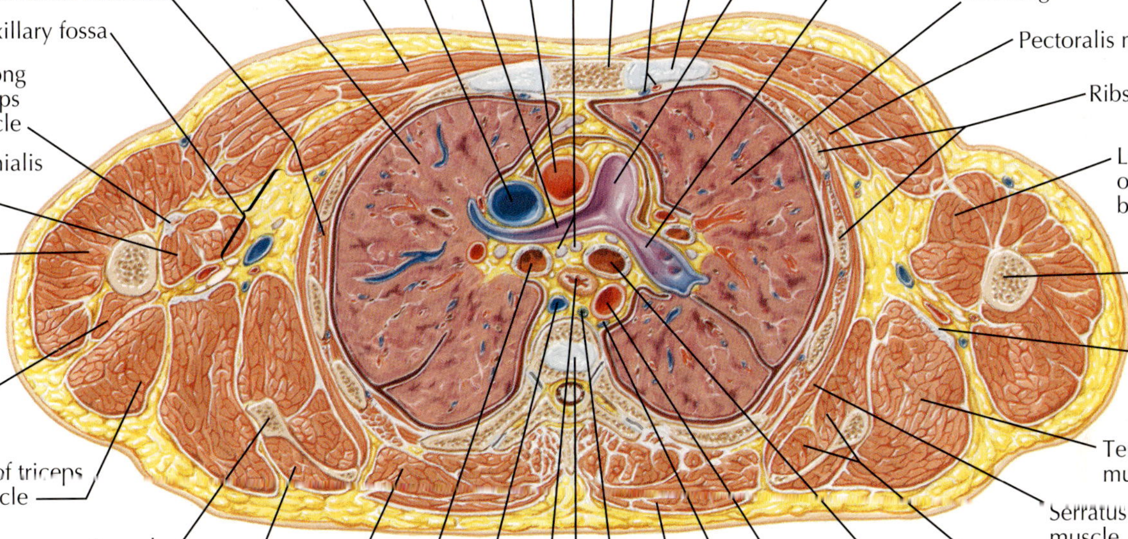

Cross Section of Thorax at T7 Level

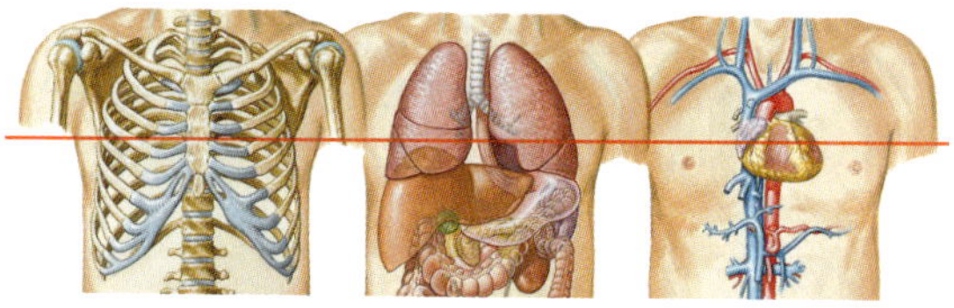

Inferior view

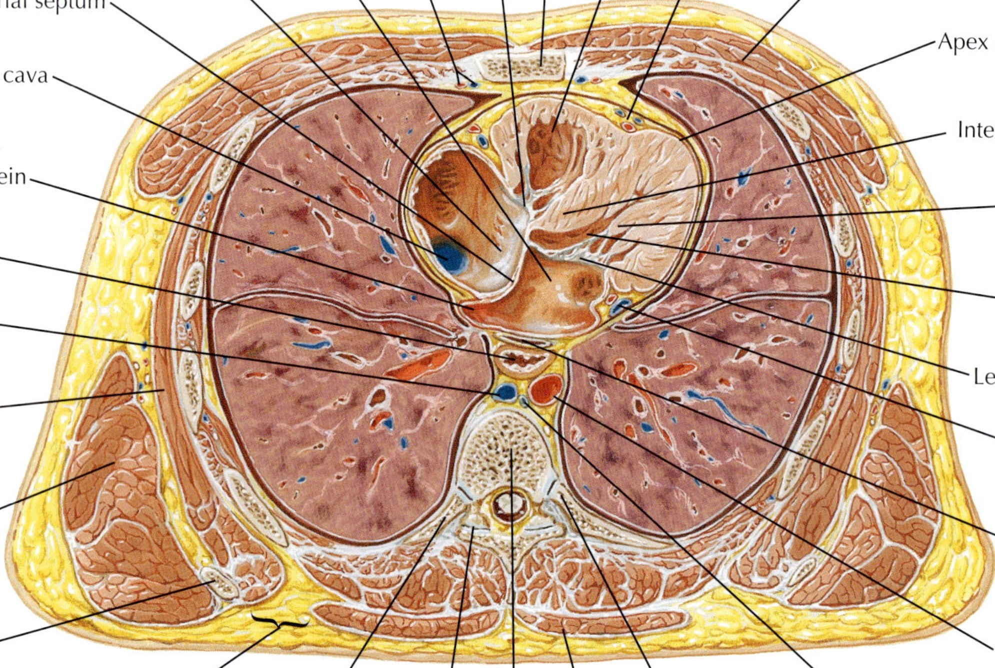

MUSCLE	PROXIMAL ATTACHMENT (ORIGIN)	DISTAL ATTACHMENT (INSERTION)	INNERVATION	MAIN ACTIONS	BLOOD SUPPLY	MUSCLE GROUP
Diaphragm	Xiphoid process, lower six costal cartilages, L1–L3 vertebrae	Converge into central tendon	Phrenic nerve	Draws central tendon down and forward during inspiration	Pericardiacophrenic, musculophrenic, superior and inferior phrenic arteries	Posterior abdominal wall
External intercostal	Lower border of ribs	Upper border of rib below rib of origin	Intercostal nerves	Supports intercostal spaces in inspiration and expiration, elevates ribs in inspiration	Posterior intercostal arteries, collateral branches of posterior intercostal arteries, costocervical trunk, anterior intercostal branches of internal thoracic artery, musculophrenic artery	Thoracic wall
Innermost intercostal	Lower border of ribs	Upper border of rib below rib of origin	Intercostal nerves	Elevates ribs	Muscular branches of anterior intercostal arteries, muscular branches of posterior intercostal arteries, intercostal branches of internal thoracic and musculophrenic arteries, costocervical trunk branches	Thoracic wall
Internal intercostal	Lower border of ribs	Costal cartilage and edge of costal groove of rib above rib of origin	Intercostal nerves	Prevents pushing out or drawing in of intercostal spaces in inspiration and expiration, lowers ribs in forced expiration	Muscular branches of anterior intercostal arteries, muscular branches of posterior intercostal arteries, intercostal branches of internal thoracic and musculophrenic arteries, costocervical trunk branches	Thoracic wall
Levator costarum	Transverse processes of C7 and T1–T11	Subjacent ribs between tubercle and angle	Dorsal ramus of lower thoracic nerves	Elevates ribs	Posterior intercostal arteries	Thoracic wall
Pectoralis major	Sternal half of clavicle, sternum to 7th rib, cartilages of true ribs, aponeurosis of external oblique muscle	Lateral lip of intertubercular sulcus of humerus	Medial and lateral pectoral nerves	Flexes and adducts arm, rotates arm medially	Pectoral branch of thoraco-acromial artery, perforating branches of internal thoracic artery	Pectoral/axilla region
Pectoralis minor	Outer surface of upper margin of ribs 3–5	Coracoid process of scapula	Medial pectoral nerve	Lowers lateral angle of scapula and protracts scapula	Pectoral branch of thoraco-acromial and intercostal lateral thoracic arteries	Pectoral/axilla region
Serratus anterior	Lateral surfaces of upper 8–9 ribs	Costal surface of medial border of scapula	Long thoracic nerve	Protracts scapula and holds it against thoracic wall	Lateral thoracic artery	Pectoral/axilla region
Serratus posterior inferior	Spinous processes of T11–L2	Inferior aspect of ribs 9–12	Ventral rami of lower thoracic nerves	Depresses ribs	Posterior intercostal arteries	Intermediate back
Serratus posterior superior	Ligamentum nuchae, spinous processes of C7–T3	Superior aspect of ribs 2–4	Ventral rami of upper thoracic nerves	Elevates ribs	Posterior intercostal arteries	Intermediate back
Subcostal	Internal surface of lower ribs near their angles	Superior borders of 2nd or 3rd rib below	Intercostal nerves	Depresses ribs	Posterior intercostal artery, musculophrenic artery	Thoracic wall
Transversus thoracis	Internal surface of costal cartilages 2–6	Posterior surface of lower sternum	Intercostal nerves	Depresses ribs and costal cartilages	Anterior intercostal arteries, internal thoracic artery	Thoracic wall

Variations in spinal nerve contributions to the innervation of muscles, their arterial supply, their attachments, and their actions are common themes in human anatomy. Therefore, expect differences between texts and realize that anatomical variation is normal.

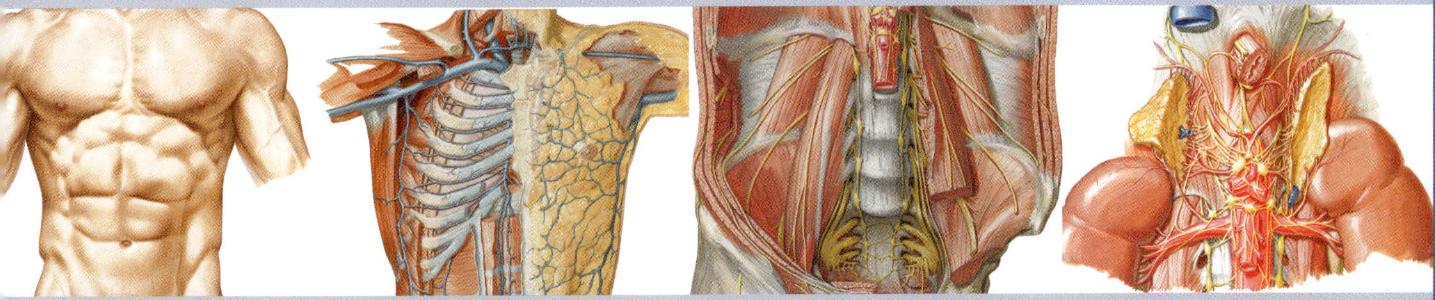

Section

4 ABDOMEN

Topographic Anatomy

Plate 242

242 Abdomen: Surface Anatomy

Body Wall

Plates 243–262

243 Bony Framework of Abdomen

244 Regions and Planes of Abdomen

245 Anterior Abdominal Wall: Superficial Dissection

246 Anterior Abdominal Wall: Intermediate Dissection

247 Anterior Abdominal Wall: Deep Dissection

248 Rectus Sheath: Cross Section

249 Anterior Abdominal Wall: Internal View

250 Posterolateral Abdominal Wall

251 Arteries of Anterior Abdominal Wall

252 Veins of Anterior Abdominal Wall

253 Nerves of Anterior Abdominal Wall

254 Thoracoabdominal Nerves

255 Inguinal Region: Dissections

256 Inguinal Canal and Spermatic Cord

257 Femoral Sheath and Inguinal Canal

258 Posterior Abdominal Wall: Internal View

259 Arteries of Posterior Abdominal Wall

260 Veins of Posterior Abdominal Wall

261 Lymph Vessels and Nodes of Posterior Abdominal Wall

262 Nerves of Posterior Abdominal Wall

Peritoneal Cavity

Plates 263–268

263 Greater Omentum and Abdominal Viscera

264 Mesenteric Relations of Intestines

265 Mesenteric Relations of Intestines (continued)

266 Omental Bursa: Stomach Reflected

267 Omental Bursa: Cross Section

268 Peritoneum of Posterior Abdominal Wall

Viscera (Gut)

Plates 269–276

269 Stomach in Situ

270 Mucosa of Stomach

271 Duodenum in Situ

272 Mucosa and Musculature of Small Intestine

273 Ileocecal Region

274 Ileocecal Region (continued)

275 (Vermiform) Appendix

276 Mucosa and Musculature of Large Intestine

Viscera (Accessory Organs)

Plates 277–282

277 Surfaces and Bed of Liver

278 Liver in Situ: Vascular and Duct Systems

279 Liver Structure: Schema

280 Gallbladder, Extrahepatic Bile Ducts, and Pancreatic Duct

281 Pancreas in Situ

282 Spleen

Visceral Vasculature

Plates 283–296

283 Arteries of Stomach, Liver, and Spleen

284 Arteries of Liver, Pancreas, Duodenum, and Spleen

285 Celiac Arteriogram and CT Angiogram

286 Arteries of Duodenum and Head of Pancreas

287 Arteries of Small Intestine

288 Arteries of Large Intestine

289 Veins of Stomach, Duodenum, Pancreas, and Spleen

290 Veins of Small Intestine

291 Veins of Large Intestine

292 Hepatic Portal Vein Tributaries: Portacaval Anastomoses

293 Lymph Vessels and Nodes of Stomach

294 Lymph Vessels and Nodes of Pancreas

295 Lymph Vessels and Nodes of Small Intestine

296 Lymph Vessels and Nodes of Large Intestine

Innervation

Pates 297–307

297 Autonomic Nerves and Ganglia of Abdomen

298 Autonomic Innervation of Stomach and Duodenum

299 Autonomic Innervation of Stomach and Duodenum (continued)

300 Autonomic Innervation of Stomach and Duodenum: Schema

301 Autonomic Innervation of Small Intestine

302 Autonomic Innervation of Large Intestine

303 Autonomic Innervation of Small and Large Intestines: Schema

304 Autonomic Reflex Pathways: Schema

305 Intrinsic Autonomic Plexuses of Intestine: Schema

306 Autonomic Innervation of Liver and Biliary Tract: Schema

307 Autonomic Innervation of Pancreas: Schema

Kidneys and Suprarenal Glands

Plates 308–320

308 Kidneys in Situ: Anterior Views

309 Kidneys in Situ: Posterior Views

310 Renal Artery and Vein in Situ

311 Gross Structure of Kidney

312 Intrarenal Arteries and Renal Segments

313 Ureters in Abdomen and Pelvis

314 Arteries of Ureters and Urinary Bladder

315 Renal Fasciae

316 Lymph Vessels and Nodes of Kidneys and Urinary Bladder
317 Autonomic Nerves of Kidneys, Ureters, and Urinary Bladder
318 Autonomic Innervation of Kidneys and Upper Ureters: Schema
319 Autonomic Nerves of Suprarenal Glands: Dissection and Schema
320 Arteries and Veins of Suprarenal Glands in Situ

Sectional Anatomy

Plates 321–328

321 Abdominal Wall and Viscera: Paramedian (Parasagittal) Section
322 Abdominal Scans: Axial CT Images
323 Abdominal Scans: Axial CT Images (continued)
324 Cross Section at T10, Esophagogastric Junction
325 Cross Section at T12, Inferior to Xiphoid
326 Cross Section at T12–L1, Intervertebral Disc
327 Cross Section at L1–2, Intervertebral Disc
328 Cross Section at L3–4

Muscle Table

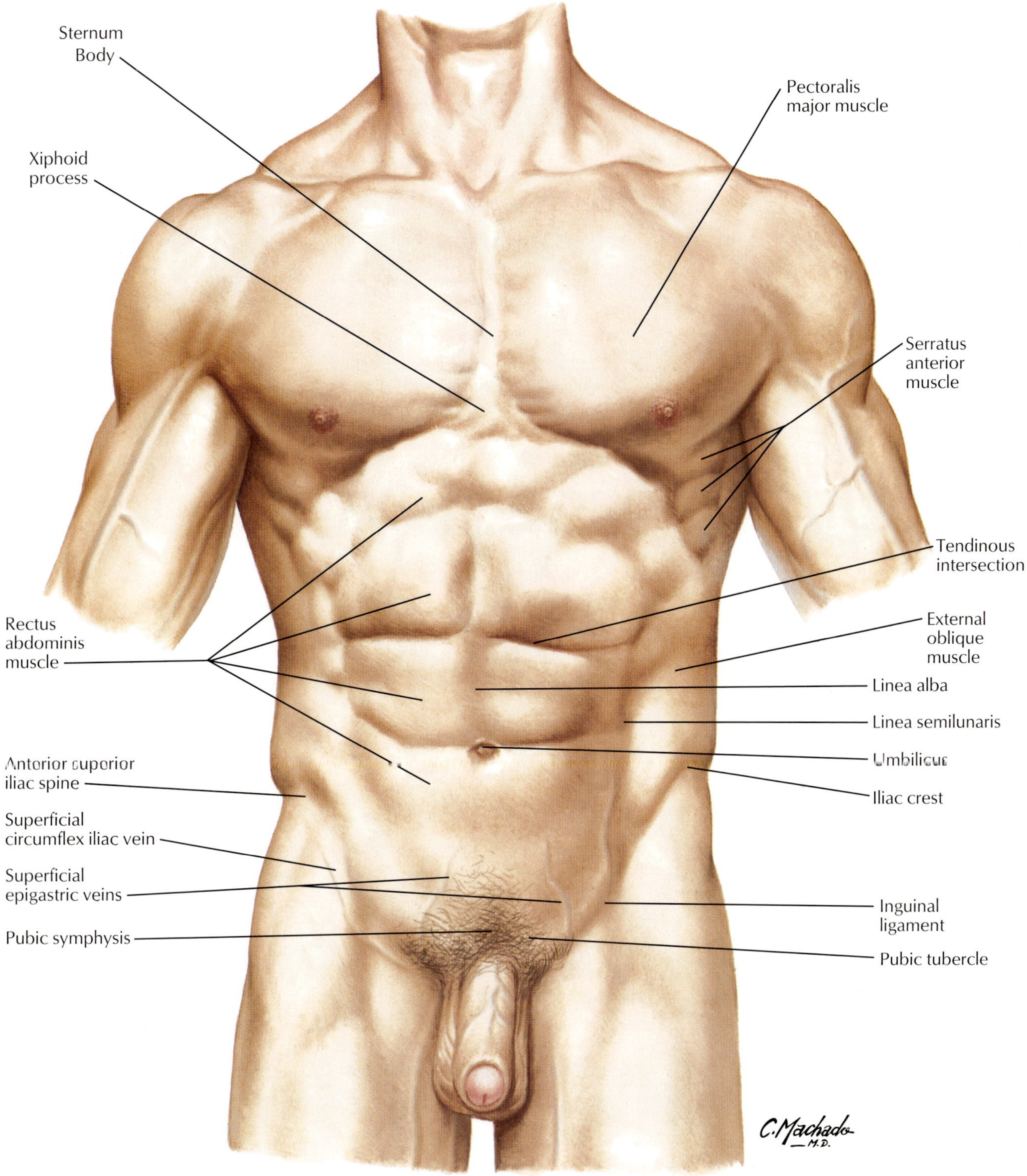
Sternum
Body
Xiphoid process
Pectoralis major muscle
Serratus anterior muscle
Tendinous intersection
Rectus abdominis muscle
External oblique muscle
Linea alba
Linea semilunaris
Anterior superior iliac spine
Umbilicus
Iliac crest
Superficial circumflex iliac vein
Superficial epigastric veins
Inguinal ligament
Pubic symphysis
Pubic tubercle
C. Machado M.D.

See also Plates 183, 332

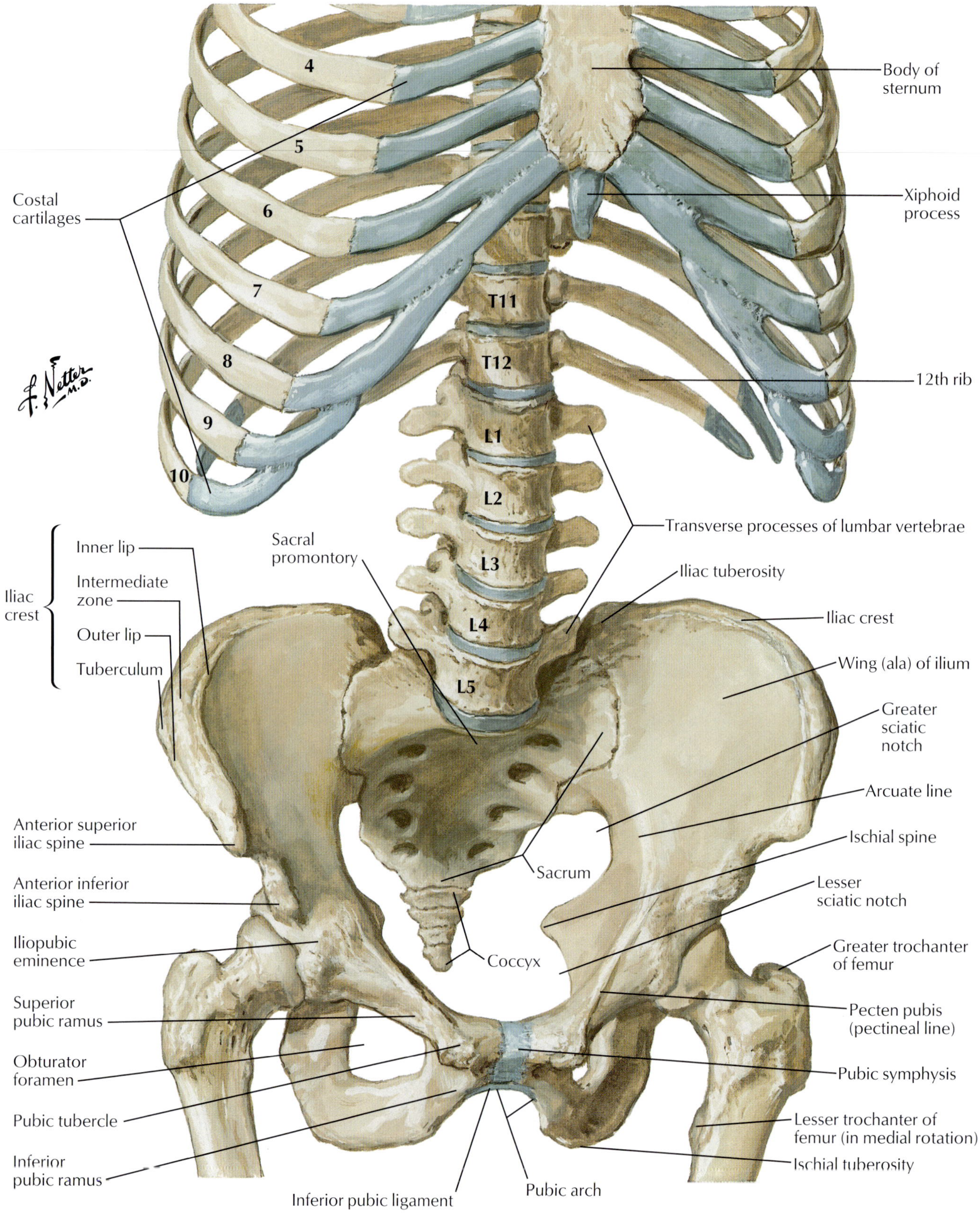

Regions and Planes of Abdomen

See also Plate 193

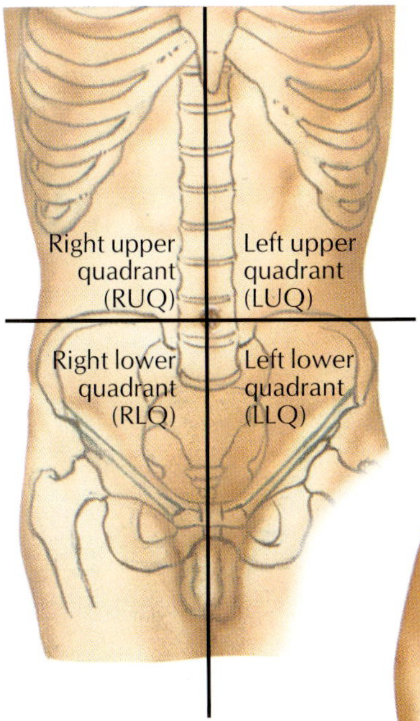

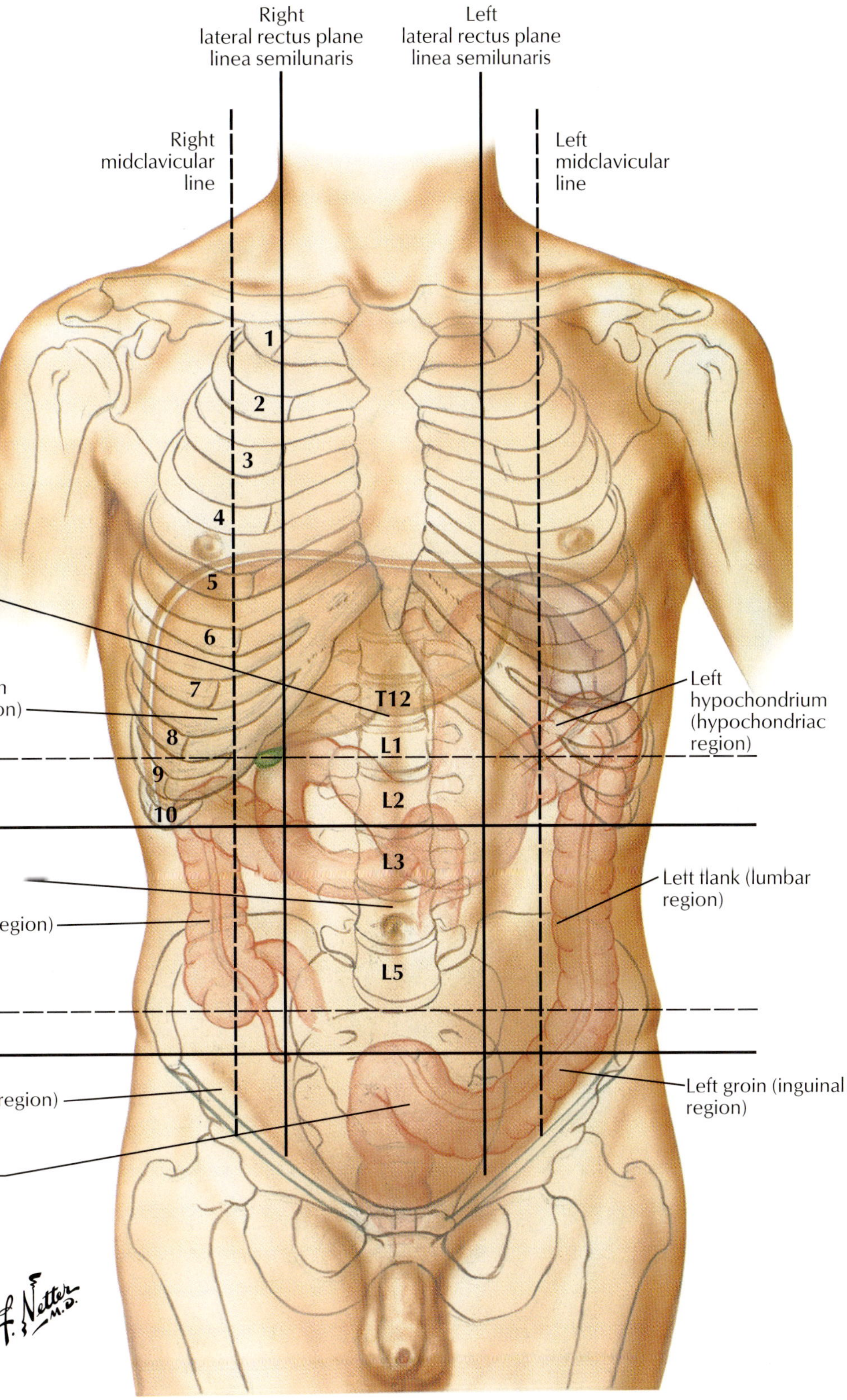

See also Plates 252, 329

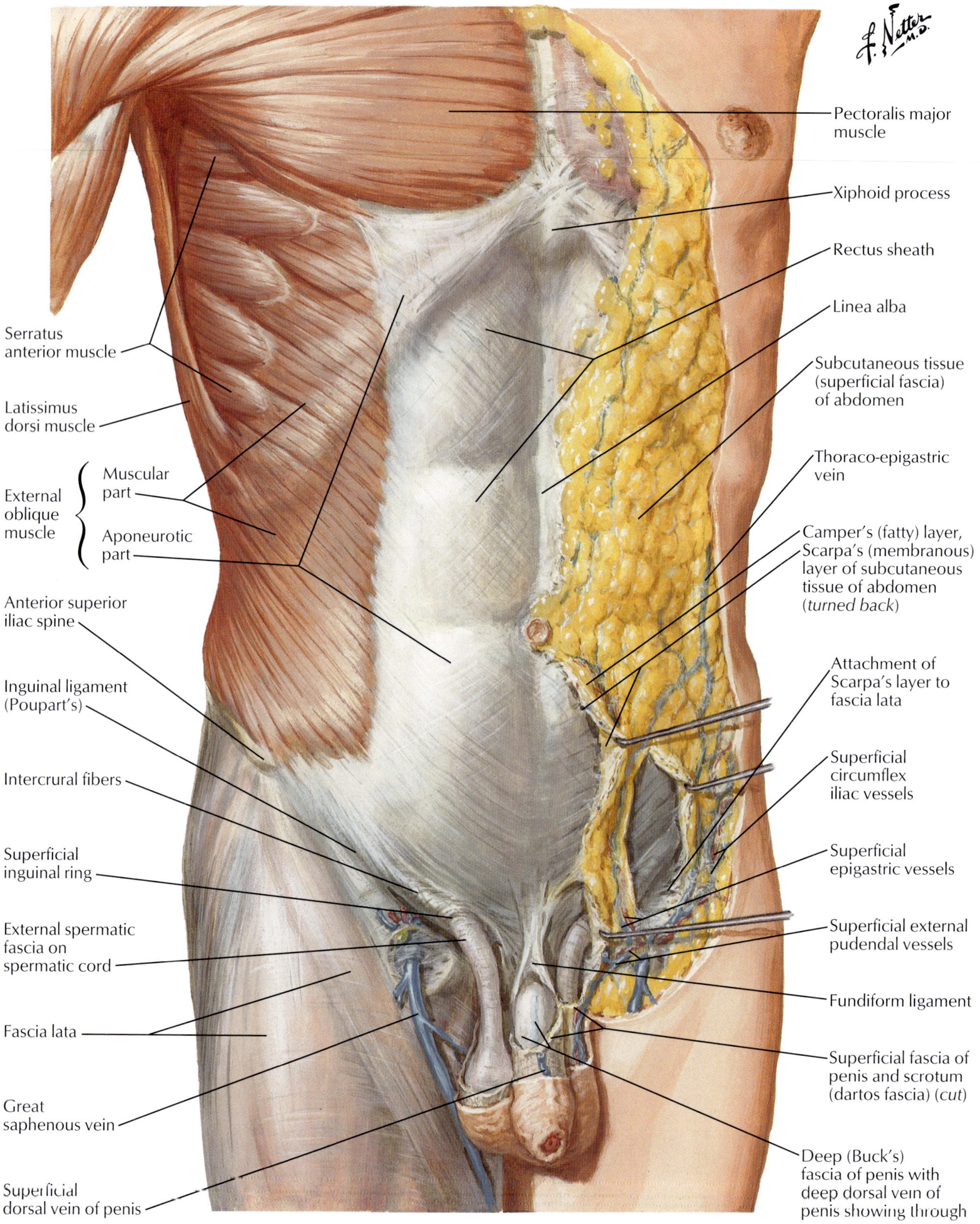

Anterior Abdominal Wall: Intermediate Dissection

See also Plates 185, 186

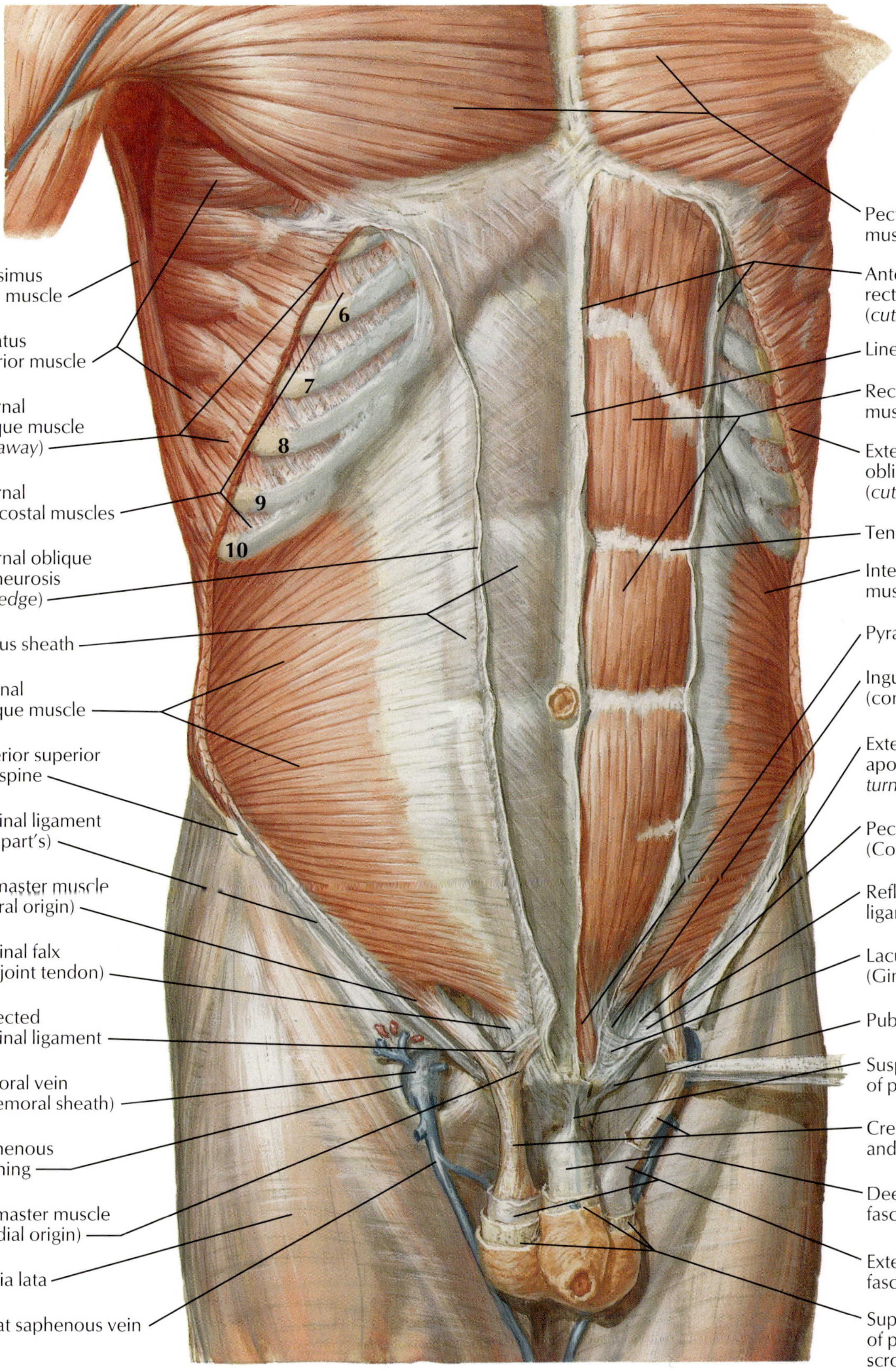

Anterior Abdominal Wall: Deep Dissection

See also Plates 186, 251

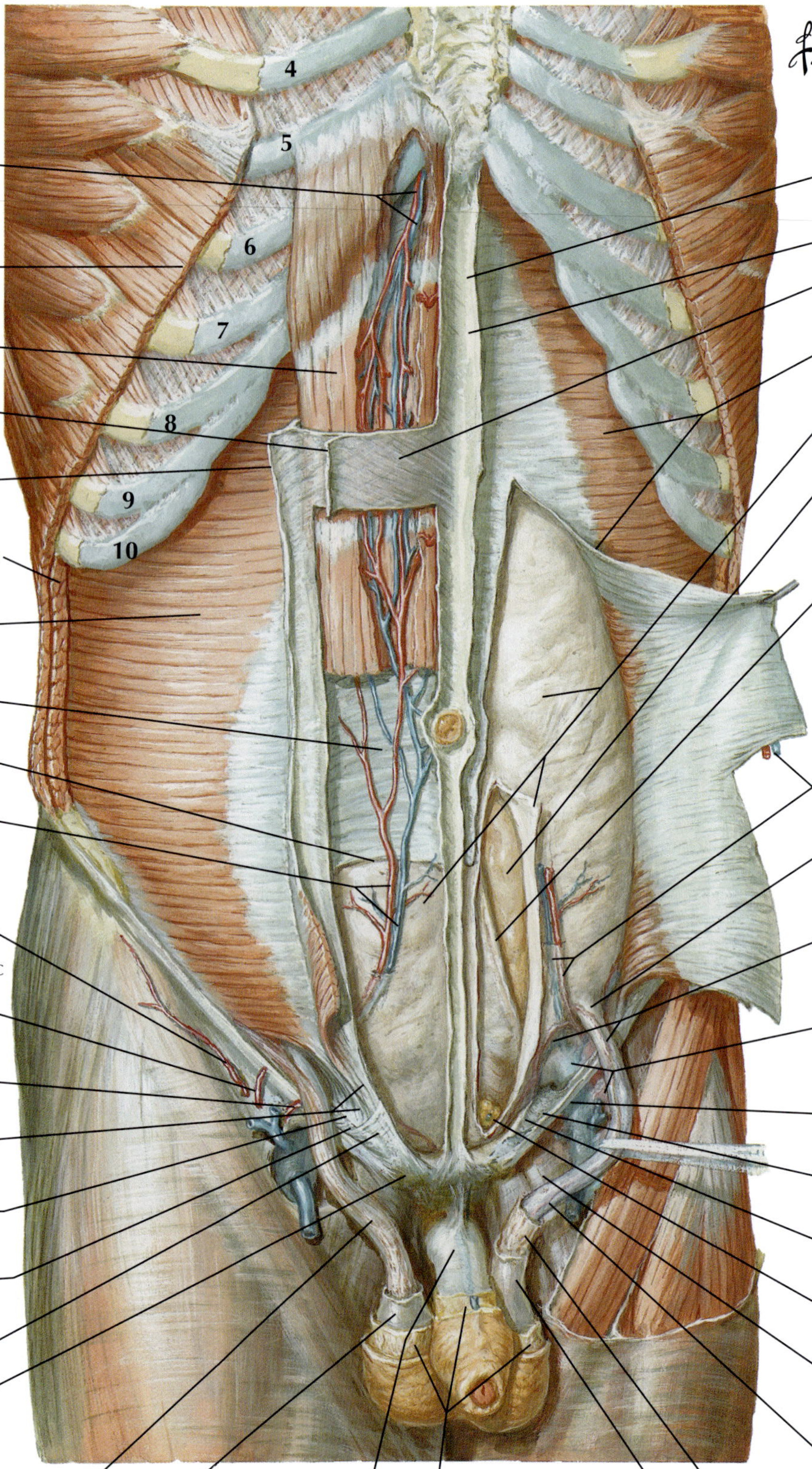

Section above arcuate line

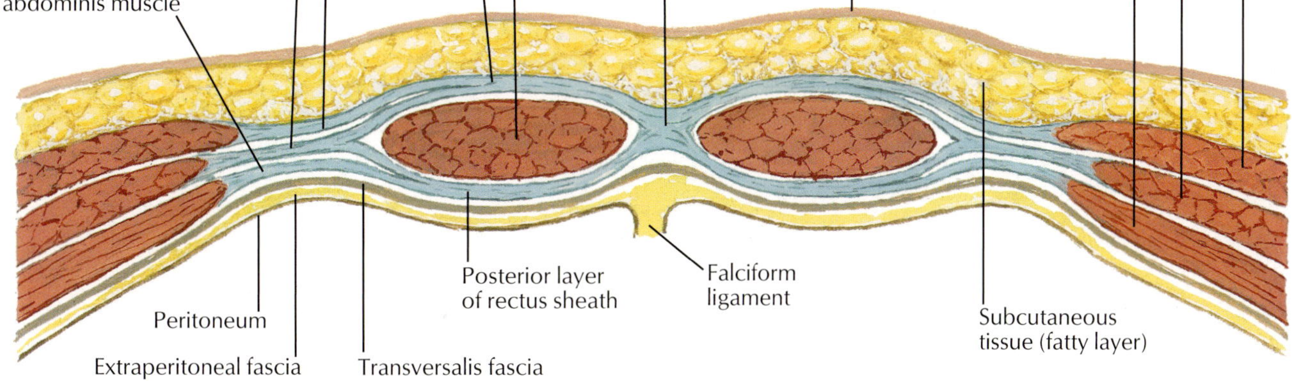

Aponeurosis of internal oblique muscle splits to form anterior and posterior layers of rectus sheath. Aponeurosis of external oblique muscle joins anterior layer of sheath; aponeurosis of transversus abdominis muscle joins posterior layer. Anterior and posterior layers of rectus sheath unite medially to form linea alba.

Section below arcuate line

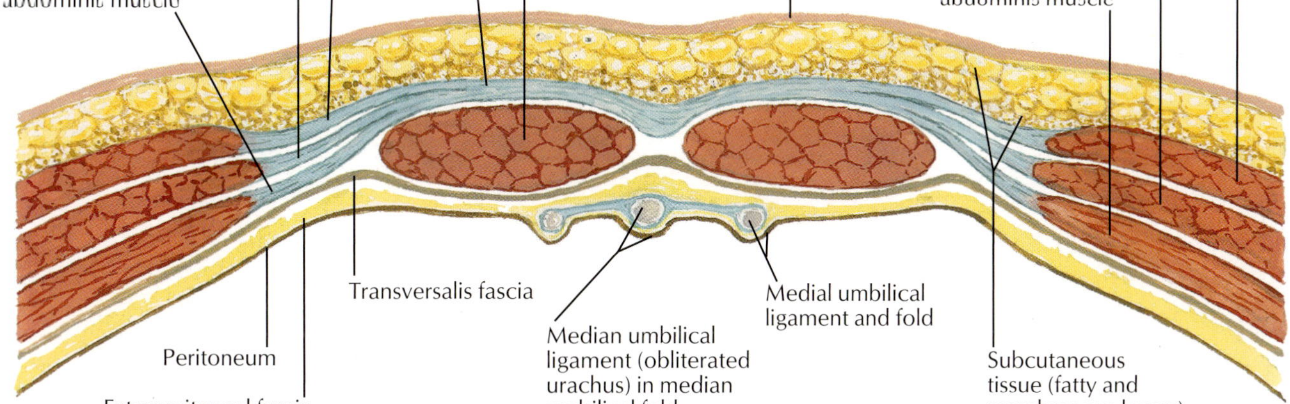

Aponeurosis of internal oblique muscle does not split at this level but passes completely anterior to rectus abdominis muscle and is fused there with both aponeurosis of external oblique muscle and that of transversus abdominis muscle. Thus, posterior wall of rectus sheath is absent below arcuate line, leaving only transversalis fascia.

See also Plates 362, 381

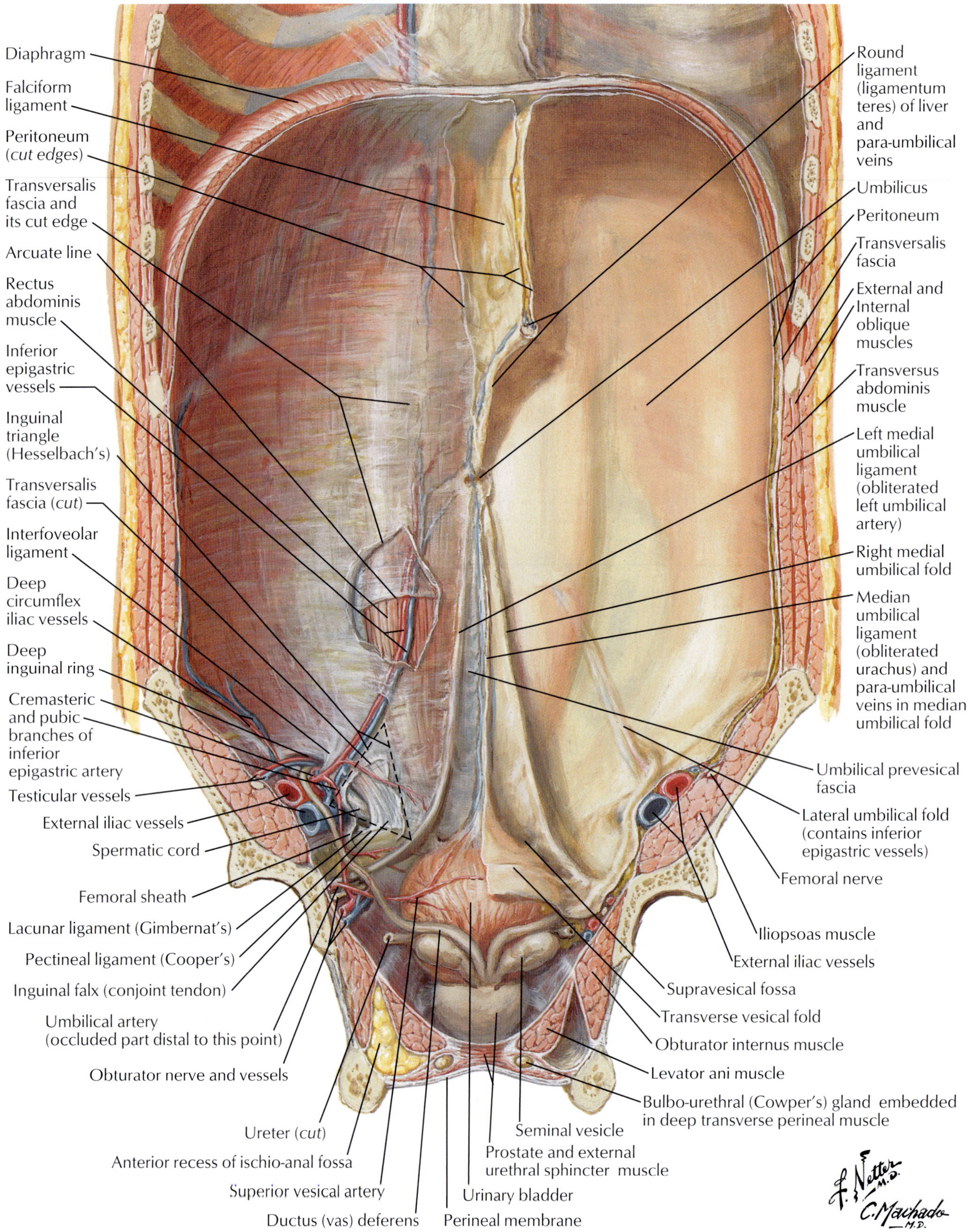

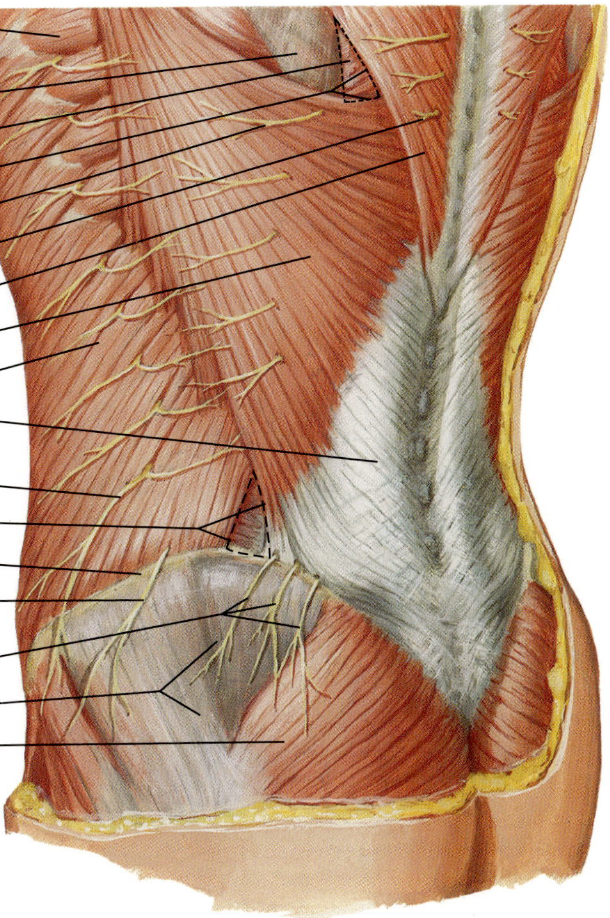
Serratus anterior muscle
Infraspinous fascia
Rhomboid major muscle
Auscultatory triangle
Lateral cutaneous branch of dorsal ramus of T7 spinal nerve
Medial cutaneous branch of dorsal ramus of T7 spinal nerve
Trapezius muscle
Latissimus dorsi muscle
External oblique muscle
Thoracolumbar fascia (posterior layer)
Lateral cutaneous branch of subcostal nerve (anterior ramus of T12)
Lumbar triangle (of Petit)
Iliac crest
Lateral cutaneous branch of iliohypogastric nerve (L1)
Superior clunial nerves (lateral cutaneous branches of posterior rami of L1–L3 spinal nerves)
Gluteal aponeurosis over gluteus medius muscle
Gluteus maximus muscle

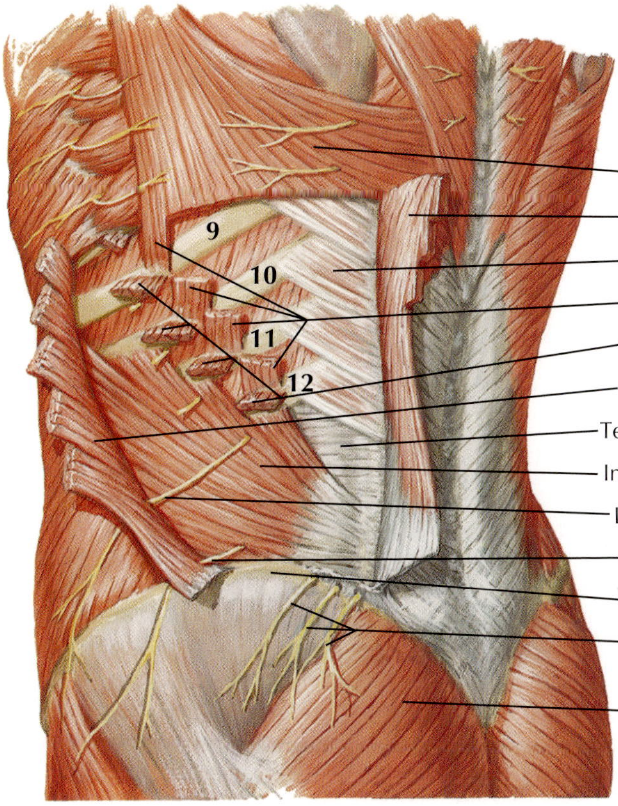
9
10
11
12
Latissimus dorsi muscle
Latissimus dorsi muscle (cut and turned back)
Serratus posterior inferior muscle
Digitations of costal origin of latissimus dorsi muscle
Digitations of costal origin of external oblique muscle
External oblique muscle (cut and turned back)
Tendon of origin of transversus abdominis muscle
Internal oblique muscle
Lateral cutaneous branch of subcostal nerve (anterior ramus of T12)
Lateral cutaneous branch of iliohypogastric nerve (L1)
Iliac crest
Superior clunial nerves (lateral cutaneous branches of posterior rami of L1–L3 spinal nerves)
Gluteus maximus muscle
F. Netter M.D.

Arteries of Anterior Abdominal Wall

See also Plate 247

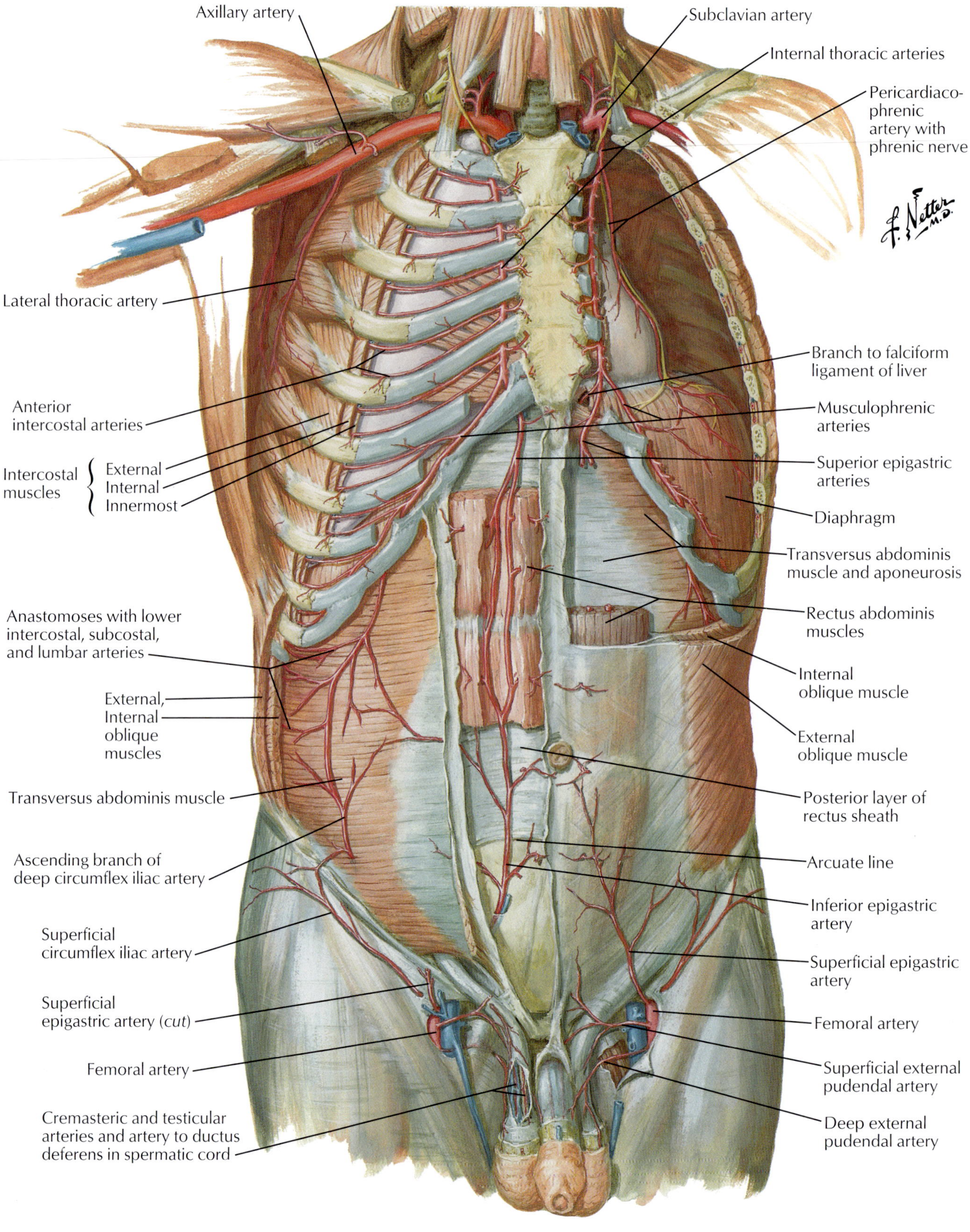

Veins of Anterior Abdominal Wall

See also **Plates 245, 248**

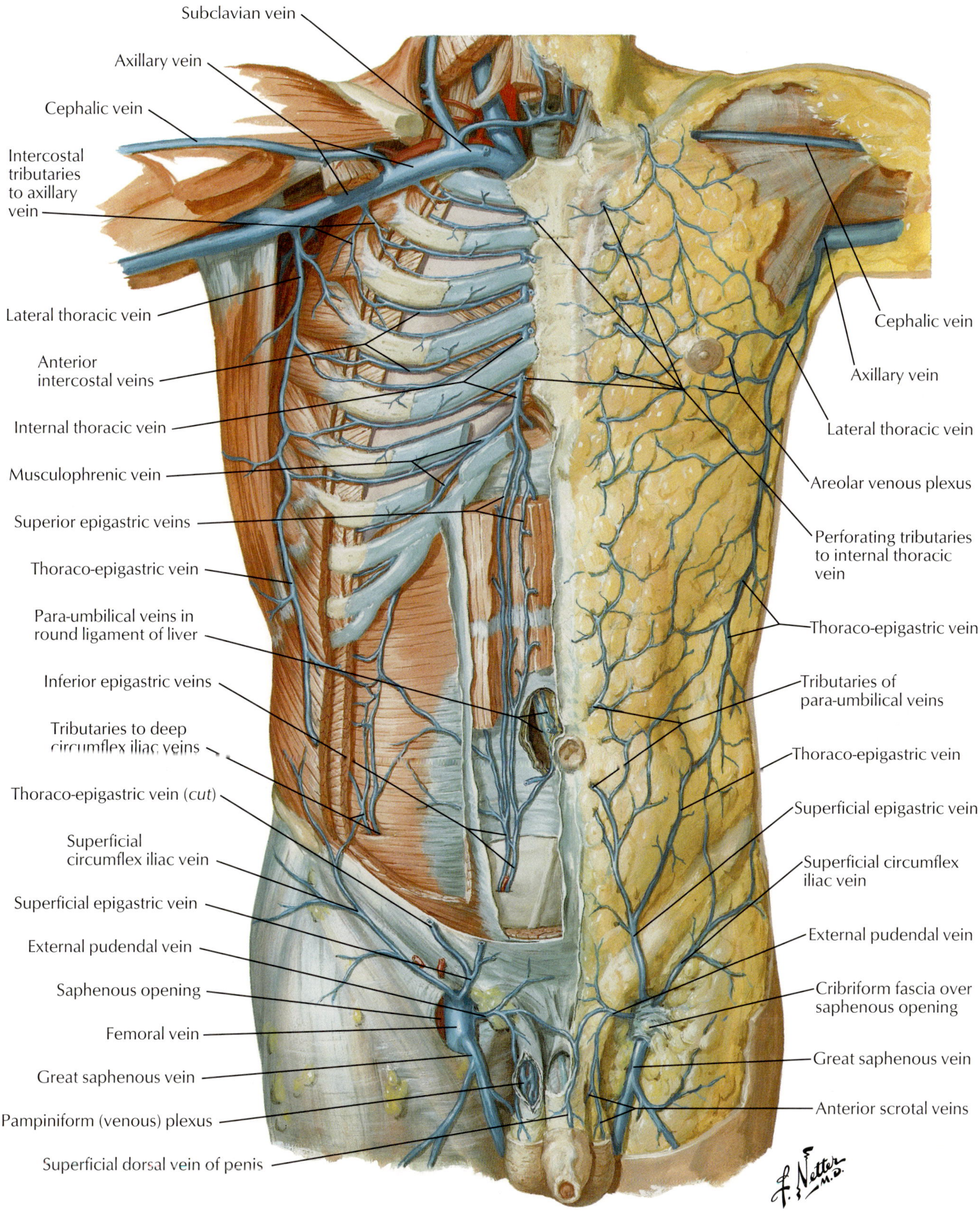

Nerves of Anterior Abdominal Wall

See also **Plates 177, 185, 254**

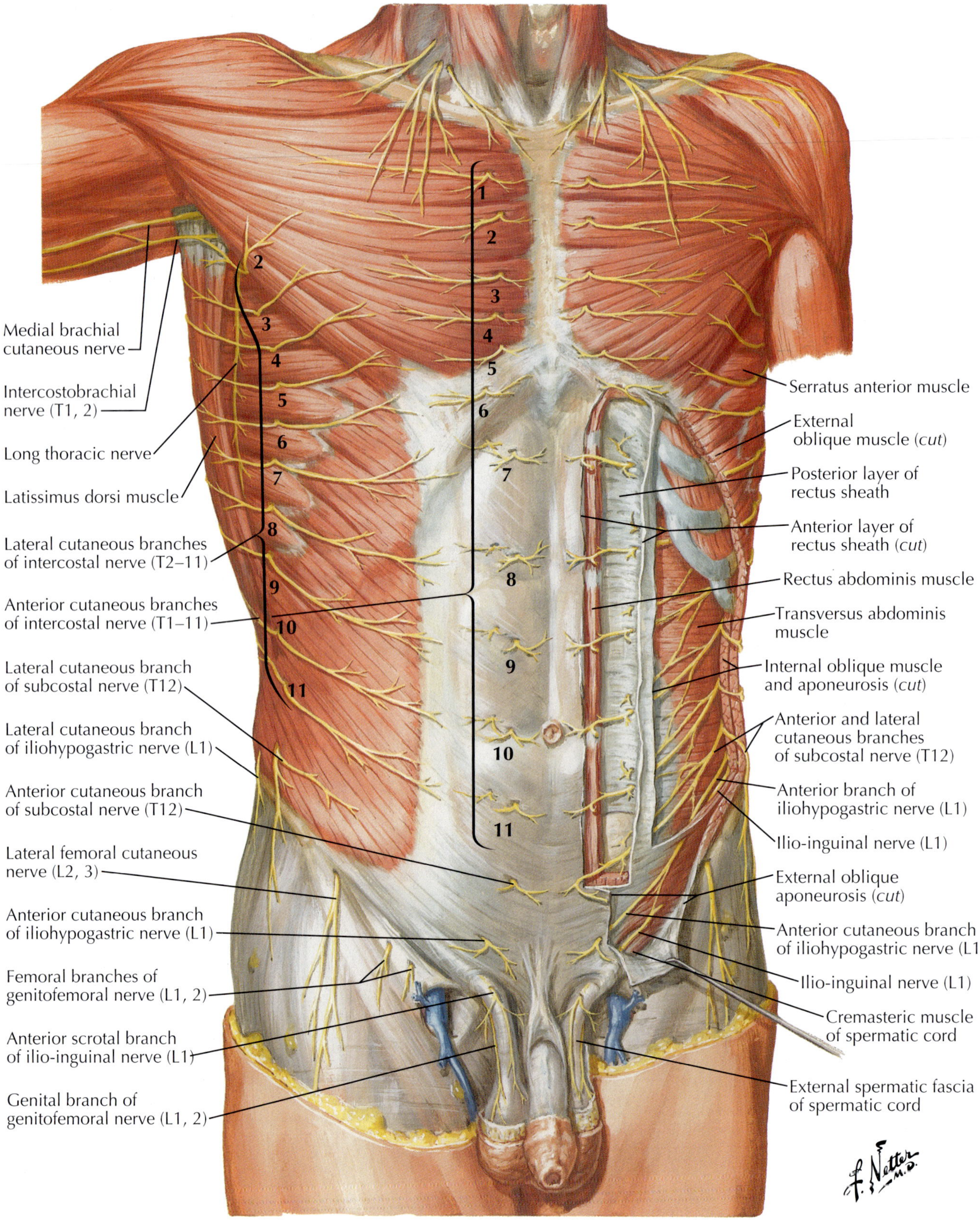

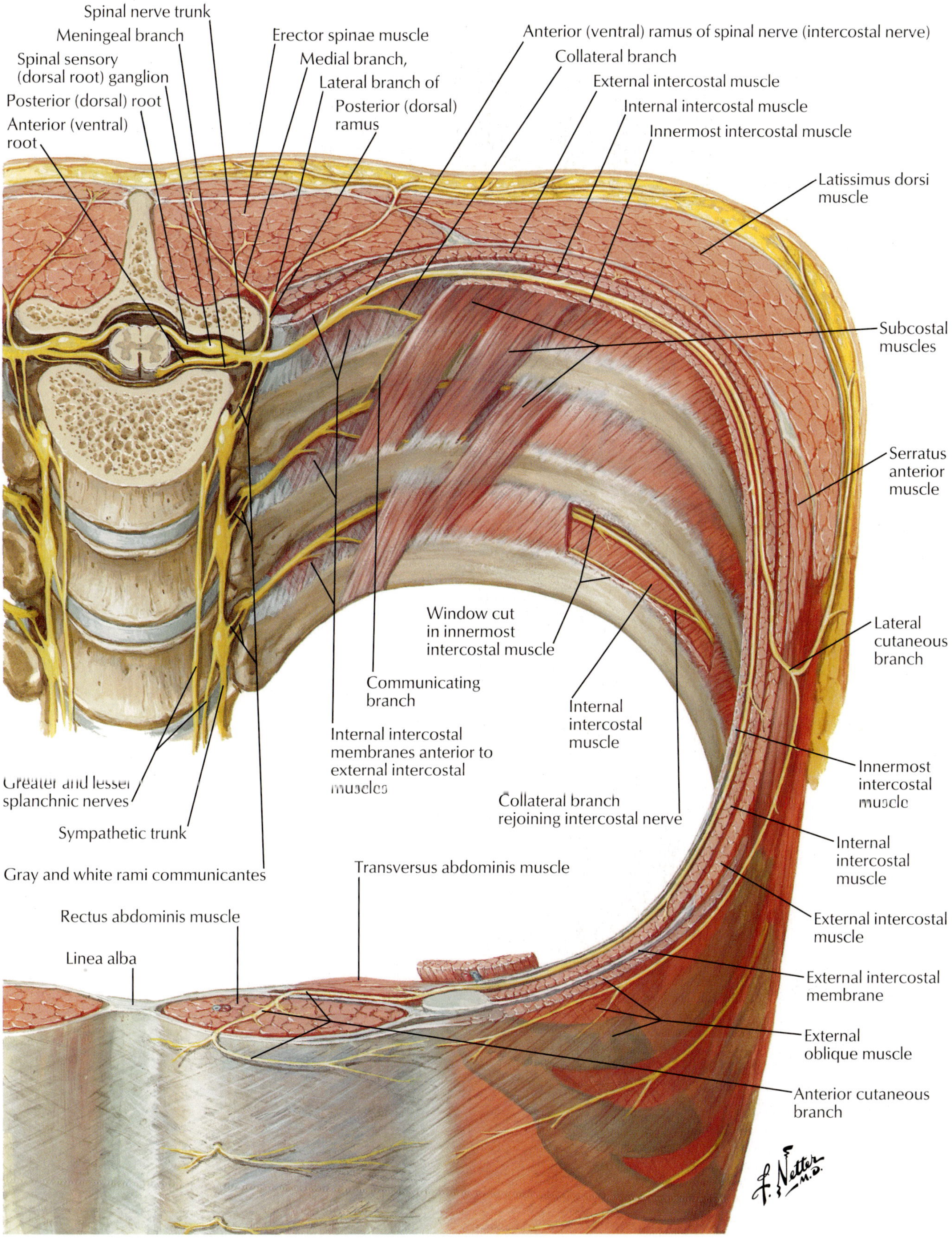
Spinal nerve trunk
Meningeal branch
Spinal sensory (dorsal root) ganglion
Posterior (dorsal) root
Anterior (ventral) root
Erector spinae muscle
Medial branch,
Lateral branch of
Posterior (dorsal) ramus
Anterior (ventral) ramus of spinal nerve (intercostal nerve)
Collateral branch
External intercostal muscle
Internal intercostal muscle
Innermost intercostal muscle
Latissimus dorsi muscle
Subcostal muscles
Serratus anterior muscle
Lateral cutaneous branch
Window cut in innermost intercostal muscle
Communicating branch
Internal intercostal muscle
Internal intercostal membranes anterior to external intercostal muscles
Greater and lesser splanchnic nerves
Sympathetic trunk
Collateral branch rejoining intercostal nerve
Innermost intercostal muscle
Internal intercostal muscle
Gray and white rami communicantes
Transversus abdominis muscle
External intercostal muscle
Rectus abdominis muscle
Linea alba
External intercostal membrane
External oblique muscle
Anterior cutaneous branch

See also Plates 247, 249

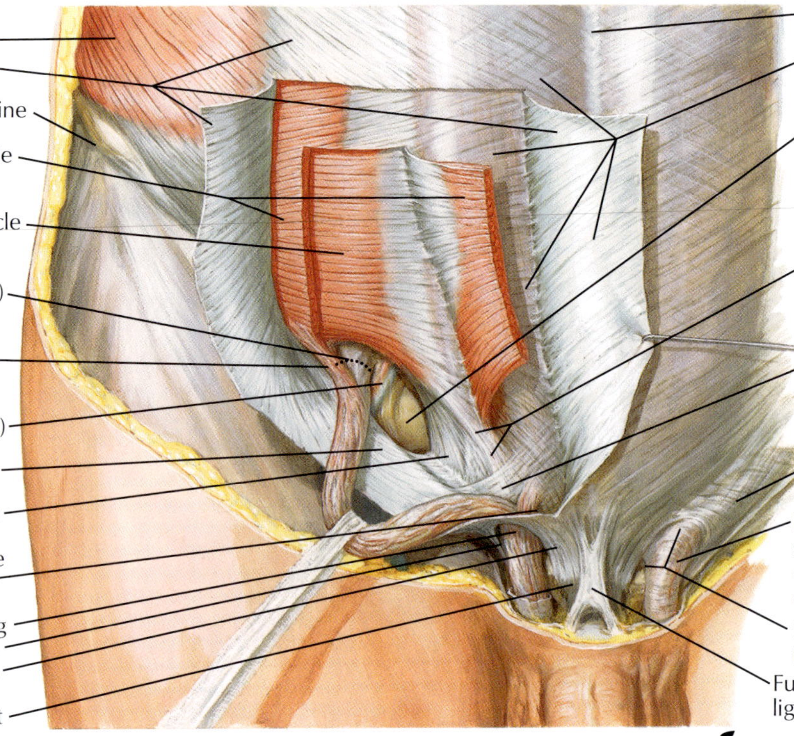

Anterior view

Posterior (internal) view

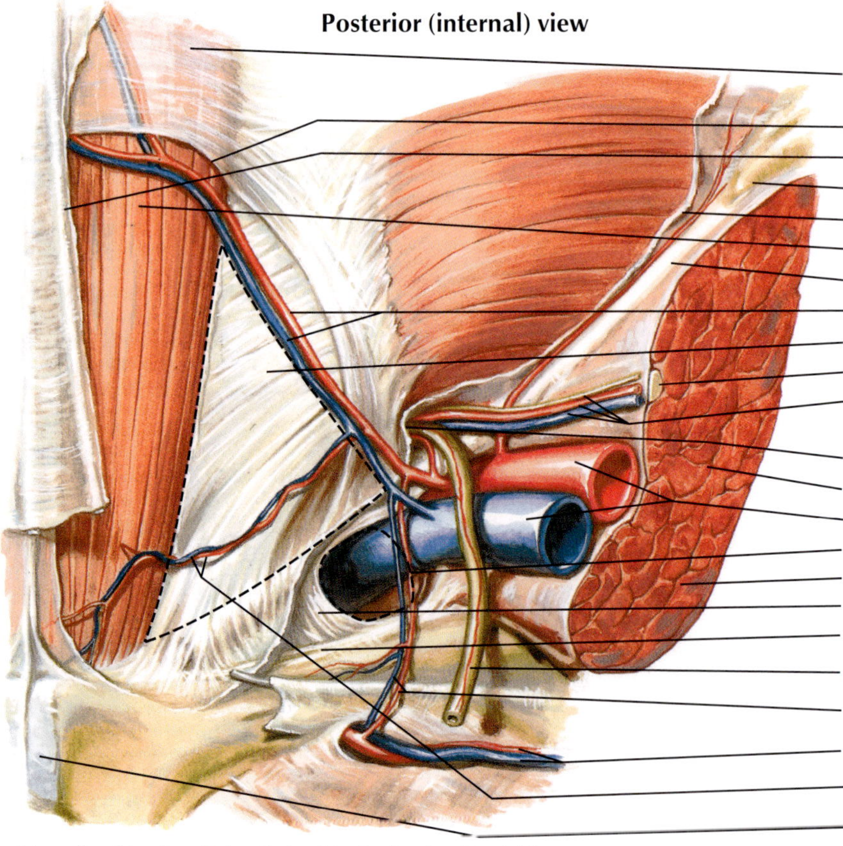

Hesselbach's triangle by Carlos Machado after Frank Netter

Inguinal Canal and Spermatic Cord

See also Plates 245, 253

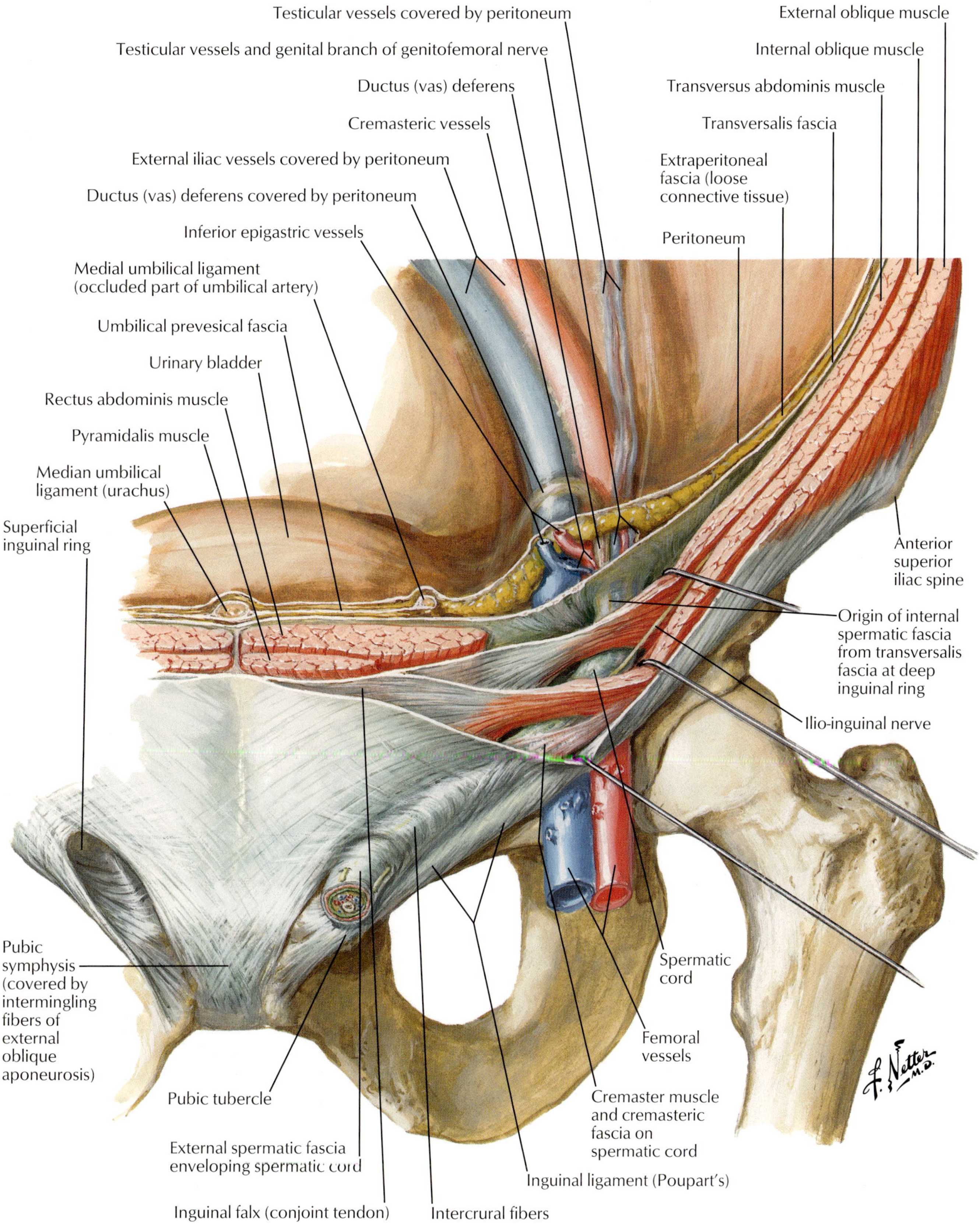

See also **Plates 246, 247, 249**

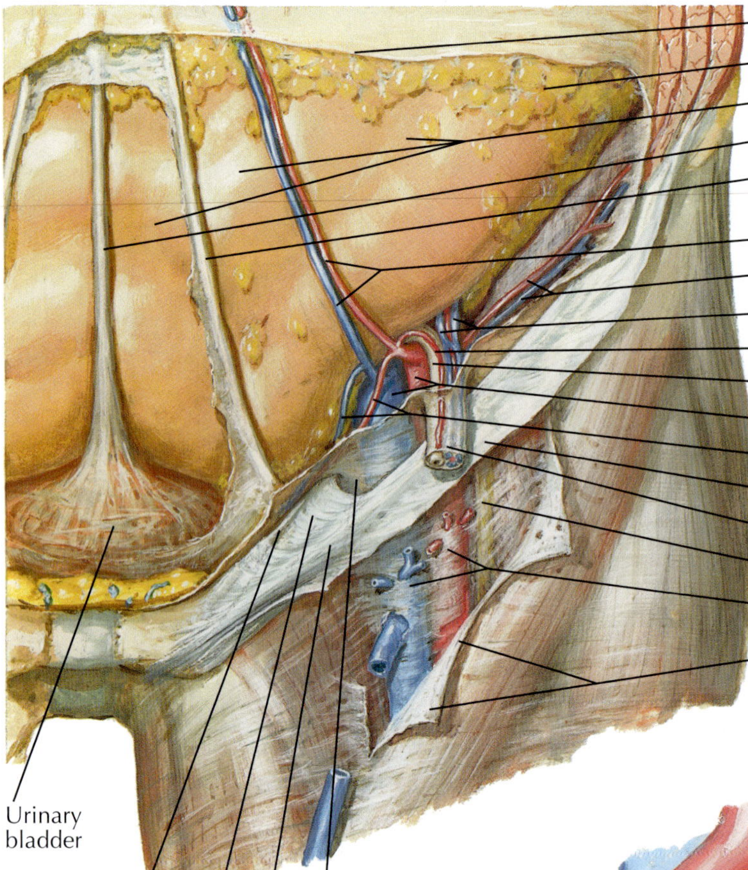

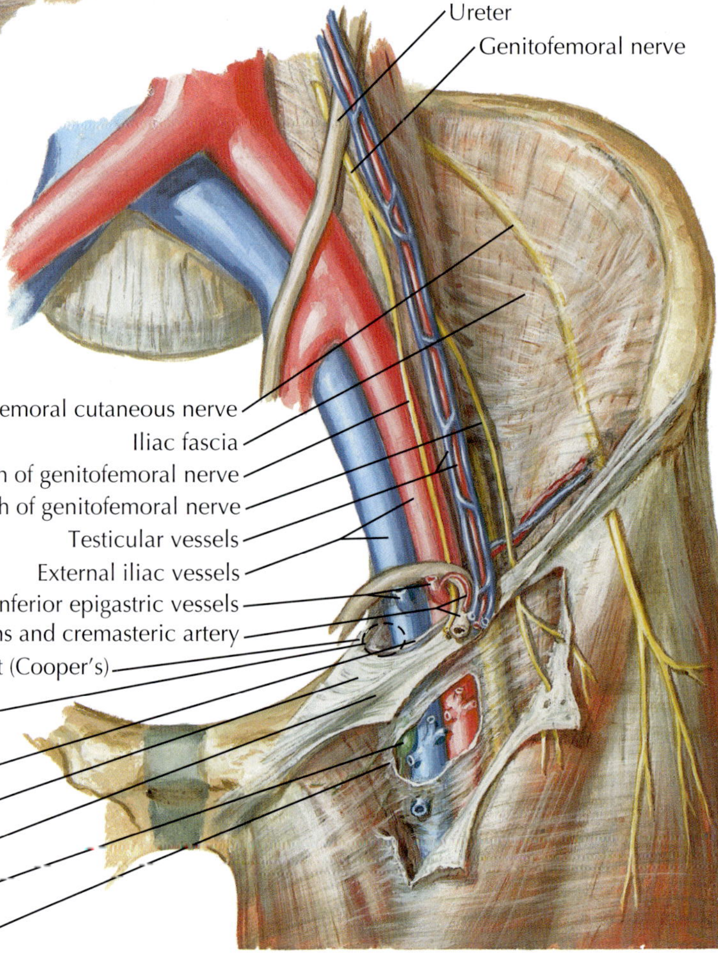

Posterior Abdominal Wall: Internal View

See also Plates 206, 236

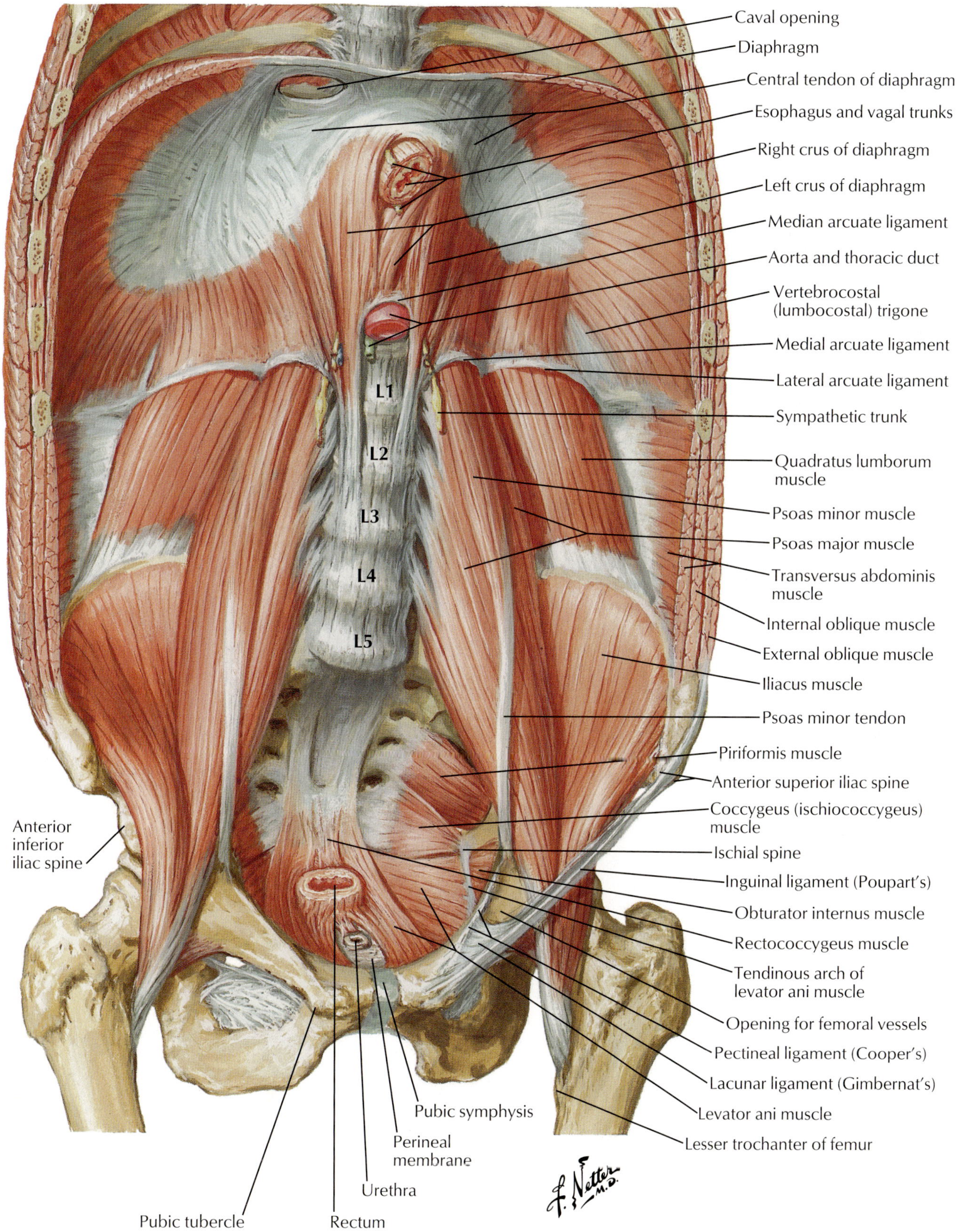

Arteries of Posterior Abdominal Wall

See also Plates 192, 379, 381

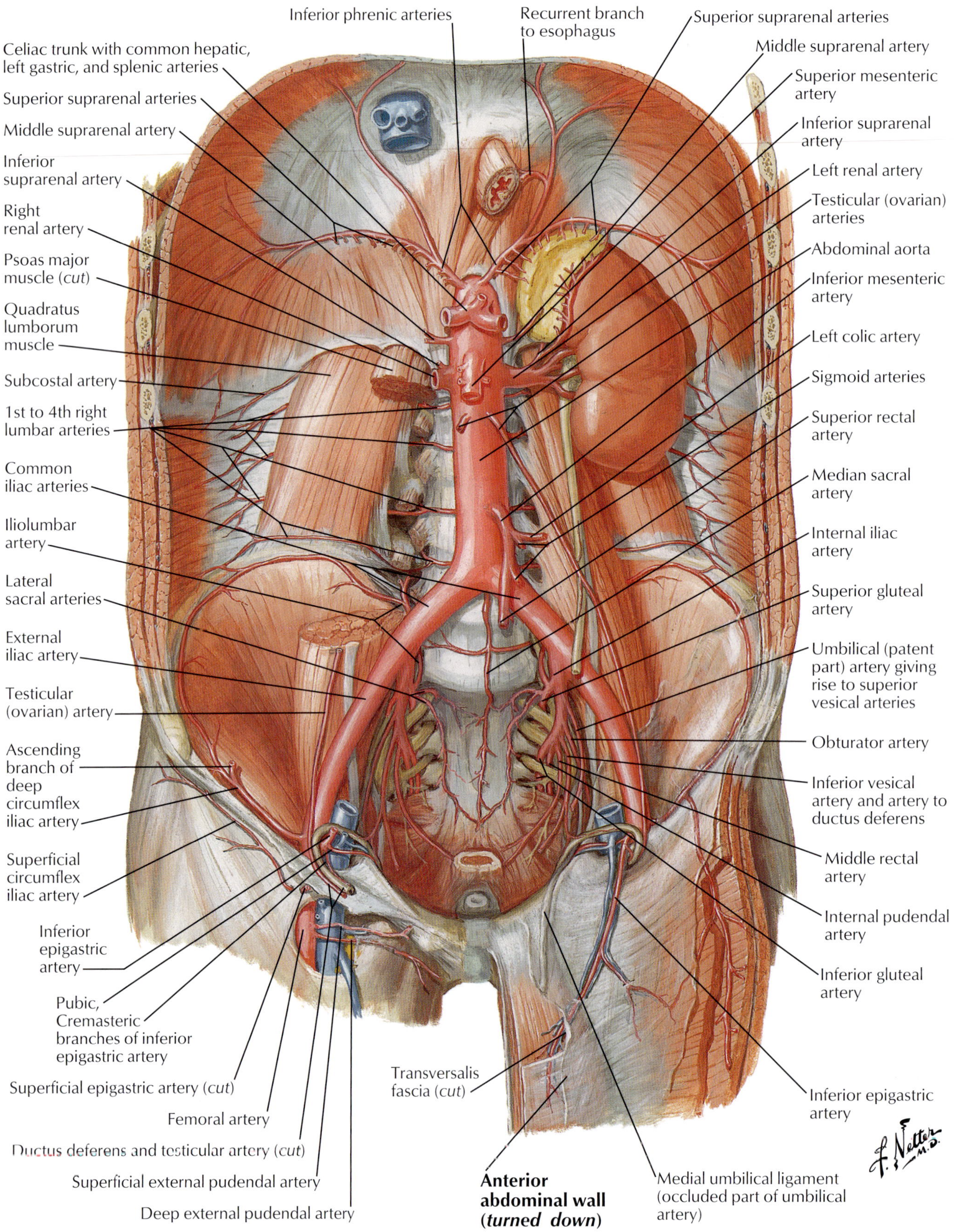

Veins of Posterior Abdominal Wall

See also Plates 379, 381

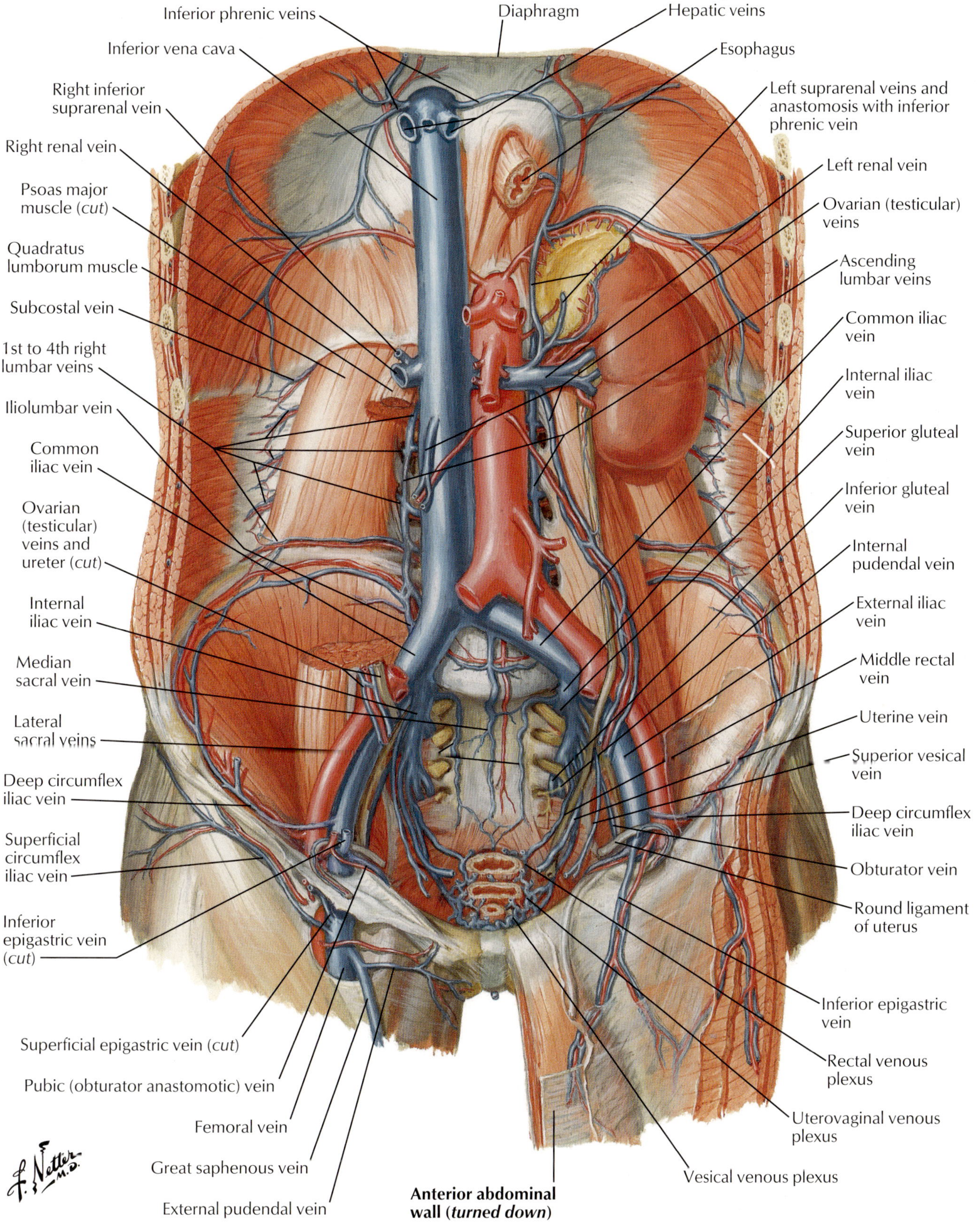

Lymph Vessels and Nodes of Posterior Abdominal Wall

See also Plates 235, 384

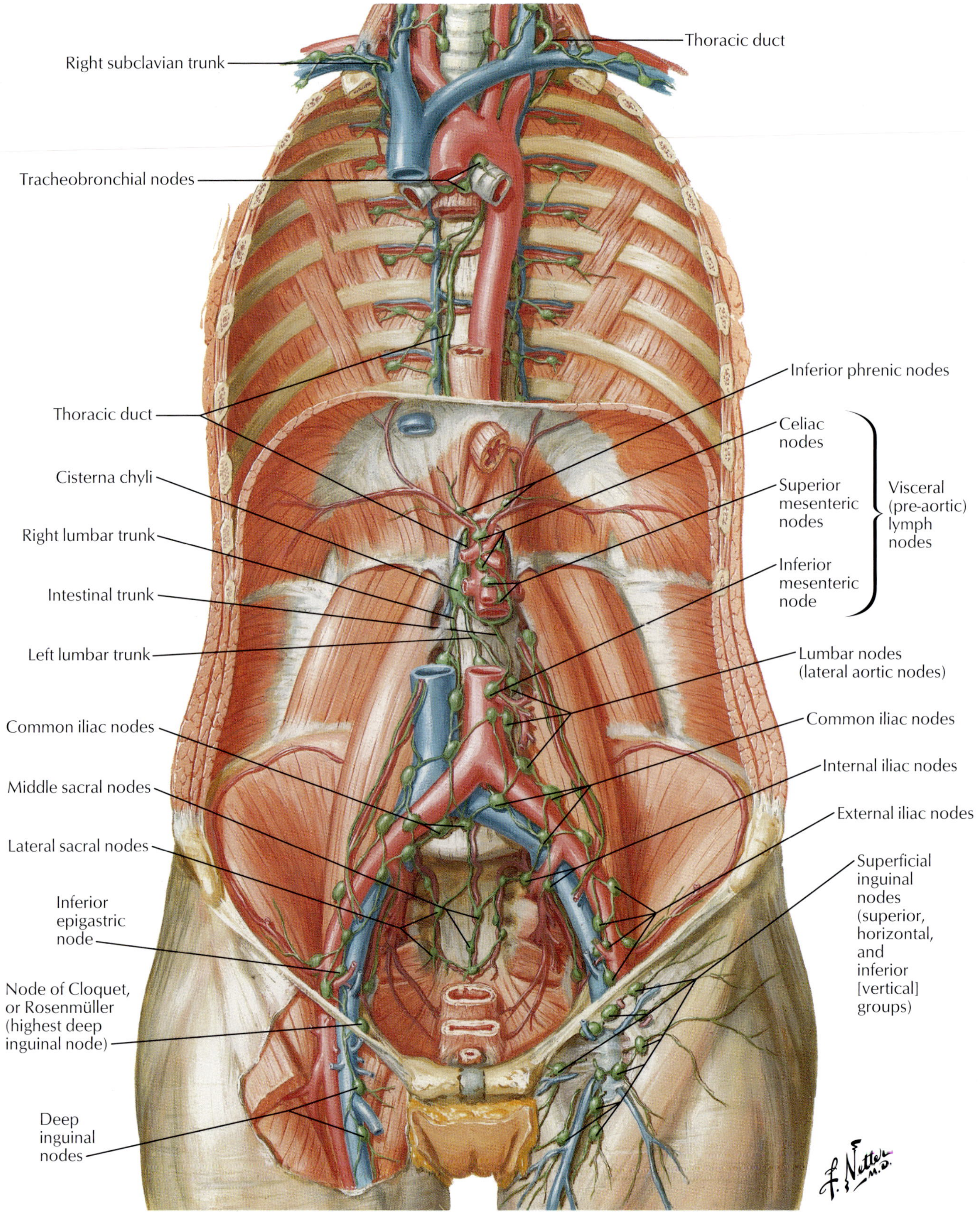

See also Plates 192, 388

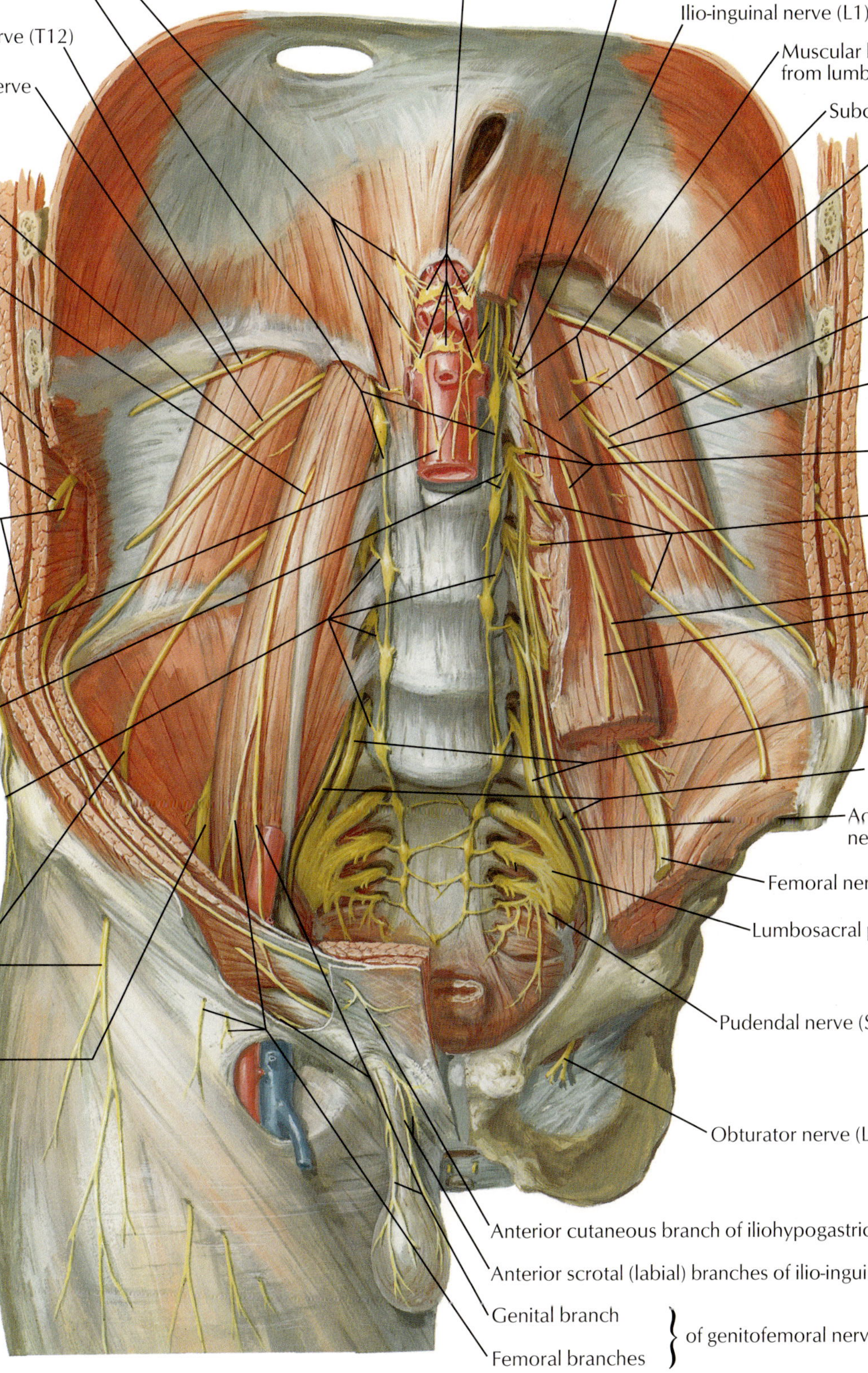

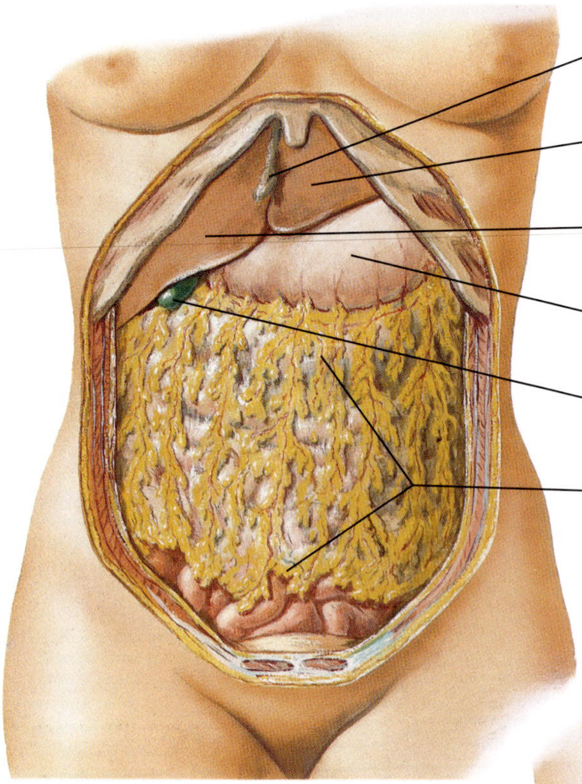

Falciform ligament
Left lobe of liver
Right lobe of liver
Stomach
Gallbladder
Greater omentum overlying transverse colon and small intestine (jejunum and ileum)

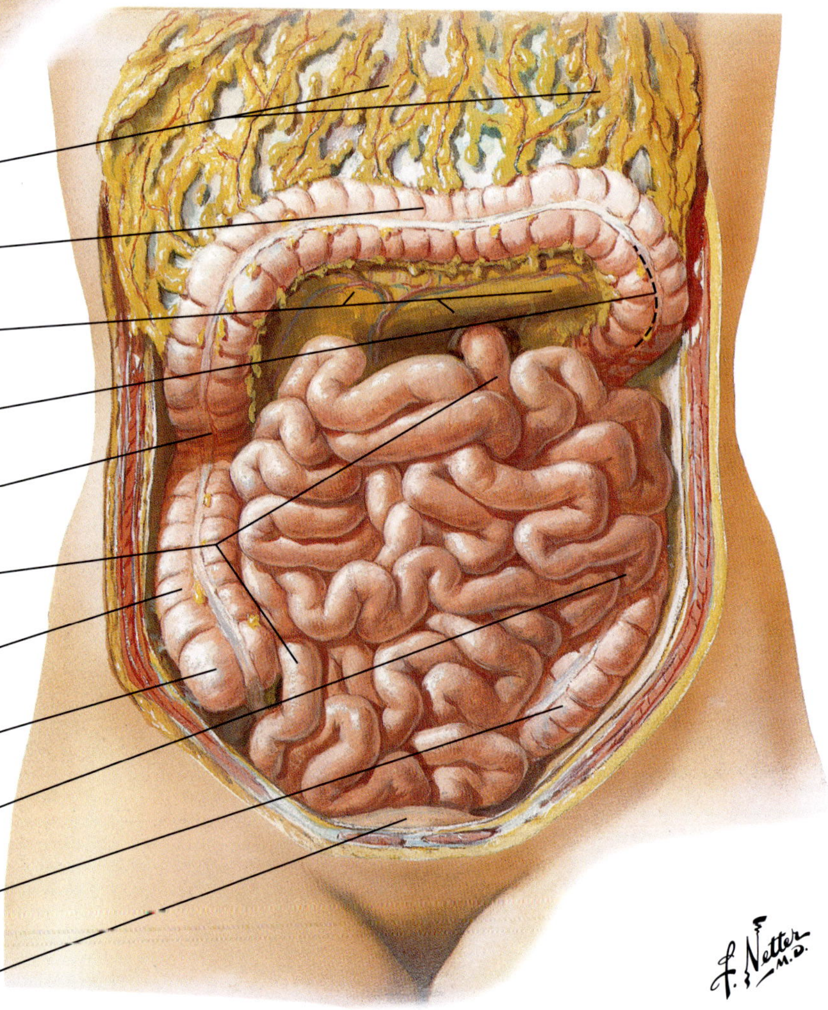

Greater omentum (turned up)
Transverse colon (turned up)
Transverse mesocolon
Left colic (splenic) flexure
Right colic (hepatic) flexure
Small intestine (jejunum and ileum)
Ascending colon
Cecum
Small intestine (covering descending colon)
Sigmoid colon
Urinary bladder

See also Plate 281

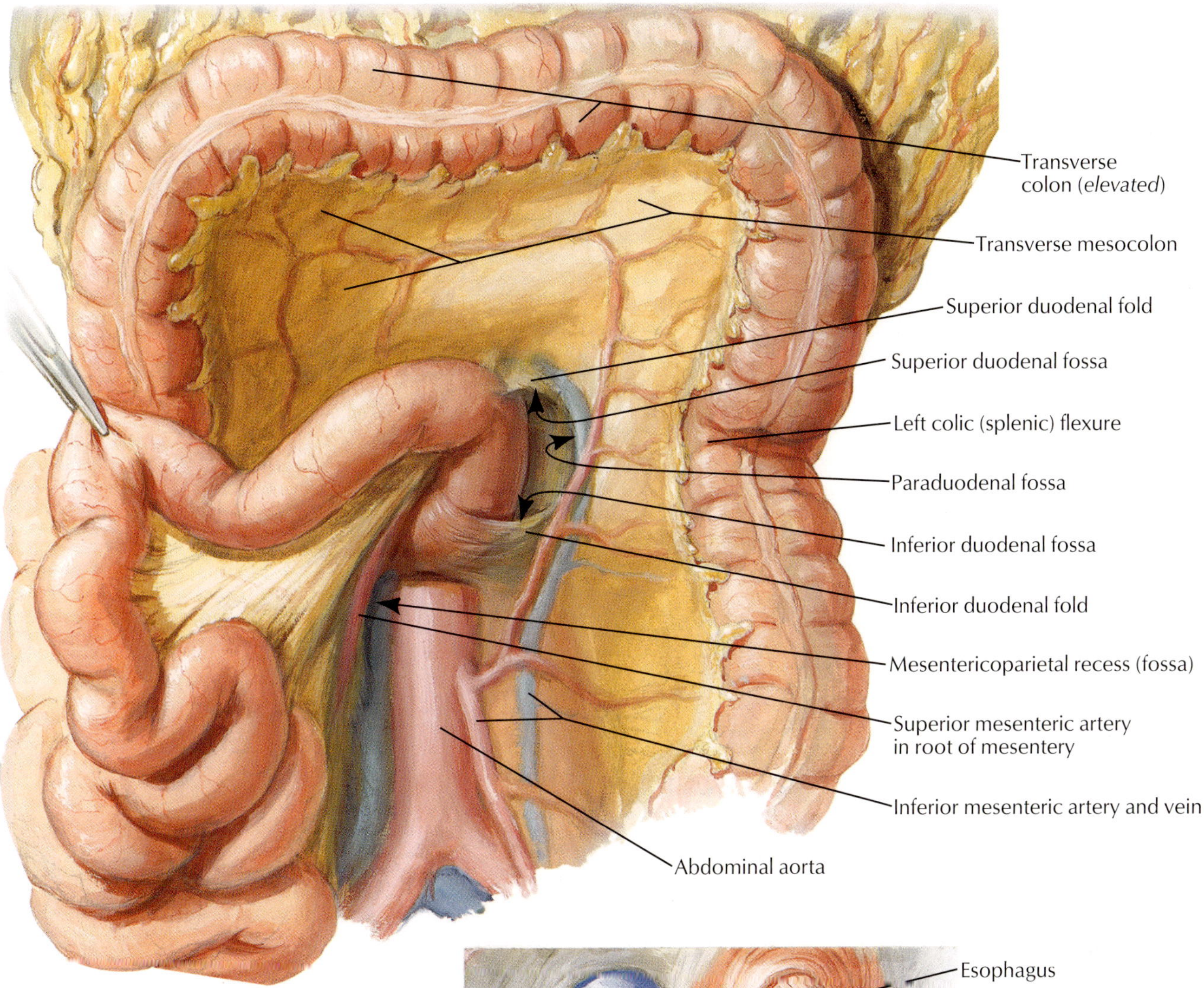

Exposure of suspensory muscle of duodenum (ligament of Treitz)

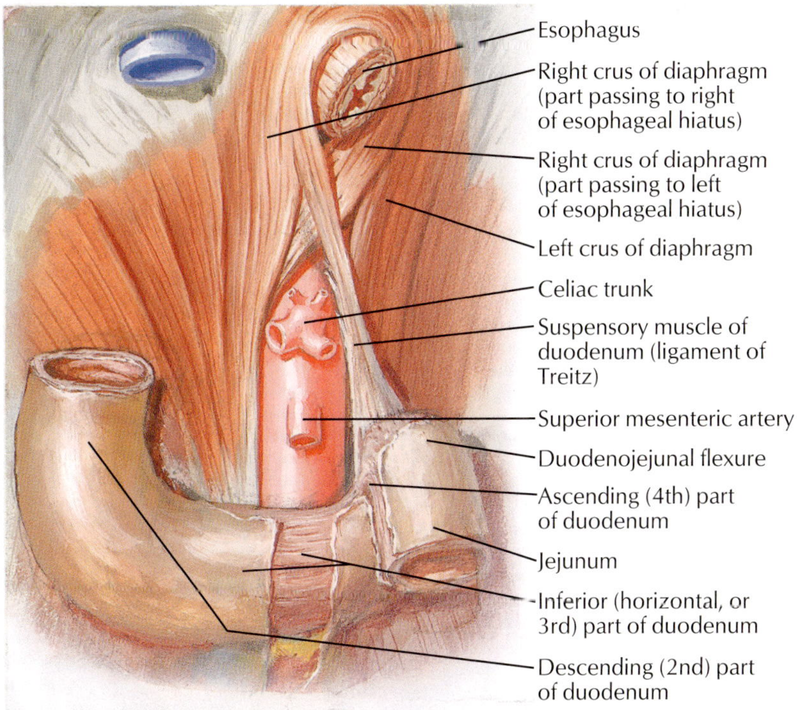

Mesenteric Relations of Intestines (continued)

See also **Plate 288**

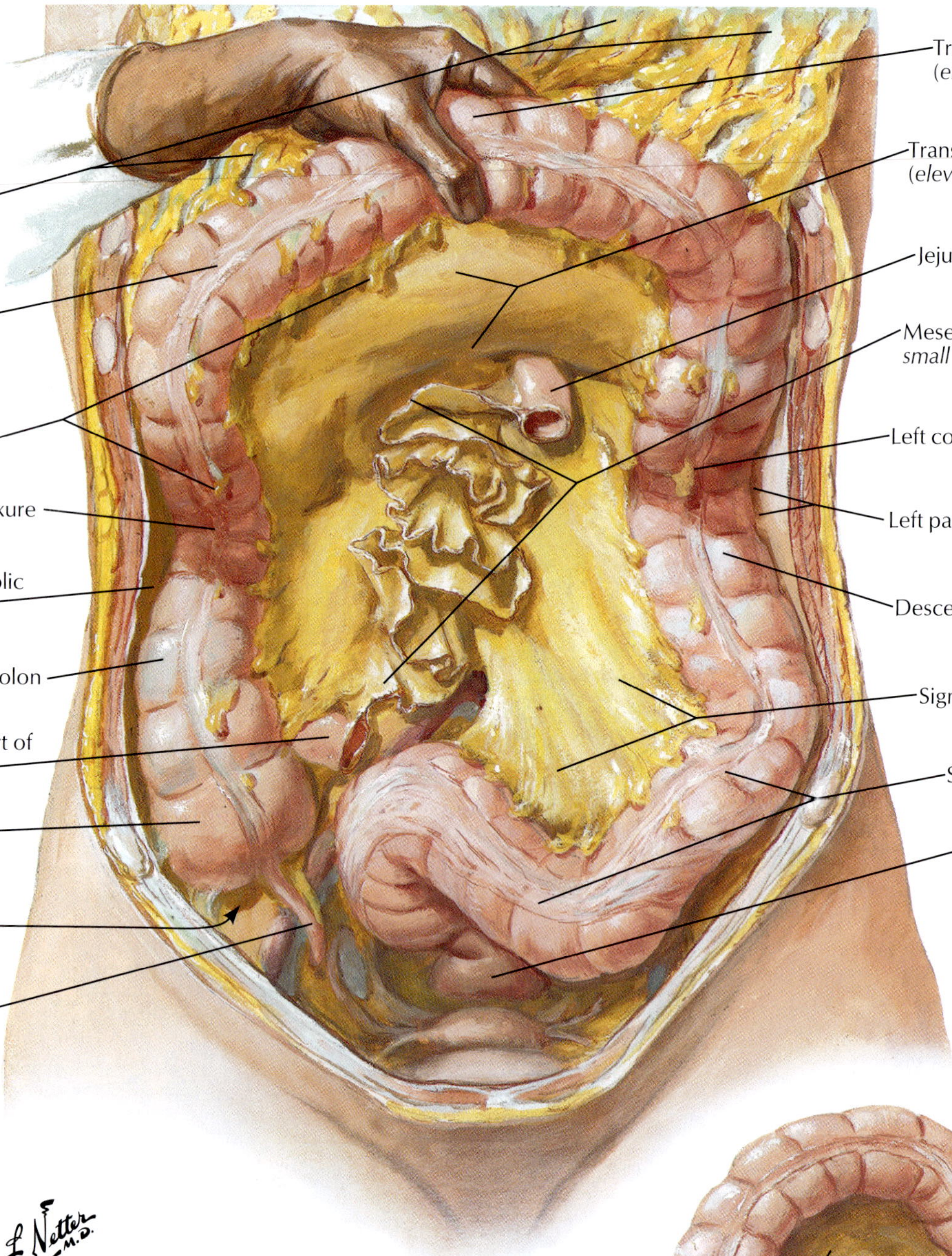

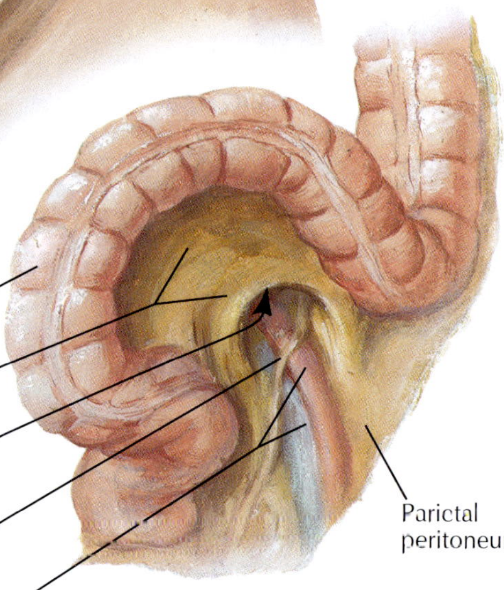

Omental Bursa: Stomach Reflected

See also Plates 281, 284

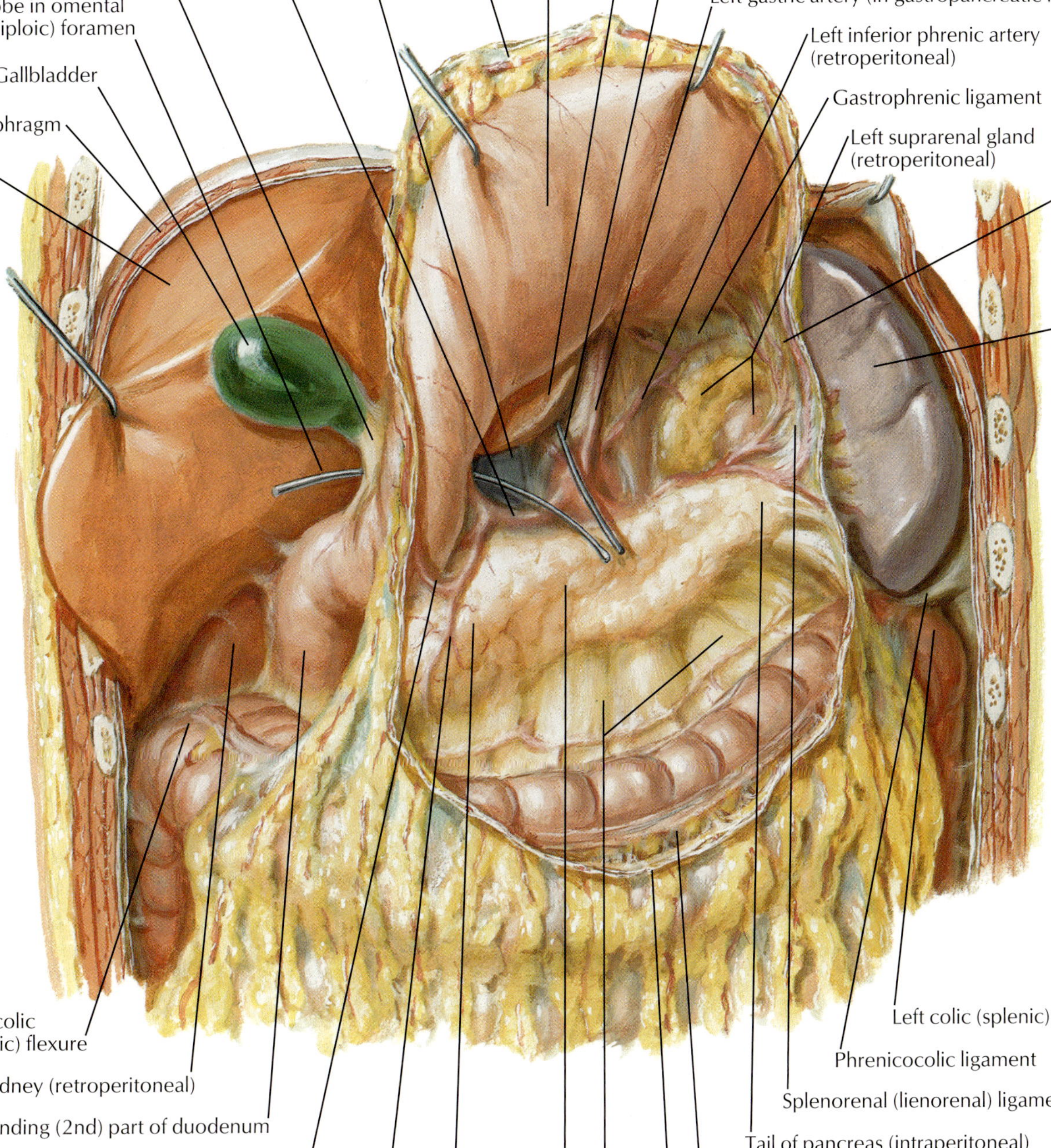

Omental Bursa: Cross Section

See also **Plate 269**

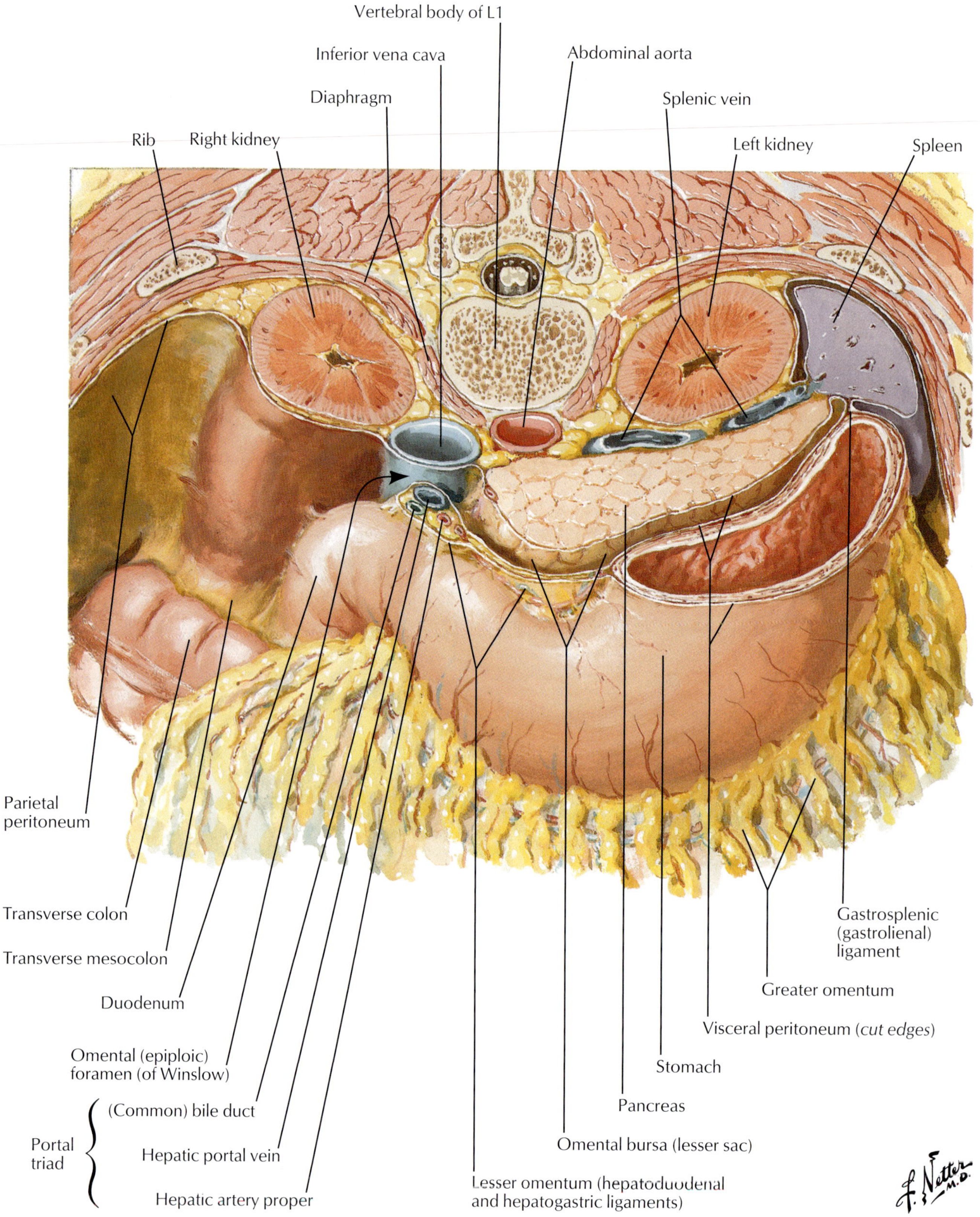

Peritoneum of Posterior Abdominal Wall

See also Plate 271

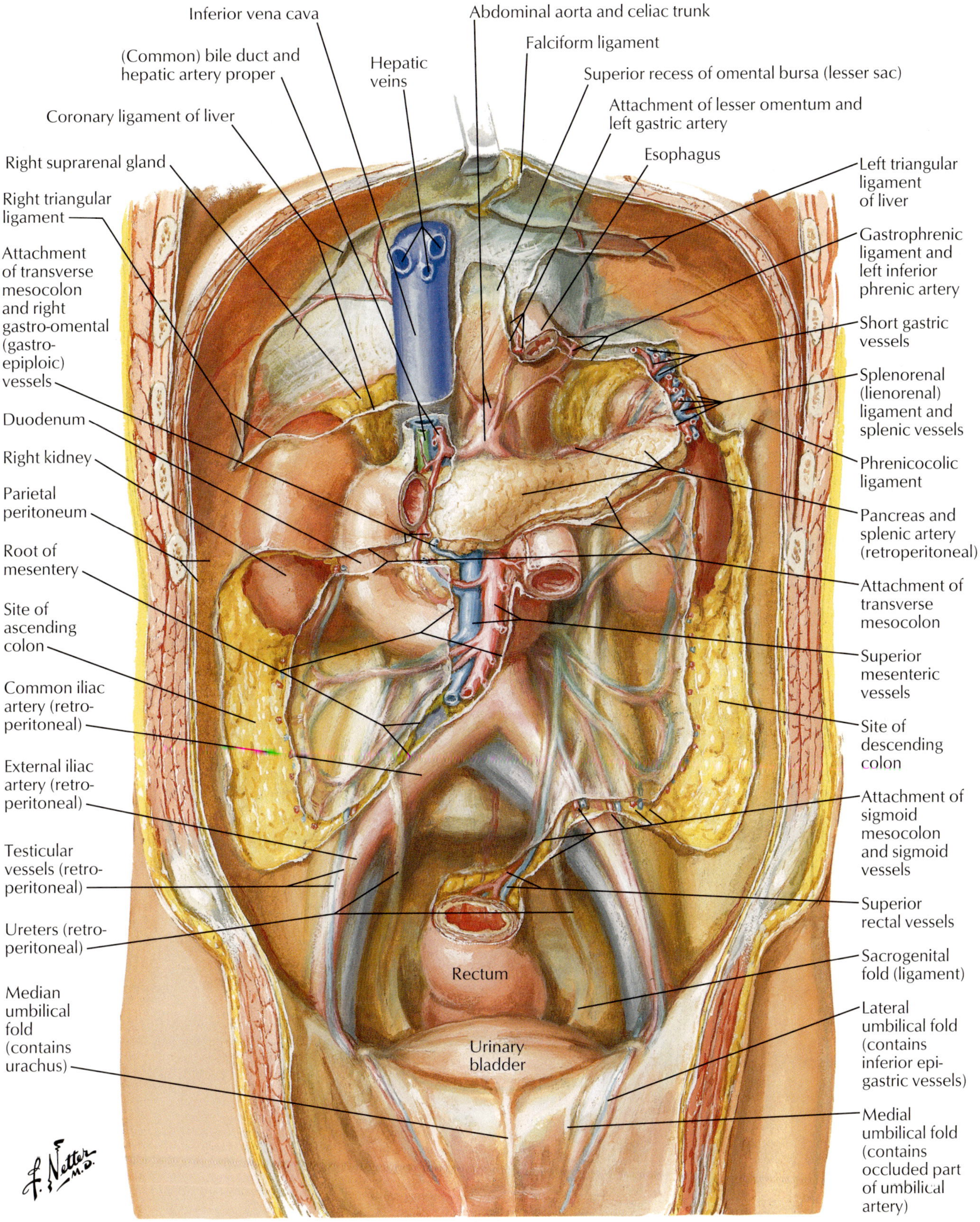

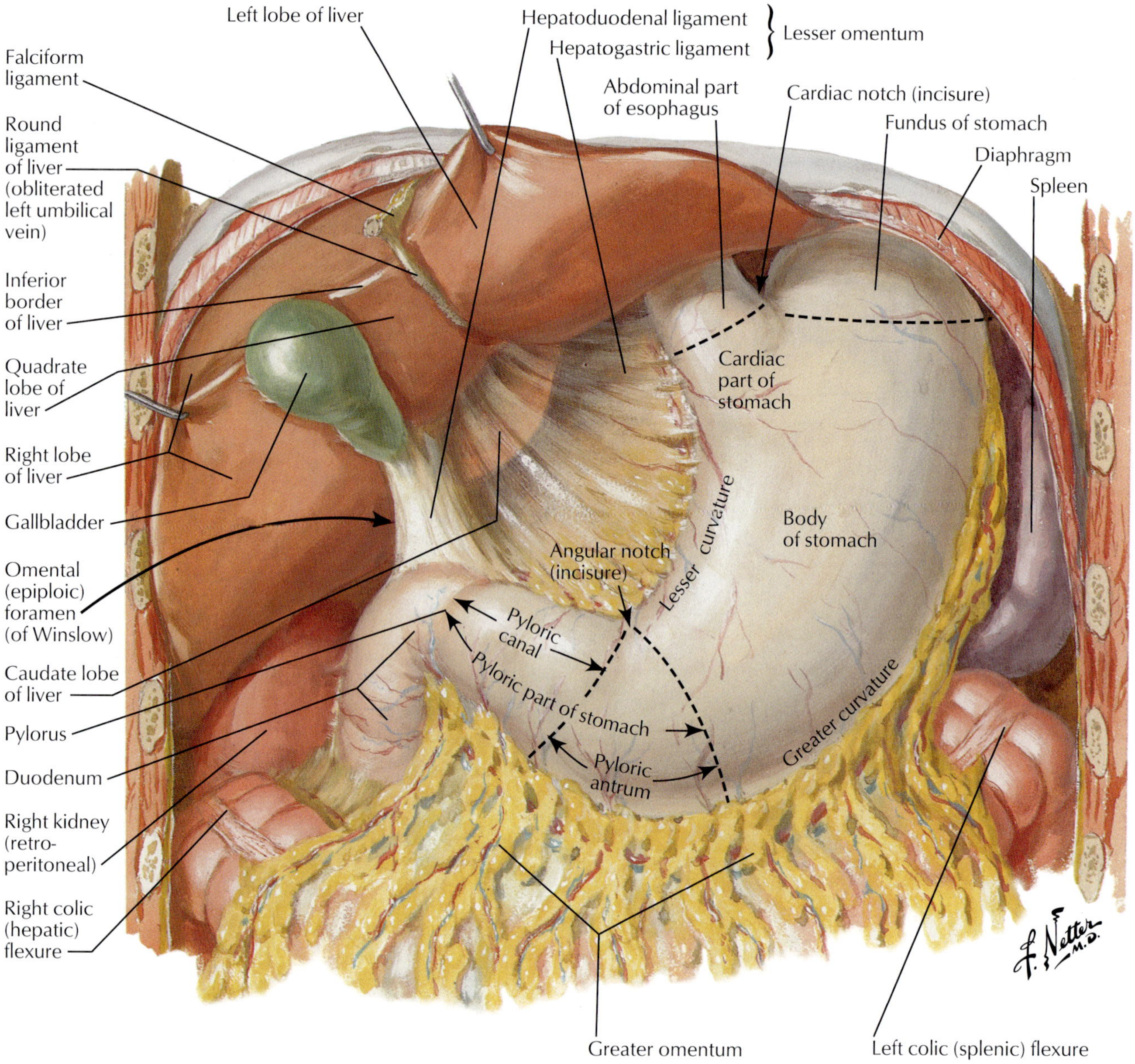

Left lobe of liver
Hepatoduodenal ligament
Hepatogastric ligament
Lesser omentum
Falciform ligament
Abdominal part of esophagus
Cardiac notch (incisure)
Fundus of stomach
Diaphragm
Spleen
Round ligament of liver (obliterated left umbilical vein)
Inferior border of liver
Cardiac part of stomach
Quadrate lobe of liver
Right lobe of liver
Lesser curvature
Gallbladder
Body of stomach
Angular notch (incisure)
Omental (epiploic) foramen (of Winslow)
Pyloric canal
Caudate lobe of liver
Pyloric part of stomach
Greater curvature
Pylorus
Duodenum
Pyloric antrum
Right kidney (retro-peritoneal)
Right colic (hepatic) flexure
Greater omentum
Left colic (splenic) flexure

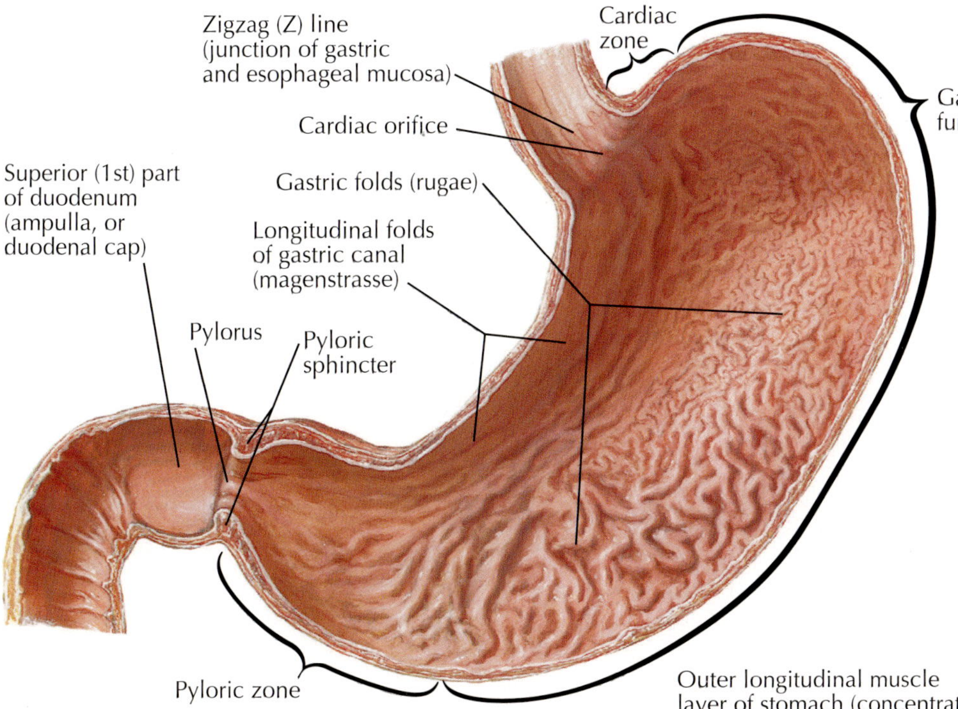
Zigzag (Z) line (junction of gastric and esophageal mucosa)
Cardiac zone
Gastric and fundic zones
Cardiac orifice
Superior (1st) part of duodenum (ampulla, or duodenal cap)
Gastric folds (rugae)
Longitudinal folds of gastric canal (magenstrasse)
Pylorus
Pyloric sphincter
Pyloric zone

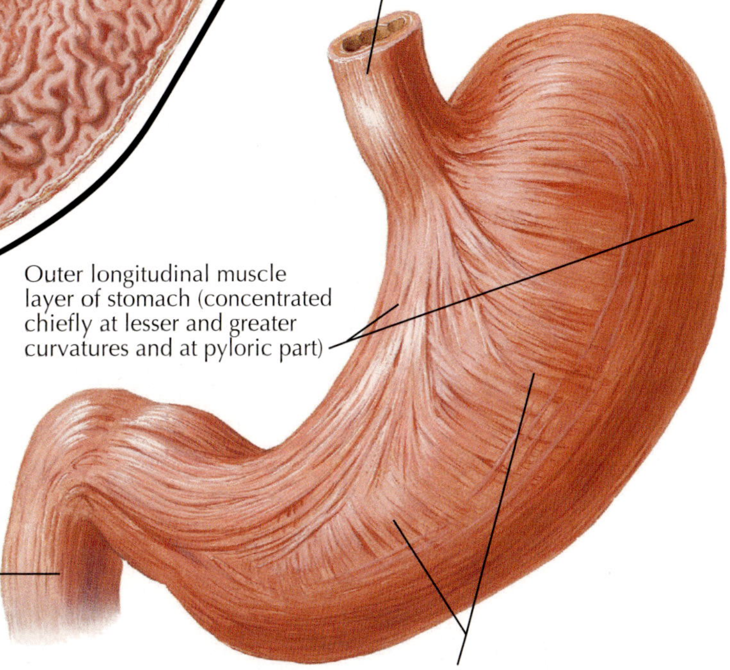
Longitudinal muscle of esophagus
Outer longitudinal muscle layer of stomach (concentrated chiefly at lesser and greater curvatures and at pyloric part)
Longitudinal muscle of duodenum
Middle circular muscle layer of stomach

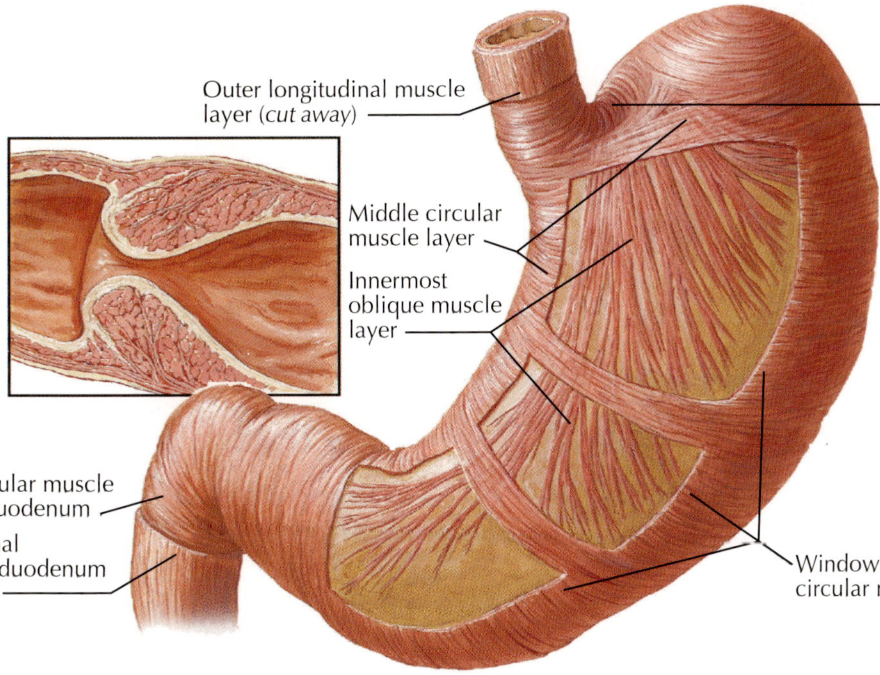
Outer longitudinal muscle layer (cut away)
Middle circular and innermost oblique fibers blend here
Longitudinal section through pyloric region (shows thickened pyloric sphincter)
Middle circular muscle layer
Innermost oblique muscle layer
Circular muscle of duodenum
Longitudinal muscle of duodenum (cut away)
Windows cut in middle circular muscle layer
F. Netter M.D.

Duodenum in Situ

See also Plate 268

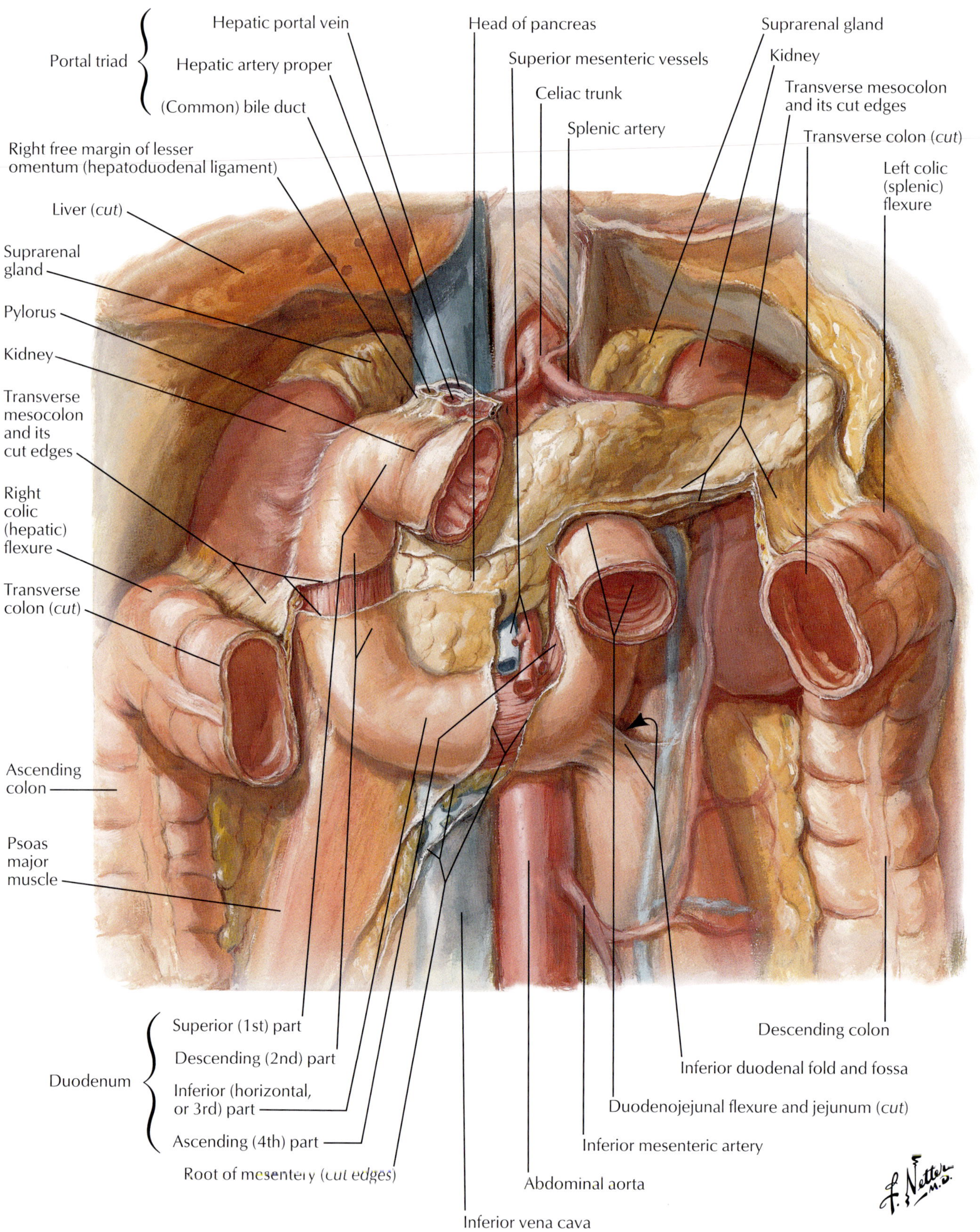

Mucosa and Musculature of Small Intestine

See also Plate 270

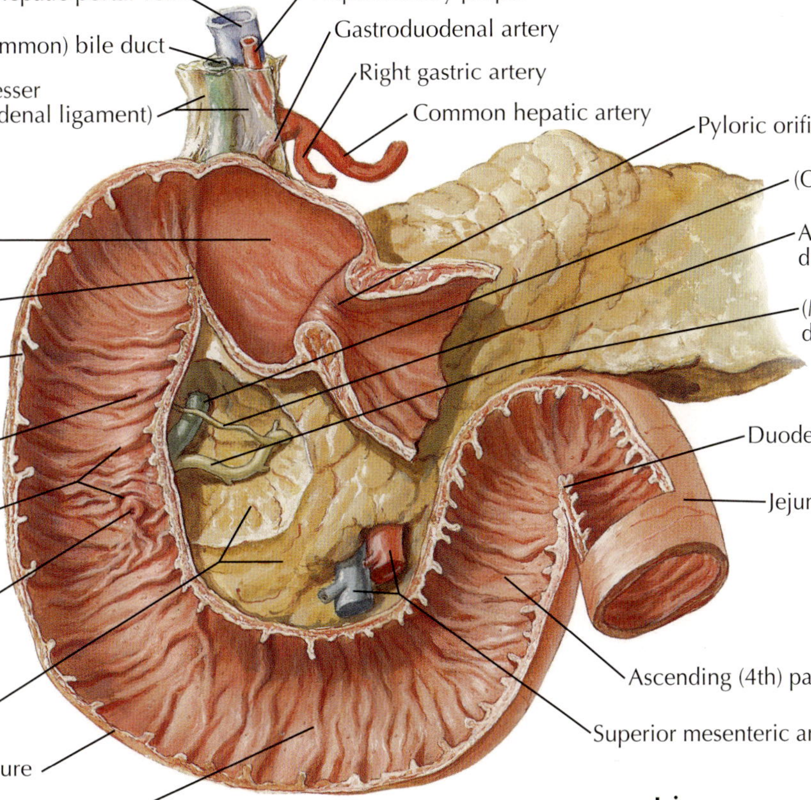

Jejunum

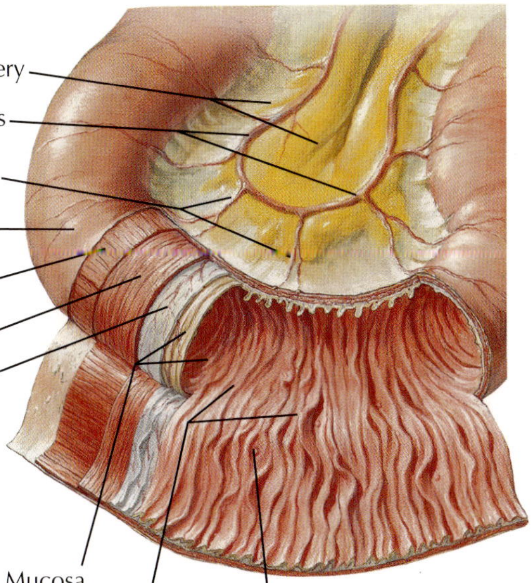

Ileum

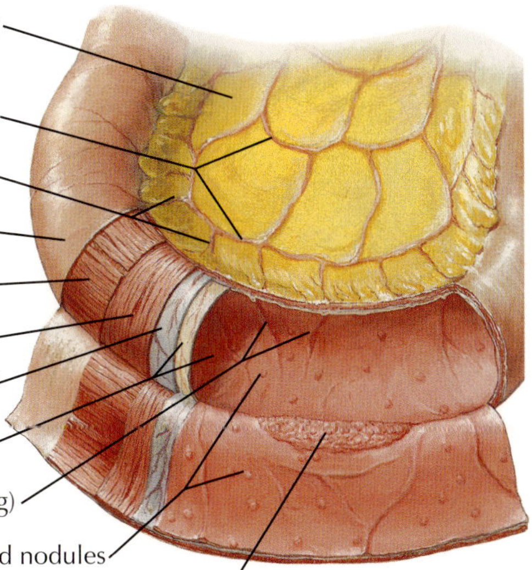

See also Plates 287, 288

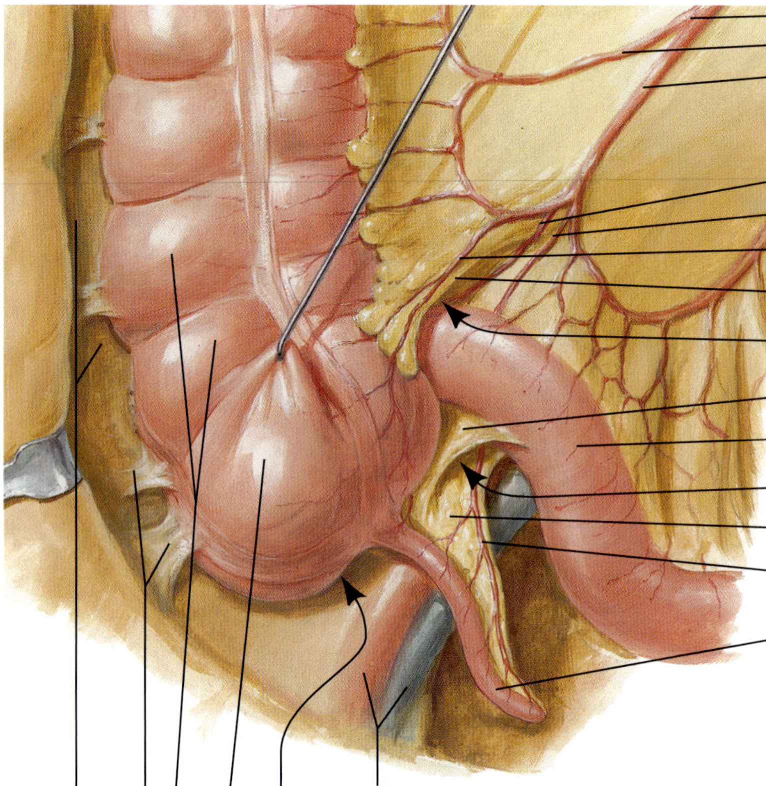

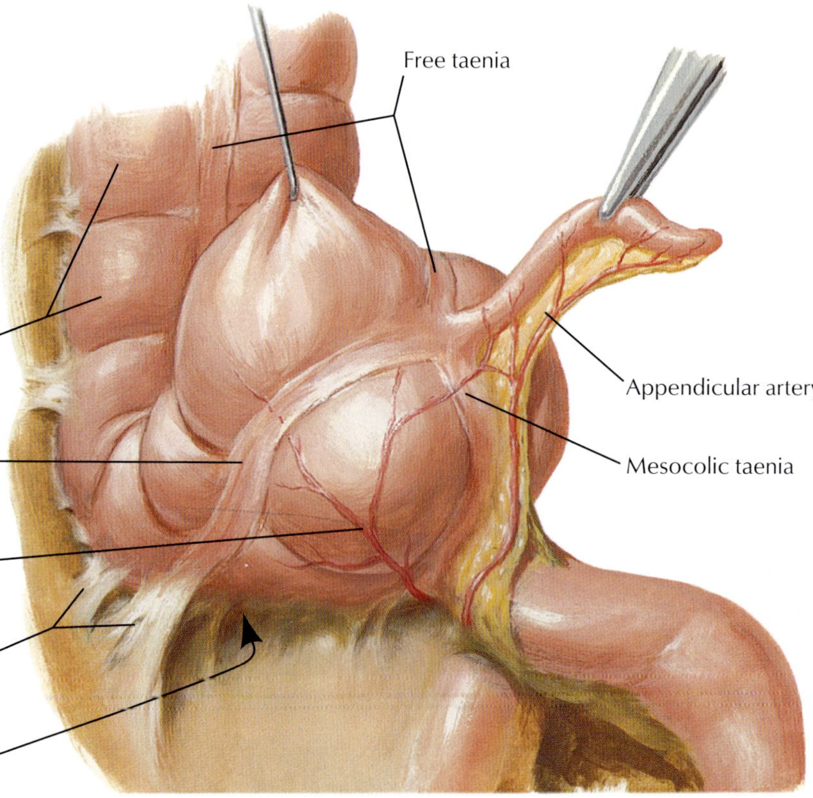

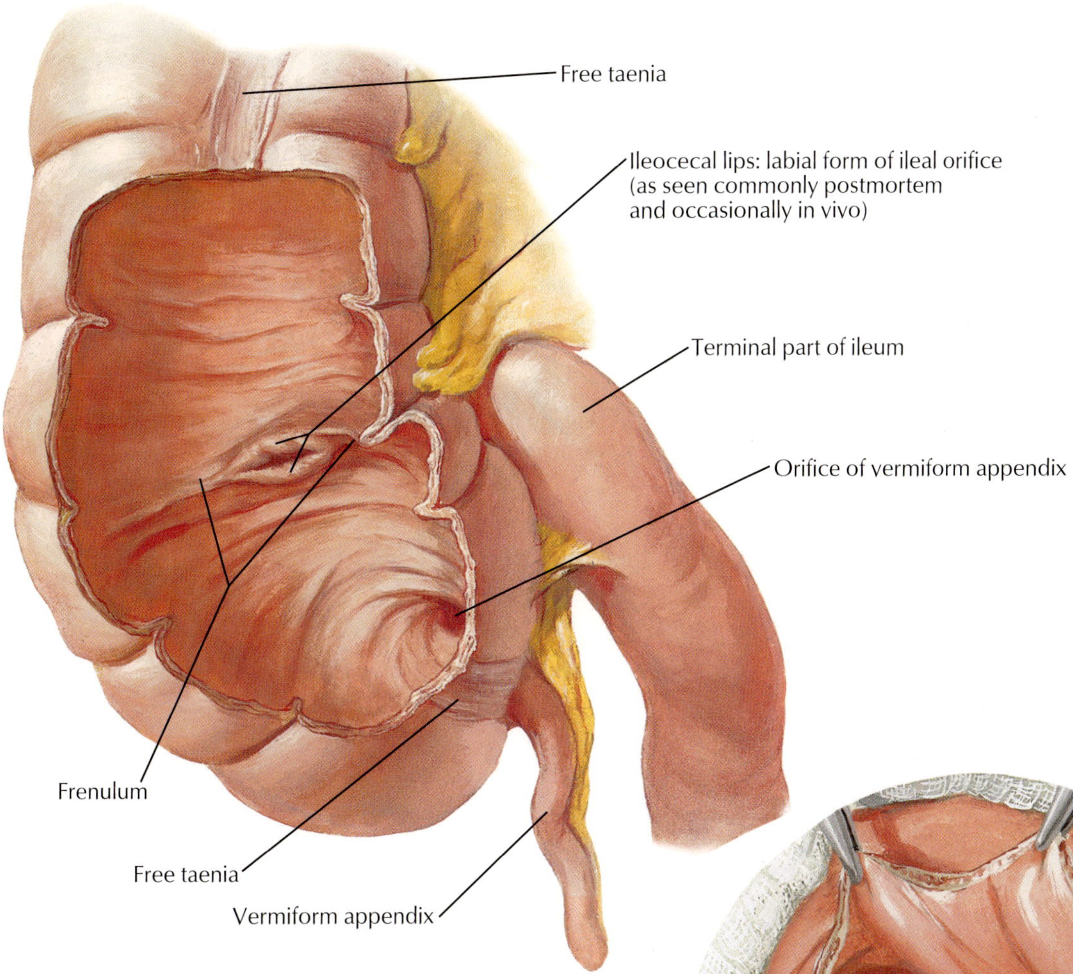

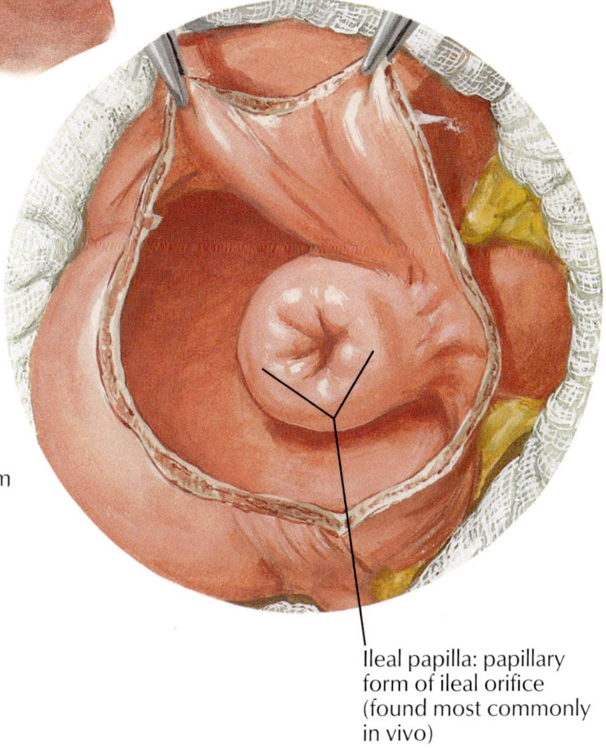

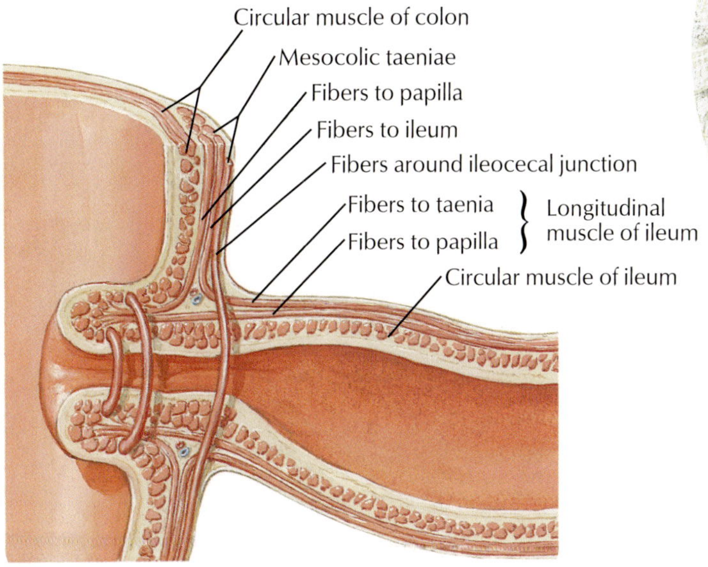

Schema of muscle fibers at ileal orifice

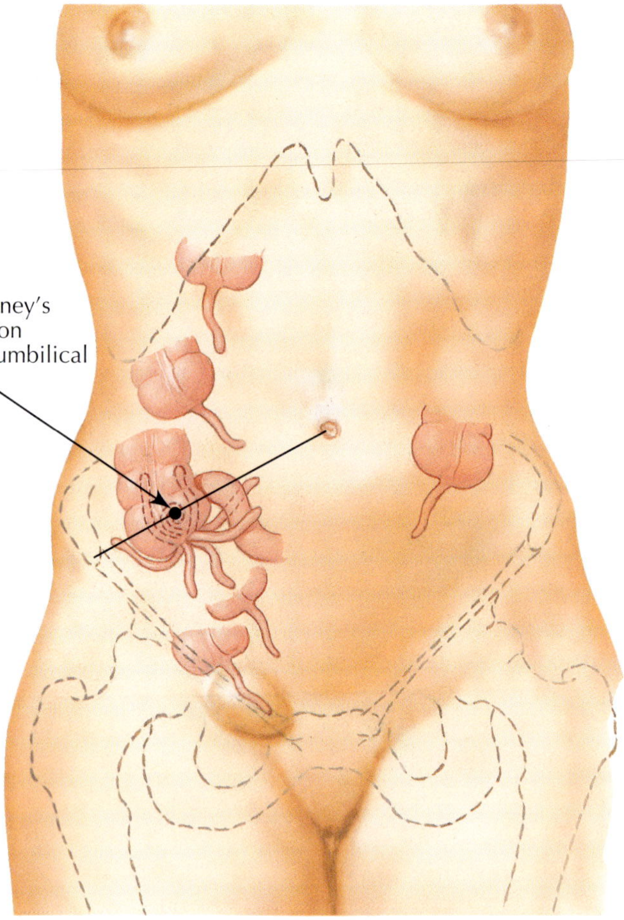

Variations in position of appendix

Coronal CT with contrast

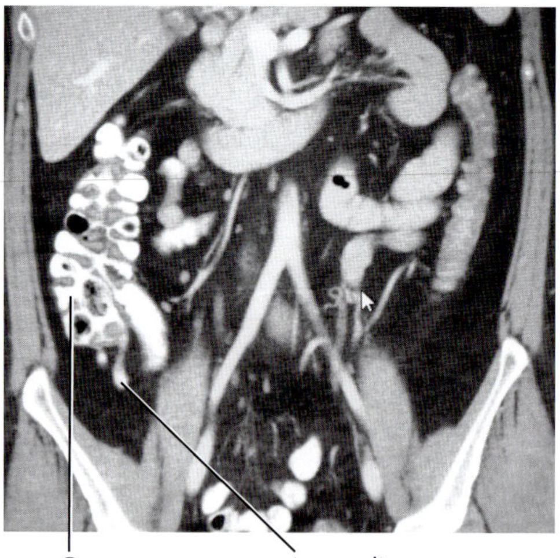

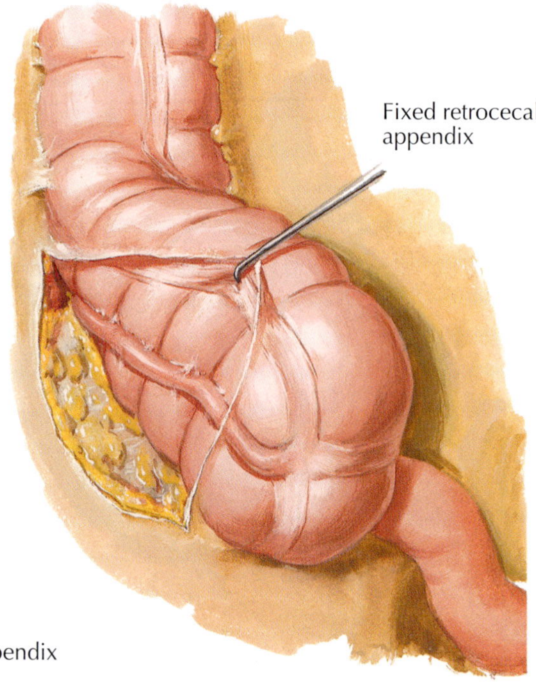

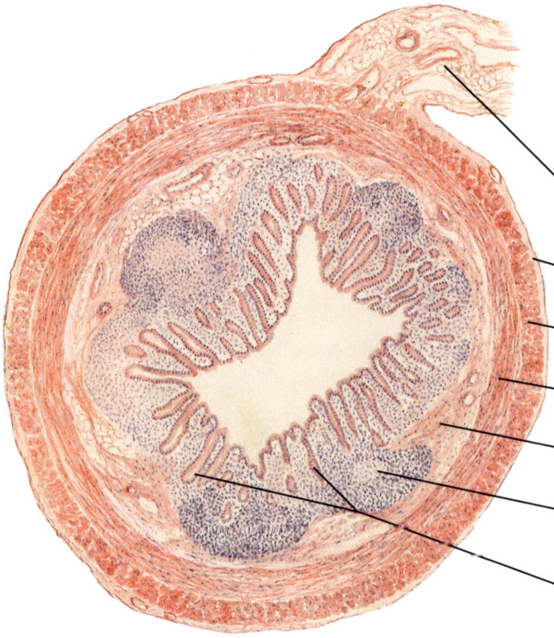

Mucosa and Musculature of Large Intestine

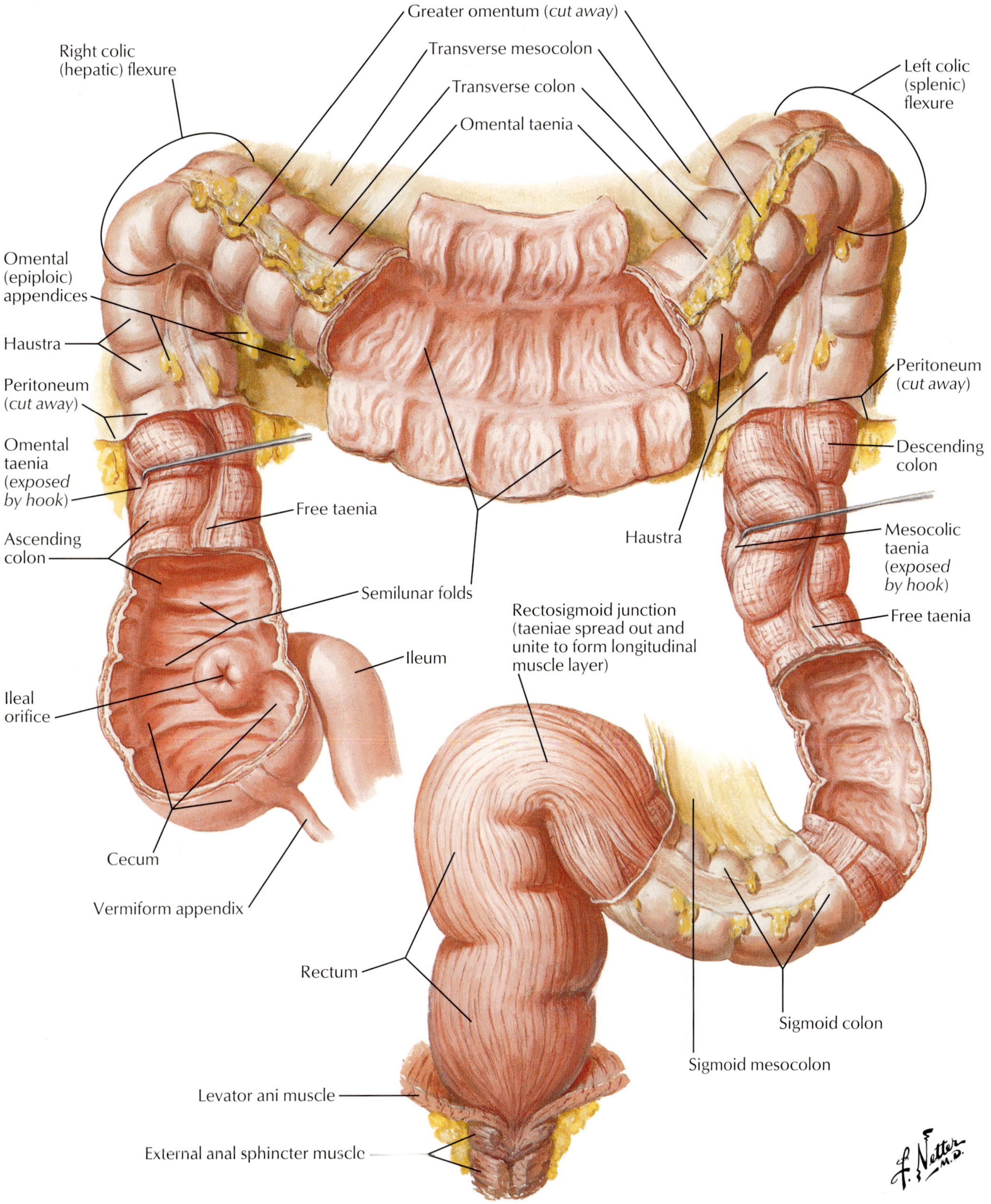

Surfaces and Bed of Liver

See also **Plate 268**

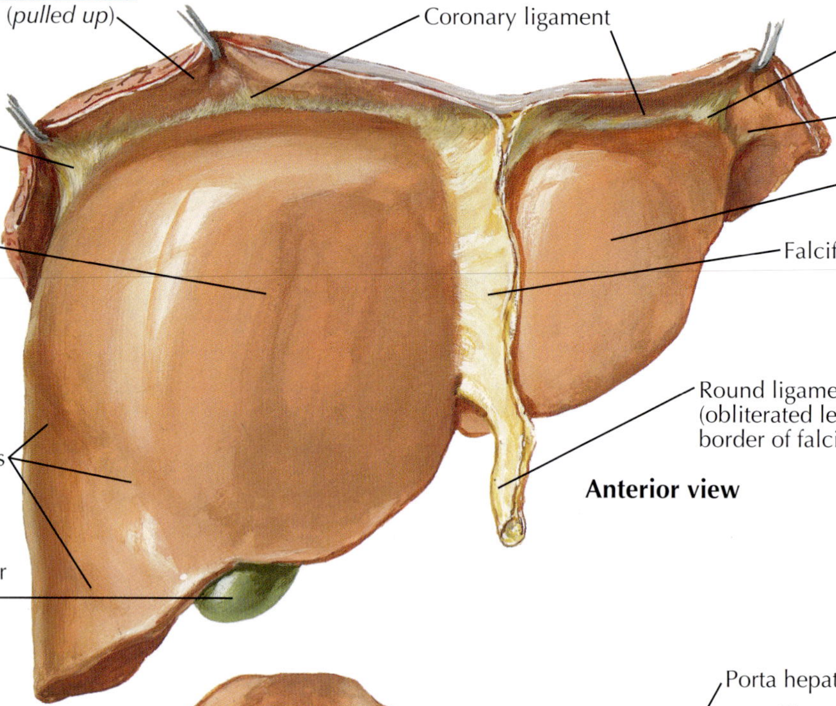

Anterior view

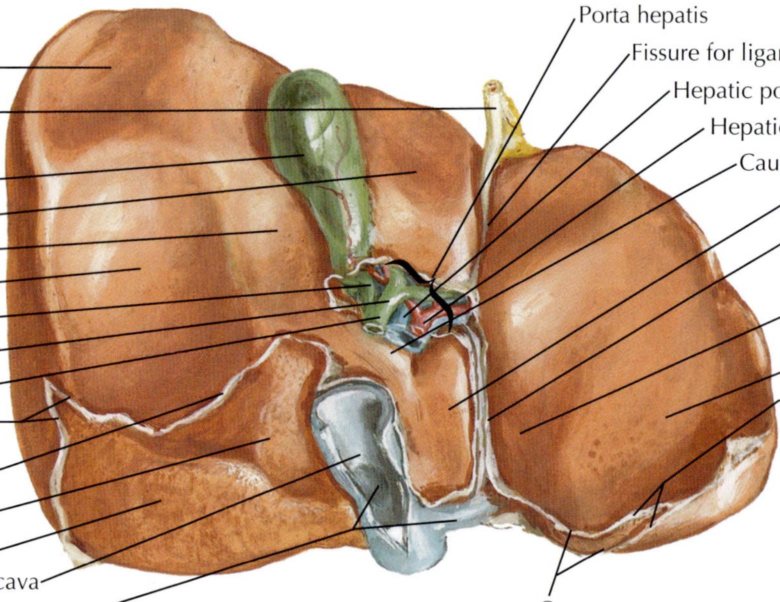

Visceral surface

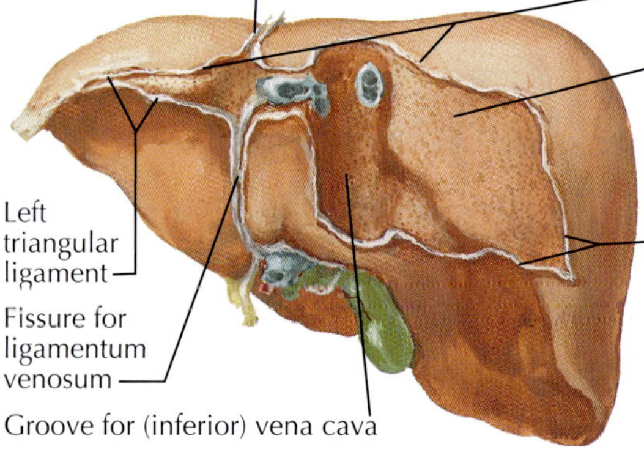

Posterior view

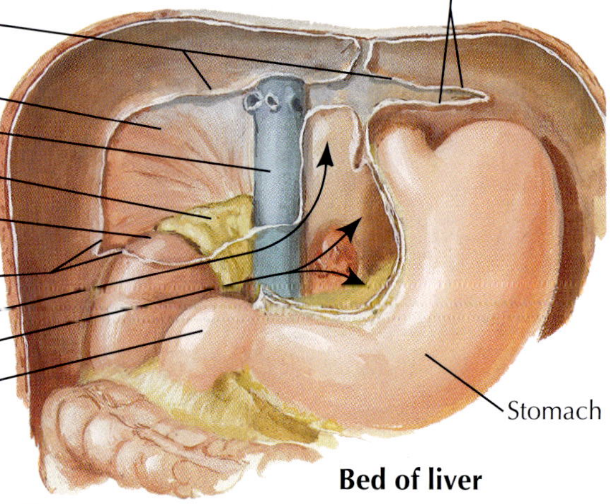

Bed of liver

Liver in Situ: Vascular and Duct Systems

See also Plate 267

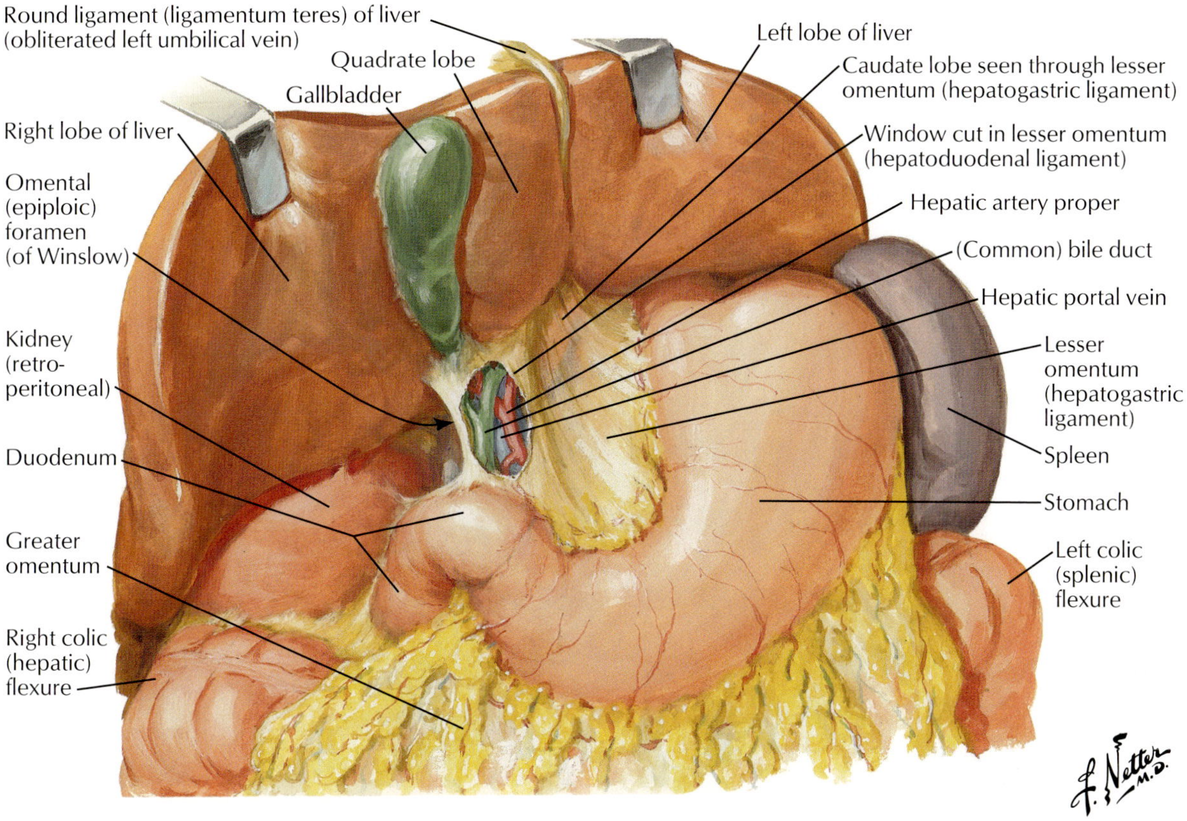

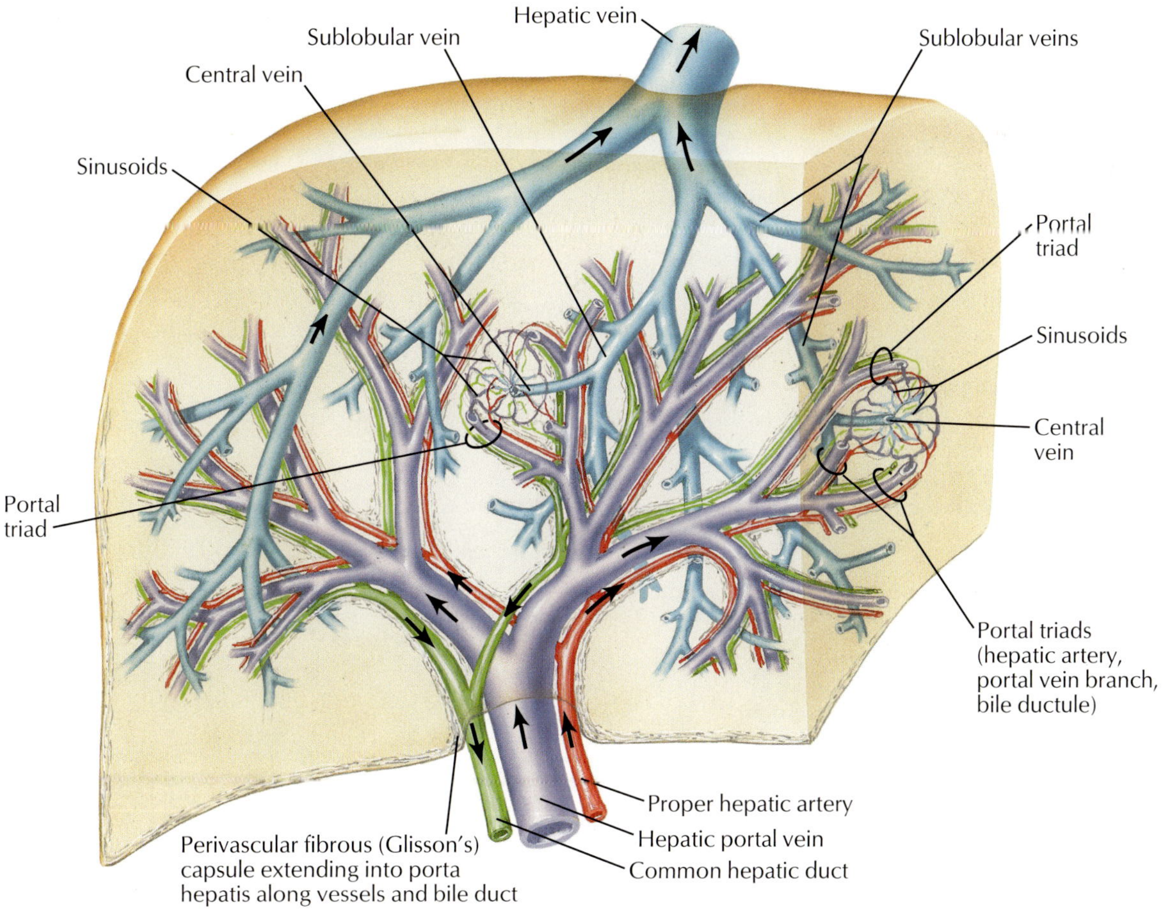

Liver Structure: Schema

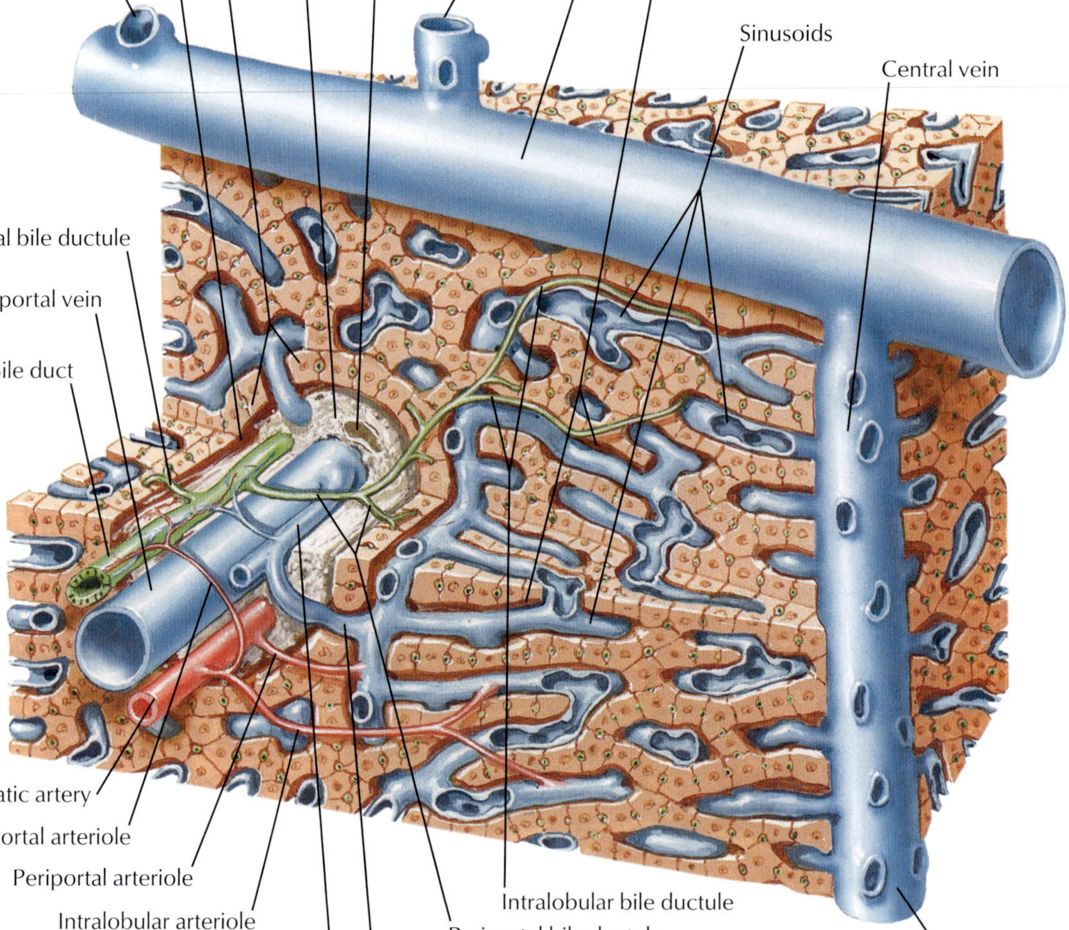

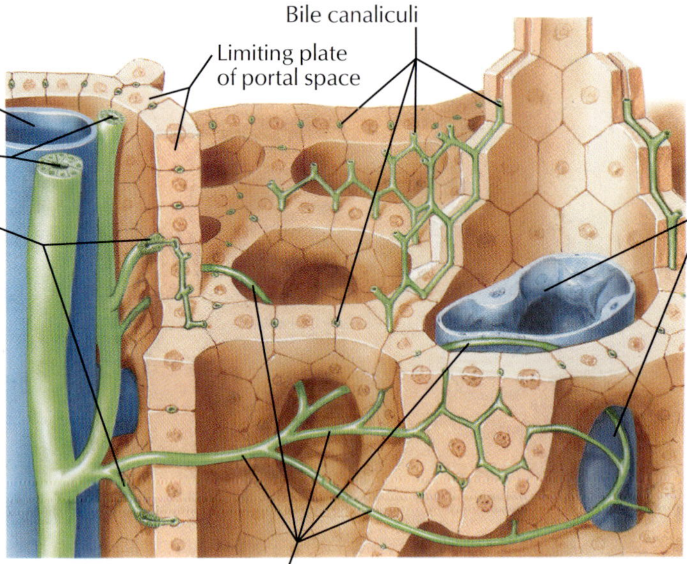

Gallbladder, Extrahepatic Bile Ducts, and Pancreatic Duct

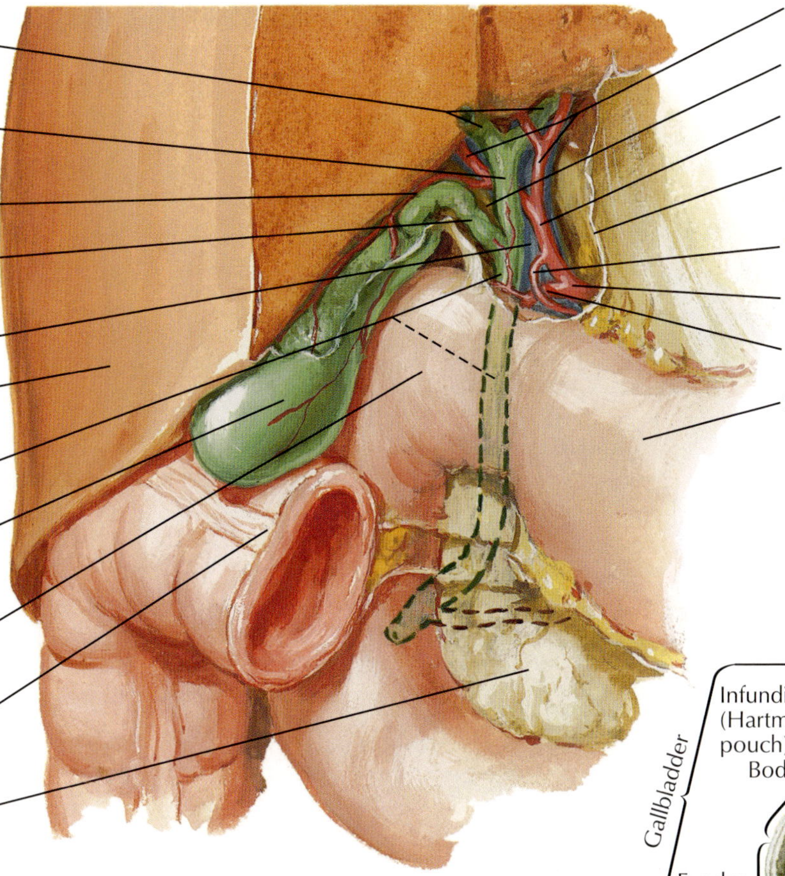

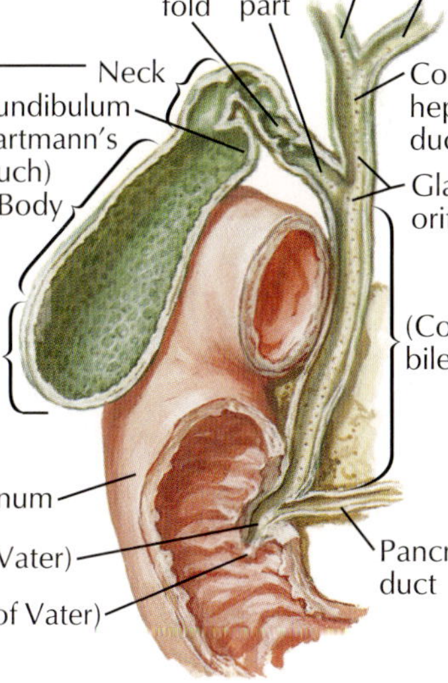

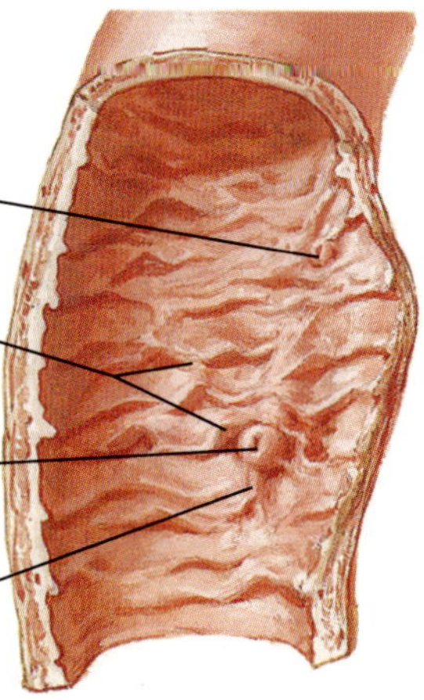

Interior of descending (2nd) part of duodenum

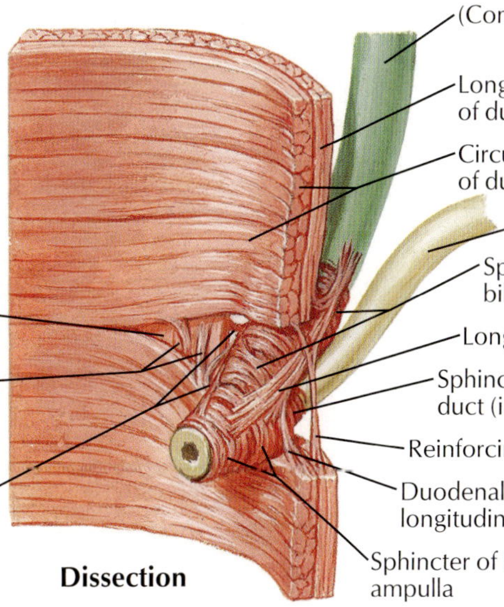

Dissection

Pancreas in Situ

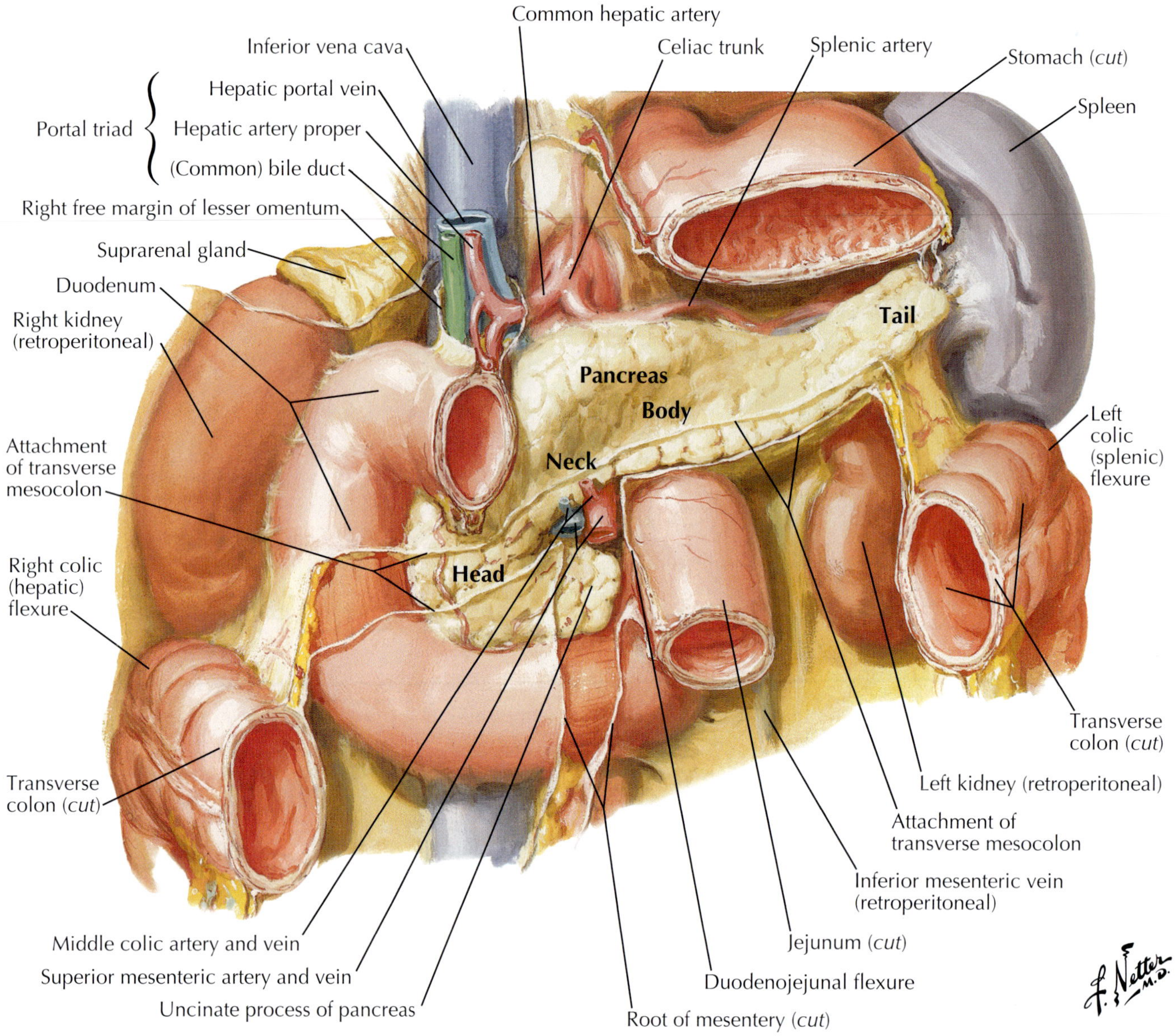

Magnetic resonance cholangiopancreatography (MRCP)

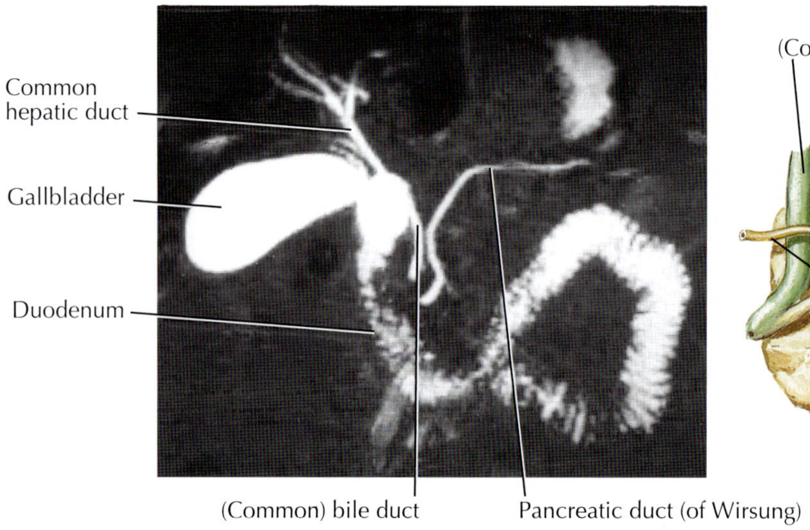

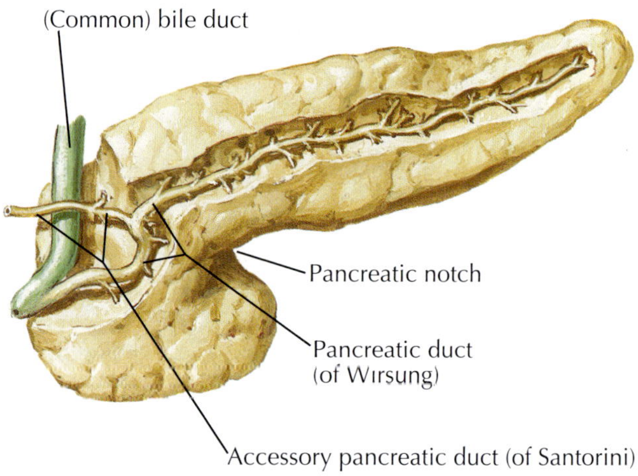

See also Plates 266

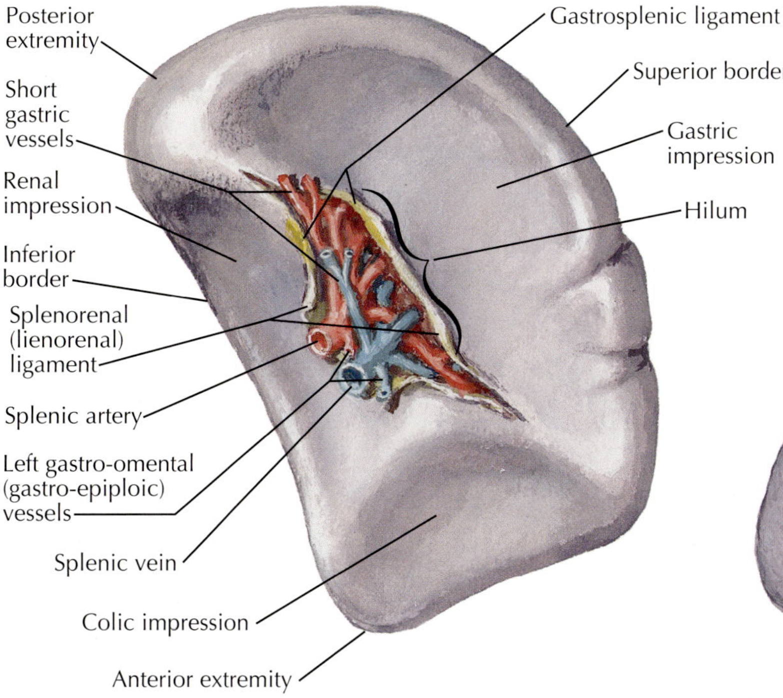

Visceral surface

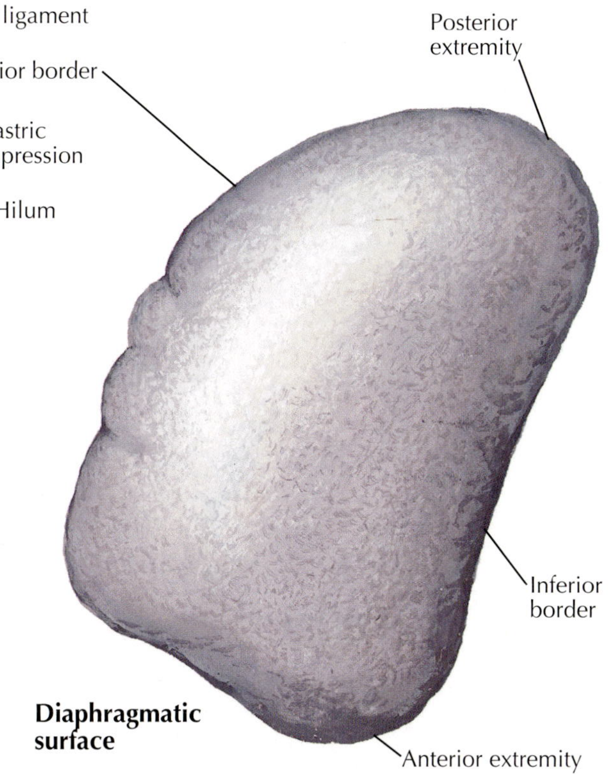

Diaphragmatic surface

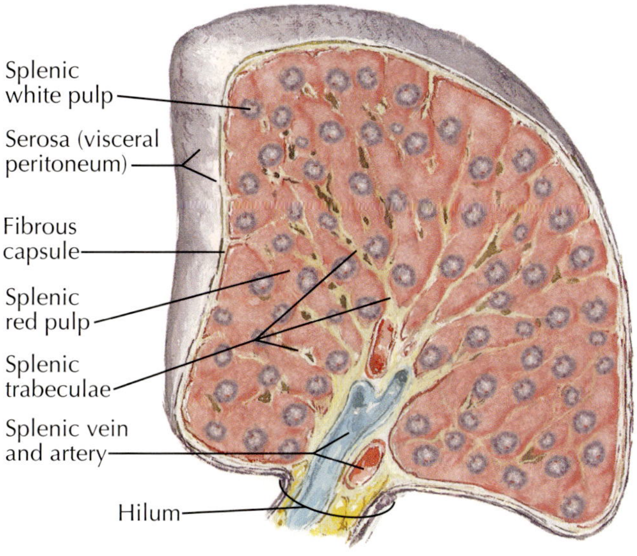

Cross section

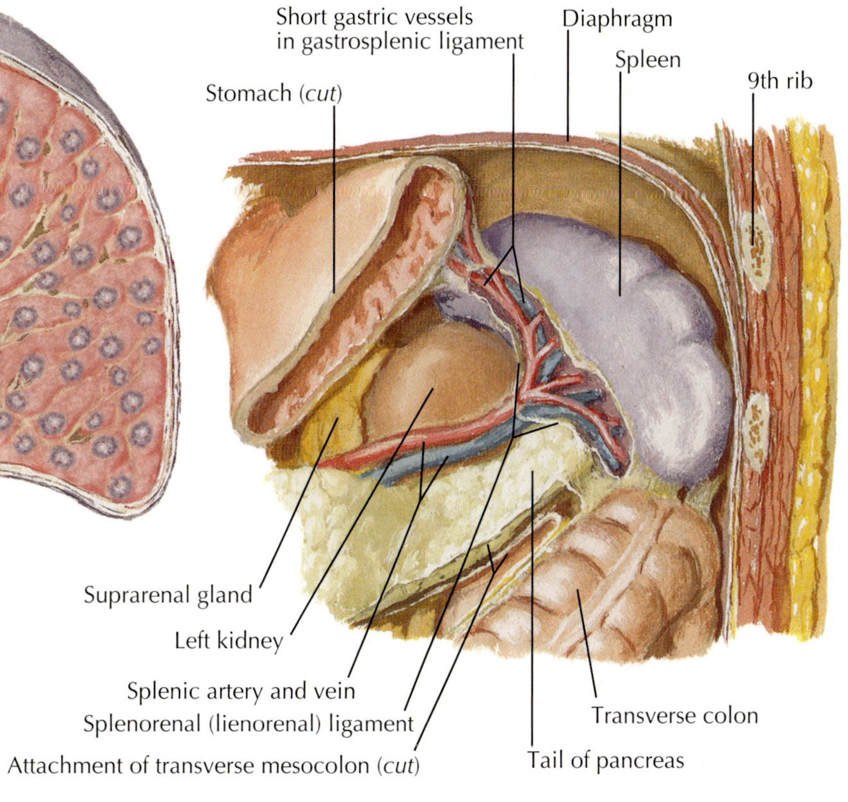

Spleen in situ

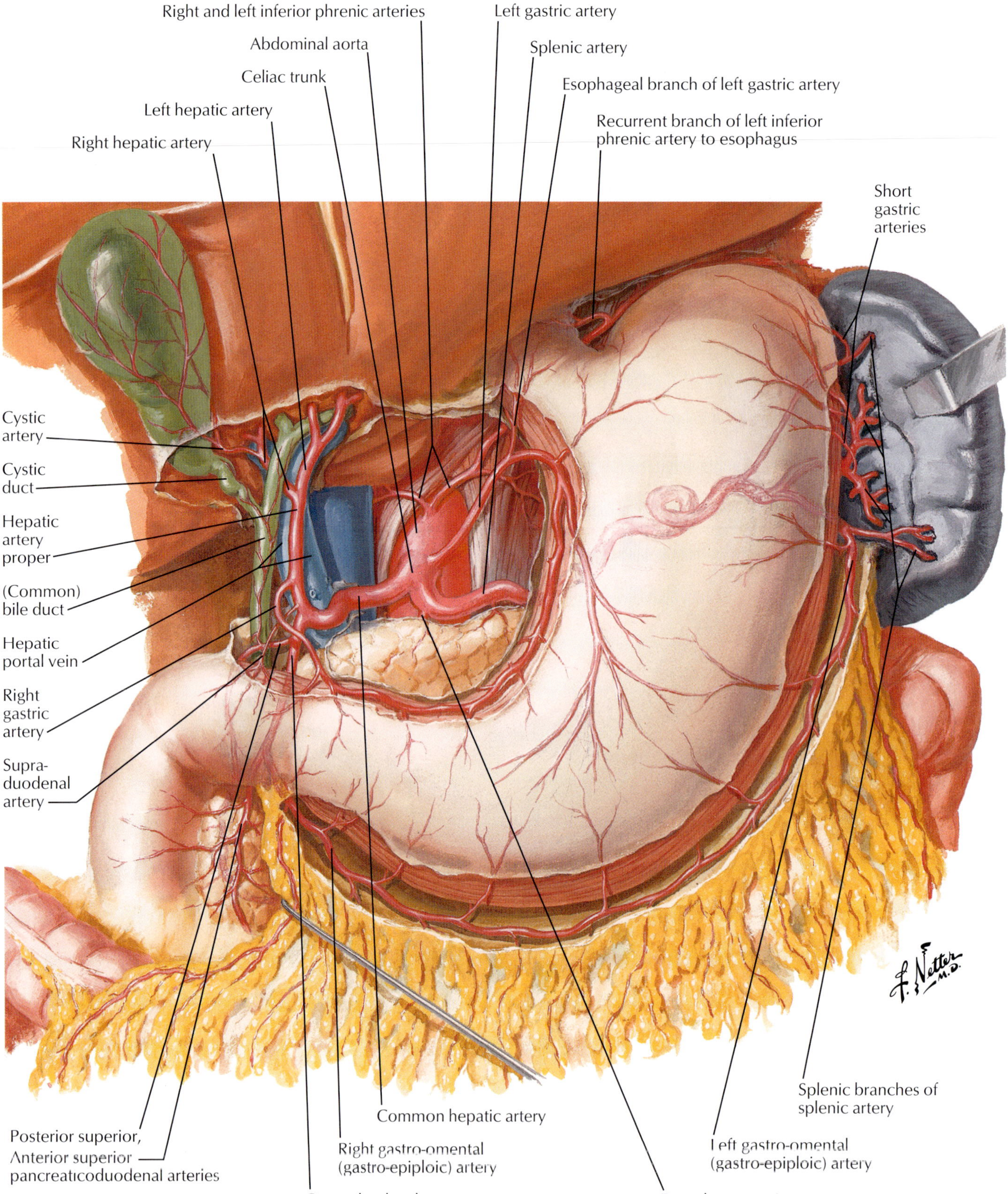
Right and left inferior phrenic arteries
Abdominal aorta
Celiac trunk
Left hepatic artery
Right hepatic artery
Left gastric artery
Splenic artery
Esophageal branch of left gastric artery
Recurrent branch of left inferior phrenic artery to esophagus
Short gastric arteries
Cystic artery
Cystic duct
Hepatic artery proper
(Common) bile duct
Hepatic portal vein
Right gastric artery
Supra-duodenal artery
Posterior superior, Anterior superior pancreaticoduodenal arteries
Gastroduodenal artery
Right gastro-omental (gastro-epiploic) artery
Common hepatic artery
Dorsal pancreatic artery
Left gastro-omental (gastro-epiploic) artery
Splenic branches of splenic artery

Arteries of Liver, Pancreas, Duodenum, and Spleen

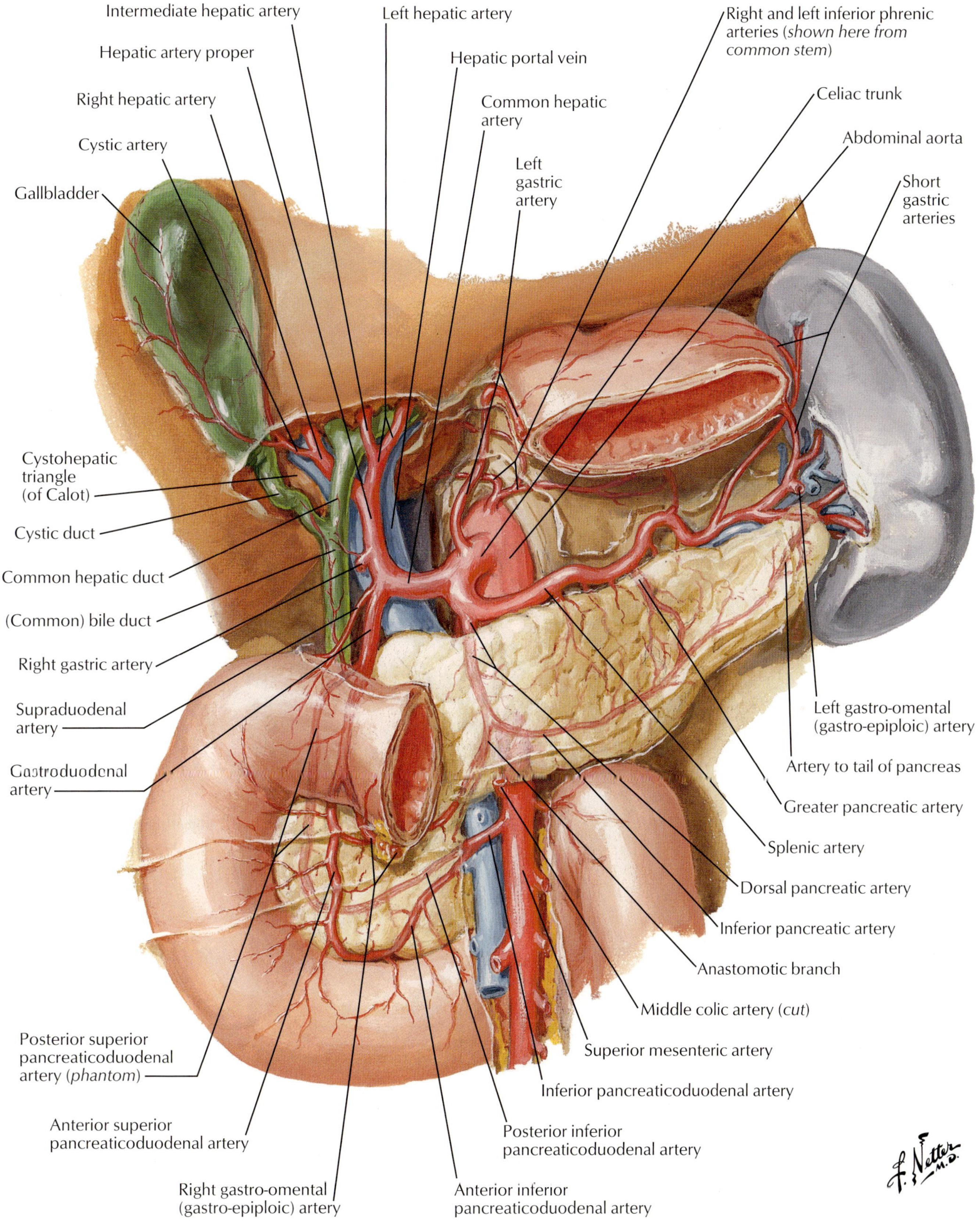

Celiac Arteriogram and CT Angiogram

See also **Plates 283, 284**

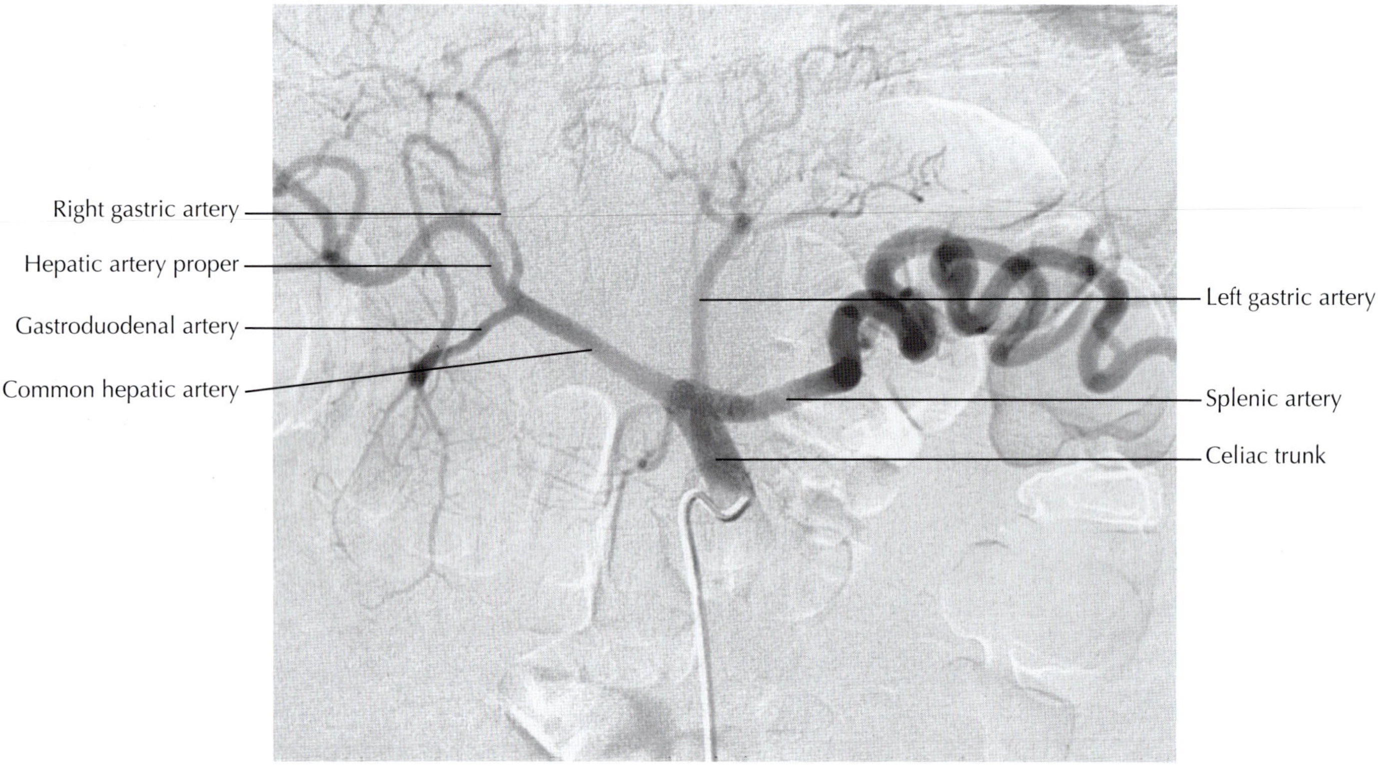

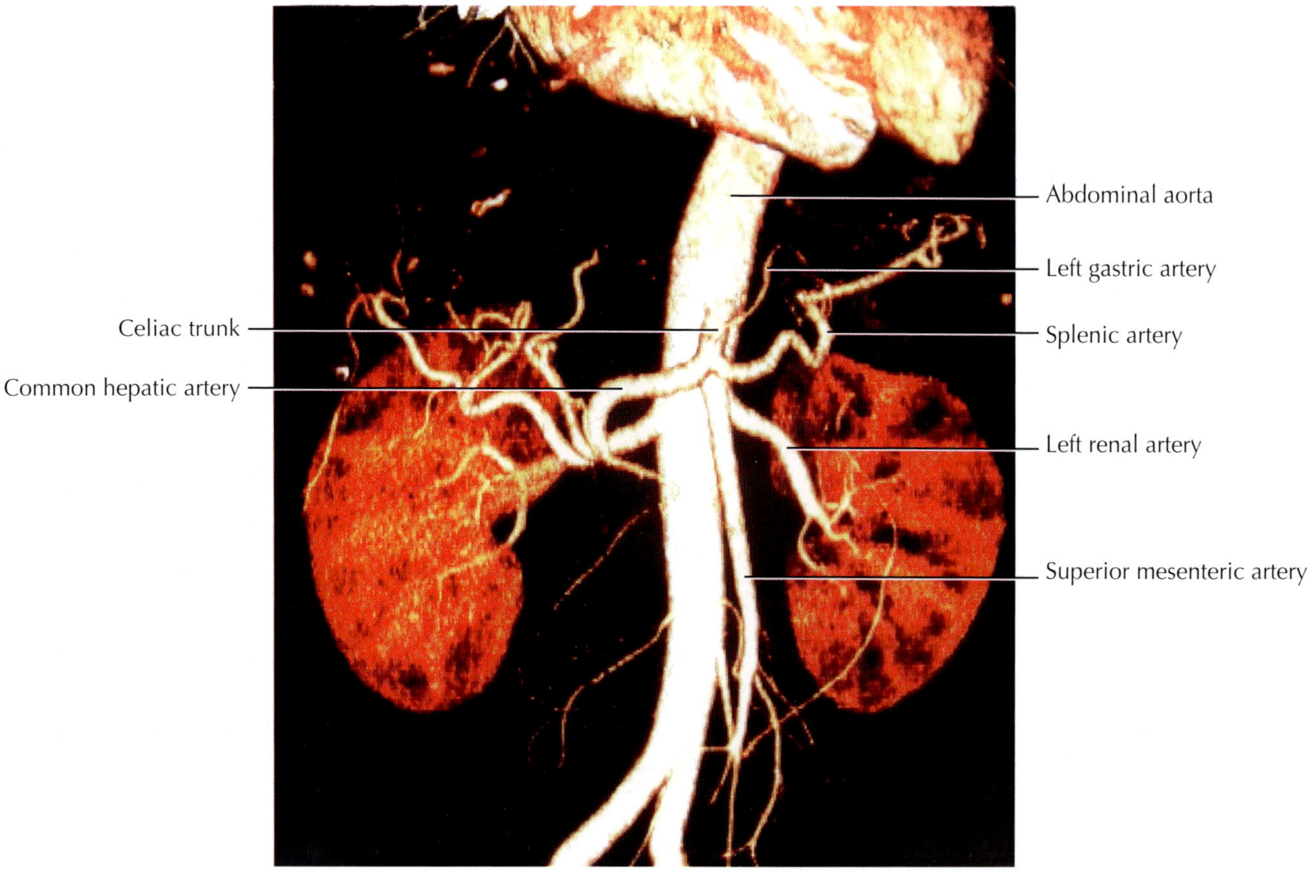

Duodenum and head of pancreas reflected to left

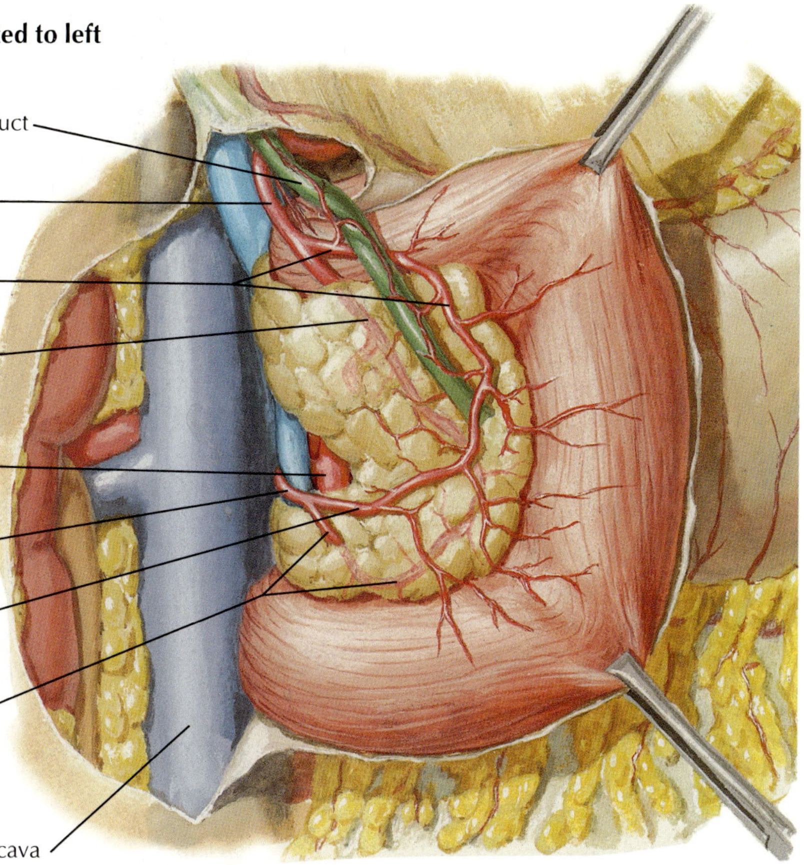

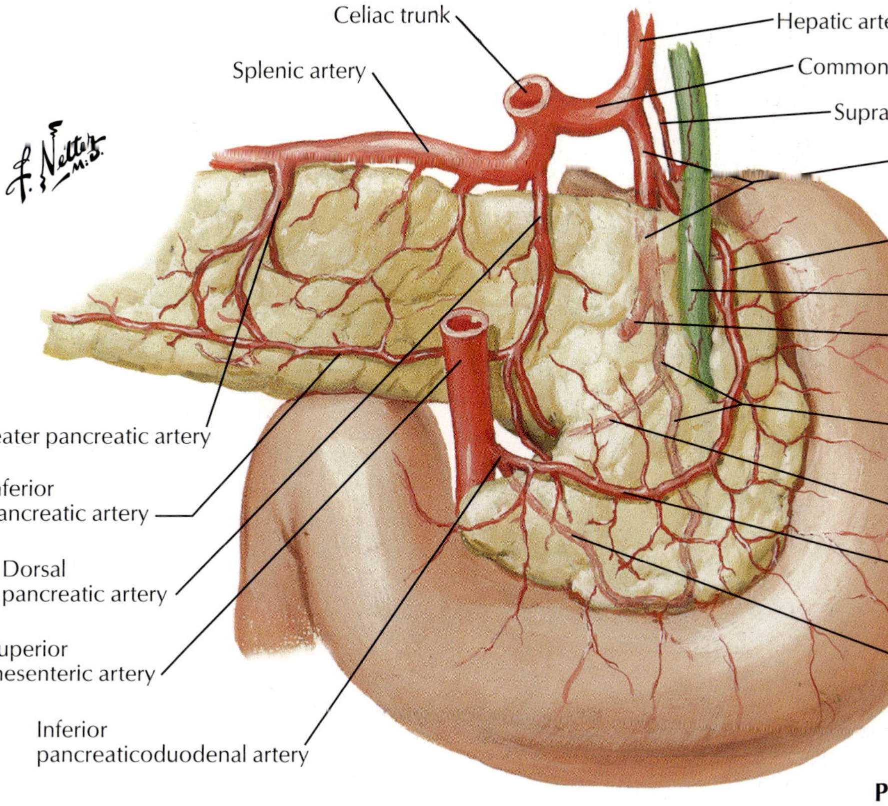

Posterior view

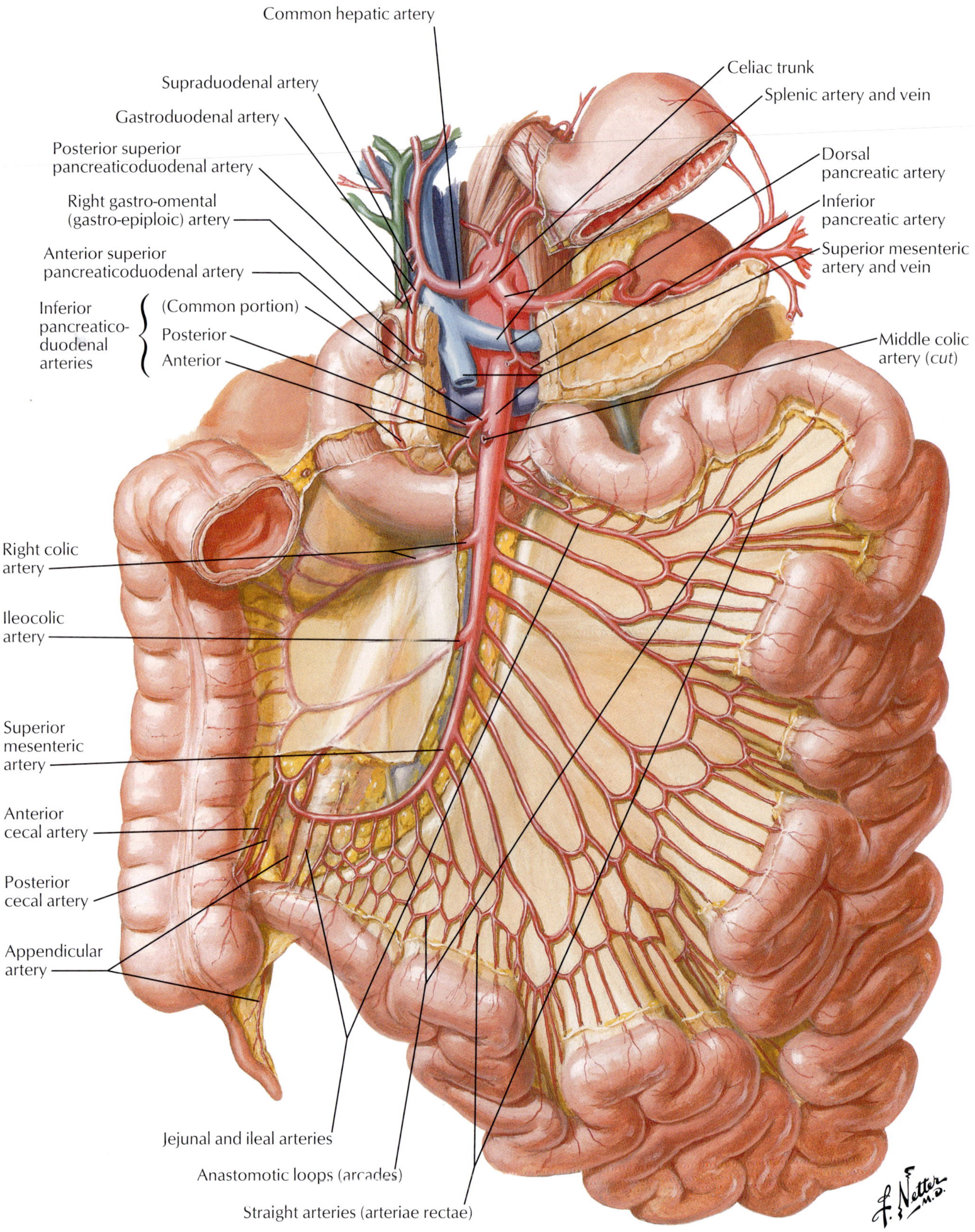
Common hepatic artery
Supraduodenal artery
Gastroduodenal artery
Posterior superior pancreaticoduodenal artery
Right gastro-omental (gastro-epiploic) artery
Anterior superior pancreaticoduodenal artery
Inferior pancreatico-duodenal arteries
(Common portion)
Posterior
Anterior
Celiac trunk
Splenic artery and vein
Dorsal pancreatic artery
Inferior pancreatic artery
Superior mesenteric artery and vein
Middle colic artery (cut)
Right colic artery
Ileocolic artery
Superior mesenteric artery
Anterior cecal artery
Posterior cecal artery
Appendicular artery
Jejunal and ileal arteries
Anastomotic loops (arcades)
Straight arteries (arteriae rectae)

Arteries of Large Intestine

For arteries of rectum see also Plate 376

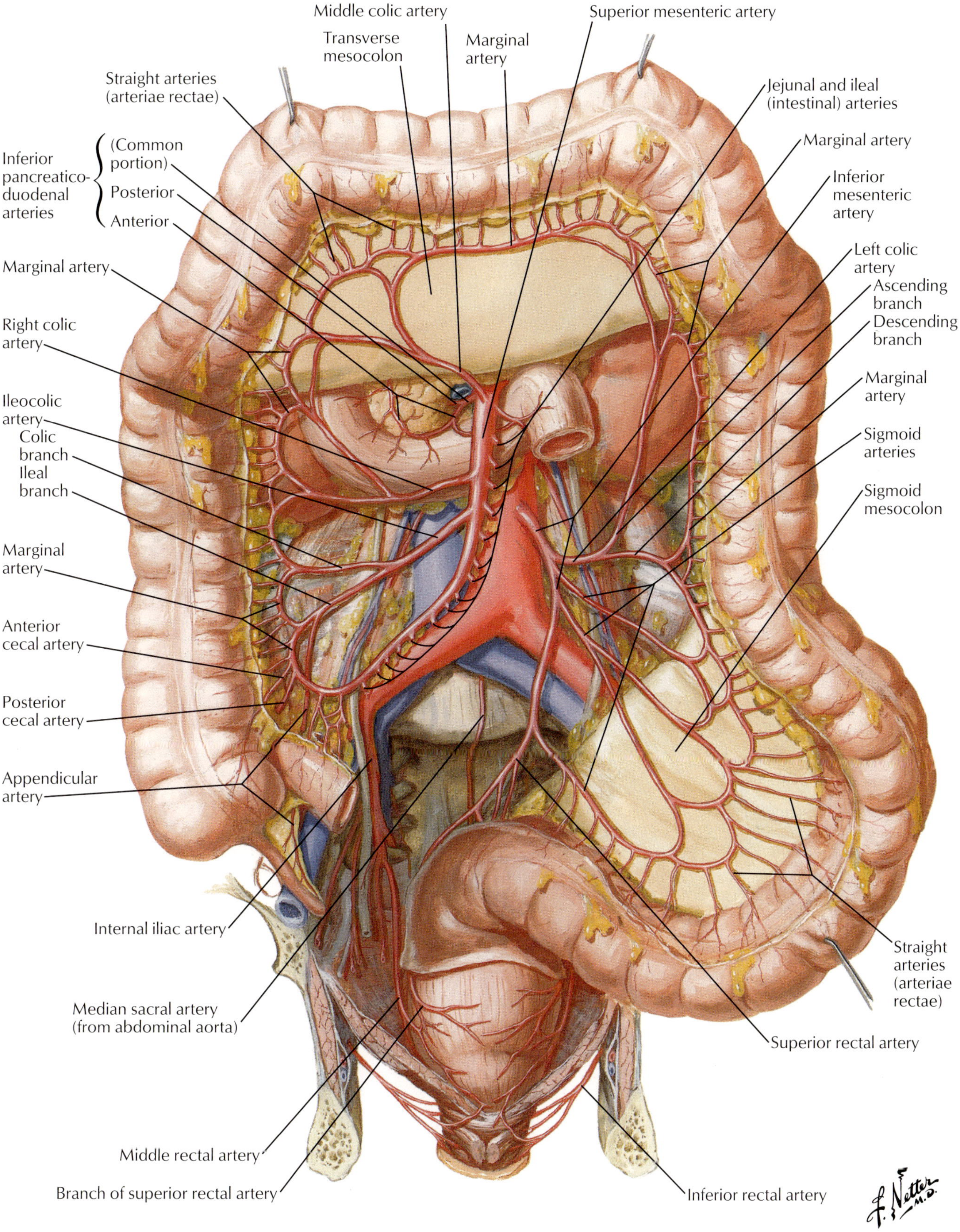

Veins of Stomach, Duodenum, Pancreas, and Spleen

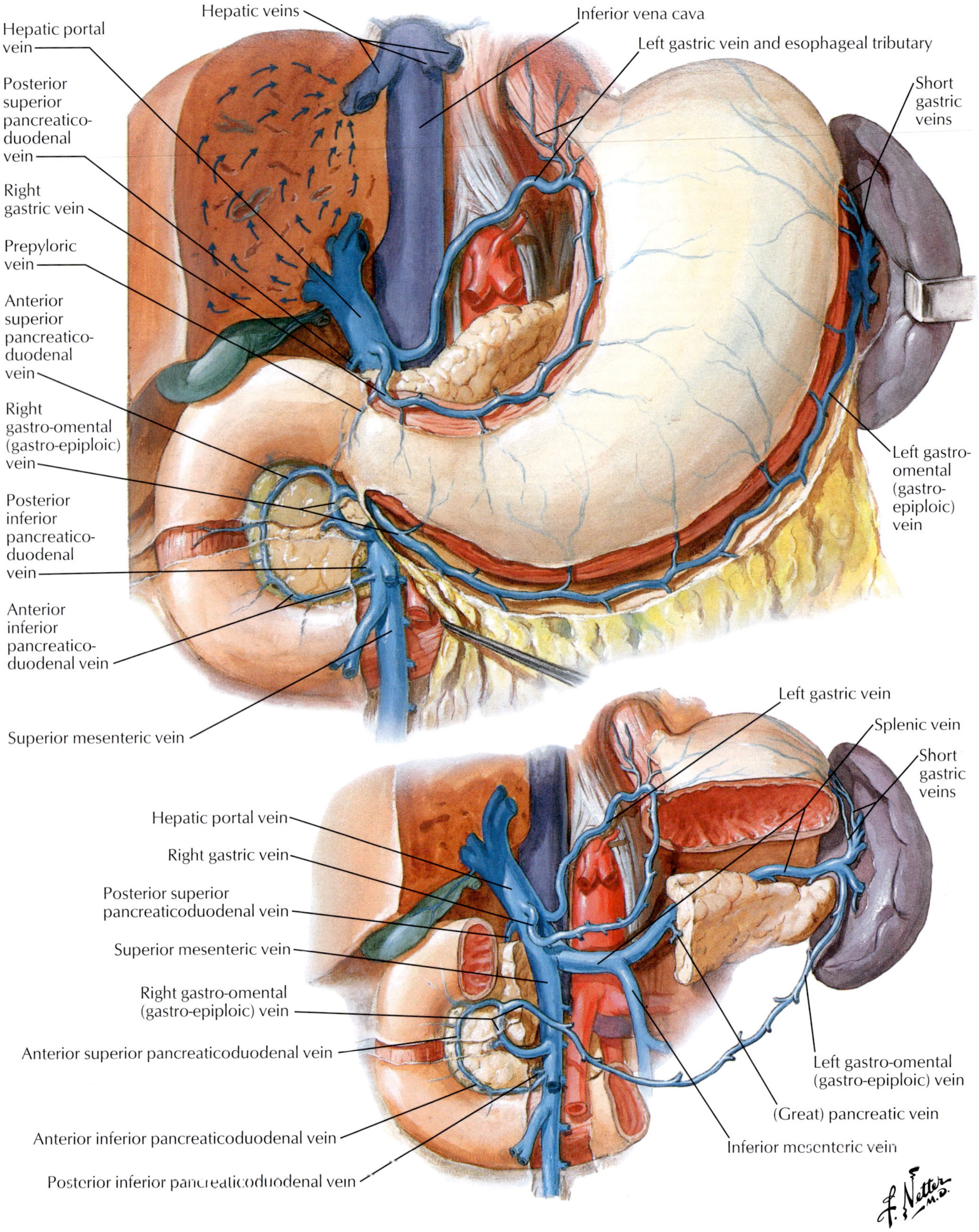

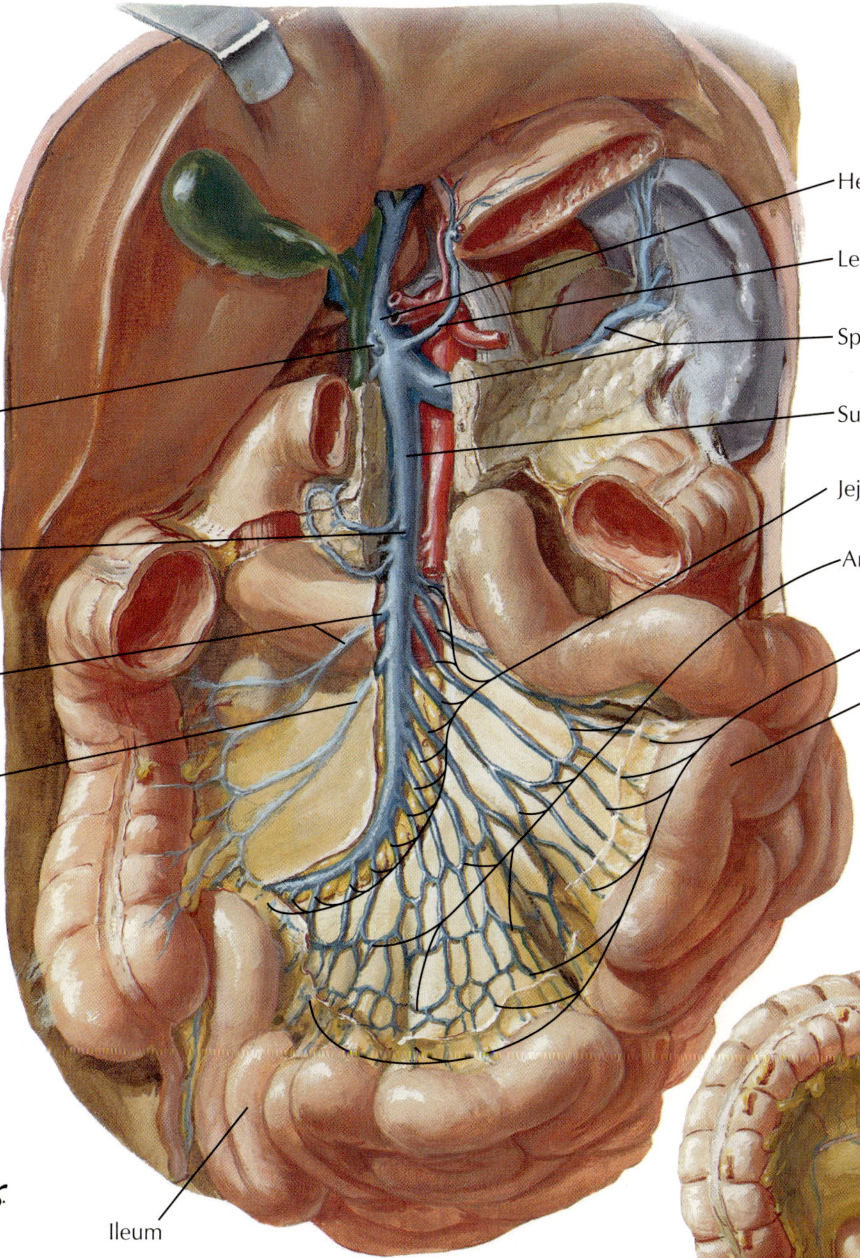

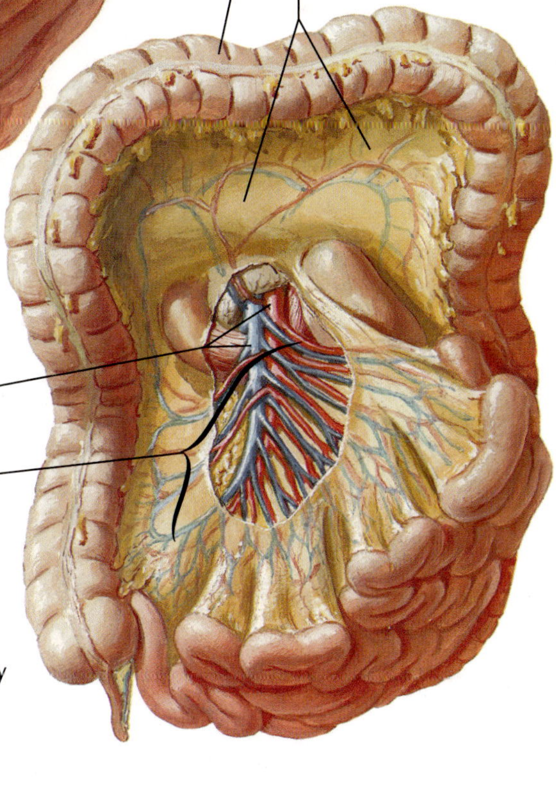

Relations of superior mesenteric vein and artery in root of mesentery

Veins of Large Intestine

For veins of rectum see also Plate 377

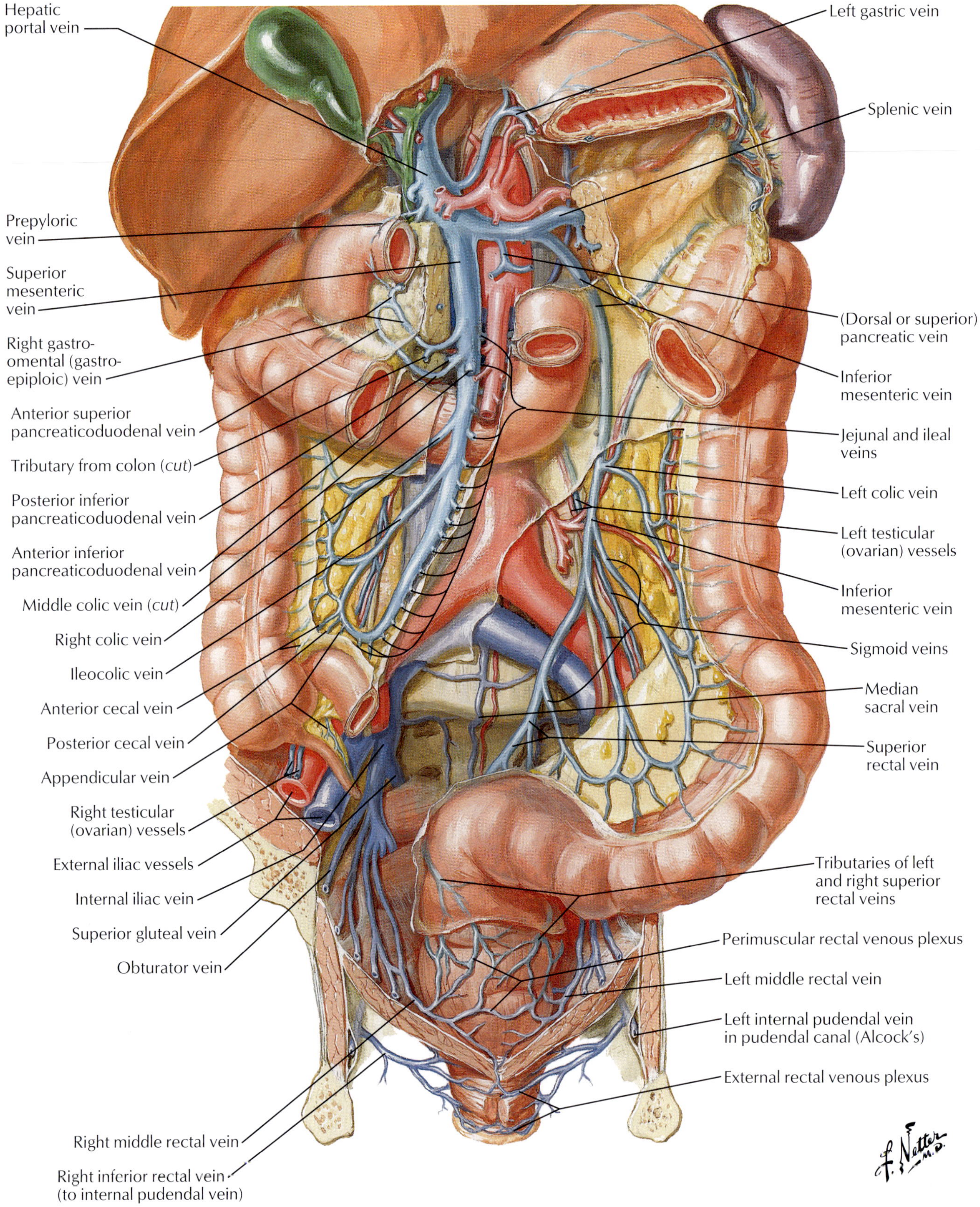

Hepatic Portal Vein Tributaries: Portacaval Anastomoses

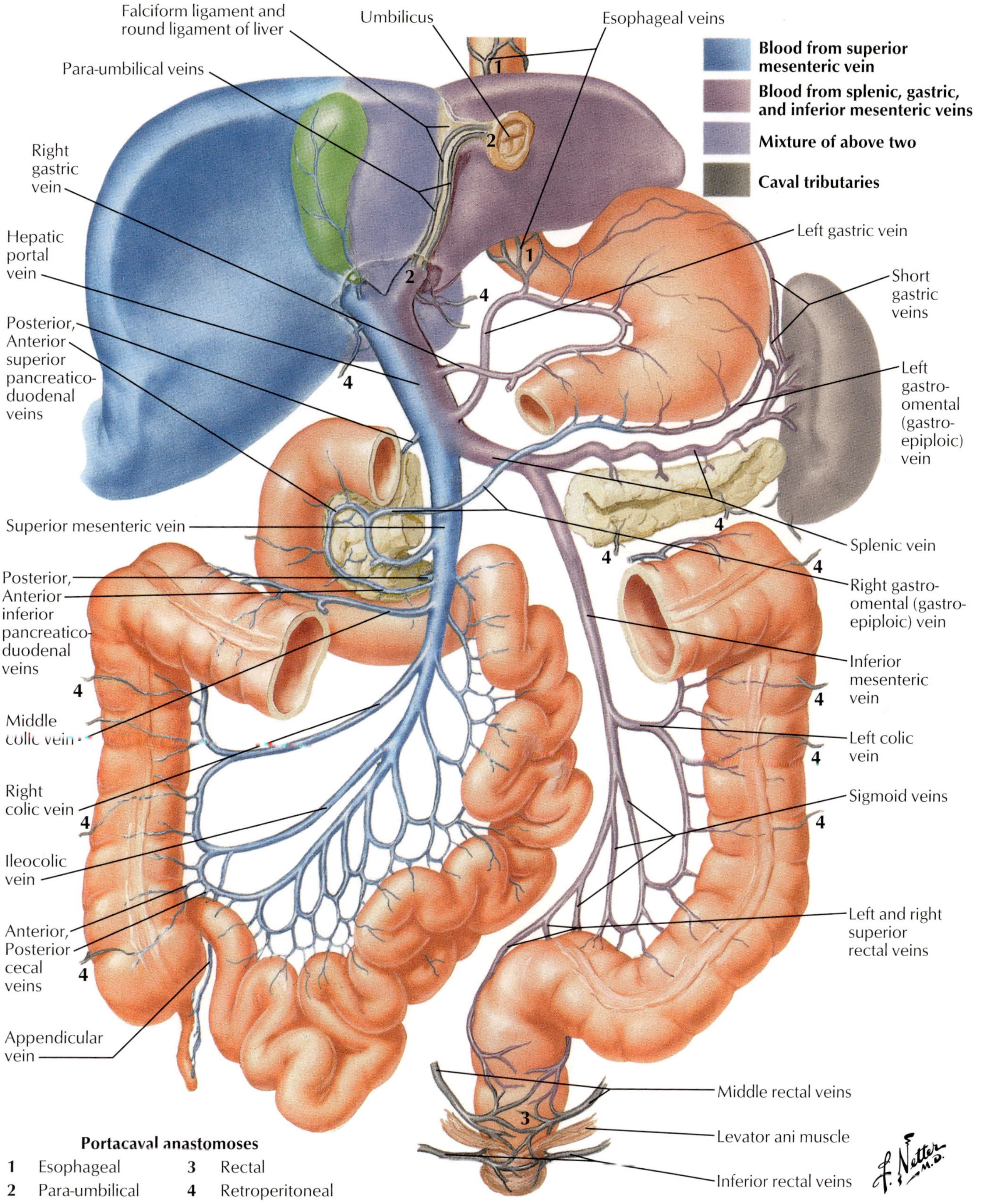

Portacaval anastomoses

1	Esophageal	3	Rectal
2	Para-umbilical	4	Retroperitoneal

Lymph Vessels and Nodes of Stomach

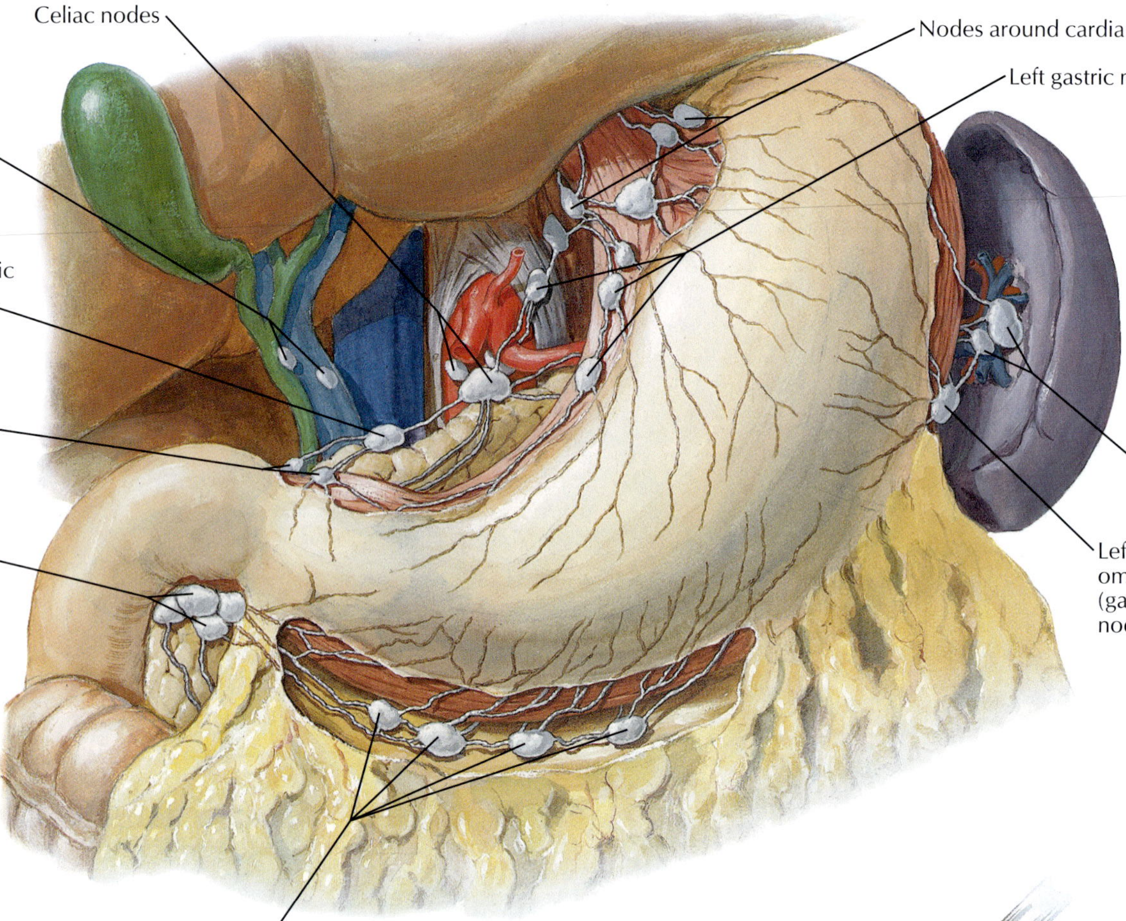

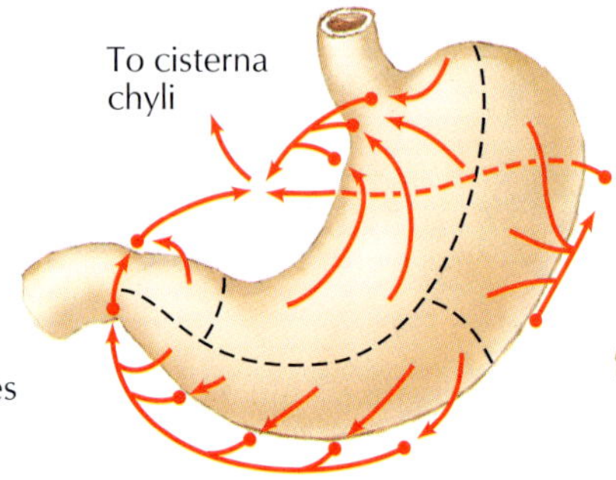

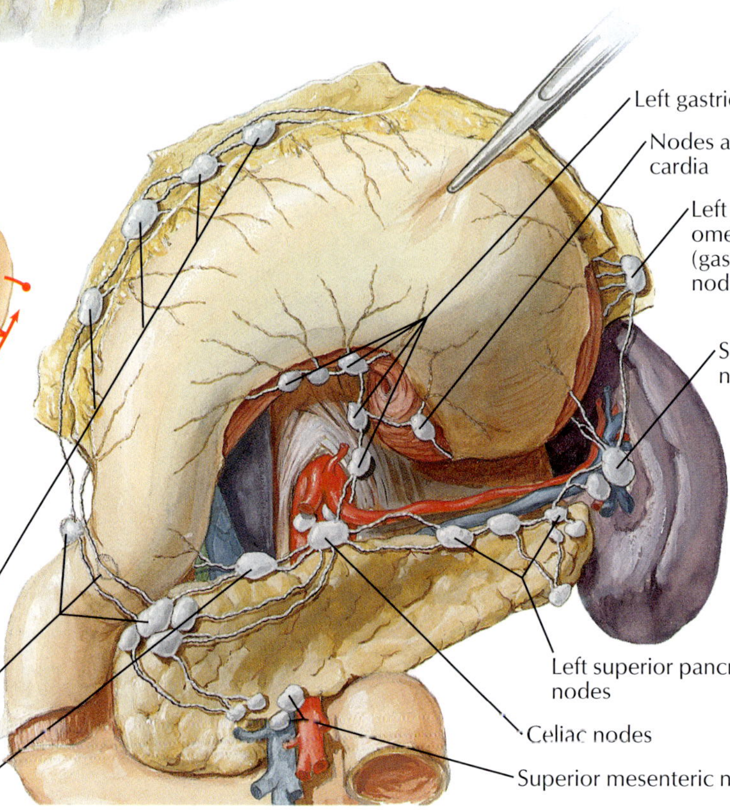

Lymph Vessels and Nodes of Pancreas

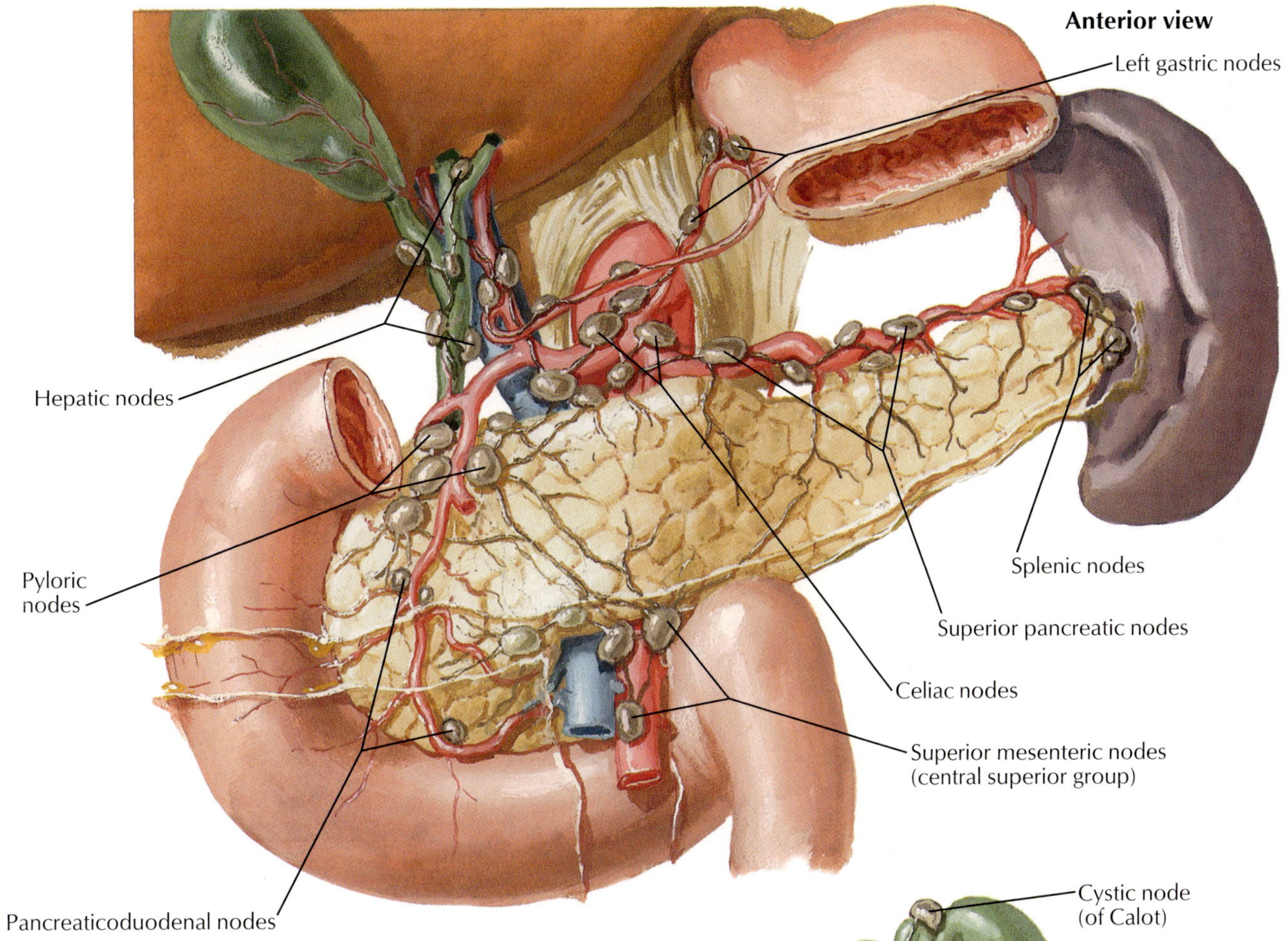

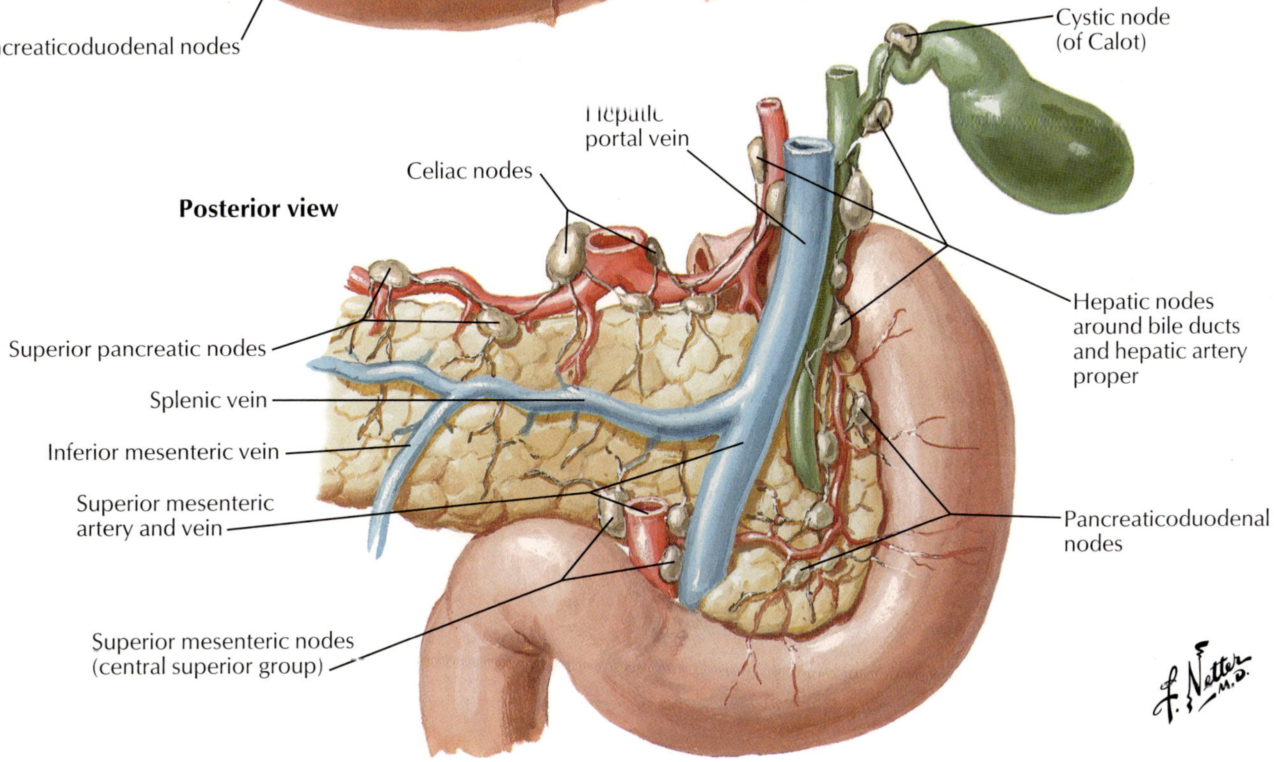

Lymph Vessels and Nodes of Small Intestine

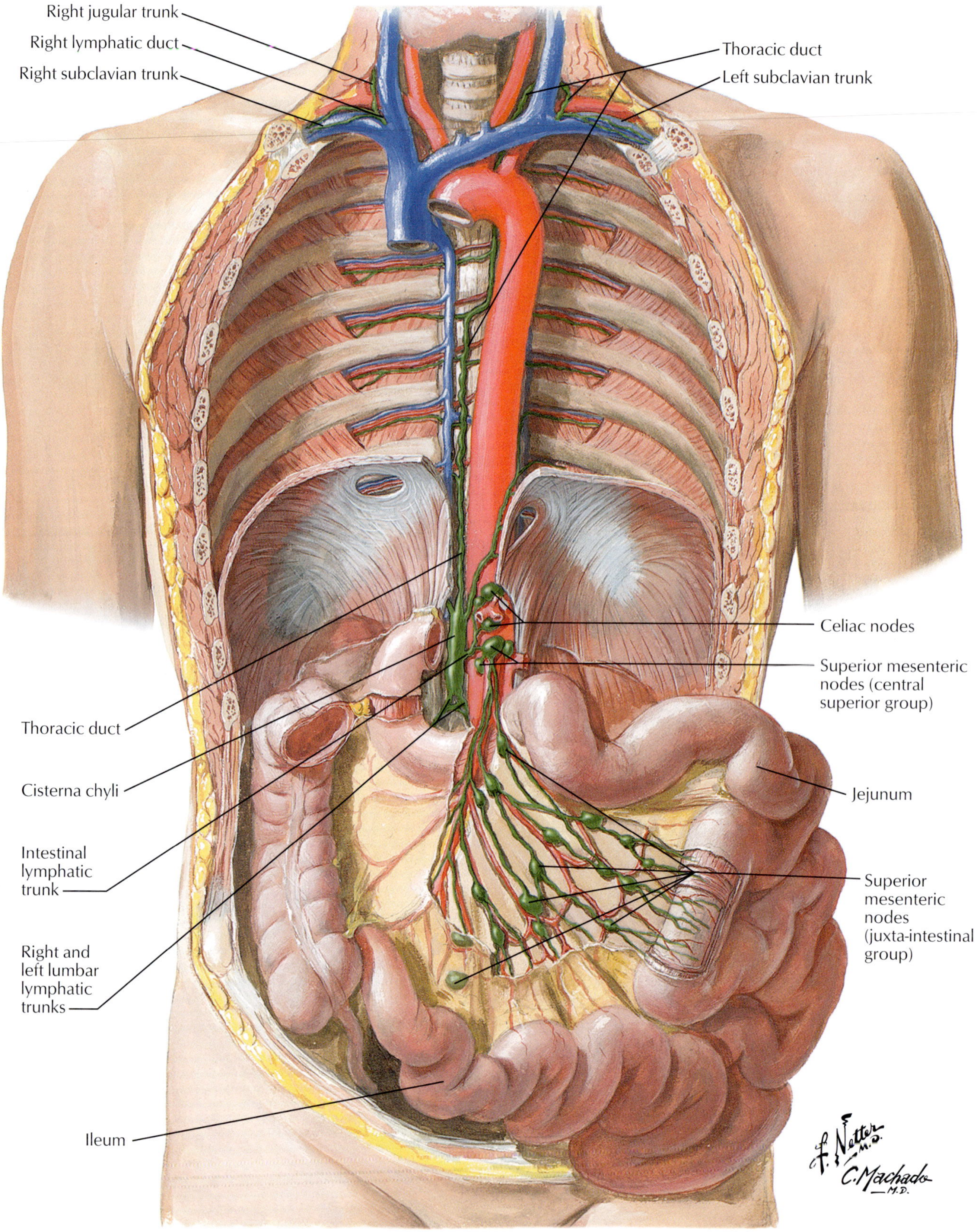

Lymph Vessels and Nodes of Large Intestine

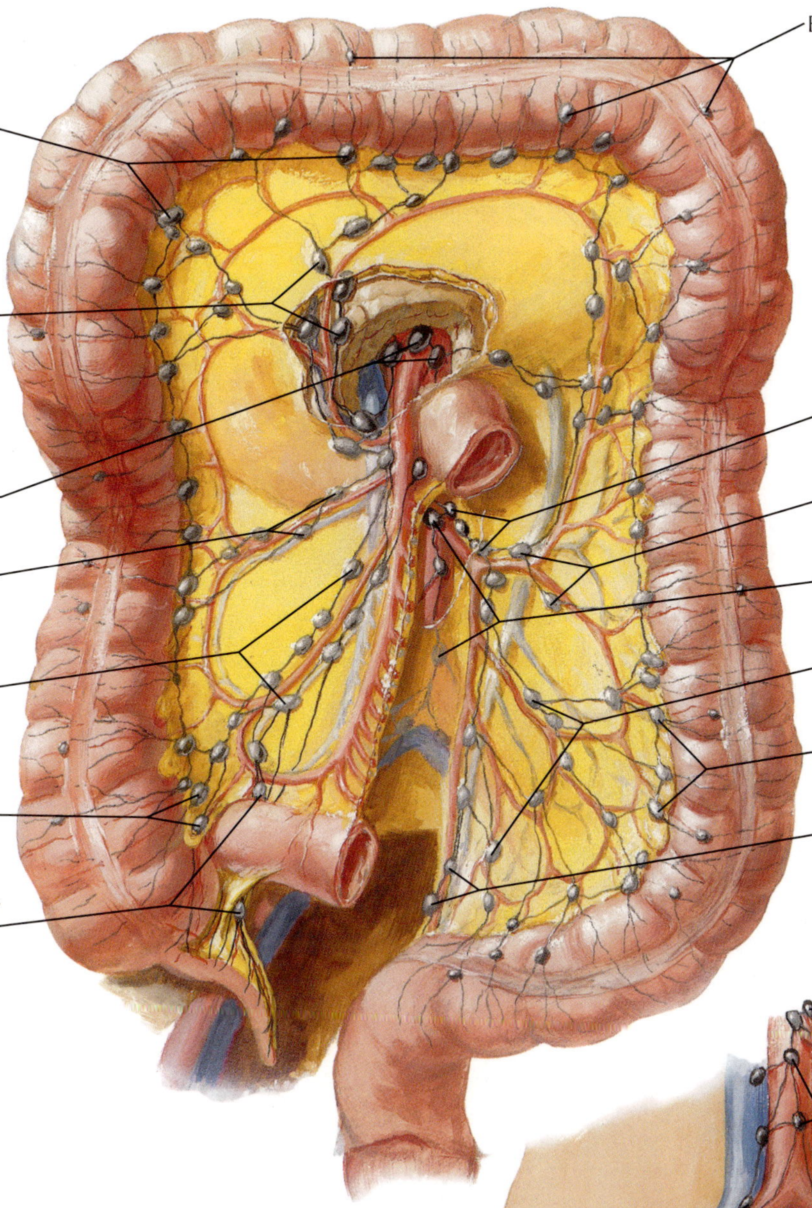

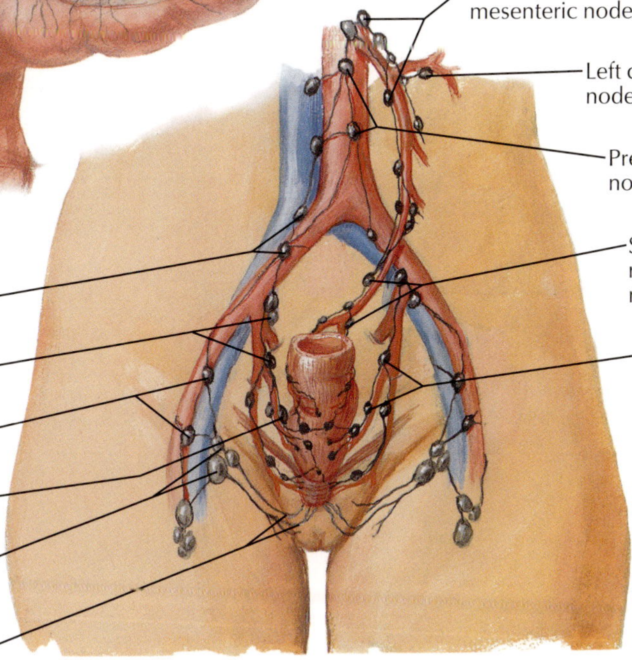

Autonomic Nerves and Ganglia of Abdomen

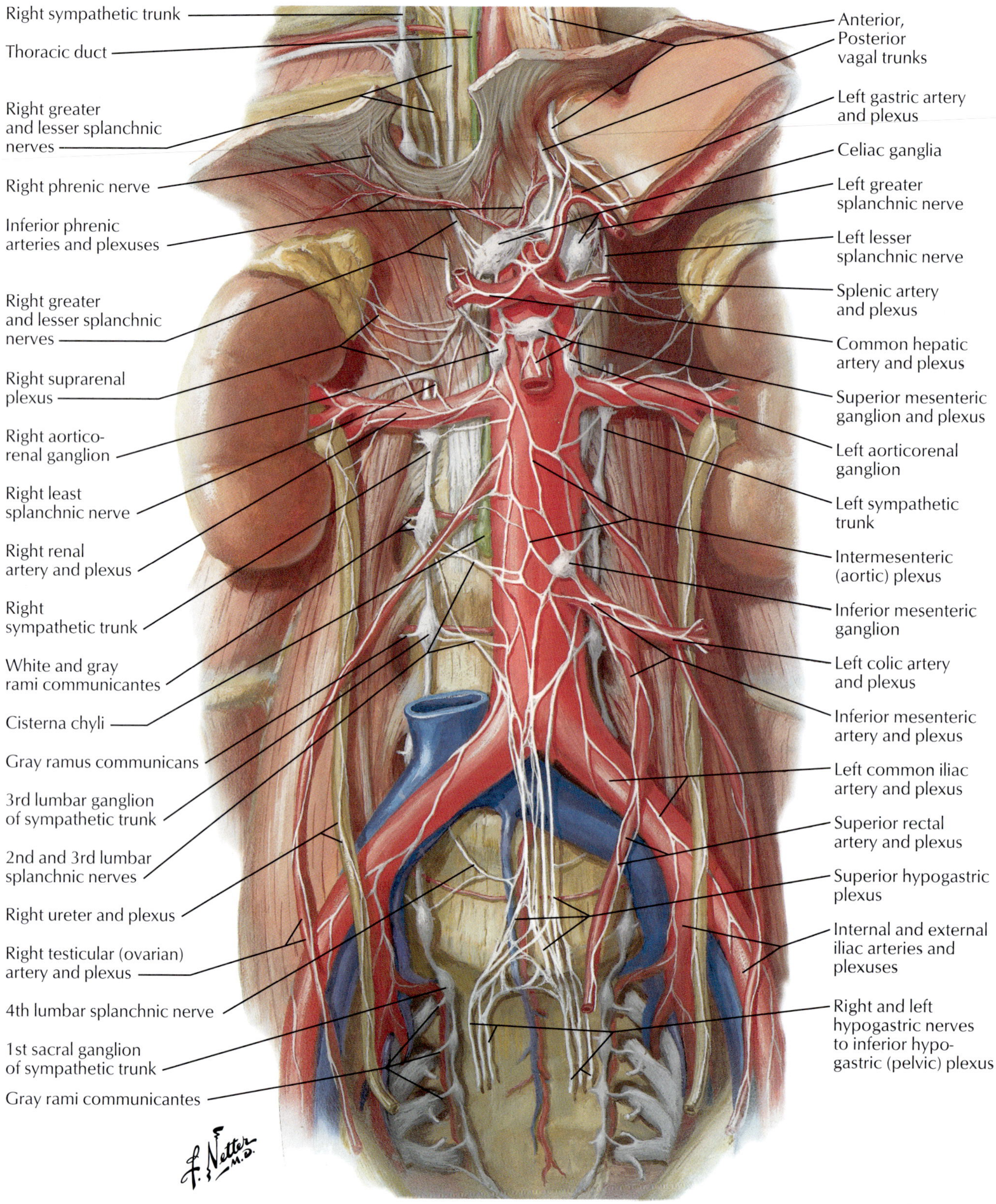

Autonomic Innervation of Stomach and Duodenum

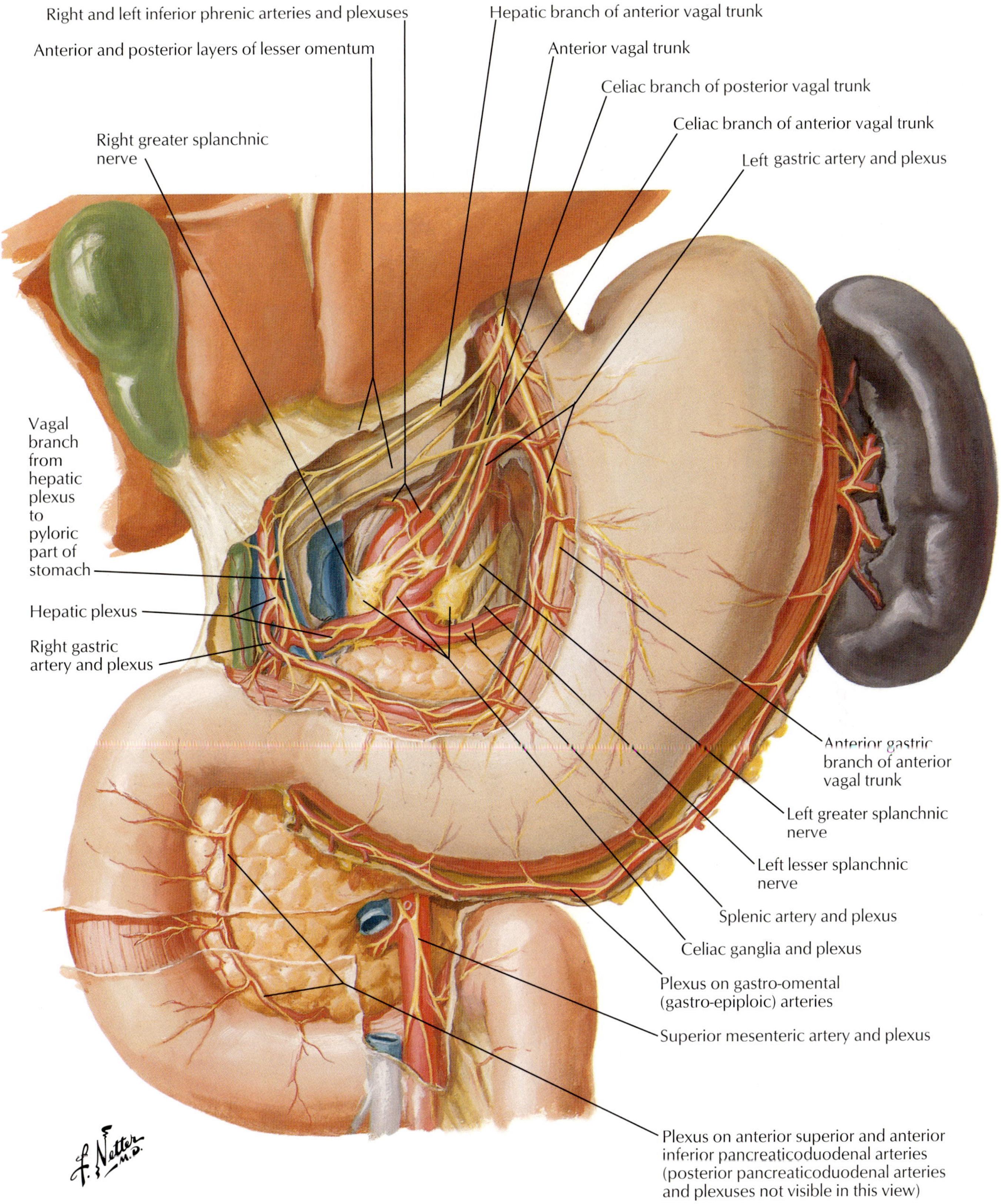

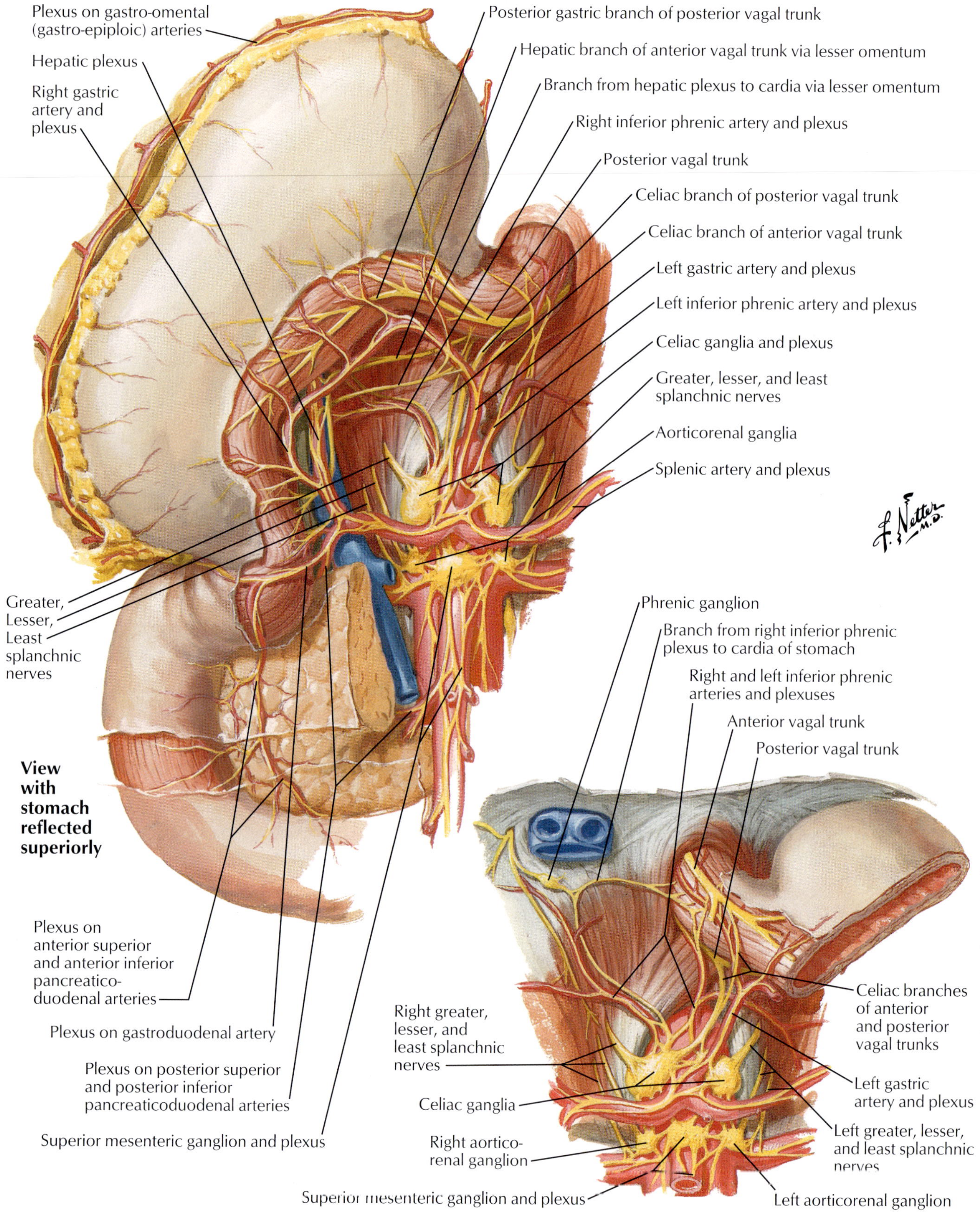
Plexus on gastro-omental (gastro-epiploic) arteries
Hepatic plexus
Right gastric artery and plexus
Posterior gastric branch of posterior vagal trunk
Hepatic branch of anterior vagal trunk via lesser omentum
Branch from hepatic plexus to cardia via lesser omentum
Right inferior phrenic artery and plexus
Posterior vagal trunk
Celiac branch of posterior vagal trunk
Celiac branch of anterior vagal trunk
Left gastric artery and plexus
Left inferior phrenic artery and plexus
Celiac ganglia and plexus
Greater, lesser, and least splanchnic nerves
Aorticorenal ganglia
Splenic artery and plexus
Greater, Lesser, Least splanchnic nerves
View with stomach reflected superiorly
Plexus on anterior superior and anterior inferior pancreaticoduodenal arteries
Plexus on gastroduodenal artery
Plexus on posterior superior and posterior inferior pancreaticoduodenal arteries
Superior mesenteric ganglion and plexus
Phrenic ganglion
Branch from right inferior phrenic plexus to cardia of stomach
Right and left inferior phrenic arteries and plexuses
Anterior vagal trunk
Posterior vagal trunk
Celiac branches of anterior and posterior vagal trunks
Right greater, lesser, and least splanchnic nerves
Left gastric artery and plexus
Celiac ganglia
Left greater, lesser, and least splanchnic nerves
Right aortico-renal ganglion
Superior mesenteric ganglion and plexus
Left aorticorenal ganglion

Autonomic Innervation of Stomach and Duodenum: Schema

See also Plates 163, 164

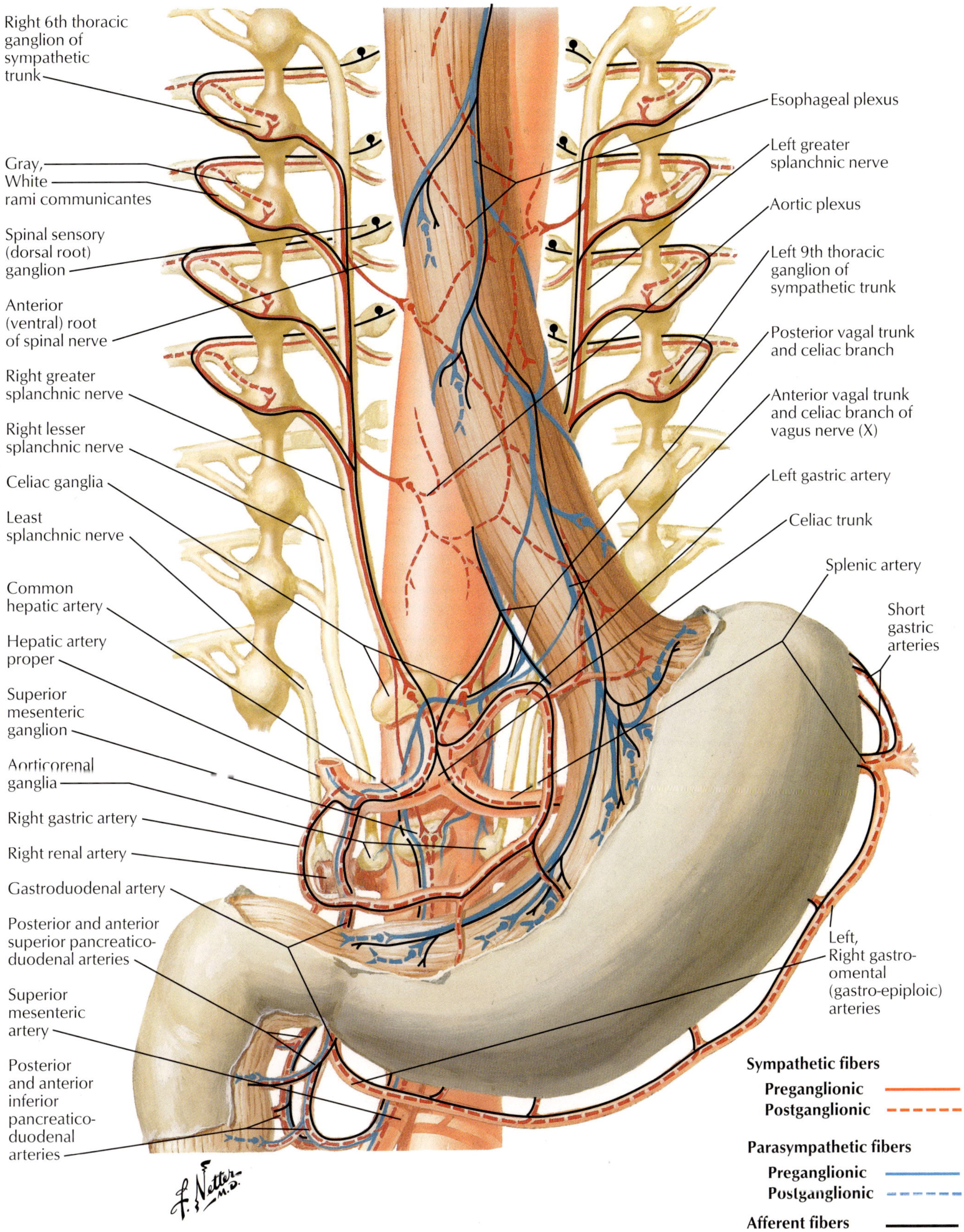

Autonomic Innervation of Small Intestine

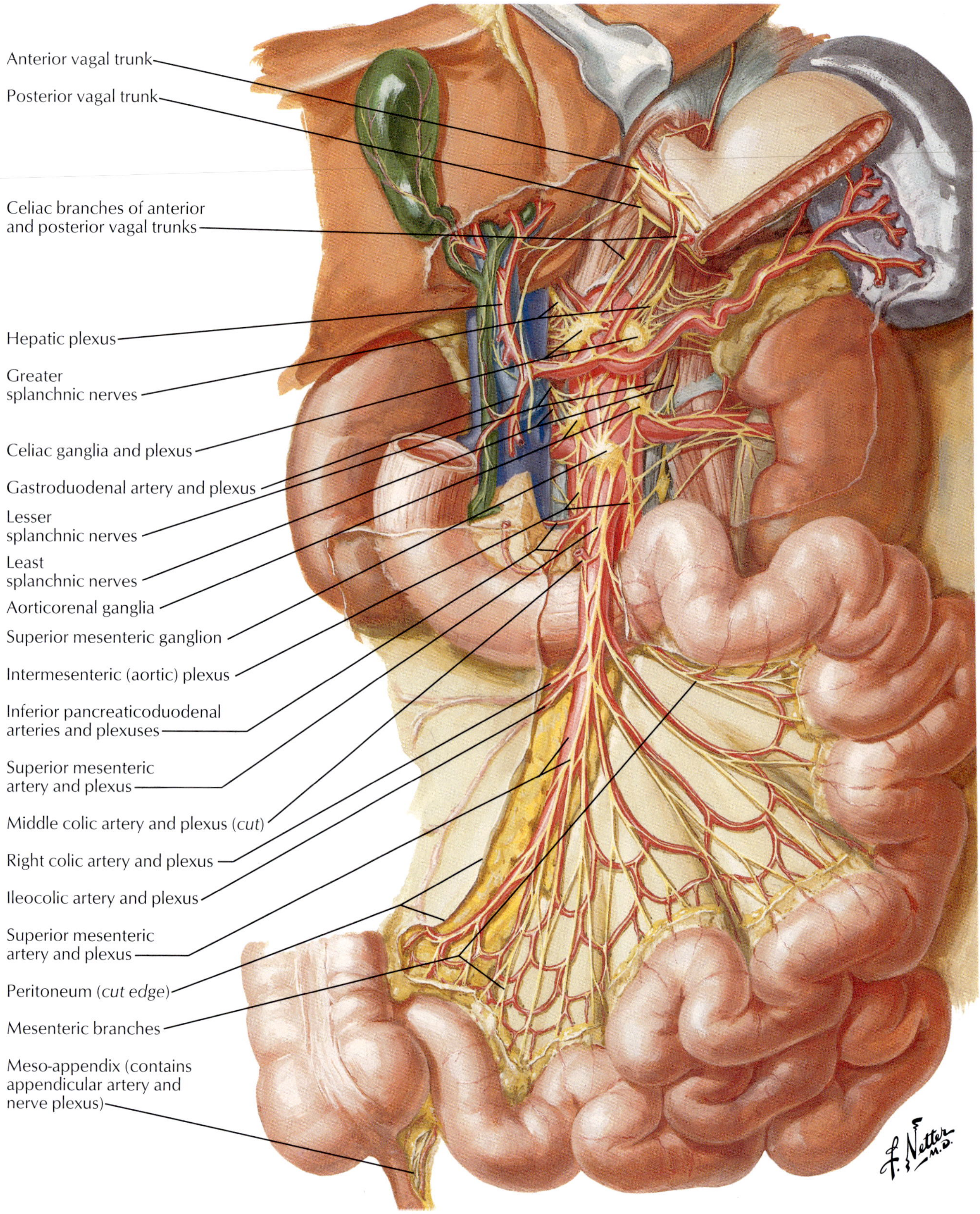

Autonomic Innervation of Large Intestine

For nerves of rectum see Plates 388–391

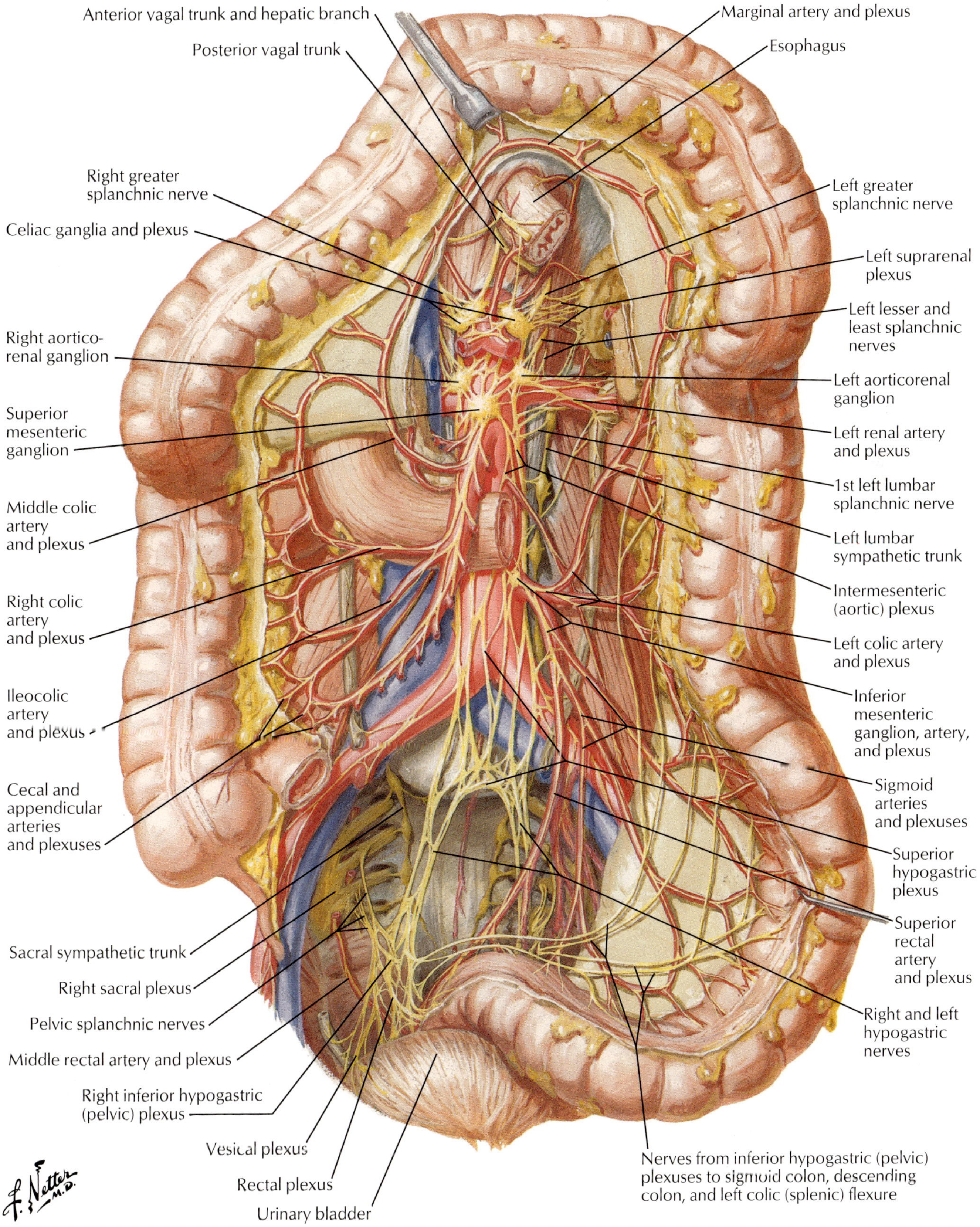

Autonomic Innervation of Small and Large Intestines: Schema

See also Plates 163, 164

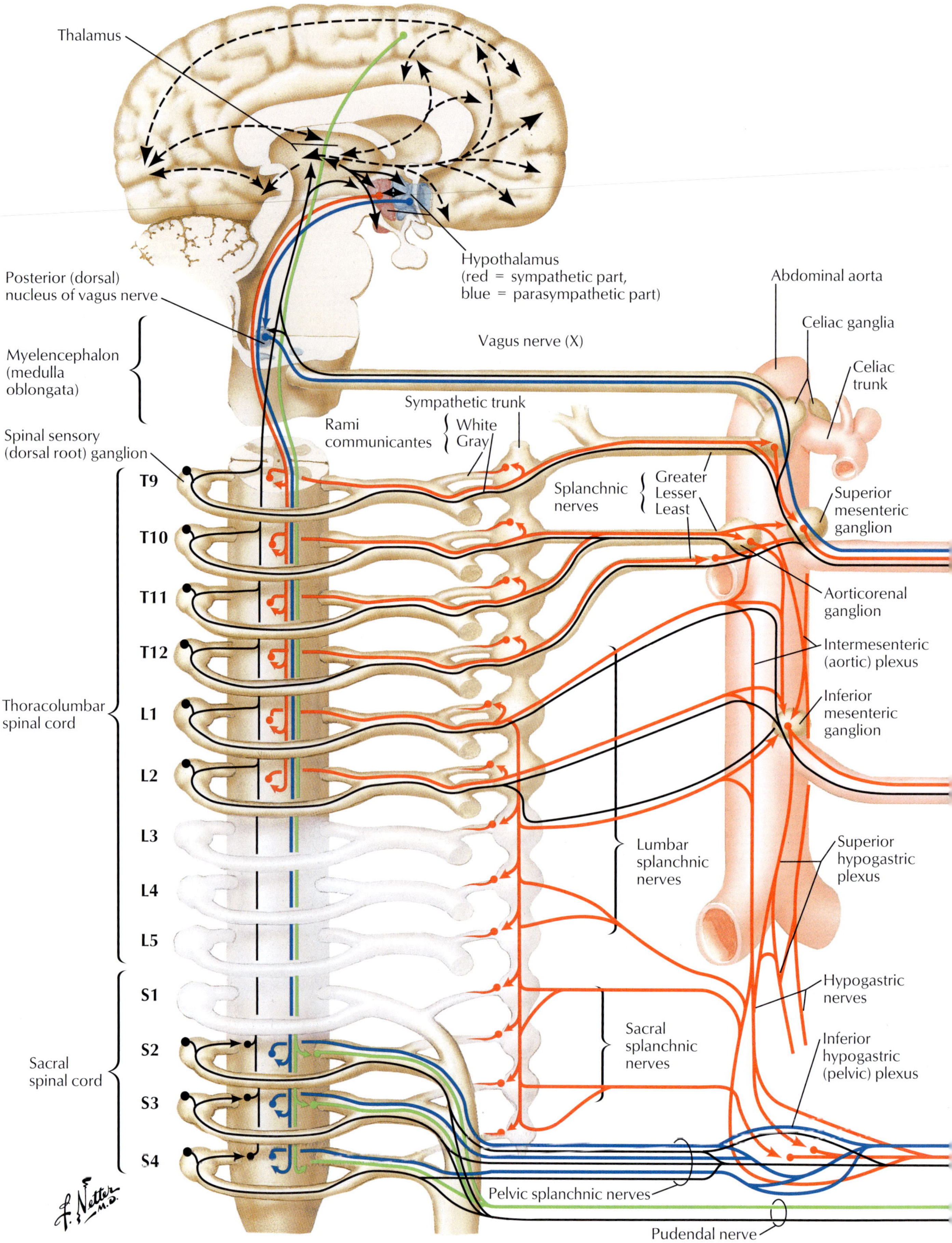

Autonomic Innervation of Small and Large Intestines: Schema

See also **Plates 163, 164**

Sympathetic efferents
Parasympathetic efferents
Somatic efferents
Afferents and CNS connections
Indefinite paths

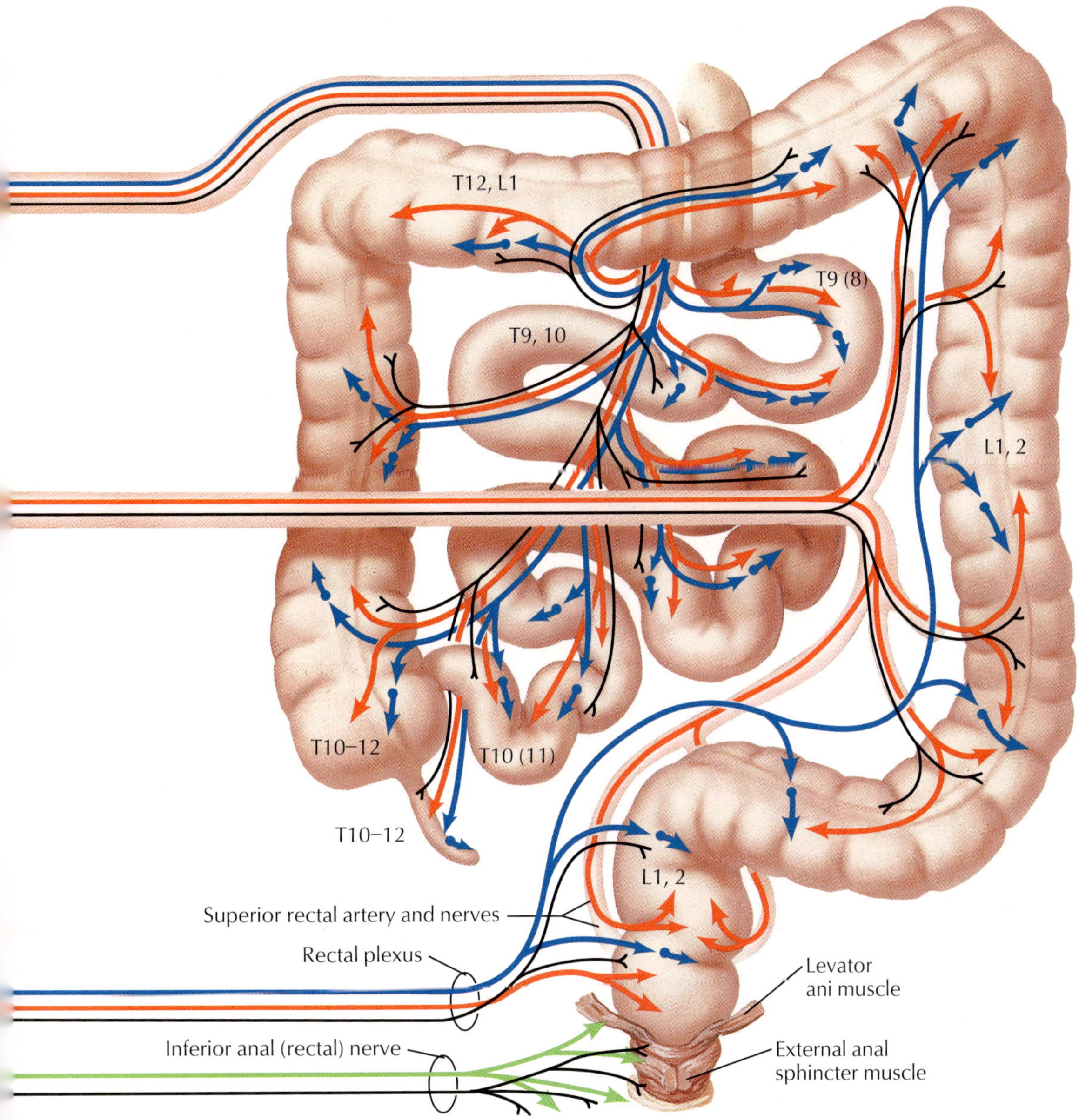

Chief segmental sources of sympathetic fibers innervating different regions of intestinal tract are indicated. Numerous afferent fibers are carried centripetally through approximately the same sympathetic splanchnic nerves that transmit preganglionic fibers.

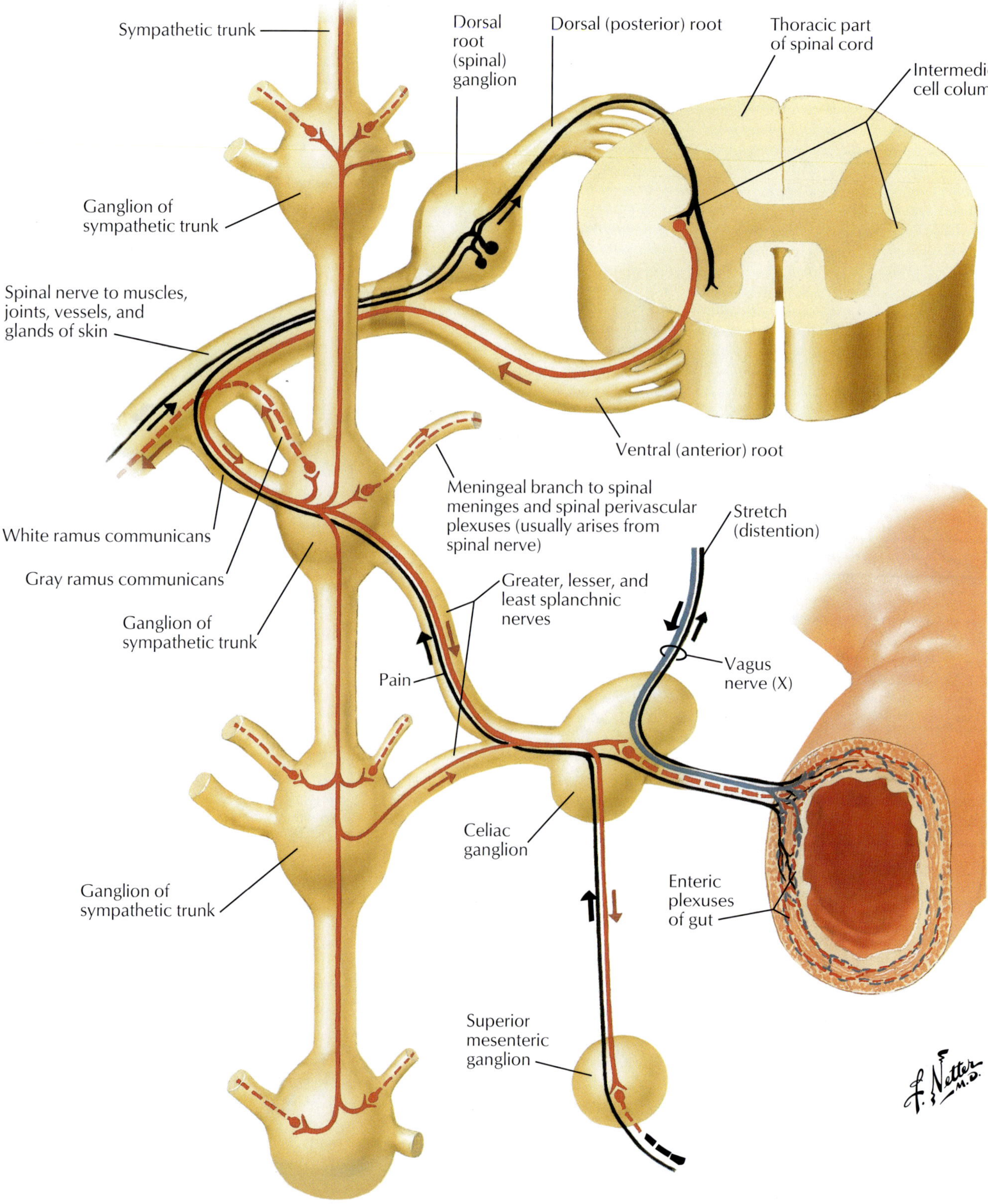

Sympathetic fibers { **Preganglionic** —— **Postganglionic** - - - -

Parasympathetic fibers { **Preganglionic** —— **Postganglionic** - - - -

Afferent fibers ——

Intrinsic Autonomic Plexuses of Intestine: Schema

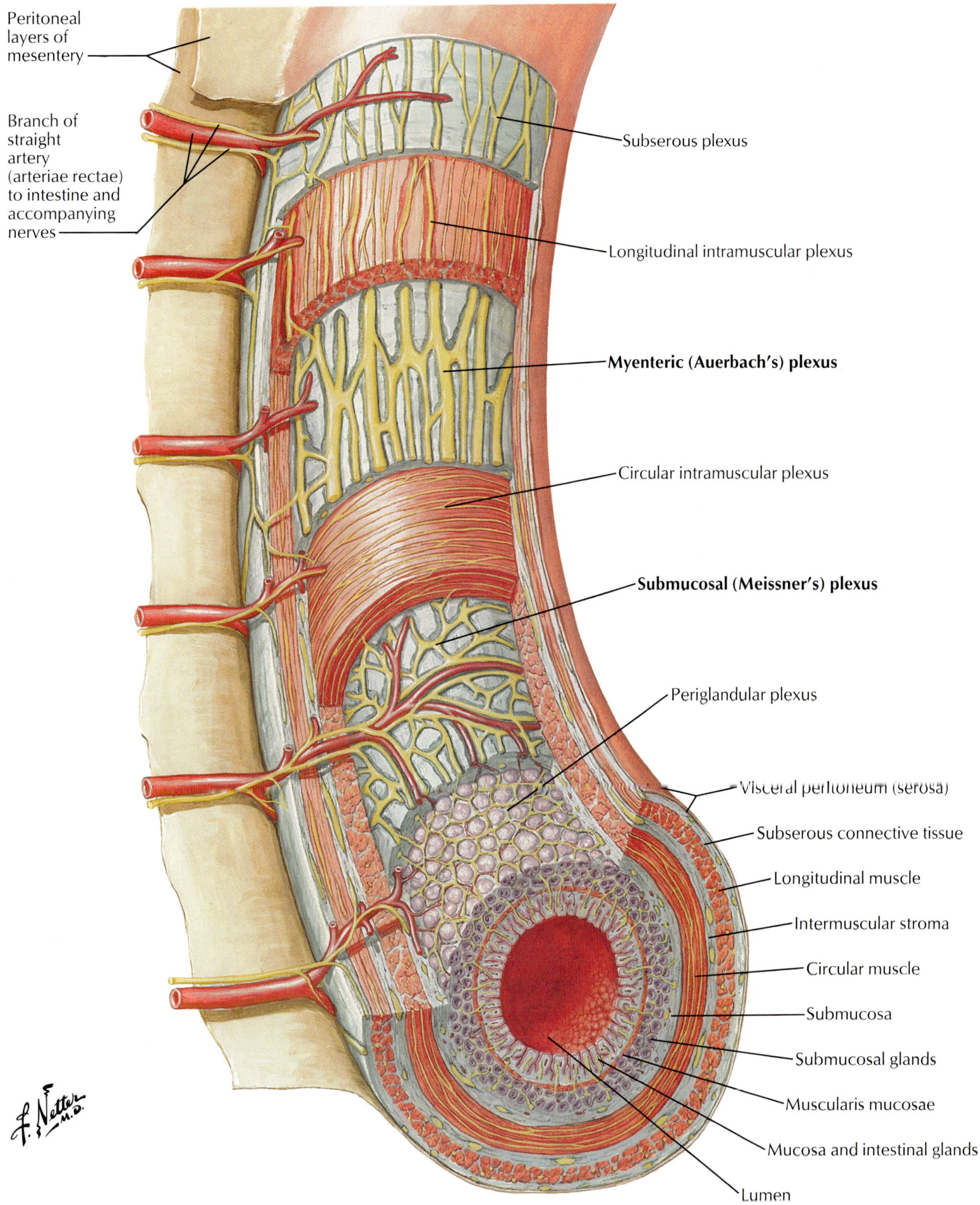

Note: Intestinal wall is shown much thicker than in actuality.

Autonomic Innervation of Liver and Biliary Tract: Schema

See also **Plates 163, 164**

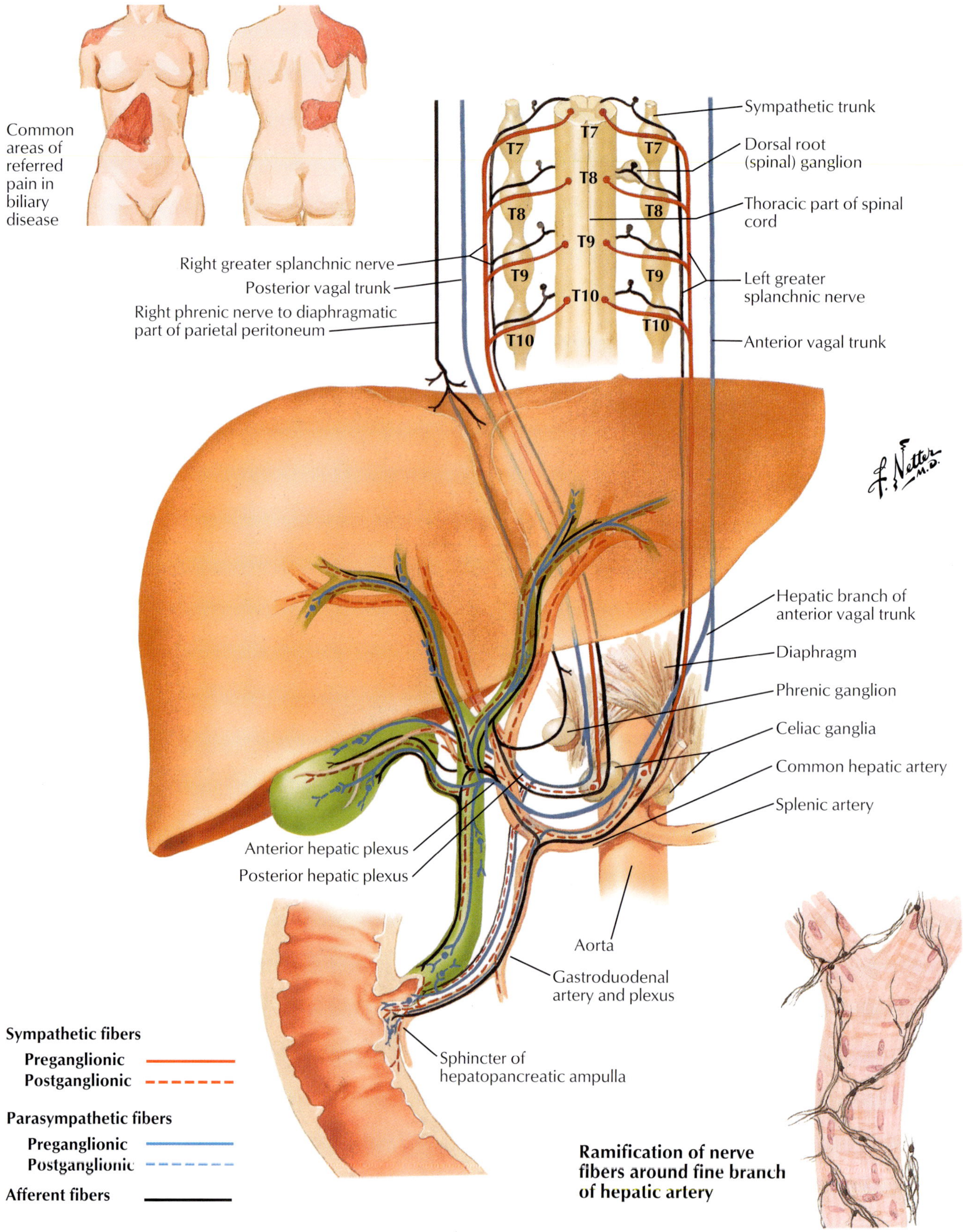

Autonomic Innervation of Pancreas: Schema

See also Plates 163, 164

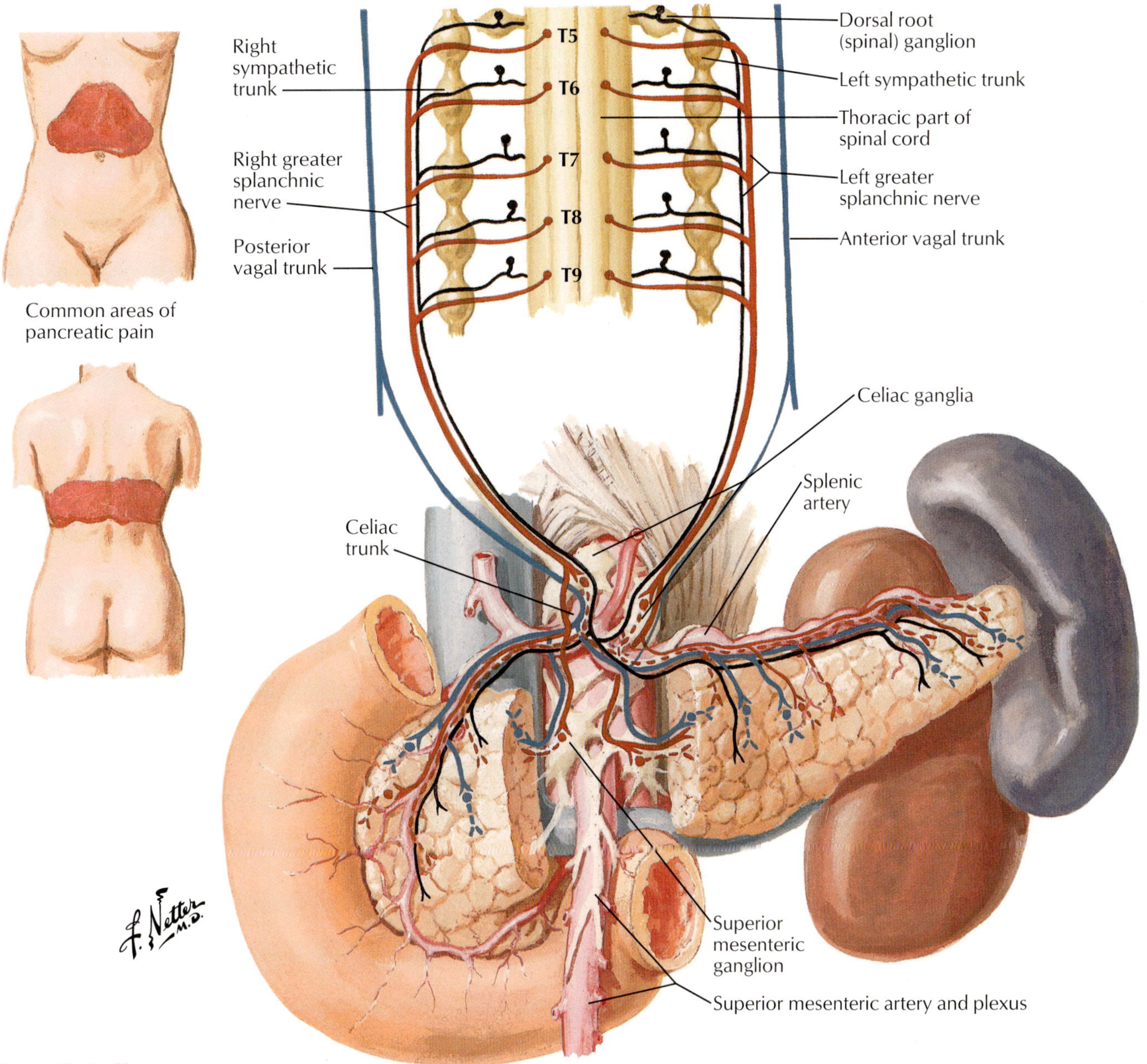

Sympathetic fibers

- **Preganglionic** ———
- **Postganglionic** - - - - -

Parasympathetic fibers

- **Preganglionic** ———
- **Postganglionic** - - - - -

Afferent fibers ———

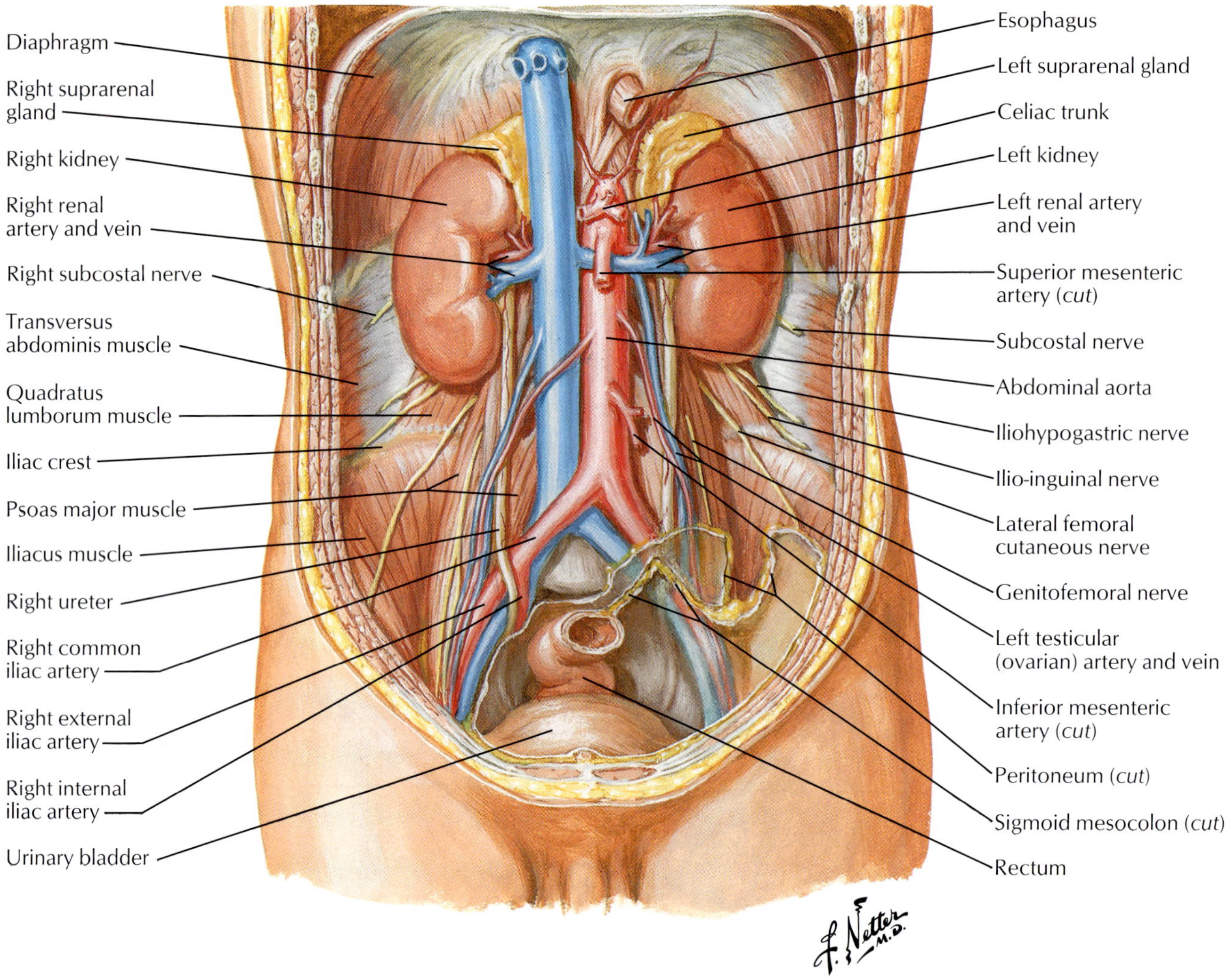

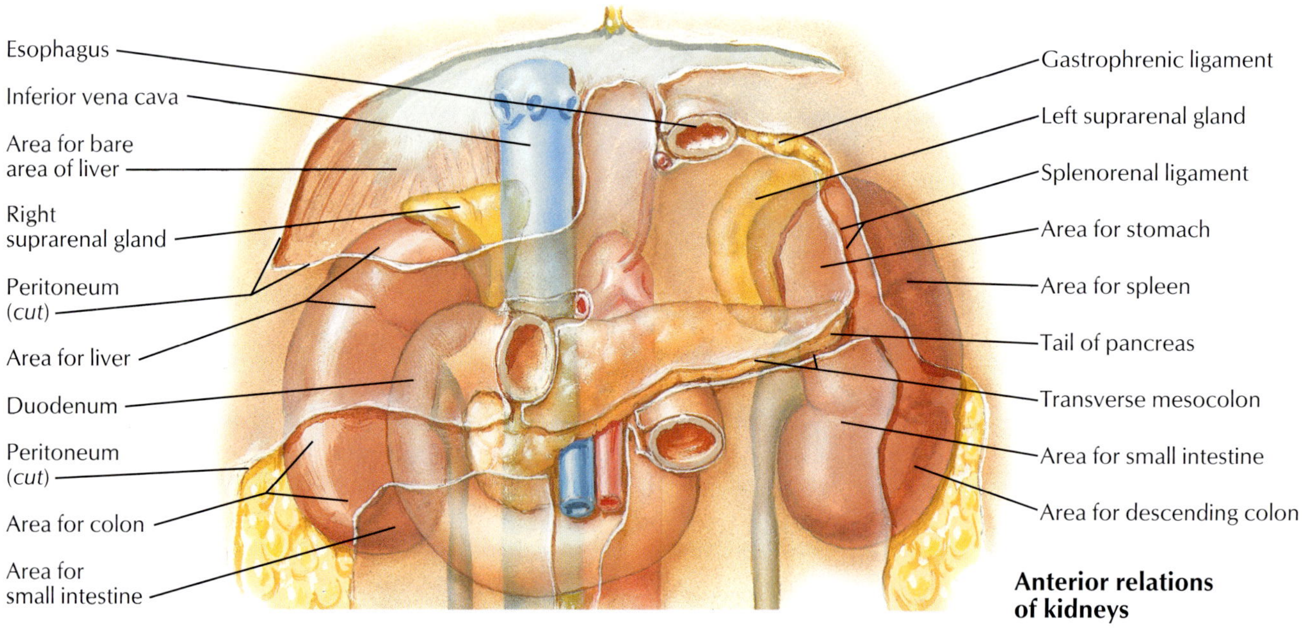

Anterior relations of kidneys

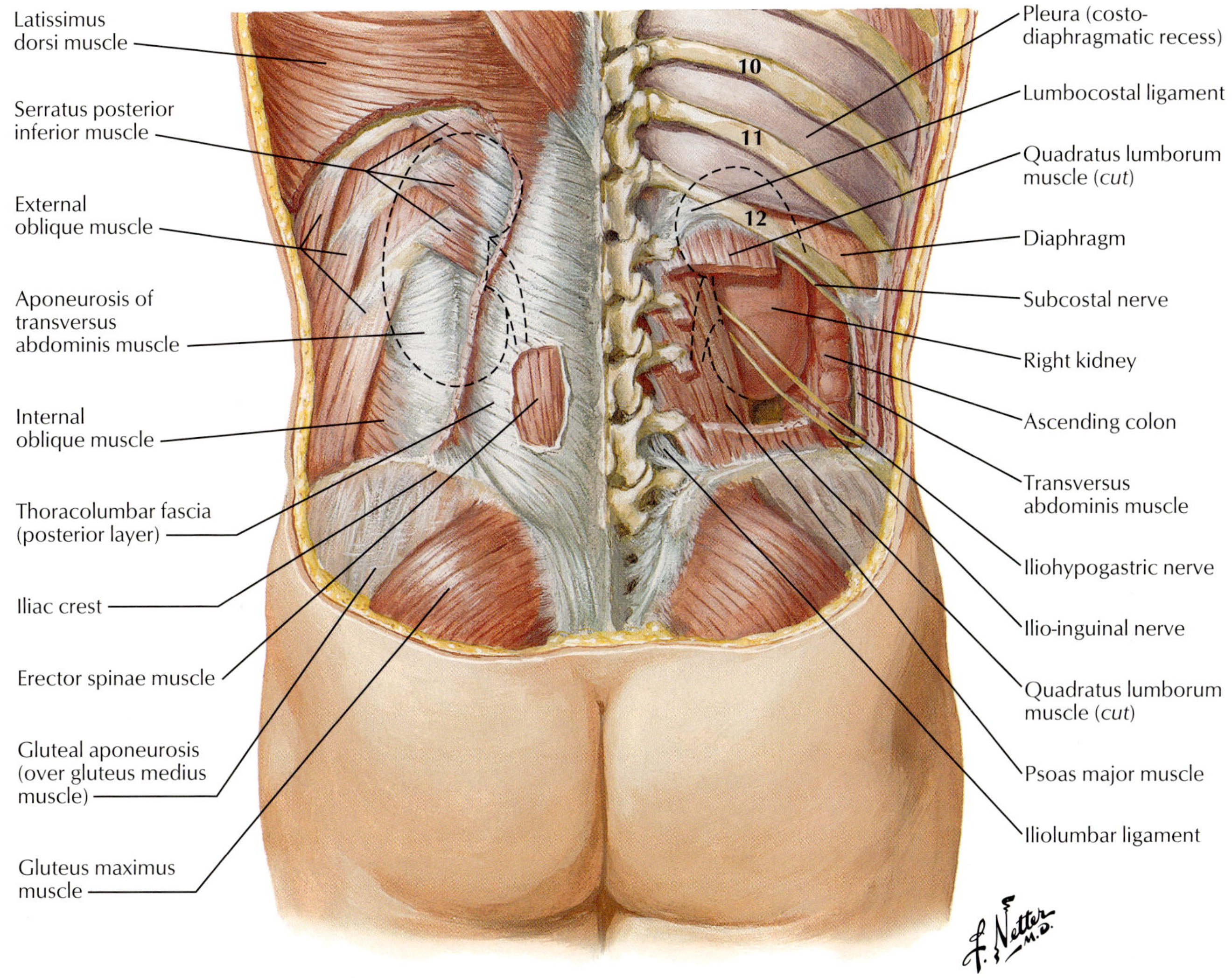

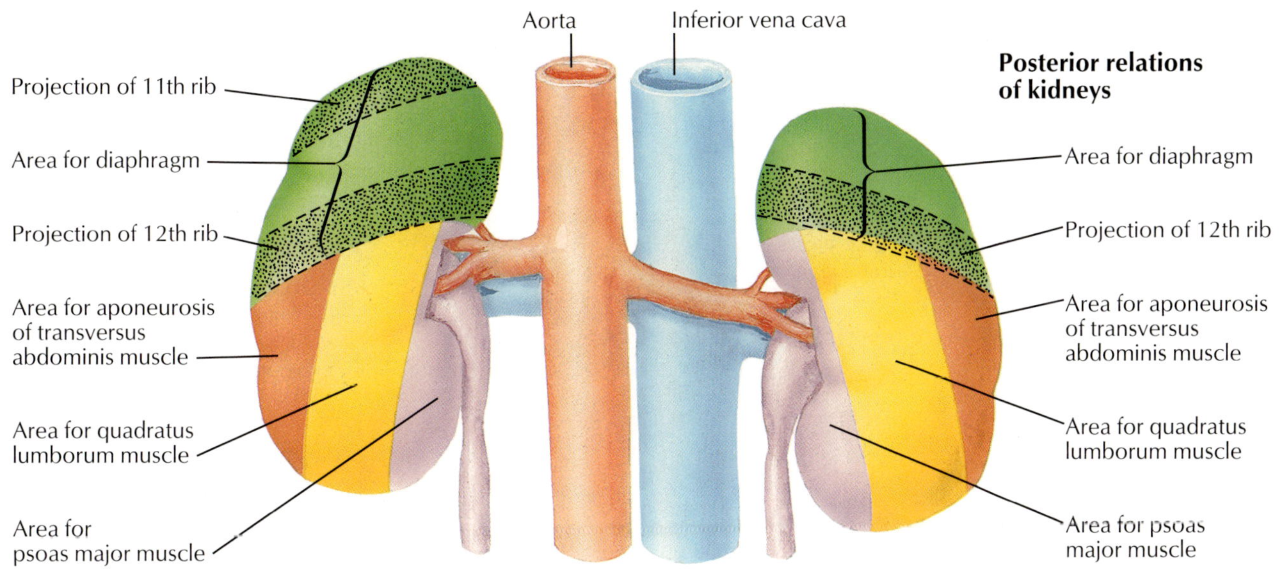

Posterior relations of kidneys

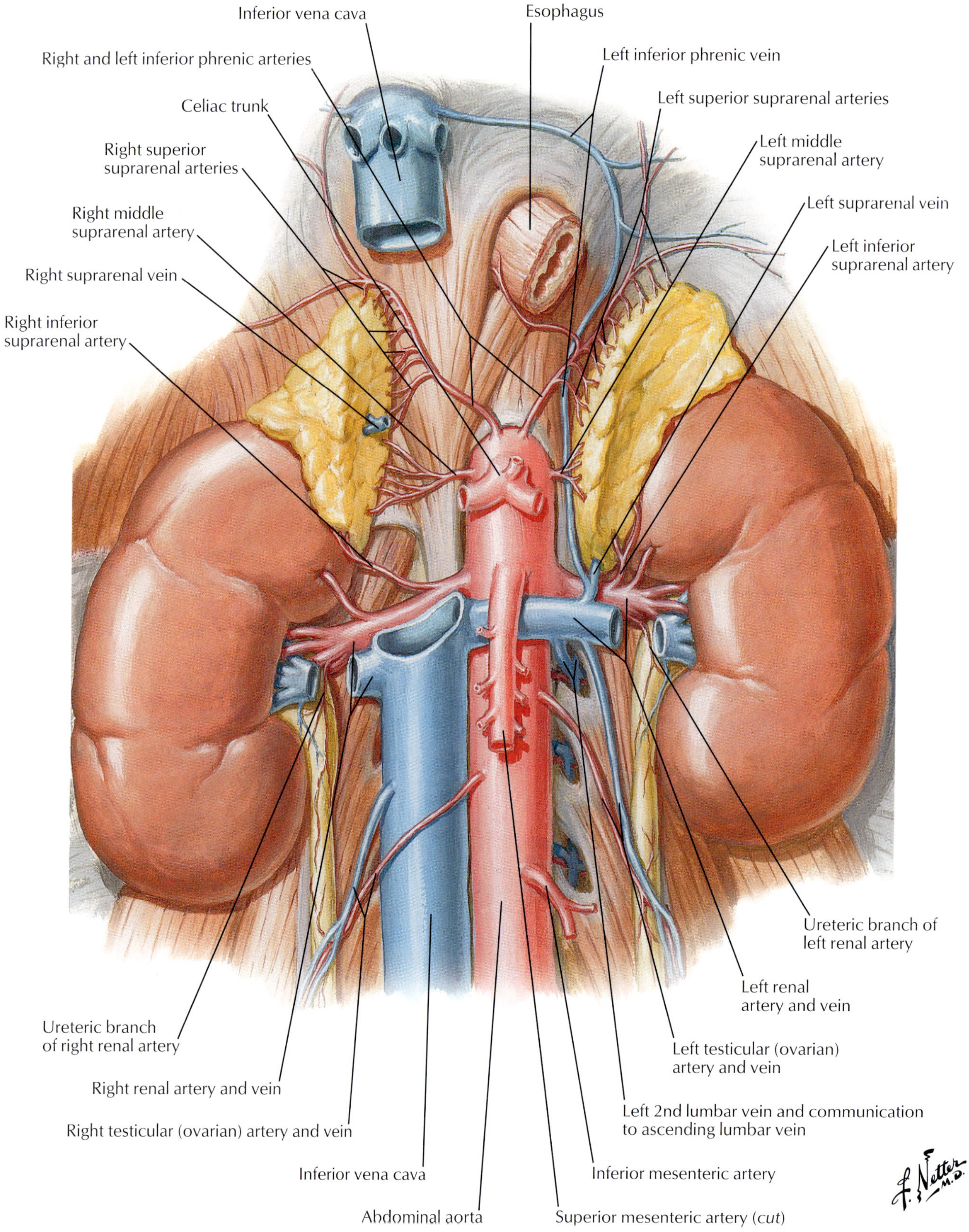

Inferior vena cava
Esophagus
Right and left inferior phrenic arteries
Left inferior phrenic vein
Celiac trunk
Left superior suprarenal arteries
Right superior suprarenal arteries
Left middle suprarenal artery
Right middle suprarenal artery
Left suprarenal vein
Right suprarenal vein
Left inferior suprarenal artery
Right inferior suprarenal artery
Ureteric branch of left renal artery
Left renal artery and vein
Ureteric branch of right renal artery
Left testicular (ovarian) artery and vein
Right renal artery and vein
Left 2nd lumbar vein and communication to ascending lumbar vein
Right testicular (ovarian) artery and vein
Inferior vena cava
Inferior mesenteric artery
Abdominal aorta
Superior mesenteric artery (*cut*)

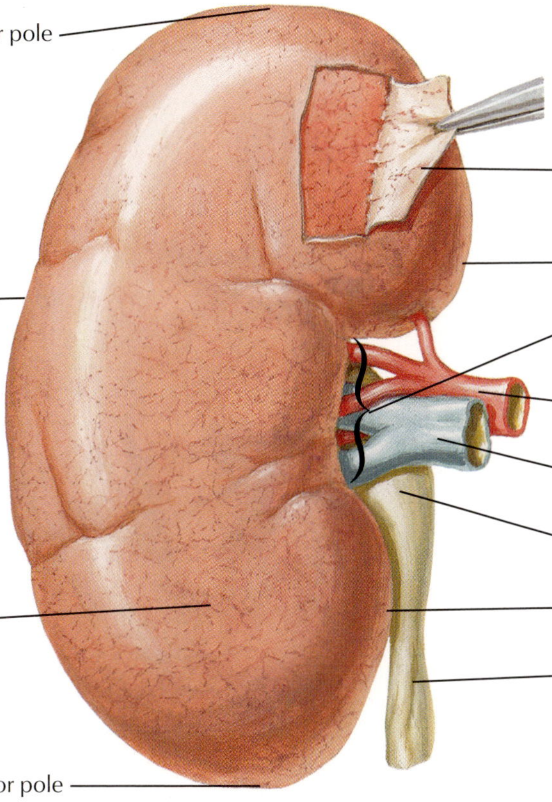

Anterior surface of right kidney

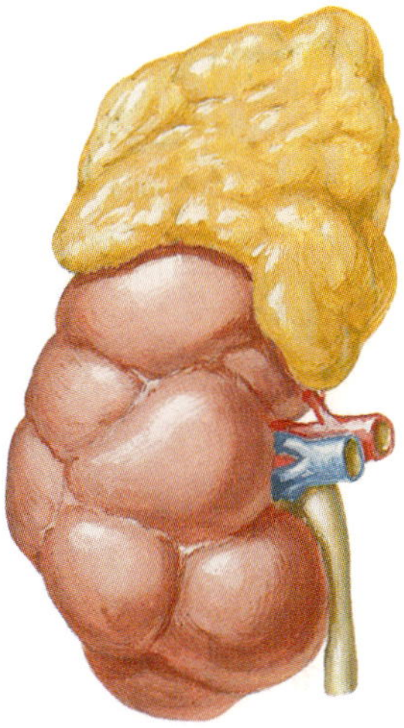

Suprarenal gland and lobulated kidney of infant

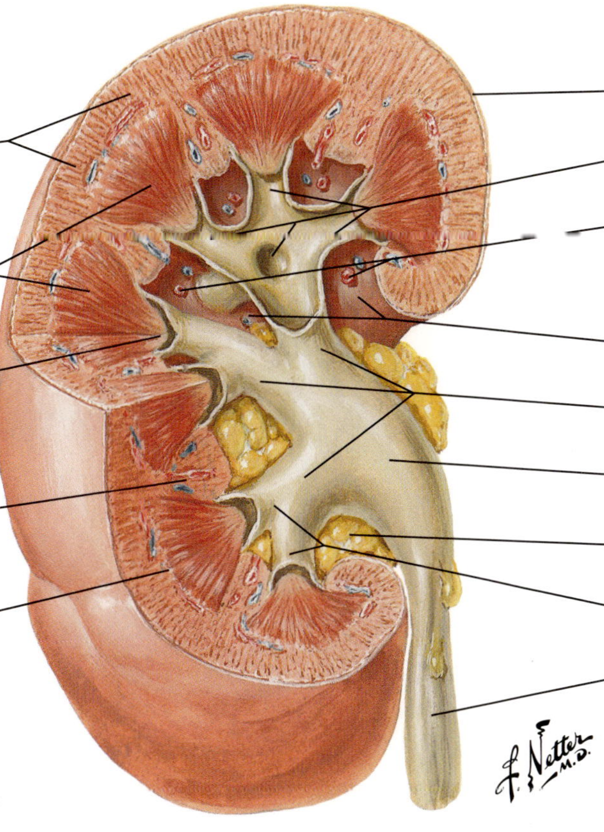

Right kidney sectioned in several planes, exposing parenchyma and renal pelvis

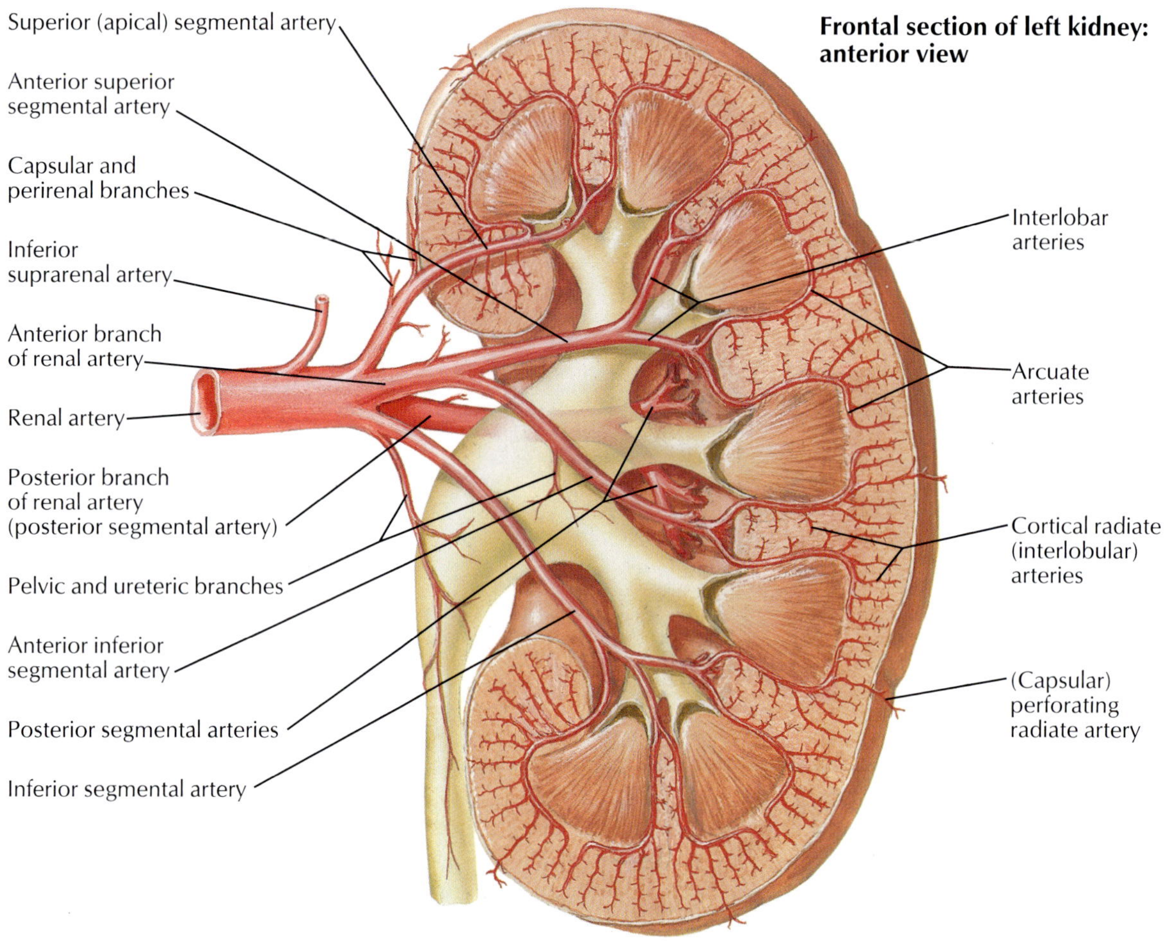
Frontal section of left kidney: anterior view
Superior (apical) segmental artery
Anterior superior segmental artery
Capsular and perirenal branches
Inferior suprarenal artery
Anterior branch of renal artery
Renal artery
Posterior branch of renal artery (posterior segmental artery)
Pelvic and ureteric branches
Anterior inferior segmental artery
Posterior segmental arteries
Inferior segmental artery
Interlobar arteries
Arcuate arteries
Cortical radiate (interlobular) arteries
(Capsular) perforating radiate artery

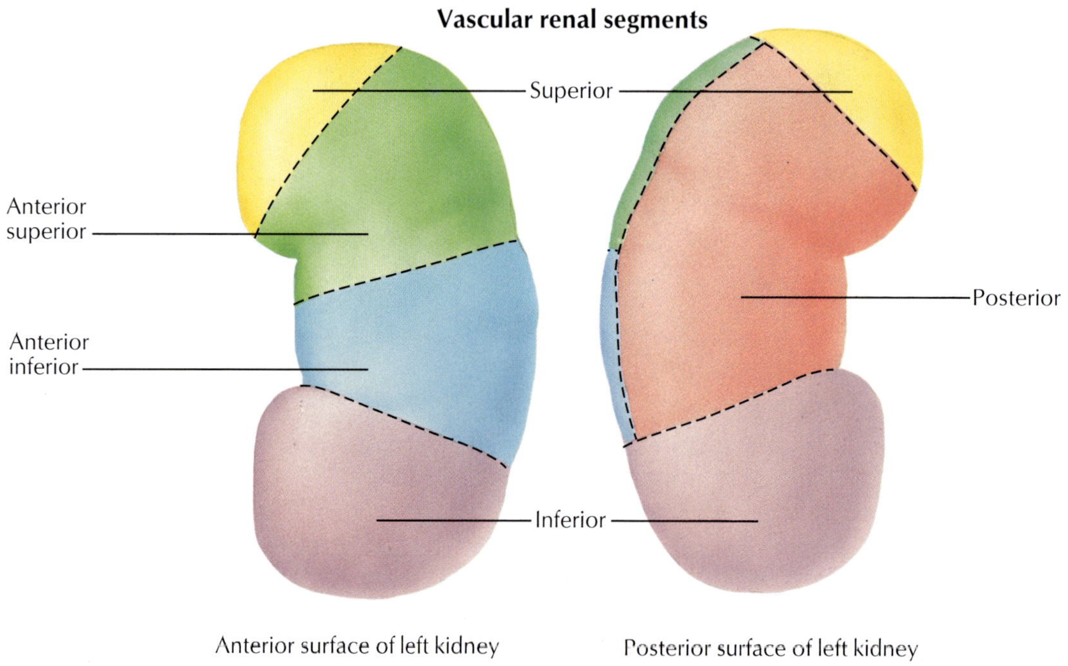
Vascular renal segments
Superior
Anterior superior
Anterior inferior
Inferior
Posterior
Anterior surface of left kidney
Posterior surface of left kidney

Ureters in Abdomen and Pelvis

See also **Plates 341, 342, 345**

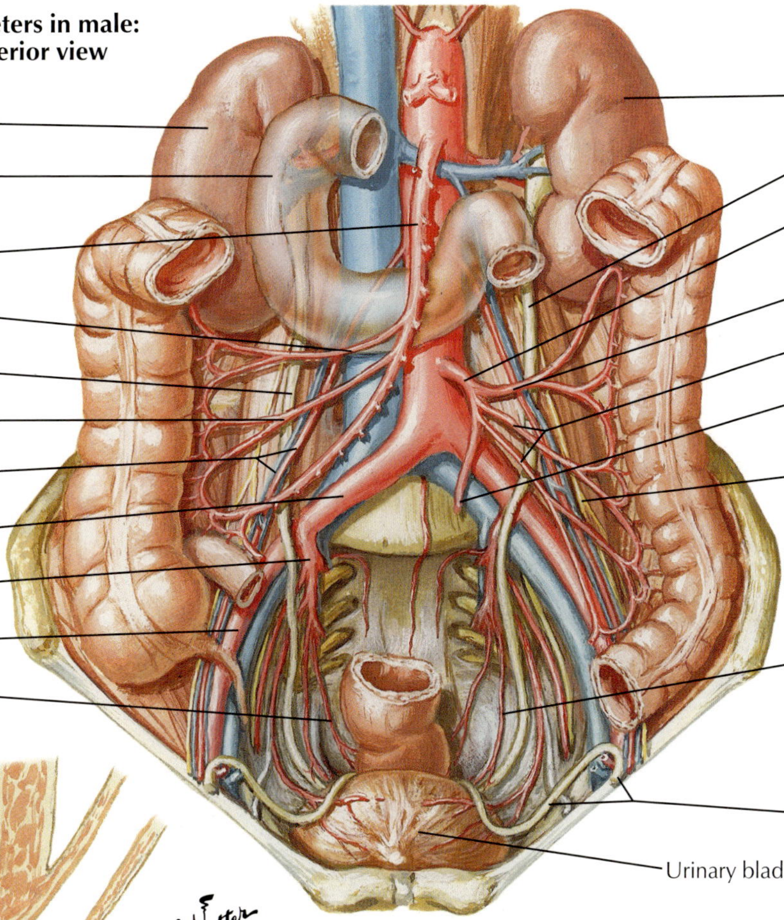

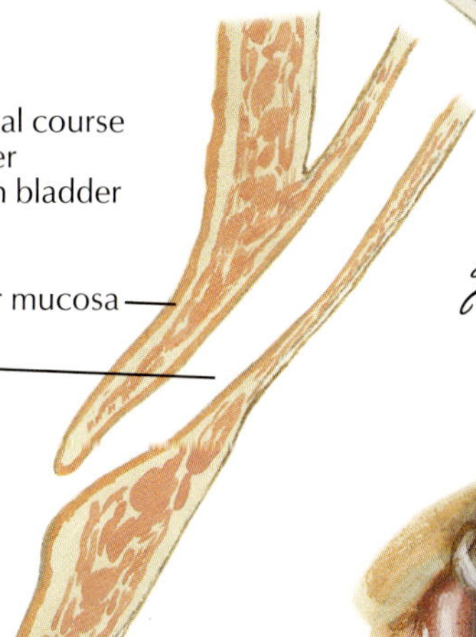

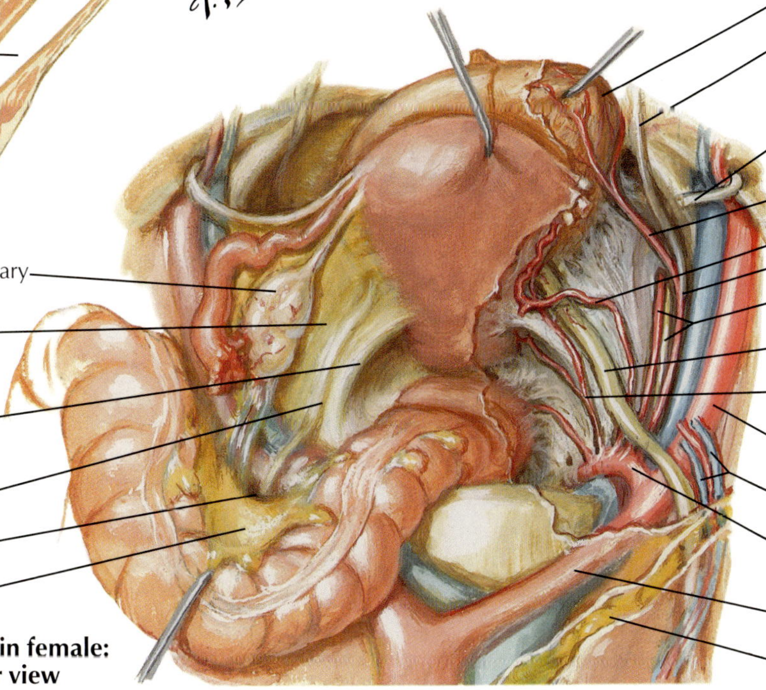

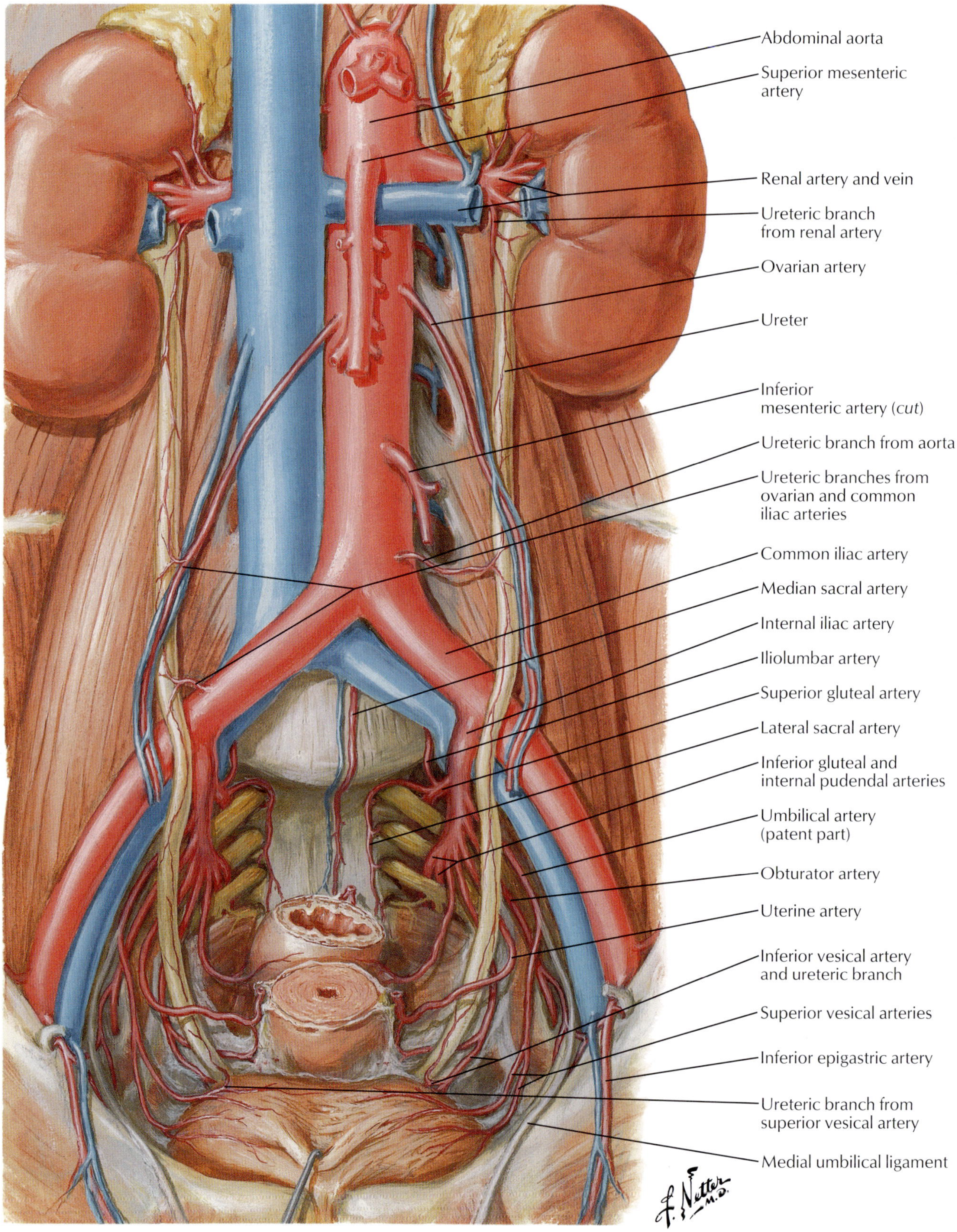
Abdominal aorta
Superior mesenteric artery
Renal artery and vein
Ureteric branch from renal artery
Ovarian artery
Ureter
Inferior mesenteric artery (*cut*)
Ureteric branch from aorta
Ureteric branches from ovarian and common iliac arteries
Common iliac artery
Median sacral artery
Internal iliac artery
Iliolumbar artery
Superior gluteal artery
Lateral sacral artery
Inferior gluteal and internal pudendal arteries
Umbilical artery (patent part)
Obturator artery
Uterine artery
Inferior vesical artery and ureteric branch
Superior vesical arteries
Inferior epigastric artery
Ureteric branch from superior vesical artery
Medial umbilical ligament

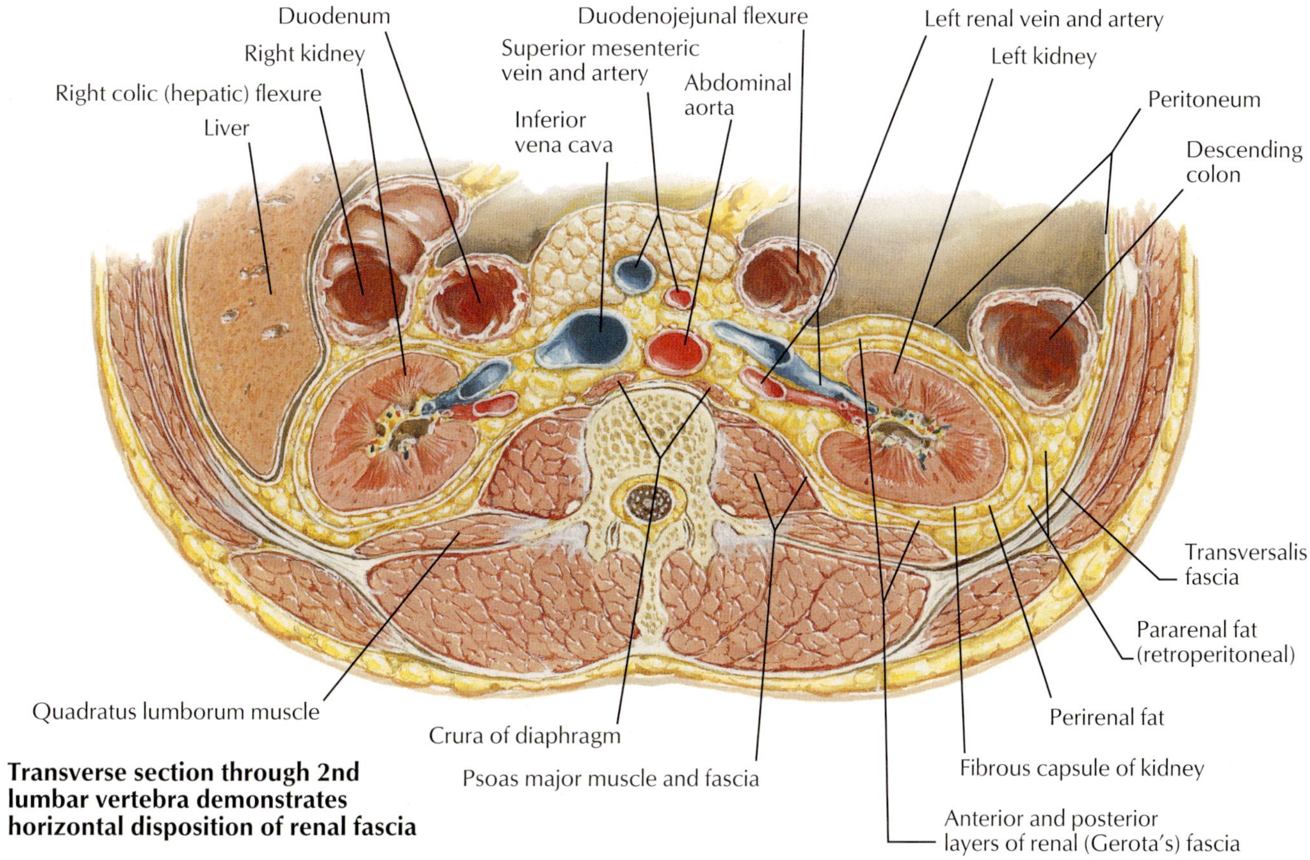

Transverse section through 2nd lumbar vertebra demonstrates horizontal disposition of renal fascia

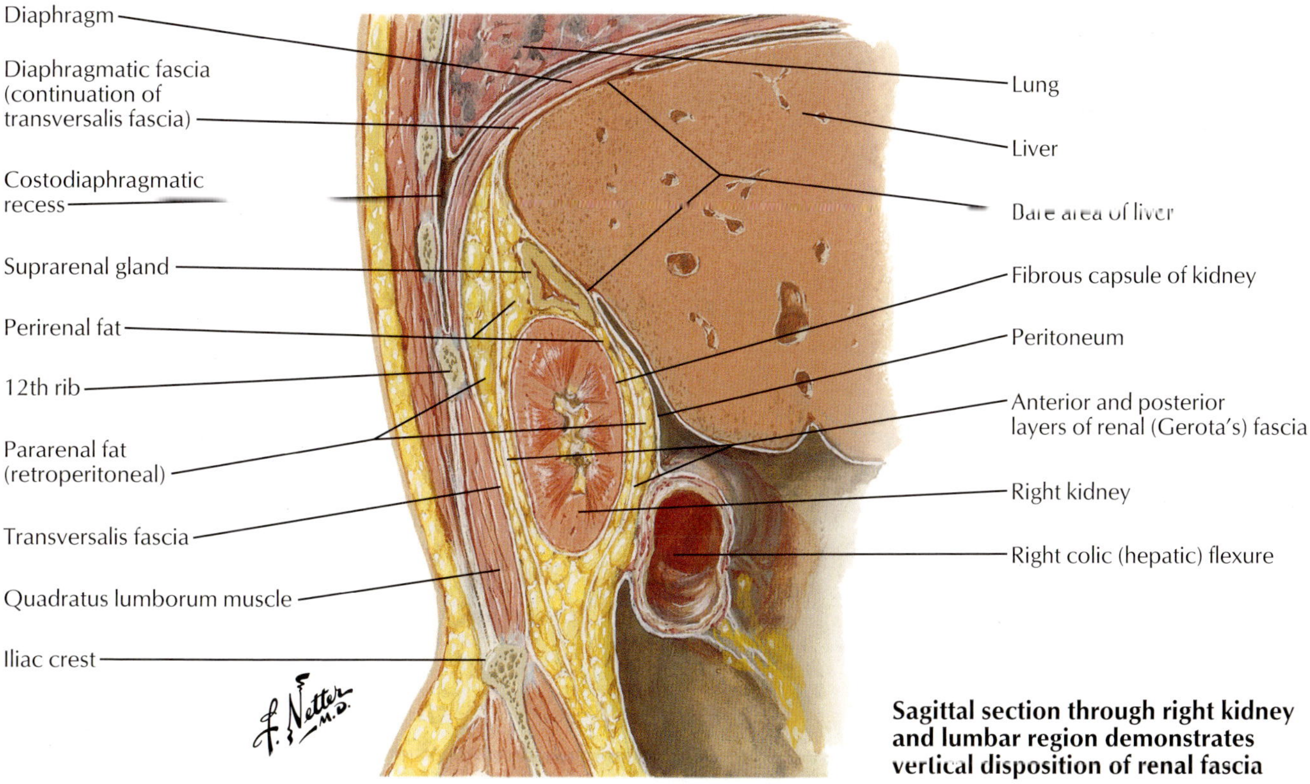

Sagittal section through right kidney and lumbar region demonstrates vertical disposition of renal fascia

Lymph Vessels and Nodes of Kidneys and Urinary Bladder

See also Plates 384, 386

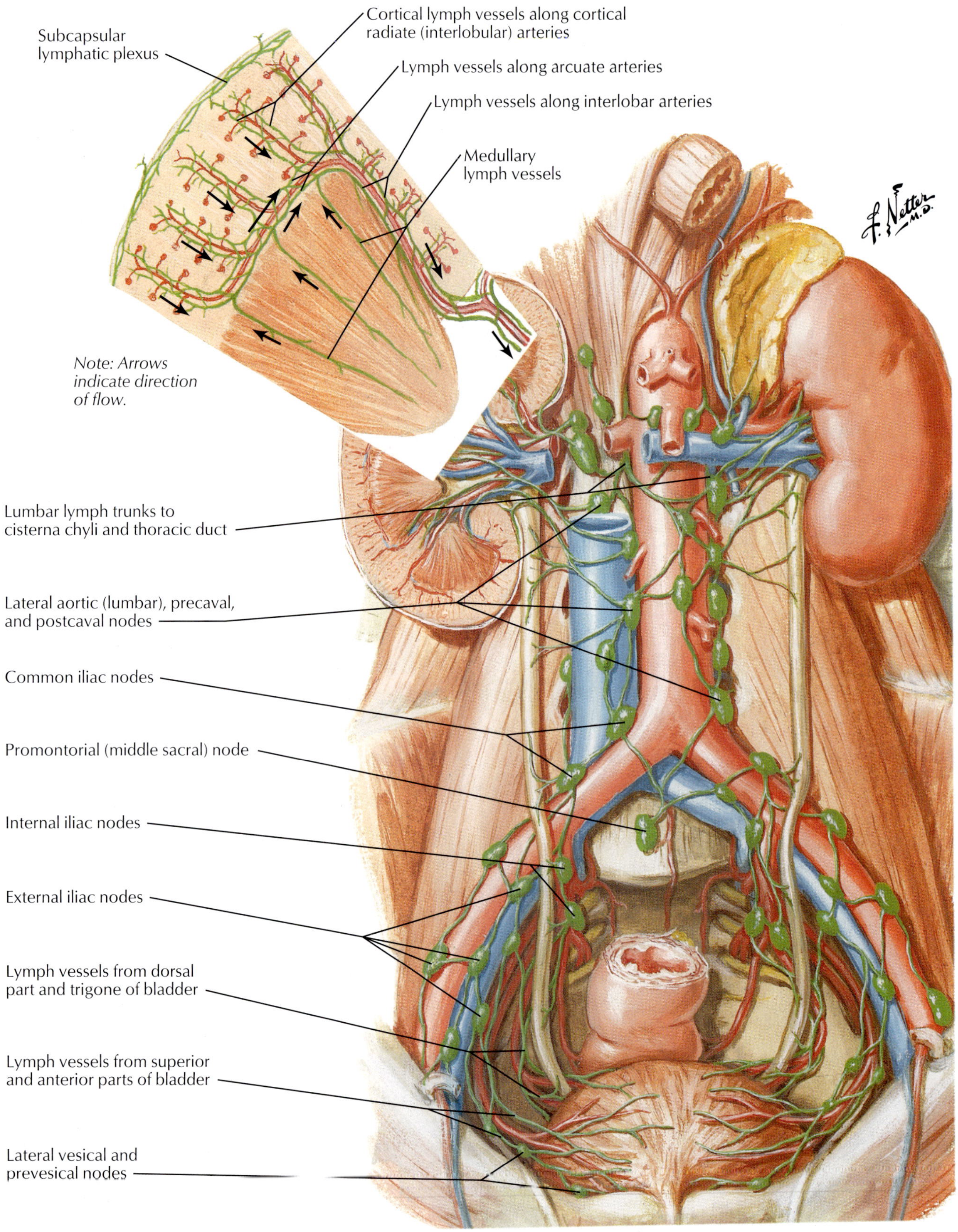

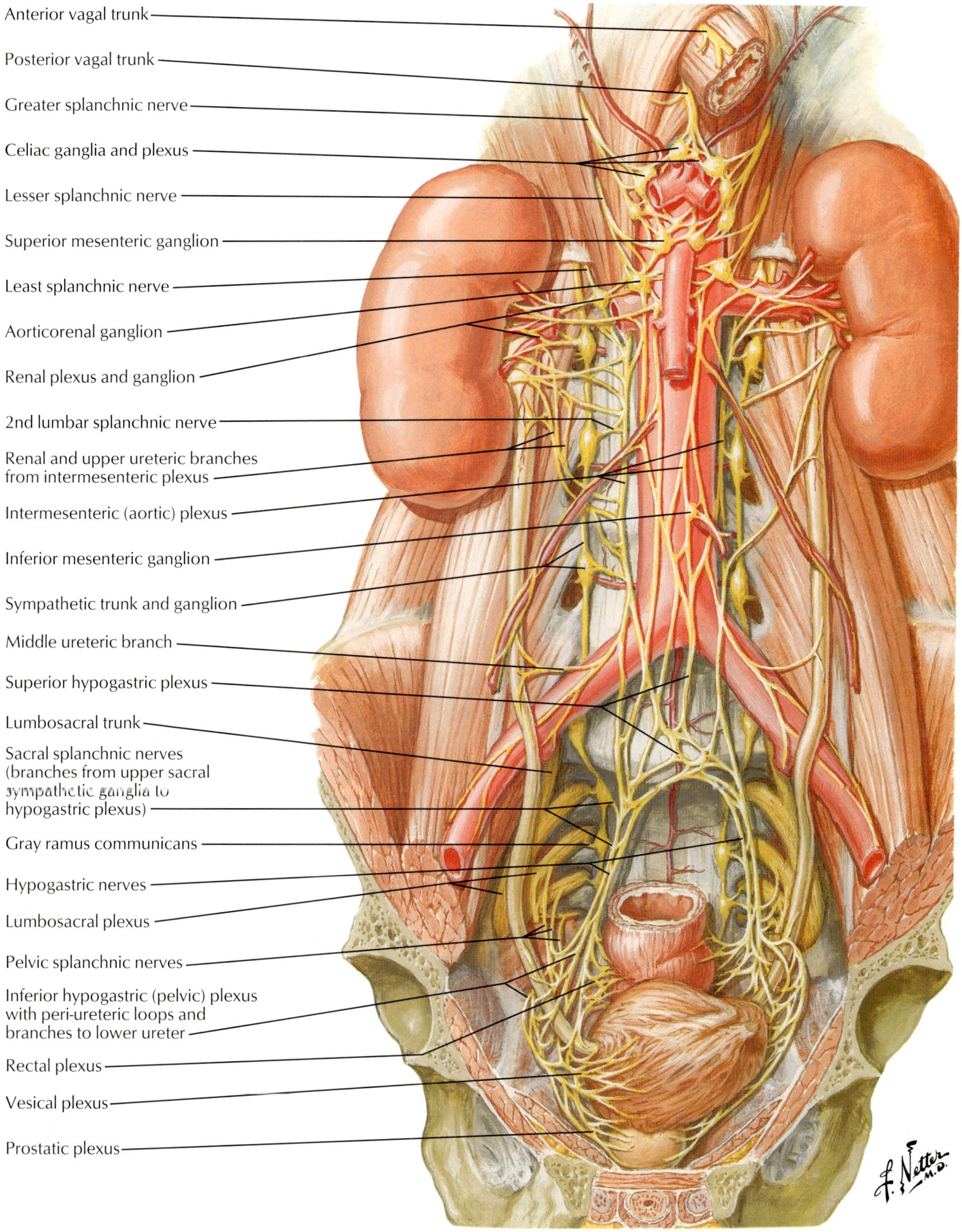
Anterior vagal trunk
Posterior vagal trunk
Greater splanchnic nerve
Celiac ganglia and plexus
Lesser splanchnic nerve
Superior mesenteric ganglion
Least splanchnic nerve
Aorticorenal ganglion
Renal plexus and ganglion
2nd lumbar splanchnic nerve
Renal and upper ureteric branches from intermesenteric plexus
Intermesenteric (aortic) plexus
Inferior mesenteric ganglion
Sympathetic trunk and ganglion
Middle ureteric branch
Superior hypogastric plexus
Lumbosacral trunk
Sacral splanchnic nerves (branches from upper sacral sympathetic ganglia to hypogastric plexus)
Gray ramus communicans
Hypogastric nerves
Lumbosacral plexus
Pelvic splanchnic nerves
Inferior hypogastric (pelvic) plexus with peri-ureteric loops and branches to lower ureter
Rectal plexus
Vesical plexus
Prostatic plexus
F. Netter M.D.

Autonomic Innervation of Kidneys and Upper Ureters: Schema

See also Plates 163, 164, 395

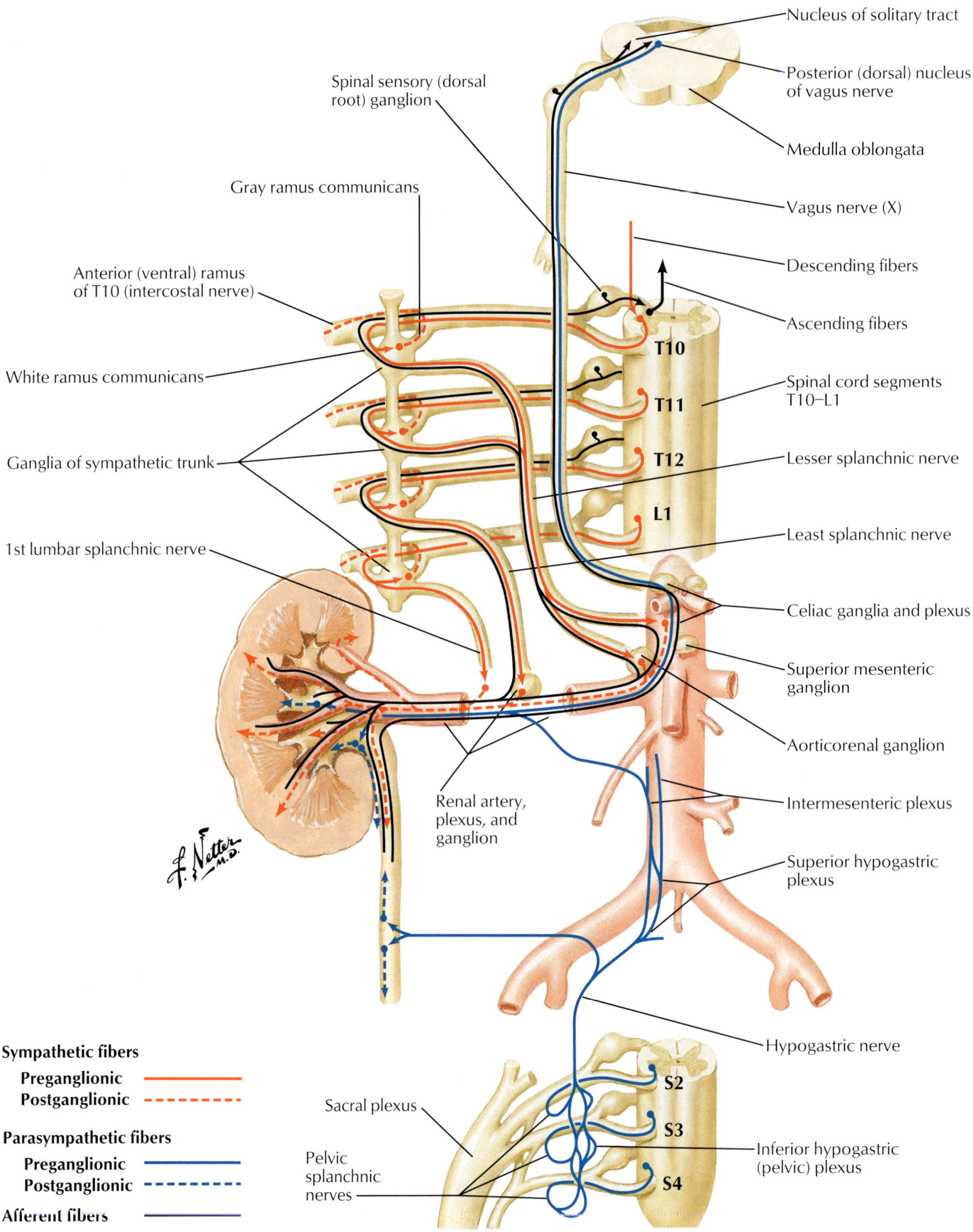

Autonomic Nerves of Suprarenal Glands: Dissection and Schema

See also Plates 163, 164

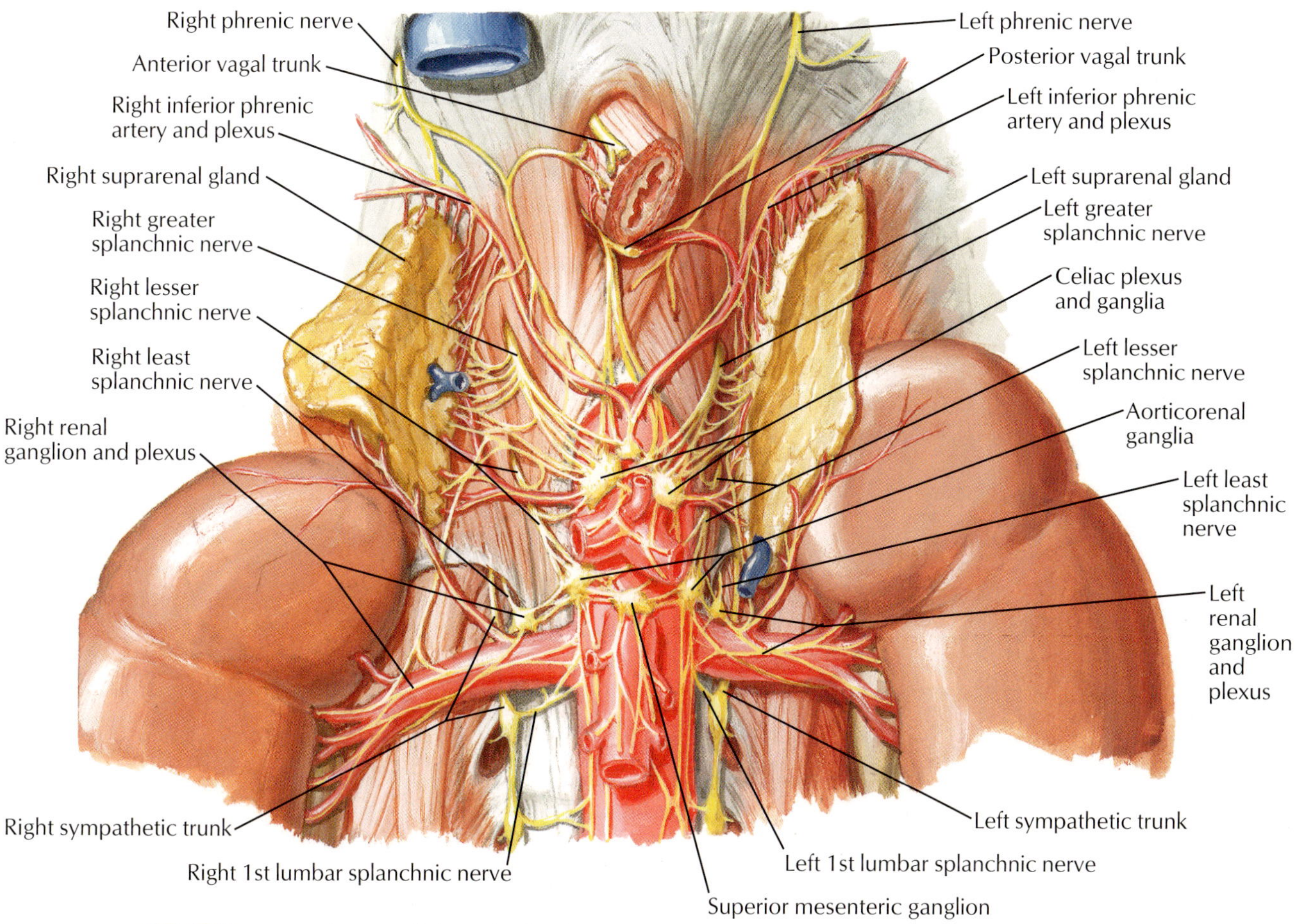

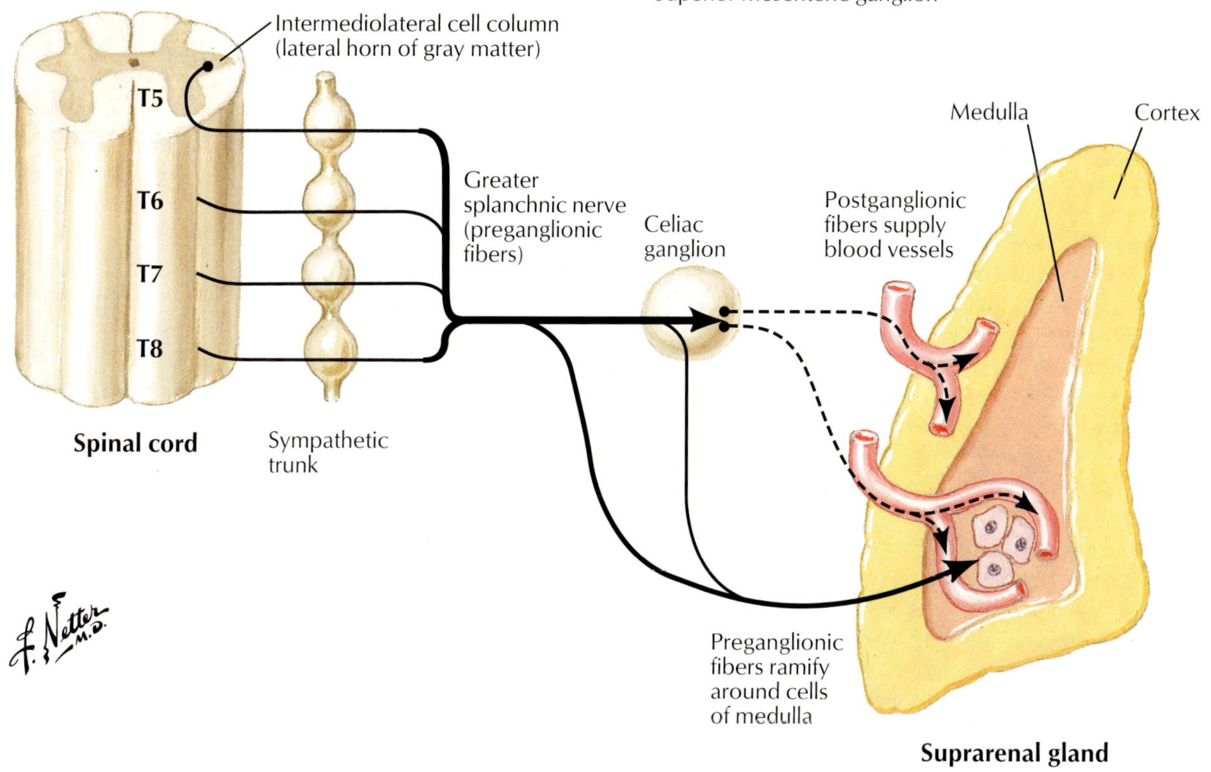

Arteries and Veins of Suprarenal Glands in Situ

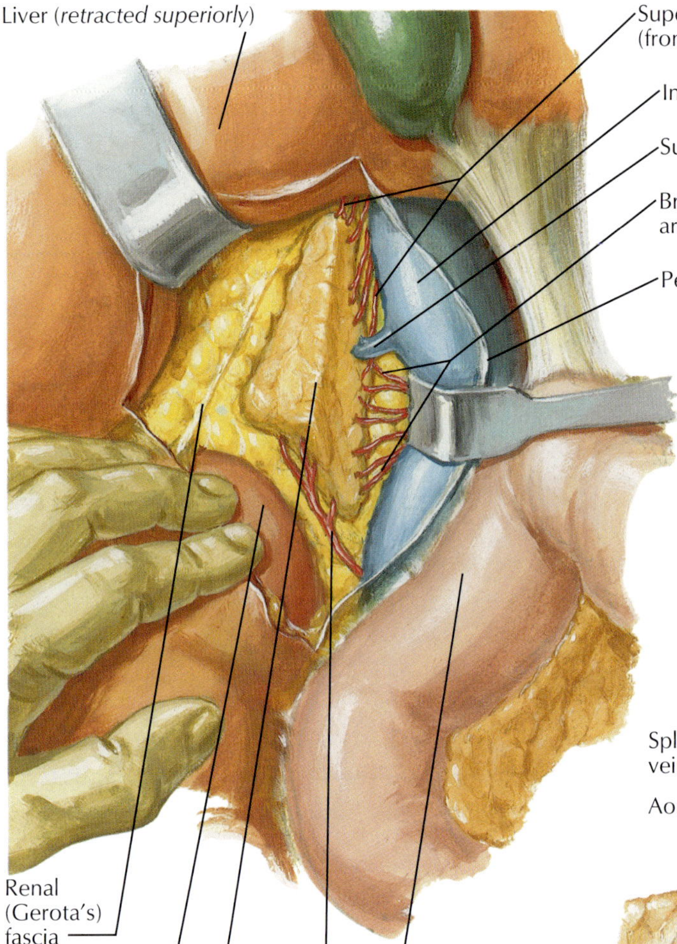

Abdominal exposure of right suprarenal gland

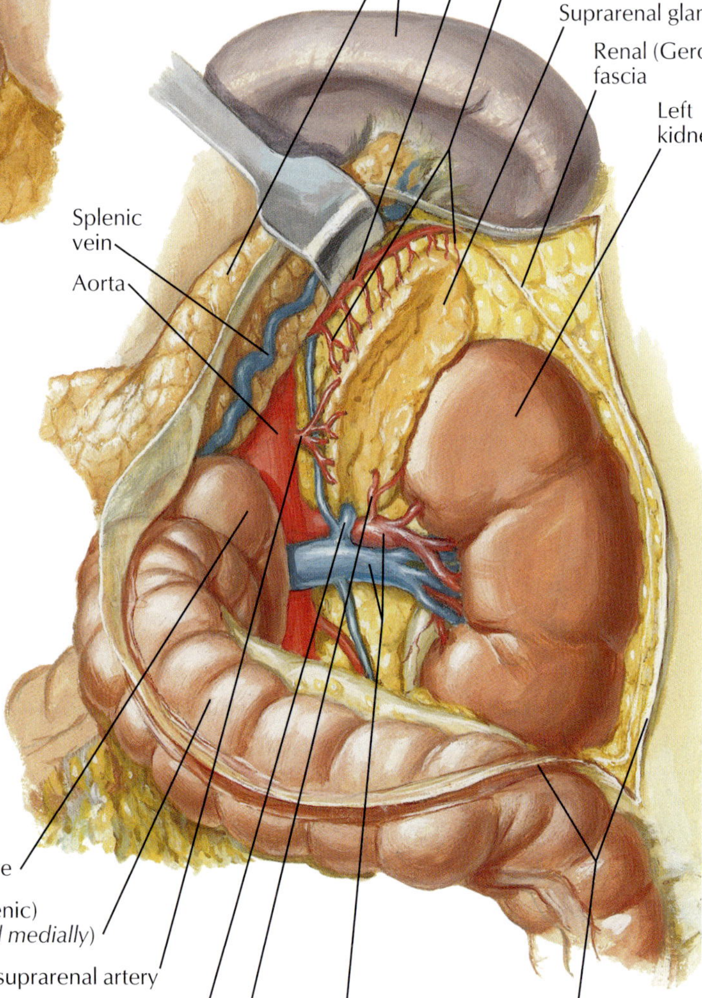

Abdominal exposure of left suprarenal gland

Cross section through suprarenal gland

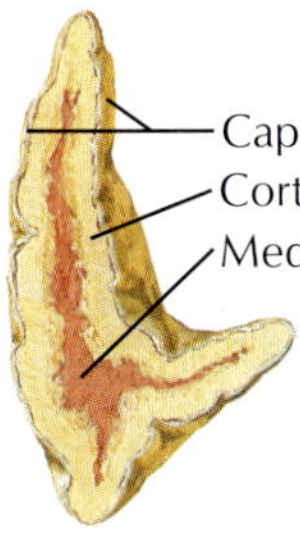

Abdominal Wall and Viscera: Paramedian (Parasagittal) Section

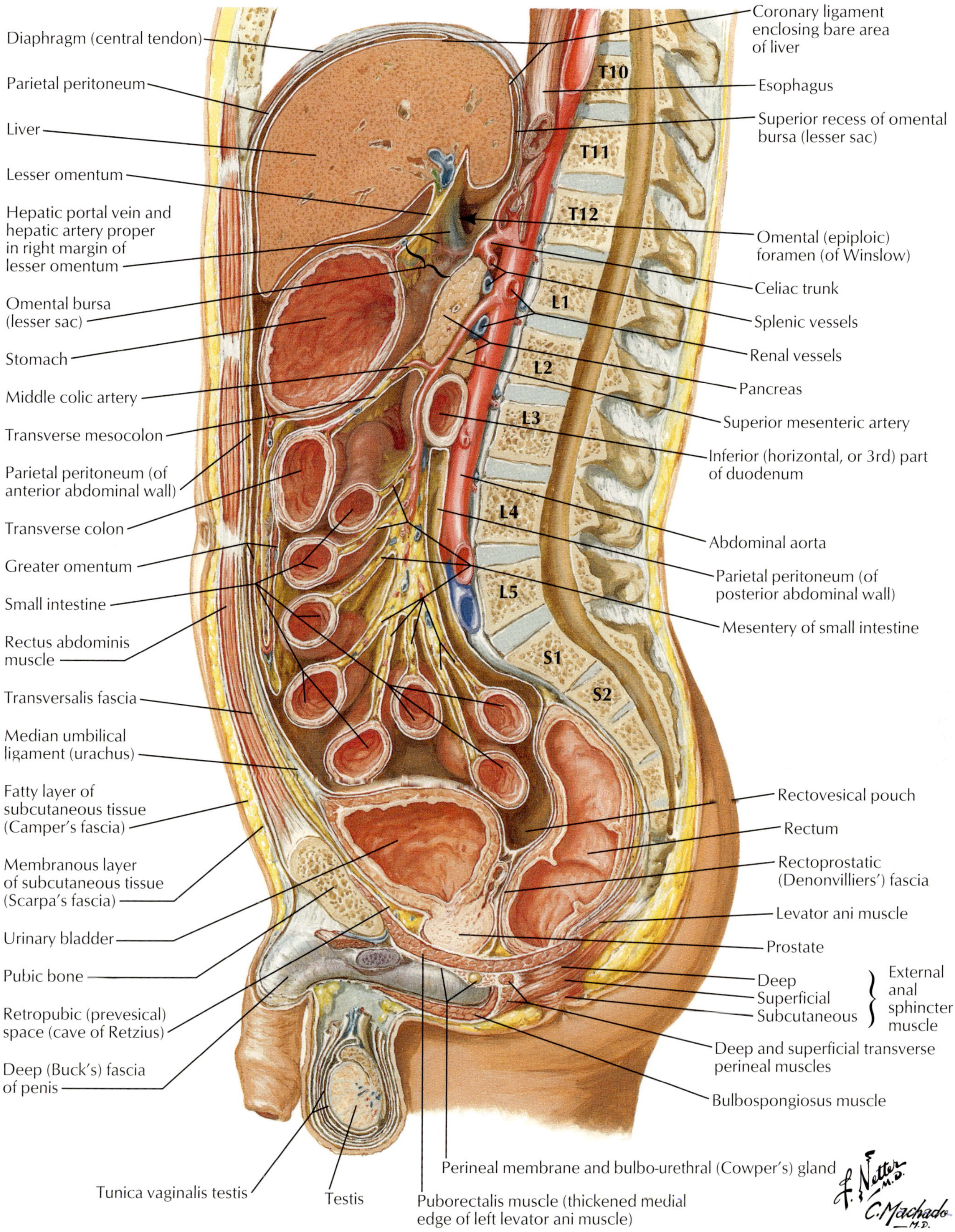

Series of abdominal axial CT images from superior (A) to inferior (C)

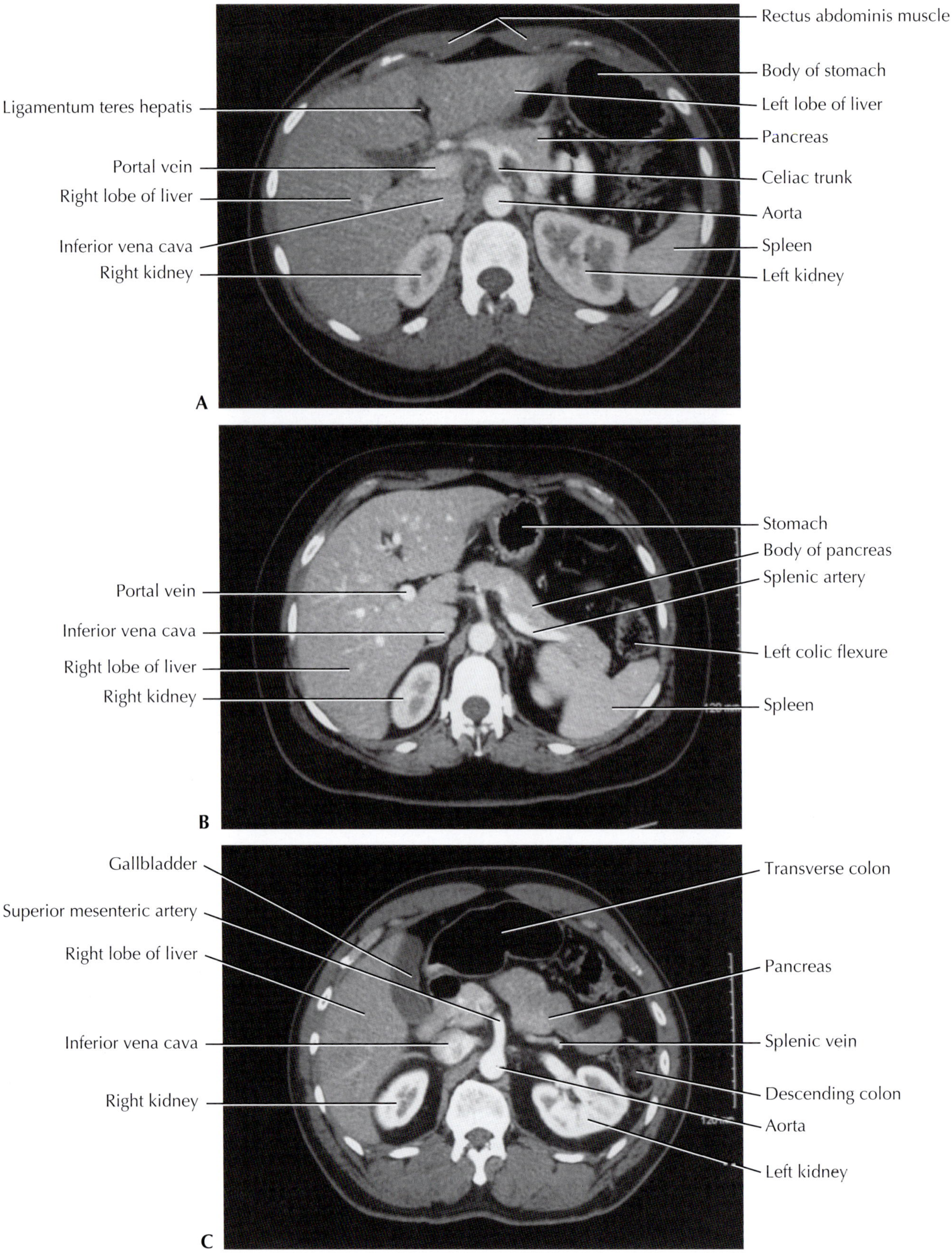

Series of abdominal axial CT images from superior (D) to inferior (E)

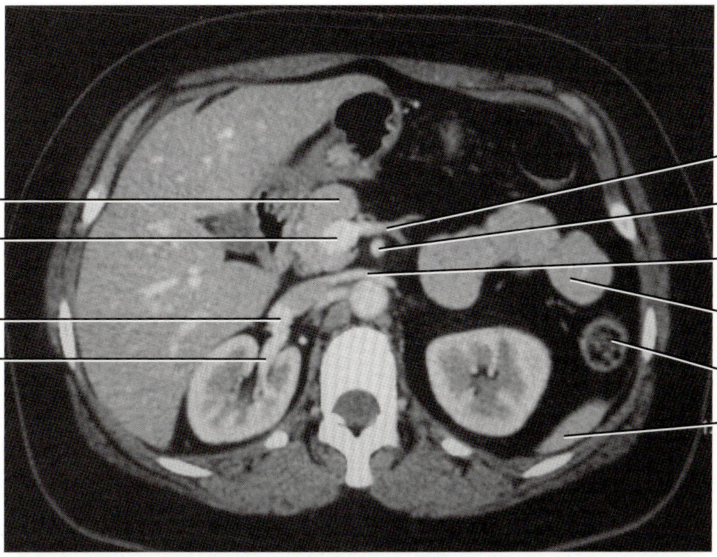

D

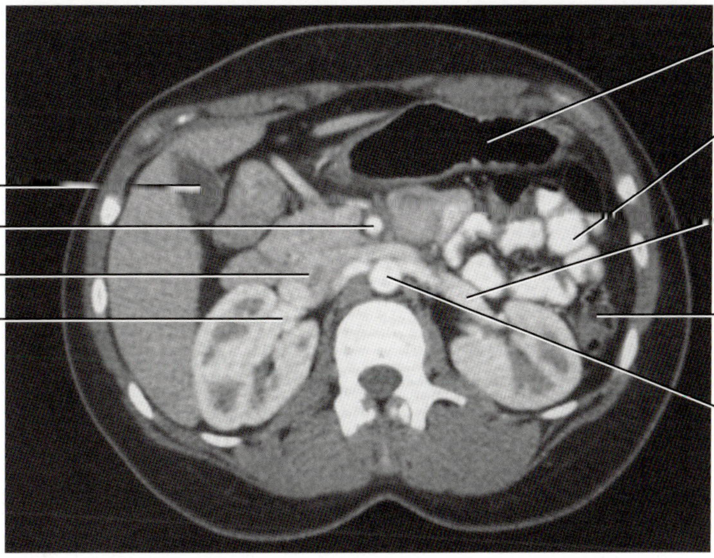

E

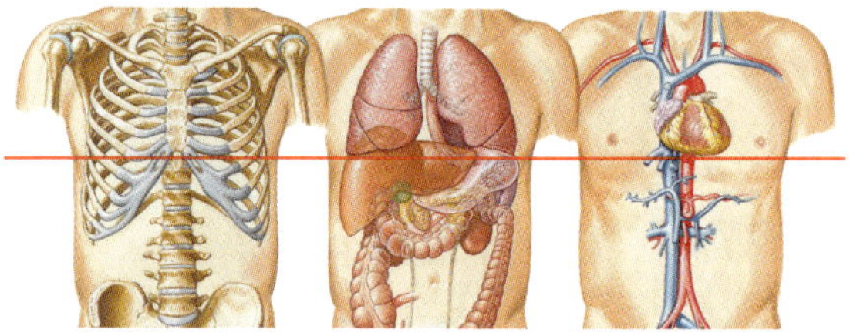

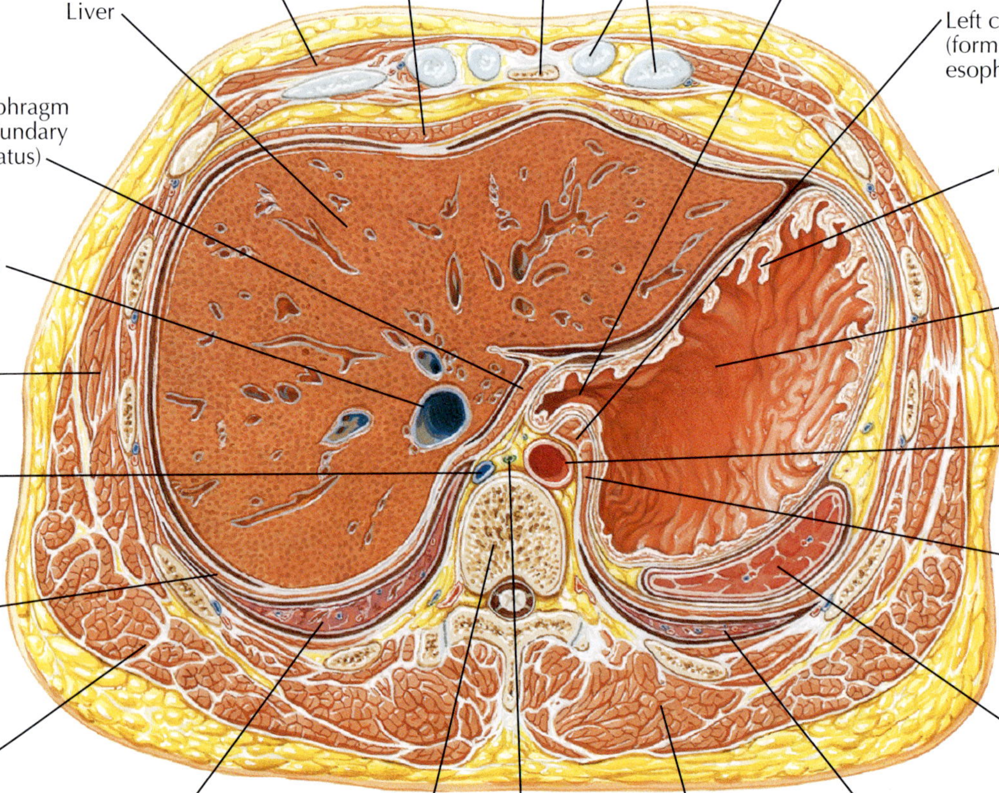

Xiphoid process
Diaphragm
Costal cartilages
Rectus abdominis muscle
Esophagogastric junction
Liver
Left crus of diaphragm (forming left boundary of esophageal hiatus)
Right crus of diaphragm (forming right boundary of esophageal hiatus)
Gastric folds (rugae)
Inferior vena cava
Fundus of stomach
Serratus anterior muscle
Thoracic aorta
Azygos vein
Left crus of diaphragm
Diaphragm
Spleen
Latissimus dorsi muscle
Inferior lobe of right lung in costodiaphragmatic recess
Inferior lobe of left lung in costodiaphragmatic recess
Body of T10 vertebra
Erector spinae muscle
Thoracic duct
C.Machado M.D.

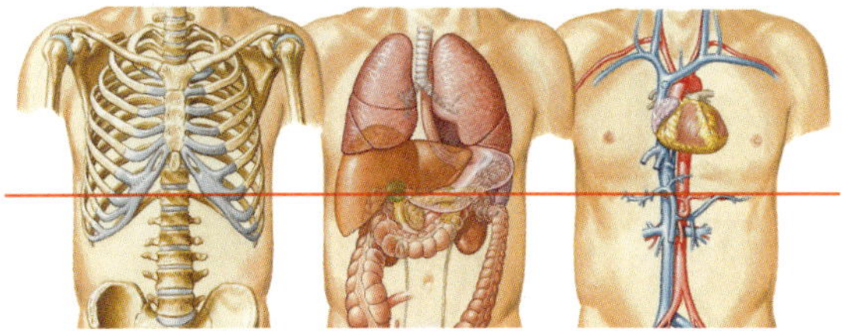

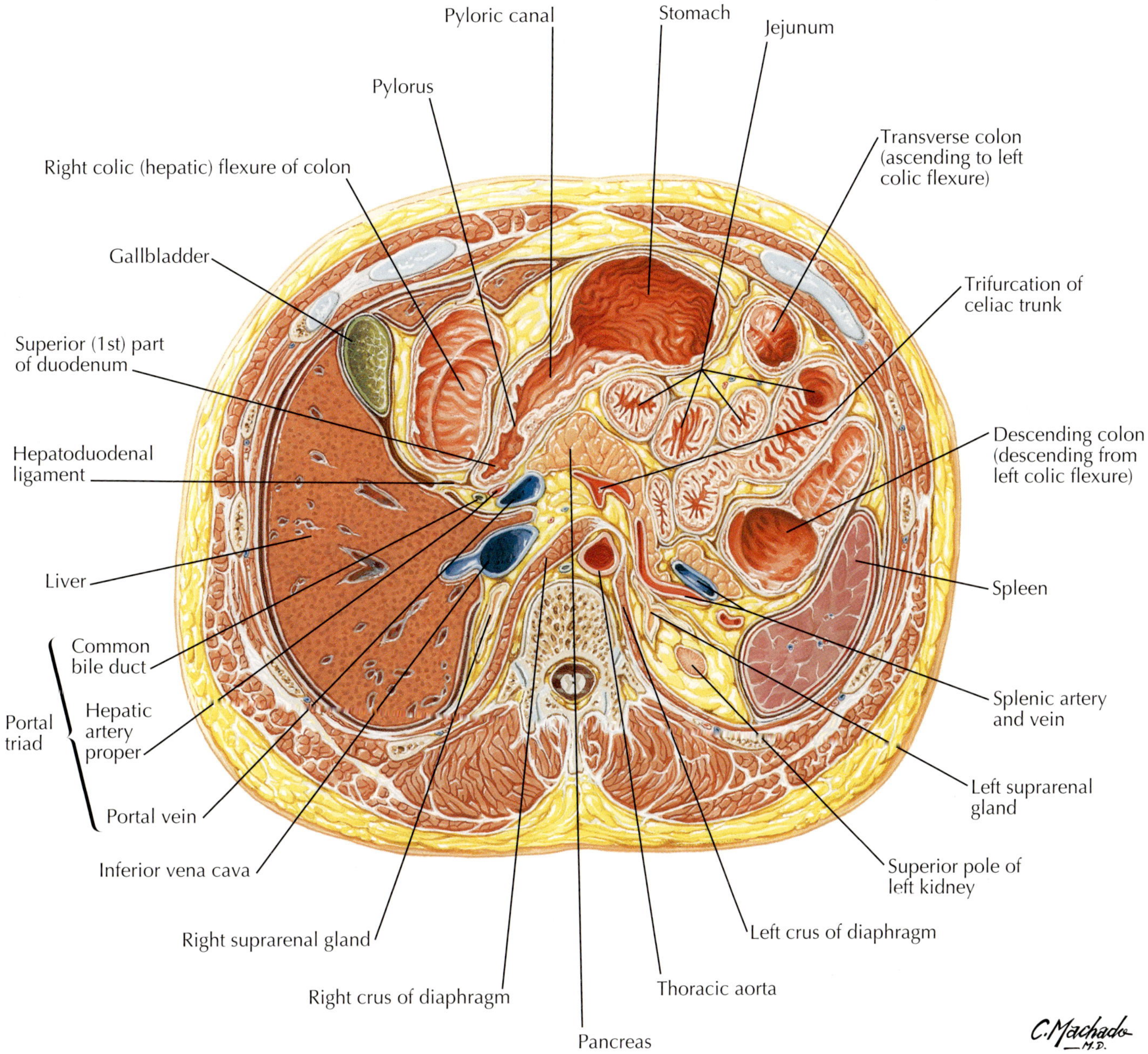
Pyloric canal
Stomach
Jejunum
Pylorus
Transverse colon (ascending to left colic flexure)
Right colic (hepatic) flexure of colon
Gallbladder
Trifurcation of celiac trunk
Superior (1st) part of duodenum
Descending colon (descending from left colic flexure)
Hepatoduodenal ligament
Liver
Spleen
Common bile duct
Portal triad
Hepatic artery proper
Splenic artery and vein
Portal vein
Left suprarenal gland
Inferior vena cava
Superior pole of left kidney
Left crus of diaphragm
Right suprarenal gland
Thoracic aorta
Right crus of diaphragm
Pancreas
C. Machado M.D.

Cross Section at T12–L1, Intervertebral Disc

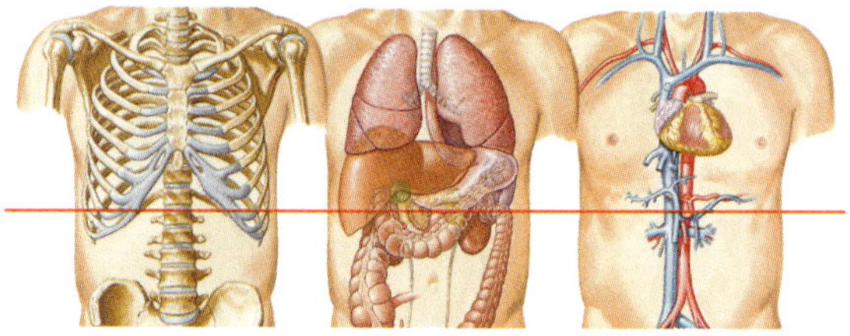

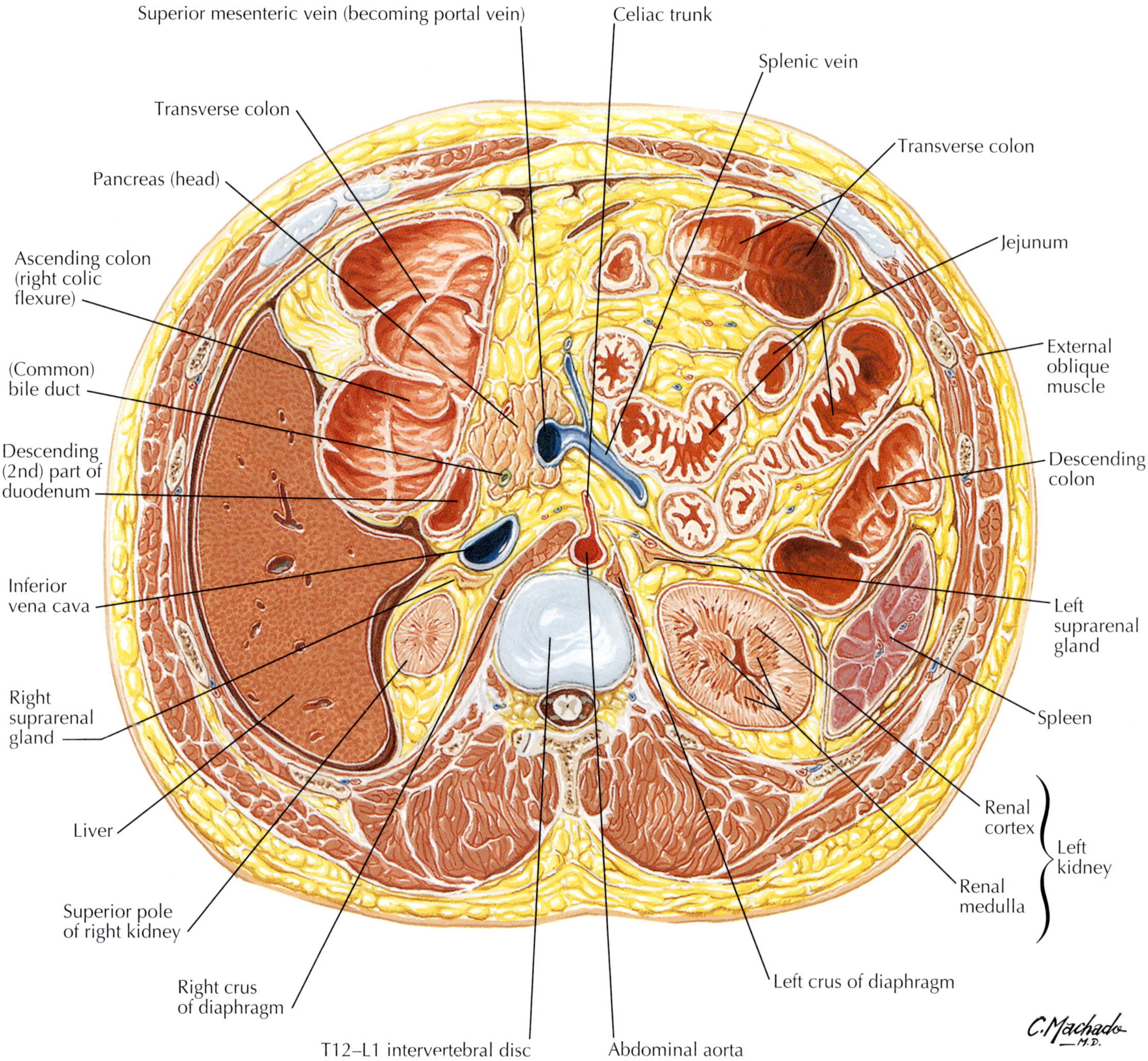

Cross Section at L1–2, Intervertebral Disc

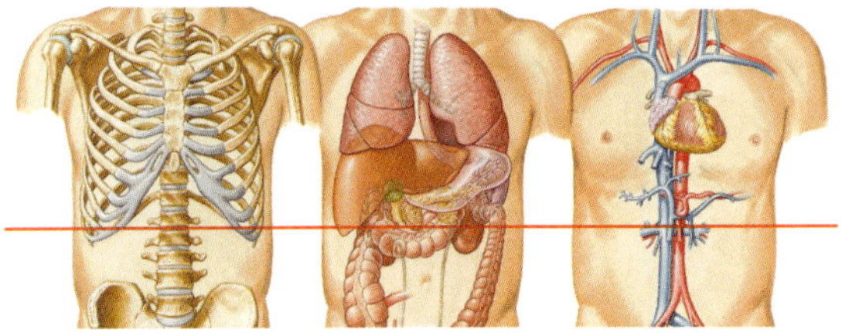

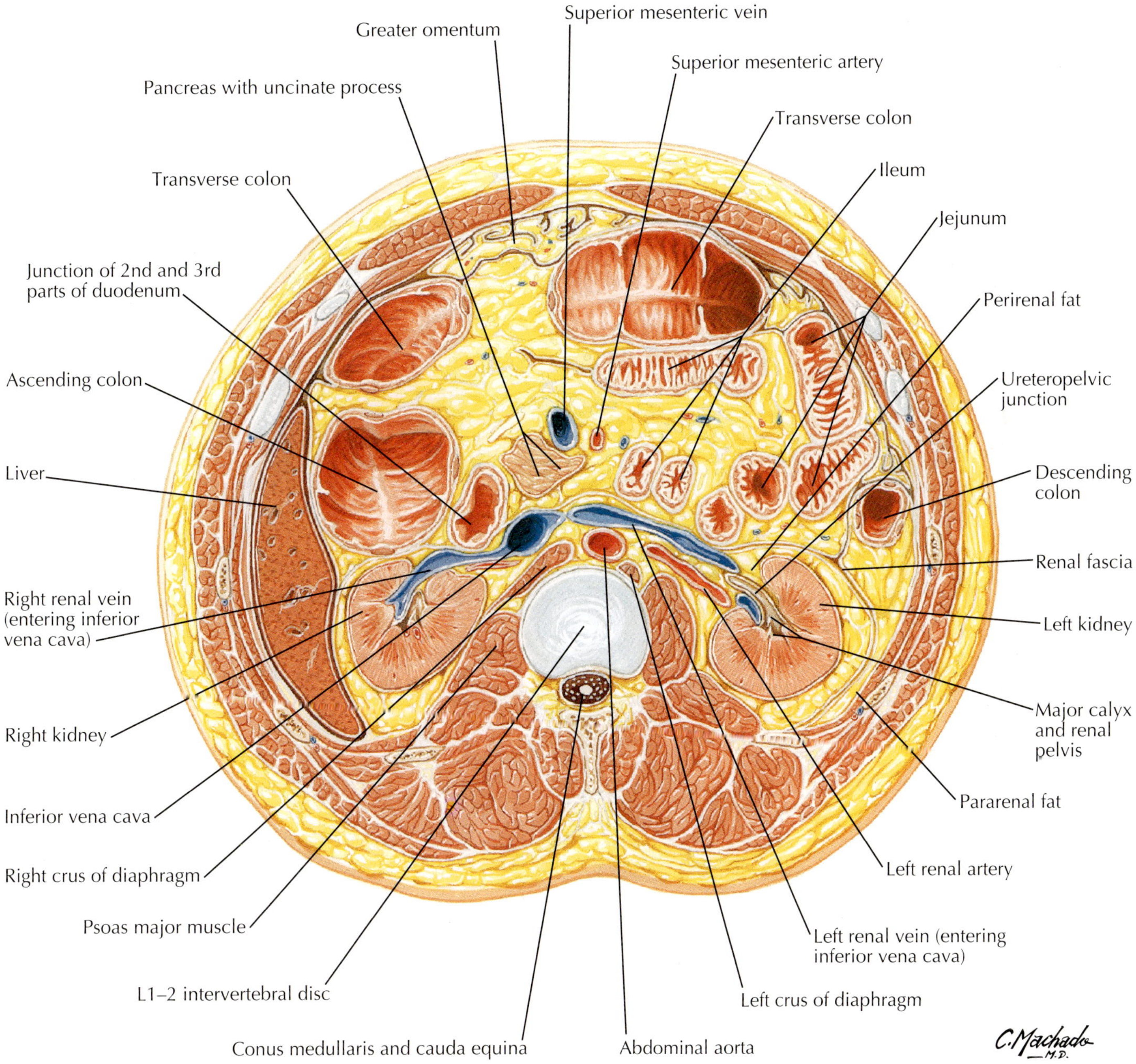

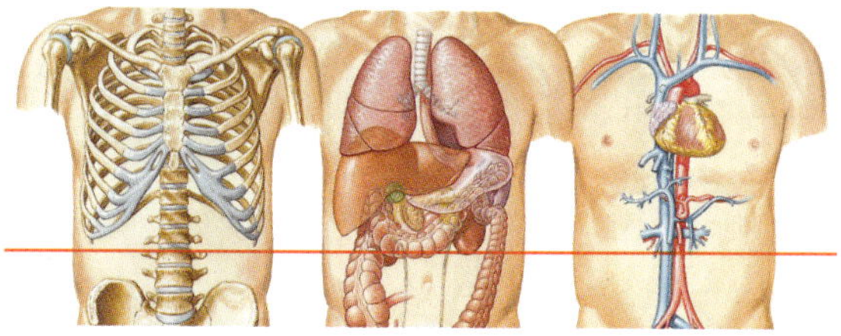

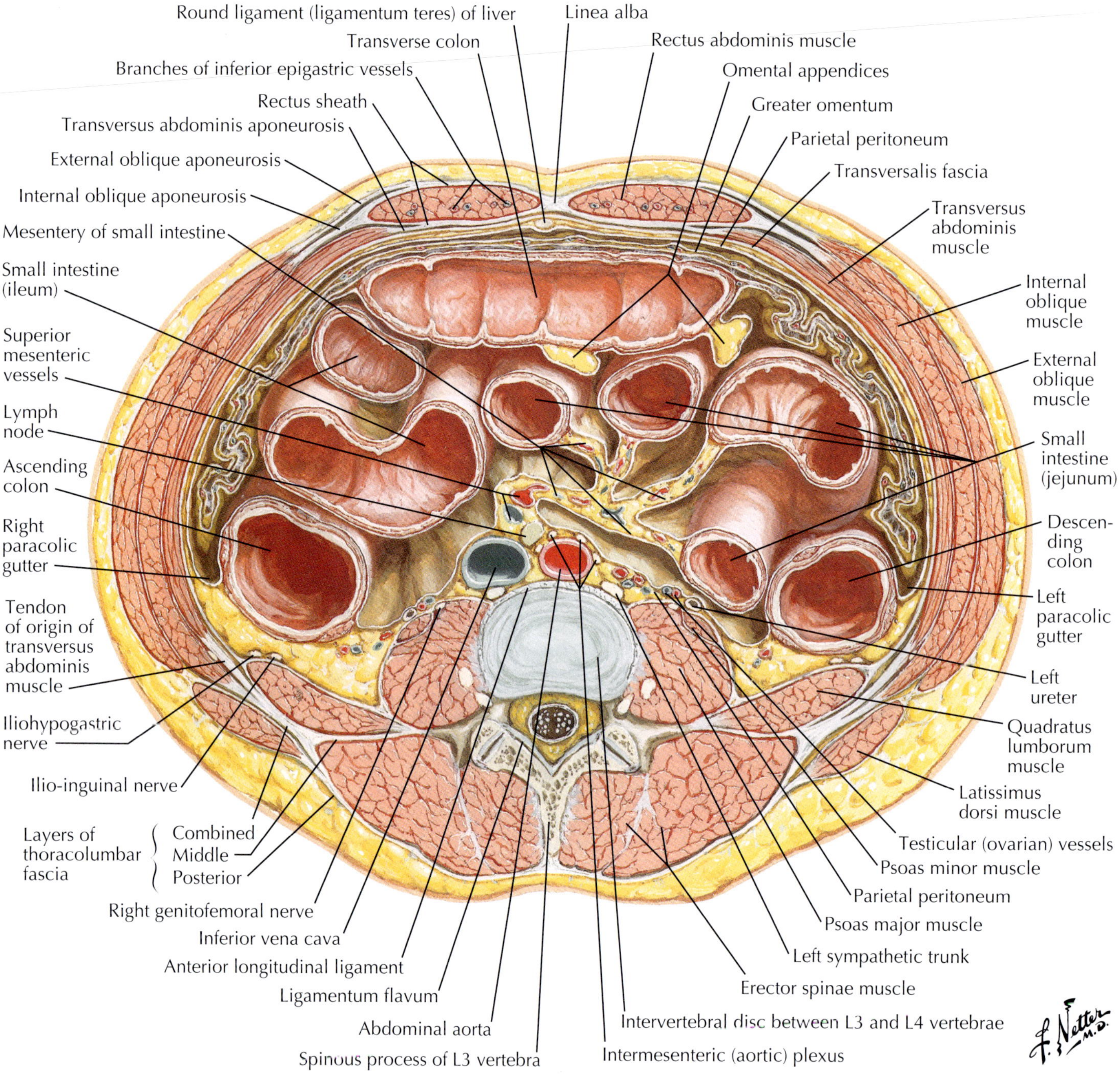
Round ligament (ligamentum teres) of liver
Linea alba
Transverse colon
Rectus abdominis muscle
Branches of inferior epigastric vessels
Omental appendices
Rectus sheath
Greater omentum
Transversus abdominis aponeurosis
Parietal peritoneum
External oblique aponeurosis
Transversalis fascia
Internal oblique aponeurosis
Transversus abdominis muscle
Mesentery of small intestine
Small intestine (ileum)
Internal oblique muscle
Superior mesenteric vessels
External oblique muscle
Lymph node
Small intestine (jejunum)
Ascending colon
Right paracolic gutter
Descending colon
Left paracolic gutter
Tendon of origin of transversus abdominis muscle
Left ureter
Iliohypogastric nerve
Quadratus lumborum muscle
Ilio-inguinal nerve
Latissimus dorsi muscle
Layers of thoracolumbar fascia
Combined
Middle
Posterior
Testicular (ovarian) vessels
Psoas minor muscle
Parietal peritoneum
Right genitofemoral nerve
Psoas major muscle
Inferior vena cava
Left sympathetic trunk
Anterior longitudinal ligament
Erector spinae muscle
Ligamentum flavum
Abdominal aorta
Intervertebral disc between L3 and L4 vertebrae
Spinous process of L3 vertebra
Intermesenteric (aortic) plexus

MUSCLE	PROXIMAL ATTACHMENT (ORIGIN)	DISTAL ATTACHMENT (INSERTION)	INNERVATION	MAIN ACTIONS	BLOOD SUPPLY	MUSCLE GROUP
Diaphragm	Xiphoid process, lower six costal cartilages, L1–L3 vertebrae	Converges into central tendon	Phrenic nerve	Draws central tendon down and forward during inspiration	Pericardiacophrenic, musculophrenic, superior and inferior phrenic arteries	Posterior abdominal wall
External oblique	External surfaces of ribs 5–12	Linea alba, pubic tubercle, anterior half of iliac crest	Ventral rami of six inferior thoracic nerves	Compresses and supports abdominal viscera, flexes and rotates trunk	Superior and inferior epigastric arteries	Abdominal wall
Iliacus	Superior 2/3 iliac fossa, ala of sacrum, anterior sacro-iliac ligaments	Lesser trochanter of femur and shaft inferior to it, and to psoas major tendon	Femoral nerve	Flexes hip and stabilizes hip joint; acts with psoas major	Iliac branches of iliolumbar artery	Posterior abdominal wall
Internal oblique	Thoracolumbar fascia, anterior 2/3 of iliac crest, lateral half of inguinal ligament	Inferior borders of ribs 10–12, linea alba, pubis via conjoint tendon	Ventral rami of six inferior thoracic and first lumbar nerves	Compresses and supports abdominal viscera, flexes and rotates trunk	Superior and inferior epigastric and deep circumflex iliac arteries	Abdominal wall
Psoas major	Transverse processes of lumbar vertebrae, sides of bodies of T12–L5 vertebrae, intervening intervertebral discs	Lesser trochanter of femur	Ventral rami of first four lumbar nerves	Acting superiorly with iliacus, flexes hip; acting inferiorly, flexes vertebral column laterally; used to balance trunk in sitting position; acting inferiorly with iliacus, flexes trunk	Lumbar branches of iliolumbar artery	Posterior abdominal wall
Psoas minor	Vertebral margins of T12–L1 vertebrae, corresponding intervertebral disc	Pectineal line, iliopectineal eminence	Ventral rami of first lumbar nerve	Flexes pelvis on vertebral column	Lumbar branch of iliolumbar artery	Posterior abdominal wall
Pyramidalis	Body of pubis, anterior to rectus abdominis	Linea alba	Iliohypogastric nerve	Tenses linea alba	Inferior epigastric artery	Abdominal wall
Quadratus lumborum	Medial half of inferior border of 12th rib, tips of lumbar transverse processes	Iliolumbar ligament, internal lip of iliac crest	Ventral rami of T12 and first four lumbar nerves	Extends and laterally flexes vertebral column, fixes 12th rib during inspiration	Iliolumbar artery	Posterior abdominal wall
Rectus abdominis	Pubic symphysis, pubic crest	Xiphoid process, costal cartilages 5–7	Ventral rami of six inferior thoracic nerves	Flexes trunk, compresses abdominal viscera	Superior and interior epigastric arteries	Abdominal wall
Transversus abdominis	Internal surfaces of costal cartilages 7–12, thoracolumbar fascia, iliac crest, lateral third of inguinal ligament	Linea alba with aponeurosis of internal oblique, pubic crest, and pecten pubis via conjoint tendon	Ventral rami of six inferior thoracic and first lumbar nerves	Compresses and supports abdominal viscera	Deep circumflex iliac and inferior epigastric arteries	Abdominal wall

Variations in spinal nerve contributions to the innervation of muscles, their arterial supply, their attachments, and their actions are common themes in human anatomy. Therefore, expect differences between texts and realize that anatomical variation is normal.

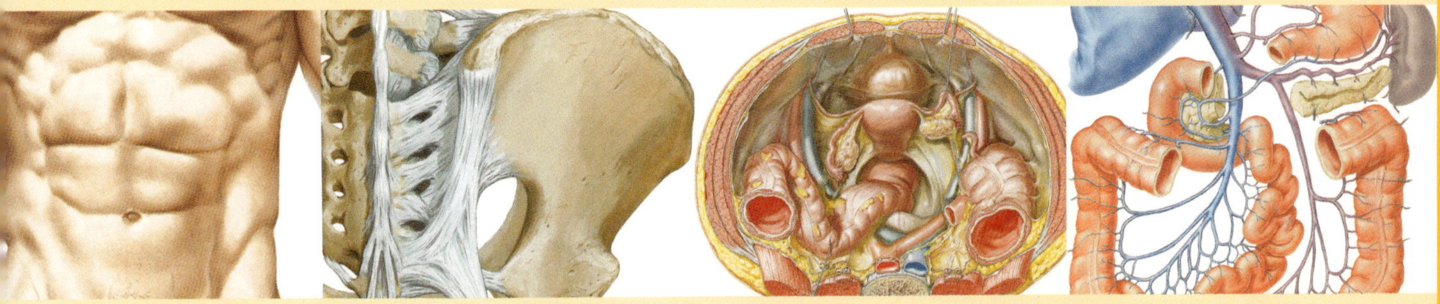

5 PELVIS AND PERINEUM

Topographic Anatomy
Plate 329

329 Pelvis and Perineum: Surface Anatomy

Bones and Ligaments
Plates 330–334

330 Bony Framework of Pelvis

331 Radiographs of Male and Female Pelvis

332 Sex Differences of Pelvis: Measurements

333 Bones and Ligaments of Pelvis

334 Bones and Ligaments of Pelvis (continued)

Pelvic Floor and Contents
Plates 335–345

335 Pelvic Diaphragm: Female

336 Pelvic Diaphragm: Female (continued)

337 Pelvic Diaphragm: Female (continued)

338 Pelvic Diaphragm: Male

339 Pelvic Diaphragm: Male (continued)

340 Pelvic Viscera and Perineum: Female

341 Pelvic Contents: Female

342 Pelvic Viscera: Female

343 Endopelvic Fascia and Potential Spaces

344 Pelvic Viscera and Perineum: Male

345 Pelvic Contents: Male

Urinary Bladder
Plates 346–348

346 Urinary Bladder: Orientation and Supports
347 Female Sphincters
348 Urinary Bladder: Female and Male

Uterus, Vagina, and Supporting Structures
Plates 349–353

349 Uterine Growth
350 Uterus, Vagina, and Supporting Structures
351 Uterus: Fascial Ligaments
352 Uterus and Adnexa
353 Pelvic Ligaments

Perineum and External Genitalia: Female
Plates 354–357

354 Female Perineum and External Genitalia (Pudendum or Vulva)
355 Female Perineum (Superficial Dissection)
356 Female Perineum and Deep Perineum
357 Female Perineal Spaces

Perineum and External Genitalia: Male
Plates 358–365

358 Male Perineum and External Genitalia (Superficial Dissection)
359 Male Perineum and External Genitalia (Deeper Dissection)
360 Penis
361 Male Perineal Spaces
362 Prostate and Seminal Vesicles
363 Urethra
364 Descent of Testis
365 Scrotum and Contents

Homologues of Genitalia
Plates 366–367

366 Homologues of External Genitalia
367 Homologues of Internal Genitalia

Testis, Epididymis, and Ductus Deferens
Plate 368

368 Testis, Epididymis, and Ductus Deferens

Rectum
Plates 369–374

369 Rectum in Situ: Female and Male
370 Ischio-anal Fossae
371 Rectum and Anal Canal
372 Anorectal Musculature
373 External Anal Sphincter Muscle: Perineal Views
374 Actual and Potential Perineopelvic Spaces

Regional Scans
Plate 375

375 Pelvic Scans: Sagittal CT Images

Vasculature
Plates 376–386

376 Arteries of Rectum and Anal Canal: Male
377 Veins of Rectum and Anal Canal: Female
378 Arteries and Veins of Pelvic Organs: Female
379 Arteries and Veins of Testis
380 Arteries of Pelvis: Female
381 Arteries and Veins of Pelvis: Male
382 Arteries and Veins of Perineum and Uterus
383 Arteries and Veins of Perineum: Male
384 Lymph Vessels and Nodes of Pelvis and Genitalia: Female
385 Lymph Vessels and Nodes of Perineum: Female
386 Lymph Vessels and Nodes of Pelvis and Genitalia: Male

Innervation

Plates 387–395

387 Nerves of External Genitalia: Male

388 Nerves of Pelvic Viscera: Male

389 Nerves of Perineum: Male

390 Nerves of Pelvic Viscera: Female

391 Nerves of Perineum and External Genitalia: Female

392 Neuropathways in Parturition

393 Innervation of Female Reproductive Organs: Schema

394 Innervation of Male Reproductive Organs: Schema

395 Innervation of Urinary Bladder and Lower Ureter: Schema

Cross-Sectional Anatomy

Plates 396–397

396 Male Pelvis: Cross Section of Bladder-Prostate Junction

397 Female Pelvis: Cross Section of Vagina-Urethra

Muscle Tables

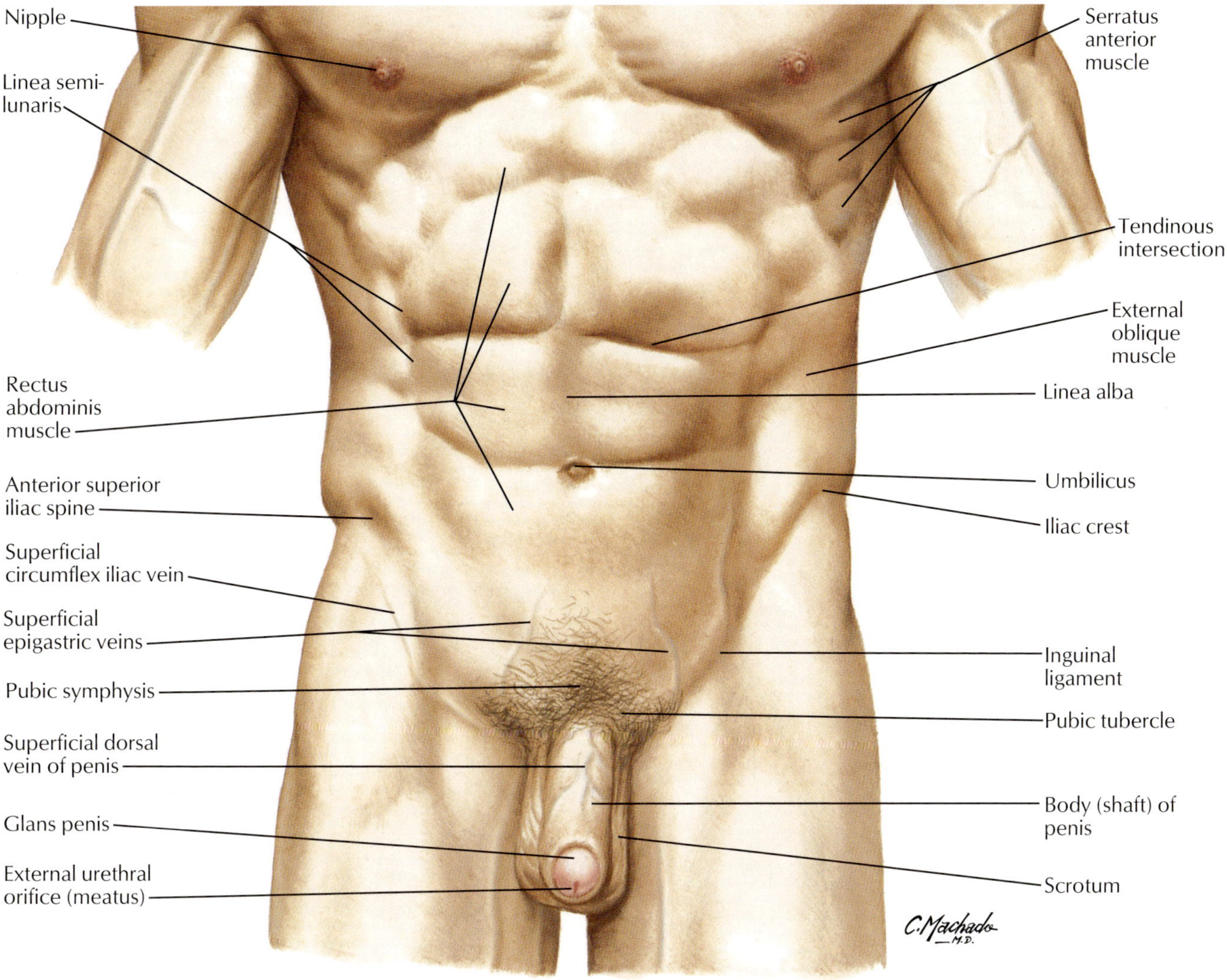
Nipple
Linea semi-lunaris
Rectus abdominis muscle
Anterior superior iliac spine
Superficial circumflex iliac vein
Superficial epigastric veins
Pubic symphysis
Superficial dorsal vein of penis
Glans penis
External urethral orifice (meatus)
Serratus anterior muscle
Tendinous intersection
External oblique muscle
Linea alba
Umbilicus
Iliac crest
Inguinal ligament
Pubic tubercle
Body (shaft) of penis
Scrotum
C. Machado M.D.

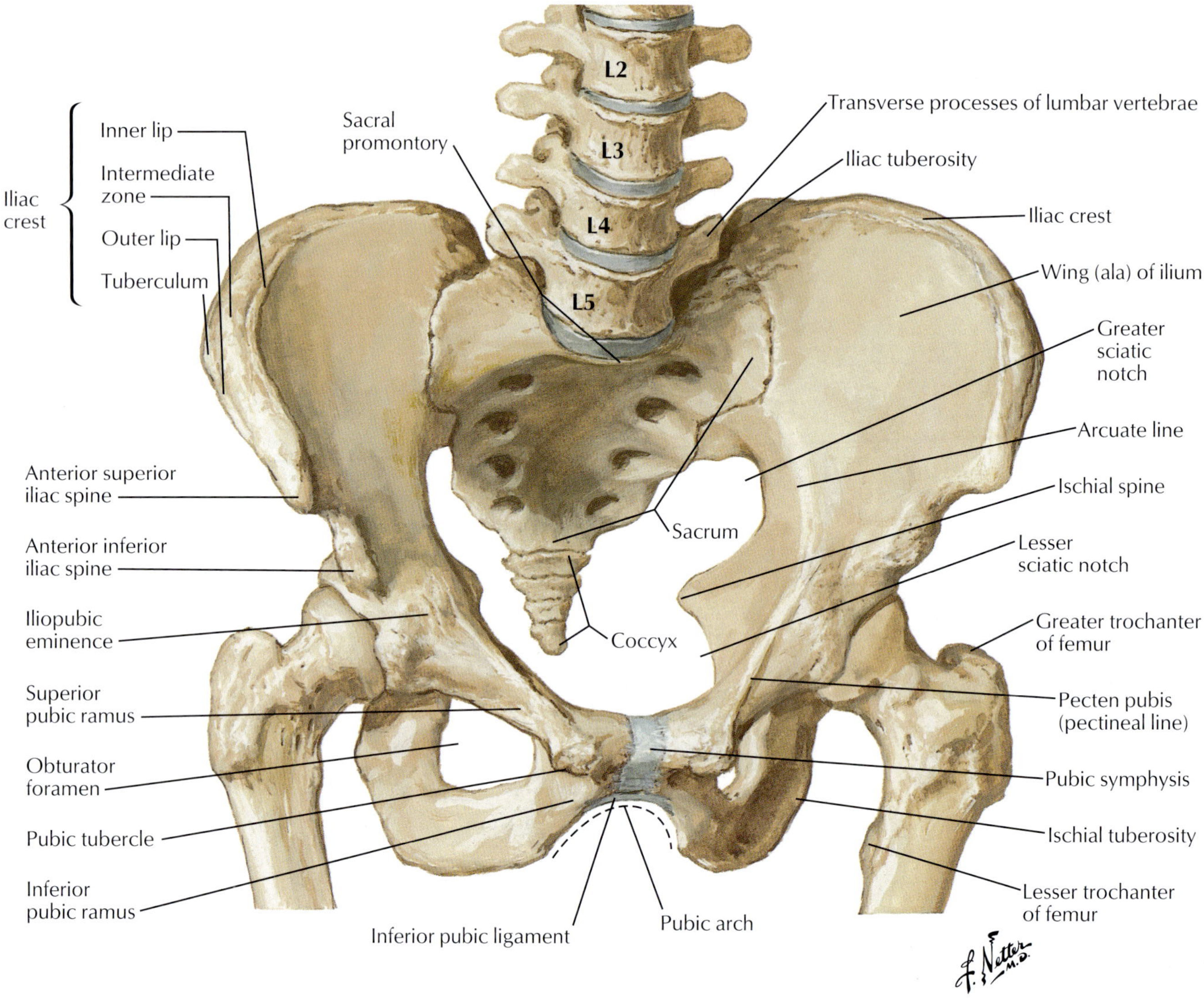

L2
L3
L4
L5
Iliac crest
Inner lip
Intermediate zone
Outer lip
Tuberculum
Sacral promontory
Transverse processes of lumbar vertebrae
Iliac tuberosity
Iliac crest
Wing (ala) of ilium
Greater sciatic notch
Arcuate line
Ischial spine
Lesser sciatic notch
Greater trochanter of femur
Pecten pubis (pectineal line)
Pubic symphysis
Ischial tuberosity
Lesser trochanter of femur
Anterior superior iliac spine
Anterior inferior iliac spine
Iliopubic eminence
Superior pubic ramus
Obturator foramen
Pubic tubercle
Inferior pubic ramus
Sacrum
Coccyx
Inferior pubic ligament
Pubic arch

Radiographs of Male and Female Pelvis

See also Plates 243, 475

Female Pelvis

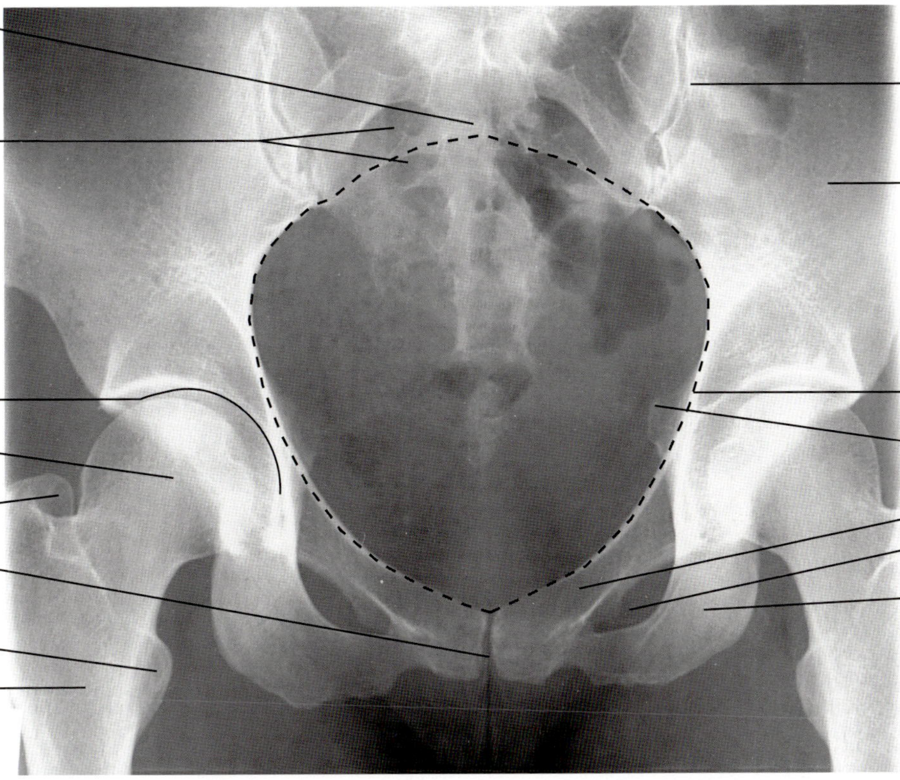

Male Pelvis

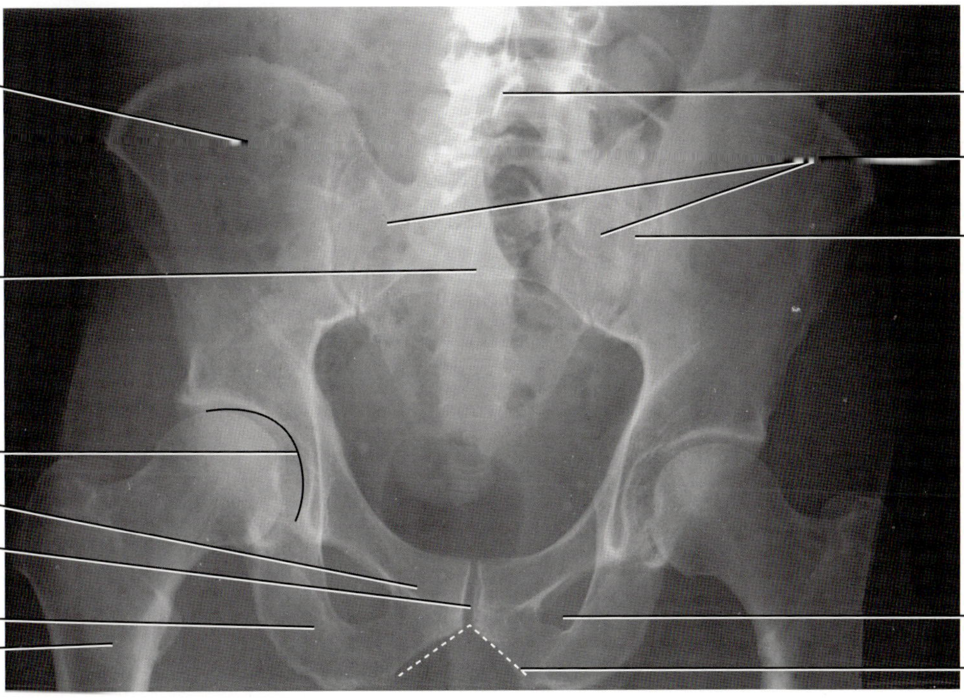

Sex Differences of Pelvis: Measurements

See also Plate 243

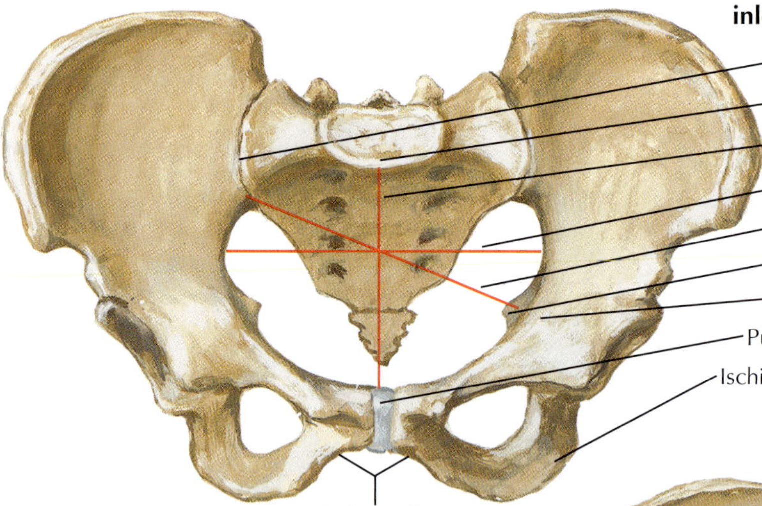

Female pelvis/female pelvic inlet: anterior view

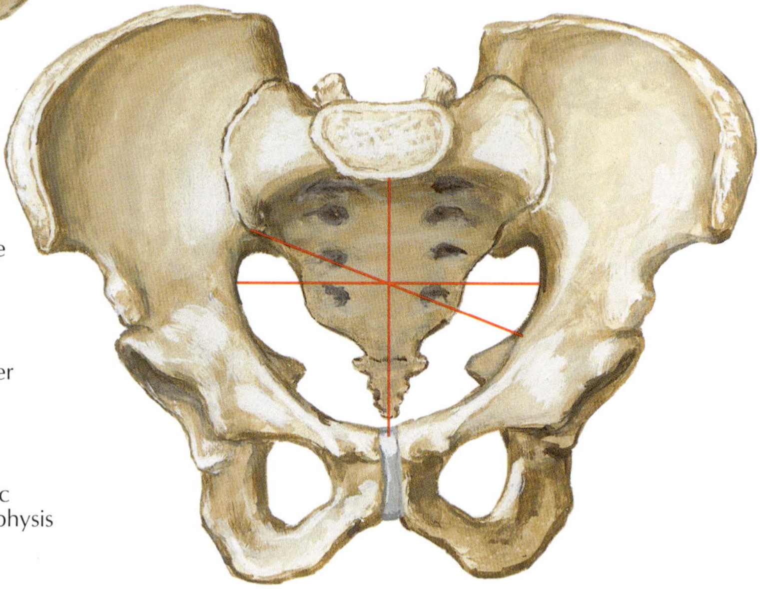

Male pelvis/male pelvic inlet: anterior view

Diagonal conjugate is only diameter of pelvic inlet that can be measured clinically

- All measurements slightly shorter in relation to body size than in female
- Pelvic inlet oriented more anteroposteriorly than in female, where it tends to be transversely oval
- Pubic symphysis deeper (taller)
- Pubic arch (subpubic angle) narrower
- Ischial tuberosities less far apart
- Iliac wings less flared

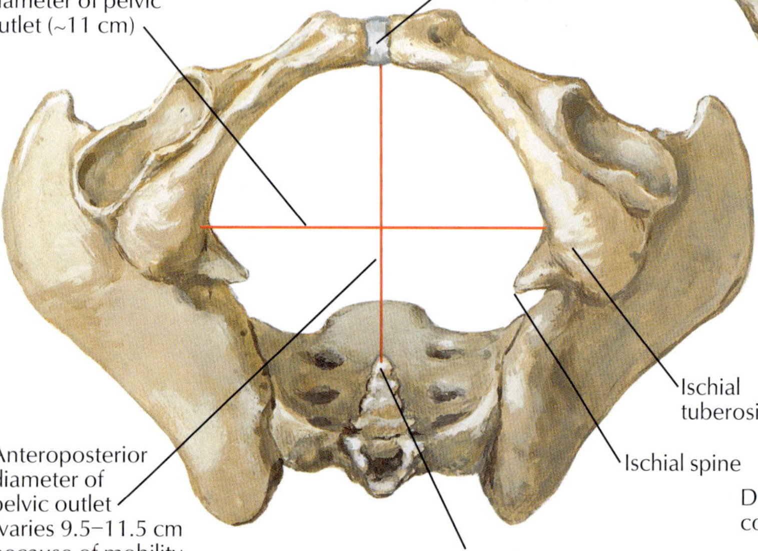

Female pelvis/female pelvic outlet: inferior view

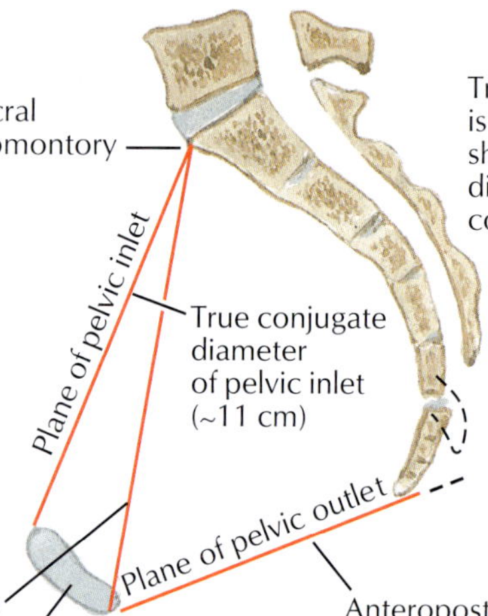

Transverse diameter is the widest distance of pelvic inlet

Female: sagittal section

See also Plate 473

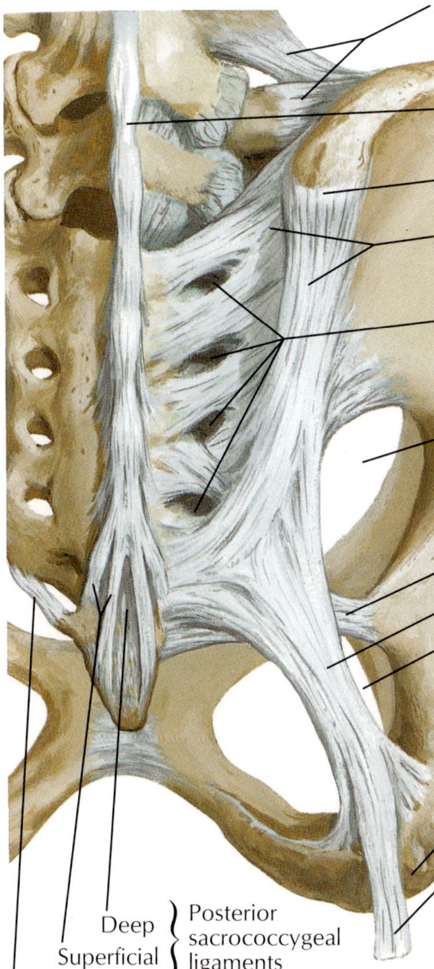

Posterior view

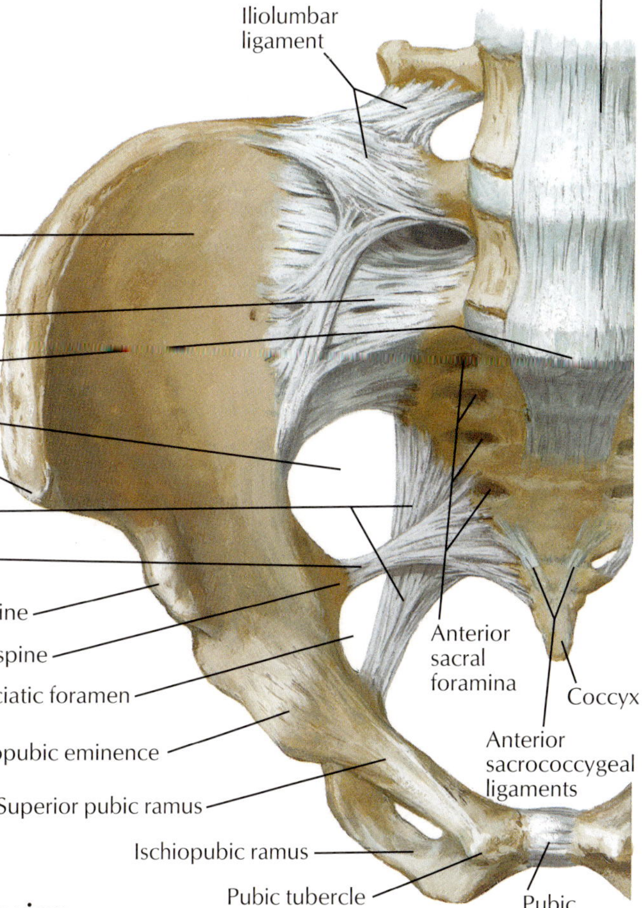

Anterior view

See also Plate 158

Median (sagittal) section

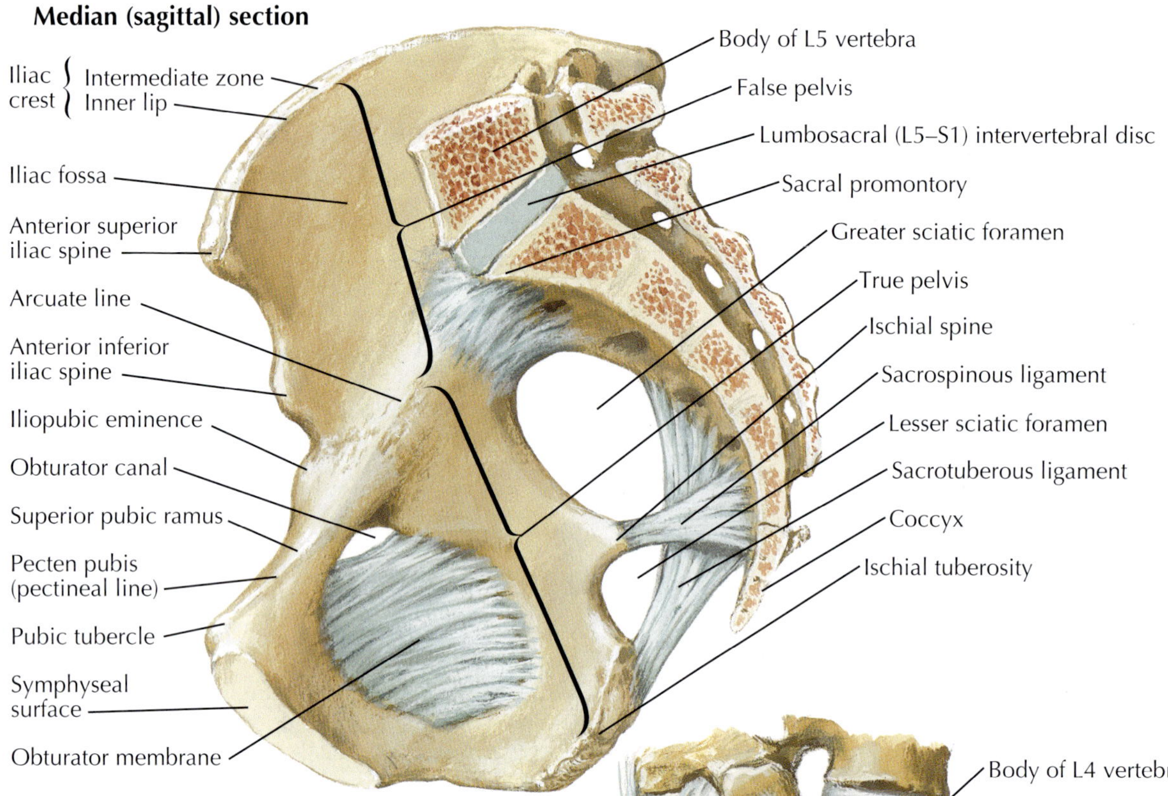

Lateral view

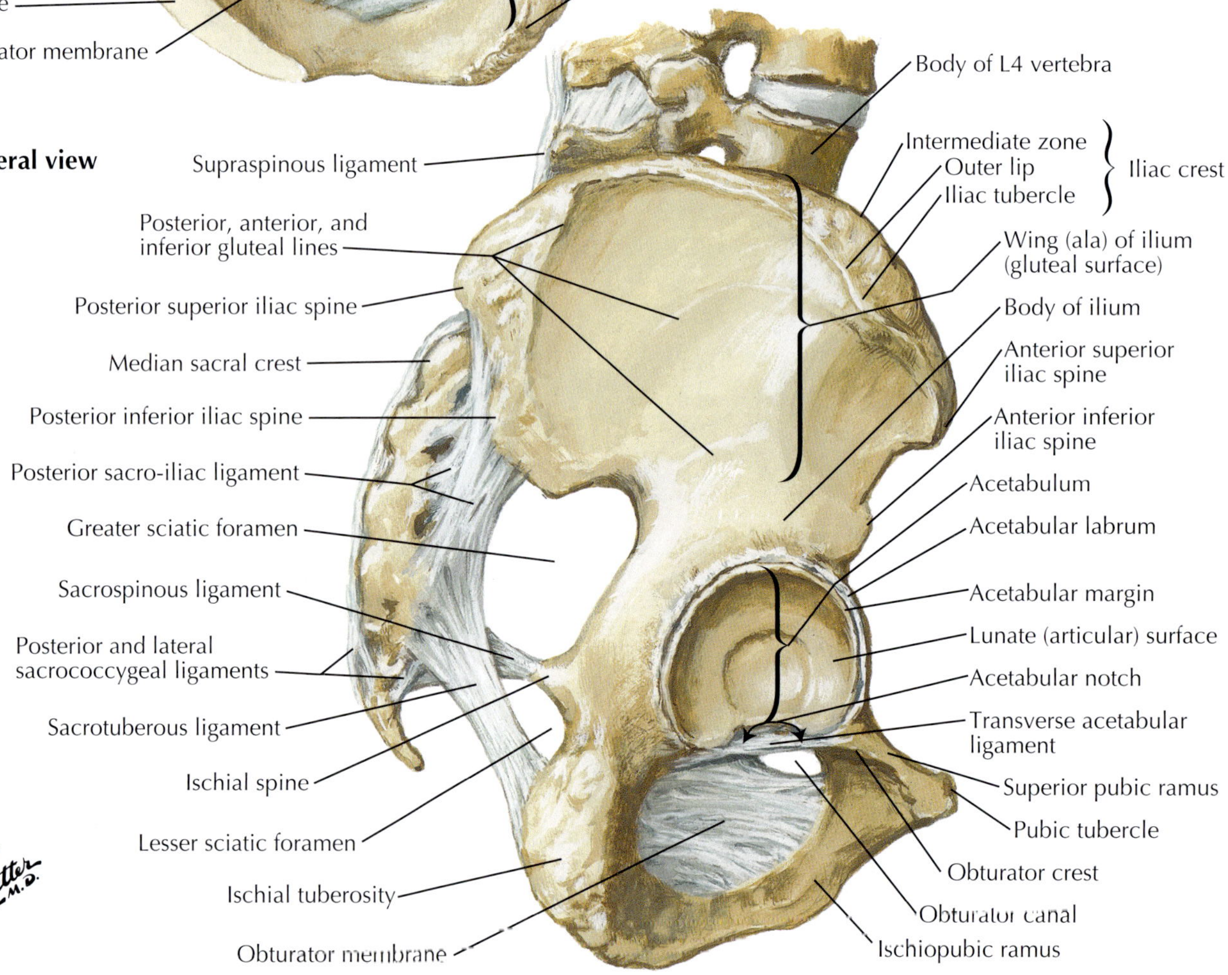

See also Plates 348, 350, 370

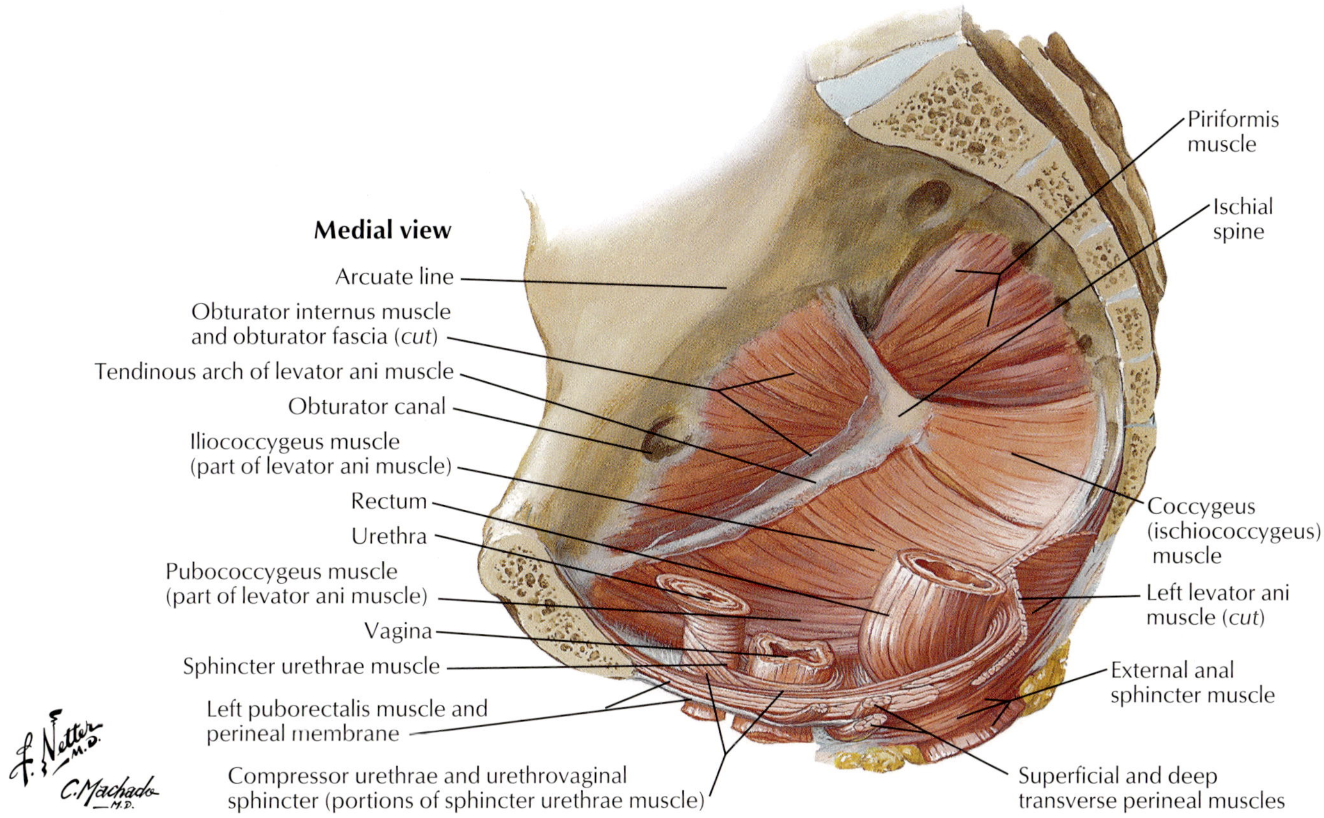

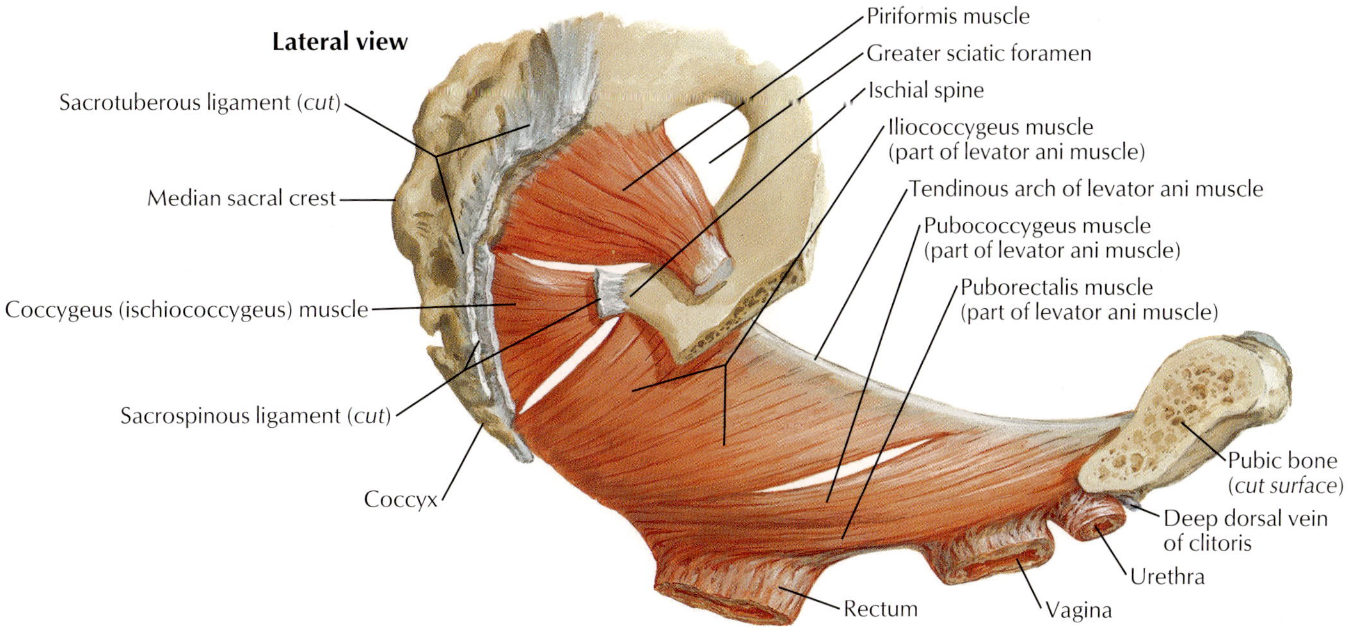

Pelvic Diaphragm: Female (continued)

For urogenital diaphragm see Plate 356

Medial view

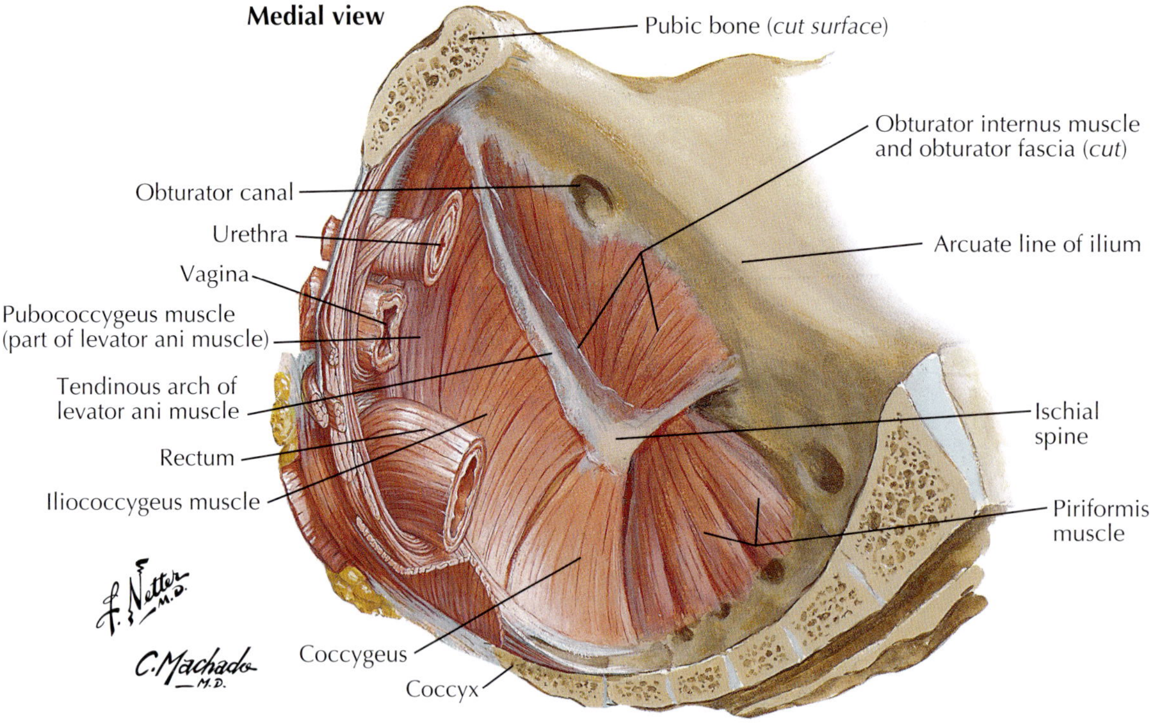

Superior view

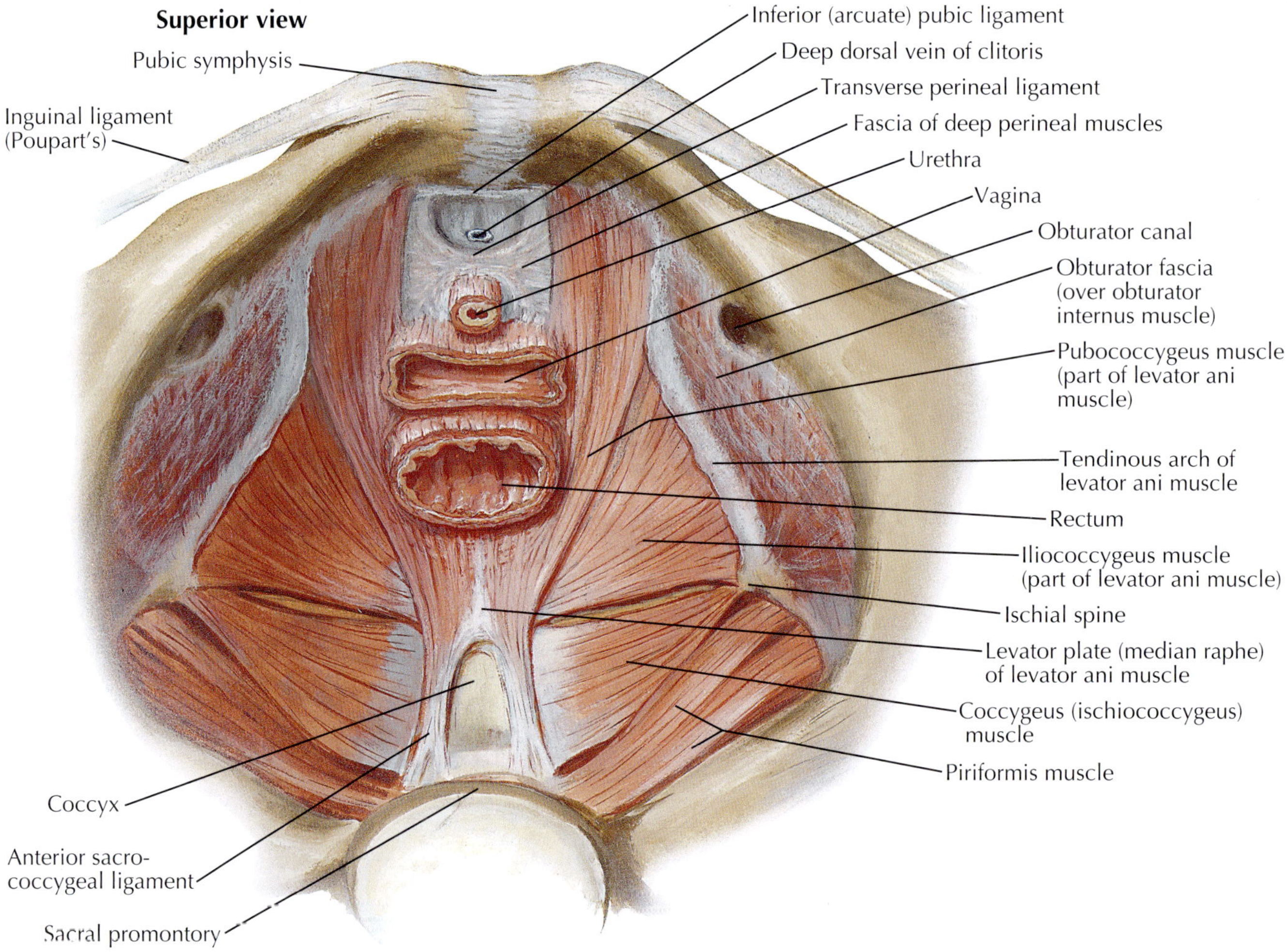

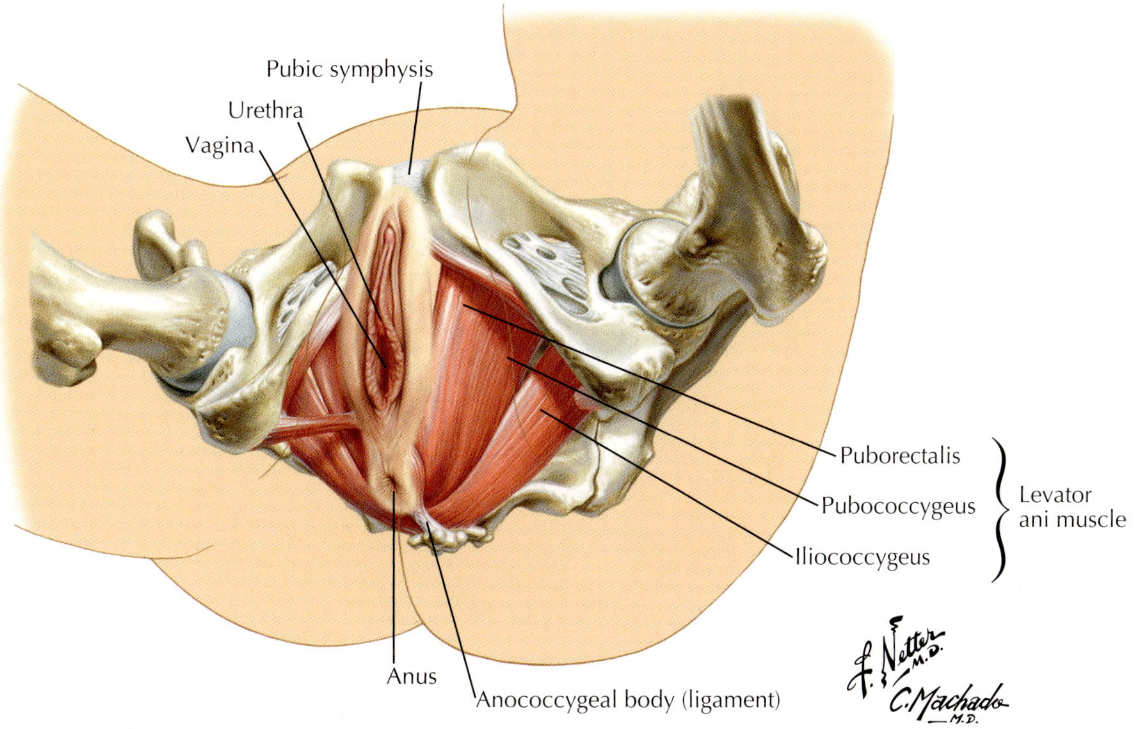

Inferior view

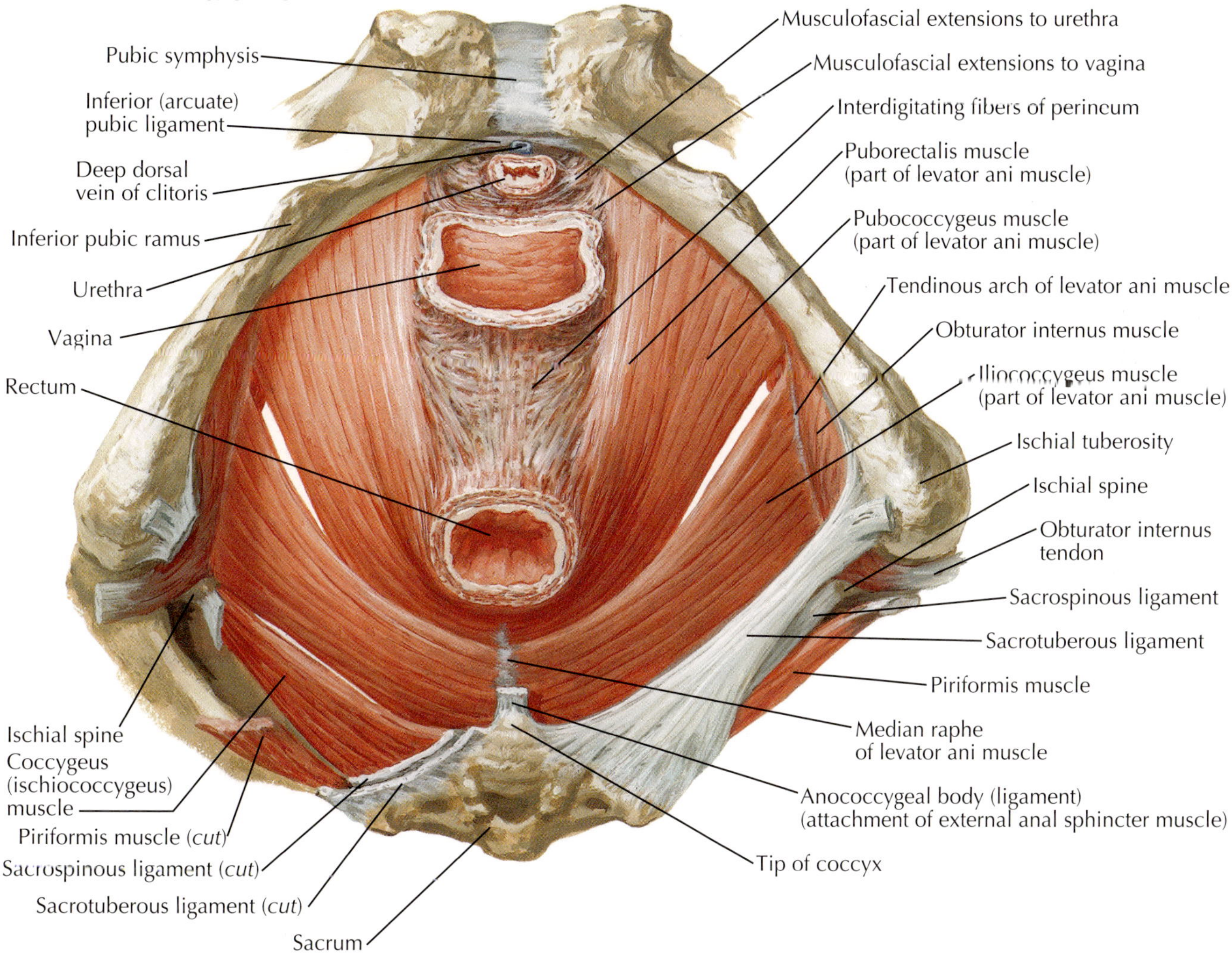

See also Plates 258, 261

Superior view
(*viscera removed*)

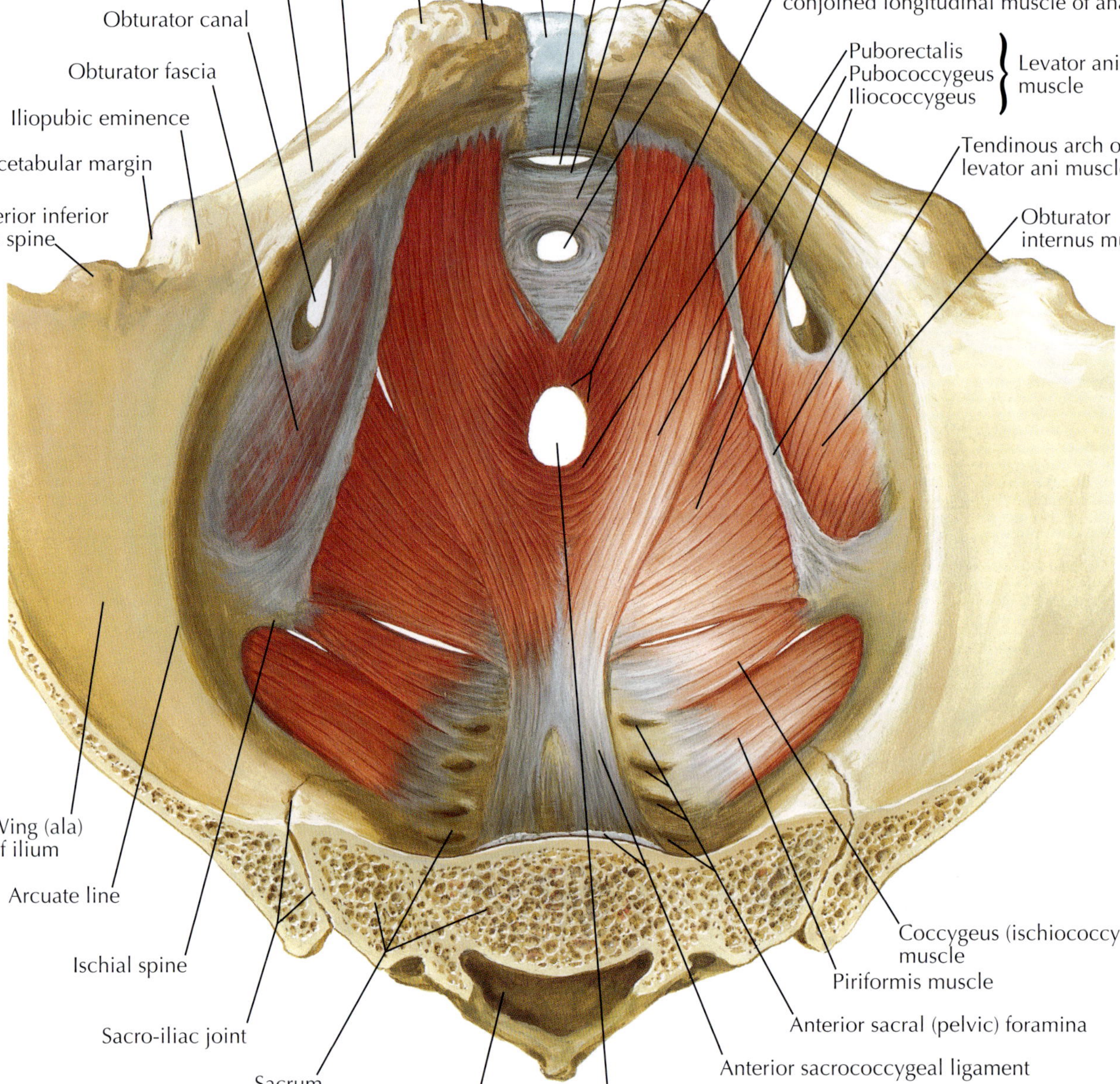

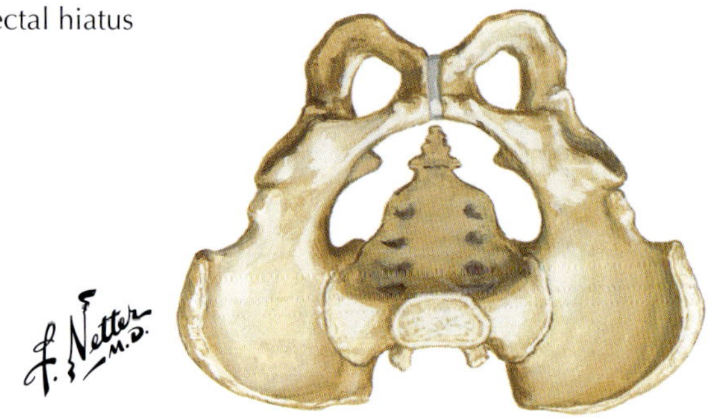

Pelvic Diaphragm: Male (continued)

For urogenital diaphragm see Plate 361

Inferior view

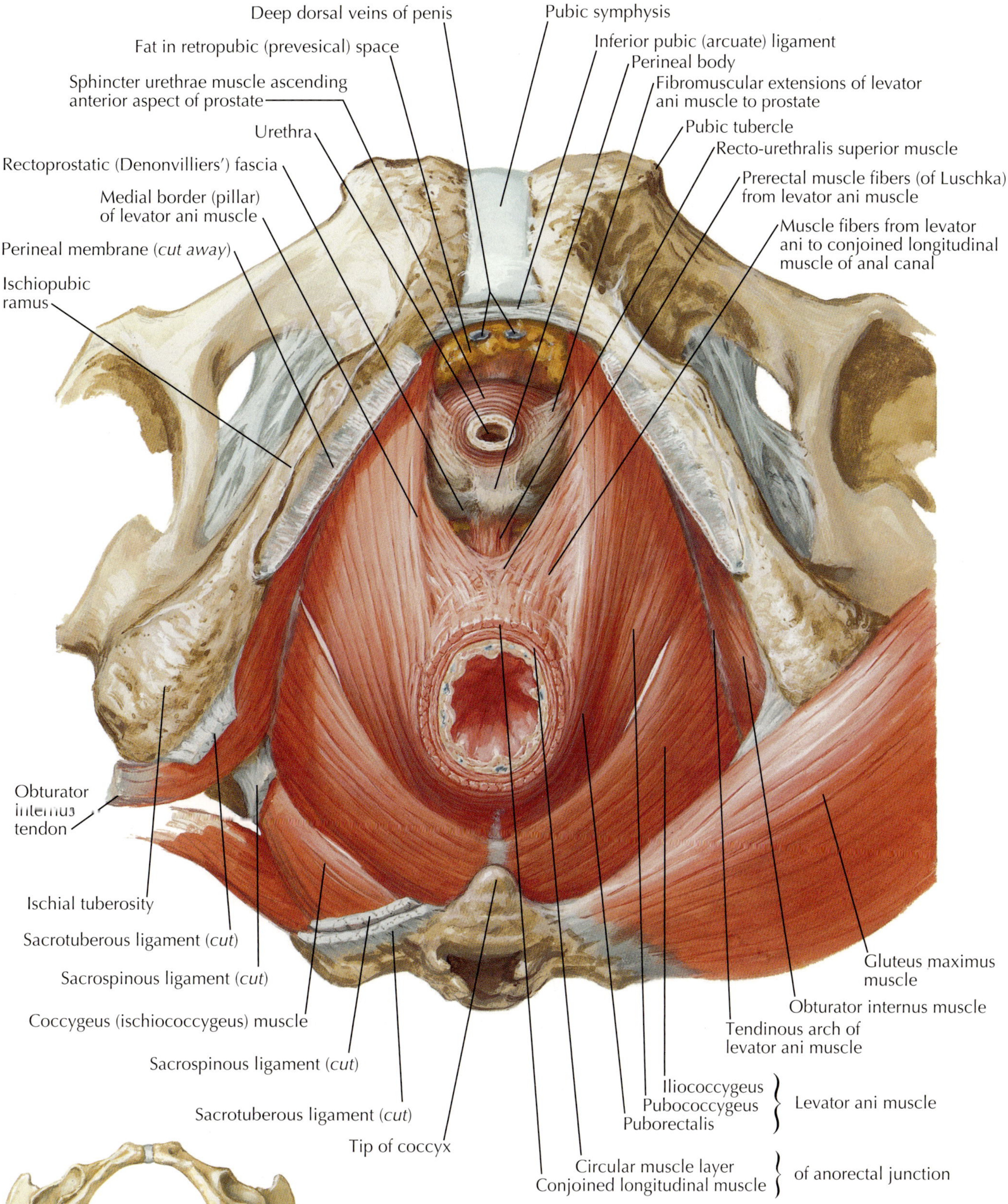

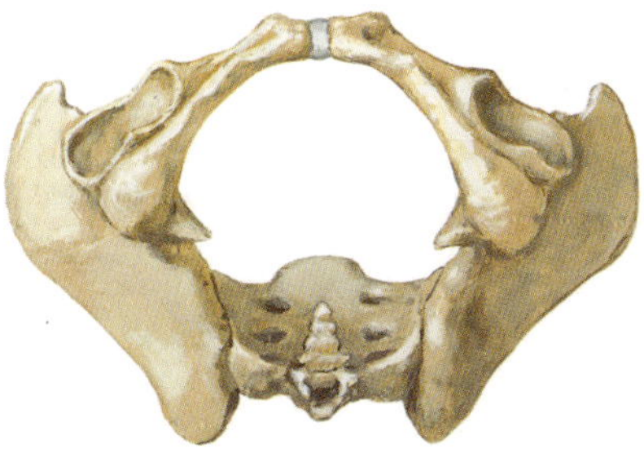

Paramedian (sagittal) dissection

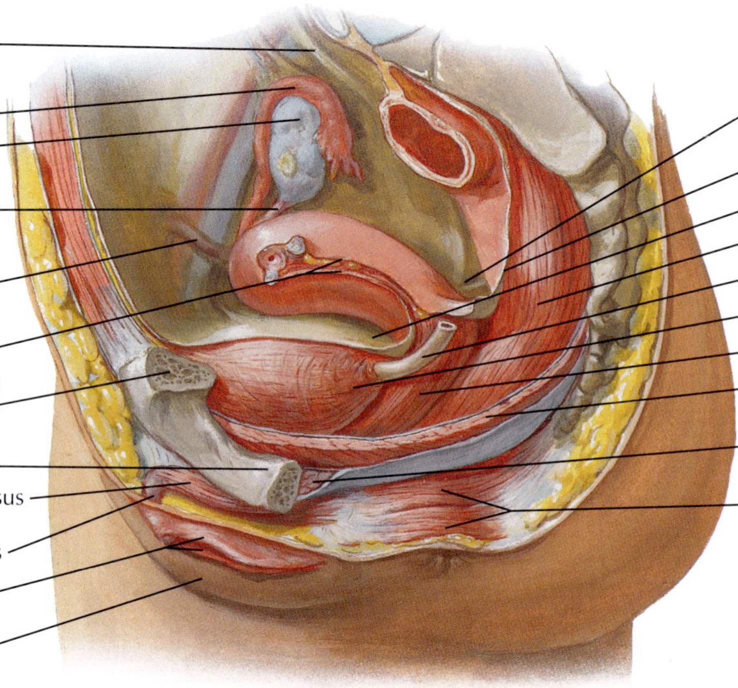

Median (sagittal) section

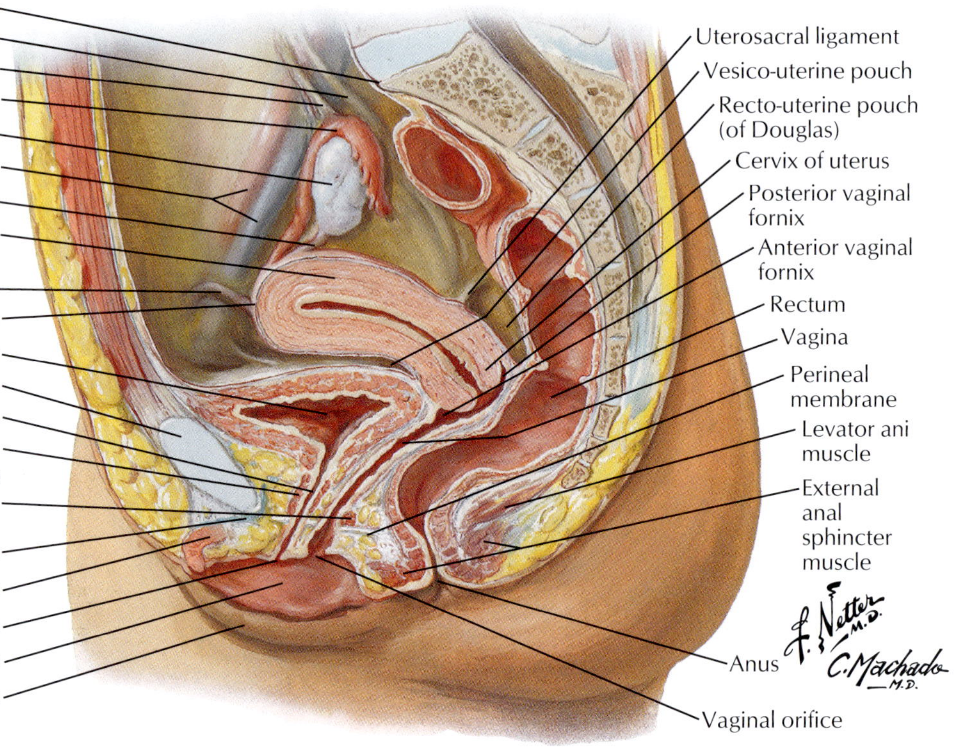

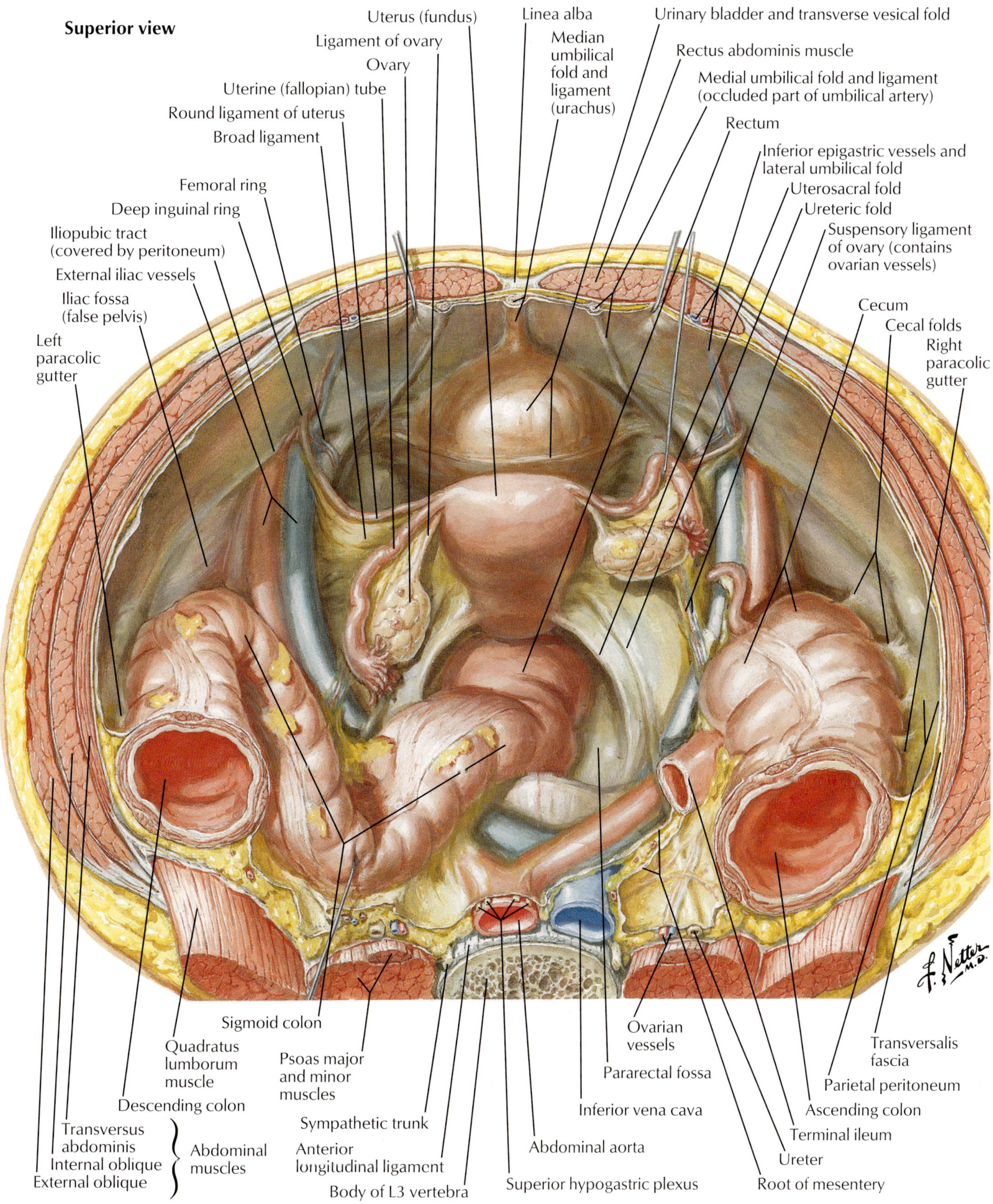
Superior view
Uterus (fundus)
Ligament of ovary
Ovary
Uterine (fallopian) tube
Round ligament of uterus
Broad ligament
Femoral ring
Deep inguinal ring
Iliopubic tract (covered by peritoneum)
External iliac vessels
Iliac fossa (false pelvis)
Left paracolic gutter
Linea alba
Median umbilical fold and ligament (urachus)
Urinary bladder and transverse vesical fold
Rectus abdominis muscle
Medial umbilical fold and ligament (occluded part of umbilical artery)
Rectum
Inferior epigastric vessels and lateral umbilical fold
Uterosacral fold
Ureteric fold
Suspensory ligament of ovary (contains ovarian vessels)
Cecum
Cecal folds
Right paracolic gutter
Sigmoid colon
Quadratus lumborum muscle
Psoas major and minor muscles
Descending colon
Transversus abdominis
Internal oblique
External oblique
Abdominal muscles
Sympathetic trunk
Anterior longitudinal ligament
Body of L3 vertebra
Abdominal aorta
Superior hypogastric plexus
Ovarian vessels
Pararectal fossa
Inferior vena cava
Transversalis fascia
Parietal peritoneum
Ascending colon
Terminal ileum
Ureter
Root of mesentery

Superior view with peritoneum intact

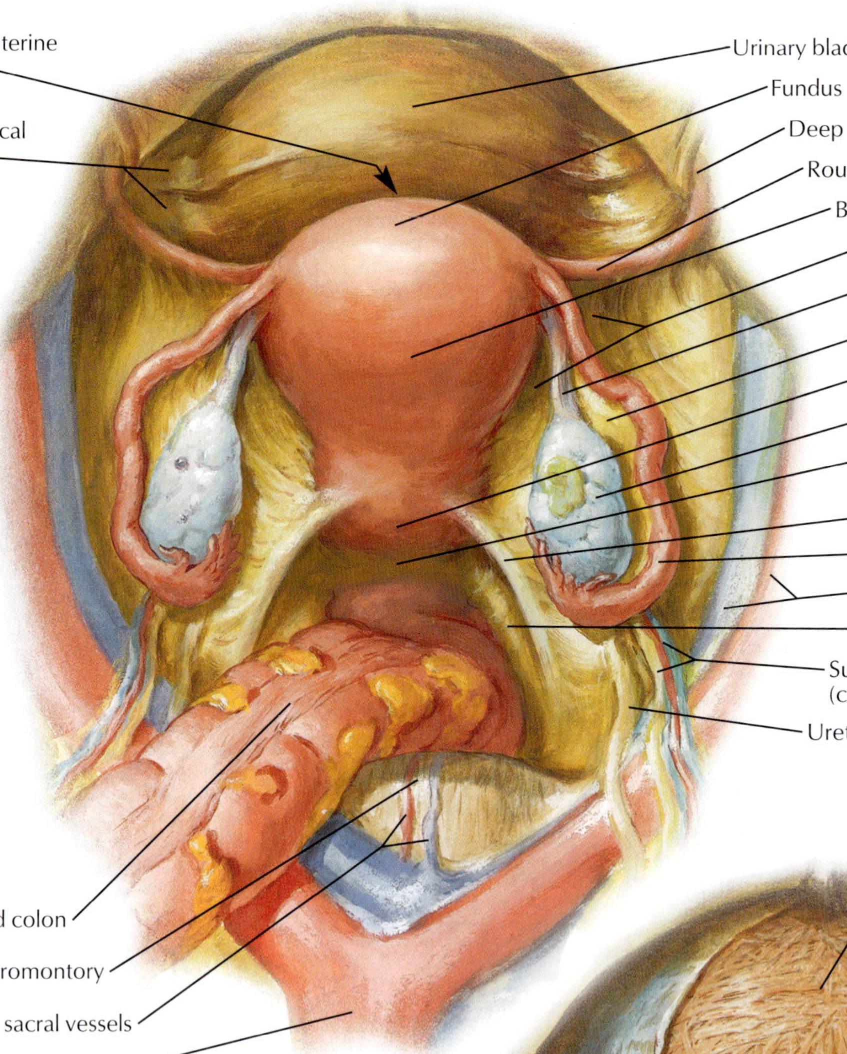

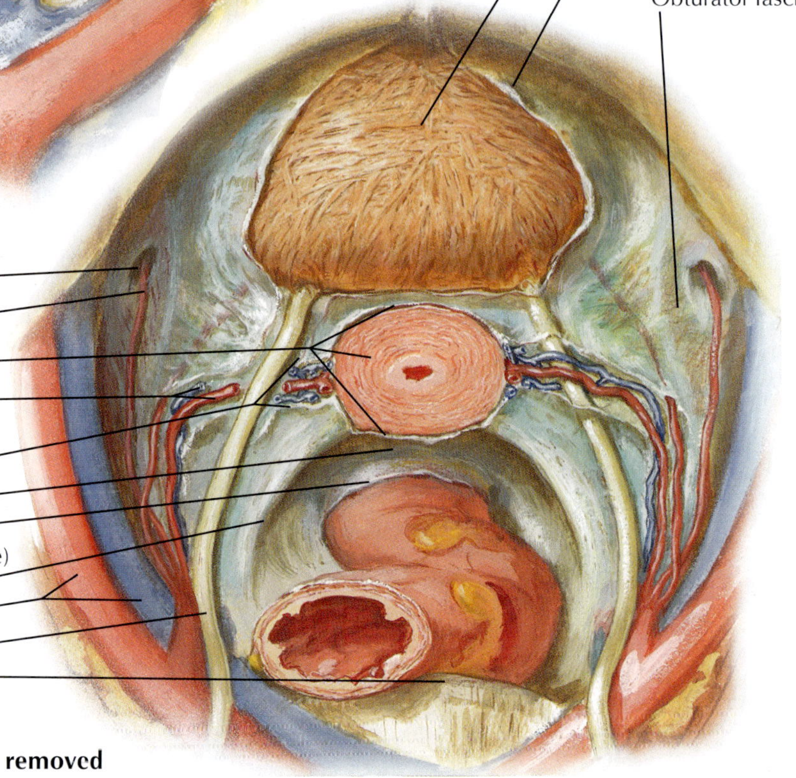

Superior view with peritoneum and uterus removed

Female: superior view (peritoneum and loose areolar tissue removed)

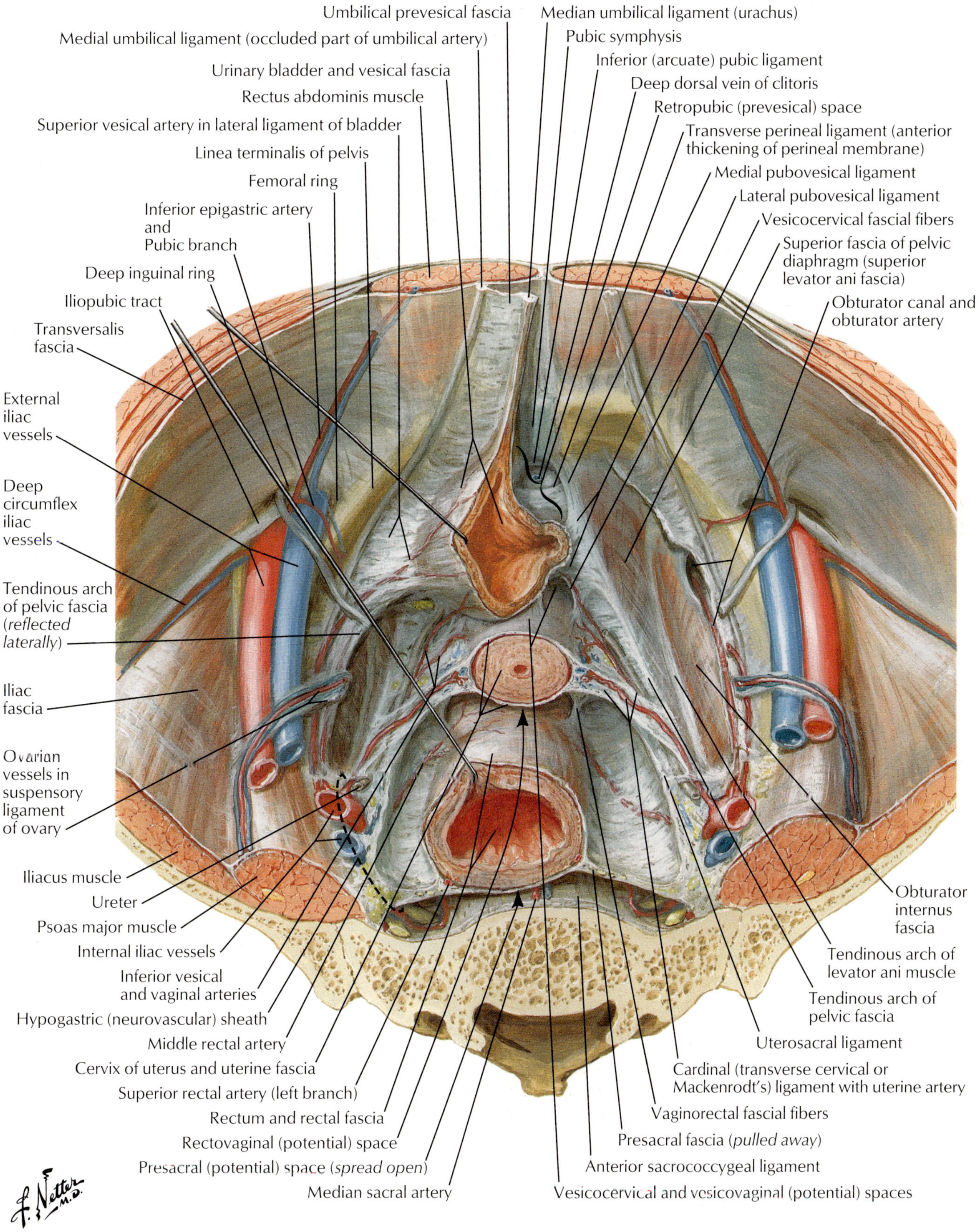

Paramedian (sagittal) dissection

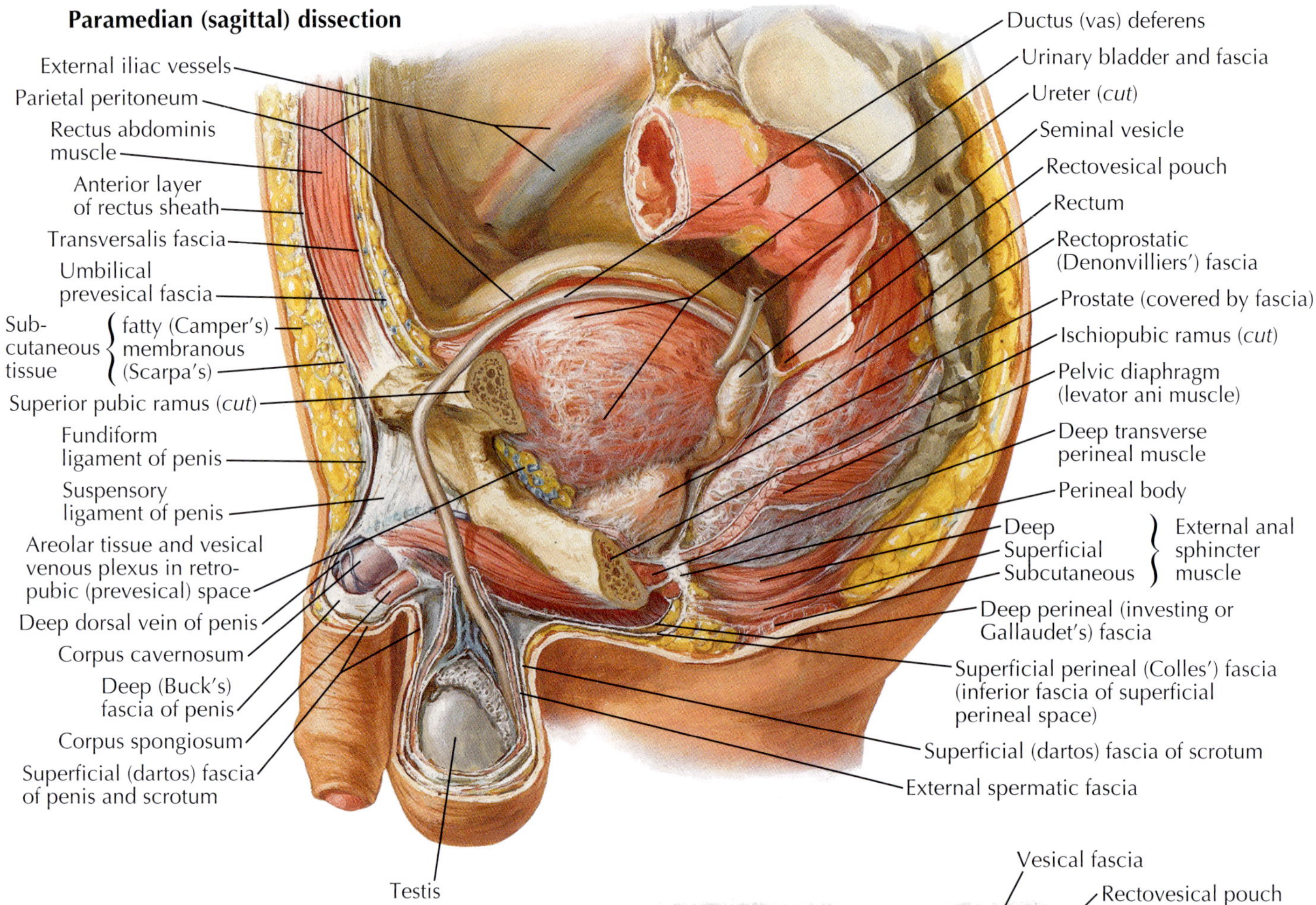

Median (sagittal) section

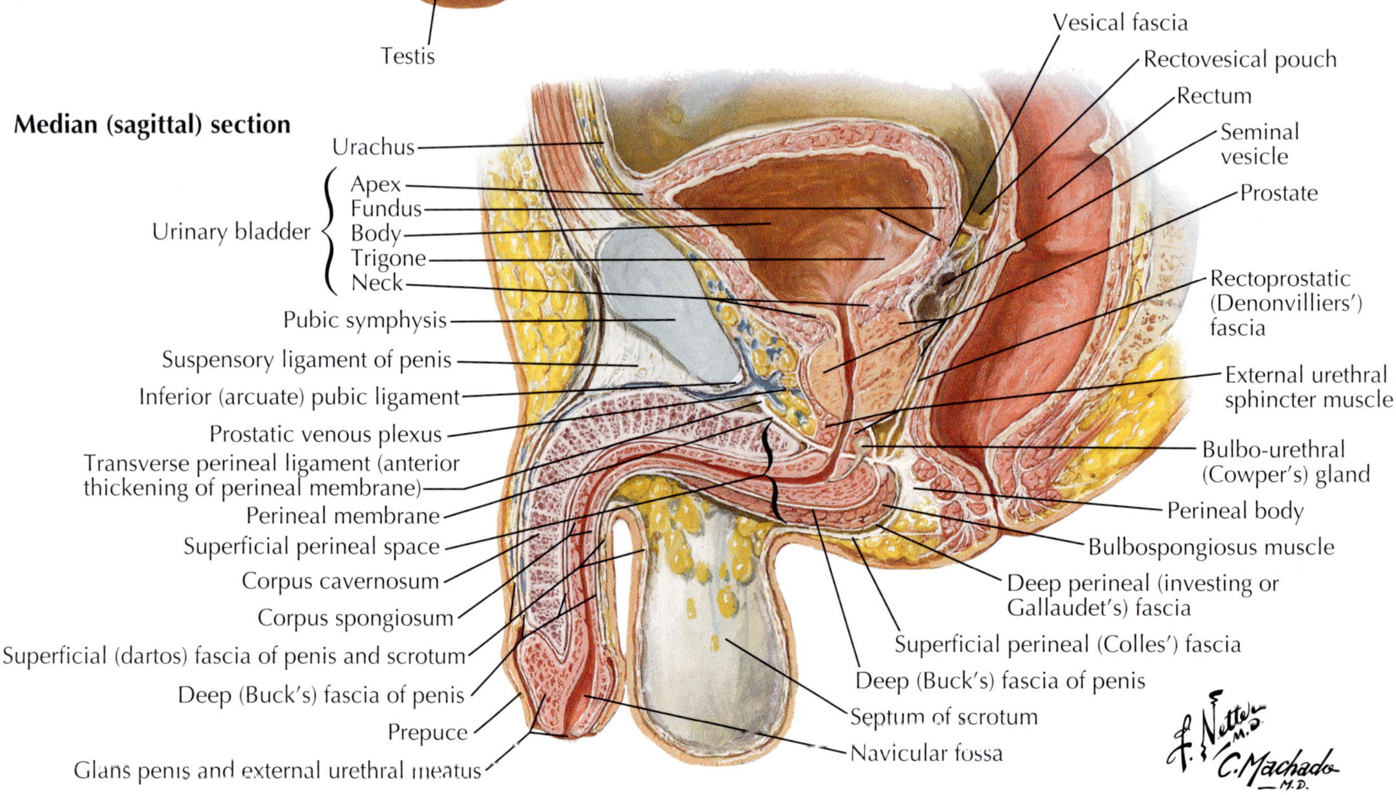

Superior view

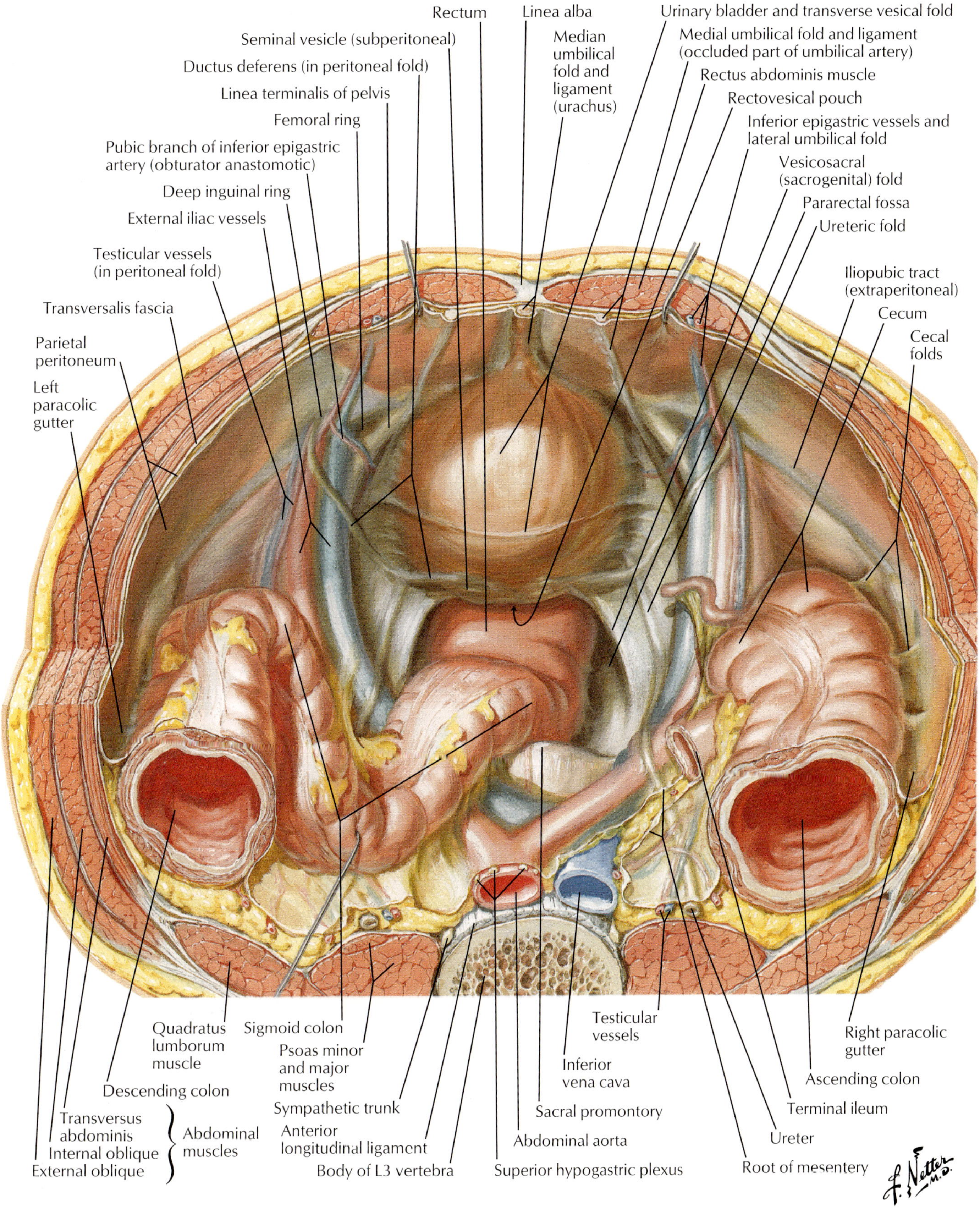

Female: midsagittal section

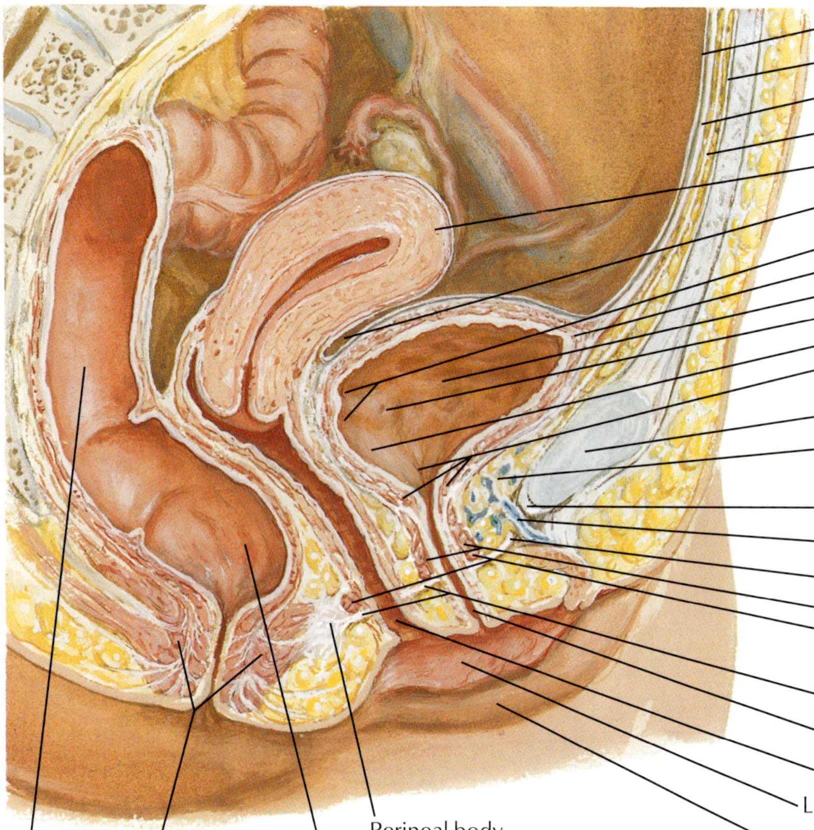

Superior view with peritoneum and vesical fascia removed

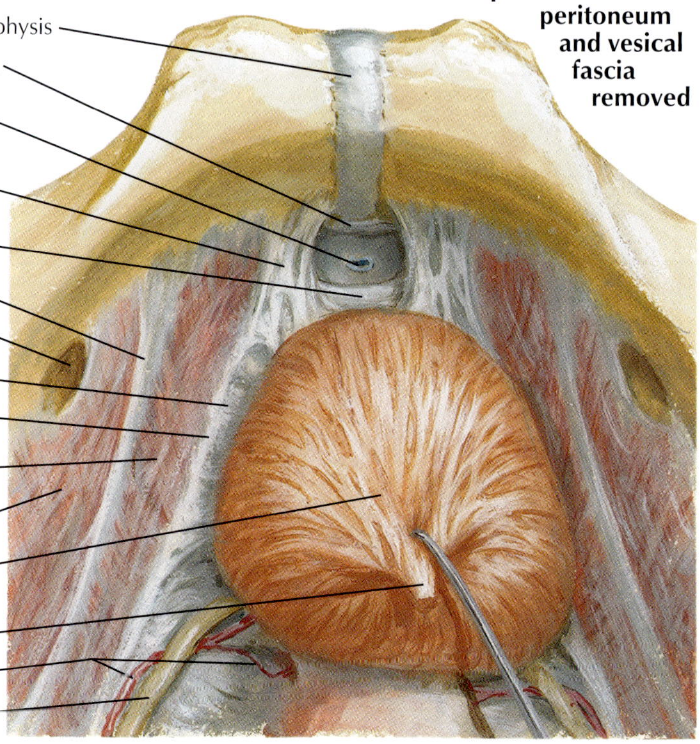

Female Sphincters

See also Plate 356

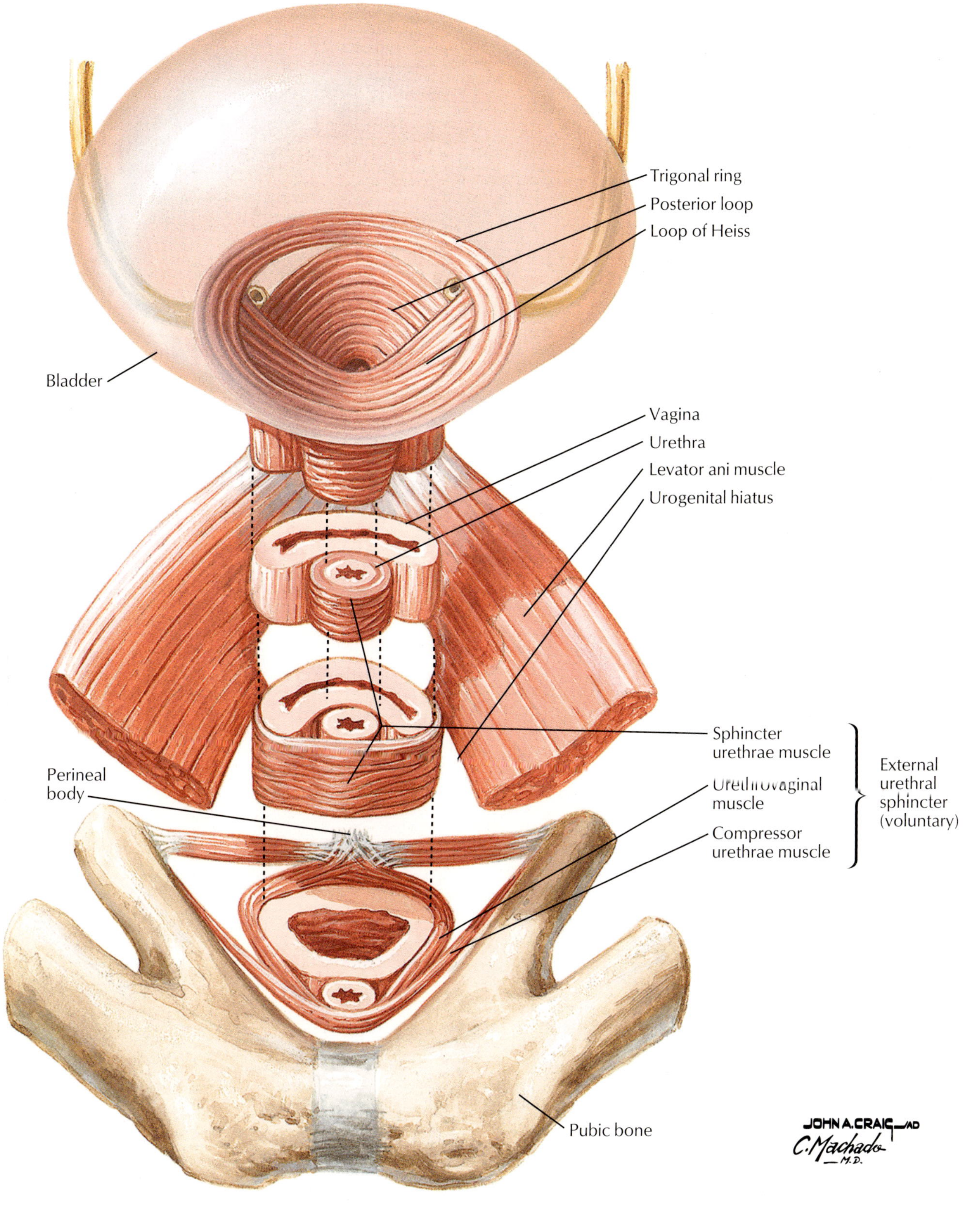

Urinary Bladder: Female and Male

See also **Plates 340, 344, 381**

Female: frontal section

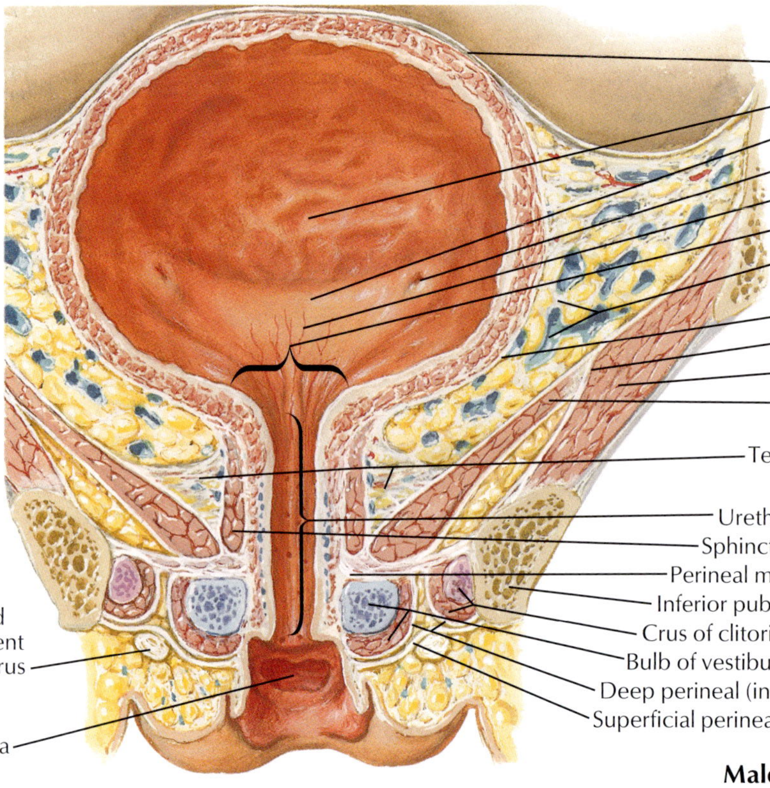

Male: frontal section

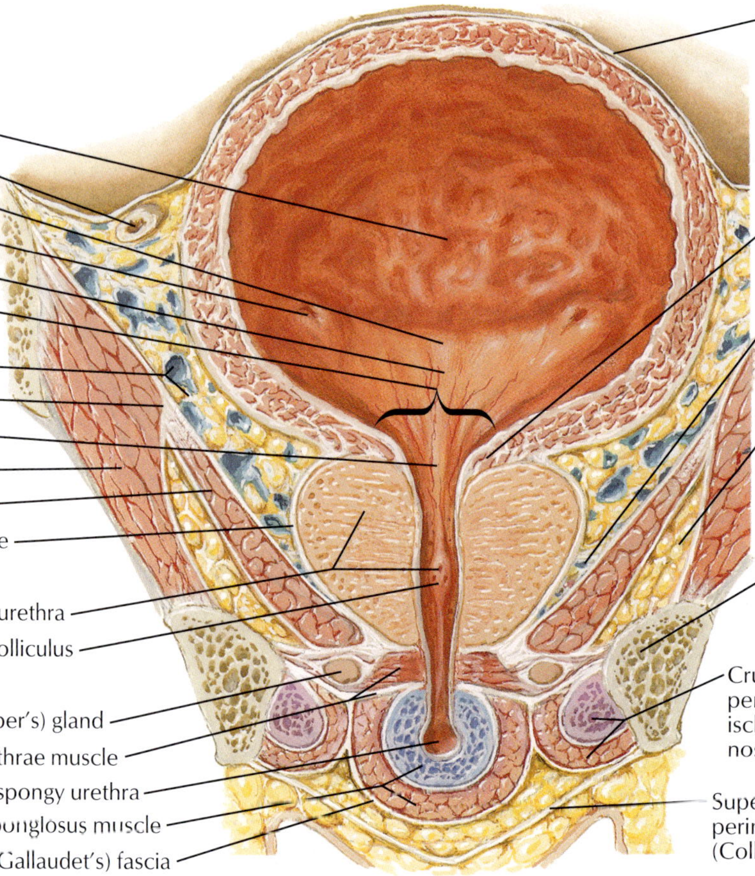

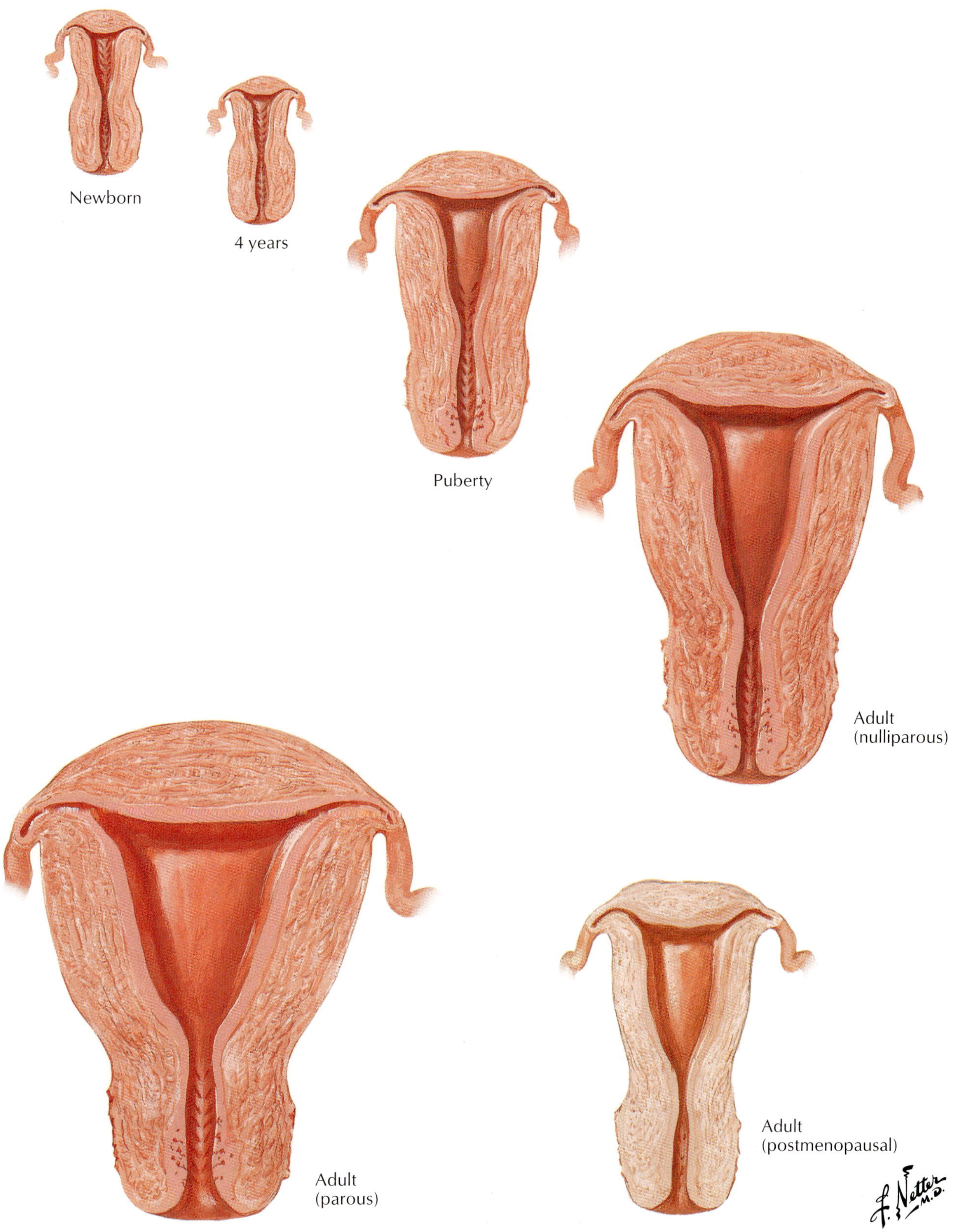
Newborn
4 years
Puberty
Adult
(nulliparous)
Adult
(parous)
Adult
(postmenopausal)
F. Netter M.D.

Uterus, Vagina, and Supporting Structures

See also **Plates 382, 384, 390**

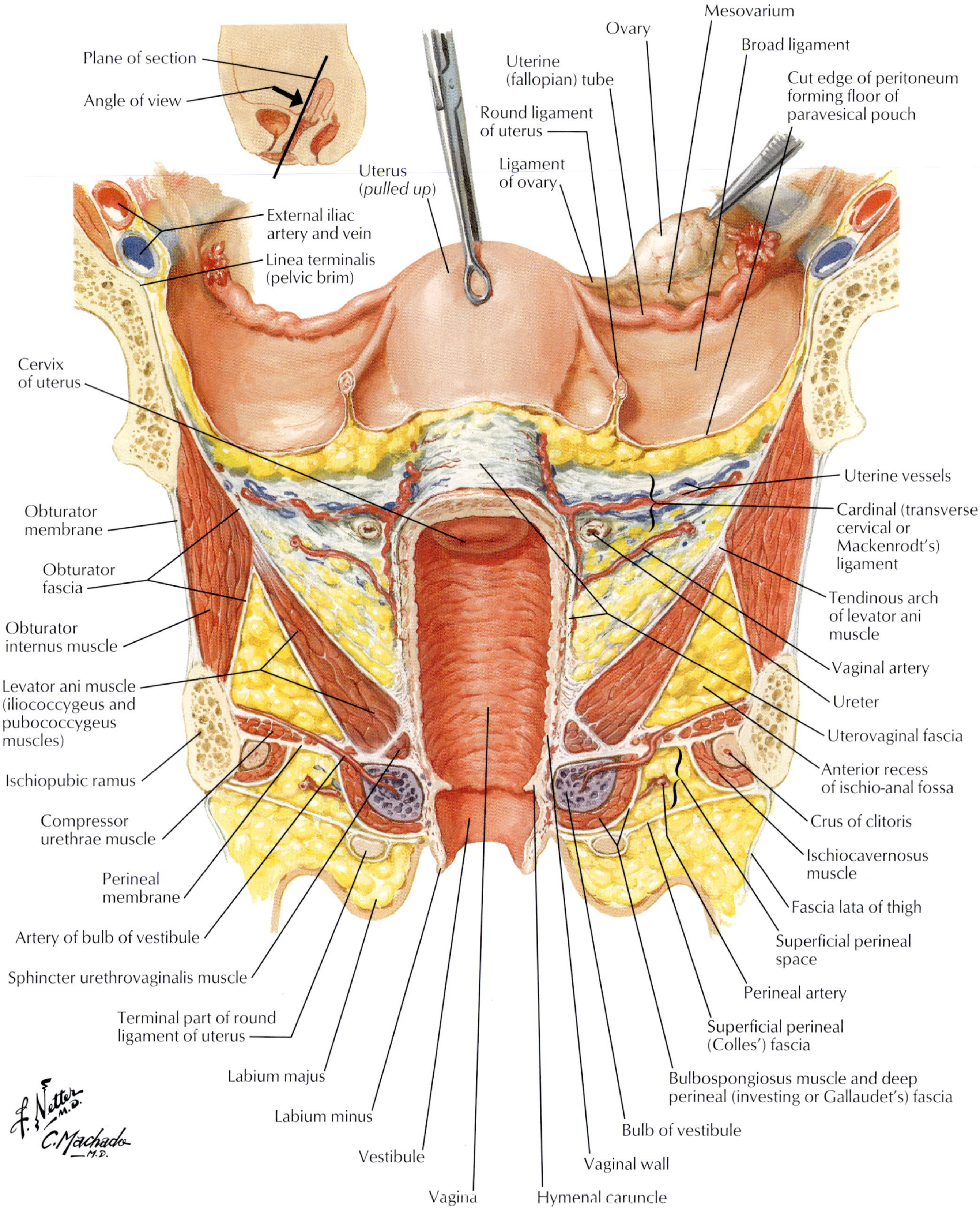

Fascial ligaments of uterus

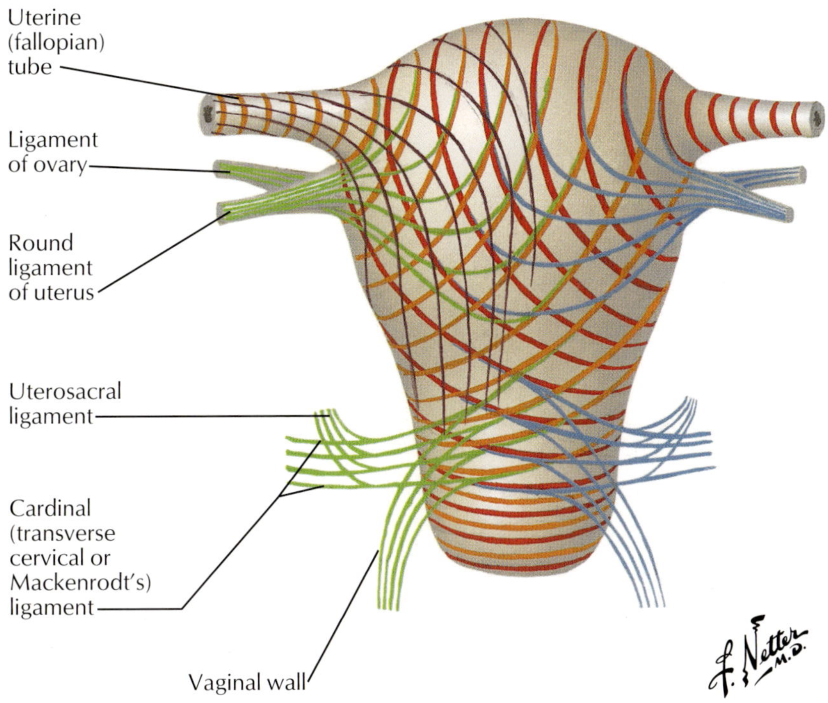

Pelvic fascia and ligaments

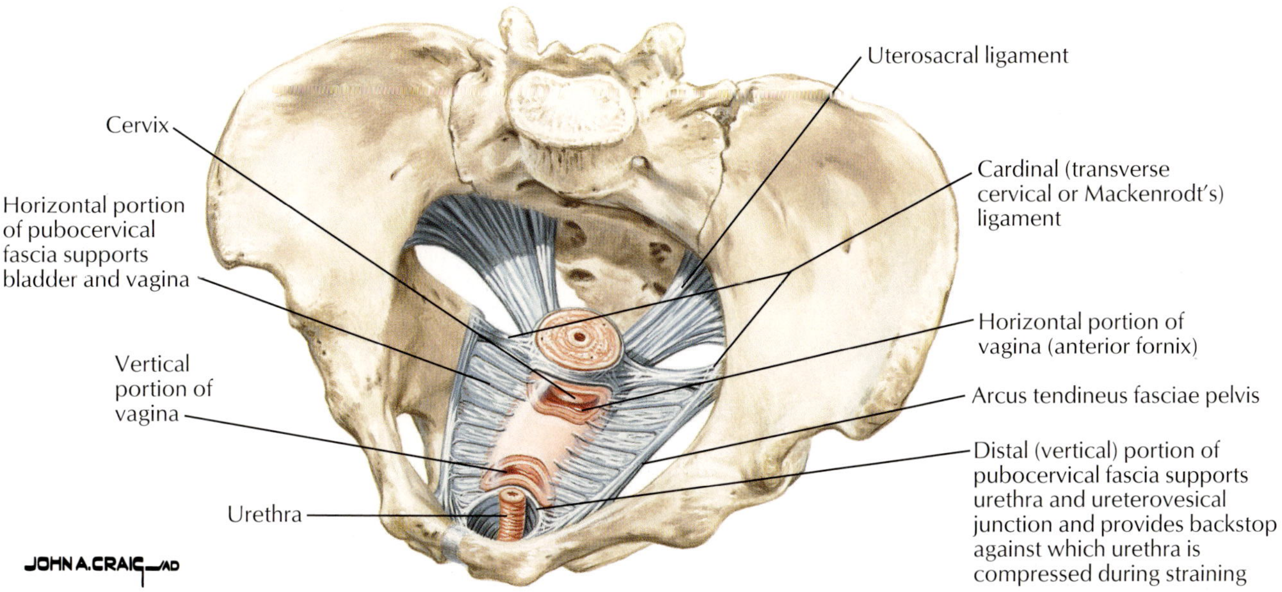

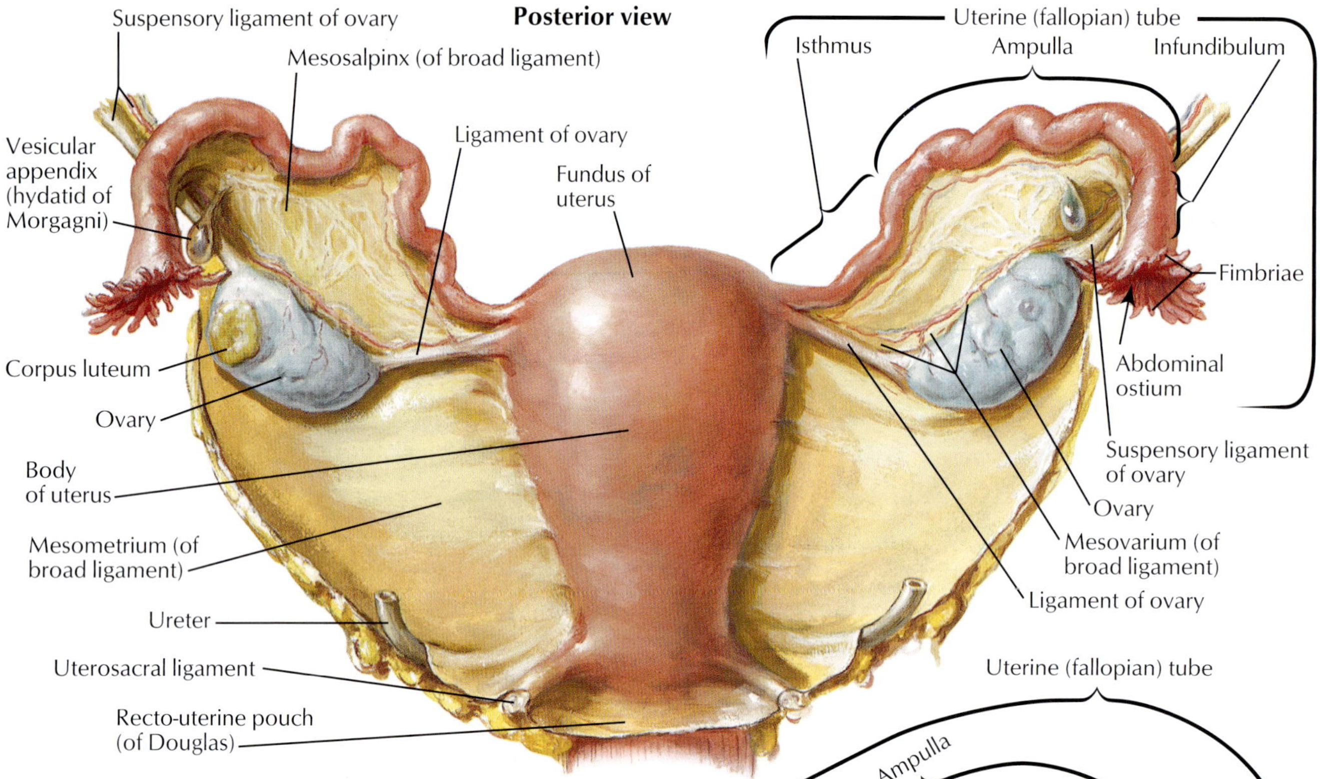

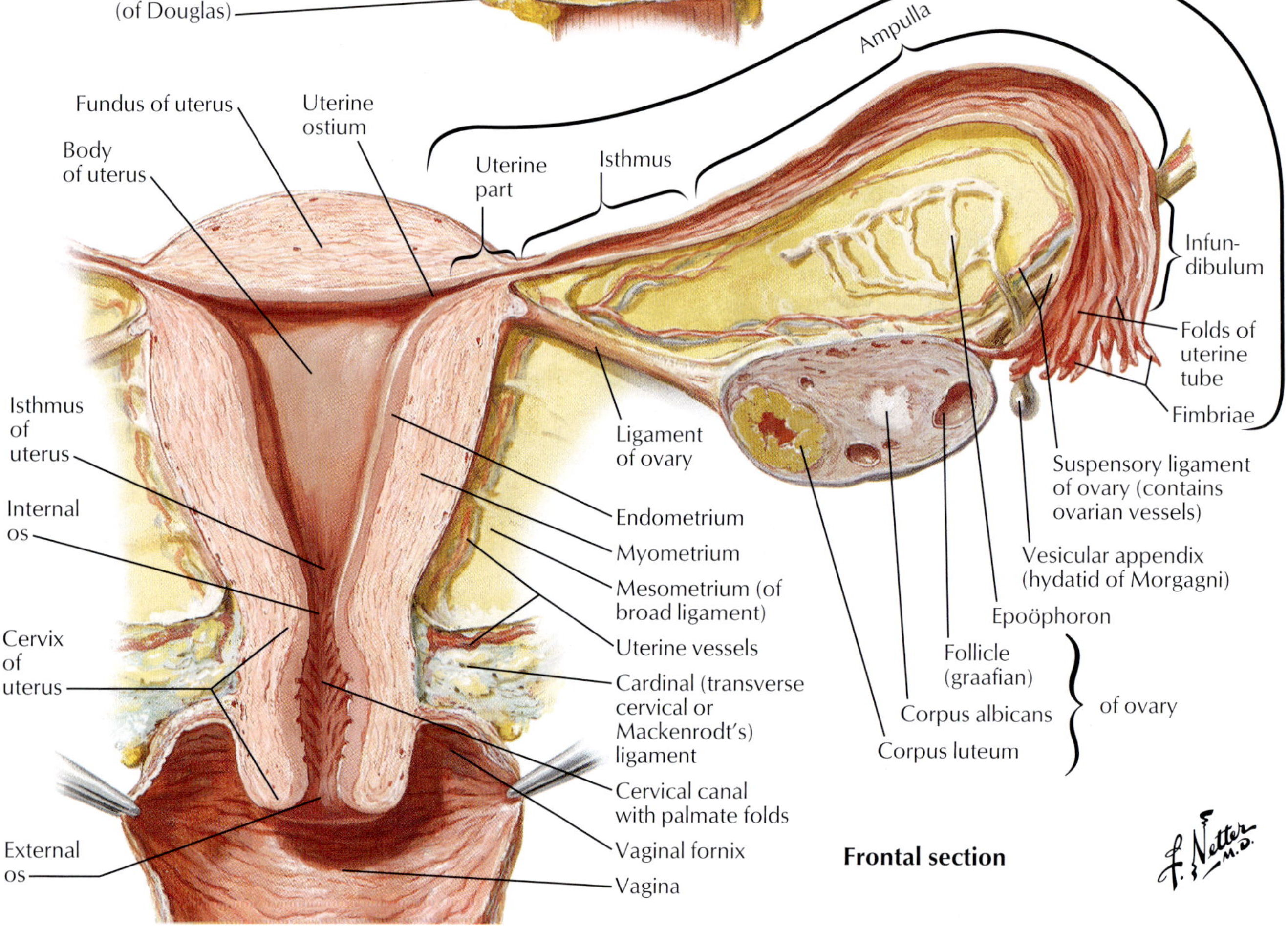

Frontal section

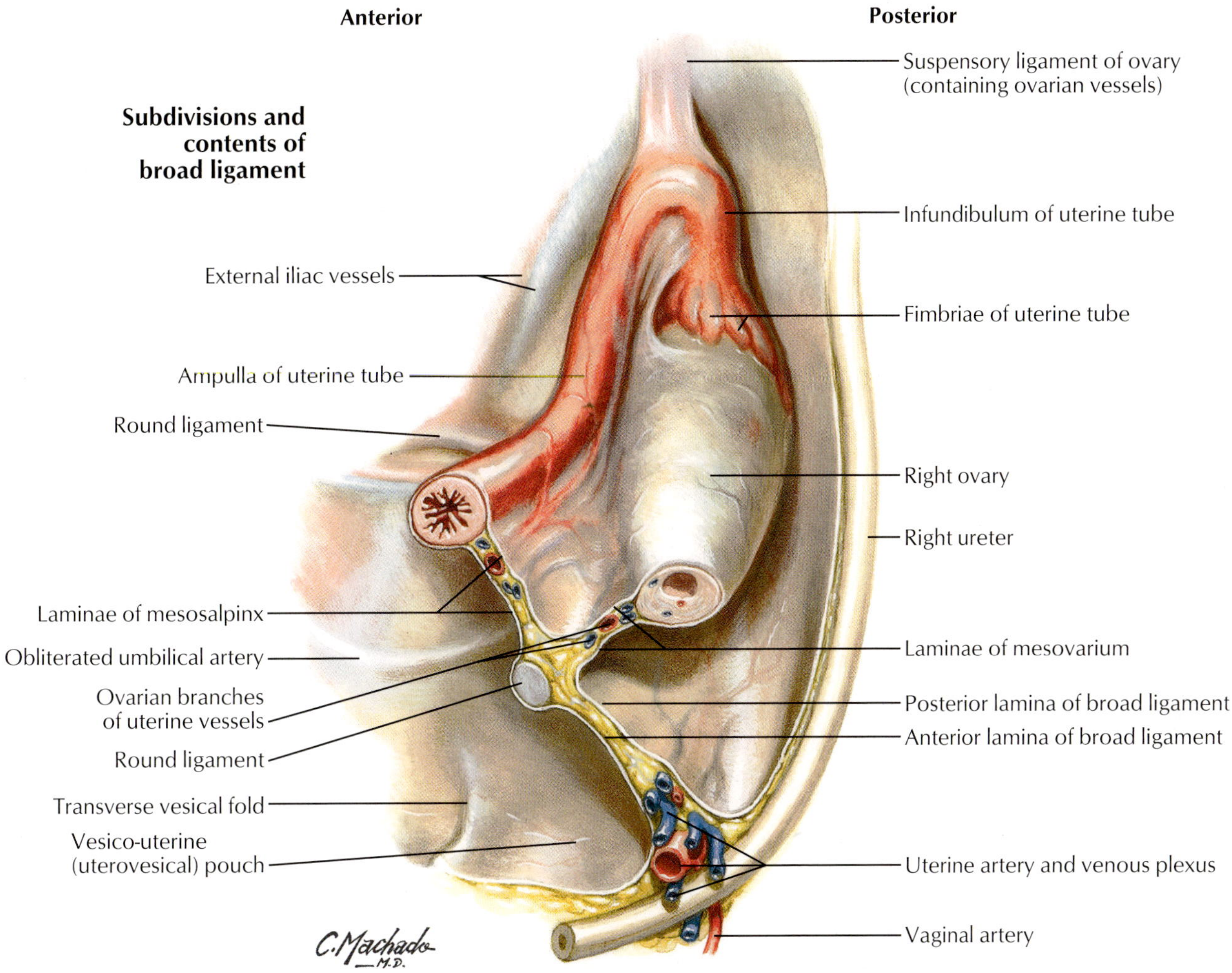
Anterior
Posterior
Subdivisions and contents of broad ligament
Suspensory ligament of ovary (containing ovarian vessels)
Infundibulum of uterine tube
External iliac vessels
Fimbriae of uterine tube
Ampulla of uterine tube
Round ligament
Right ovary
Right ureter
Laminae of mesosalpinx
Obliterated umbilical artery
Laminae of mesovarium
Ovarian branches of uterine vessels
Posterior lamina of broad ligament
Anterior lamina of broad ligament
Round ligament
Transverse vesical fold
Vesico-uterine (uterovesical) pouch
Uterine artery and venous plexus
Vaginal artery
C. Machado M.D.

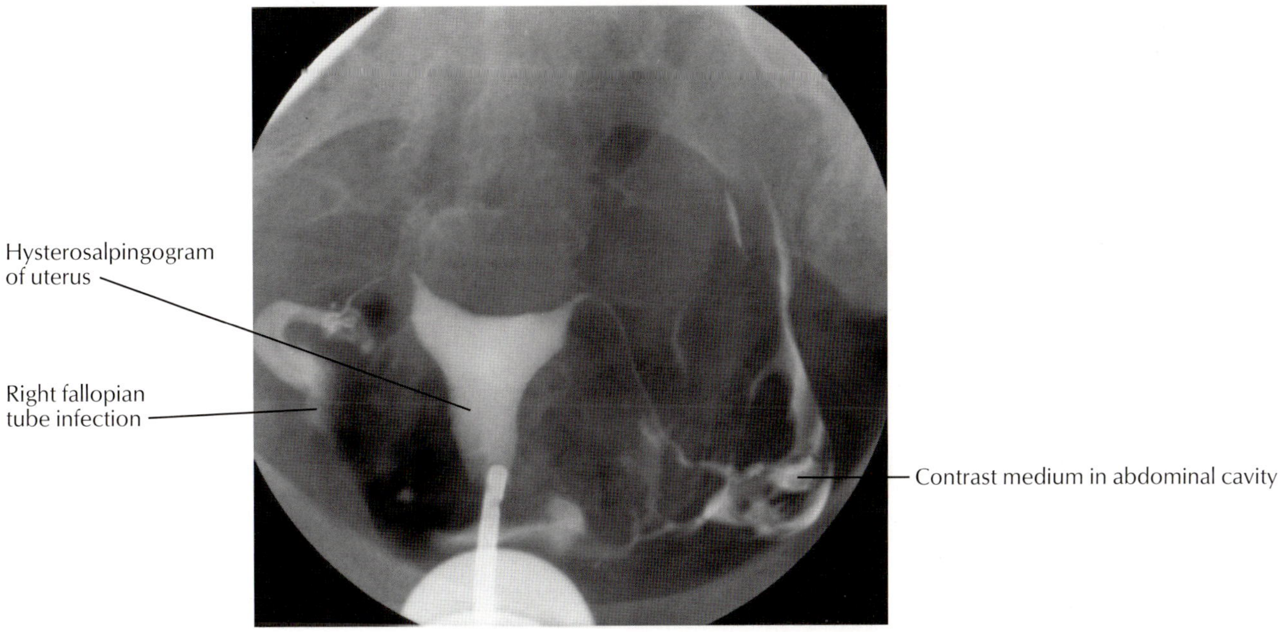
Hysterosalpingogram of uterus
Right fallopian tube infection
Contrast medium in abdominal cavity

See also Plates 382, 385, 391

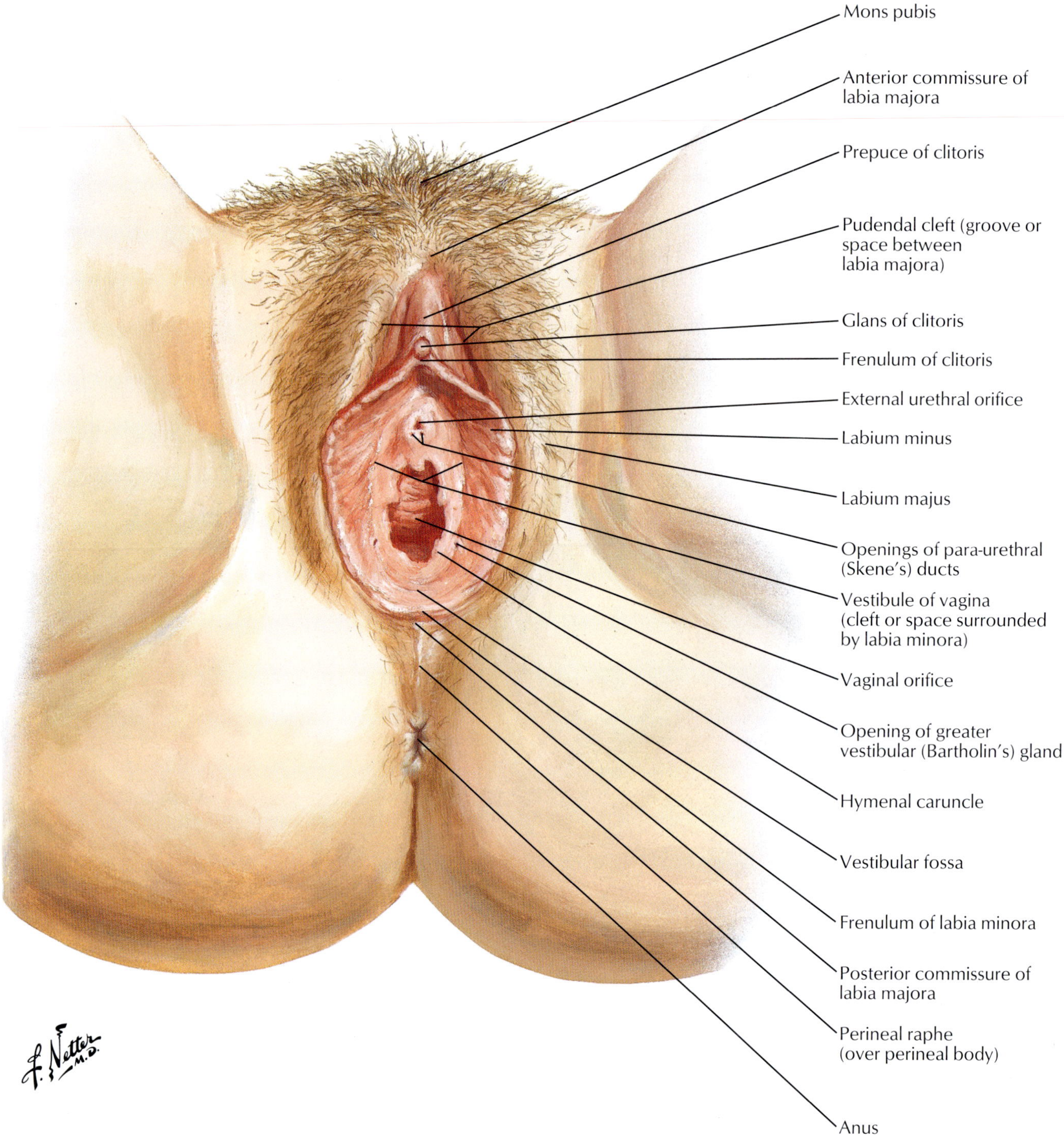

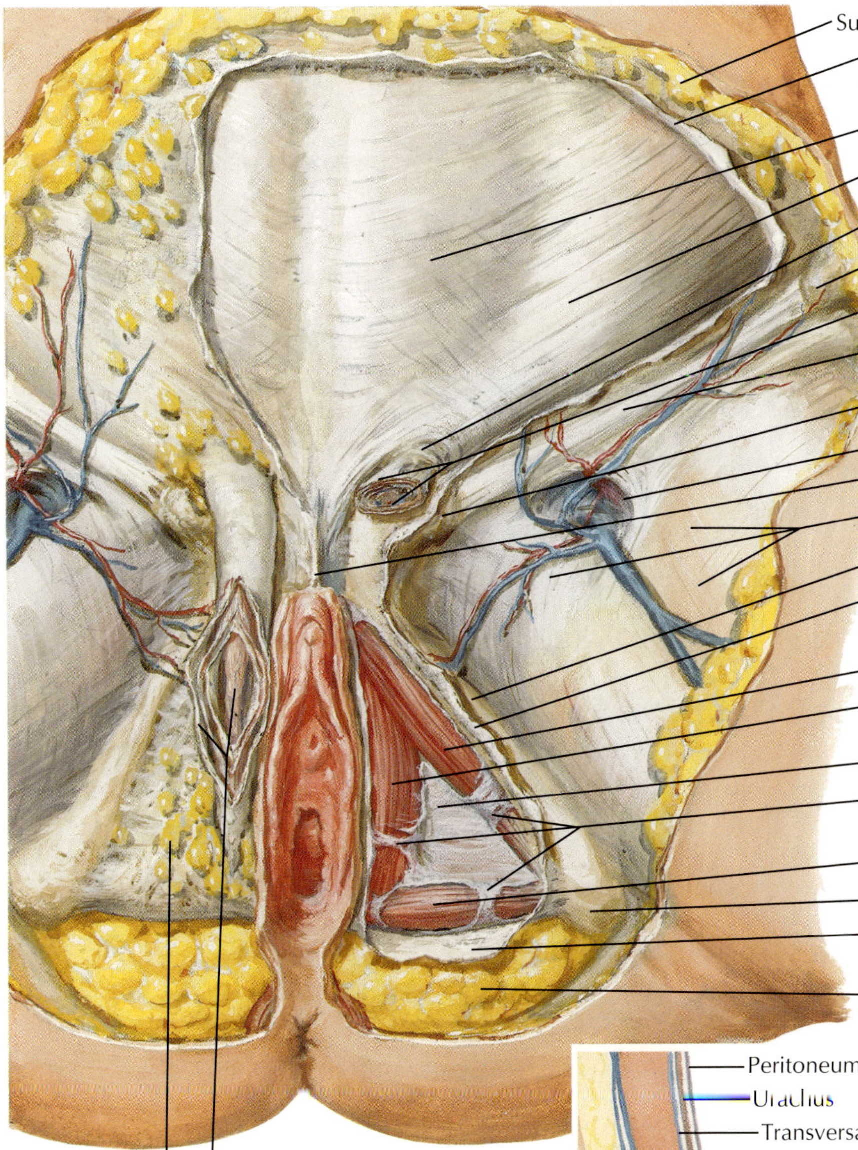
Superficial fatty (Camper's) layer
Deeper membranous (Scarpa's) layer
Subcutaneous tissue
Rectus sheath (anterior layer)
Aponeurosis of external oblique muscle
Superficial inguinal ring
Anterior superior iliac spine
Round ligament of uterus and coverings (*cut*)
Inguinal ligament (Poupart's)
Pubic tubercle
Saphenous opening
Suspensory ligament of clitoris
Fascia lata of thigh
Ischiopubic ramus
Superficial perineal (Colles') fascia (*cut away*) to open superficial perineal space
Ischiocavernosus muscle
Bulbospongiosus muscle (covers bulb of vestibule)
Perineal membrane
Deep perineal (investing or Gallaudet's) fascia (*partially cut away*)
Superficial transverse perineal muscle
Ischial tuberosity
Superficial perineal (Colles') fascia (*cut edge turned down*)
Fat body of ischio-anal fossa
Superficial perineal (Colles') fascia
Round ligament of uterus and coverings

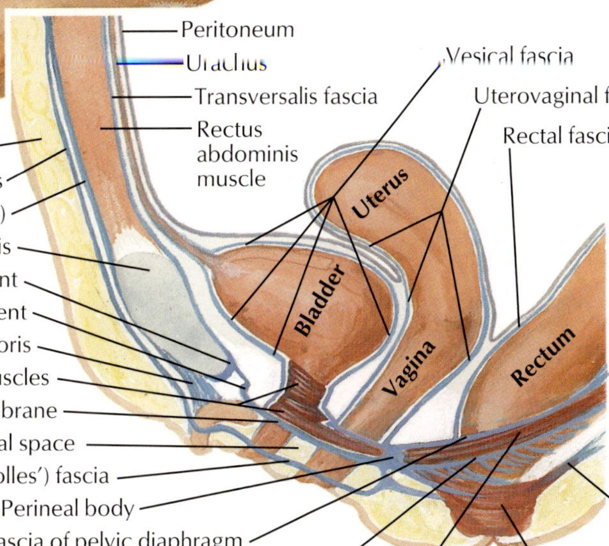
Peritoneum
Urachus
Transversalis fascia
Rectus abdominis muscle
Vesical fascia
Uterovaginal fascia
Rectal fascia
Uterus
Bladder
Vagina
Rectum
Subcutaneous tissue
Fatty
Membranous
Rectus sheath (anterior layer)
Pubic symphysis
Inferior (arcuate) pubic ligament
Transverse perineal ligament
Suspensory ligament of clitoris
Sphincter urethrae and sphincter urethrovaginalis muscles
Perineal membrane
Superficial perineal space
Superficial perineal (Colles') fascia
Perineal body
Superior fascia of pelvic diaphragm
Inferior fascia of pelvic diaphragm
Levator ani muscle
Anococcygeal body
External anal sphincter muscle

Female Perineum and Deep Perineum

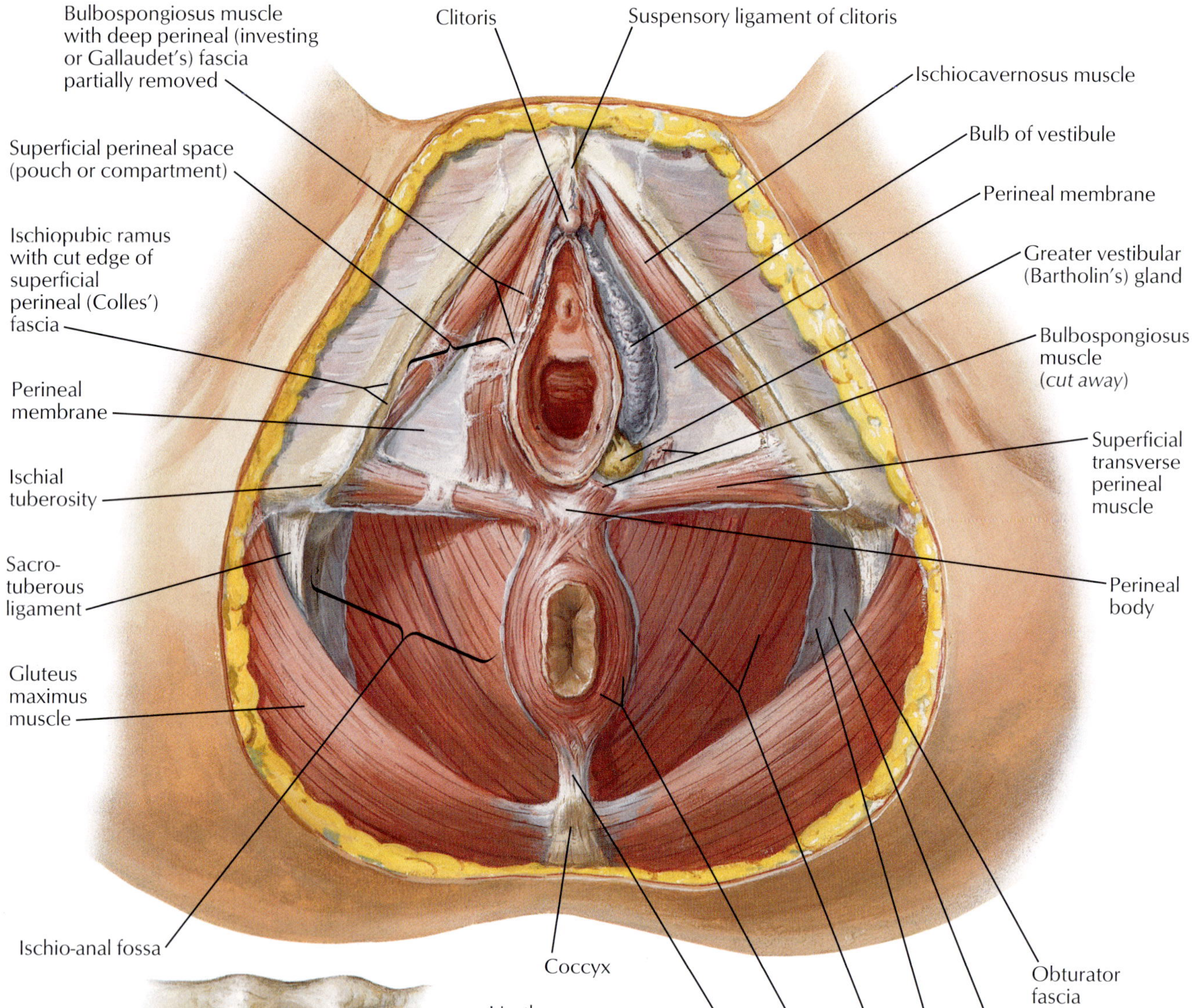

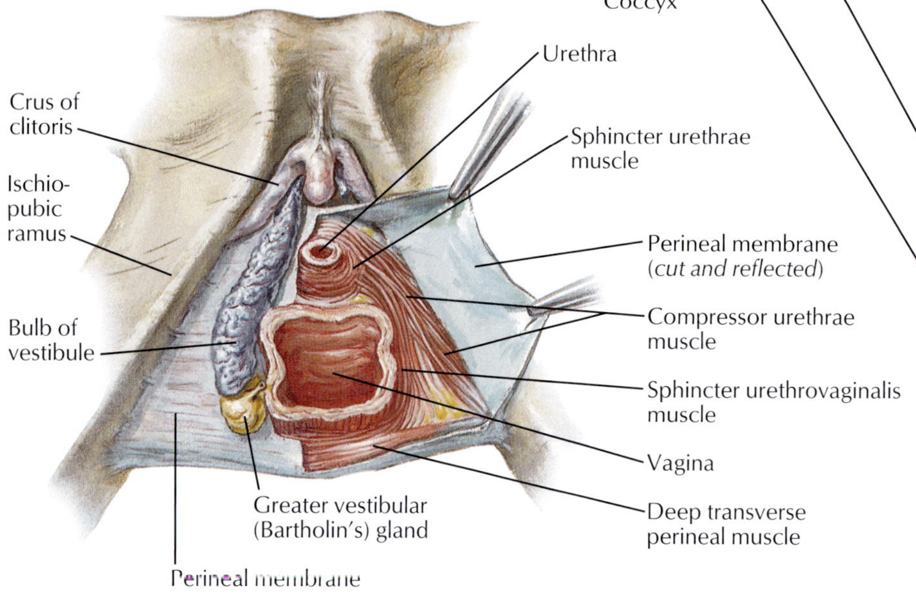

See also Plates 382, 391

Superficial perineal space

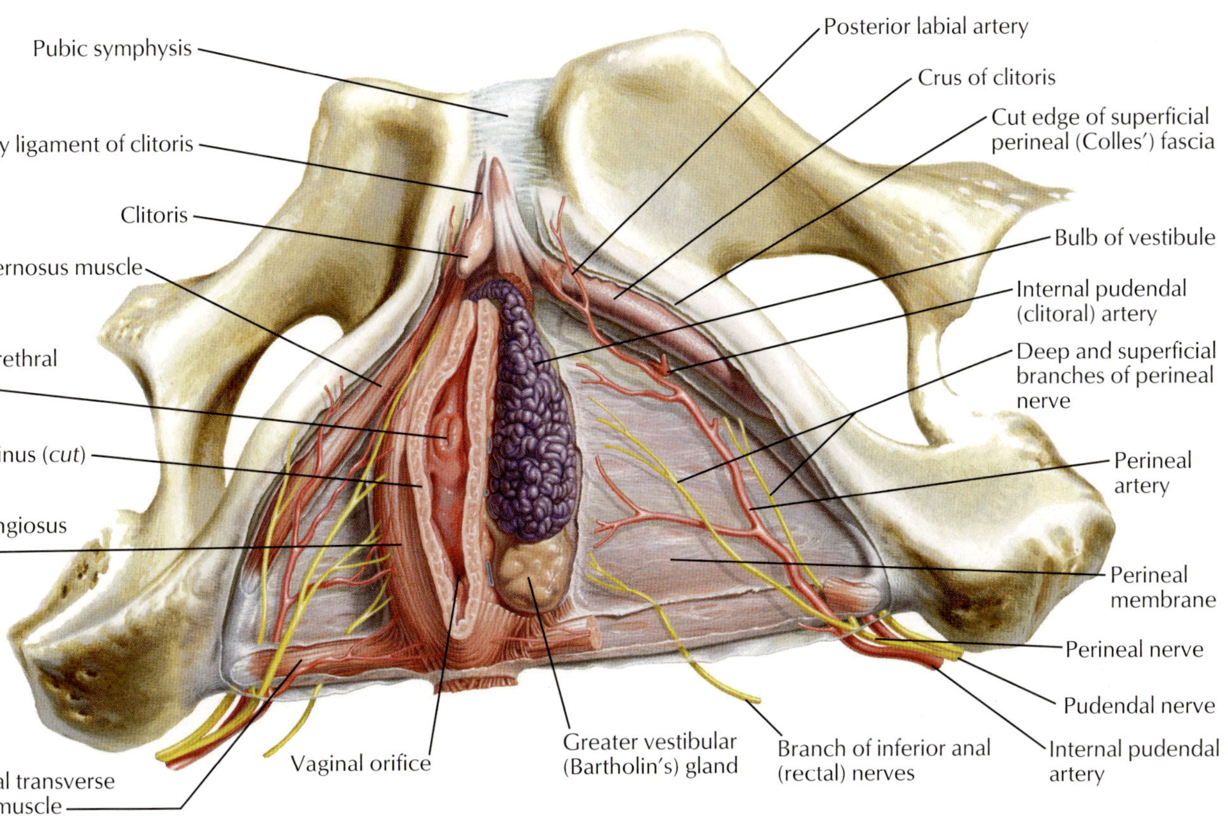

Deep perineal space

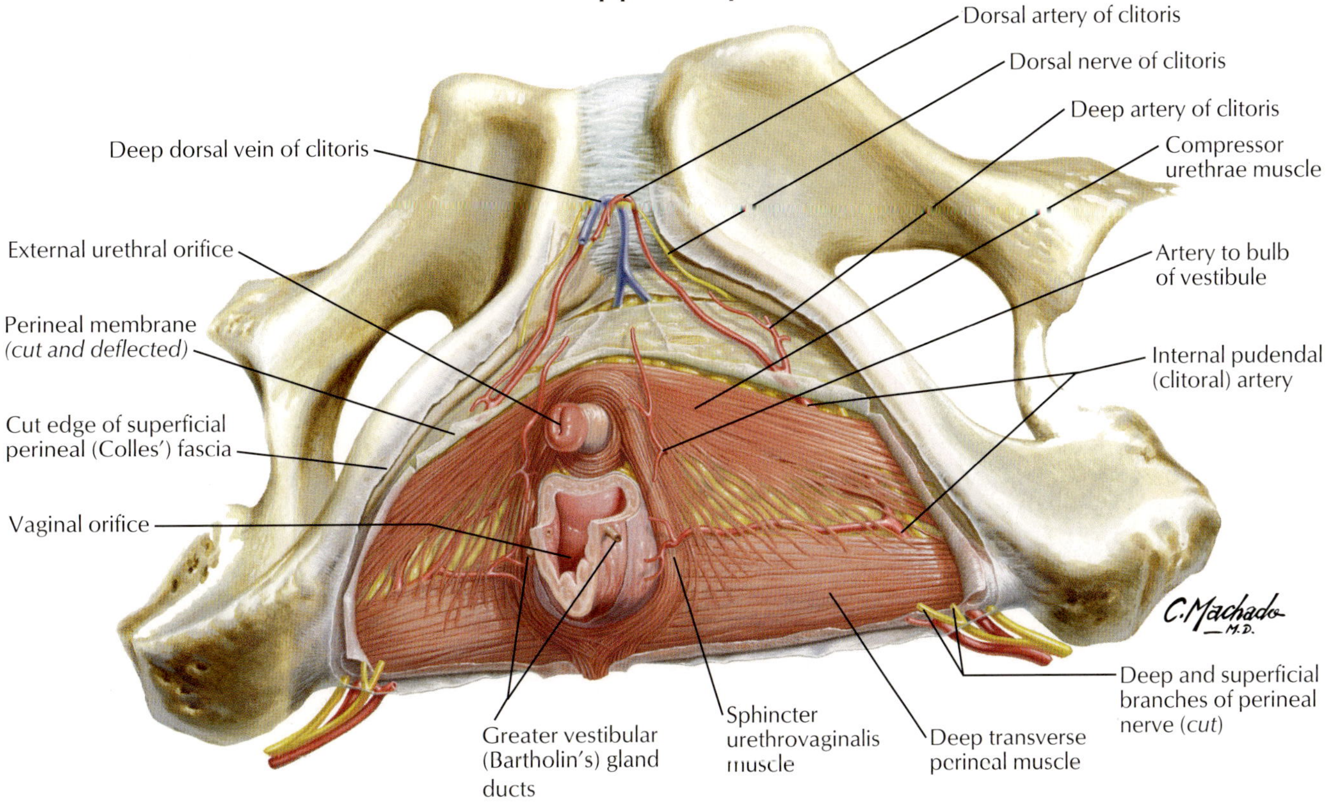

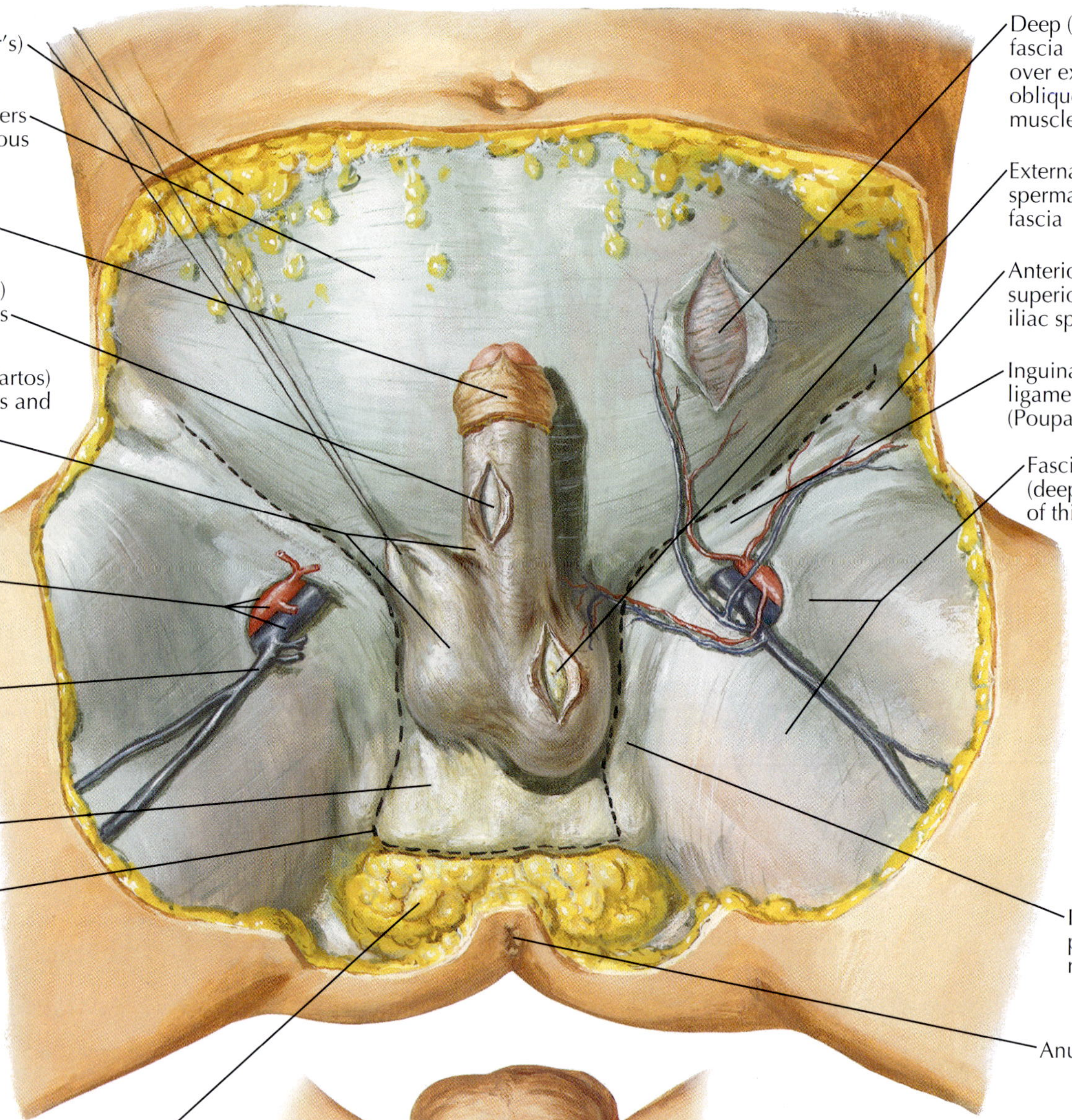

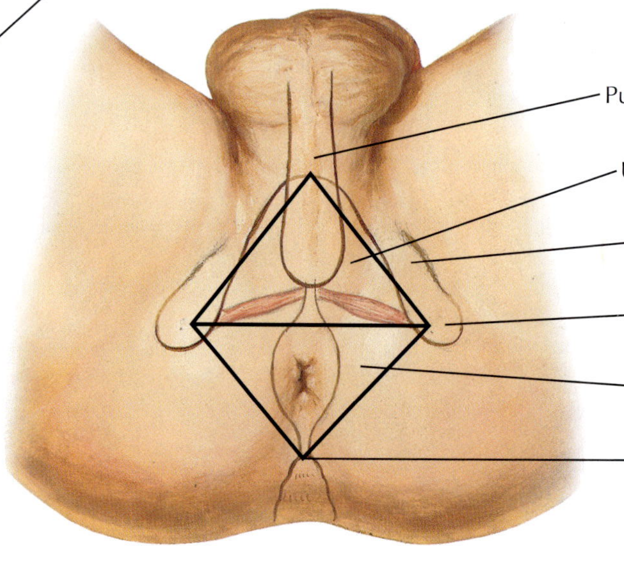

Regions (triangles) of perineum: surface topography

Male Perineum and External Genitalia (Deeper Dissection)

See also Plates 378, 380, 383

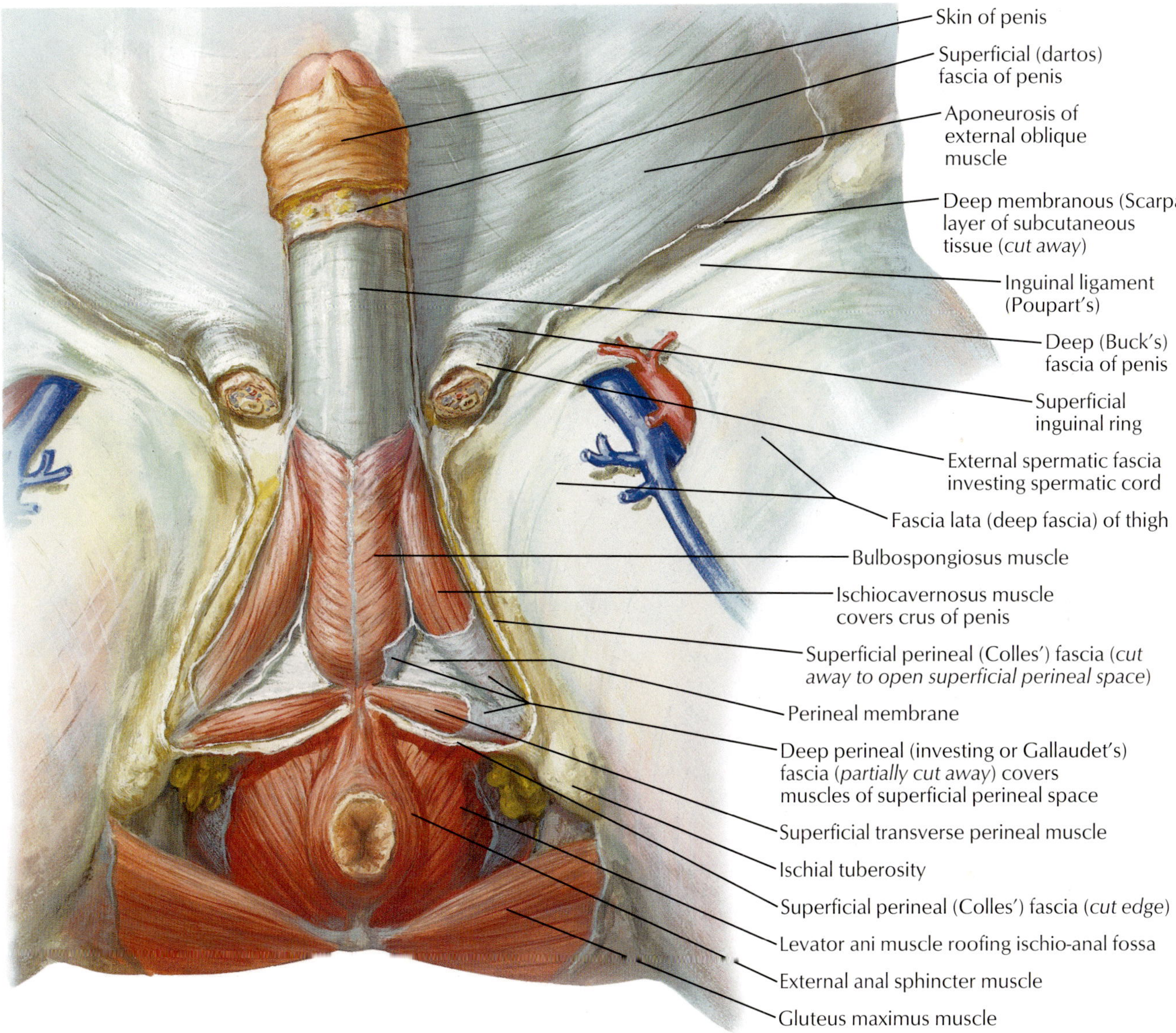

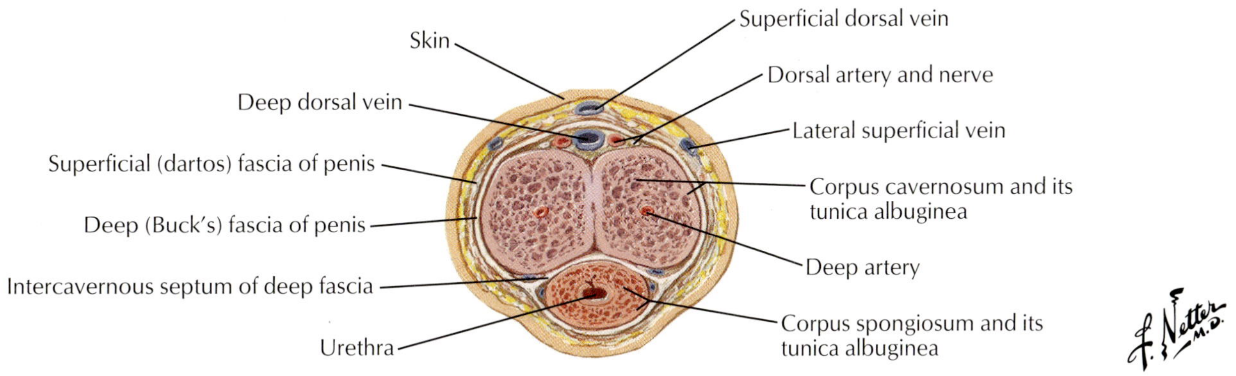

Transverse section through body of penis

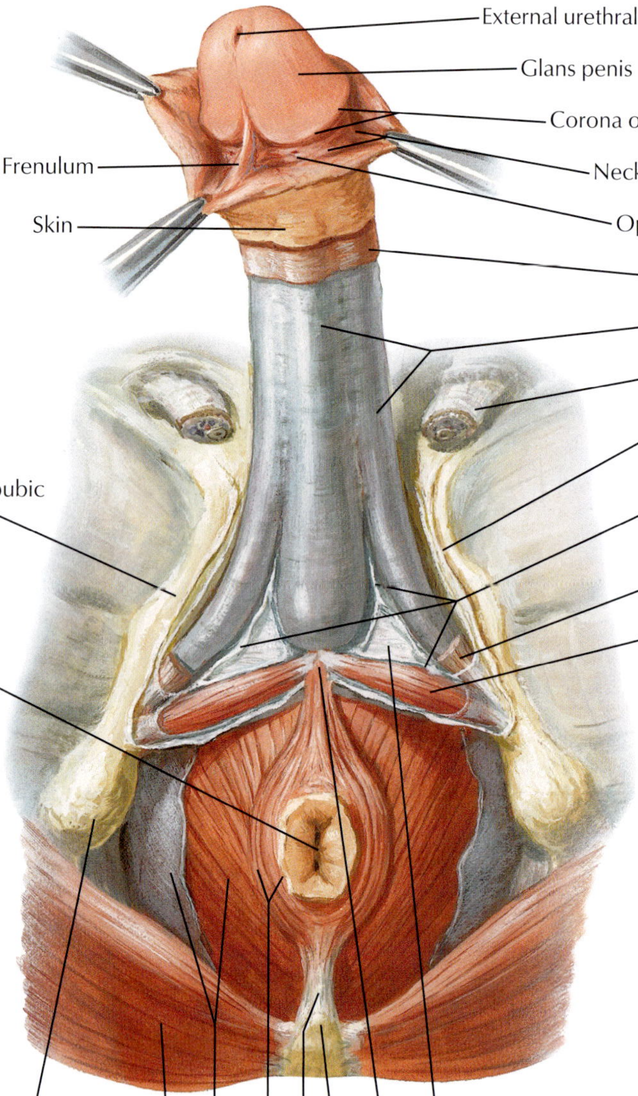
External urethral orifice (meatus)
Glans penis
Corona of glans
Neck of glans
Opening of preputial (Tyson's) gland
Superficial (dartos) fascia of penis
Deep (Buck's) fascia of penis
External spermatic fascia investing spermatic cord (*cut*)
Superficial perineal (Colles') fascia (*cut away to open superficial perineal space*)
Deep perineal (investing or Gallaudet's) fascia (*cut away*) over muscles of superficial perineal space
Ischiocavernosus muscle (*cut away*)
Superficial transverse perineal muscle
Frenulum
Skin
Ischiopubic ramus
Anus
Ischial tuberosity
Gluteus maximus muscle
Levator ani muscle and inferior fascia of pelvic diaphragm roofing ischio-anal fossa
External anal sphincter muscle
Anococcygeal ligament
Tip of coccyx
Perineal body
Perineal membrane

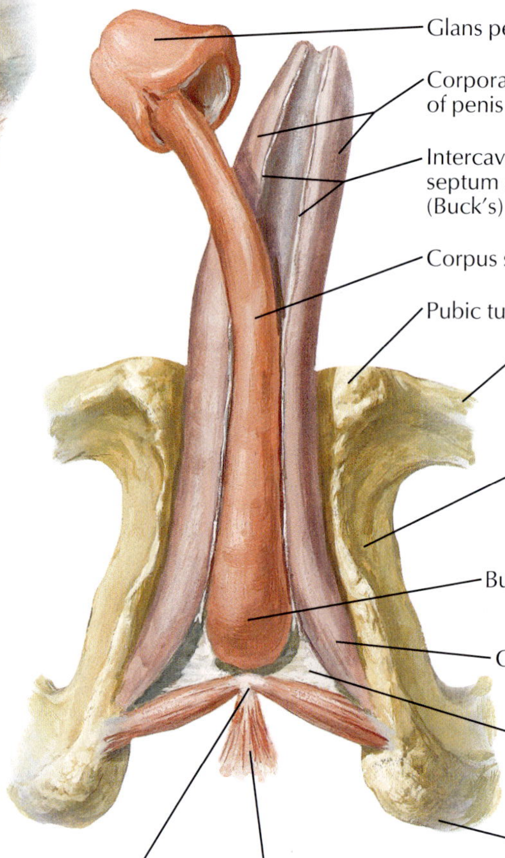
Glans penis
Corpora cavernosa of penis
Intercavernous septum of deep (Buck's) fascia
Corpus spongiosum
Pubic tubercle
Superior pubic ramus
Ischiopubic ramus
Bulb of penis
Crus of penis
Perineal membrane
Ischial tuberosity
Perineal body
External anal sphincter muscle

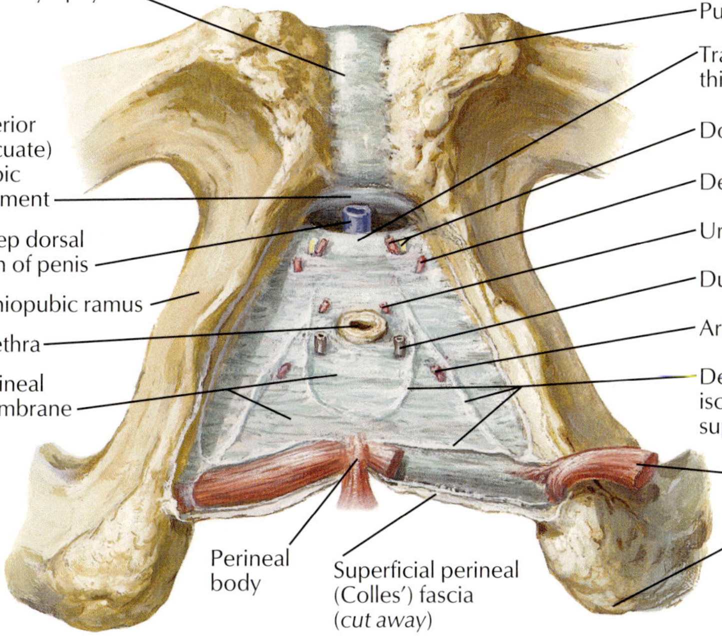

Inferior views

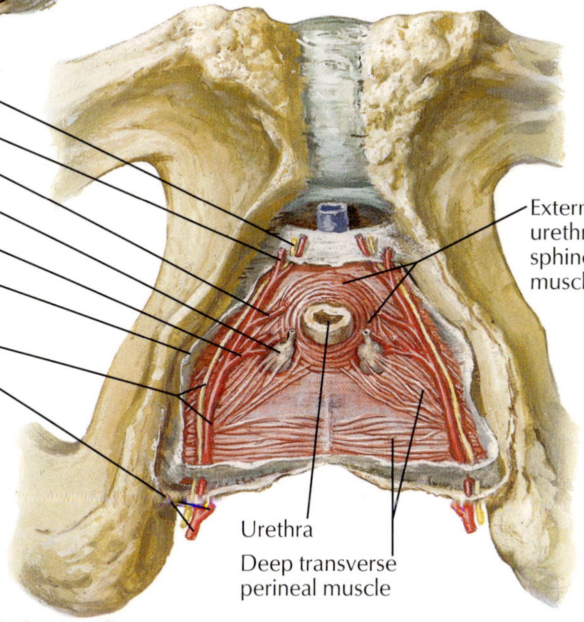

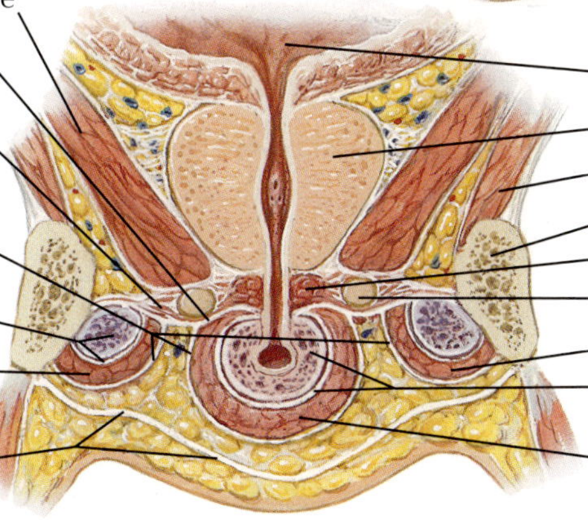

Frontal section, anterior view of perineum: schema

Prostate and Seminal Vesicles

See also **Plates 344, 348, 381**

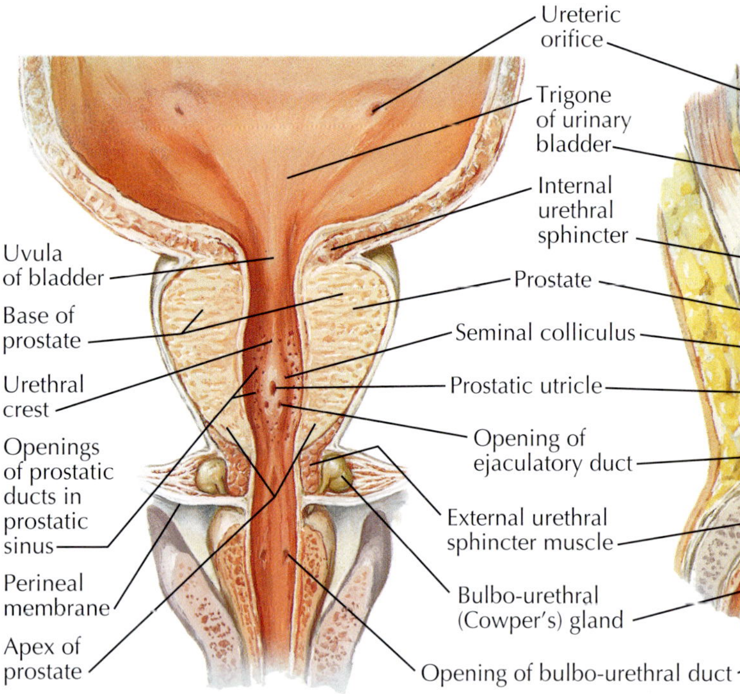

Frontal section, anterior view of bulbous portion of spongy urethra schematically extended

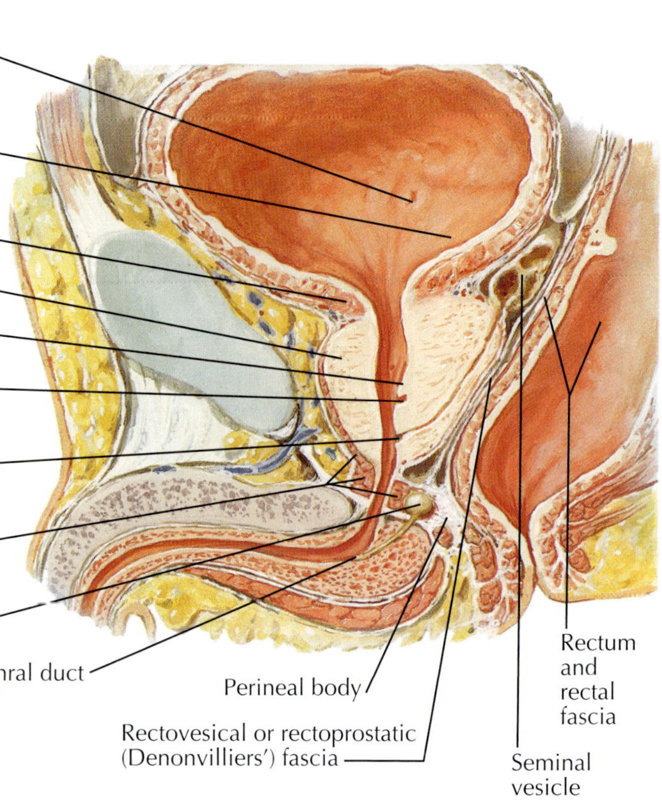

Sagittal section

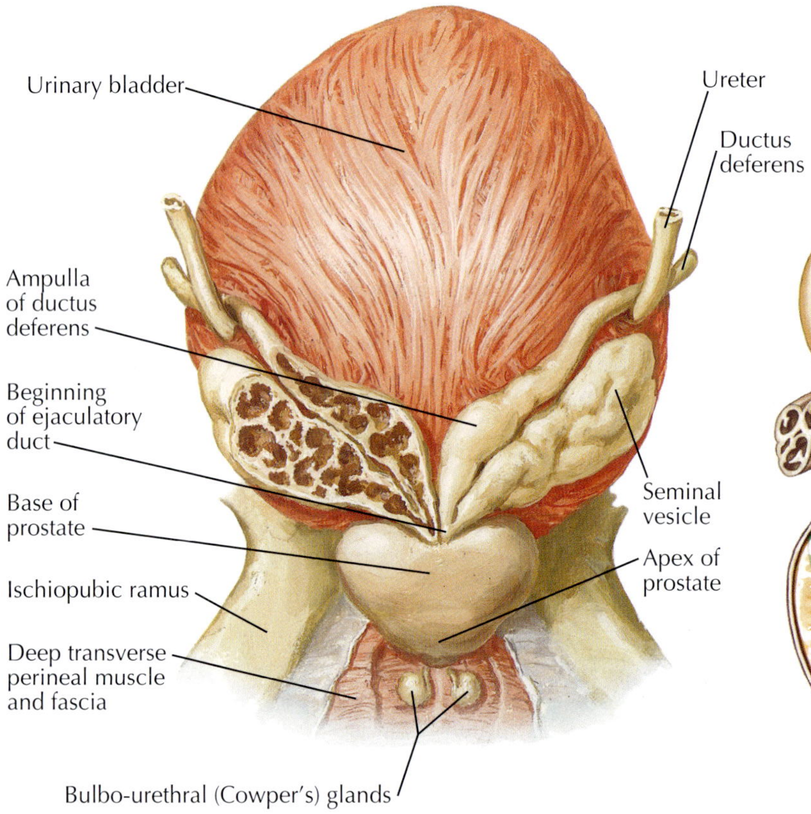

Posterior view

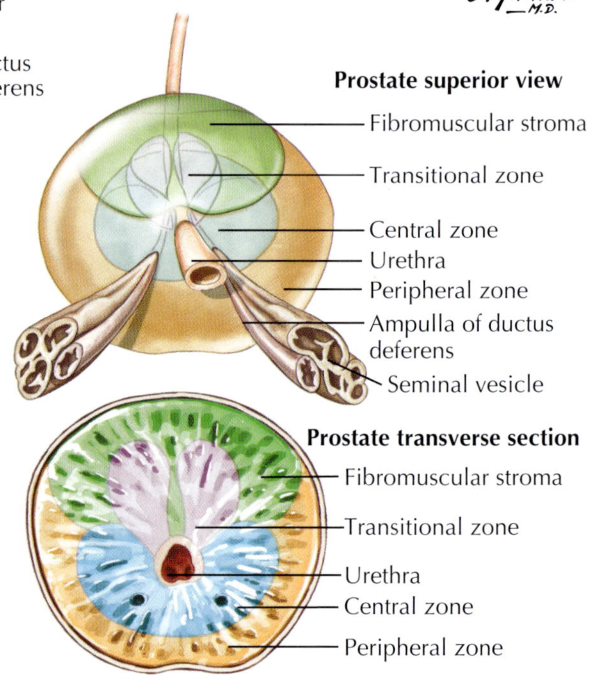

Posterior view

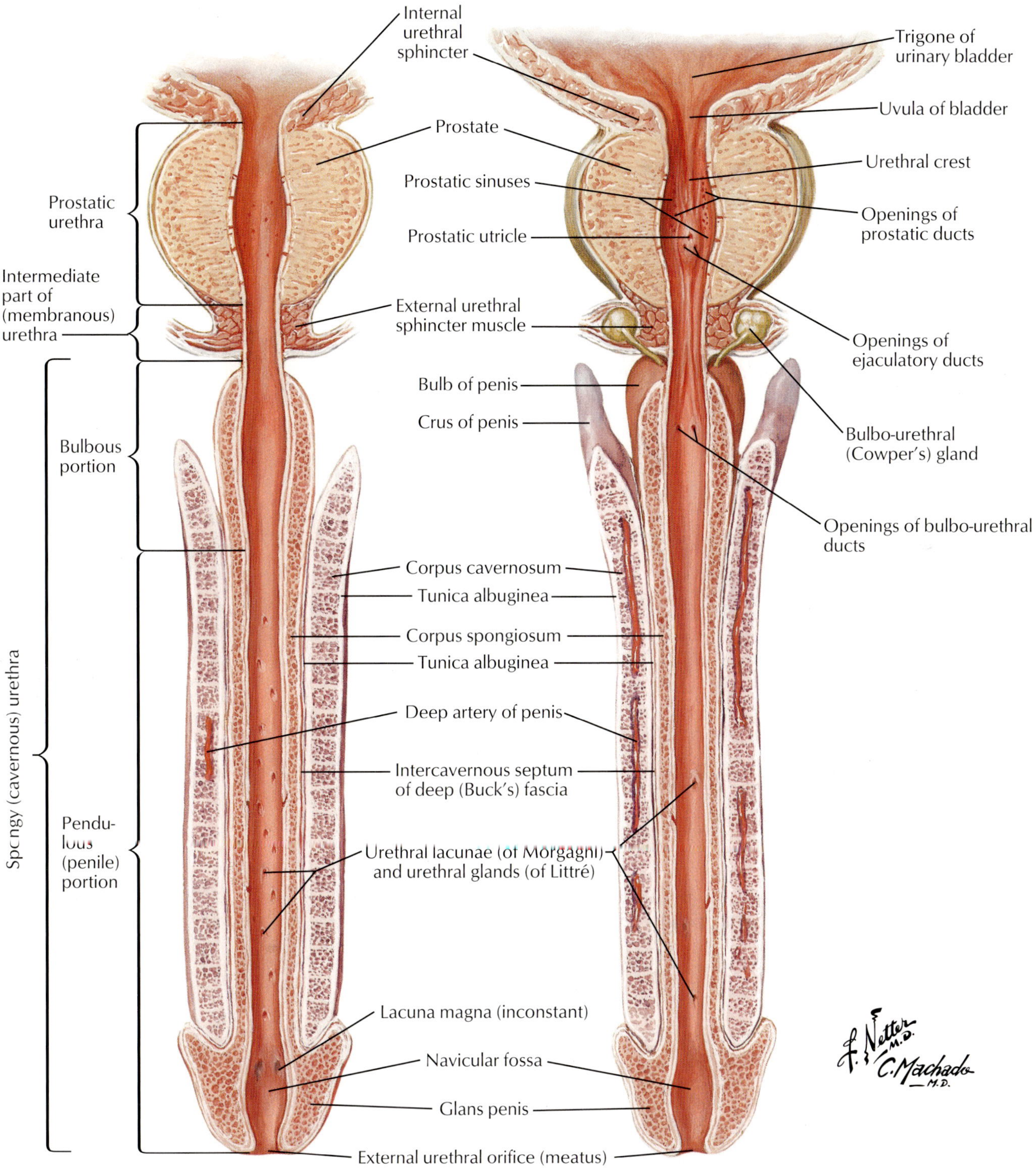

Roof of urethra

Floor of urethra

Descent of Testis

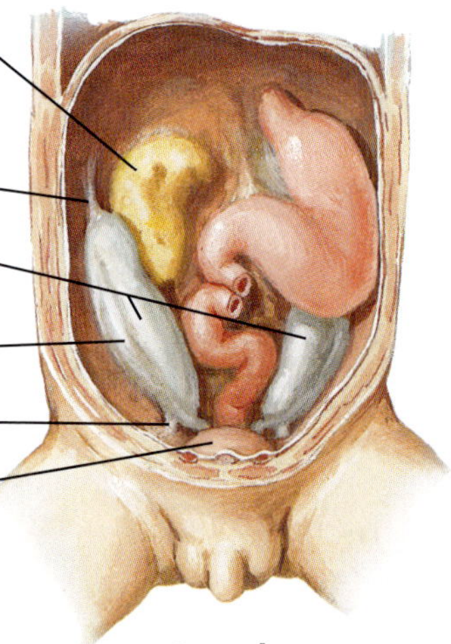

8 weeks (22.5-mm crown–rump)

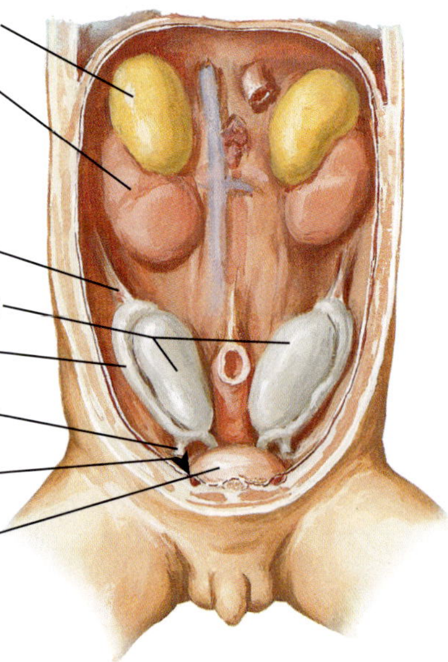

11 weeks (43-mm crown–rump)

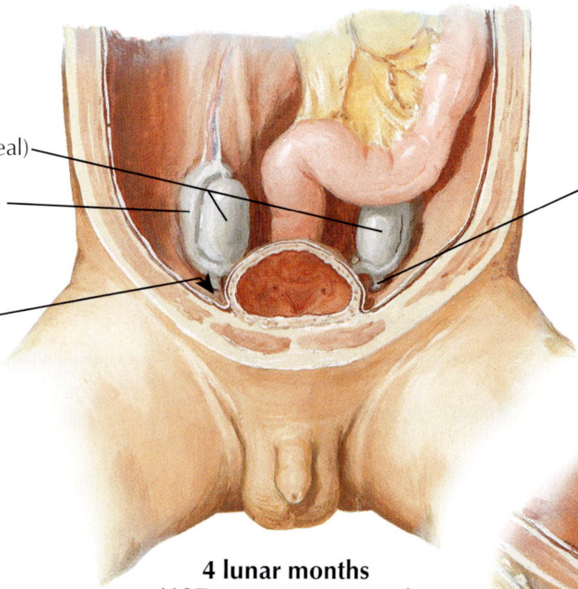

4 lunar months (107-mm crown–rump)

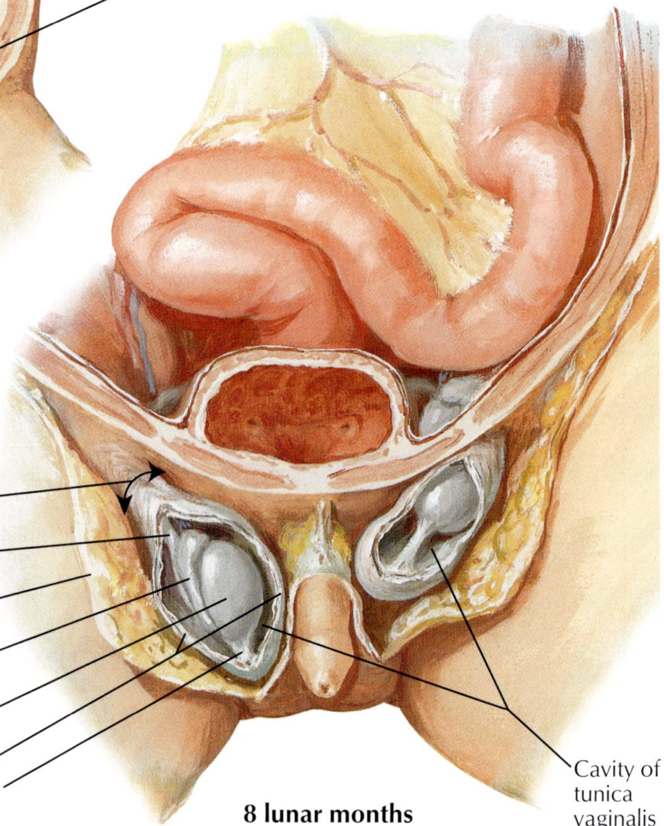

8 lunar months (26-cm crown–rump)

See also Plates 321, 344

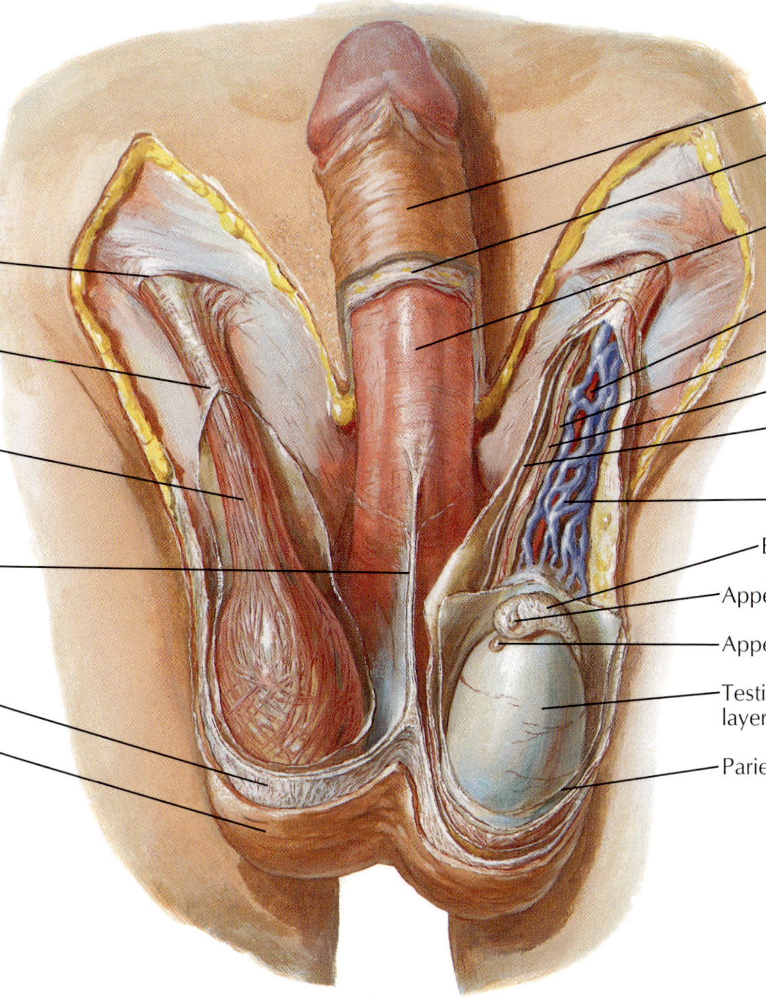

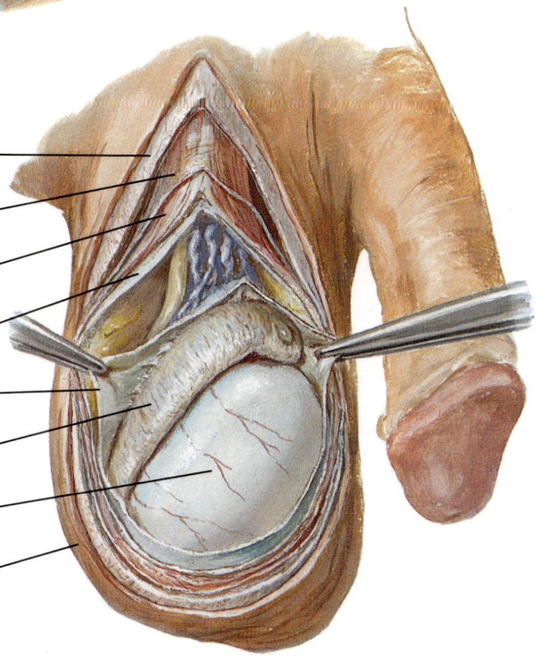

Homologues of External Genitalia

See also Plate 354

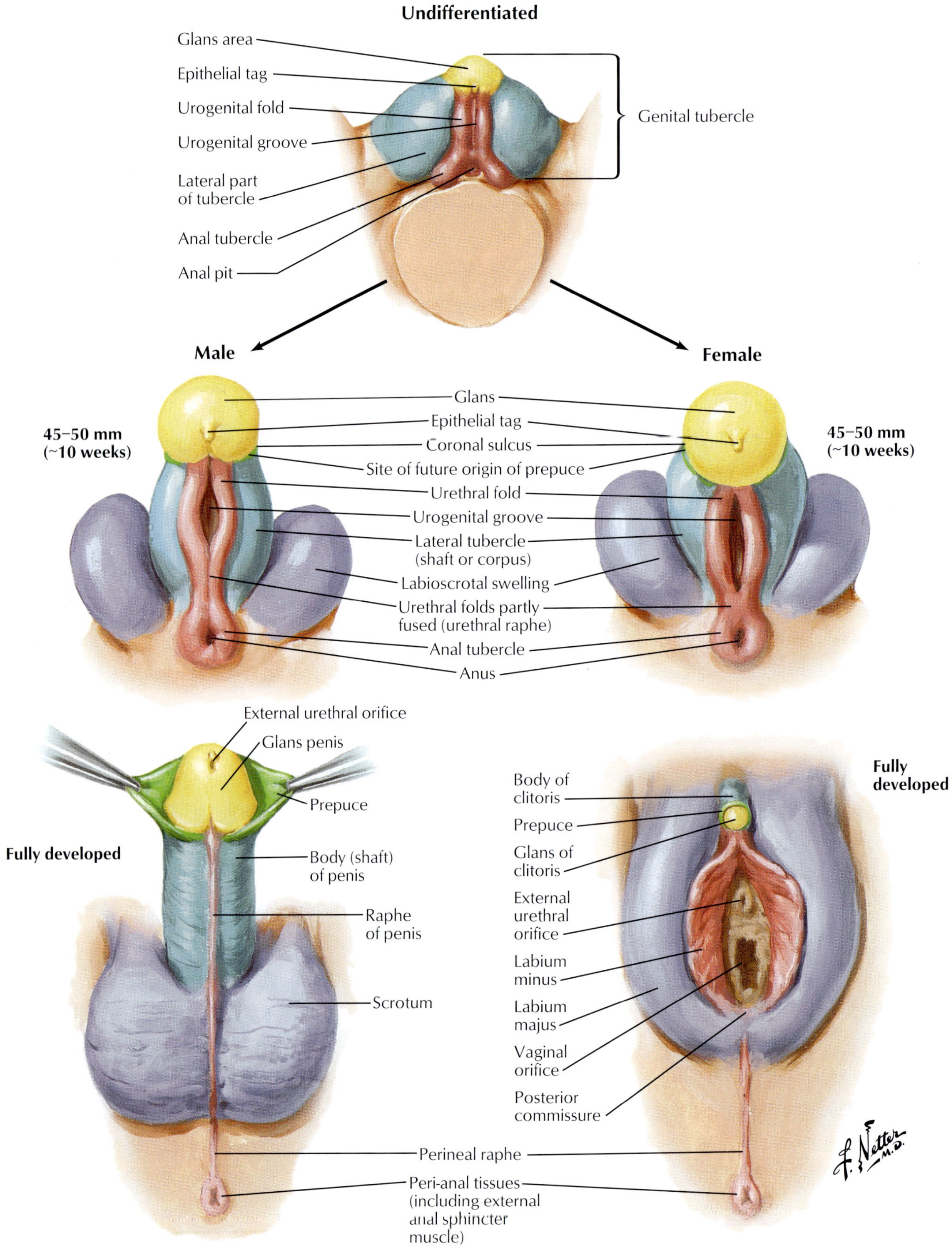

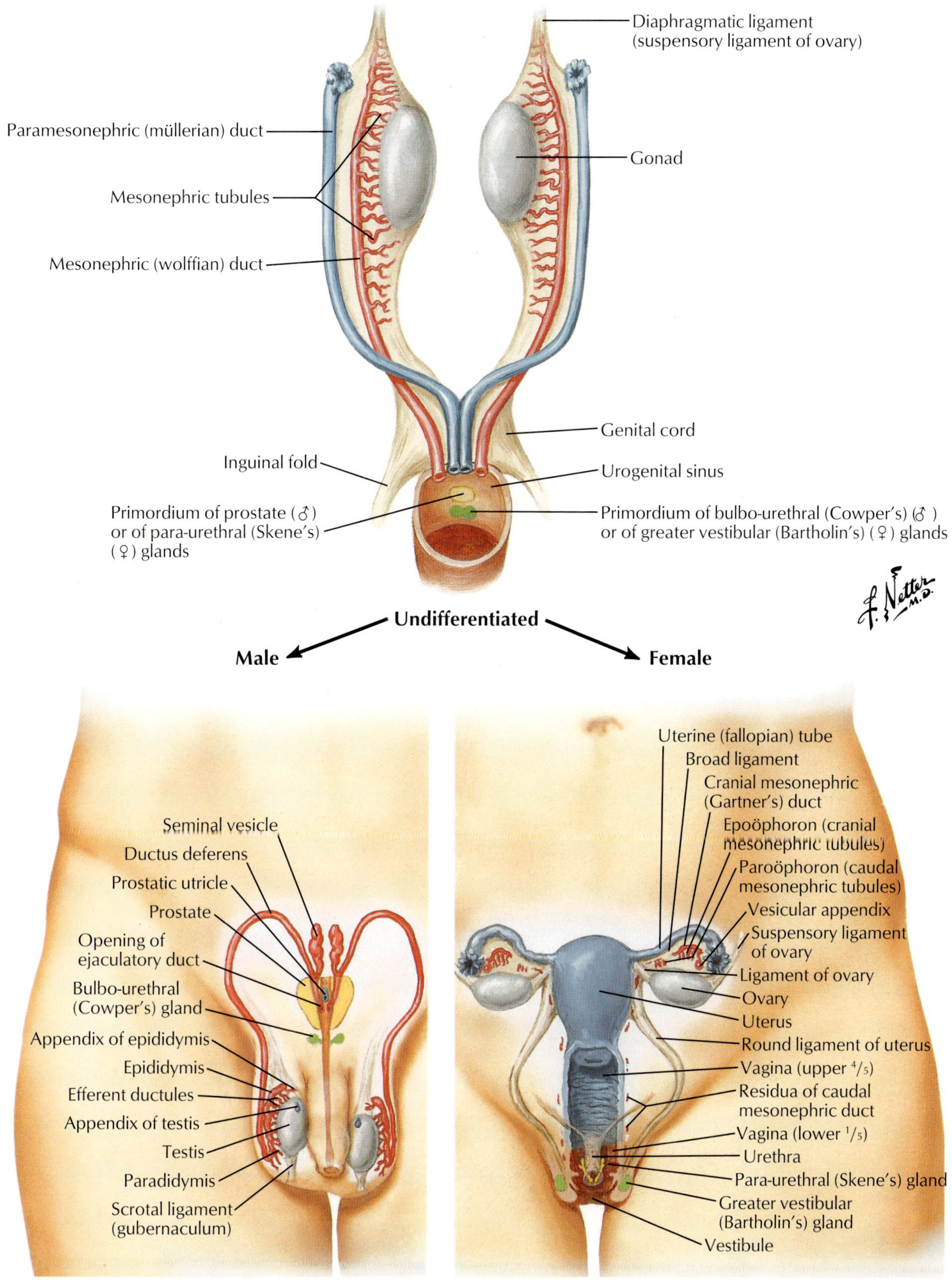
Diaphragmatic ligament (suspensory ligament of ovary)
Paramesonephric (müllerian) duct
Gonad
Mesonephric tubules
Mesonephric (wolffian) duct
Genital cord
Inguinal fold
Urogenital sinus
Primordium of prostate (♂) or of para-urethral (Skene's) (♀) glands
Primordium of bulbo-urethral (Cowper's) (♂) or of greater vestibular (Bartholin's) (♀) glands
Undifferentiated
Male
Female
Seminal vesicle
Ductus deferens
Prostatic utricle
Prostate
Opening of ejaculatory duct
Bulbo-urethral (Cowper's) gland
Appendix of epididymis
Epididymis
Efferent ductules
Appendix of testis
Testis
Paradidymis
Scrotal ligament (gubernaculum)
Uterine (fallopian) tube
Broad ligament
Cranial mesonephric (Gartner's) duct
Epoöphoron (cranial mesonephric tubules)
Paroöphoron (caudal mesonephric tubules)
Vesicular appendix
Suspensory ligament of ovary
Ligament of ovary
Ovary
Uterus
Round ligament of uterus
Vagina (upper 4/5)
Residua of caudal mesonephric duct
Vagina (lower 1/5)
Urethra
Para-urethral (Skene's) gland
Greater vestibular (Bartholin's) gland
Vestibule

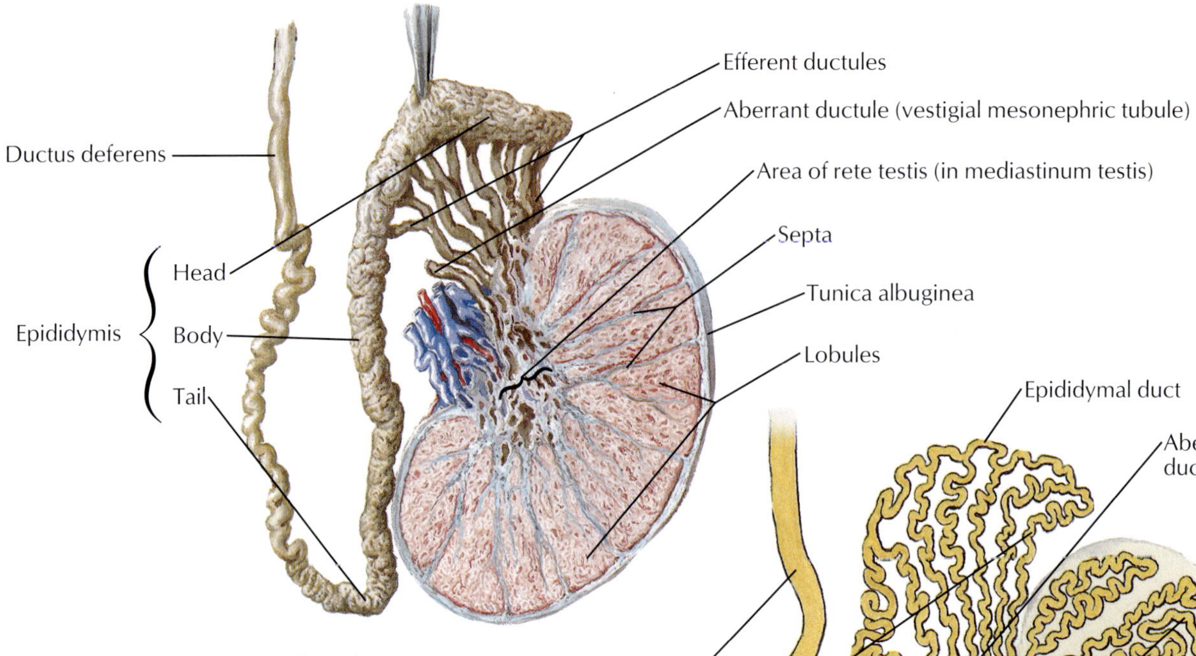

Frontal section

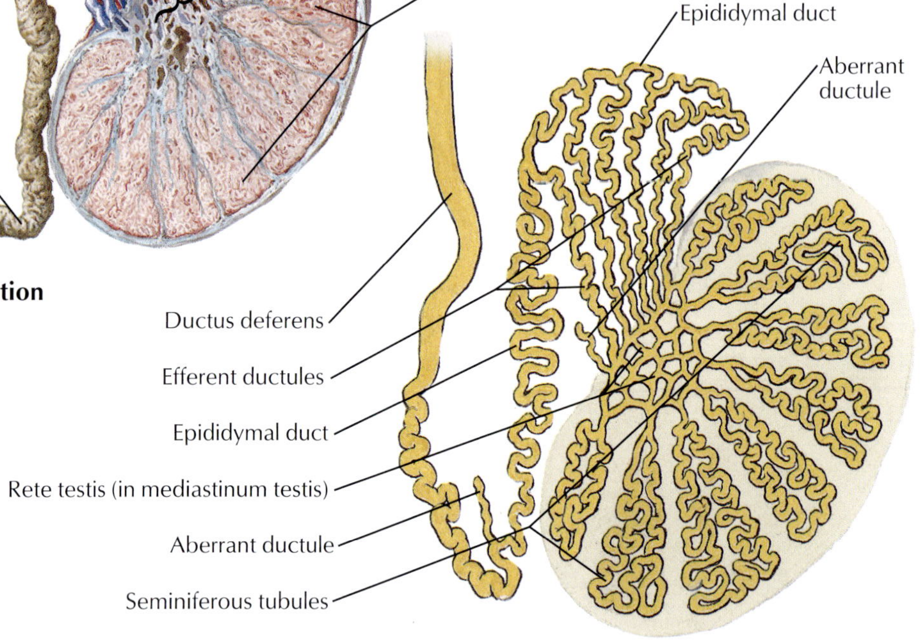

Schema

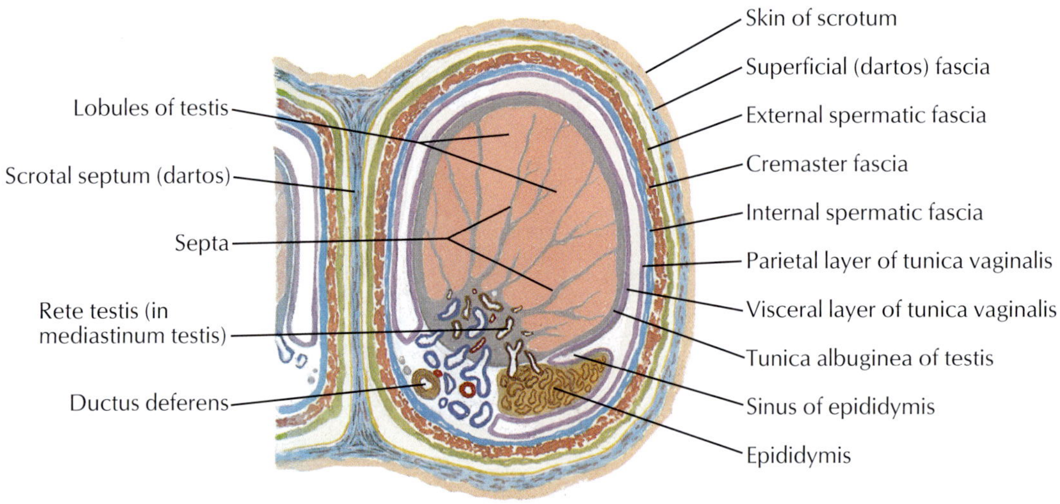

Cross section through scrotum and testis

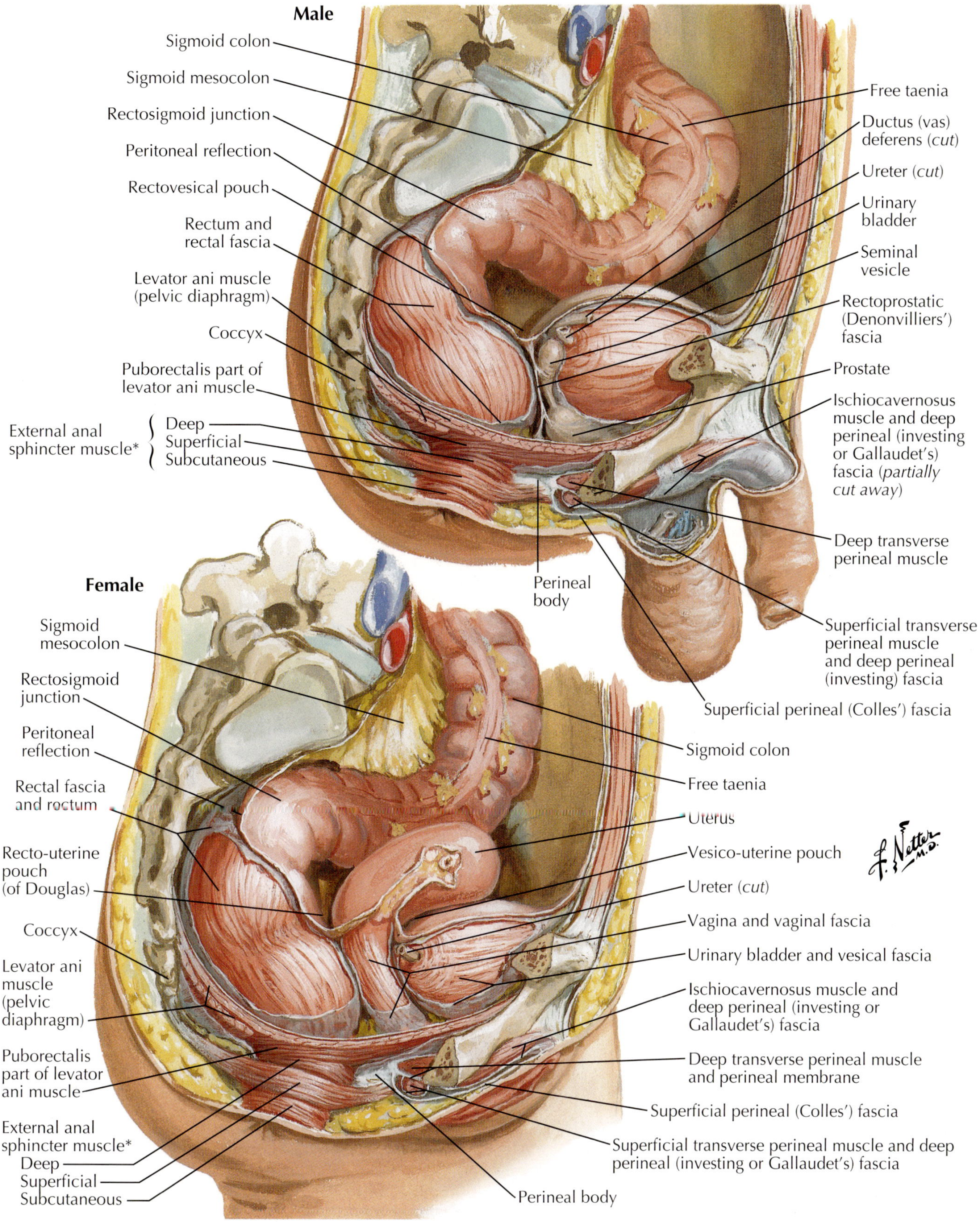

*Parts variable and often indistinct

Ischio-anal Fossae

See also Plates 296, 388

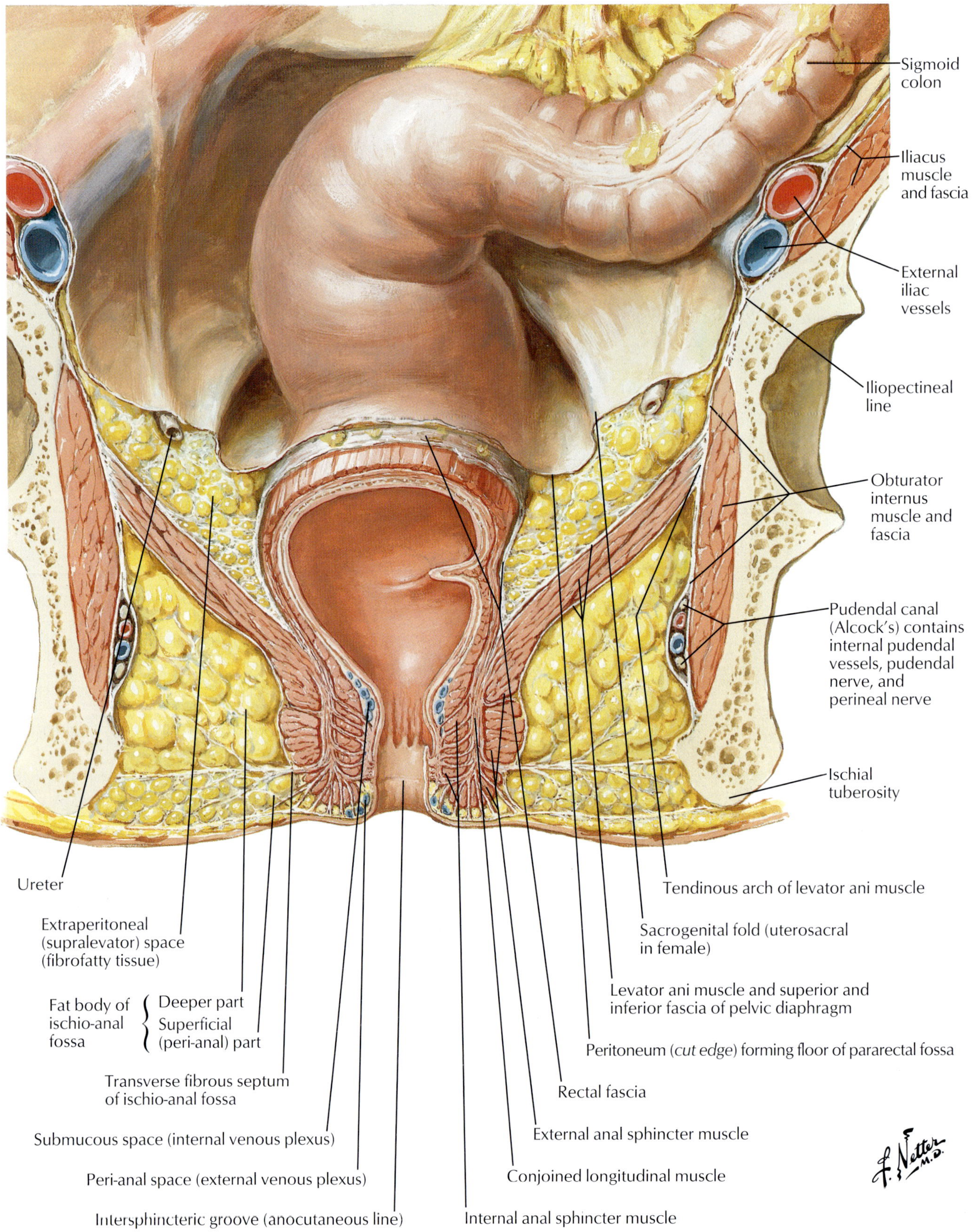

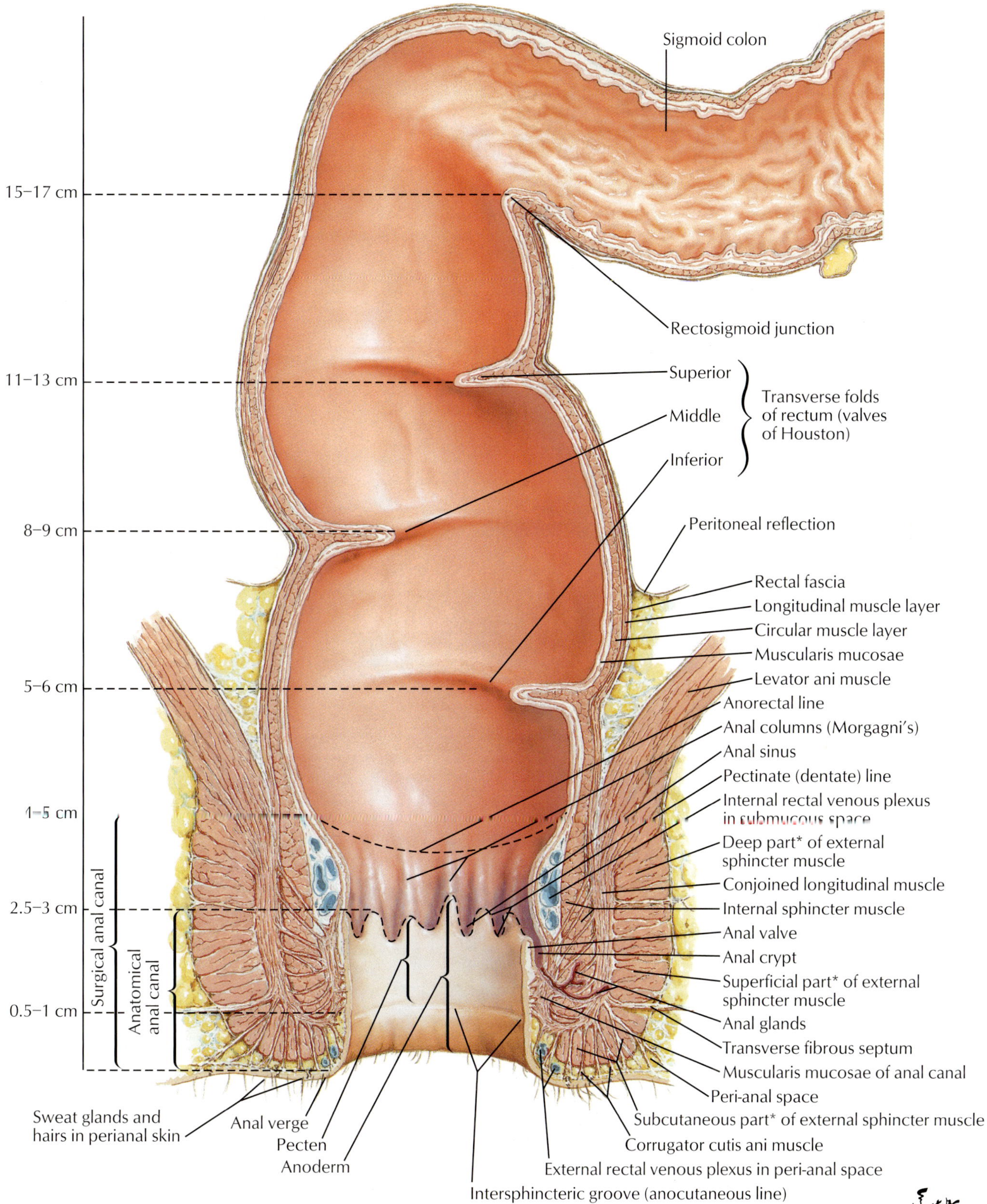

*Parts variable and often indistinct

Anorectal Musculature

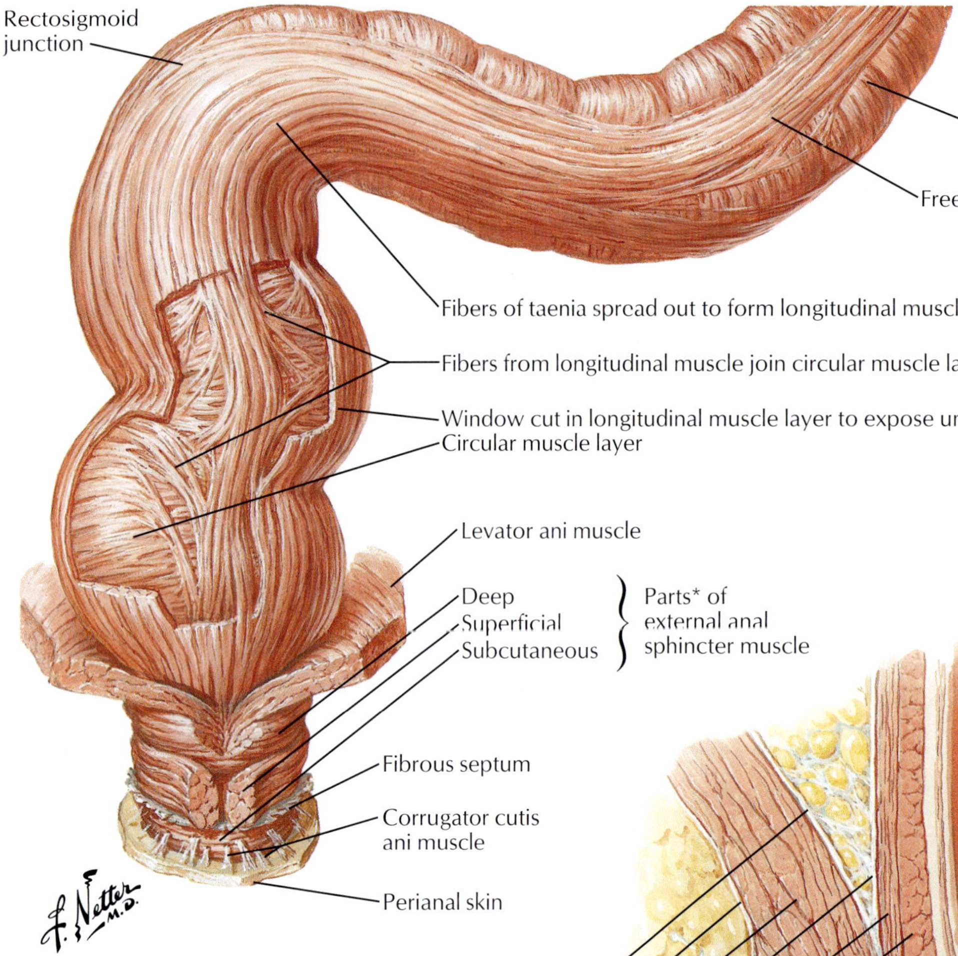

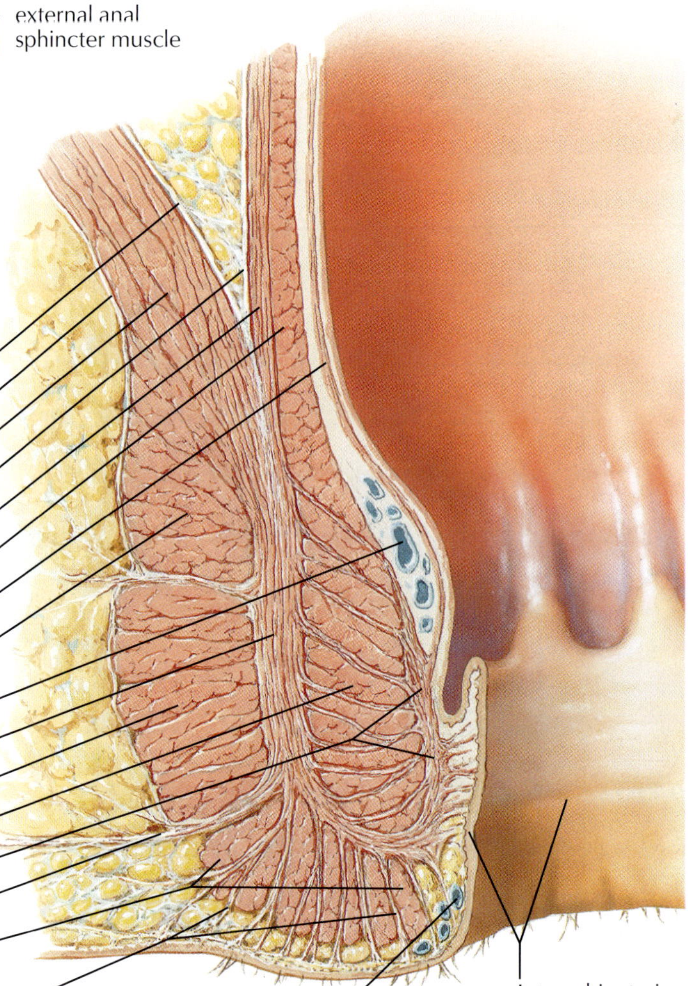

*Parts variable and often indistinct

External Anal Sphincter Muscle: Perineal Views

See also Plates 356, 359

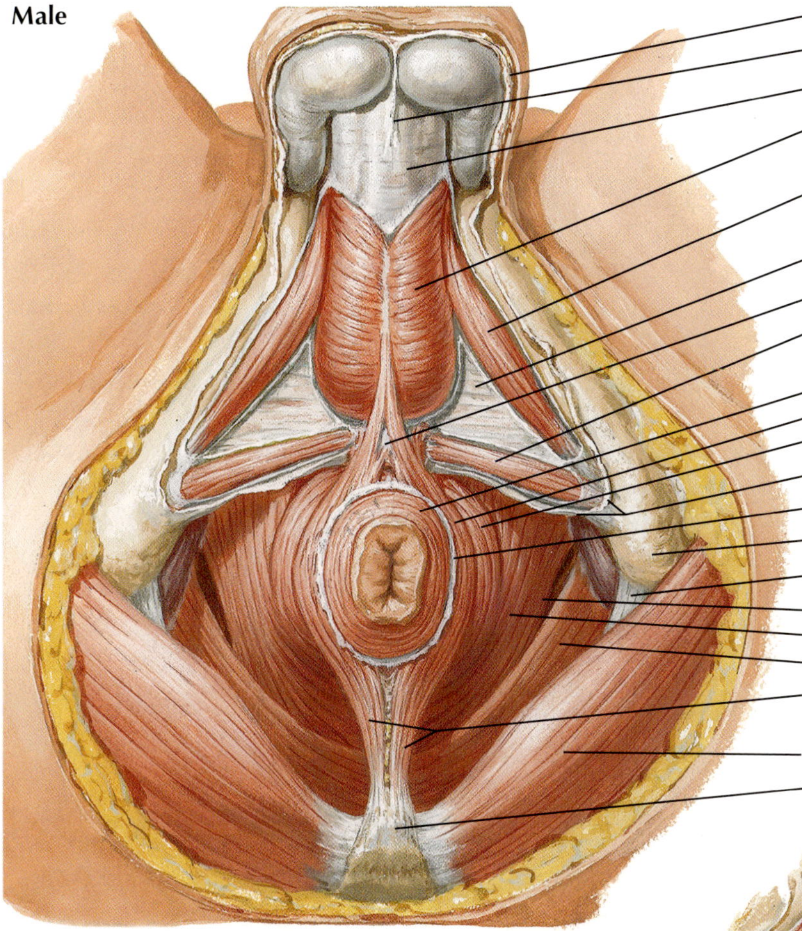

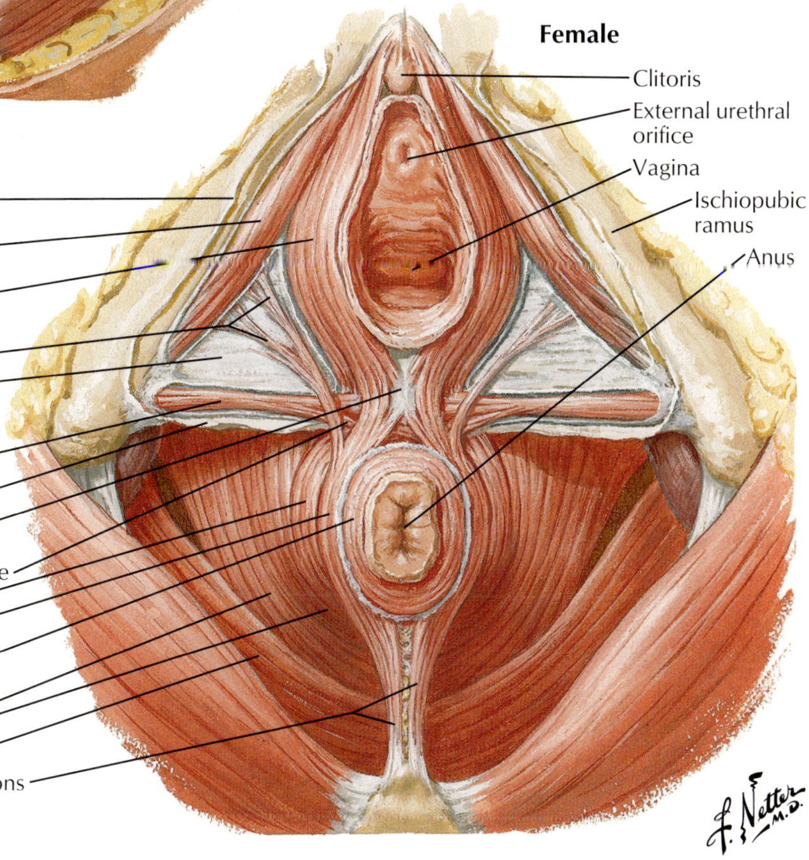

*Parts variable and often indistinct

Actual and Potential Perineopelvic Spaces

Sagittal section

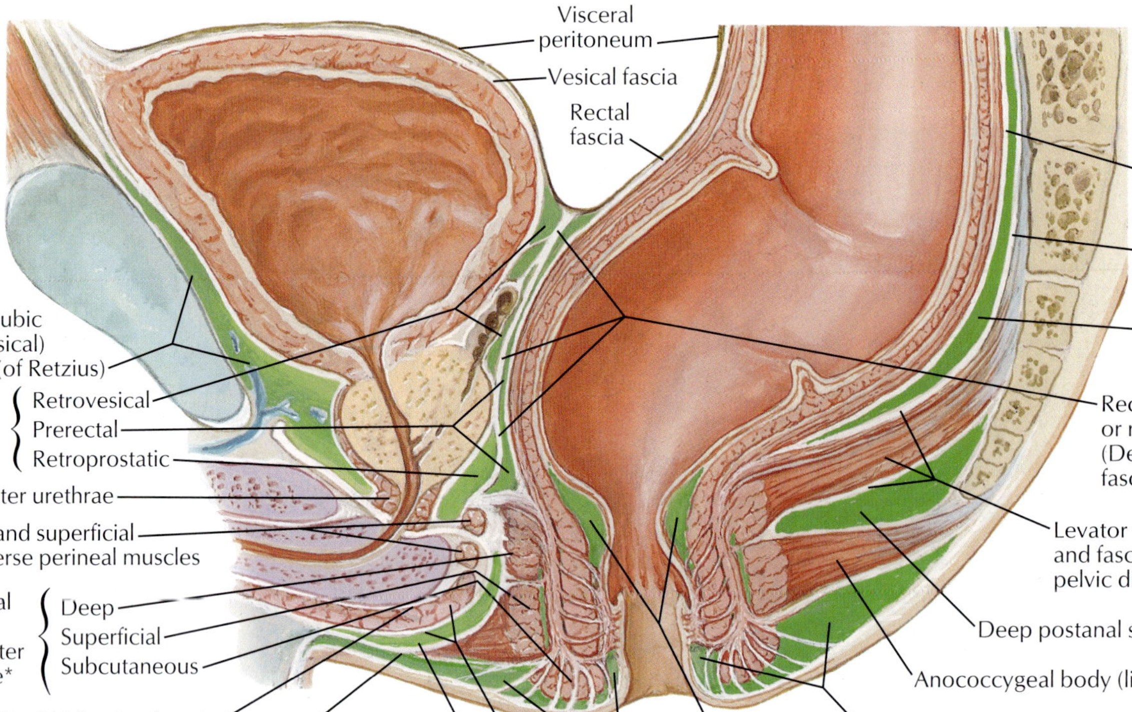

*Parts variable and often indistinct

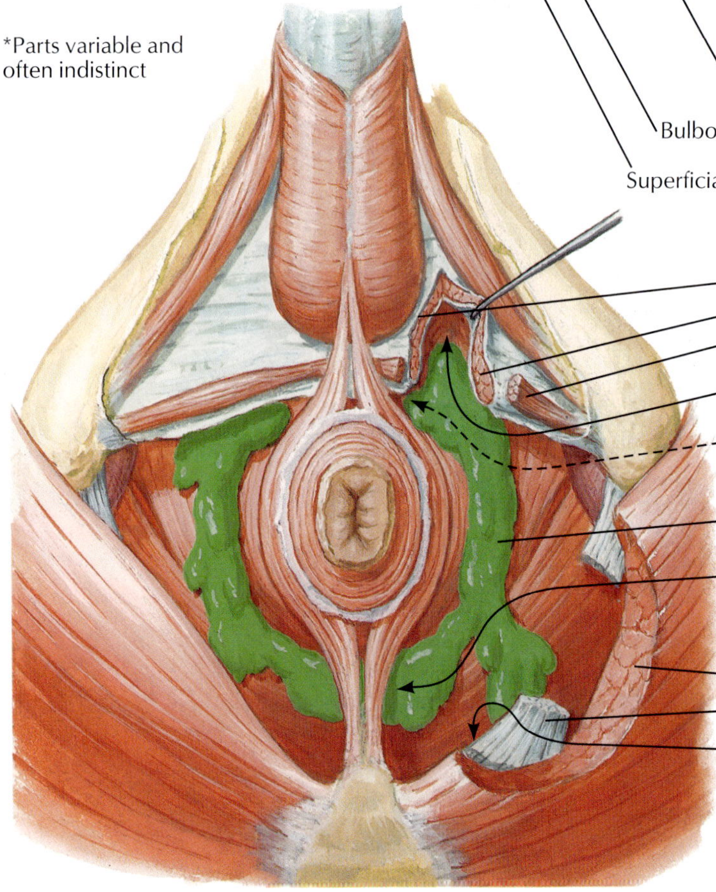

Perineal view

Spread of perineal abscess in perineal spaces

Female

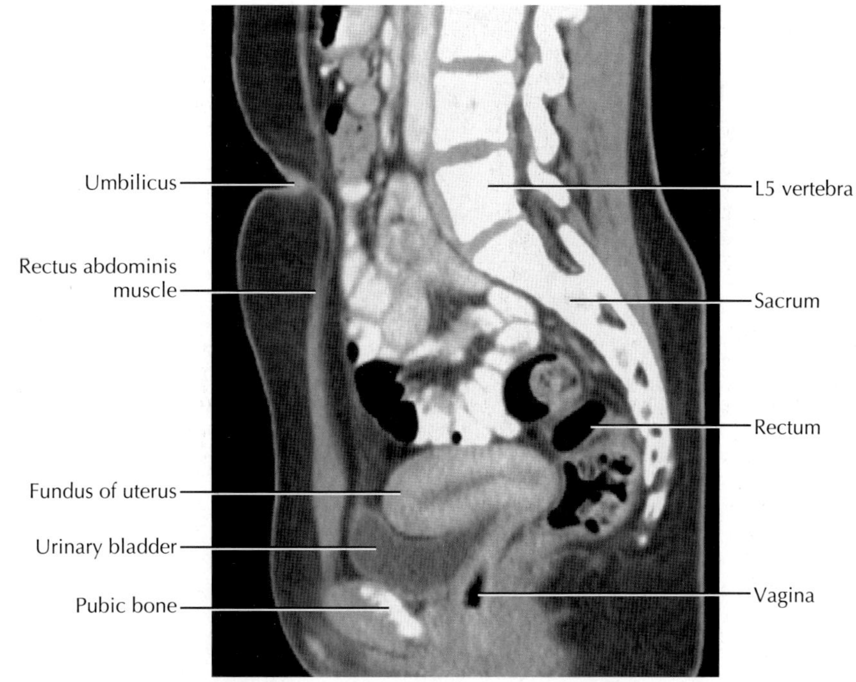
Umbilicus
Rectus abdominis muscle
Fundus of uterus
Urinary bladder
Pubic bone
L5 vertebra
Sacrum
Rectum
Vagina

Male

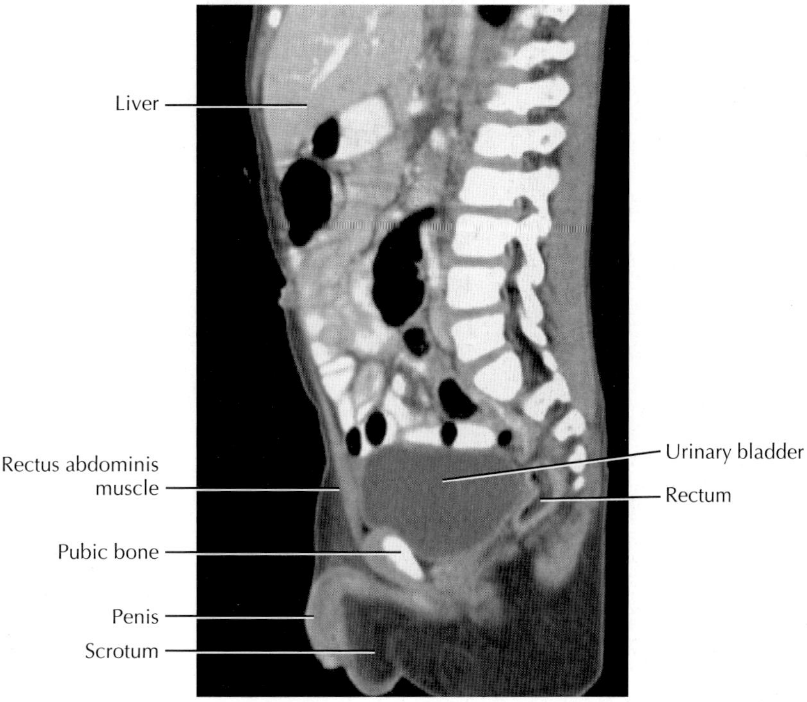
Liver
Rectus abdominis muscle
Pubic bone
Penis
Scrotum
Urinary bladder
Rectum

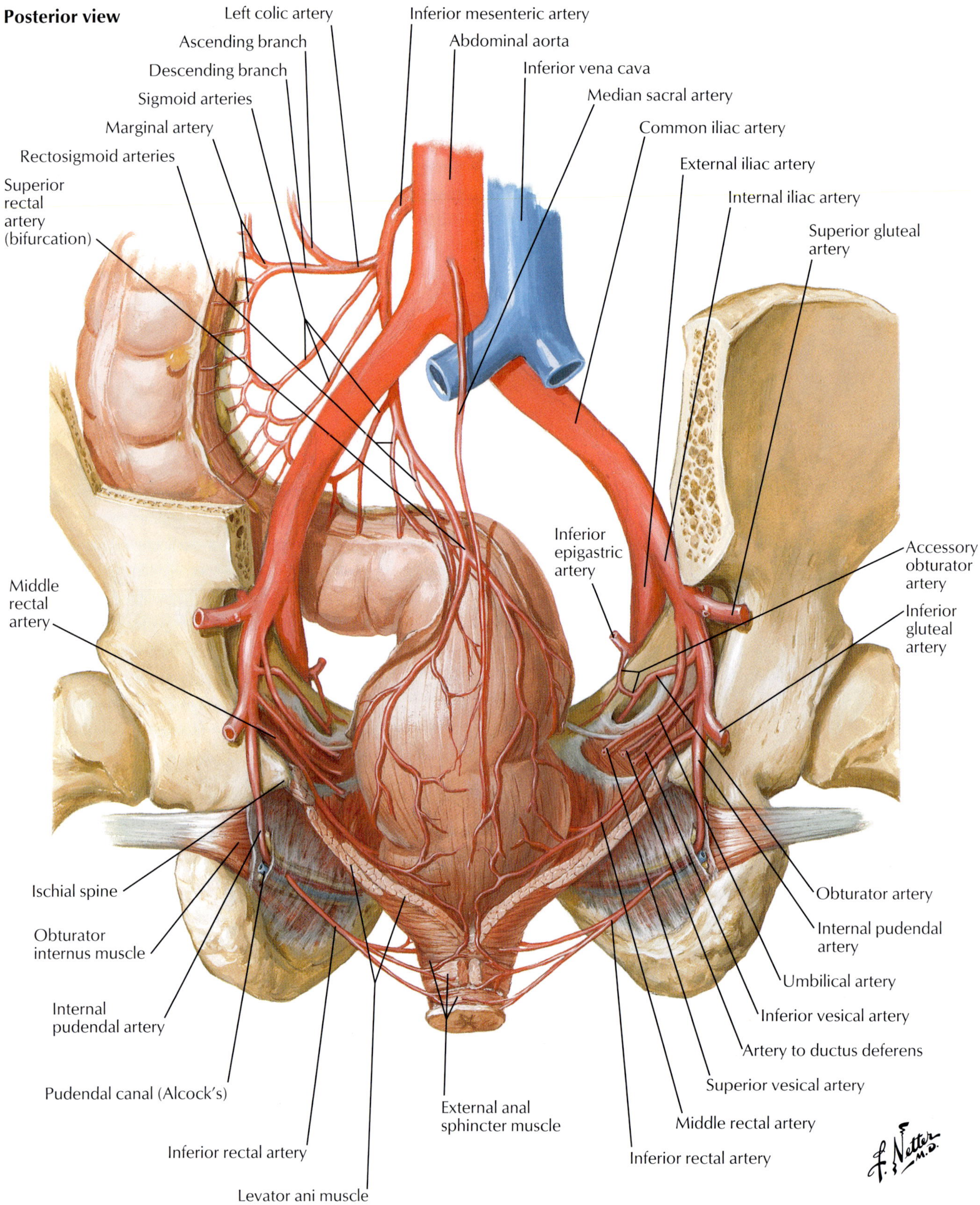
Posterior view
Left colic artery
Ascending branch
Descending branch
Sigmoid arteries
Marginal artery
Rectosigmoid arteries
Superior rectal artery (bifurcation)
Inferior mesenteric artery
Abdominal aorta
Inferior vena cava
Median sacral artery
Common iliac artery
External iliac artery
Internal iliac artery
Superior gluteal artery
Inferior epigastric artery
Accessory obturator artery
Inferior gluteal artery
Middle rectal artery
Ischial spine
Obturator internus muscle
Internal pudendal artery
Pudendal canal (Alcock's)
Inferior rectal artery
Levator ani muscle
External anal sphincter muscle
Obturator artery
Internal pudendal artery
Umbilical artery
Inferior vesical artery
Artery to ductus deferens
Superior vesical artery
Middle rectal artery
Inferior rectal artery

Anterior view

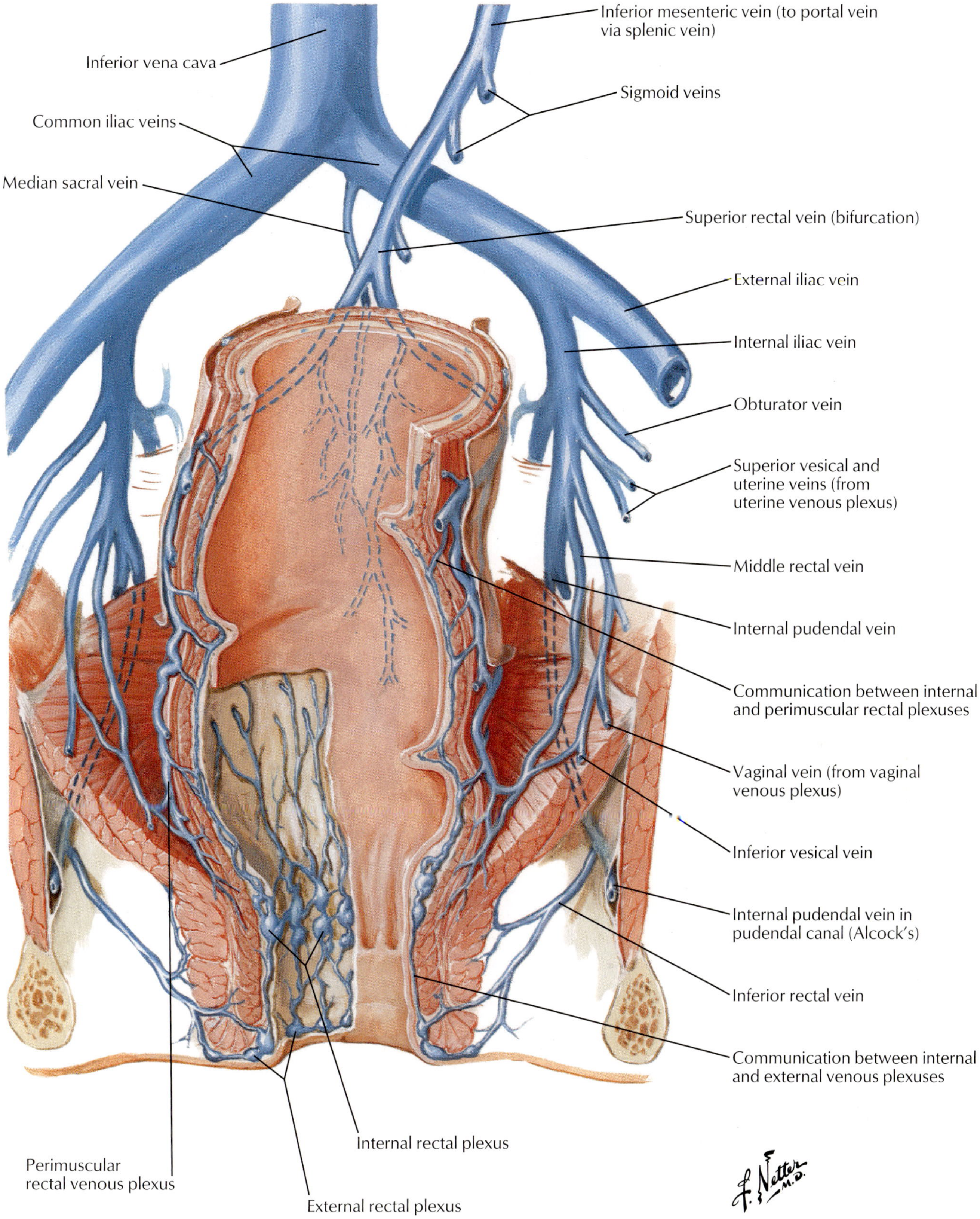

Arteries and Veins of Pelvic Organs: Female

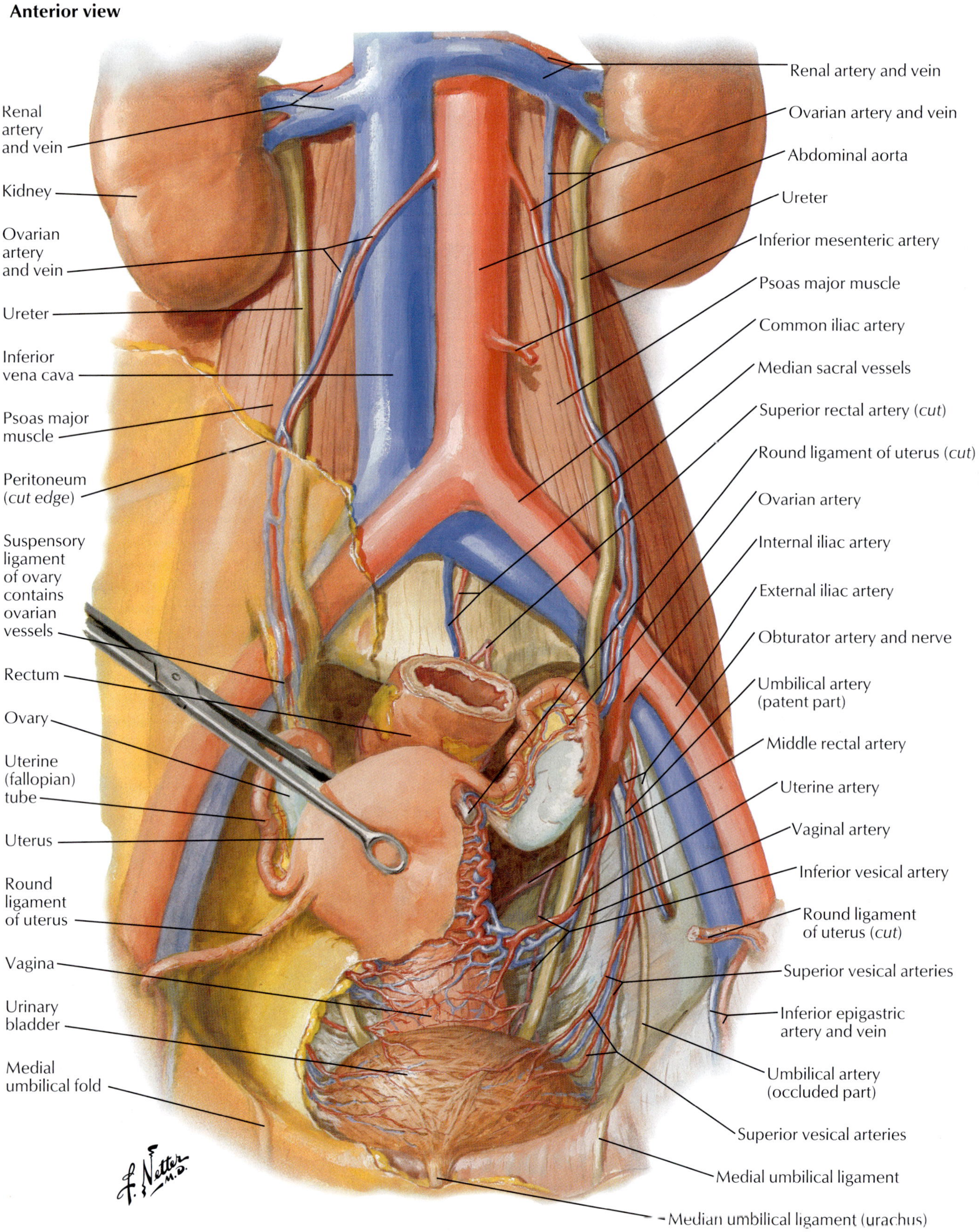

Arteries and Veins of Testis

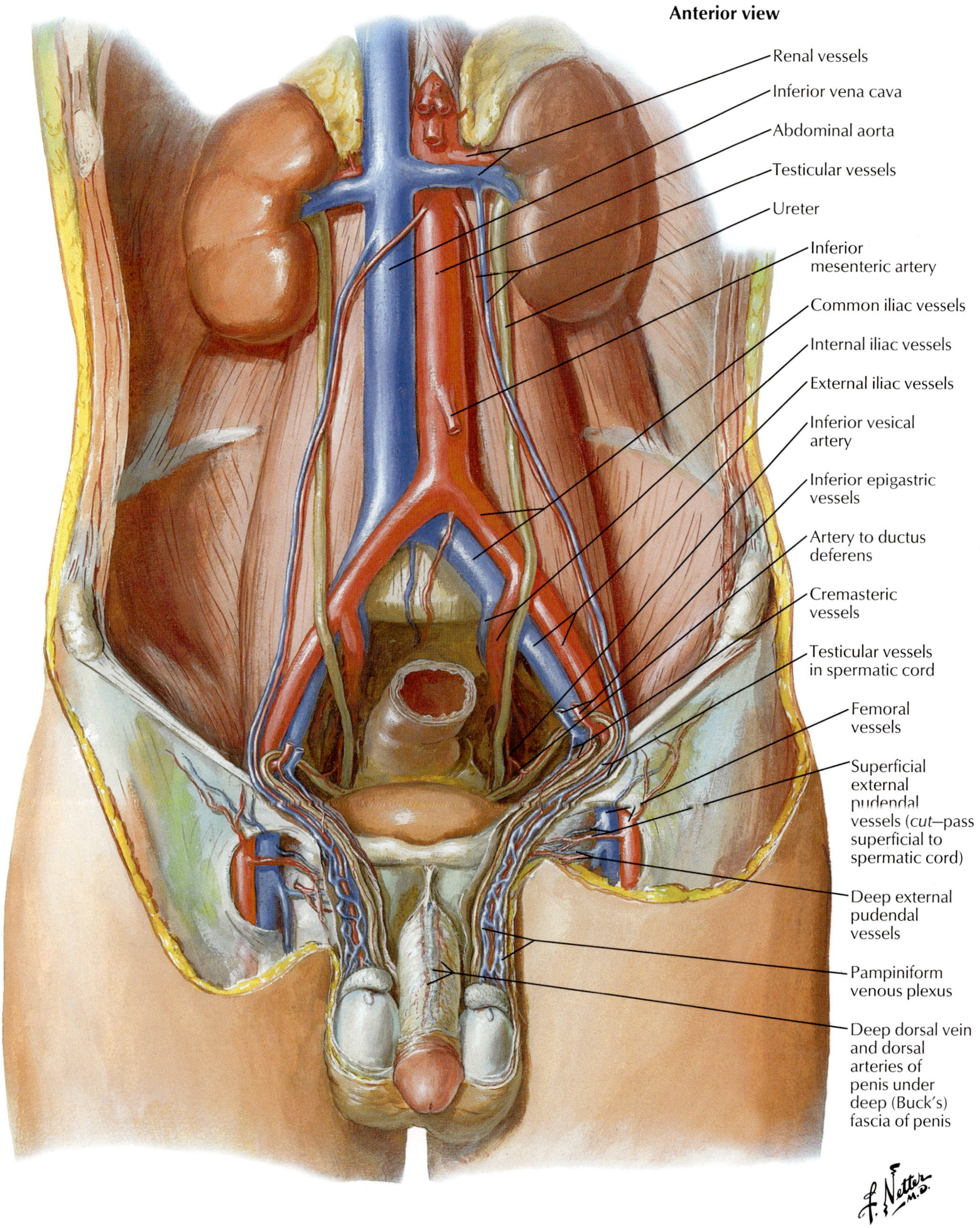

Arteries of Pelvis: Female

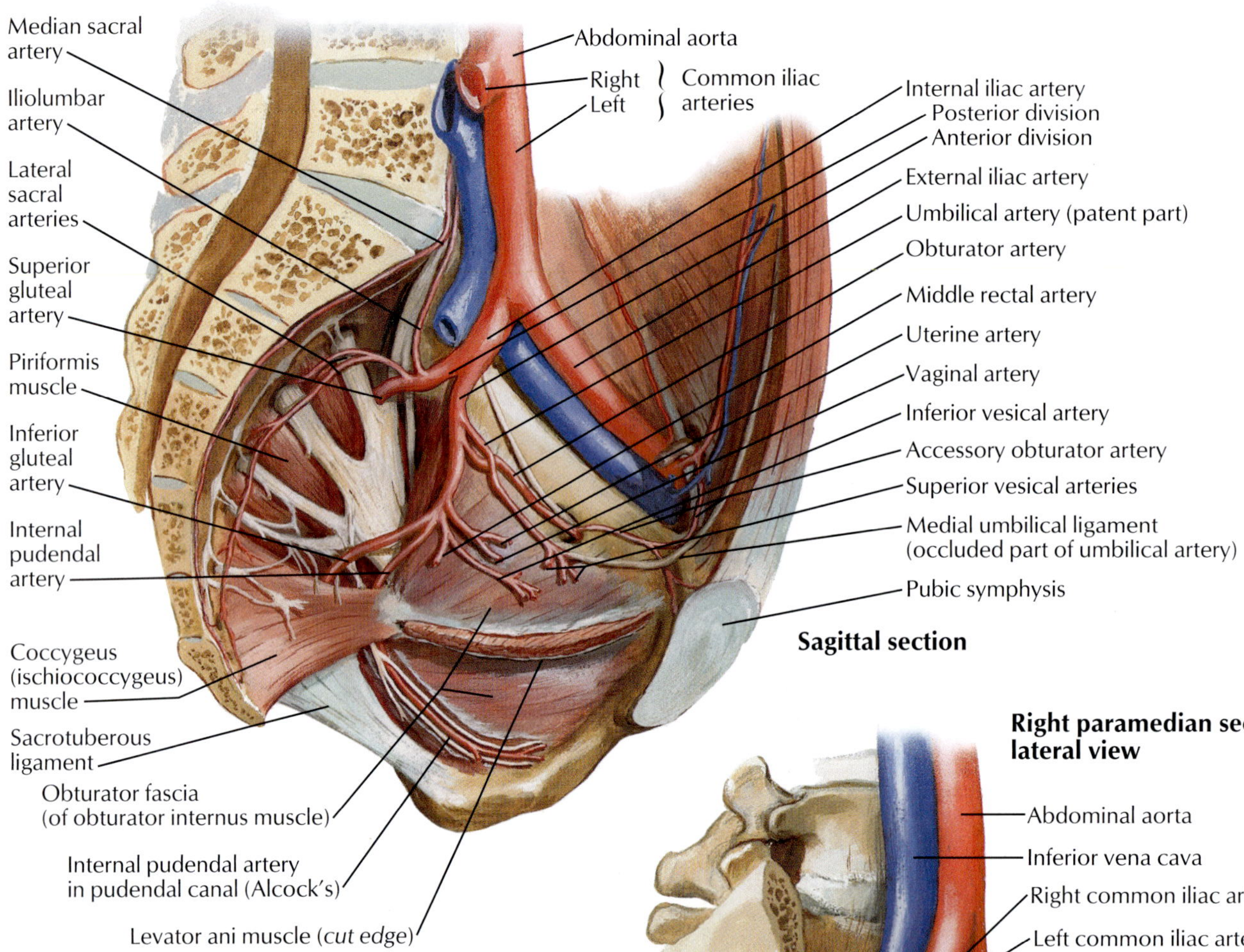

Sagittal section

Right paramedian section: lateral view

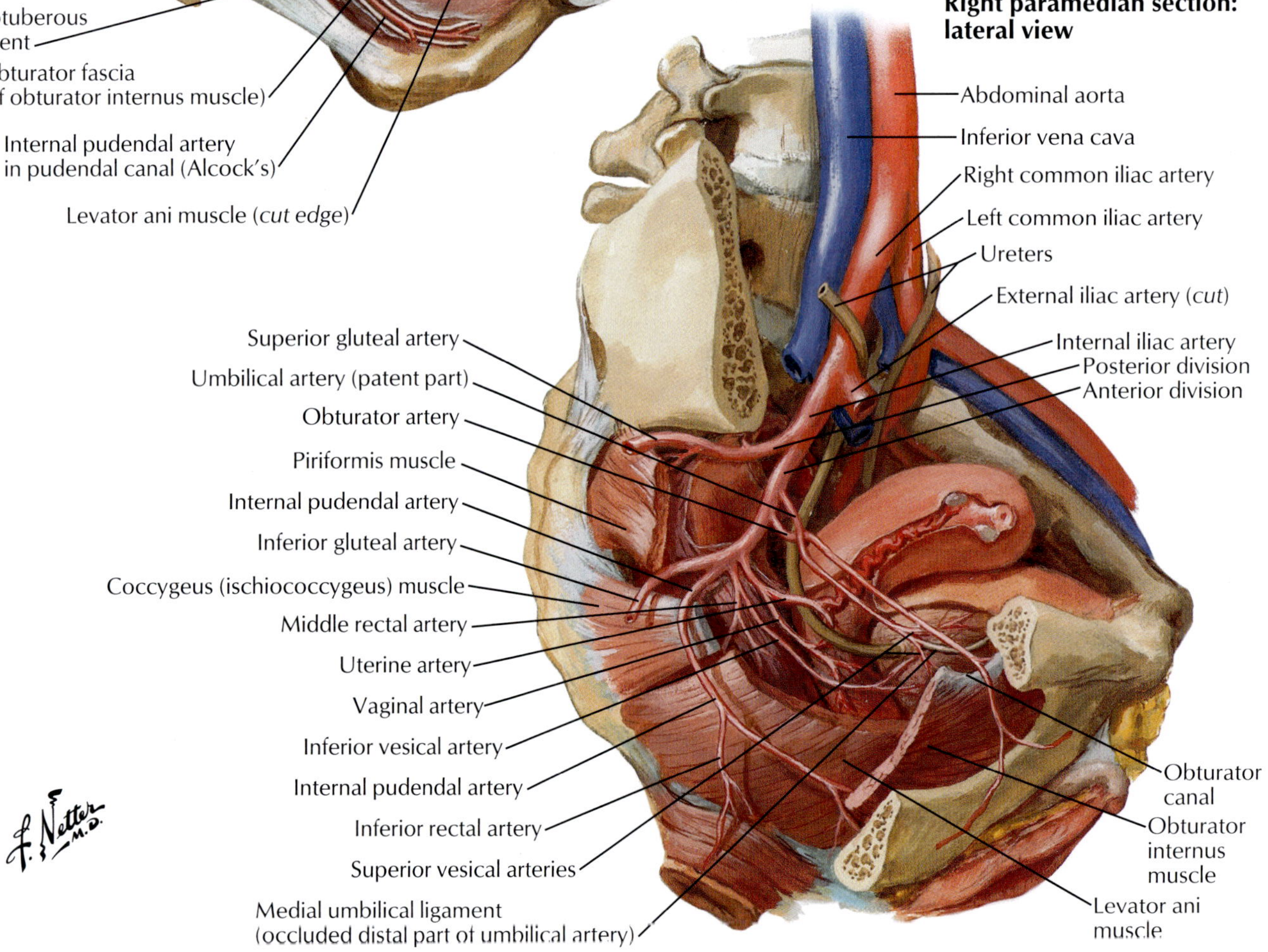

Left paramedian section: lateral view

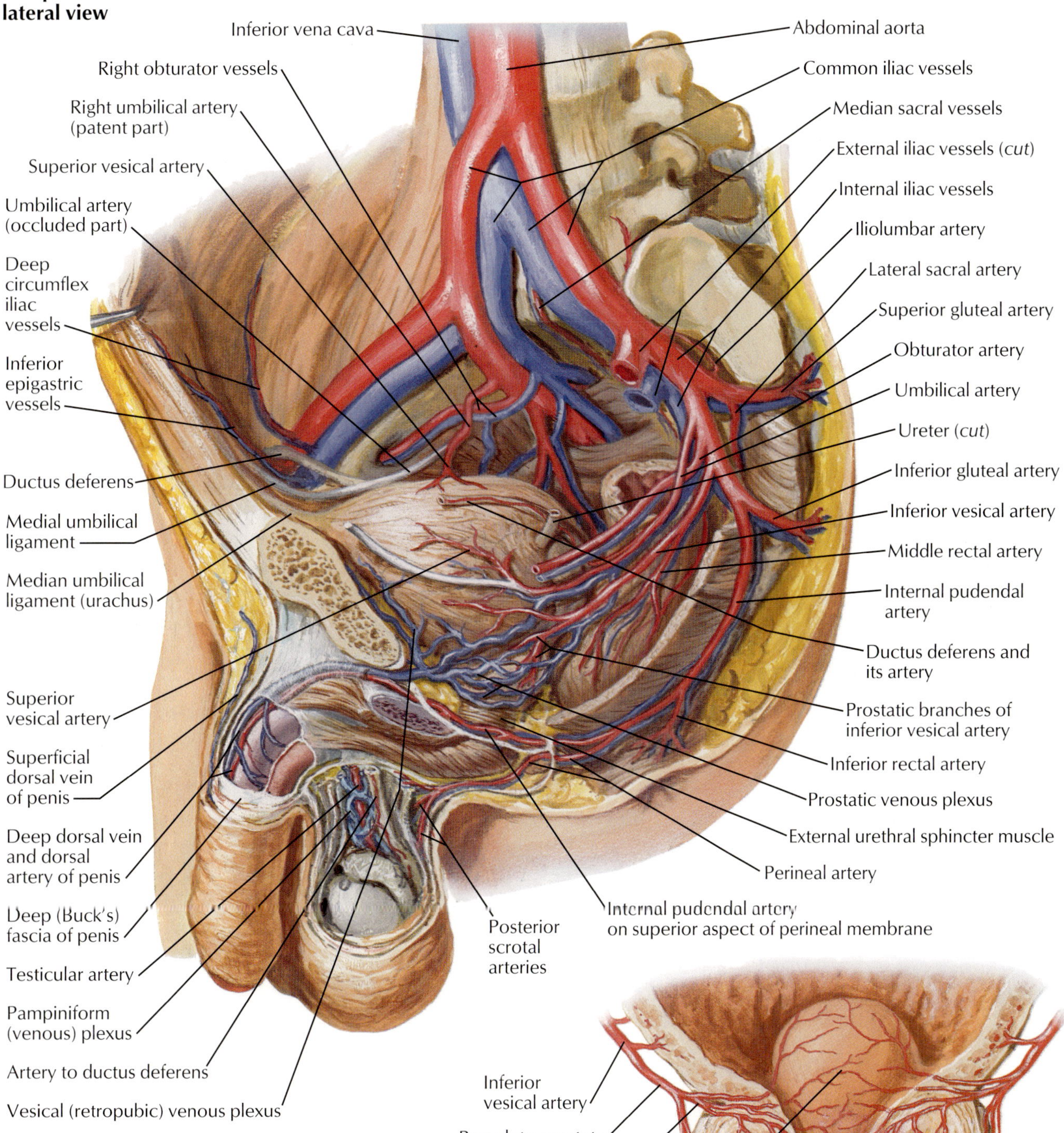

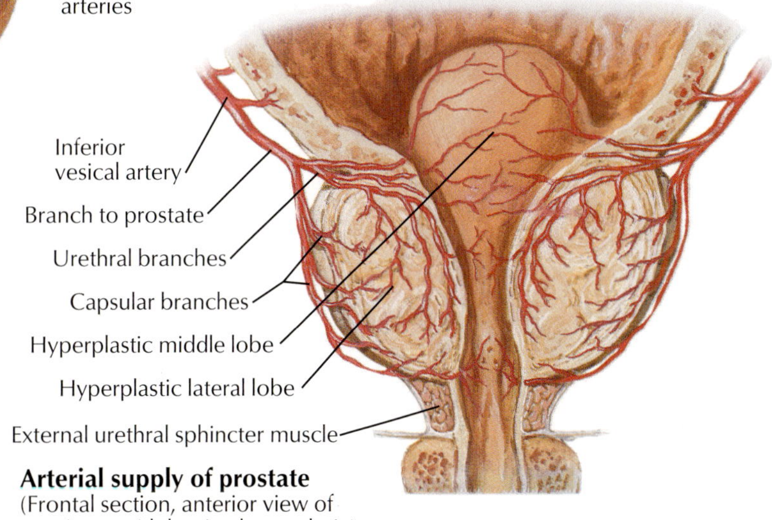

Arterial supply of prostate
(Frontal section, anterior view of specimen with benign hyperplasia)

Arteries and Veins of Perineum and Uterus

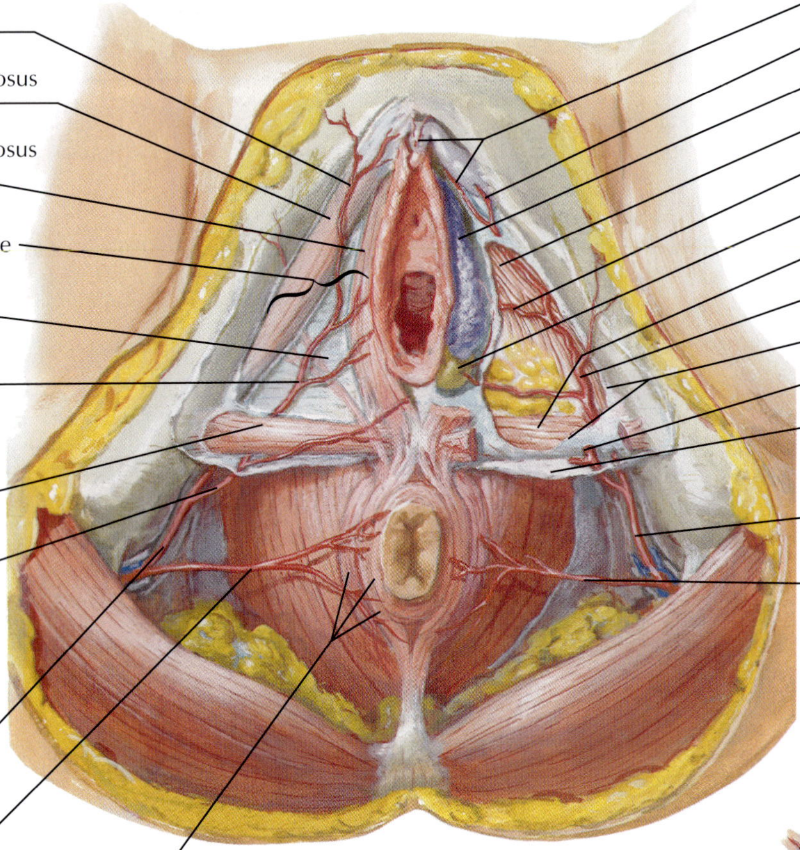

Note: Deep perineal (investing or Gallaudet's) fascia removed from muscles of superficial perineal space

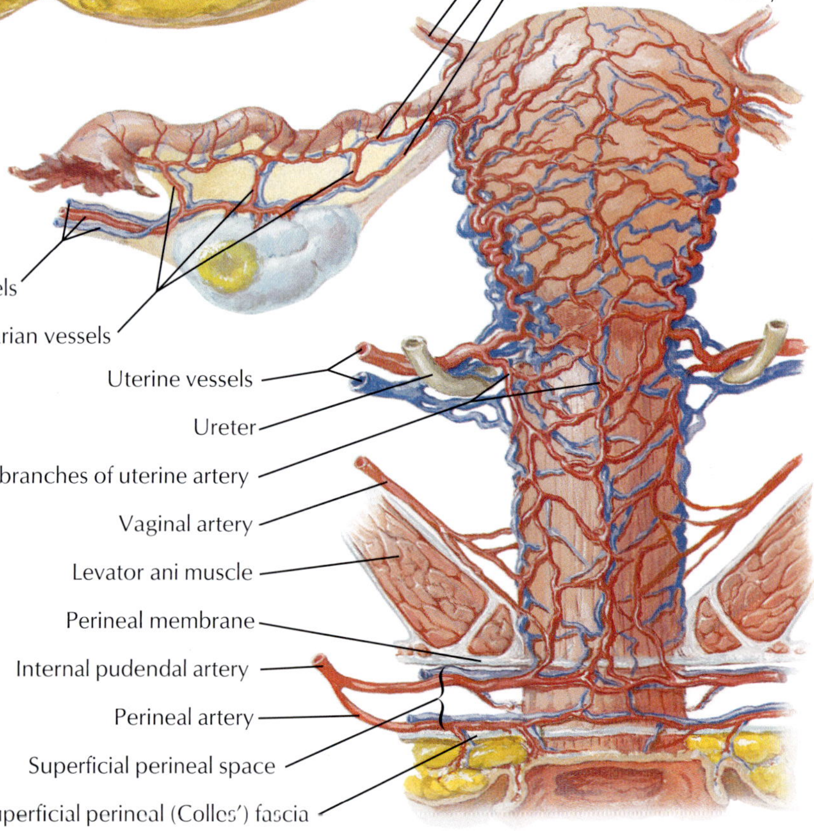

F. Netter M.D.
C. Machado M.D.

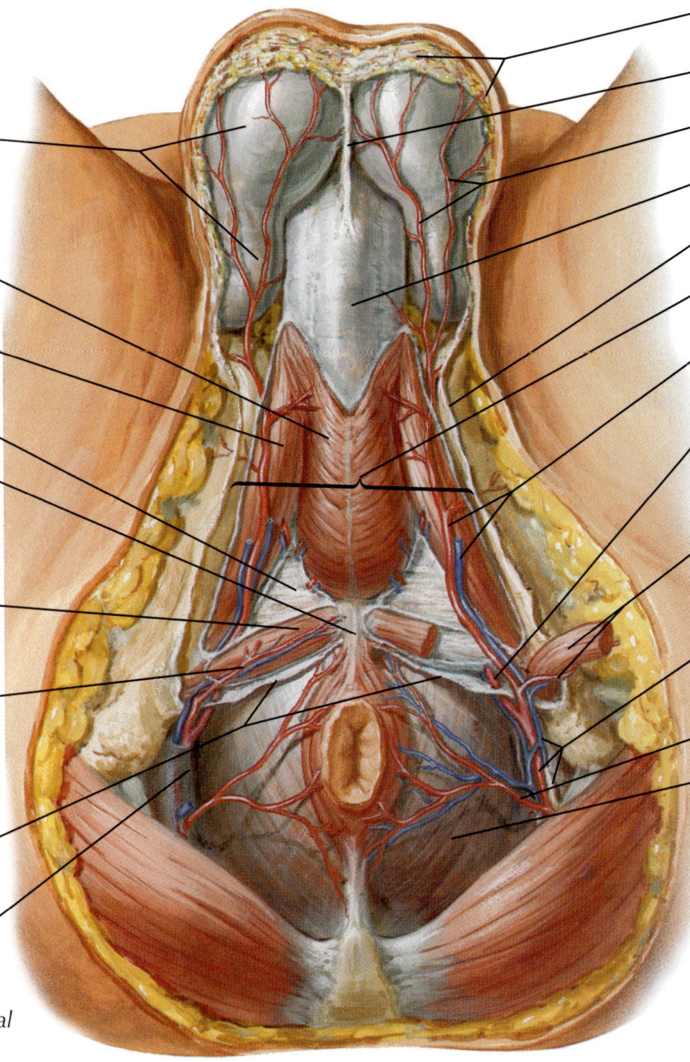

Note: Deep perineal (investing or Gallaudet's) fascia removed from muscles of superficial perineal space

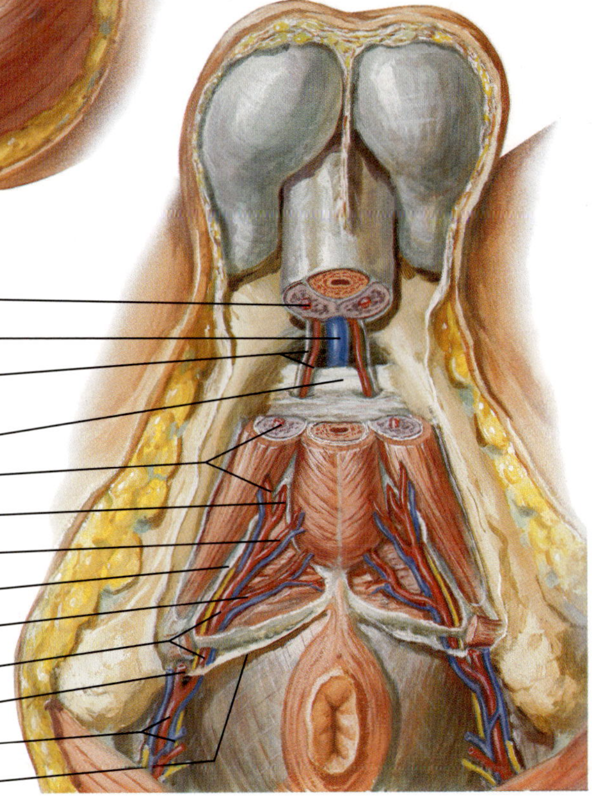

F. Netter M.D.

Lymph Vessels and Nodes of Pelvis and Genitalia: Female

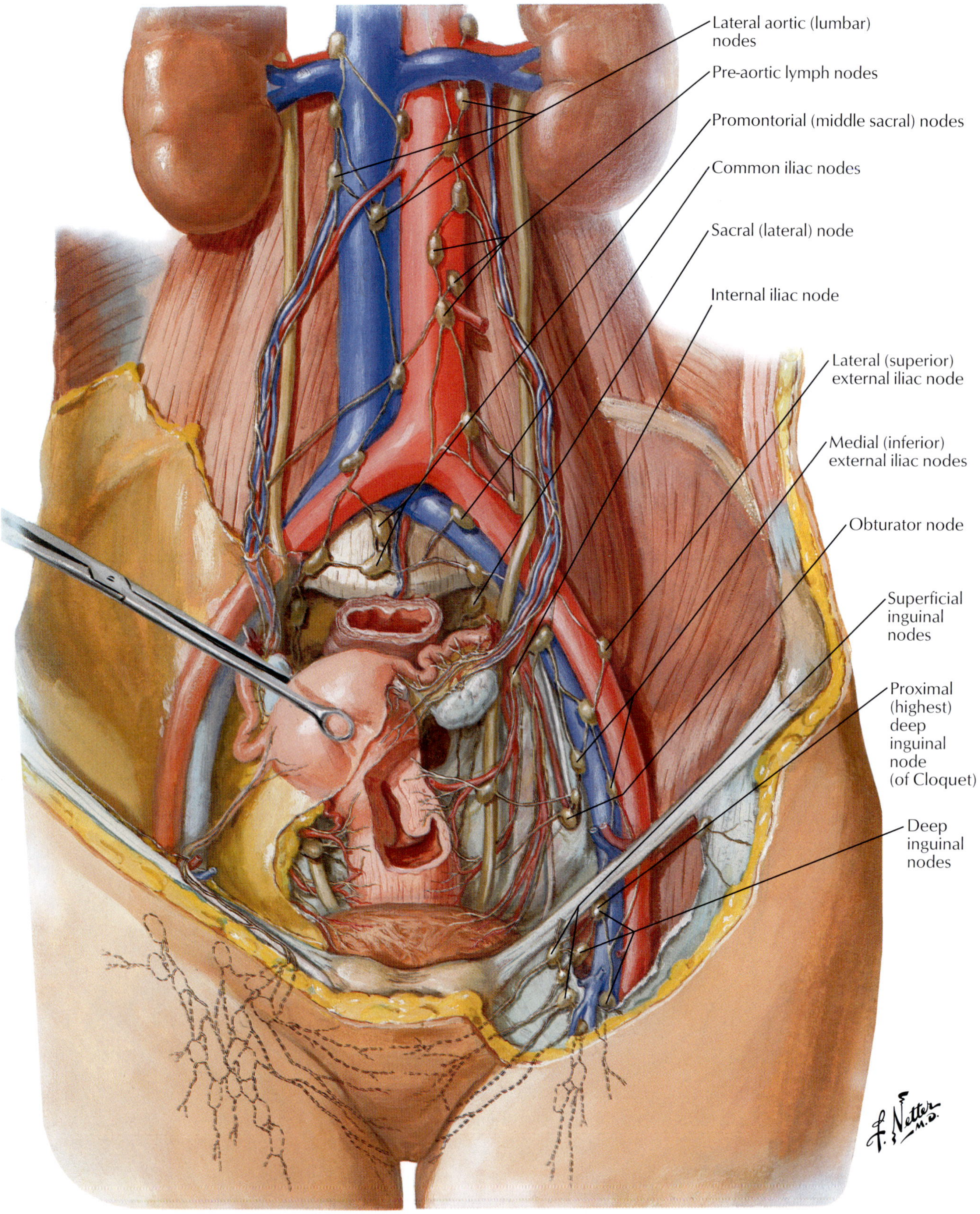

Lymph Vessels and Nodes of Perineum: Female

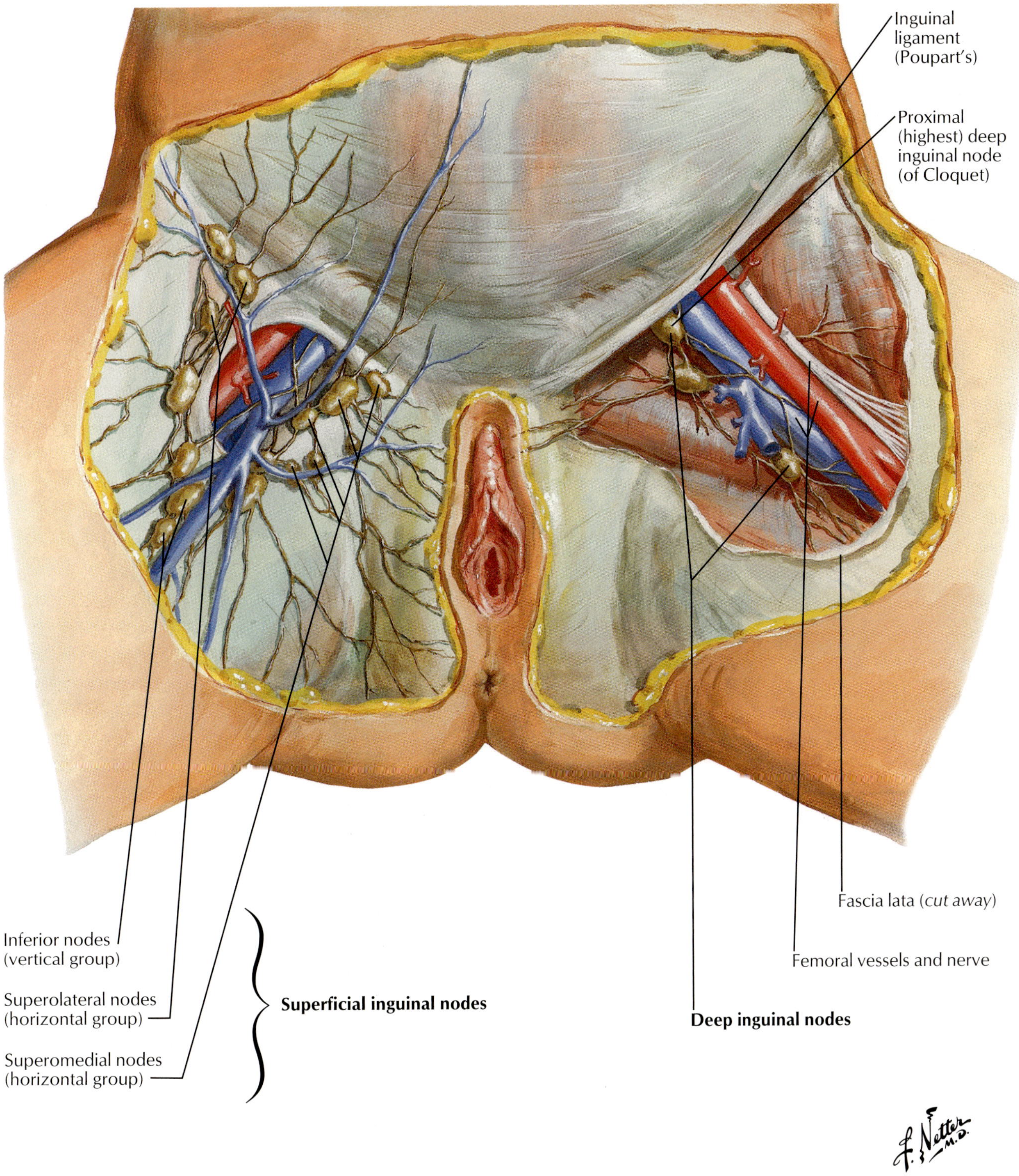

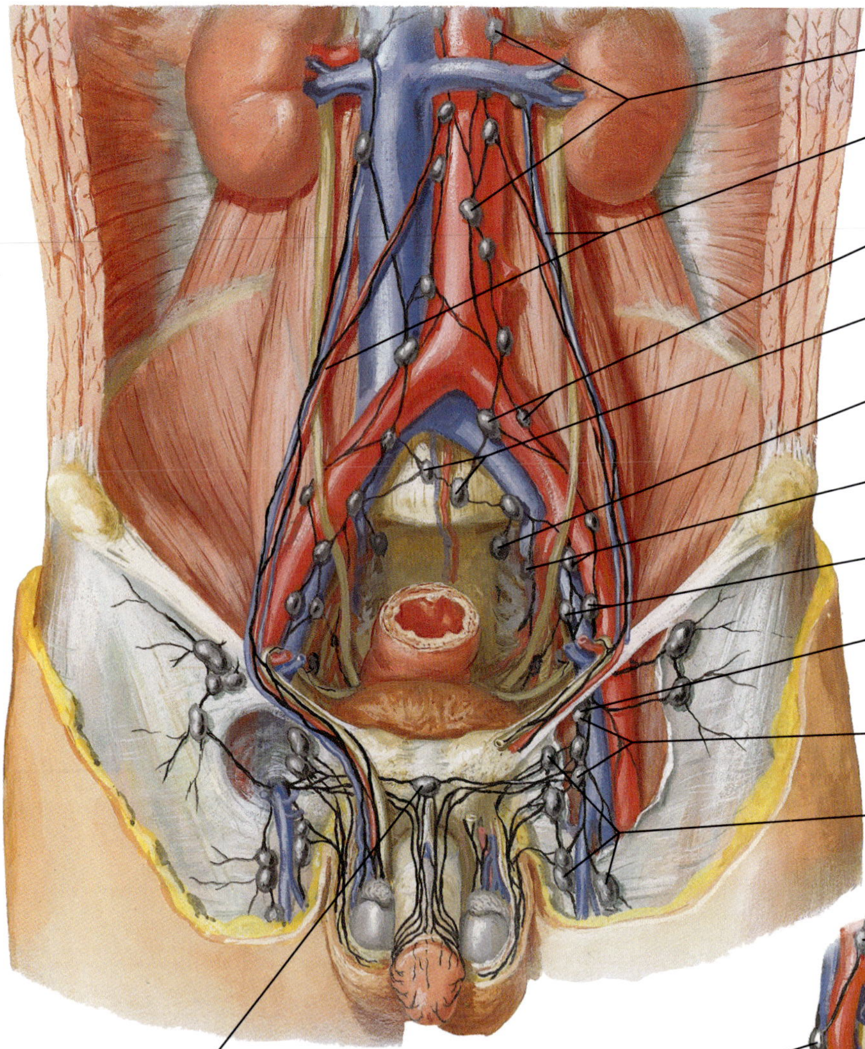

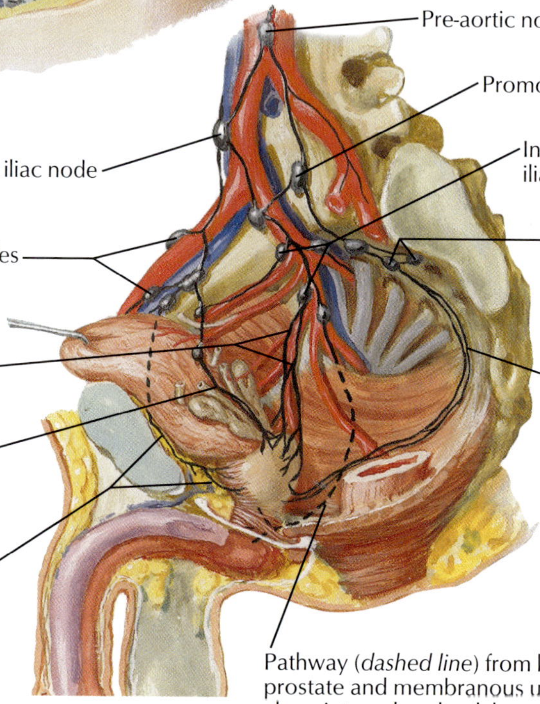

Lymphatic drainage from prostate

F. Netter M.D.
C. Machado M.D.

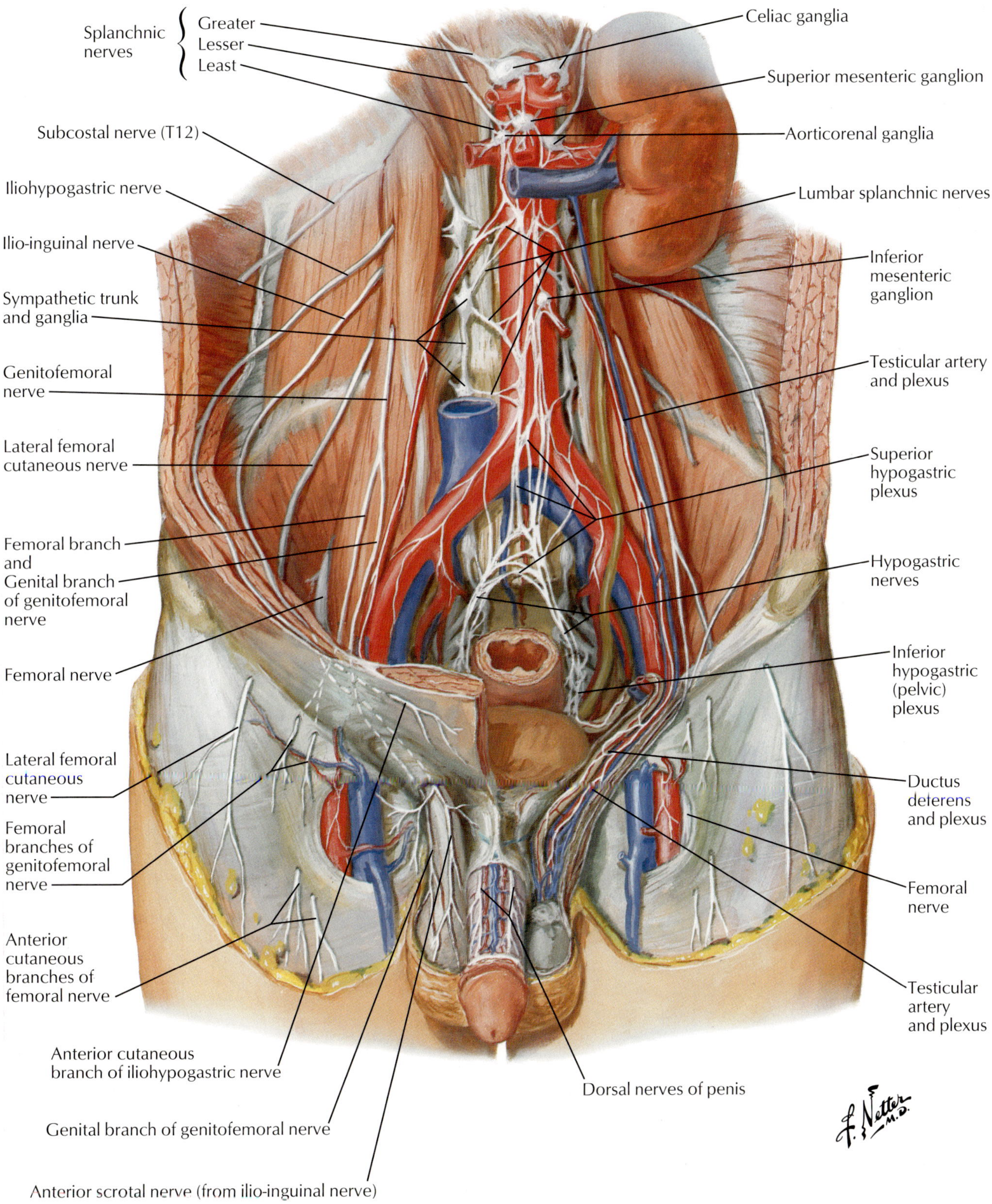
Splanchnic nerves
Greater
Lesser
Least
Celiac ganglia
Superior mesenteric ganglion
Subcostal nerve (T12)
Aorticorenal ganglia
Iliohypogastric nerve
Lumbar splanchnic nerves
Ilio-inguinal nerve
Inferior mesenteric ganglion
Sympathetic trunk and ganglia
Genitofemoral nerve
Testicular artery and plexus
Lateral femoral cutaneous nerve
Superior hypogastric plexus
Femoral branch and Genital branch of genitofemoral nerve
Hypogastric nerves
Femoral nerve
Inferior hypogastric (pelvic) plexus
Lateral femoral cutaneous nerve
Ductus deferens and plexus
Femoral branches of genitofemoral nerve
Femoral nerve
Anterior cutaneous branches of femoral nerve
Testicular artery and plexus
Anterior cutaneous branch of iliohypogastric nerve
Dorsal nerves of penis
Genital branch of genitofemoral nerve
Anterior scrotal nerve (from ilio-inguinal nerve)

Nerves of Pelvic Viscera: Male

See also Plate 297

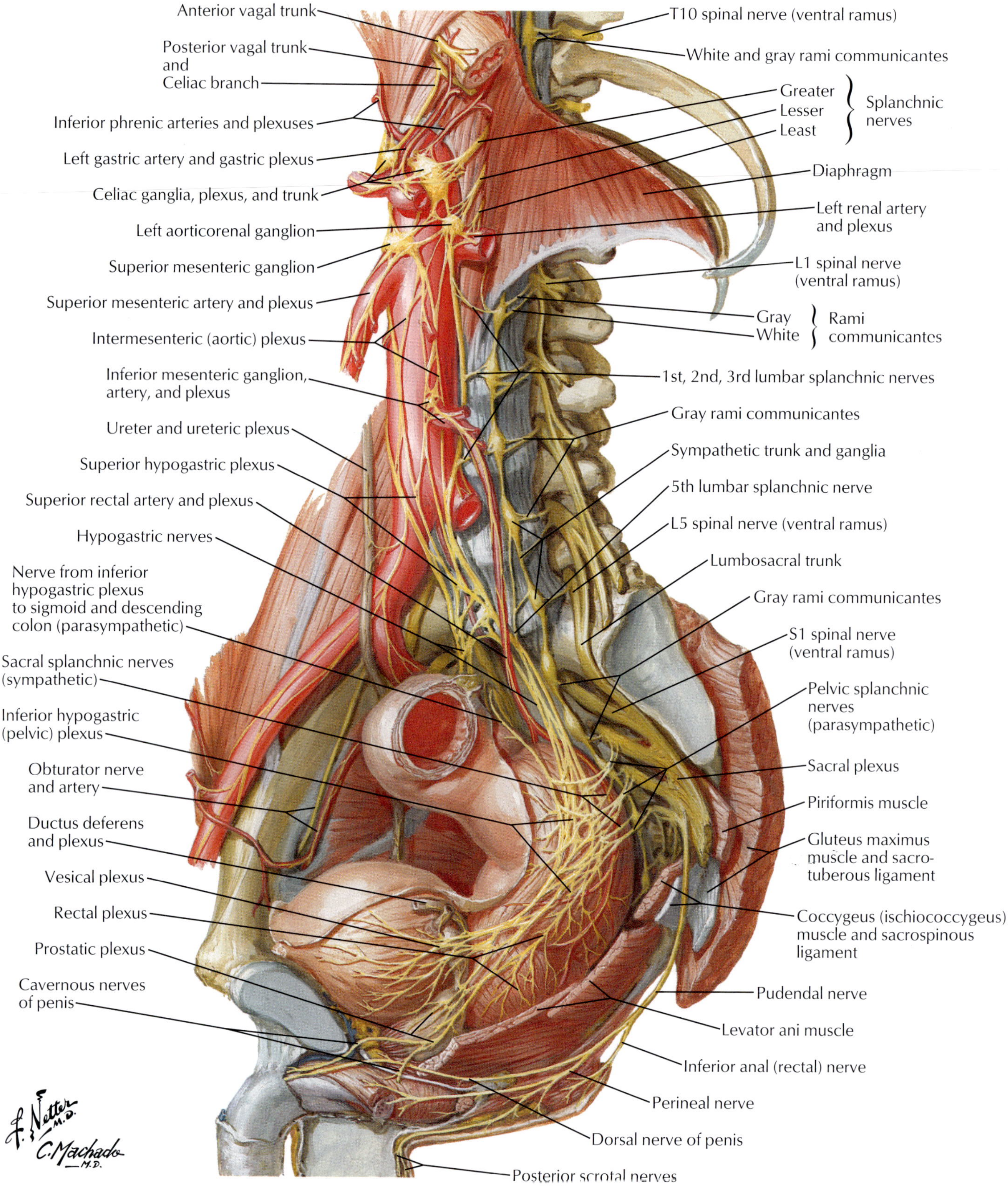

Nerves of Perineum: Male

See also Plate 394

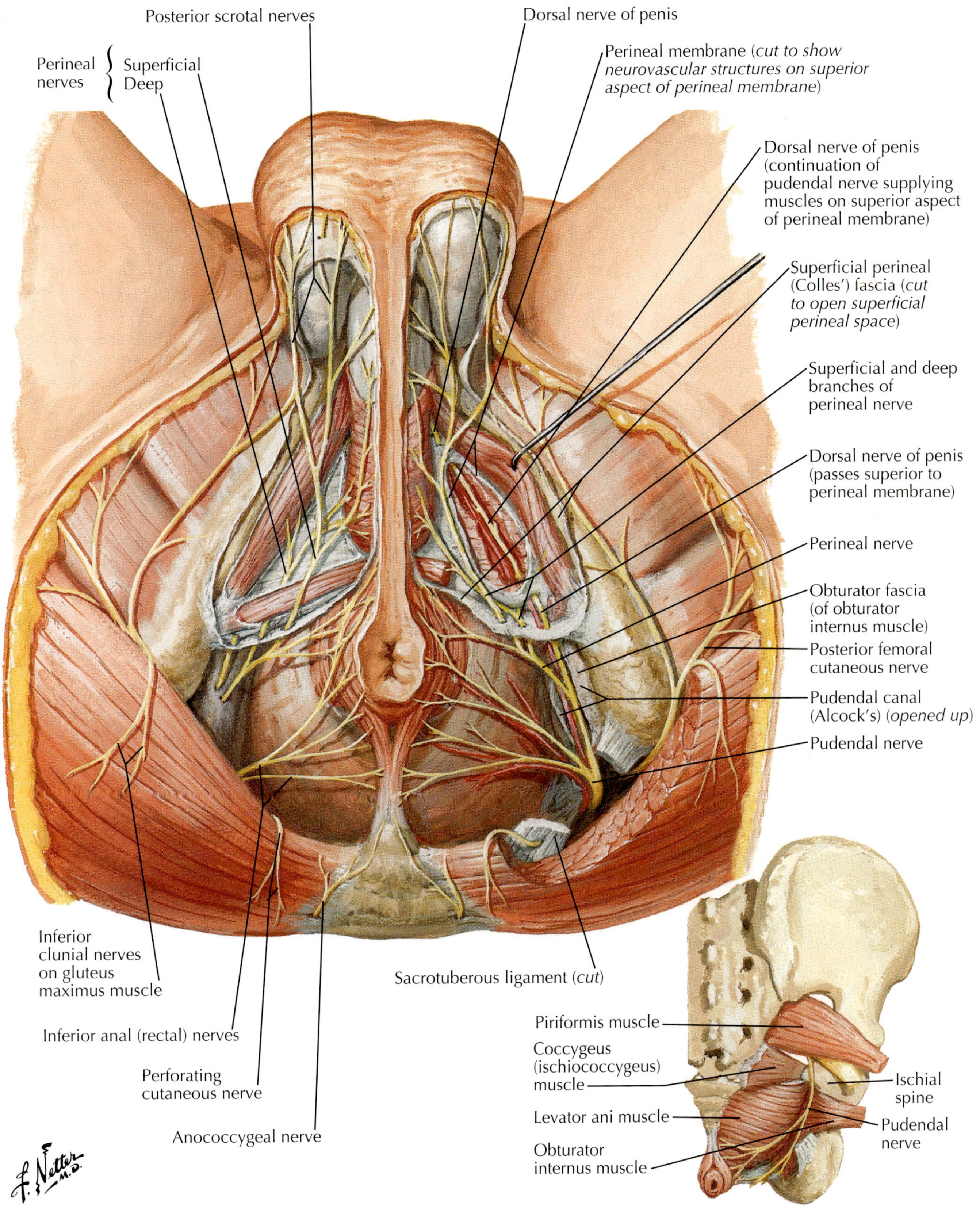

Nerves of Pelvic Viscera: Female

See also Plate 297

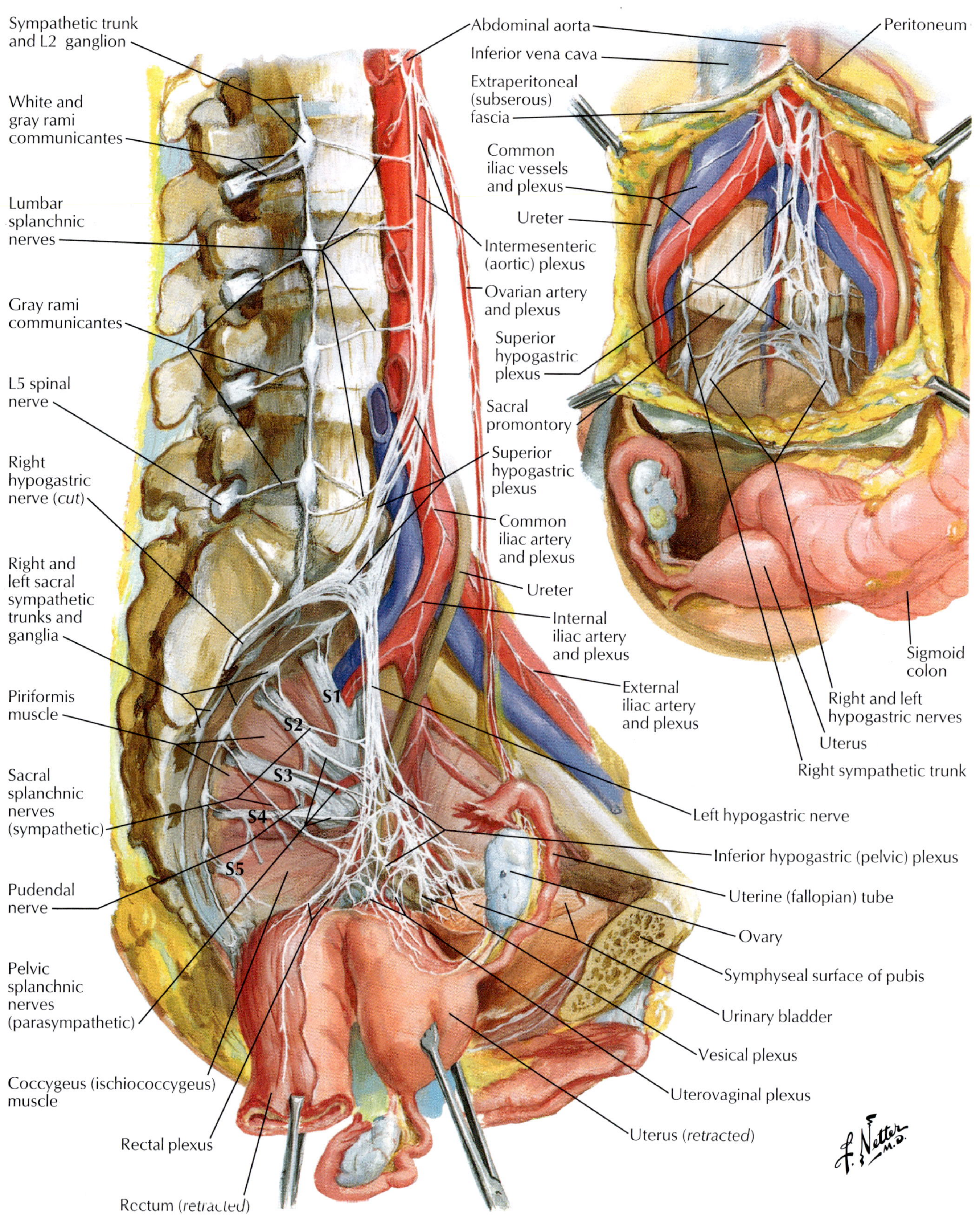

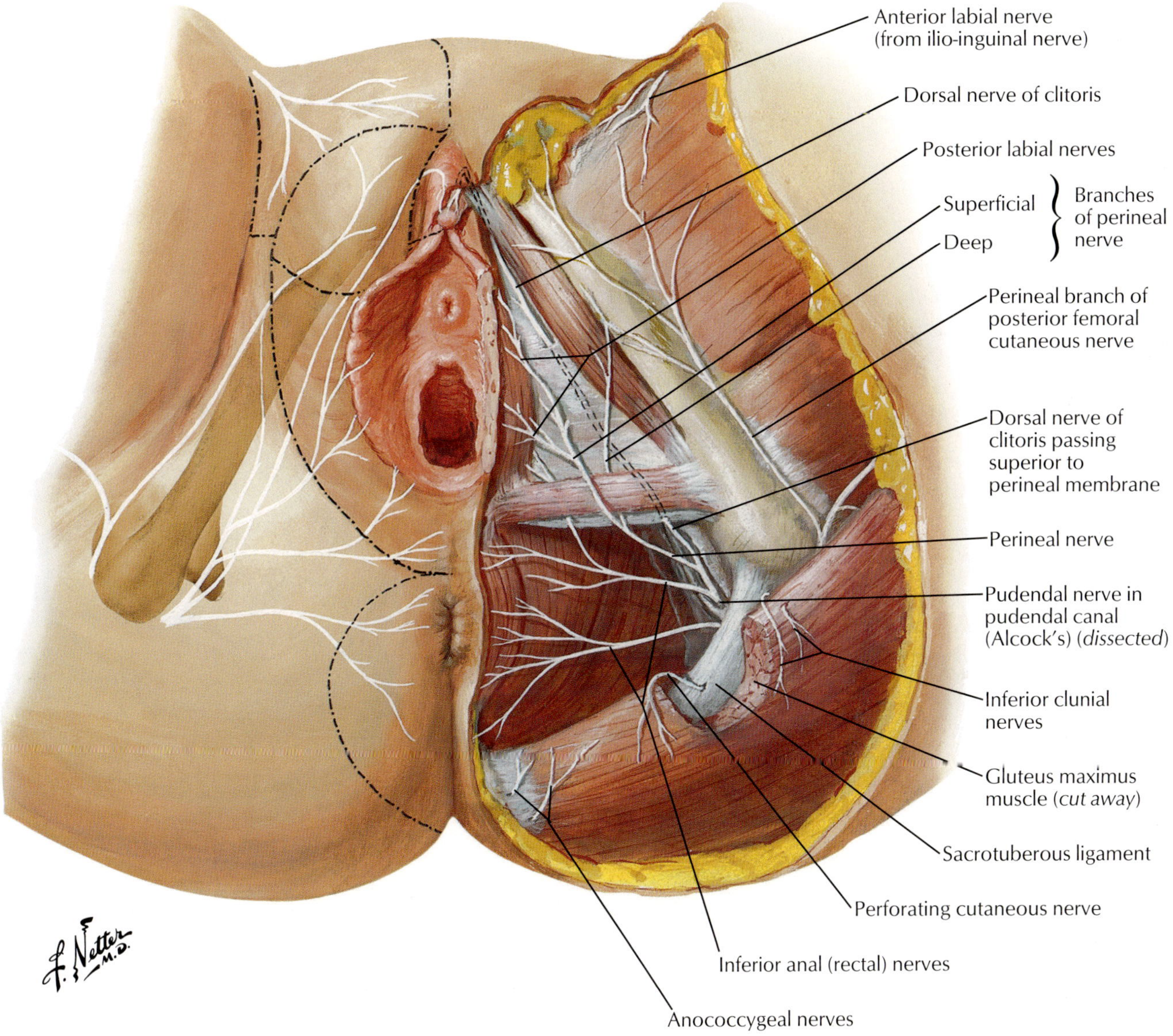
Anterior labial nerve (from ilio-inguinal nerve)
Dorsal nerve of clitoris
Posterior labial nerves
Superficial
Deep
Branches of perineal nerve
Perineal branch of posterior femoral cutaneous nerve
Dorsal nerve of clitoris passing superior to perineal membrane
Perineal nerve
Pudendal nerve in pudendal canal (Alcock's) (dissected)
Inferior clunial nerves
Gluteus maximus muscle (cut away)
Sacrotuberous ligament
Perforating cutaneous nerve
Inferior anal (rectal) nerves
Anococcygeal nerves
F. Netter M.D.

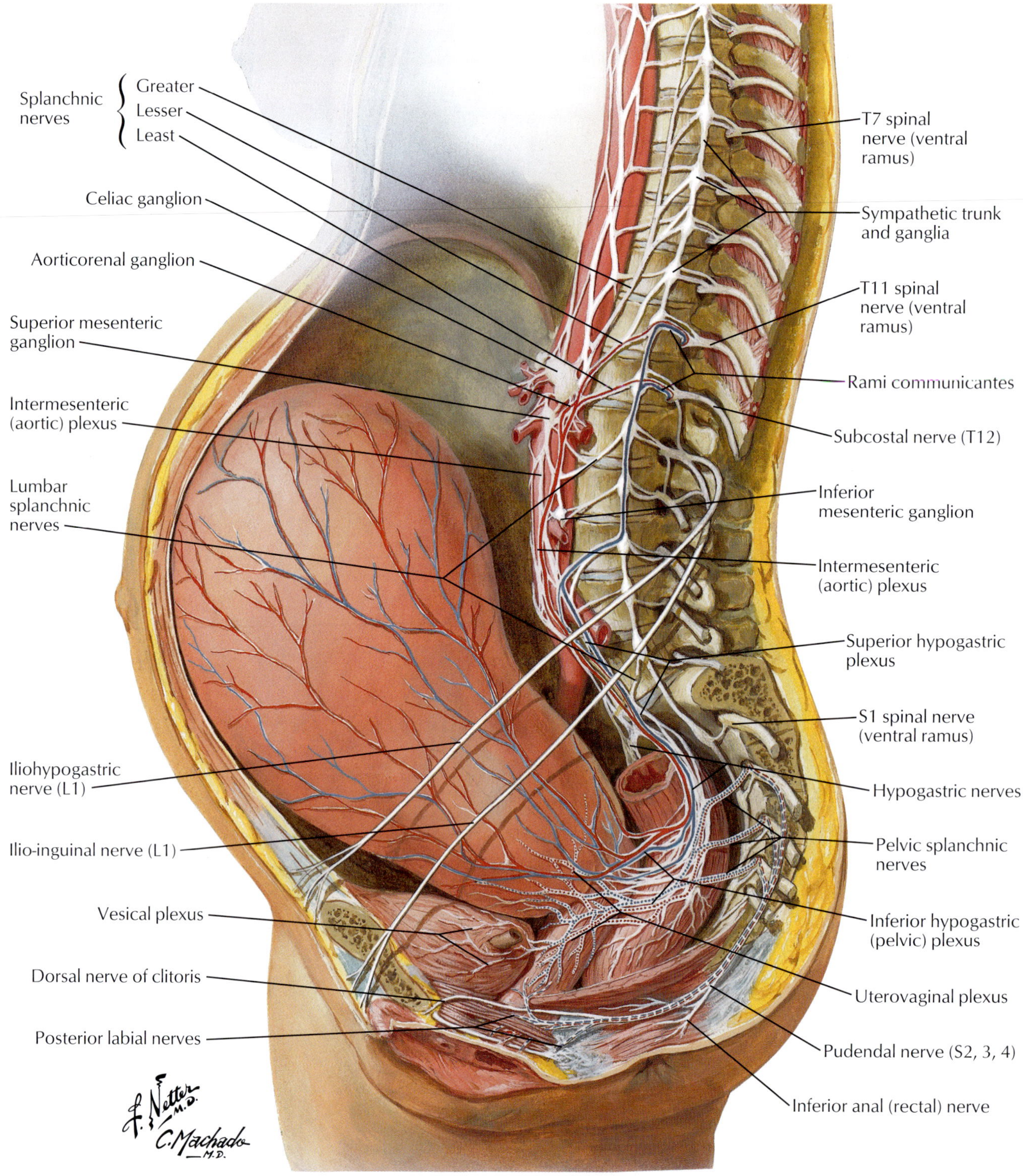

Sensory fibers from uterine body and fundus accompany sympathetic fibers via hypogastric plexuses to T11, 12 (L1?)

Motor fibers to uterine body and fundus (sympathetic)

Sensory fibers from cervix and upper vagina accompany pelvic splanchnic nerves (parasympathetic) to S2, 3, 4

Motor fibers to lower uterine segment, cervix, and upper vagina (parasympathetic)

Sensory fibers from lower vagina and perineum accompany somatic fibers via pudendal nerve to S2, 3, 4

Motor fibers to lower vagina and perineum via pudendal nerve (somatic)

Innervation of Female Reproductive Organs: Schema

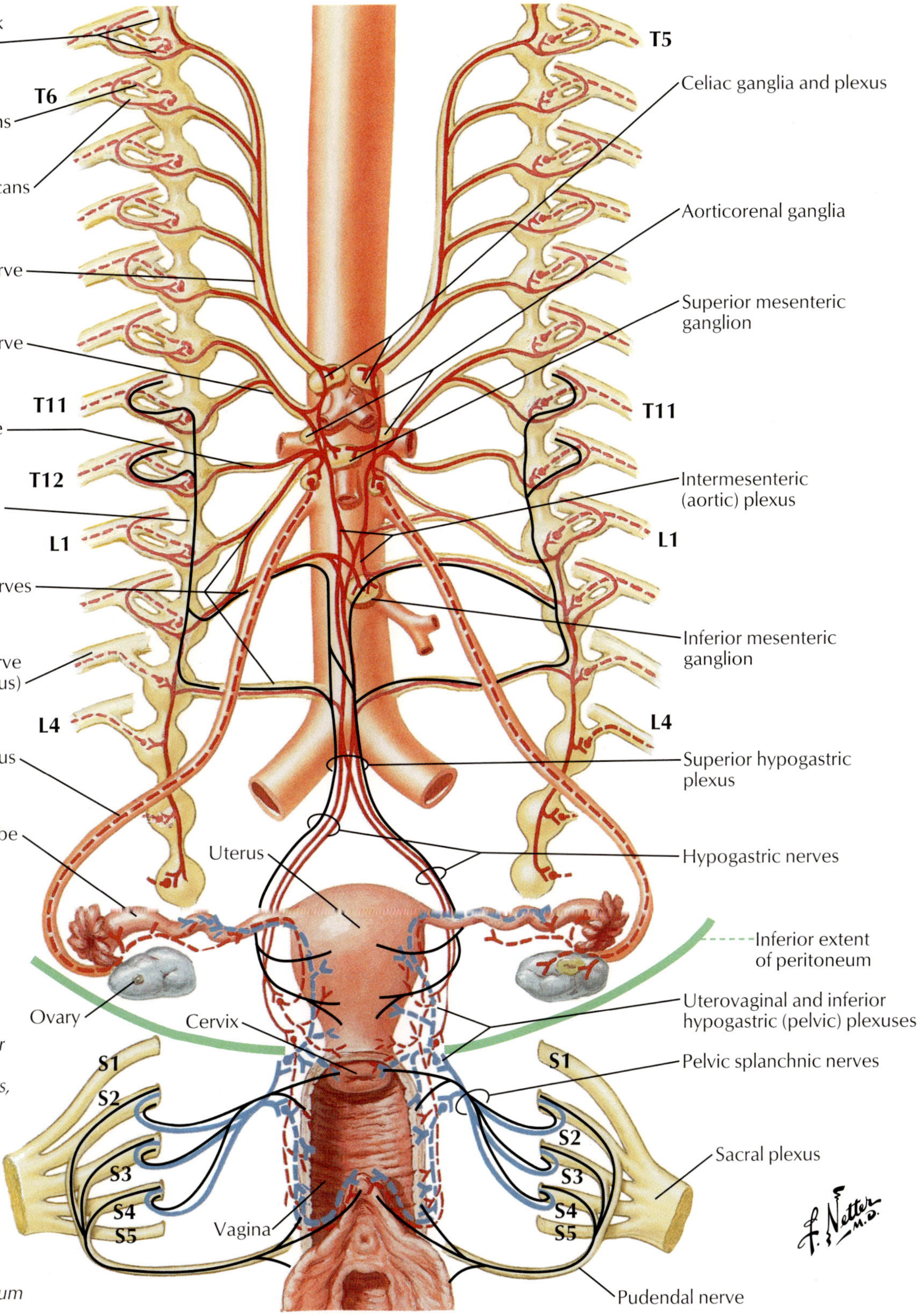

Note: Pain from intraperitoneal pelvic viscera (e.g., uterine contractions) goes via uterovaginal and pelvic plexuses, hypogastric nerves, superior hypogastric plexus, lower aortic plexus, lower lumbar splanchnic nerves, sympathetic trunk from L4 to L5 to spinal nerves T11, 12. Pain from subperitoneal pelvic viscera (e.g., cervical dilation and upper vagina) goes via pelvic splanchnic nerves to S2, 3, 4. Afferent fibers from lower vagina and perineum go via pudendal nerves to S2, 3, 4.

Sympathetic fibers { **Preganglionic** —— **Postganglionic** - - - -

Parasympathetic fibers { **Preganglionic** —— **Postganglionic** - - - -

Afferent fibers ——

Innervation of Male Reproductive Organs: Schema

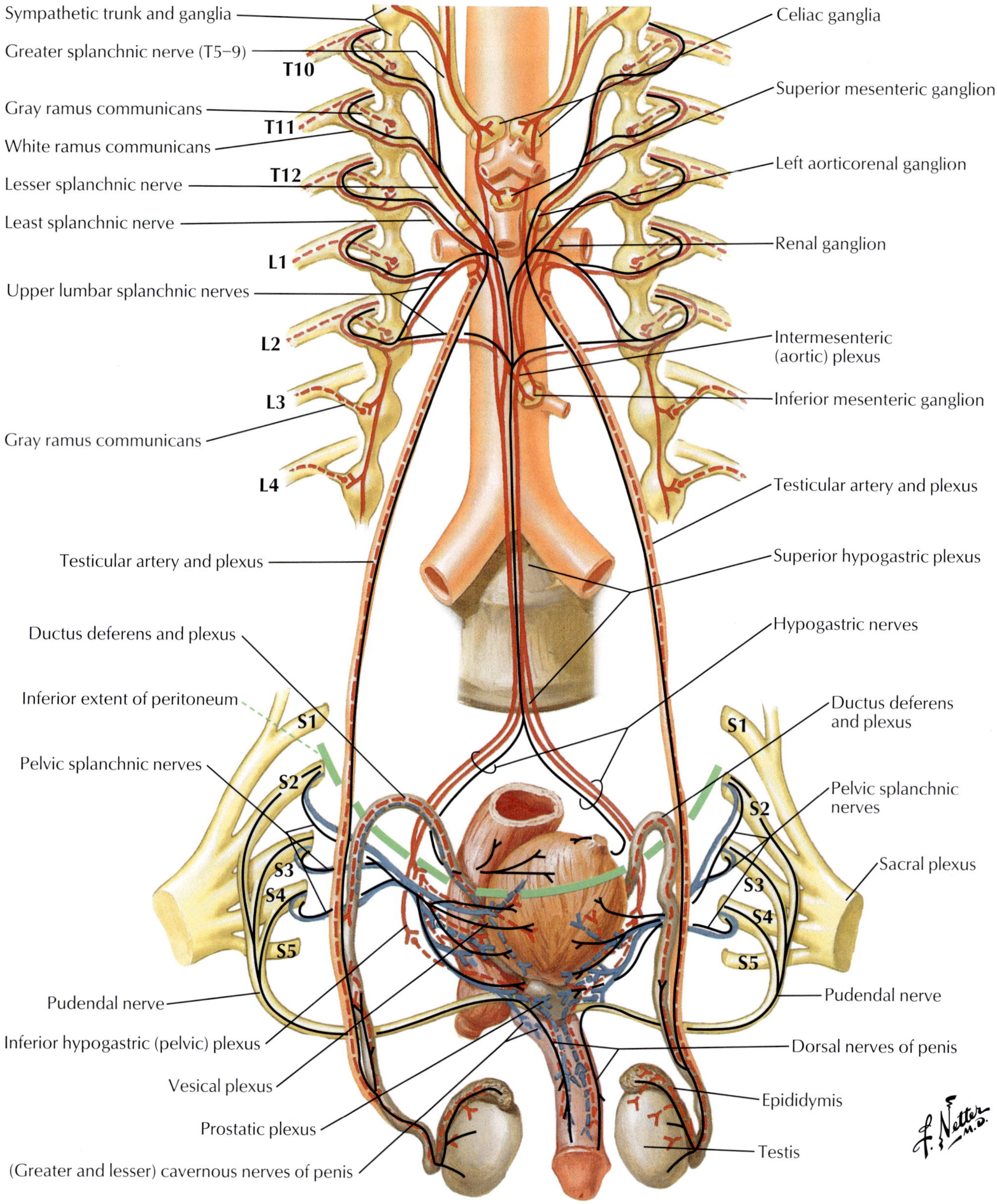

Sympathetic fibers { Preganglionic ——— Postganglionic - - - -

Parasympathetic fibers { Preganglionic ——— Postganglionic - - - -

Afferent fibers ———

Innervation of Urinary Bladder and Lower Ureter: Schema

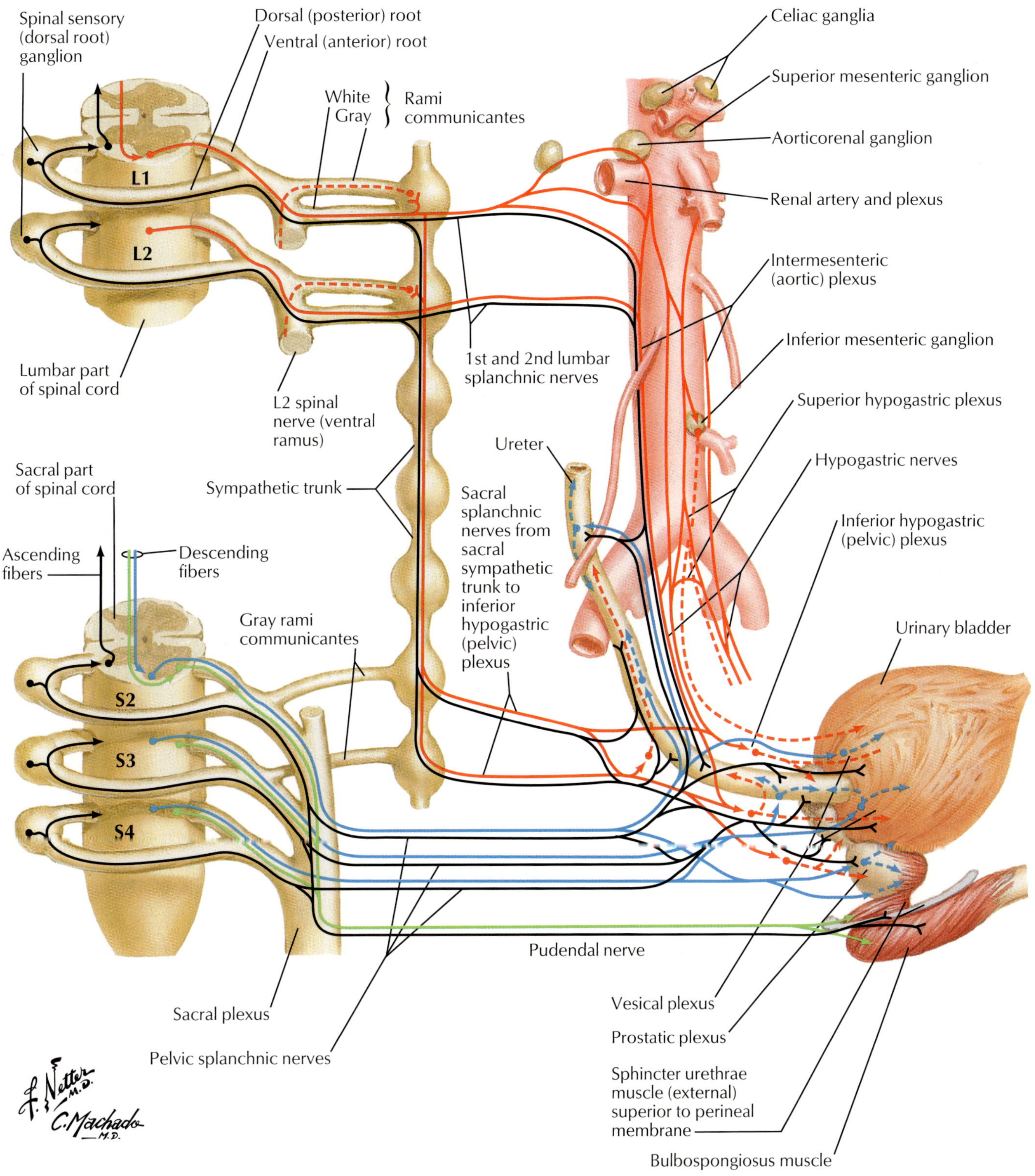

Sympathetic fibers { **Preganglionic** ——— / **Postganglionic** – – – –

Parasympathetic fibers { **Preganglionic** ——— / **Postganglionic** – – – –

Somatic efferent fibers ———

Afferent fibers ———

Male Pelvis: Cross Section of Bladder-Prostate Junction

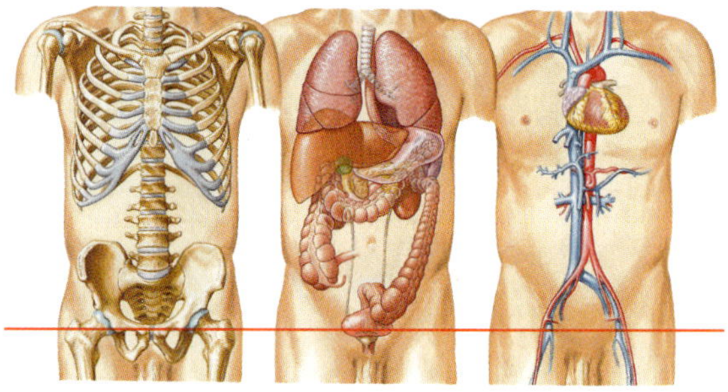

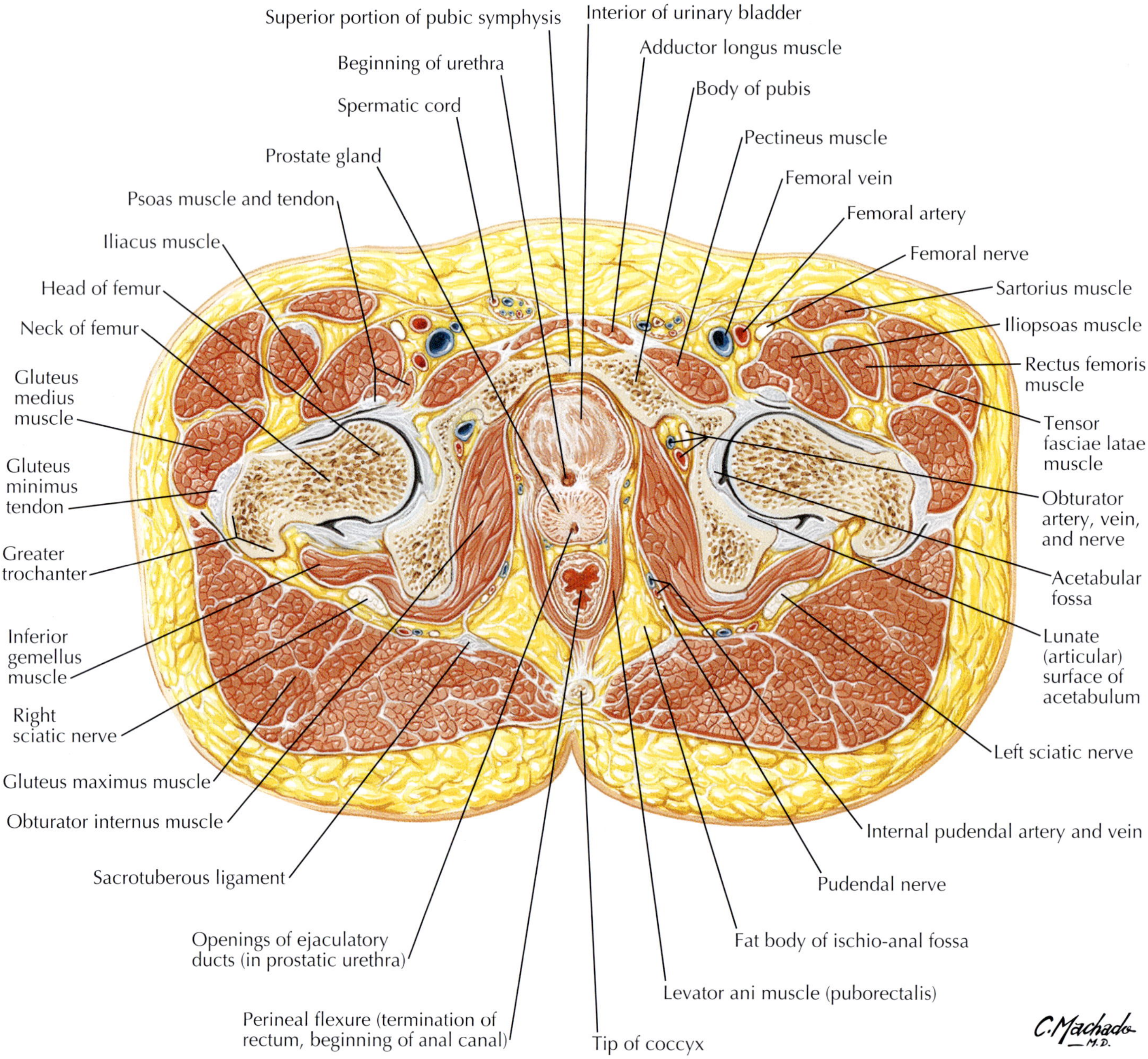

Female Pelvis: Cross Section of Vagina-Urethra

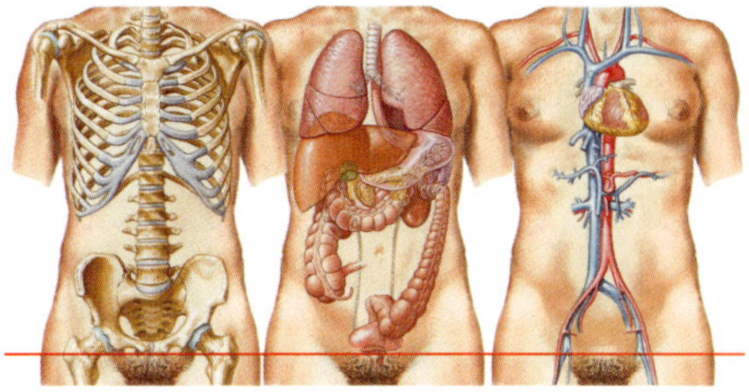

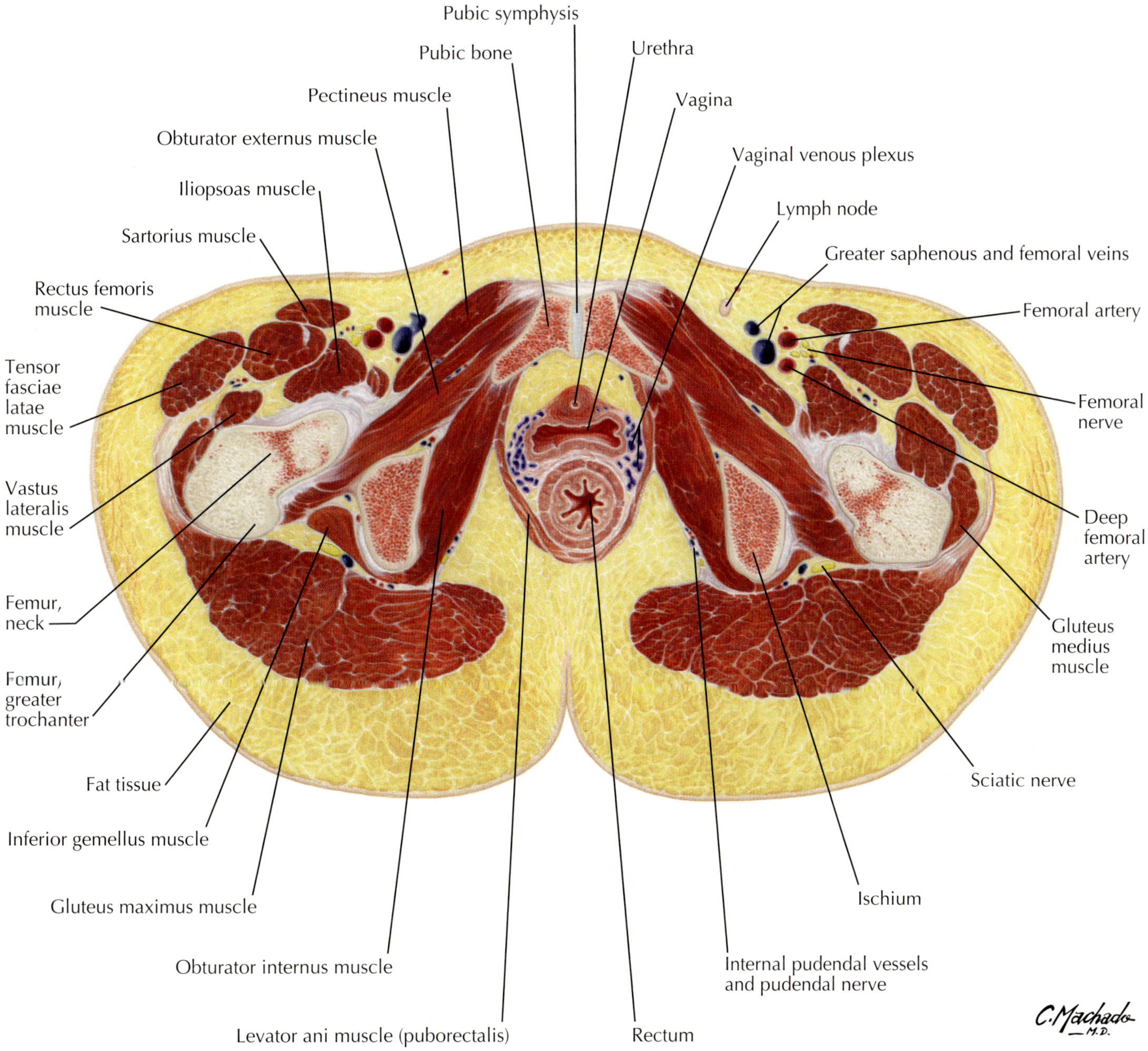

MUSCLE	PROXIMAL ATTACHMENT (ORIGIN)	DISTAL ATTACHMENT (INSERTION)	INNERVATION	MAIN ACTIONS	BLOOD SUPPLY	MUSCLE GROUP
Bulbospongiosus	*Male:* median raphe, bulb of penis, perineal body *Female:* perineal body	*Male:* perineal membrane, corpus cavernosum, bulb of penis *Female:* dorsum of clitoris, inferior fascia of urogenital diaphragm, bulb of vestibule, pubic arch	Deep branch of perineal nerve from pudendal nerve	*Male:* compresses bulb of penis, forces blood into body of penis during erection, removes urine from urethra and semen during ejaculation *Female:* constricts vaginal orifice, assists in expressing secretions of greater vestibular gland, forces blood into body of clitoris	Internal pudendal artery and its branch (perineal artery)	Perineal
Coccygeus (ischiococcygeus)	Ischial spine, sacrospinous ligament	Inferior sacrum, coccyx	Ventral rami of lower sacral nerves	Supports pelvic viscera, draws coccyx forward	Inferior gluteal artery	Pelvic floor
Compressor urethrae (female only)	Ischiopubic ramus	Anterior aspect of urethra	Perineal branches of pudendal nerve	Sphincter of urethra	Perineal branch of internal pudendal artery	Perineal
Cremaster	Lower edge of internal oblique and middle of inguinal ligament	Pubic tubercle, crest of pubis	Genital branch of genitofemoral nerve	Retracts testicle	Cremasteric branch of inferior epigastric artery	Spermatic cord
Deep transverse perineal	Inner surface of inferior ischial rami	*Male:* medial tendinous raphe and perineal body *Female:* sides of vagina	Perineal branches of pudendal nerve	Stabilizes perineal body, supports prostate/vagina	Perineal branch of internal pudendal artery	Perineal
External anal sphincter	Tip of coccyx, anococcygeal ligament	Deeper fibers surround anal canal, attach posteriorly to coccyx and anteriorly to central point of perineum	Perineal and inferior rectal branches of pudendal nerve	Closes anal orifice	Inferior rectal and transverse perineal artery	Perineal
Iliacus	Superior 2/3 of iliac fossa, ala of sacrum, anterior sacro-iliac ligaments	Lesser trochanter of femur and shaft inferior to it, to psoas major tendon	Femoral nerve	Flexes thigh at hips and stabilizes hip joint, acts with psoas major	Iliac branches of iliolumbar artery	Anterior thigh
Ischiocavernosus	Inferior internal surface of ischiopubic ramus, ischial tuberosity	Crus of penis or clitoris	Deep branch of perineal nerve from pudendal nerve	Forces blood into body of penis and clitoris during erection	Internal pudendal artery and its branch (perineal artery)	Perineal
Levator ani (iliococcygeus, pubococcygeus, and puborectalis)	Body of pubis, tendinous arch of obturator fascia, ischial spine	Perineal body, coccyx, anococcygeal raphe, walls of prostate or vagina, rectum, anal canal	Ventral rami of lower sacral nerves, perineal nerve	Supports pelvic viscera, raises pelvic floor	Inferior gluteal artery, internal pudendal artery and its branches (inferior rectal and perineal arteries)	Pelvic floor
Obturator internus	Pelvic surface of obturator membrane and surrounding bone	Medial surface of greater trochanter of femur	Nerve to obturator internus	Laterally rotates extended thigh, abducts flexed thigh at hip	Internal pudendal and obturator arteries	Gluteal region

Variations in spinal nerve contributions to the innervation of muscles, their arterial supply, their attachments, and their actions are common themes in human anatomy. Therefore, expect differences between texts and realize that anatomical variation is normal.

MUSCLE	PROXIMAL ATTACHMENT (ORIGIN)	DISTAL ATTACHMENT (INSERTION)	INNERVATION	MAIN ACTIONS	BLOOD SUPPLY	MUSCLE GROUP
Piriformis	Anterior surface of sacral segments 2–4, sacrotuberous ligament	Superior border of greater trochanter of femur	Ventral rami of L5, S1, S2	Laterally rotates extended thigh, abducts flexed thigh at hip	Superior and inferior gluteal arteries, internal pudendal artery	Gluteal region
Sphincter urethrae	External fibers from junction of inferior pubic and ischial rami and adjacent fascia; internal fibers pass medially to surround membranous urethra	*Male:* median raphe in front and behind urethra *Female:* encloses urethra, attaches to sides of vagina	Perineal branches of pudendal nerve	Compresses urethra at end of micturition; in female also compresses the distal vagina	Perineal branch of internal pudendal artery	Perineal
Sphincter urethrovaginalis (female only)	Perineal body	Passes forward and anterior around urethra	Perineal branches of pudendal nerve	Sphincter of urethra and vagina	Perineal branch of pudendal artery	Perineal
Superficial transverse perineal	Ischial rami and tuberosities	Central tendon (perineal body)	Perineal branches of pudendal nerve	Stabilizes central tendon	Perineal branch of internal pudendal artery	Perineal

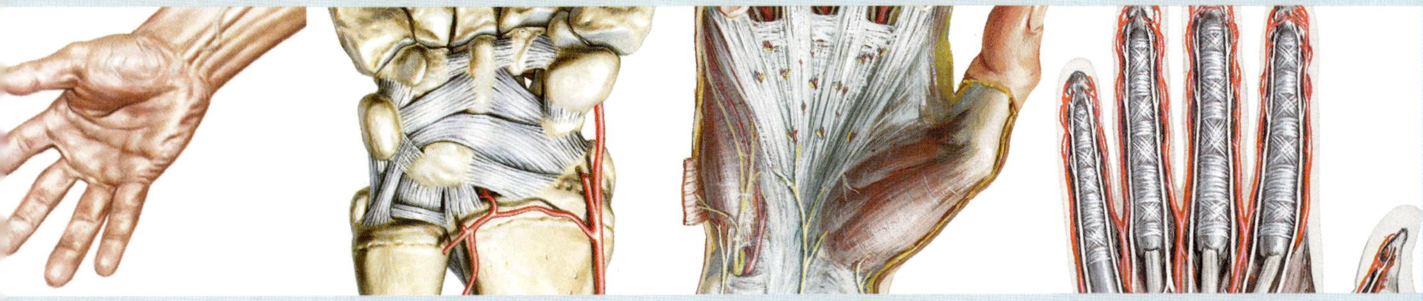

6 UPPER LIMB

Topographic Anatomy

Plate 398

398 Upper Limb: Surface Anatomy

Cutaneous Anatomy

Plates 399–403

399 Dermatomes of Upper Limb

400 Cutaneous Innervation of Upper Limb

401 Cutaneous Nerves and Superficial Veins of Shoulder and Arm

402 Cutaneous Nerves and Superficial Veins of Forearm

403 Lymph Vessels and Nodes of Upper Limb

Shoulder and Axilla

Plates 404–416

404 Clavicle and Sternoclavicular Joint

405 Humerus and Scapula: Anterior Views

406 Humerus and Scapula: Posterior View

407 Shoulder: Anteroposterior Radiograph

408 Shoulder (Glenohumeral Joint)

409 Muscles of Shoulder

410 Axilla: Posterior Wall

411 Muscles of Rotator Cuff

412 Pectoral, Clavipectoral, and Axillary Fasciae

413 Scapulothoracic and Scapulohumeral Dissection

414 Axillary Artery and Anastomoses around Scapula

415 Axilla (Dissection): Anterior View
416 Brachial Plexus: Schema

Arm

Plates 417–421

417 Muscles of Arm: Anterior Views
418 Muscles of Arm: Posterior Views
419 Brachial Artery in Situ
420 Arteries of Arm and Proximal Forearm
421 Arm: Serial Cross Sections

Elbow and Forearm

Plates 422–438

422 Bones of Elbow
423 Elbow: Radiographs
424 Ligaments of Elbow
425 Bones of Forearm
426 Individual Muscles of Forearm: Rotators of Radius
427 Individual Muscles of Forearm: Extensors of Wrist and Digits
428 Individual Muscles of Forearm: Flexors of Wrist
429 Individual Muscles of Forearm: Flexors of Digits
430 Muscles of Forearm (Superficial Layer): Posterior View
431 Muscles of Forearm (Deep Layer): Posterior View
432 Muscles of Forearm (Superficial Layer): Anterior View
433 Muscles of Forearm (Intermediate Layer): Anterior View
434 Muscles of Forearm (Deep Layer): Anterior View
435 Arteries of Forearm
436 Forearm: Serial Cross Sections, Anterior View
437 Attachments of Muscles of Forearm: Anterior View
438 Attachments of Muscles of Forearm: Posterior View

Wrist and Hand

Plates 439–458

439 Carpal Bones
440 Movements of Wrist
441 Ligaments of Wrist
442 Ligaments of Wrist (continued)
443 Bones of Wrist and Hand
444 Wrist and Hand: Radiographs
445 Metacarpophalangeal and Interphalangeal Ligaments
446 Wrist and Hand: Superficial Palmar Dissections
447 Wrist and Hand: Deeper Palmar Dissections
448 Lumbrical Muscles and Bursae, Spaces, and Sheaths: Schema
449 Flexor Tendons, Arteries, and Nerves at Wrist
450 Bursae, Spaces, and Tendon Sheaths of Hand
451 Flexor and Extensor Tendons in Fingers
452 Intrinsic Muscles of Hand
453 Arteries and Nerves of Hand: Palmar Views
454 Wrist and Hand: Superficial Radial Dissection
455 Wrist and Hand: Superficial Dorsal Dissection
456 Wrist and Hand: Deep Dorsal Dissection
457 Extensor Tendons at Wrist
458 Fingers

Neurovasculature

Plates 459–466

459 Cutaneous Innervation of Wrist and Hand
460 Arteries and Nerves of Upper Limb
461 Nerves of Upper Limb
462 Musculocutaneous Nerve
463 Median Nerve
464 Ulnar Nerve
465 Radial Nerve in Arm and Nerves of Posterior Shoulder
466 Radial Nerve in Forearm

Regional Scans

Plate 467

467 Shoulder MRI, CT Scan, and Arthrogram

Muscle Tables

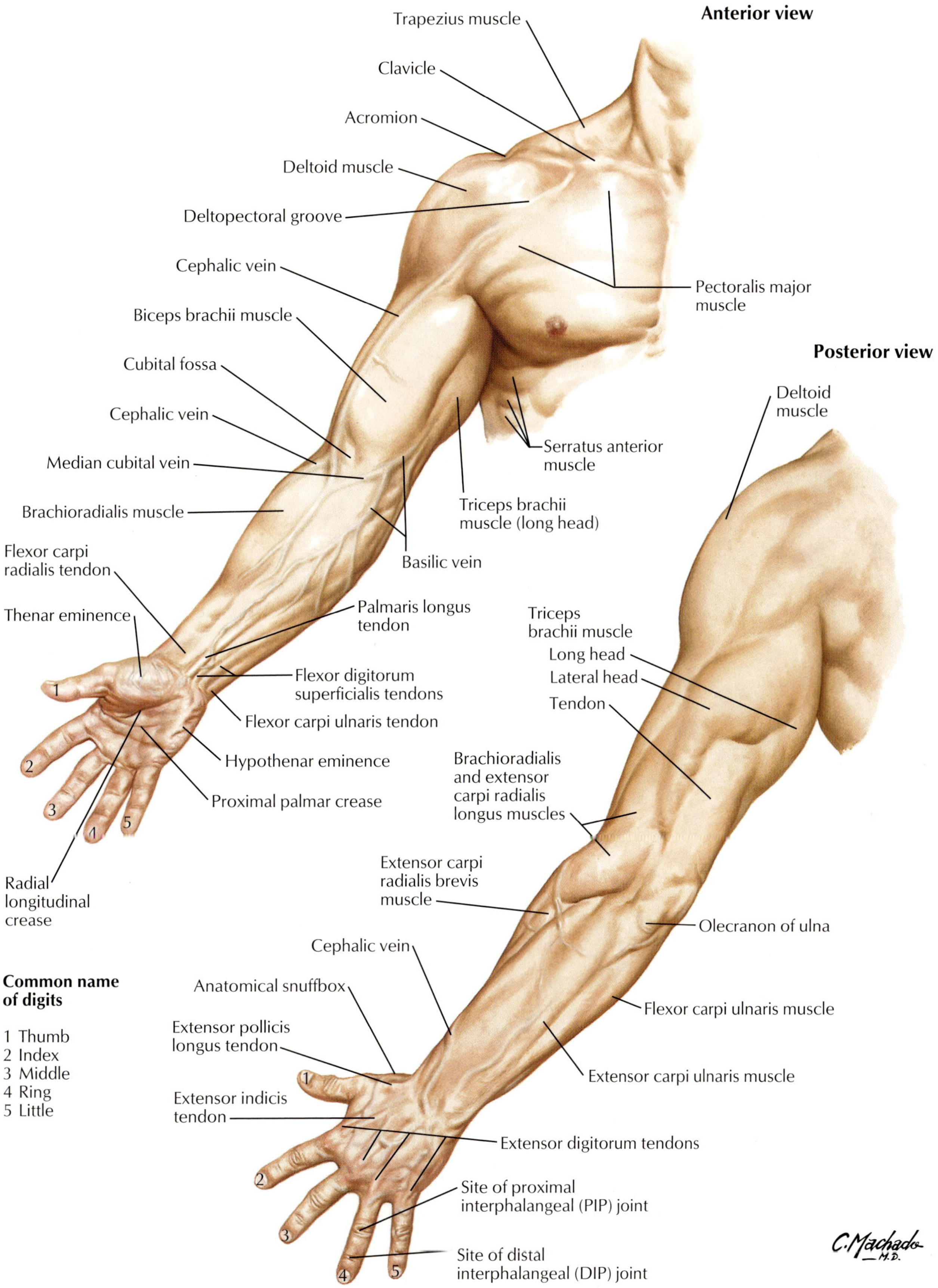

Common name of digits

1 Thumb
2 Index
3 Middle
4 Ring
5 Little

See also Plate 162

Note: Schematic demarcation of dermatomes (according to Keegan and Garrett) shown as distinct segments. There is actually considerable overlap between adjacent dermatomes.

Anterior view

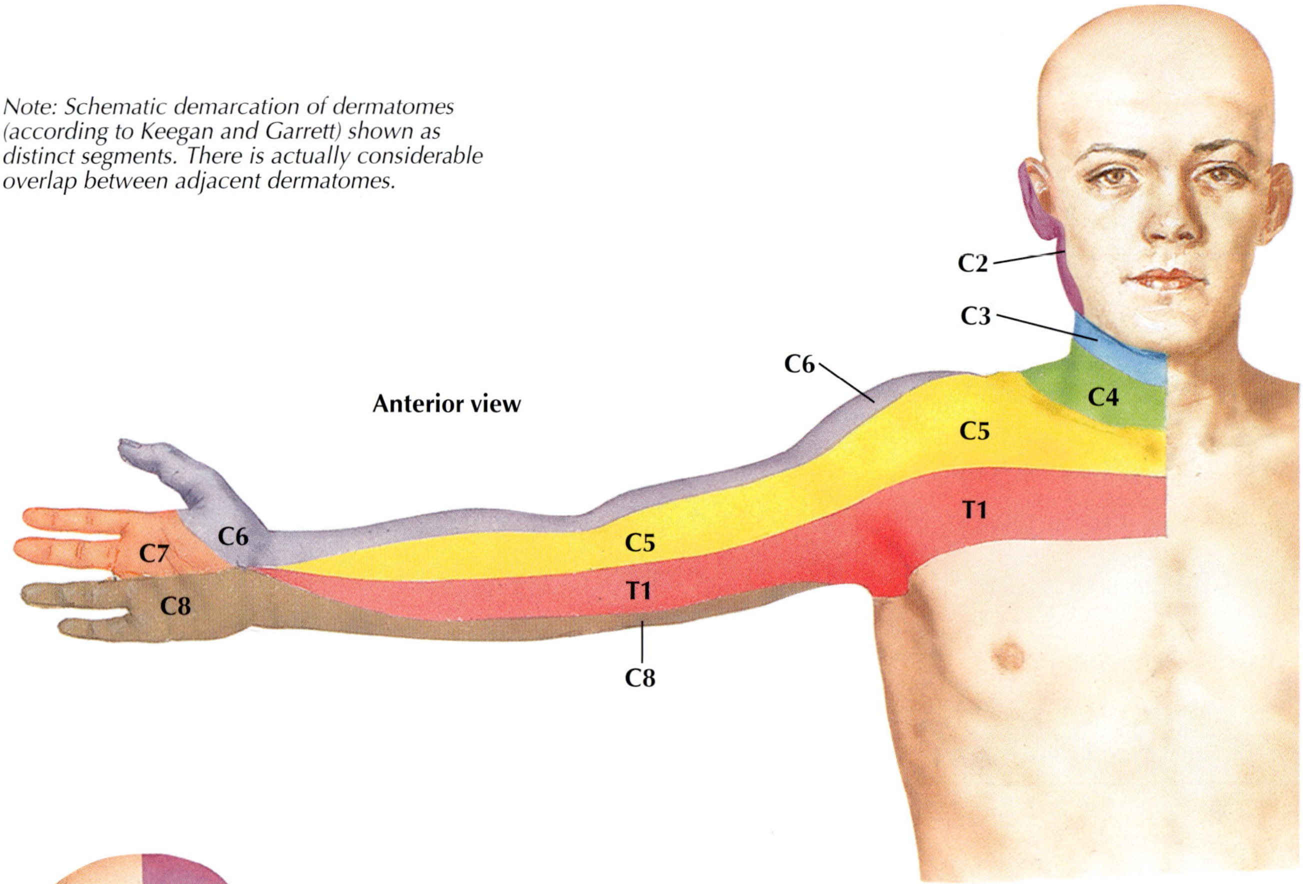

Posterior view

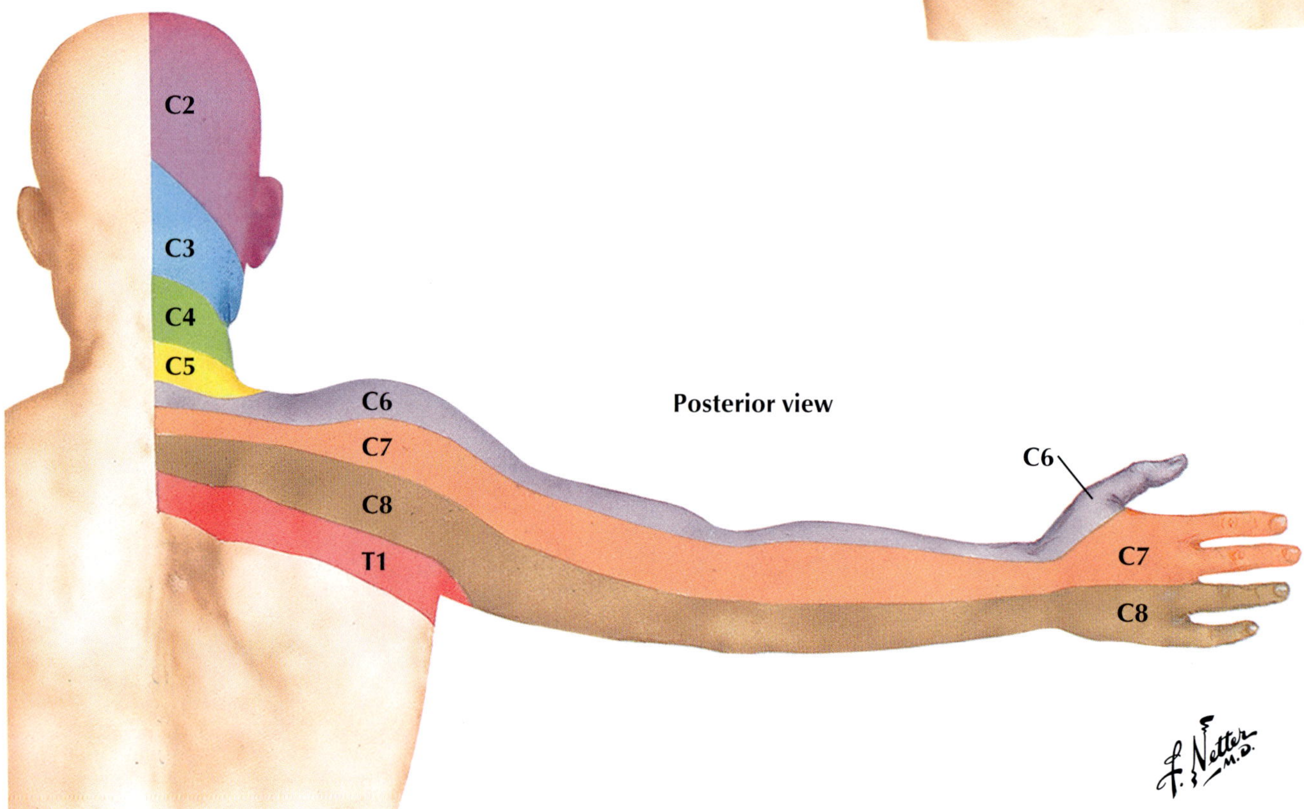

Cutaneous Innervation of Upper Limb

See also Plates 459, 461, 463

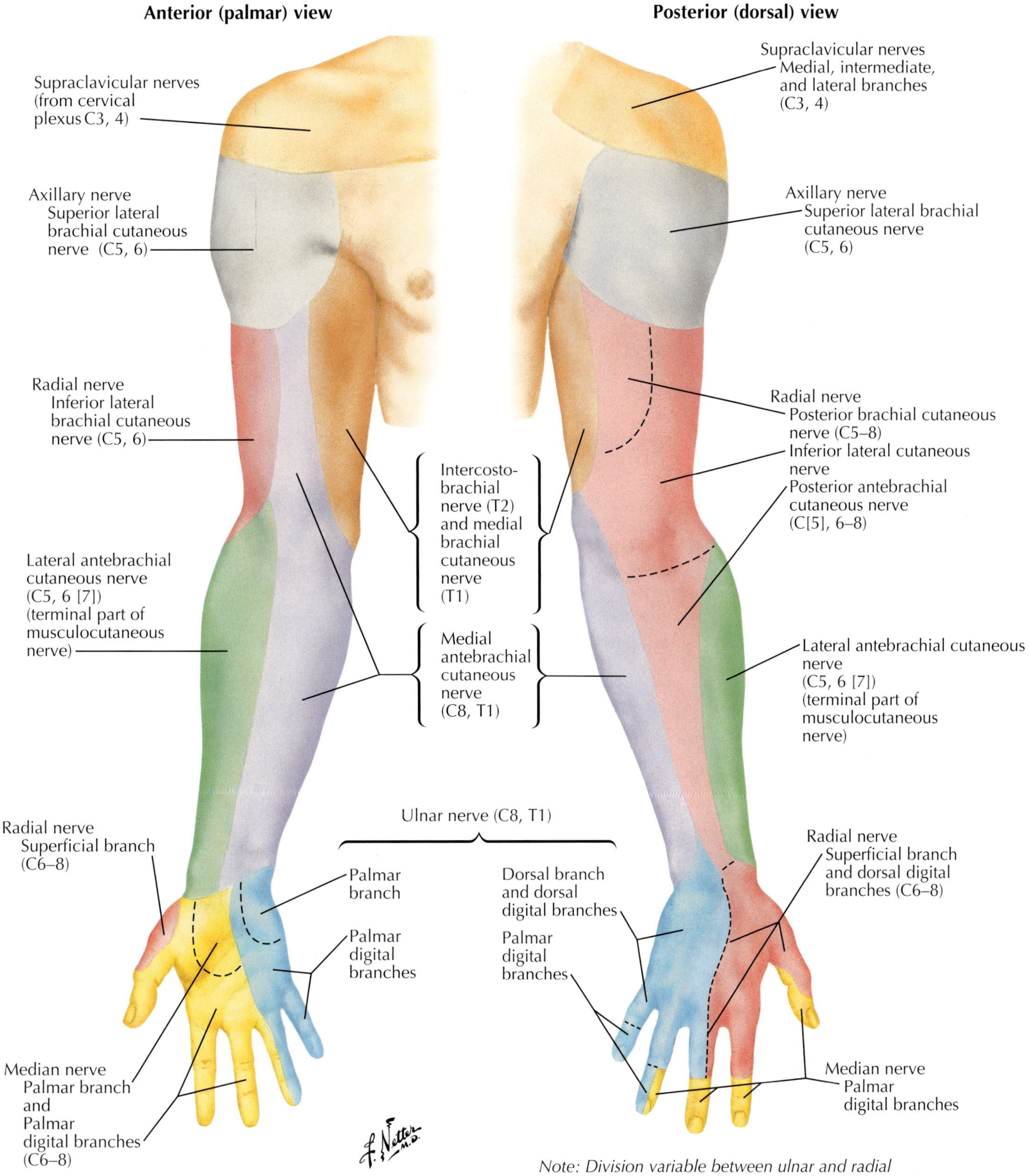

Note: Division variable between ulnar and radial innervation on dorsum of hand and often aligns with middle of 4th digit instead of 3rd digit as shown.

Cutaneous Nerves and Superficial Veins of Shoulder and Arm

See also Plates 252, 419

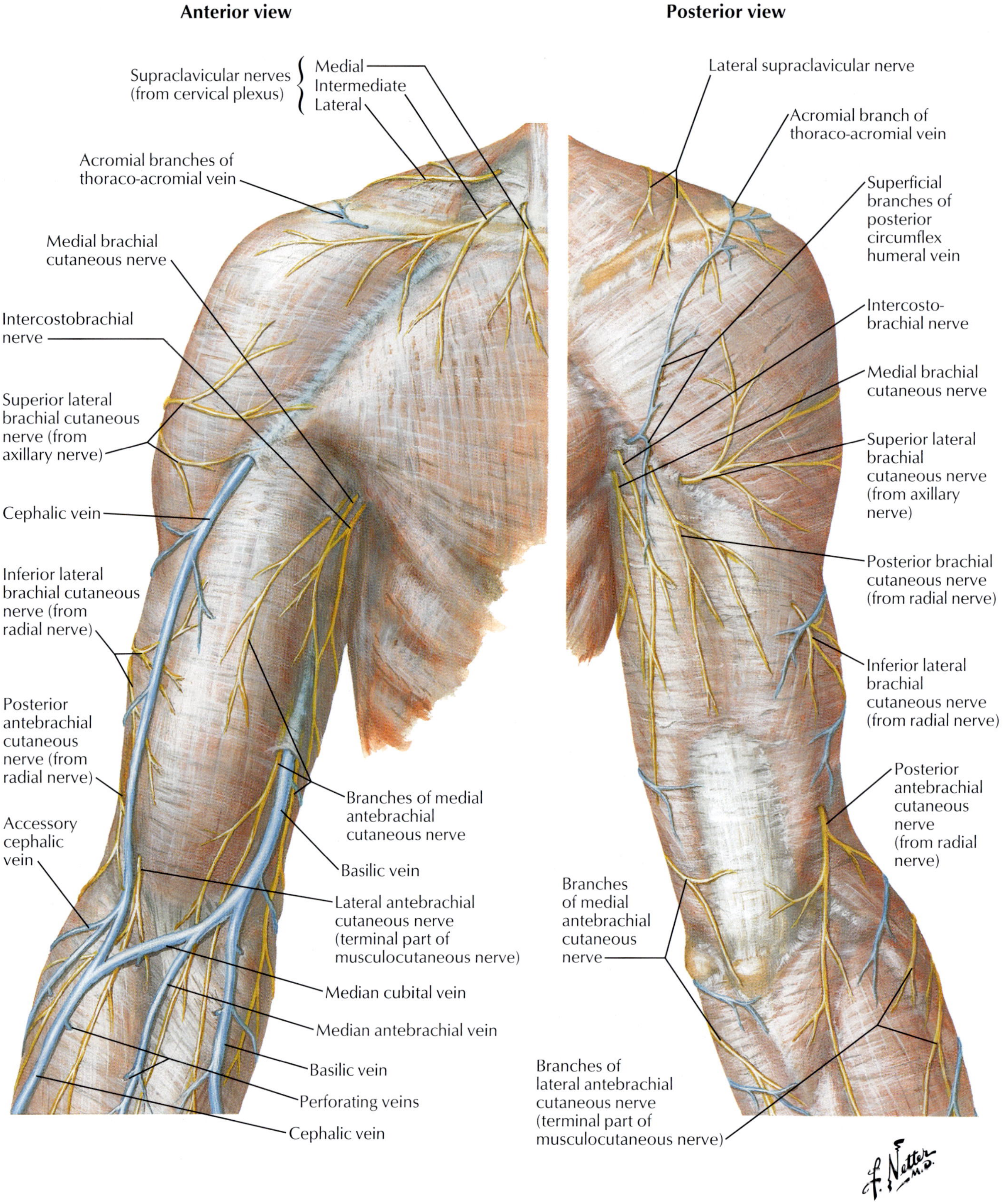

Cutaneous Nerves and Superficial Veins of Forearm

See also Plates 431, 455

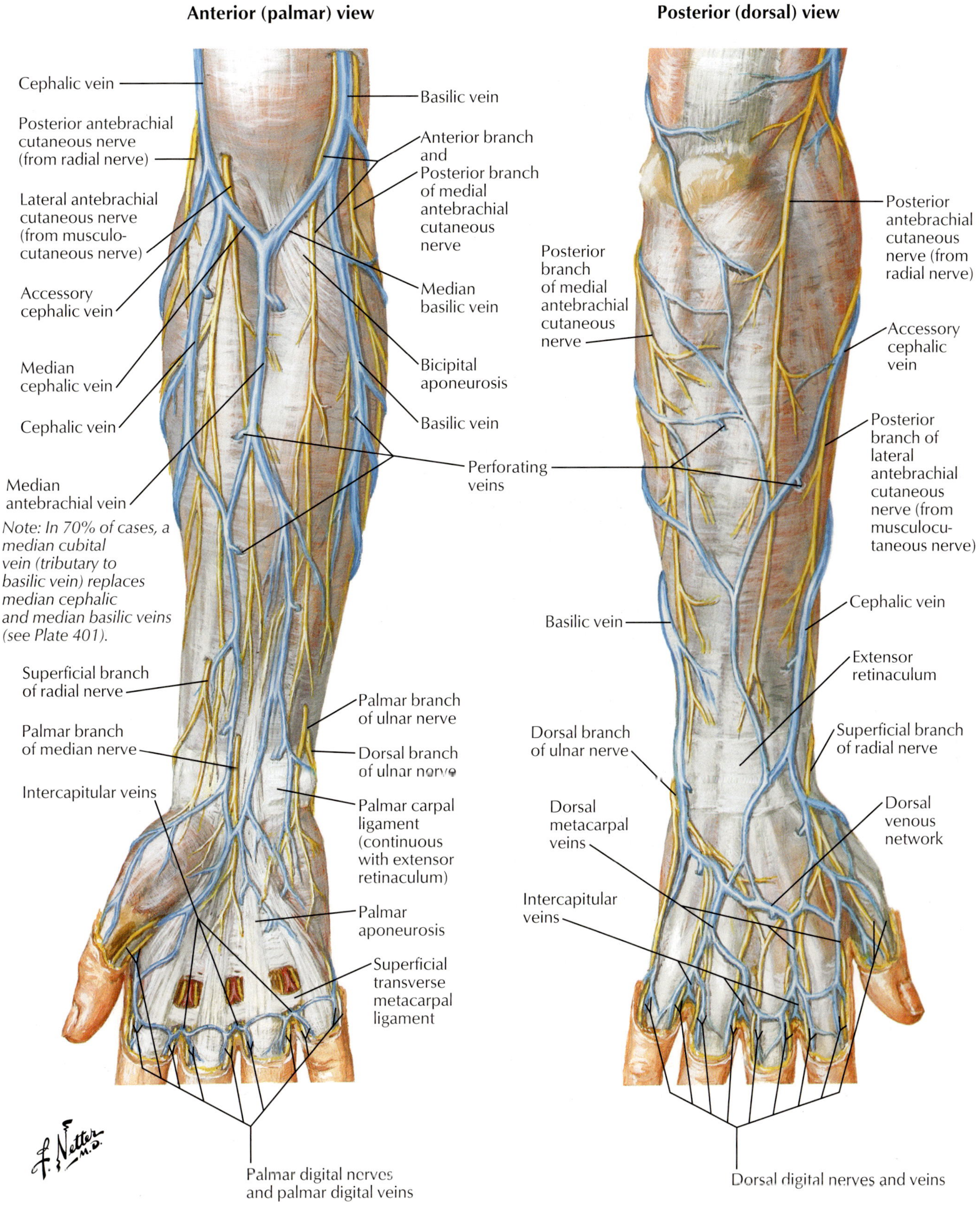

Lymph Vessels and Nodes of Upper Limb

See also Plates 181, 455

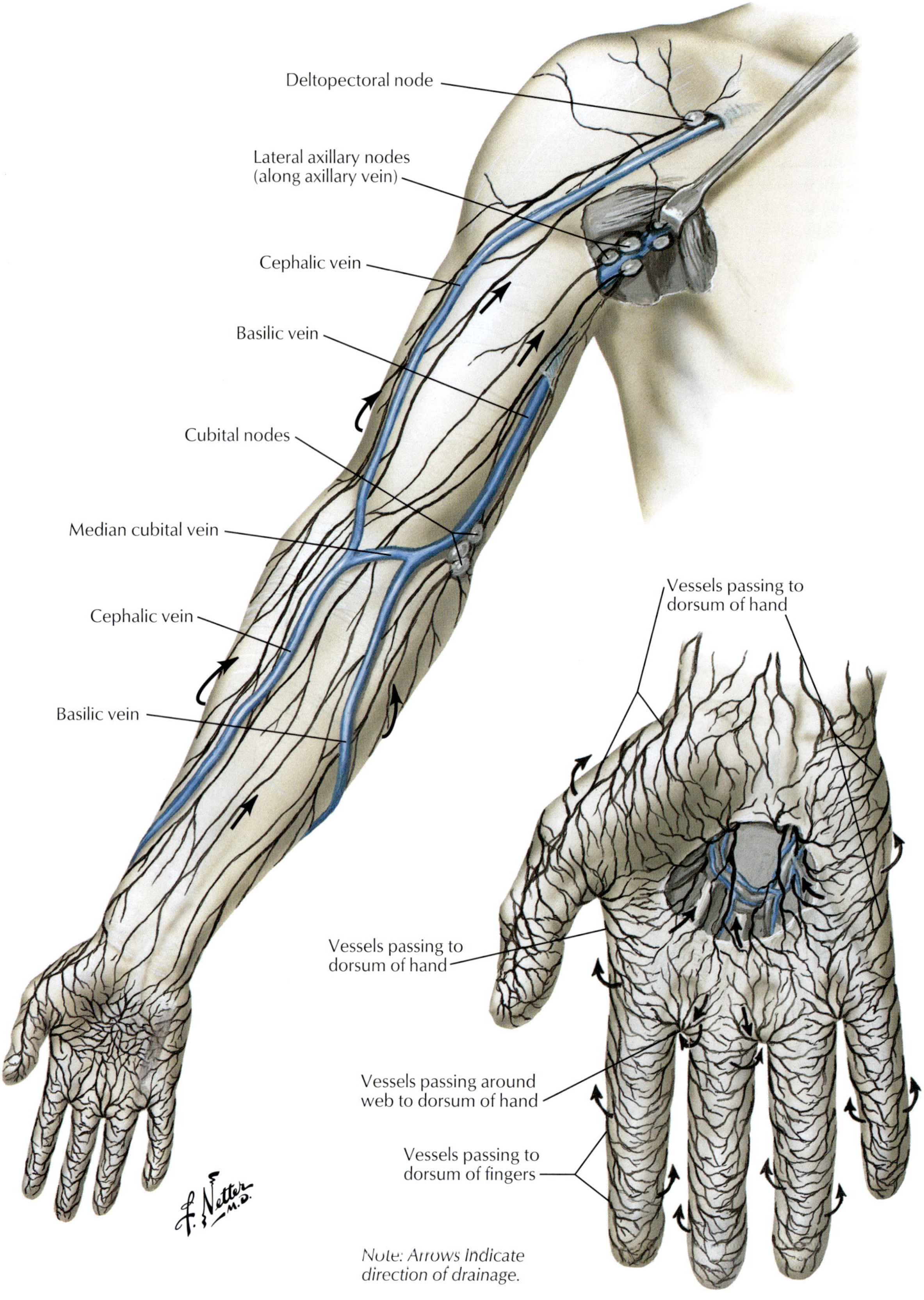

See also Plates 183, 186

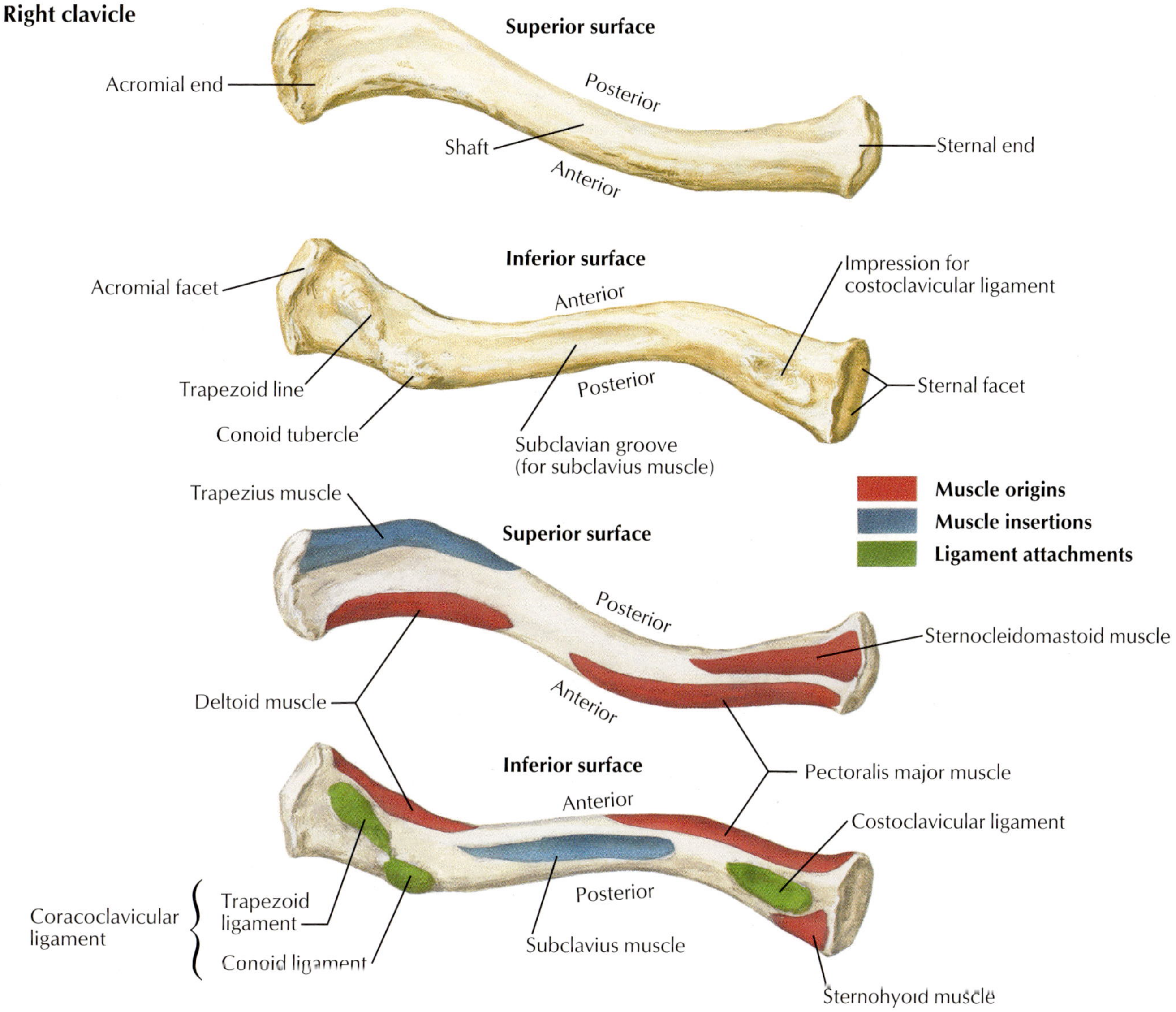

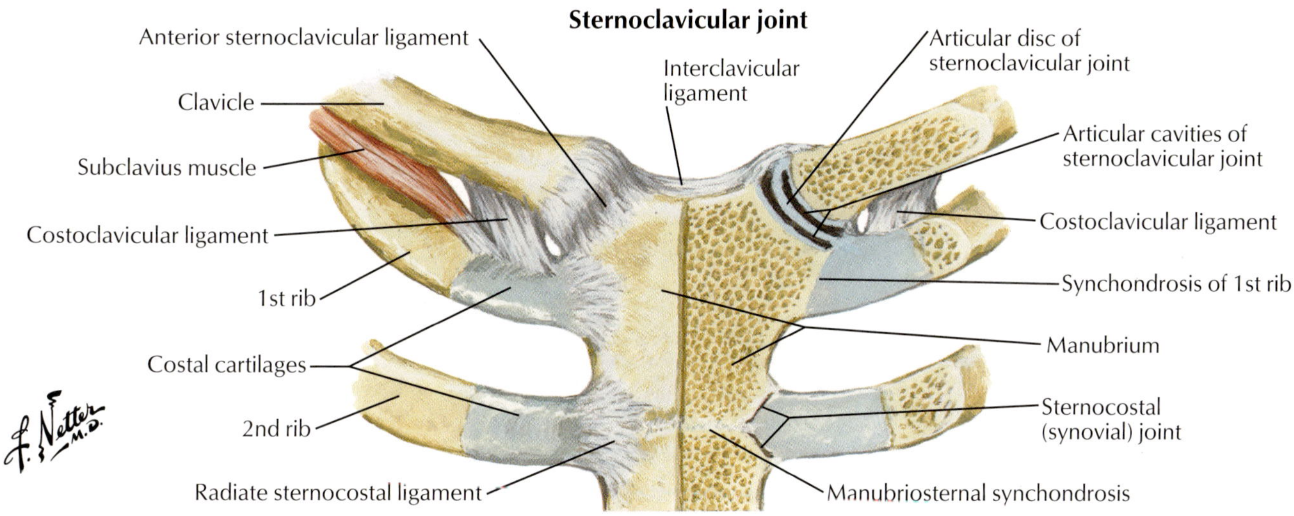

Humerus and Scapula: Anterior Views

See also Plates 183, 407, 422

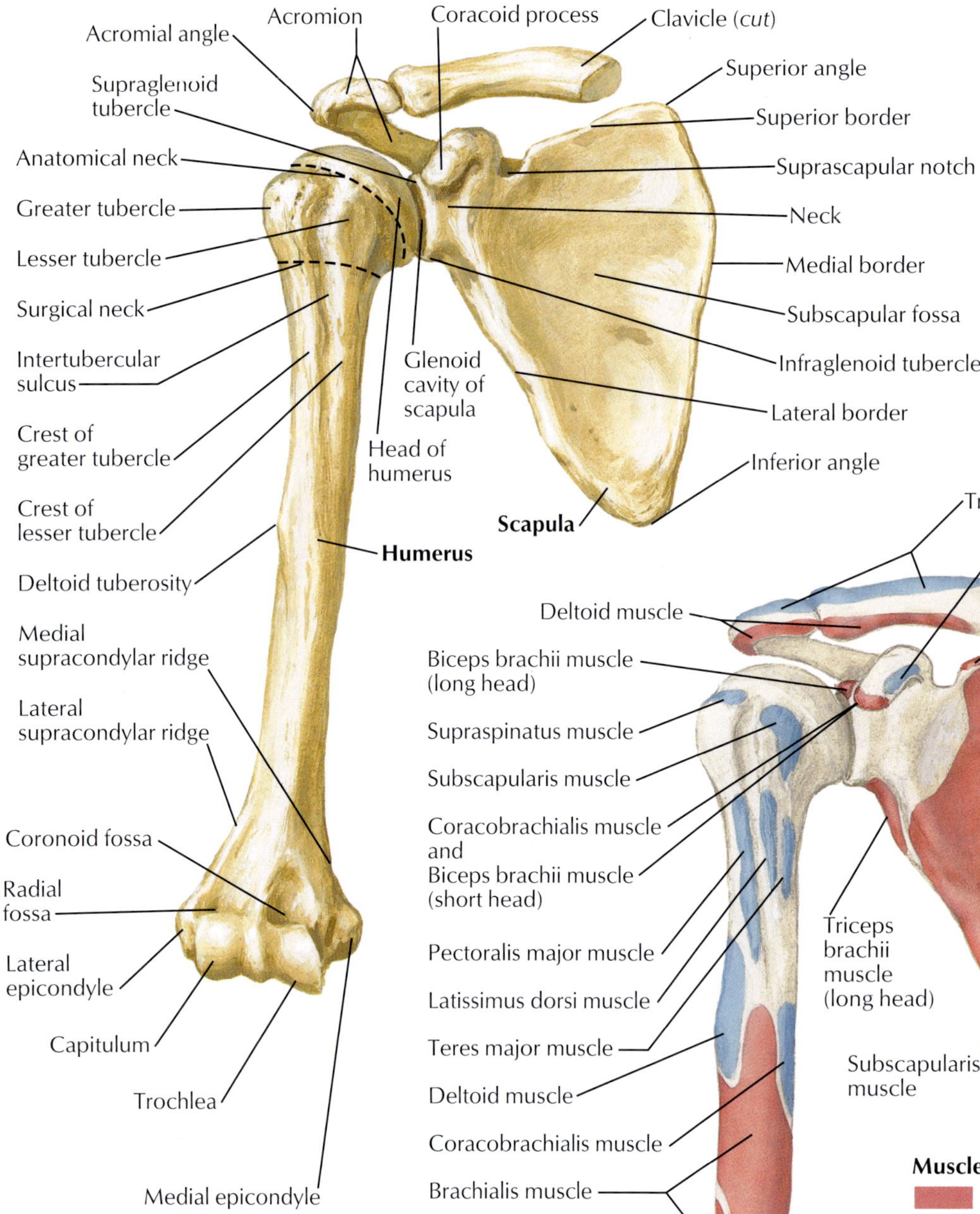

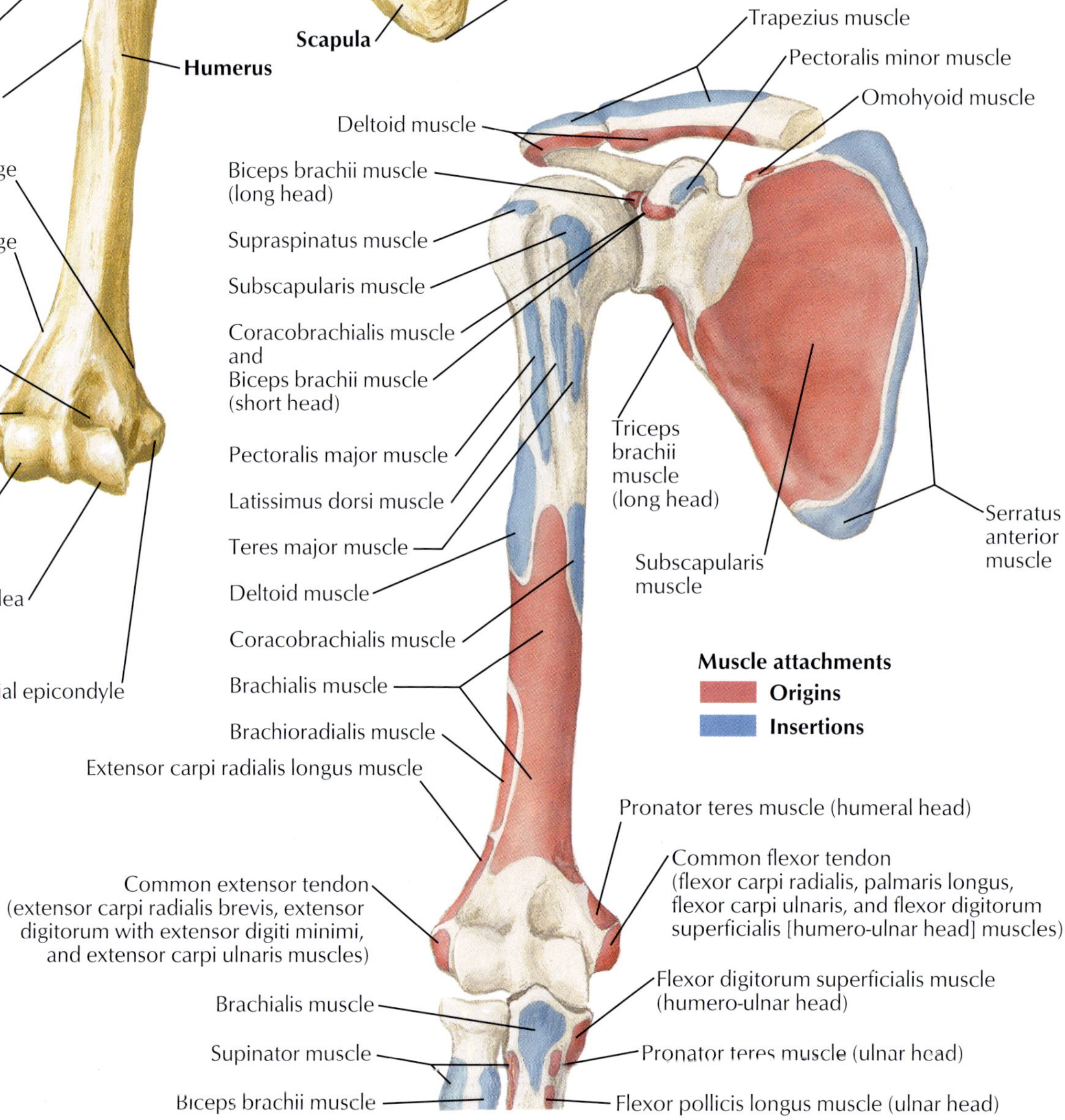

Humerus and Scapula: Posterior View

See also **Plate 183**

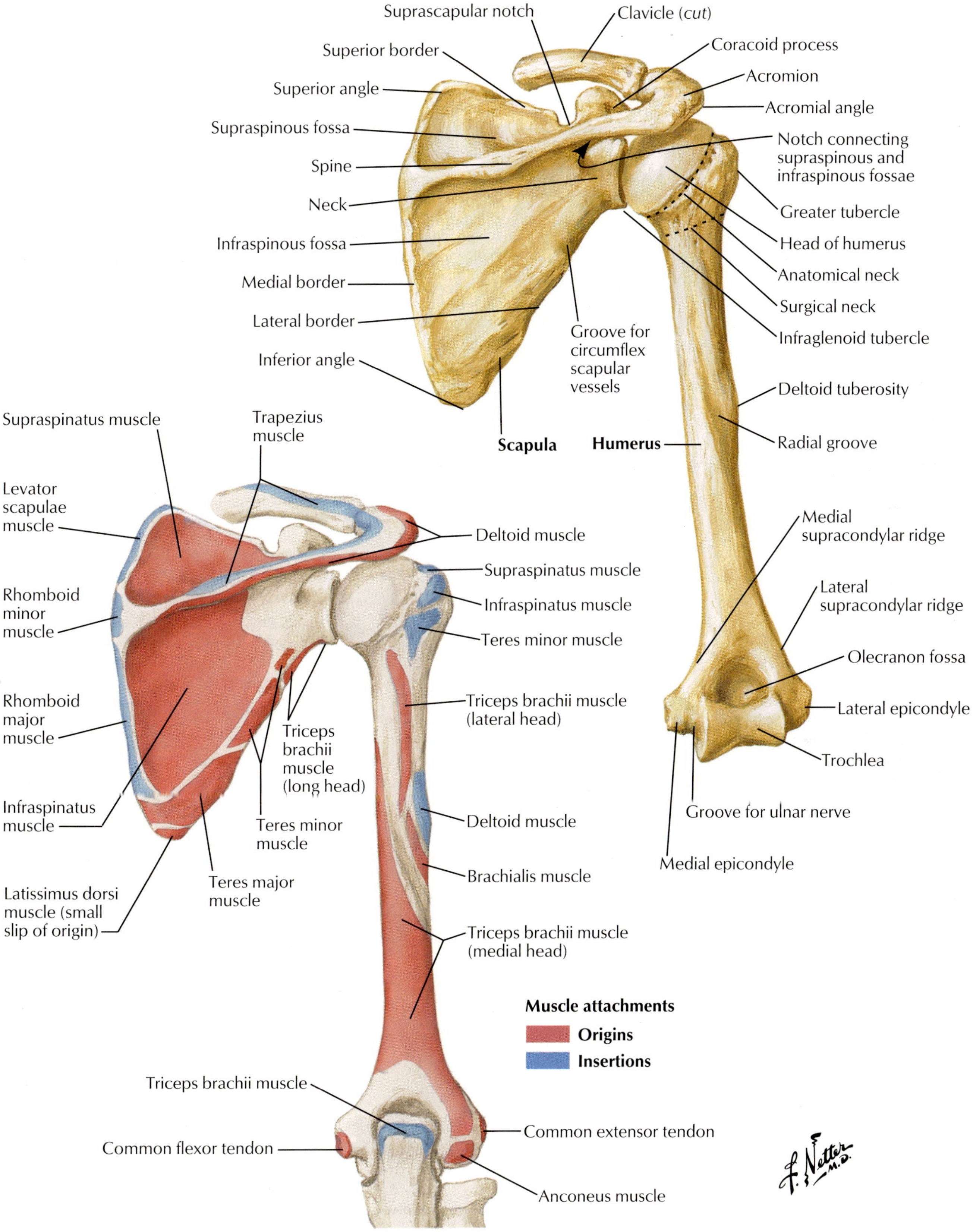

Shoulder: Anteroposterior Radiograph

See also **Plate 405**

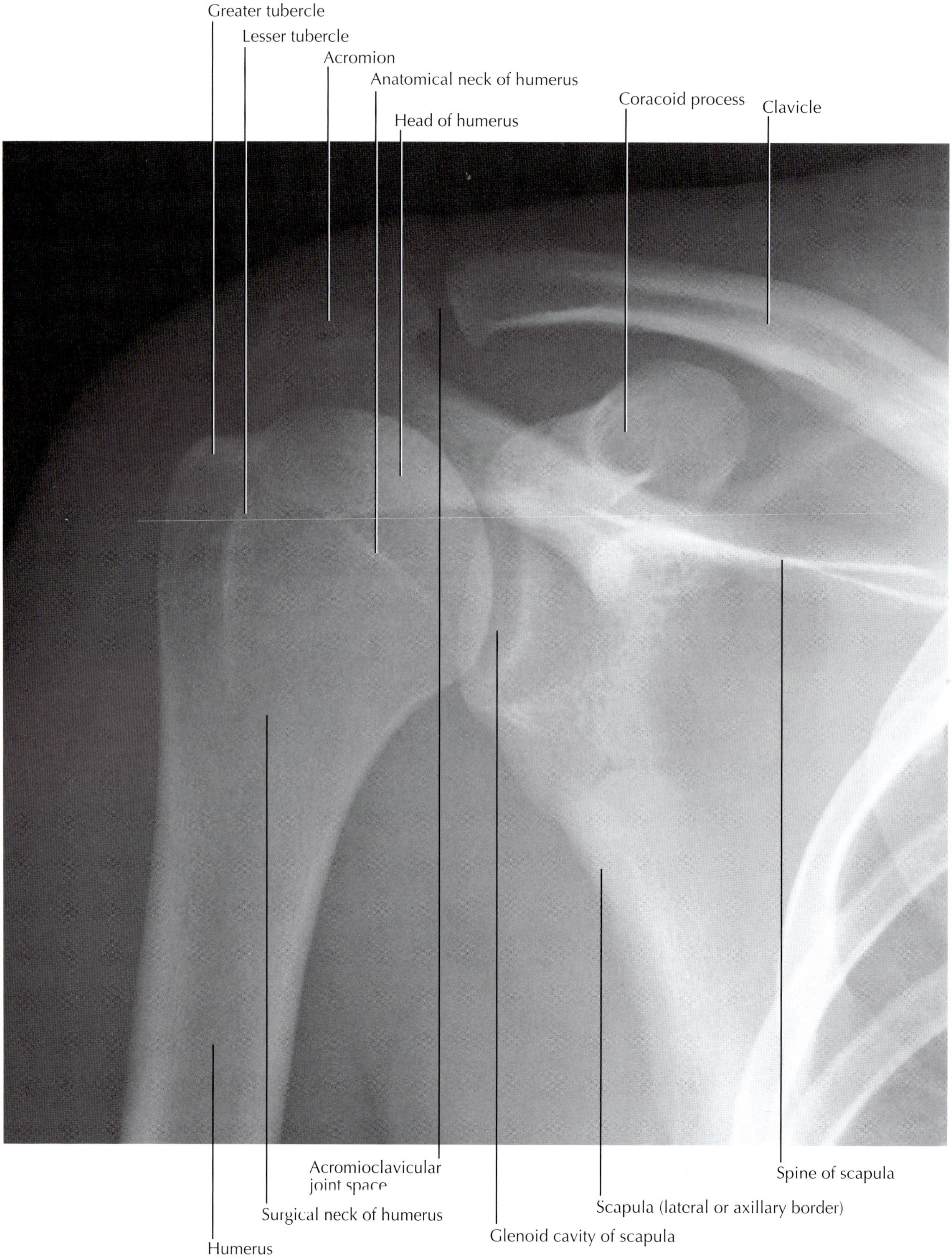

See also **Plates 411, 468**

Anterior view

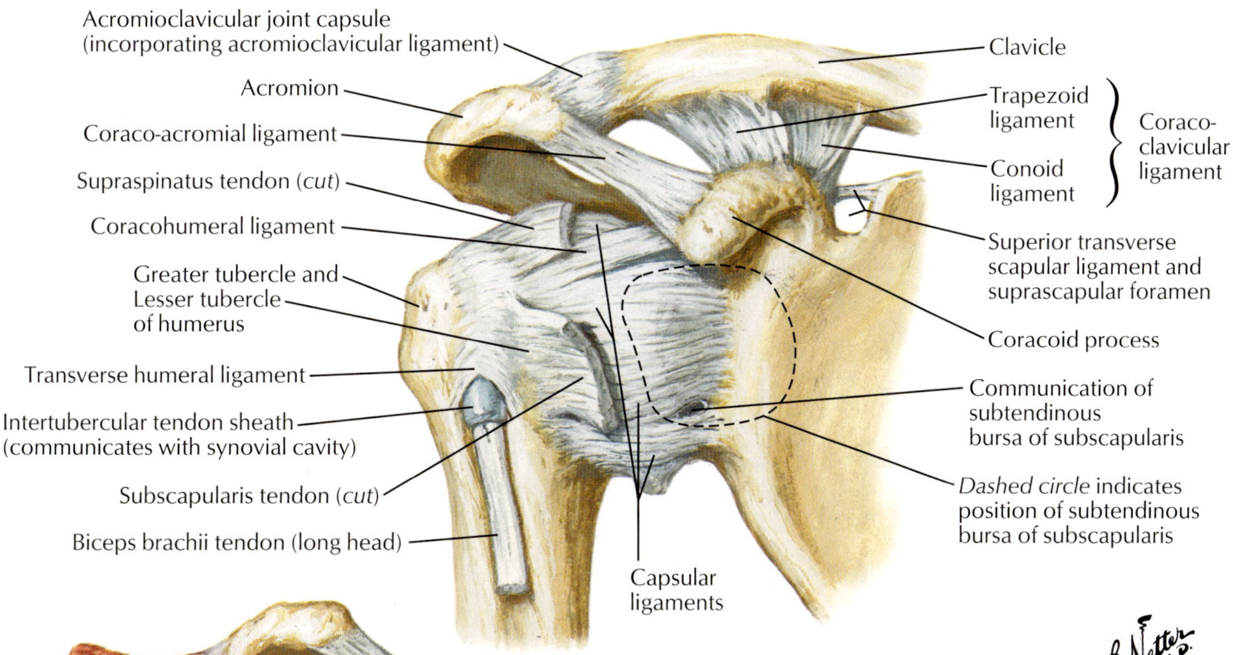

Anterior view

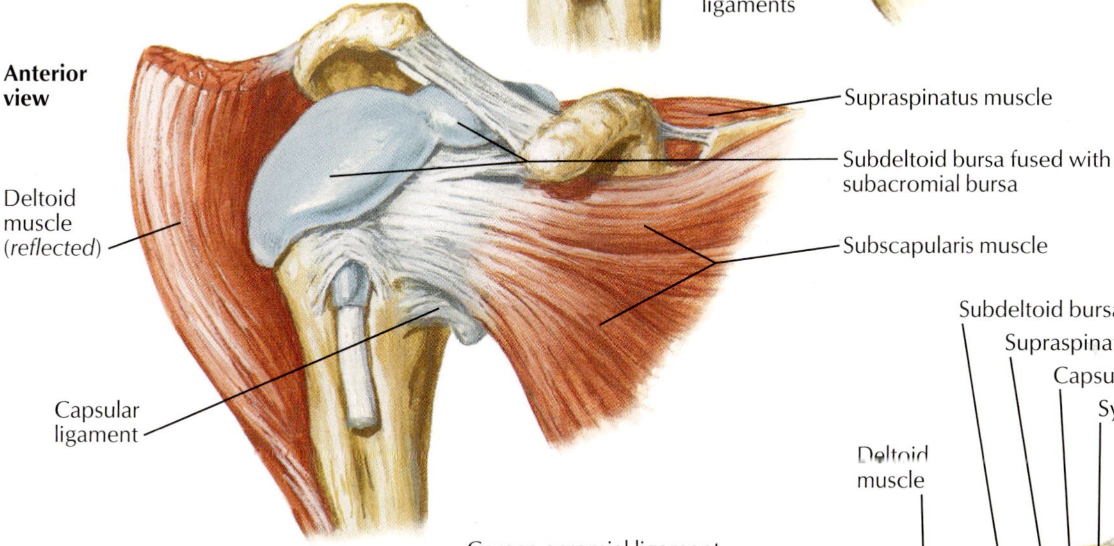

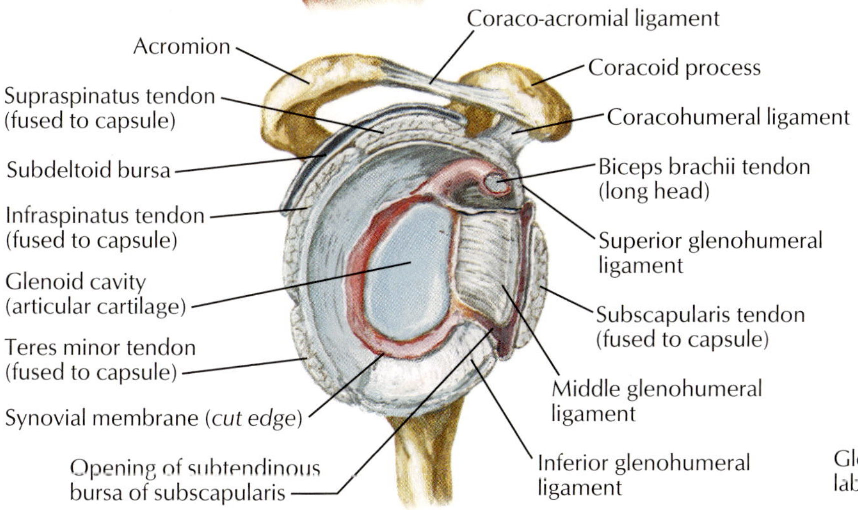

Joint opened: lateral view

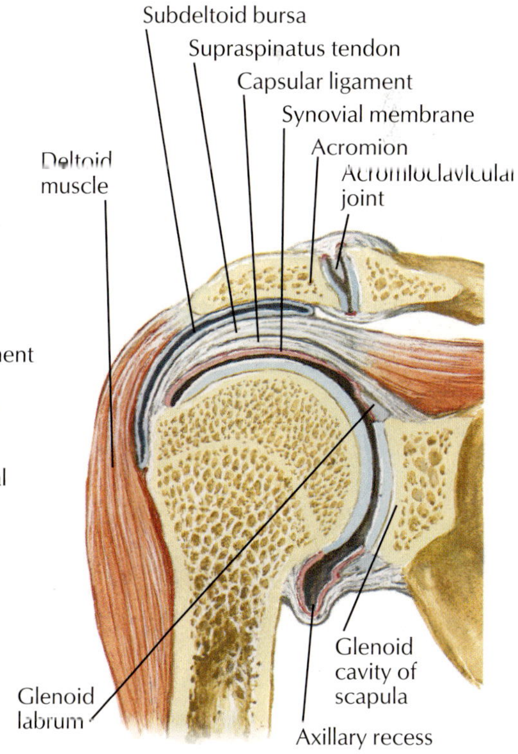

Coronal section through joint

See also Plates 29, 171, 185

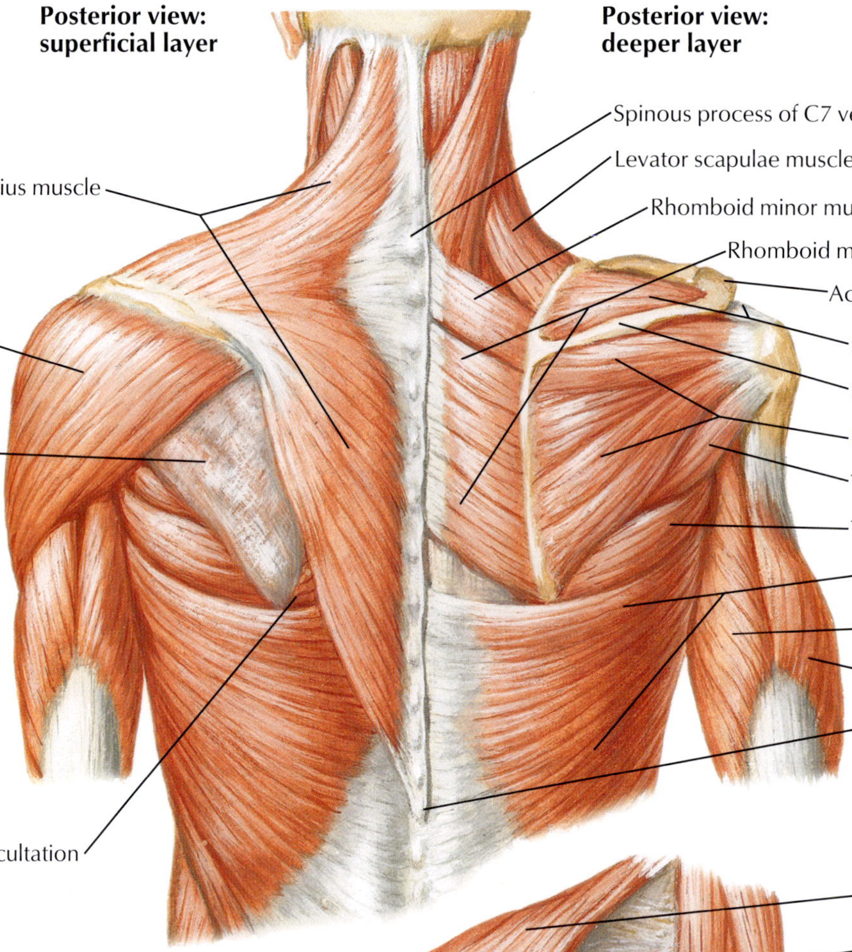

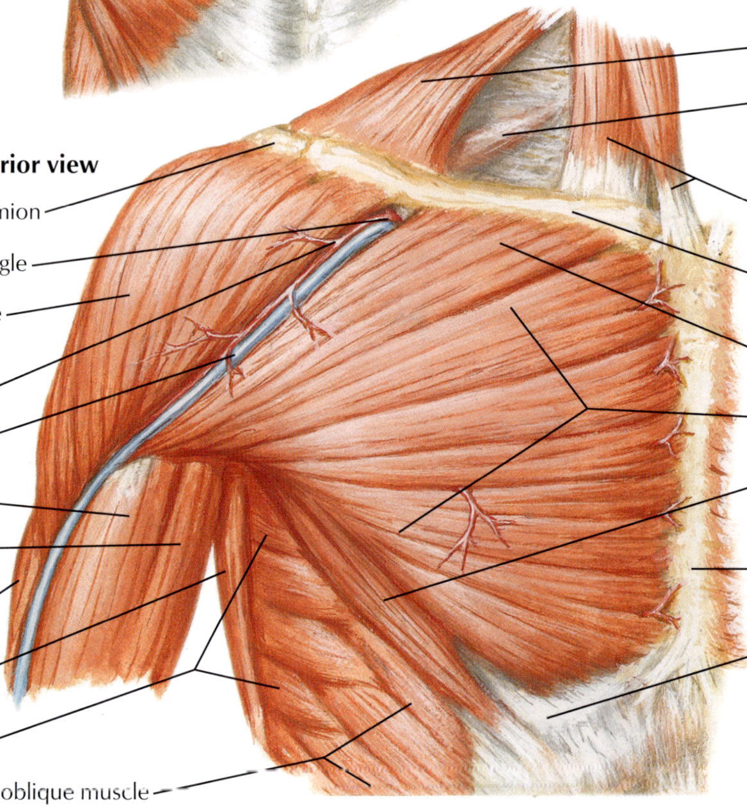

Axilla: Posterior Wall

See also **Plates 415, 416, 461**

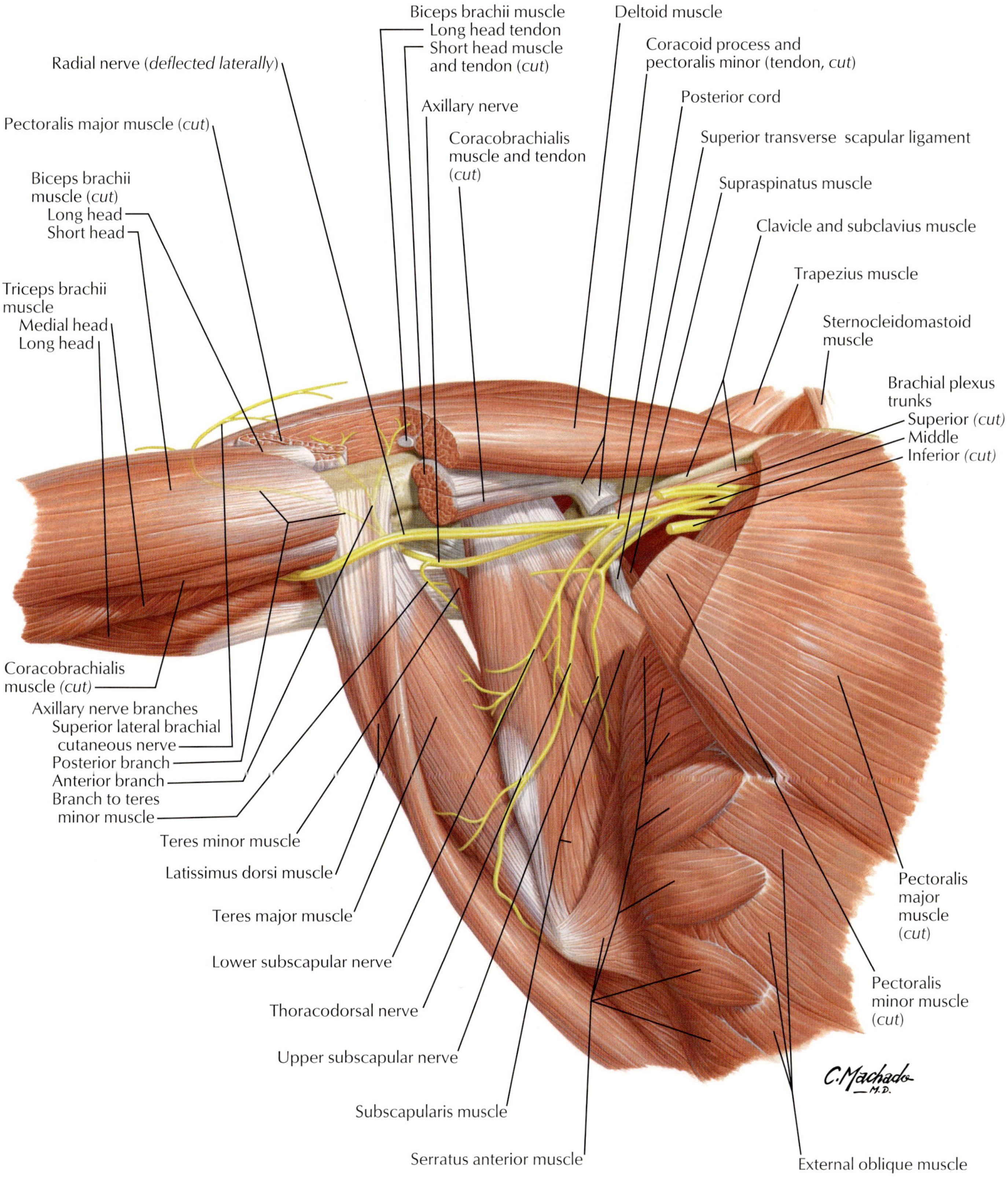

Muscles of Rotator Cuff

See also **Plates 408, 417, 418**

Superior view

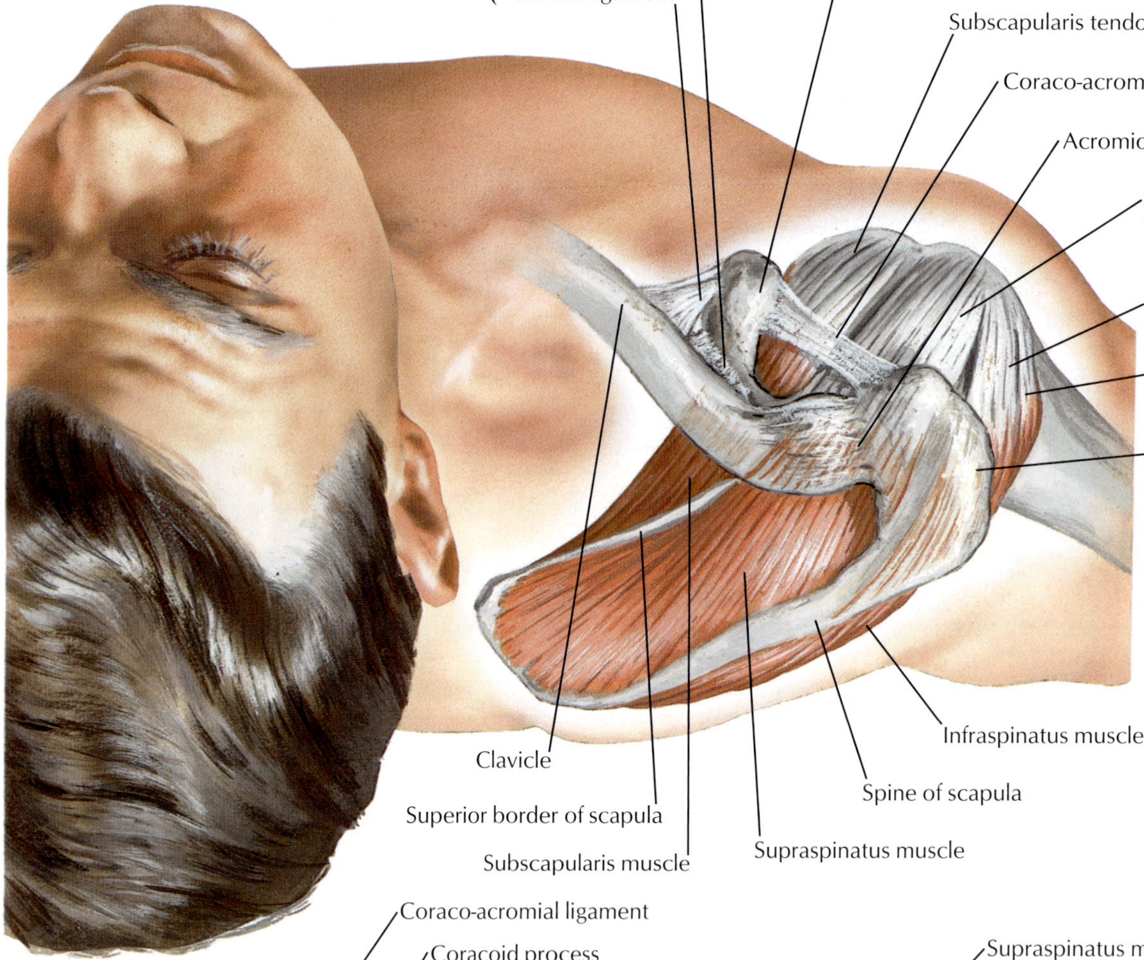

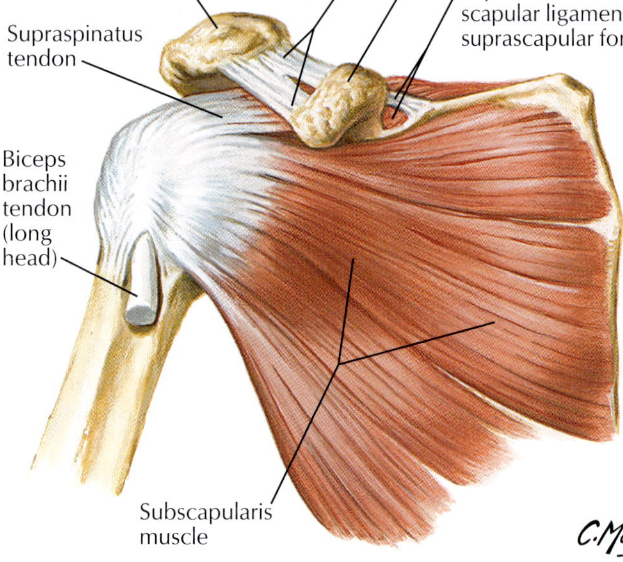

Anterior view

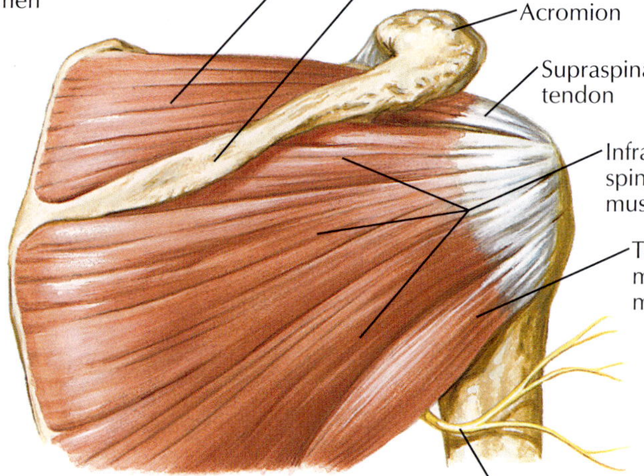

Posterior view

Pectoral, Clavipectoral, and Axillary Fasciae

See also Plates 181, 185

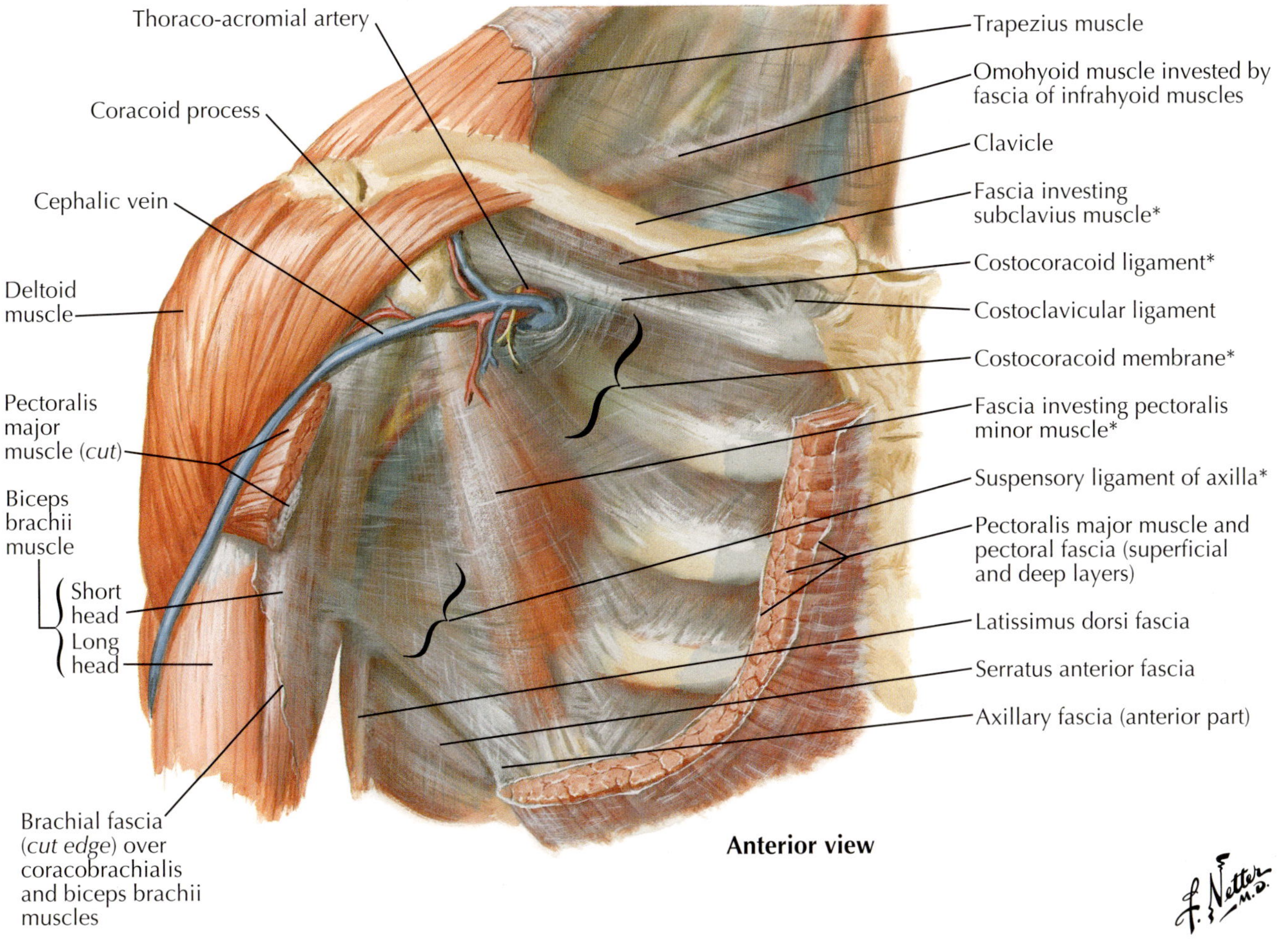

Anterior view

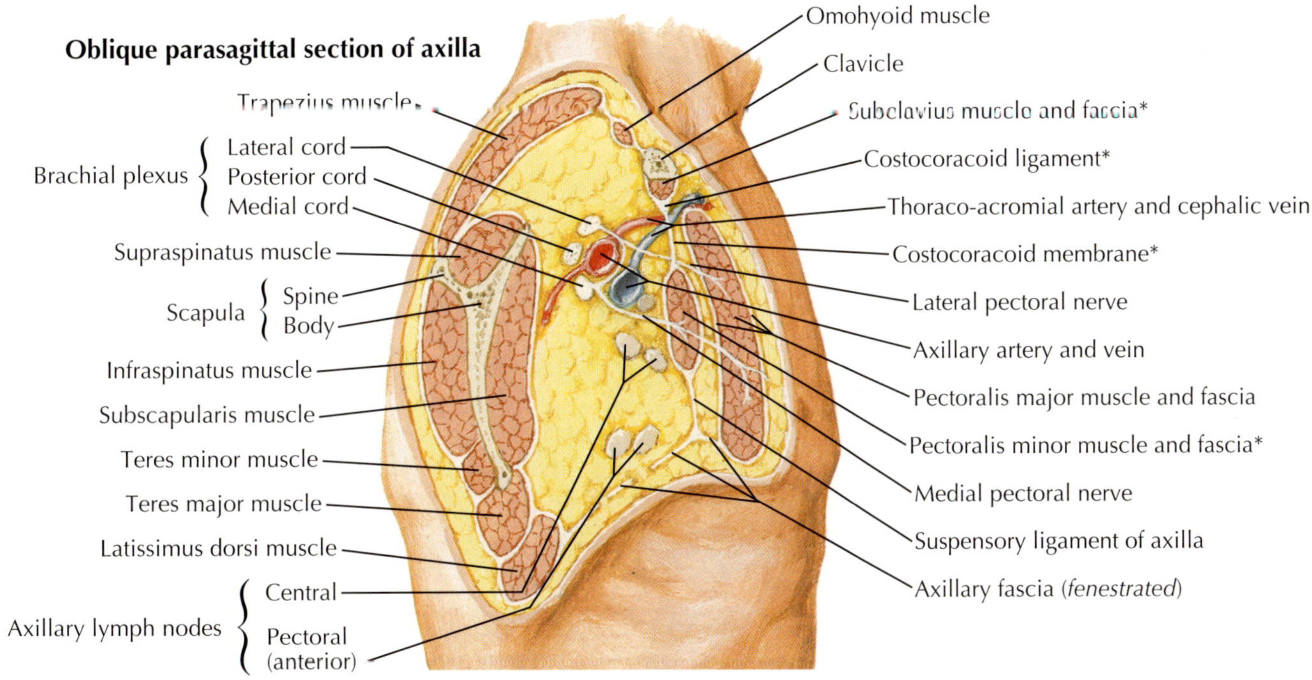

*Components of clavipectoral fascia

Scapulothoracic and Scapulohumeral Dissection

See also Plates 415, 465

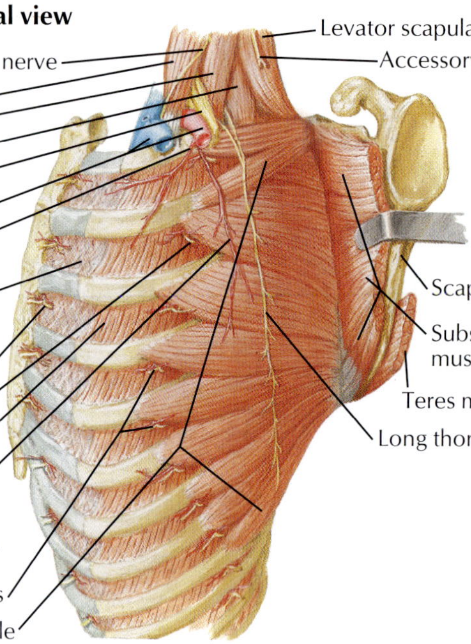

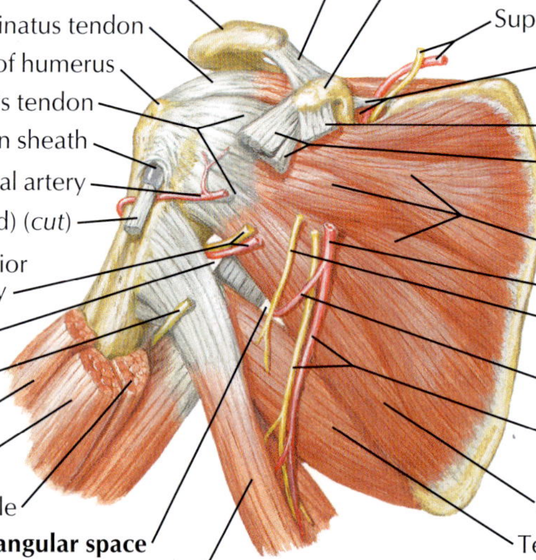

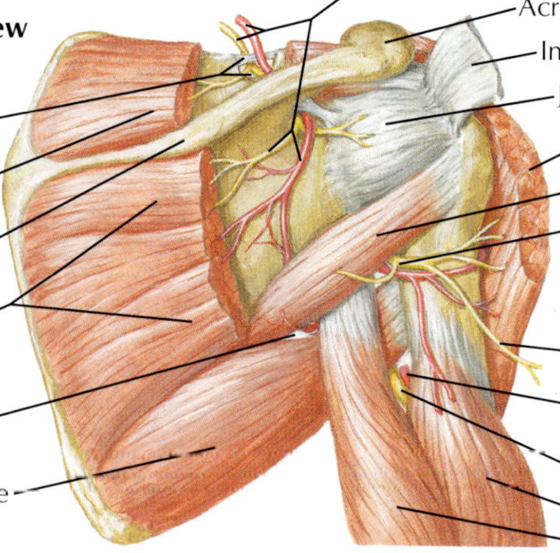

Axillary Artery and Anastomoses around Scapula

See also Plates 33, 420

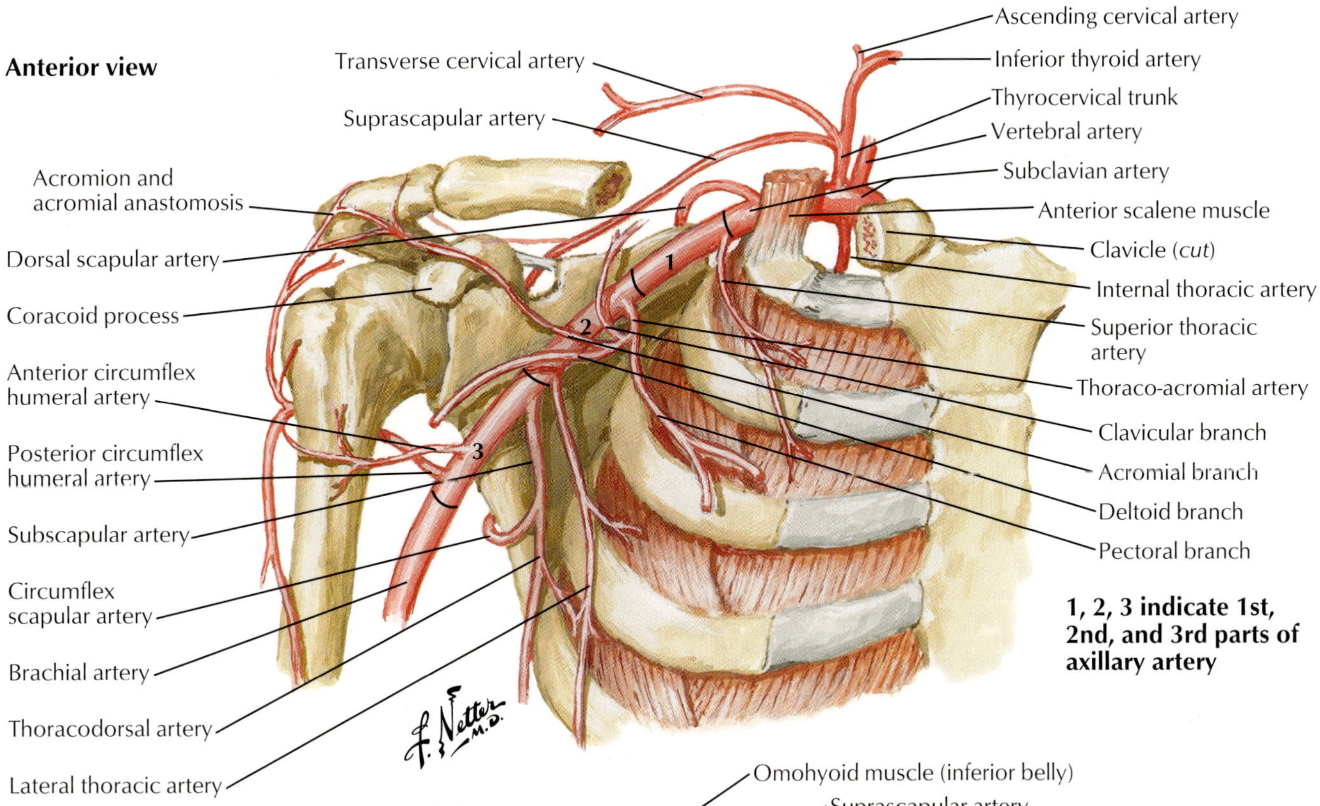

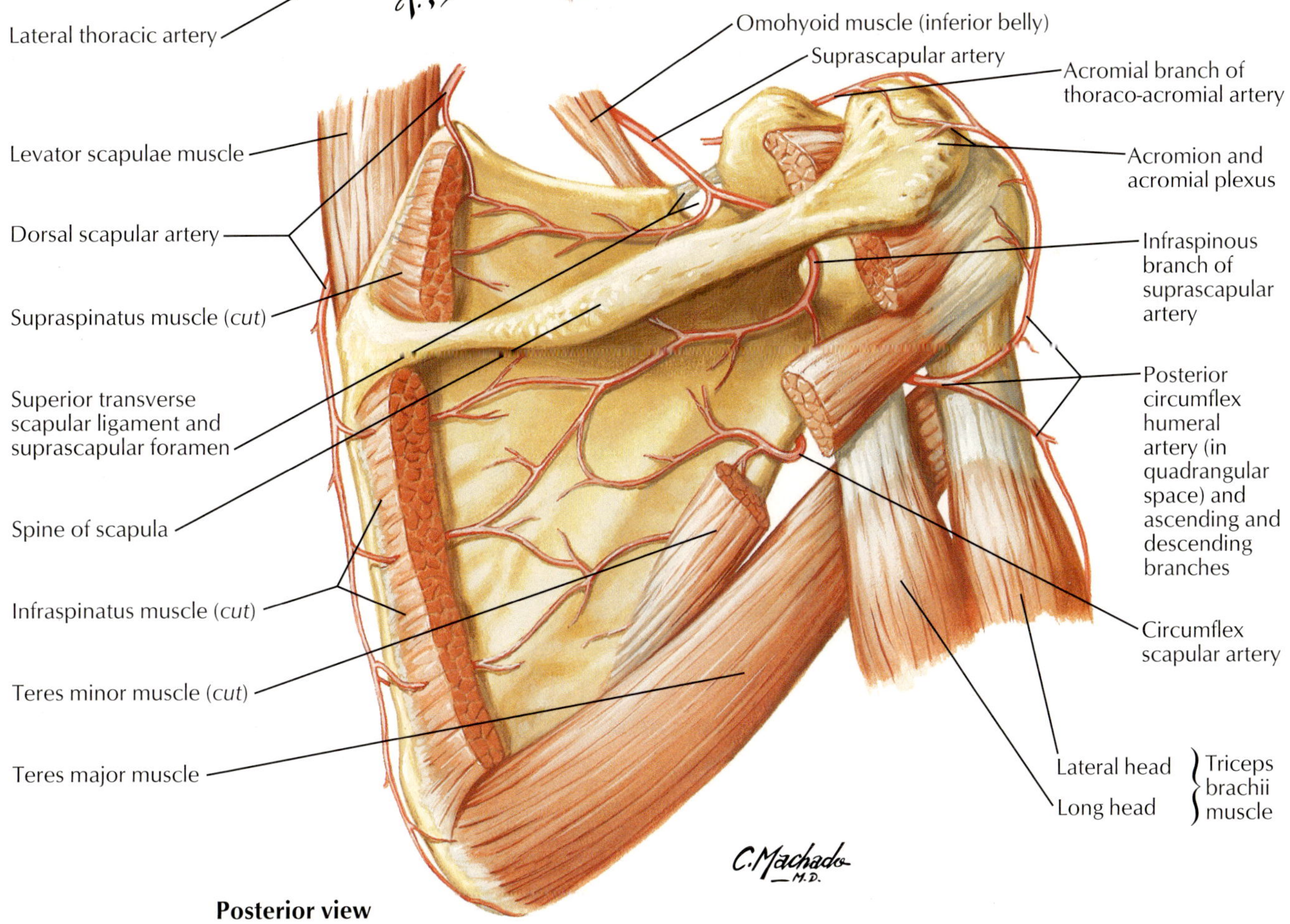

Axilla (Dissection): Anterior View

See also Plates 410, 413

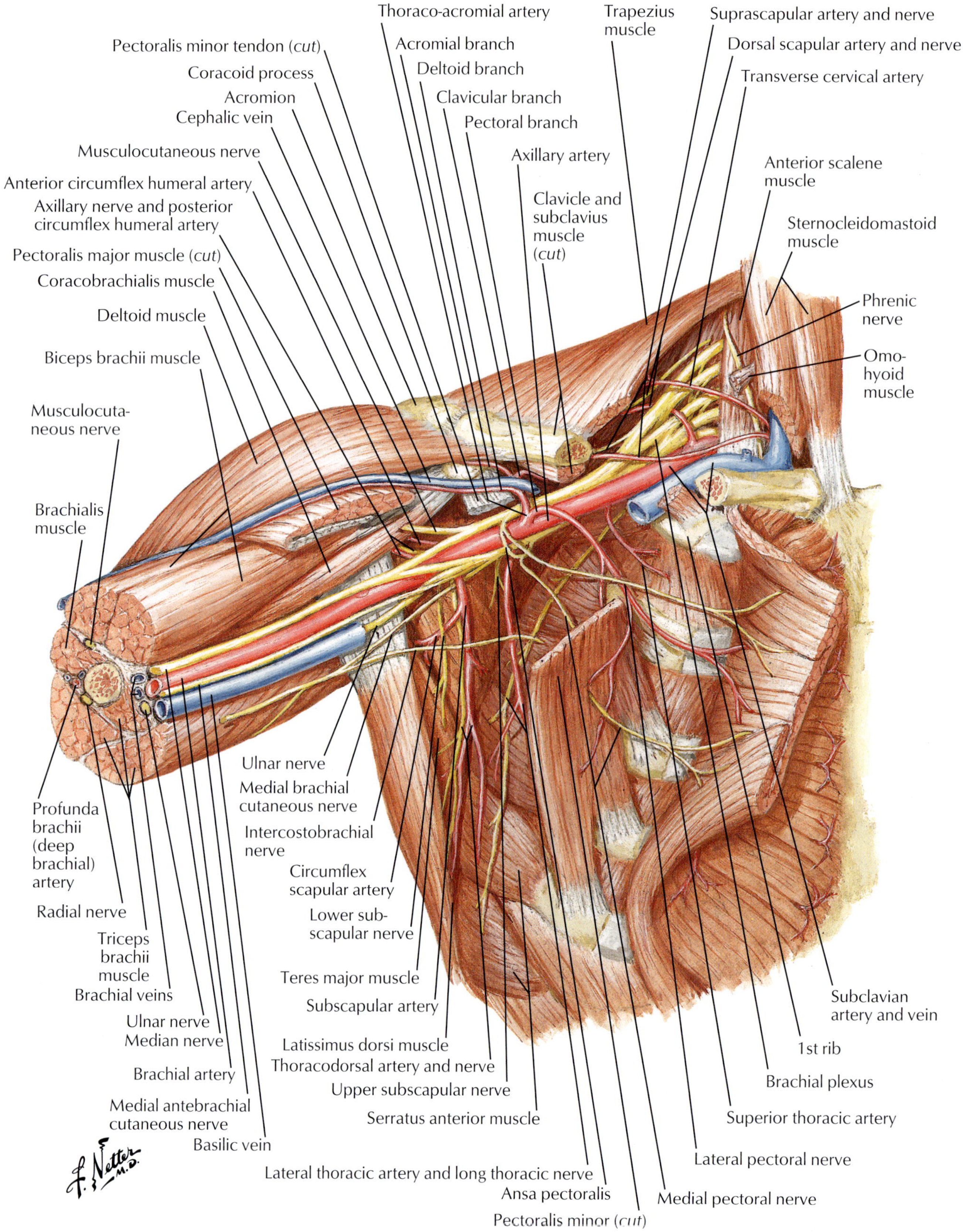

Brachial Plexus: Schema

See also Plates 410, 460, 461

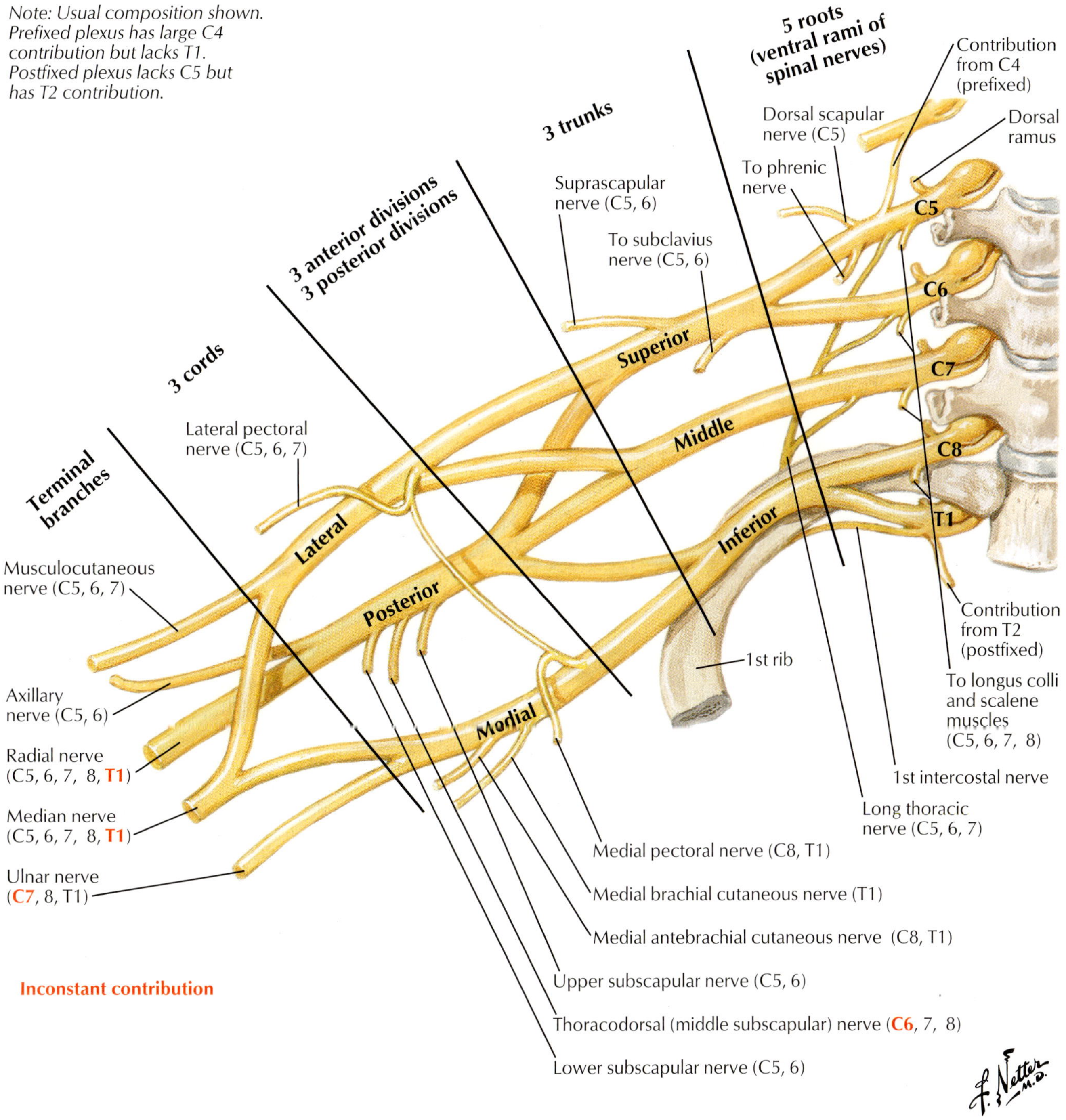

See also Plates 411, 462

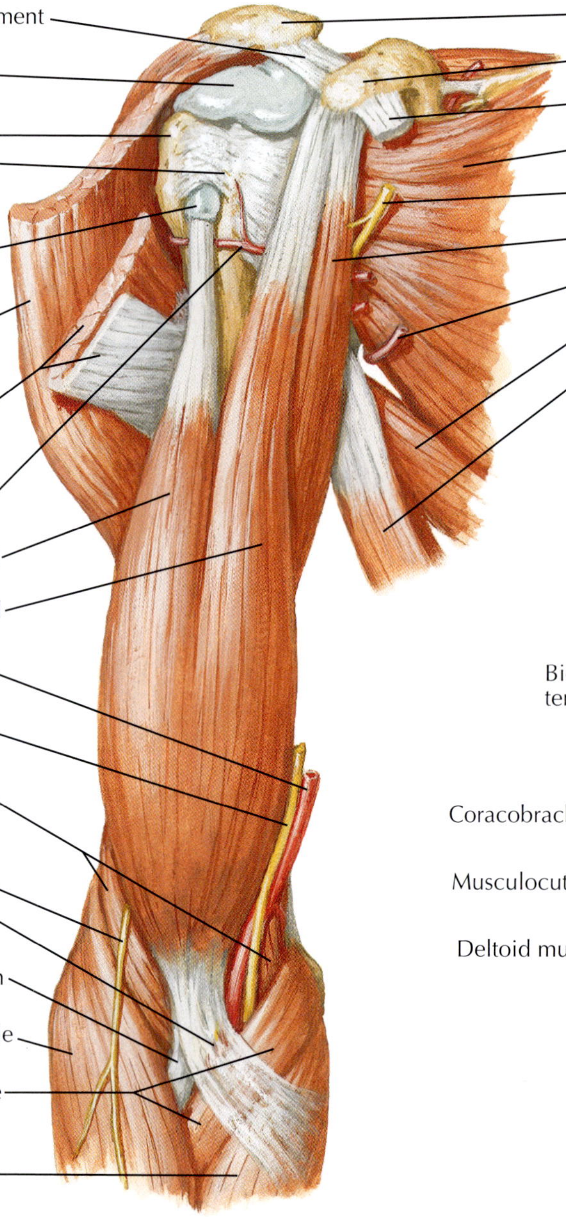

Superficial layer

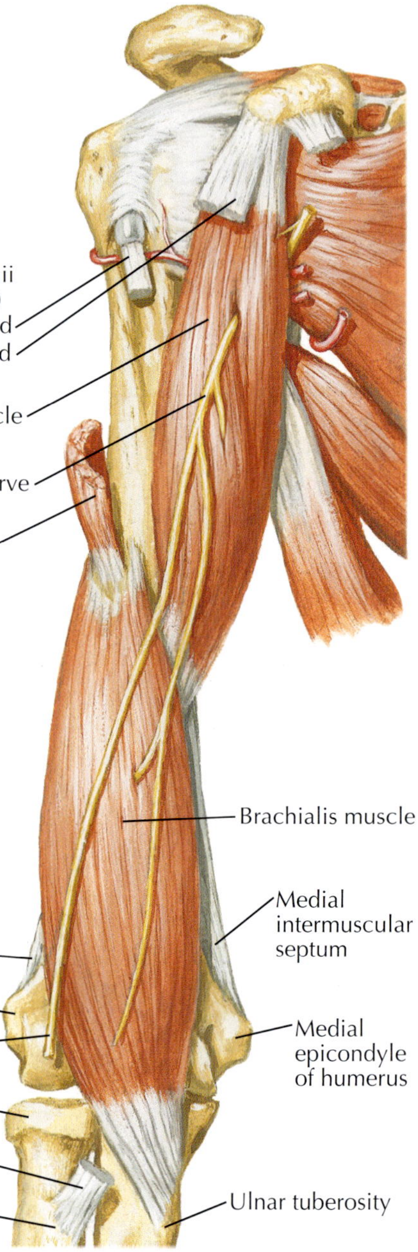

Deep layer

Muscles of Arm: Posterior Views

See also **Plates 411, 465**

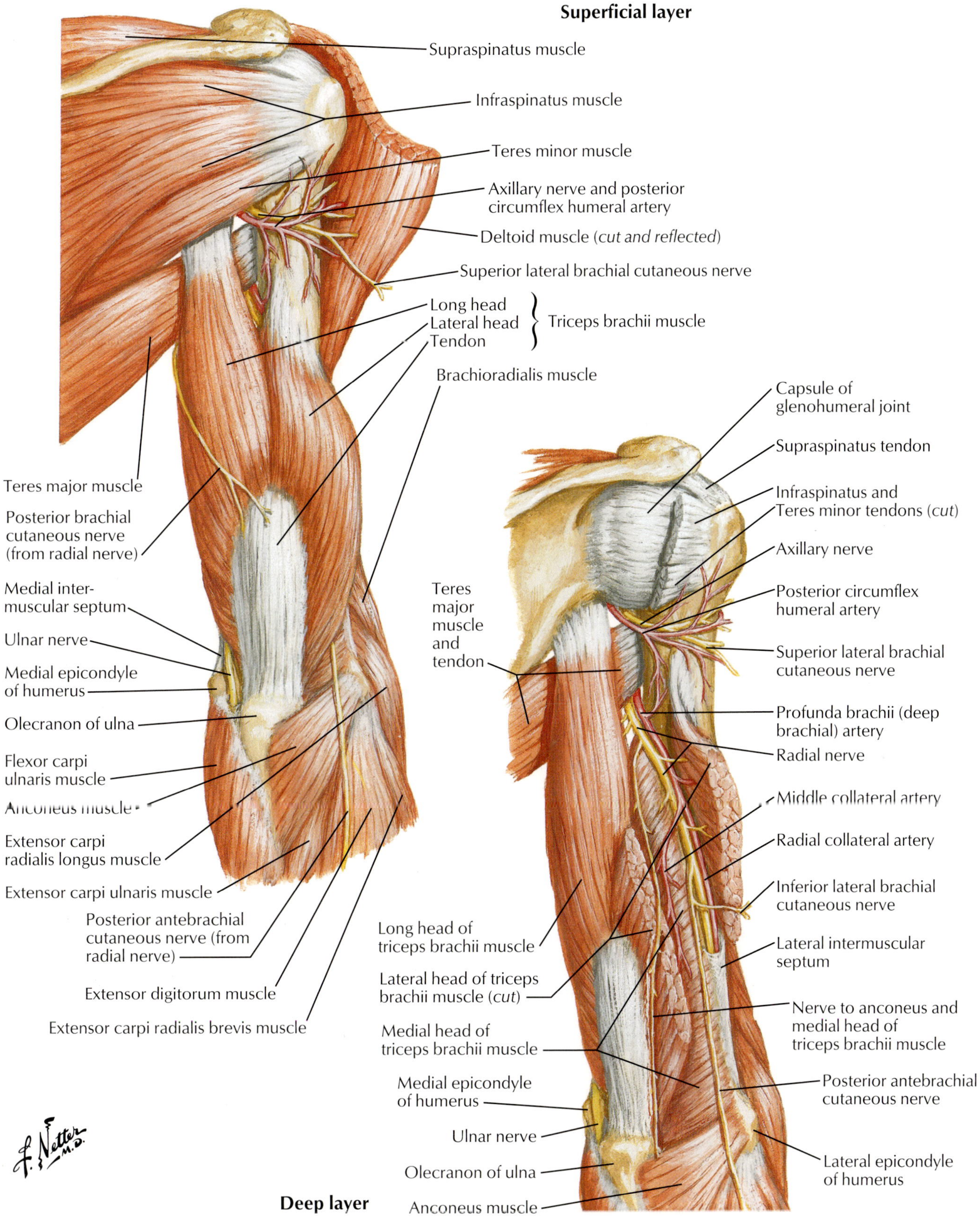

Brachial Artery in Situ

See also Plate 401

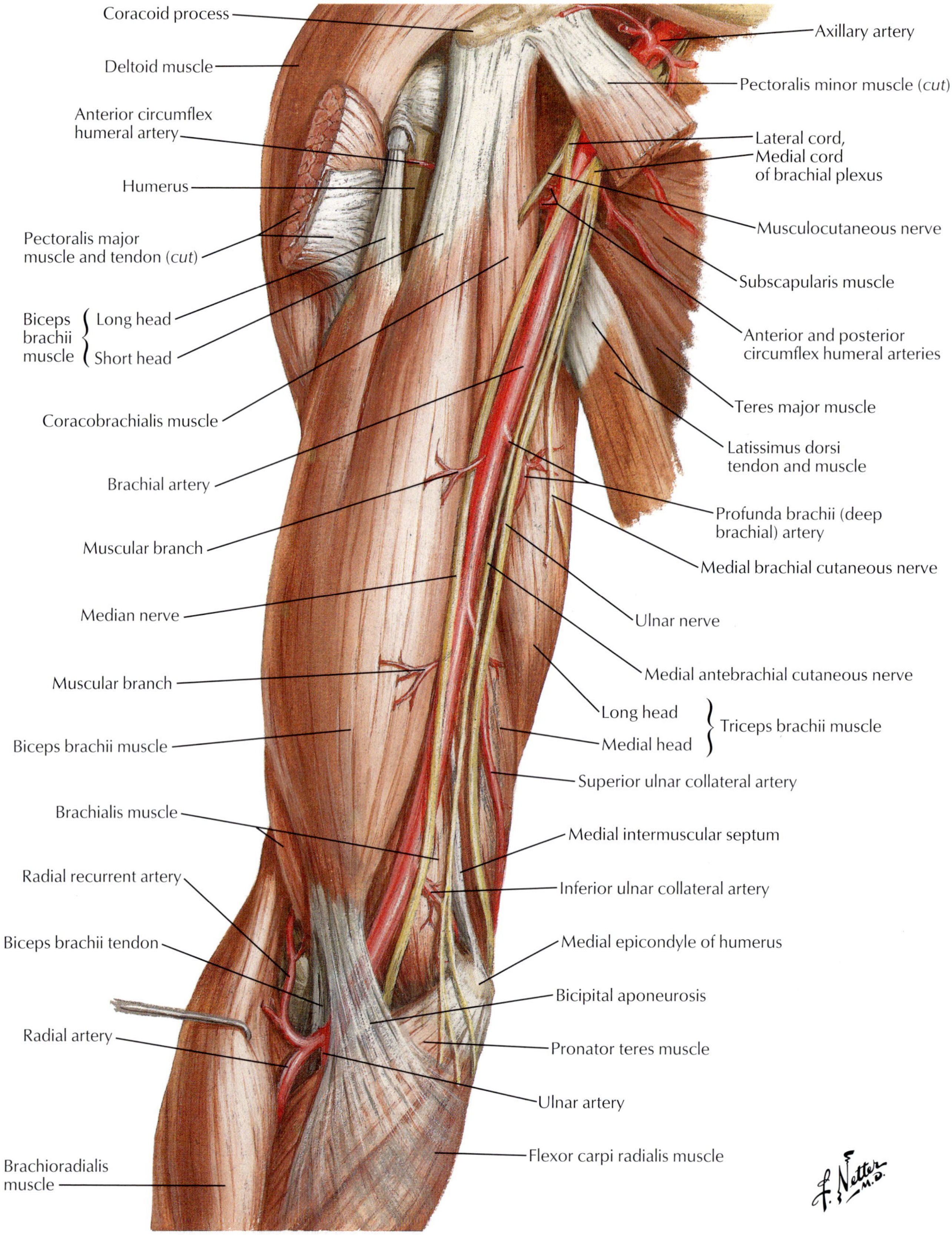

Arteries of Arm and Proximal Forearm

See also Plates 414, 433, 453

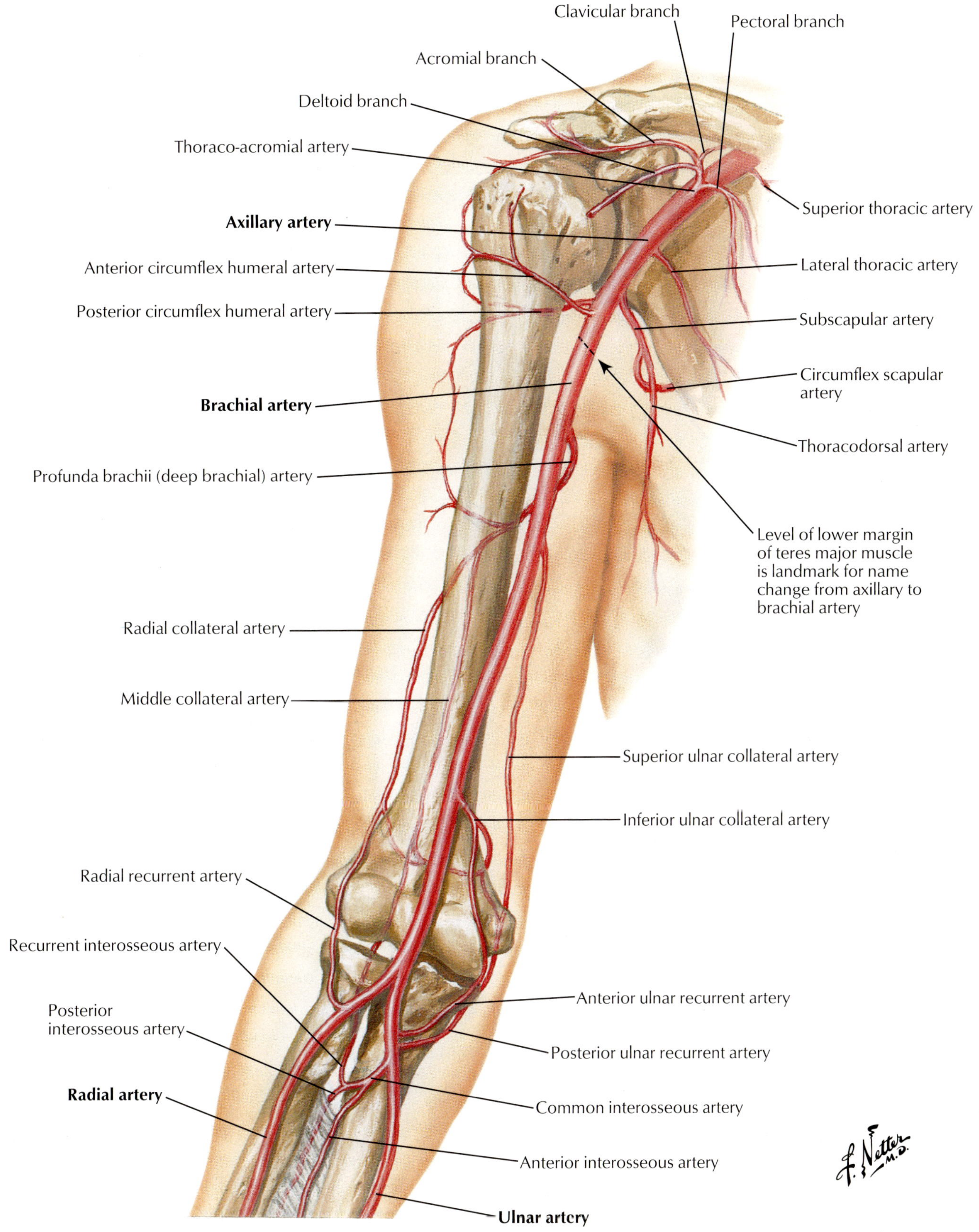

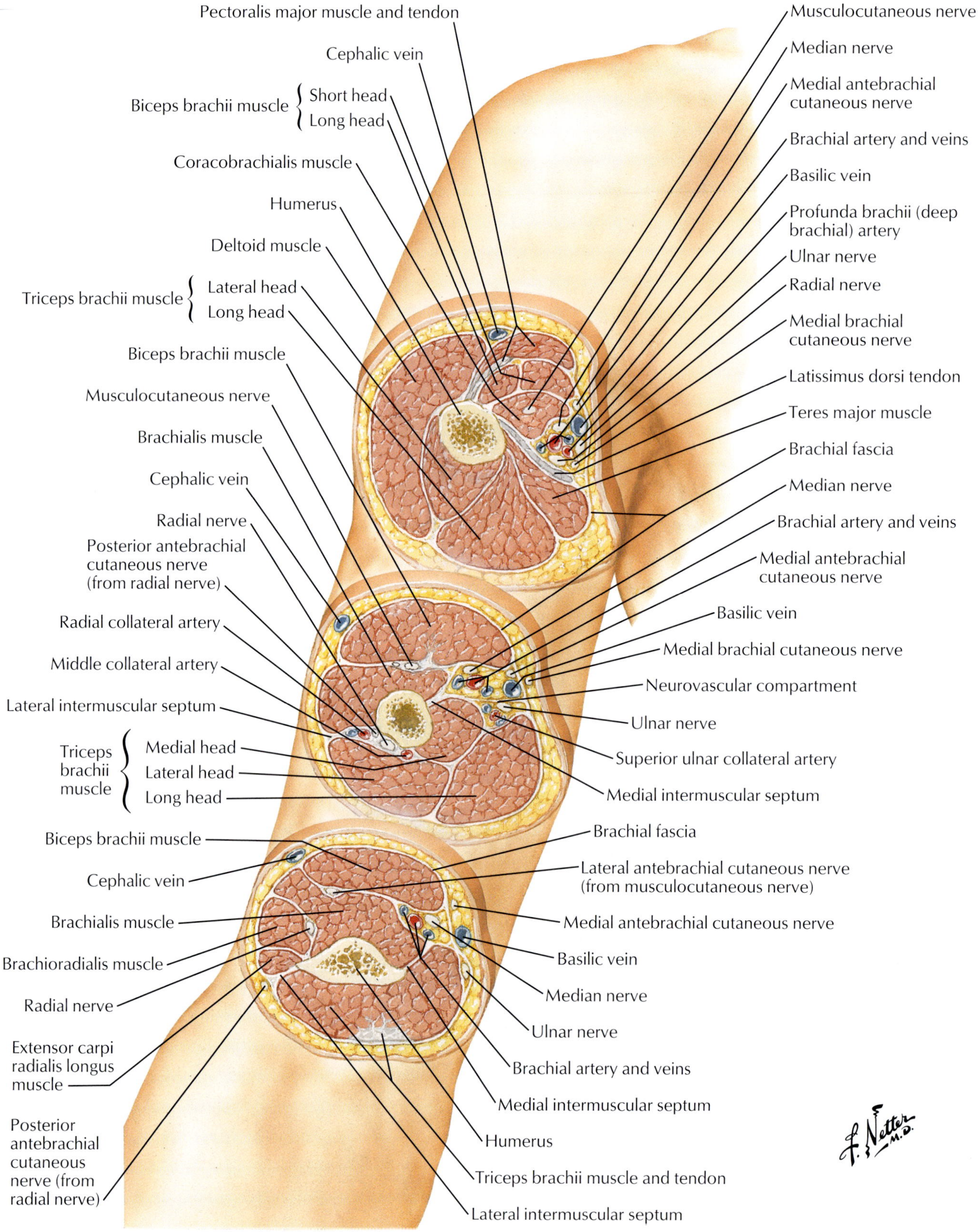

Pectoralis major muscle and tendon
Cephalic vein
Biceps brachii muscle
Short head
Long head
Coracobrachialis muscle
Humerus
Deltoid muscle
Triceps brachii muscle
Lateral head
Long head
Biceps brachii muscle
Musculocutaneous nerve
Brachialis muscle
Cephalic vein
Radial nerve
Posterior antebrachial cutaneous nerve (from radial nerve)
Radial collateral artery
Middle collateral artery
Lateral intermuscular septum
Triceps brachii muscle
Medial head
Lateral head
Long head
Biceps brachii muscle
Cephalic vein
Brachialis muscle
Brachioradialis muscle
Radial nerve
Extensor carpi radialis longus muscle
Posterior antebrachial cutaneous nerve (from radial nerve)
Musculocutaneous nerve
Median nerve
Medial antebrachial cutaneous nerve
Brachial artery and veins
Basilic vein
Profunda brachii (deep brachial) artery
Ulnar nerve
Radial nerve
Medial brachial cutaneous nerve
Latissimus dorsi tendon
Teres major muscle
Brachial fascia
Median nerve
Brachial artery and veins
Medial antebrachial cutaneous nerve
Basilic vein
Medial brachial cutaneous nerve
Neurovascular compartment
Ulnar nerve
Superior ulnar collateral artery
Medial intermuscular septum
Brachial fascia
Lateral antebrachial cutaneous nerve (from musculocutaneous nerve)
Medial antebrachial cutaneous nerve
Basilic vein
Median nerve
Ulnar nerve
Brachial artery and veins
Medial intermuscular septum
Humerus
Triceps brachii muscle and tendon
Lateral intermuscular septum
F. Netter M.D.

See also Plate 437

Right elbow

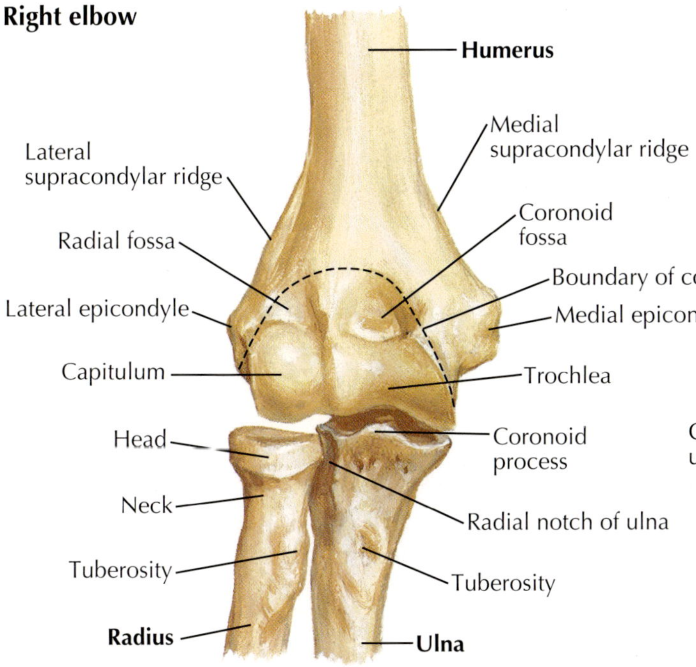

In extension: anterior view

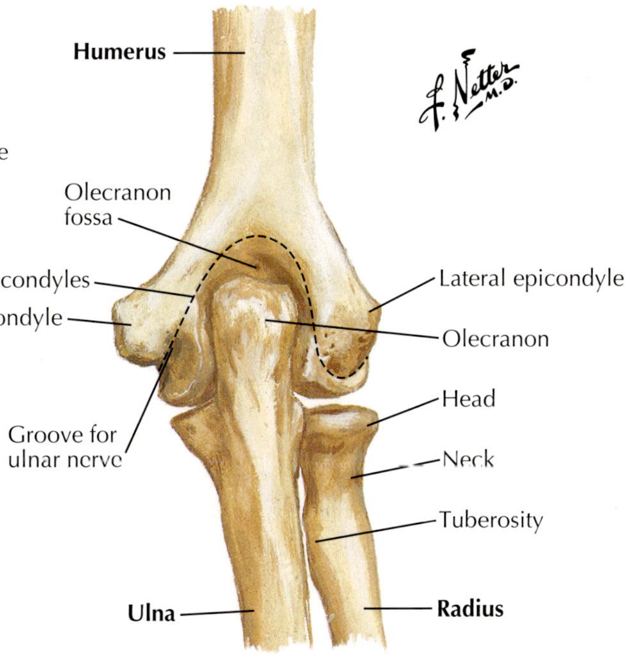

In extension: posterior view

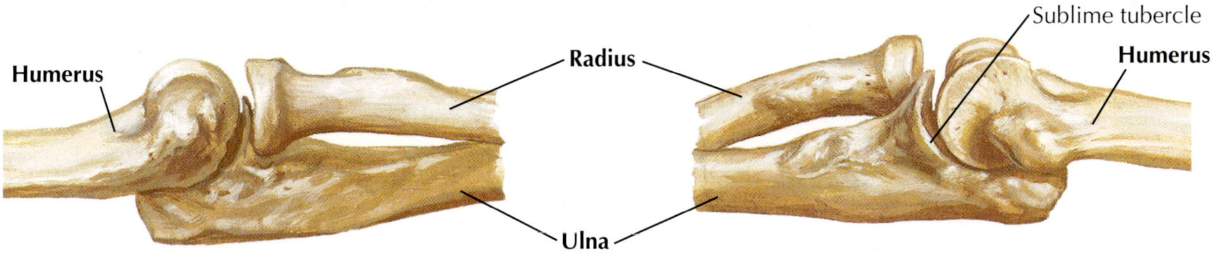

In extension: lateral view

In extension: medial view

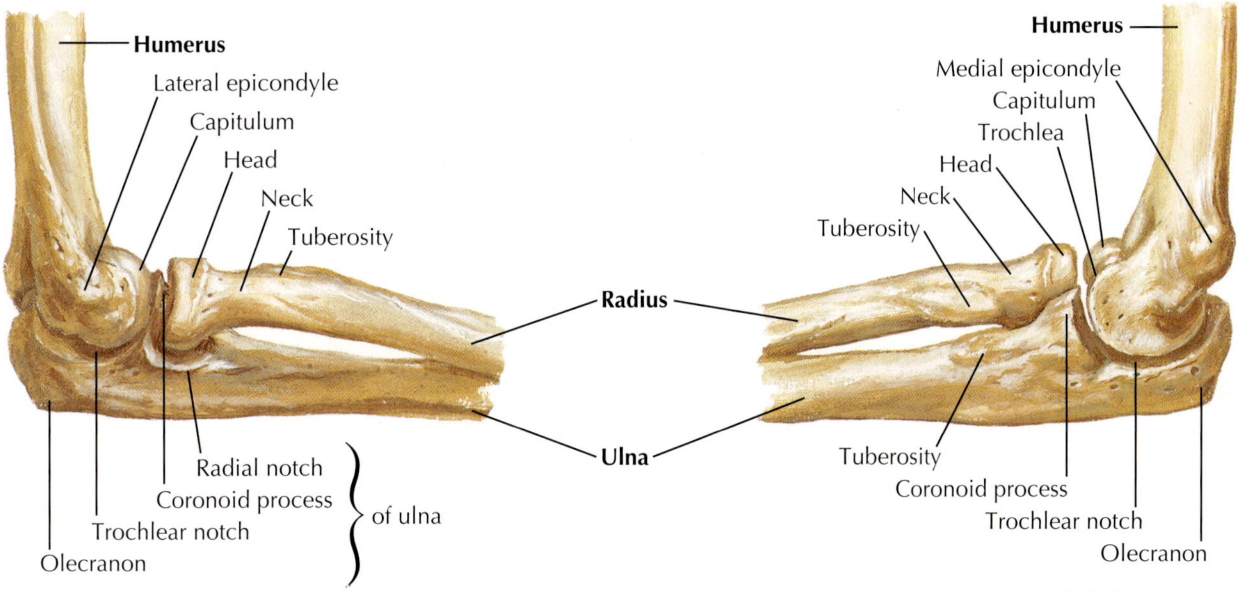

In 90° flexion: lateral view

In 90° flexion: medial view

Anteroposterior radiograph

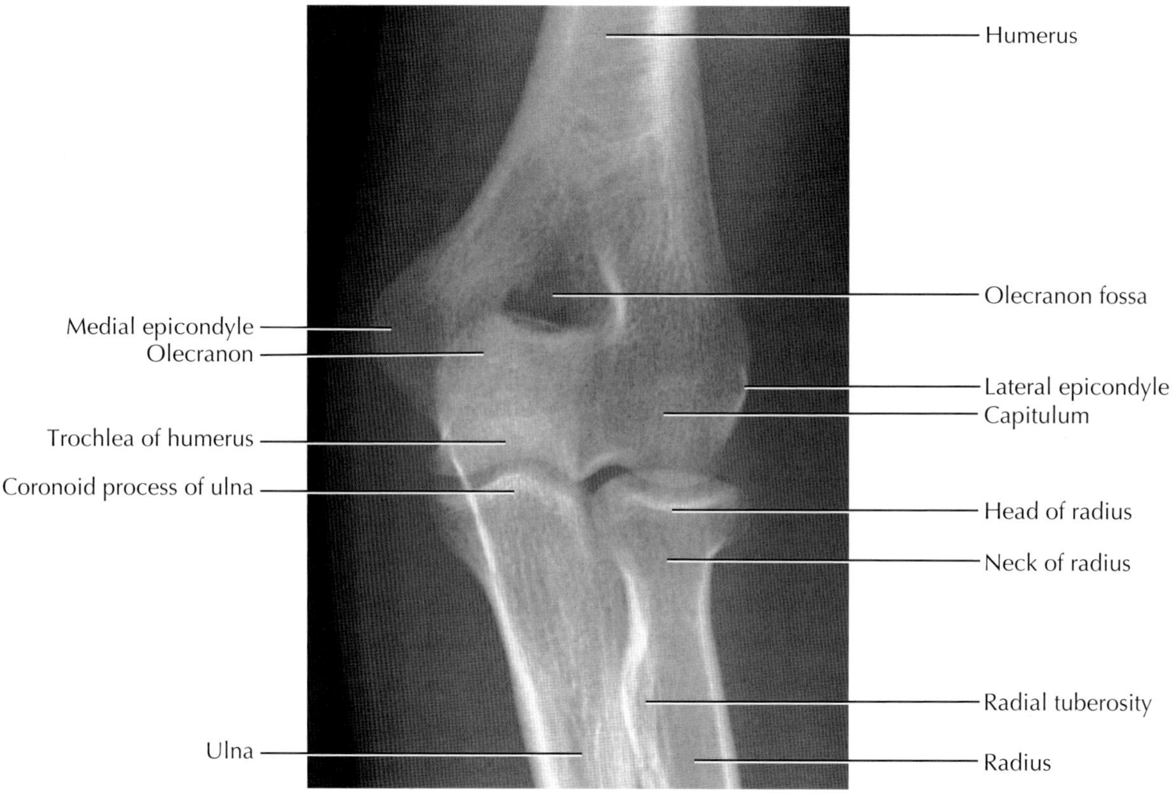

Lateral radiograph

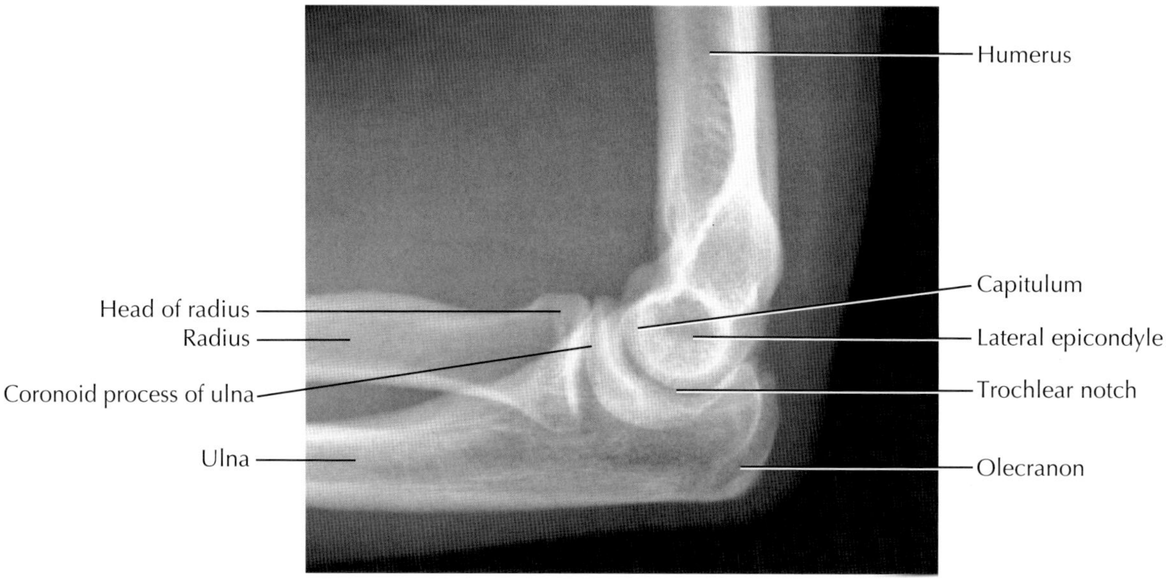

Right elbow: anterior view

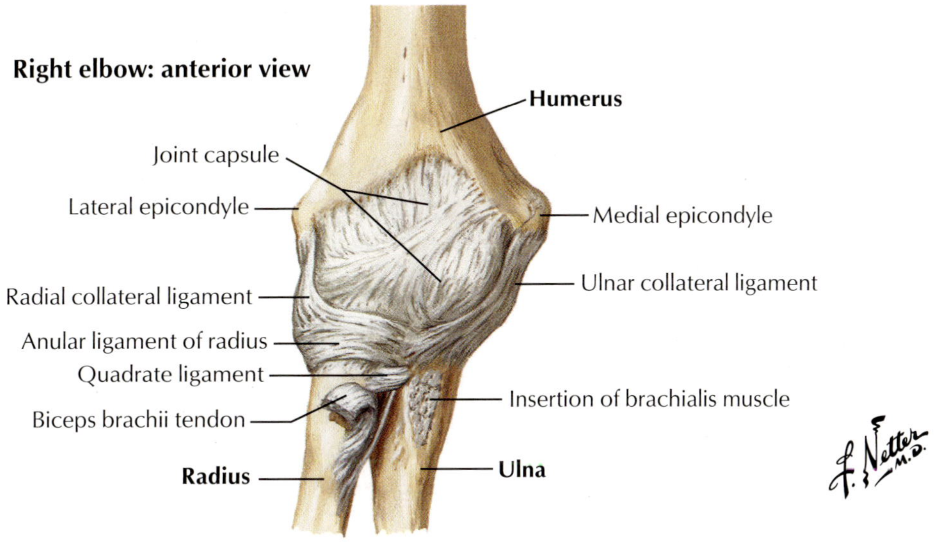

In 90° flexion: lateral view

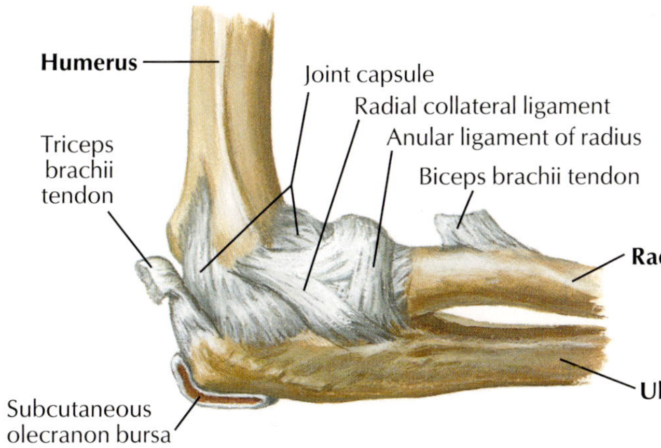

In 90° flexion: medial view

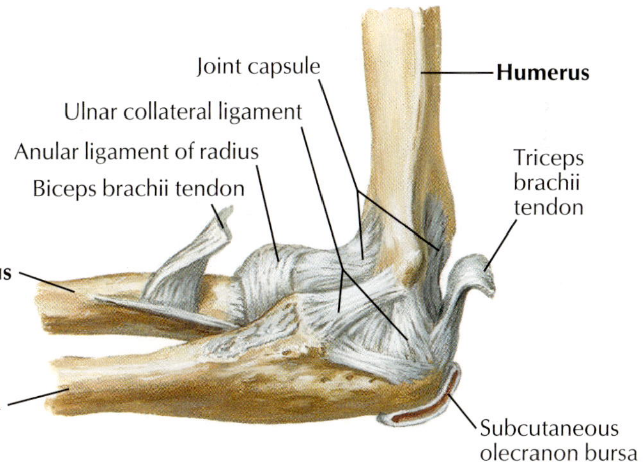

Opened joint: anterior view

Opened joint: posterior view

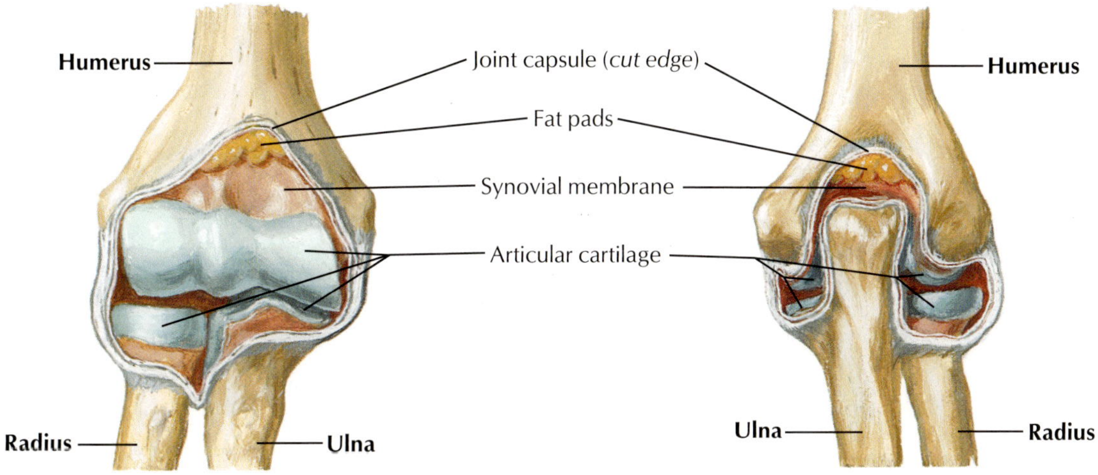

Bones of Forearm

See also Plates 439, 442

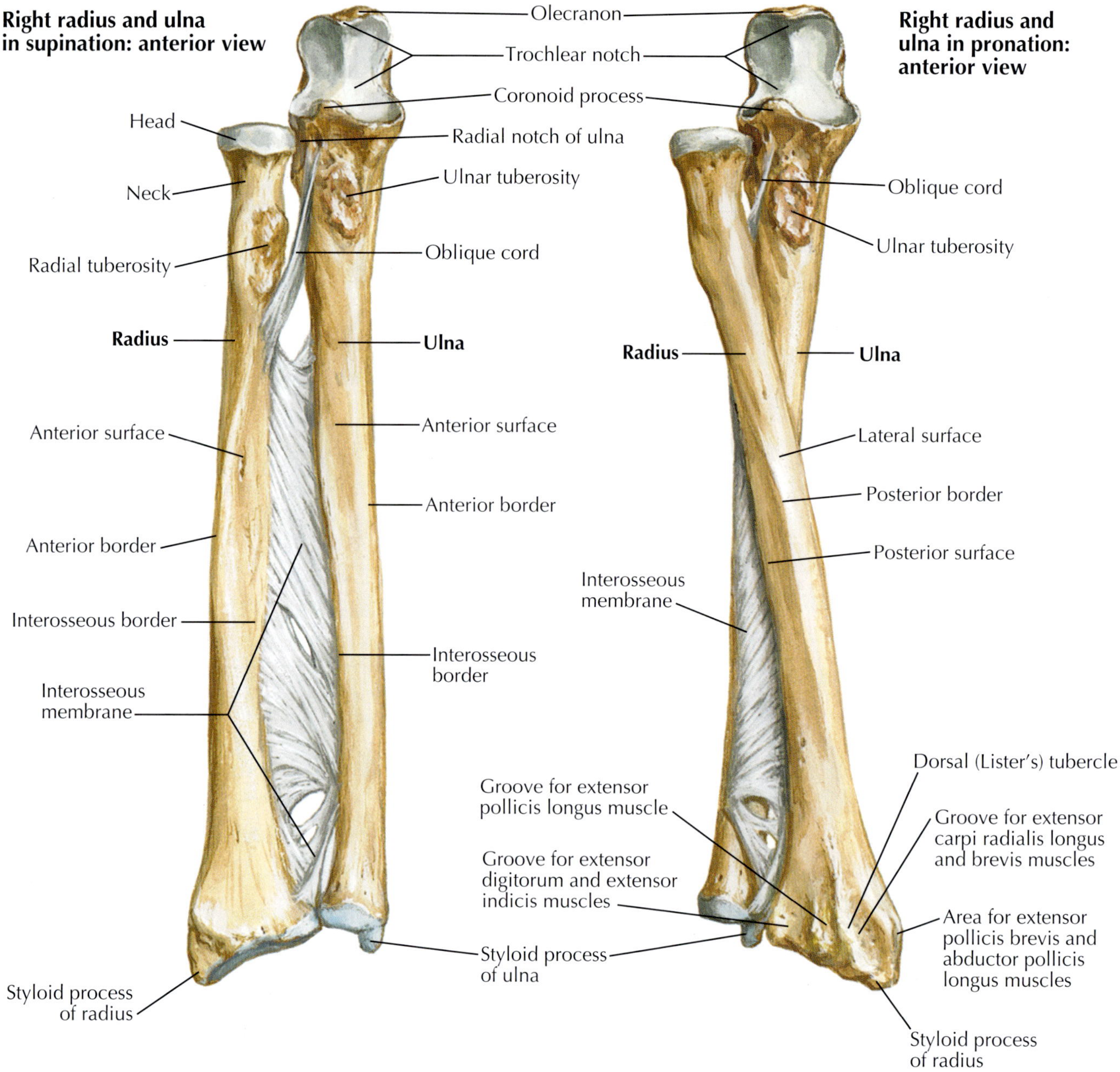

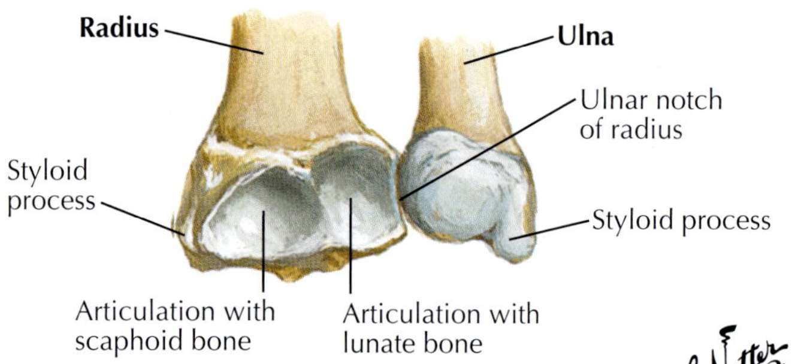

Carpal articular surface

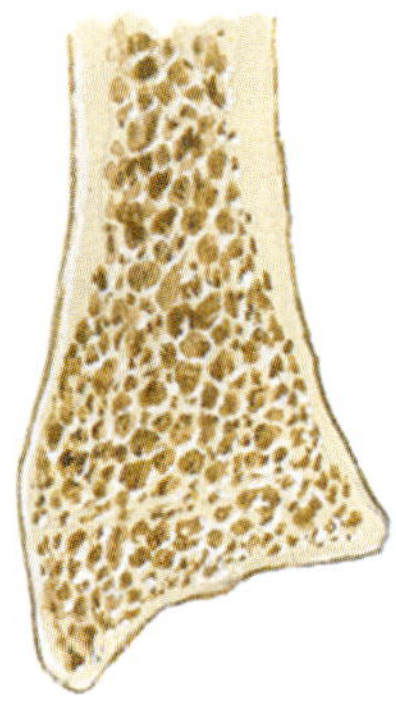

Coronal section of radius demonstrates how thickness of cortical bone of shaft diminishes to thin layer over cancellous bone at distal end

Individual Muscles of Forearm: Rotators of Radius

See also Plate 434

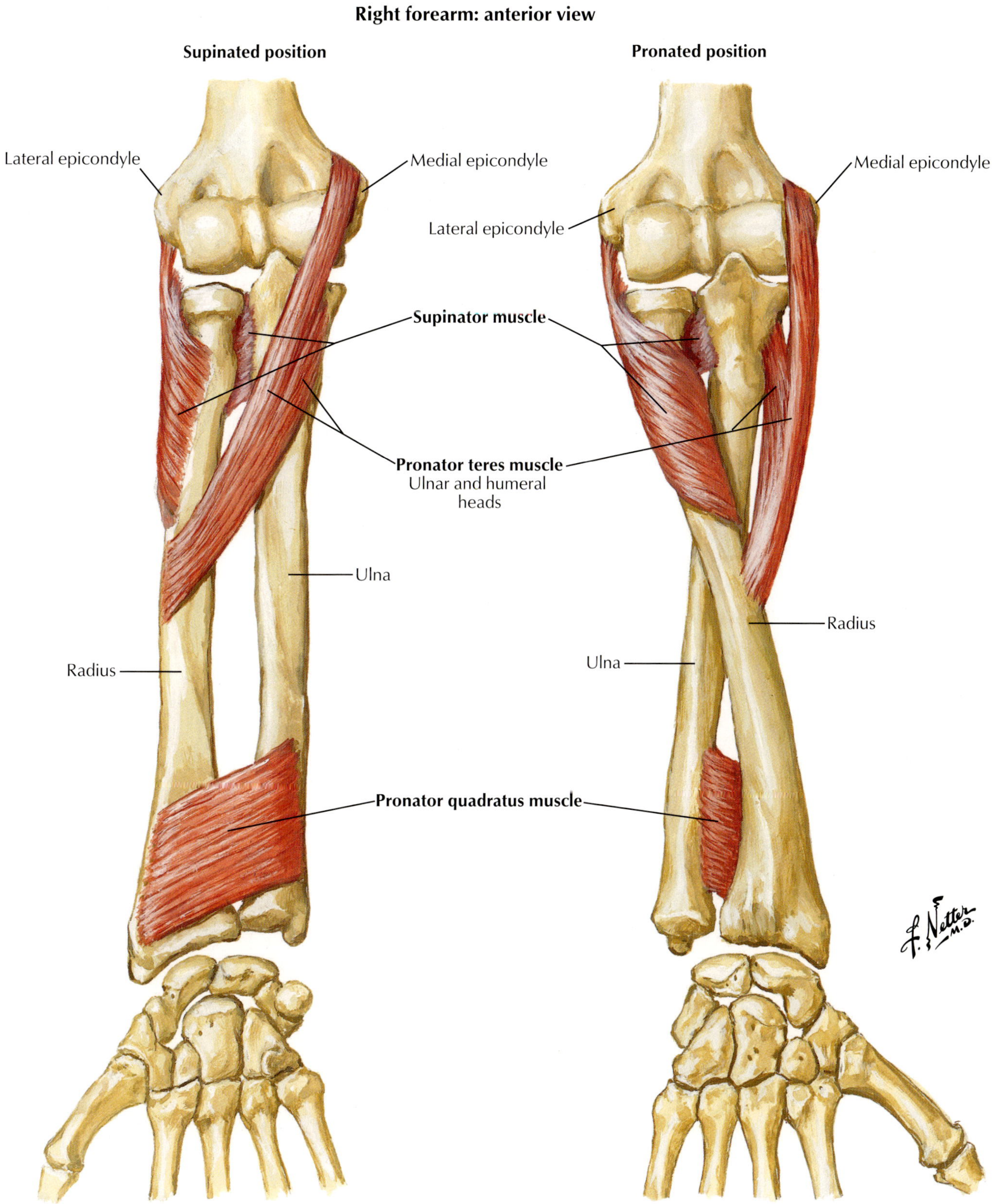

Individual Muscles of Forearm: Extensors of Wrist and Digits

See also Plate 438

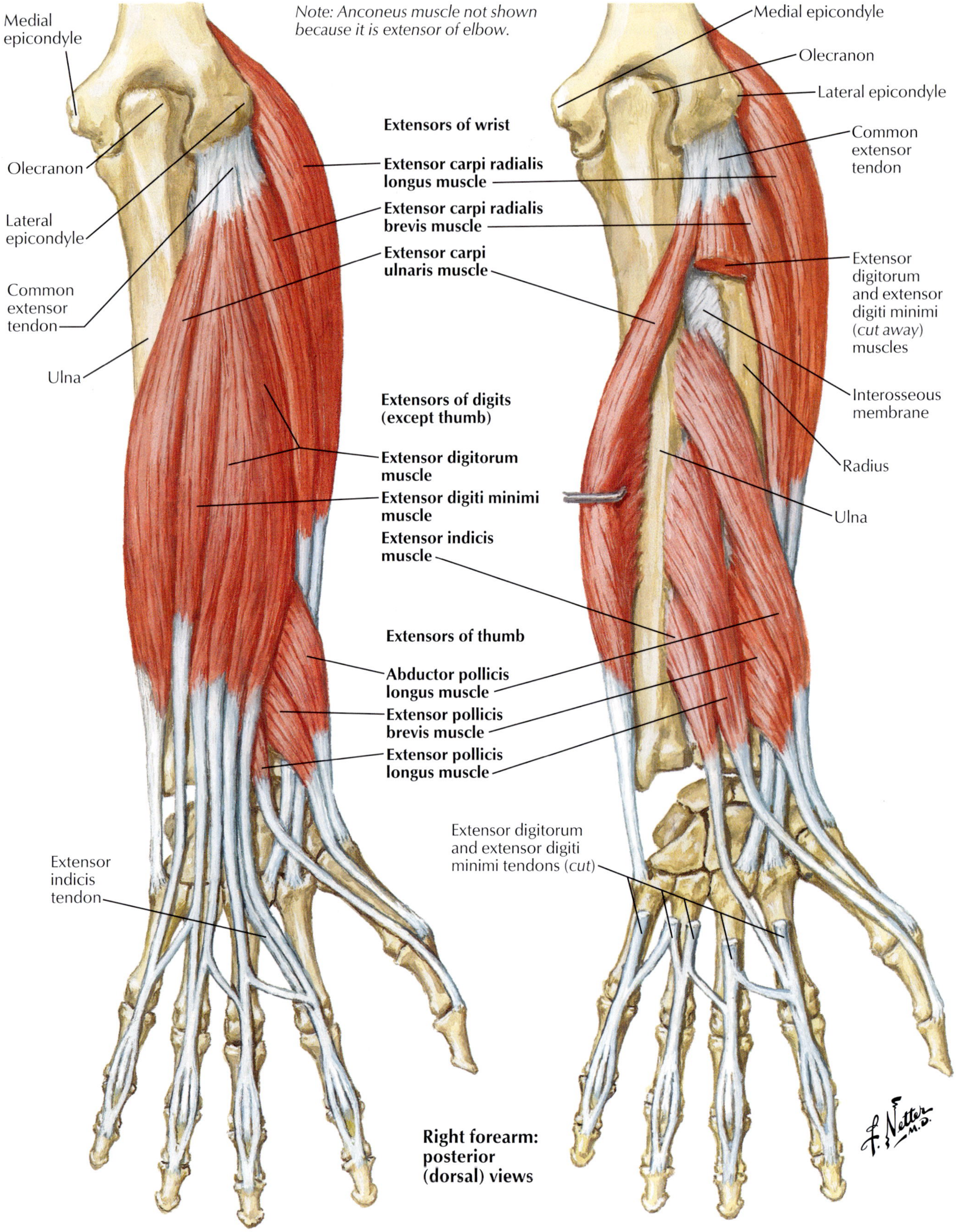

Right forearm: posterior (dorsal) views

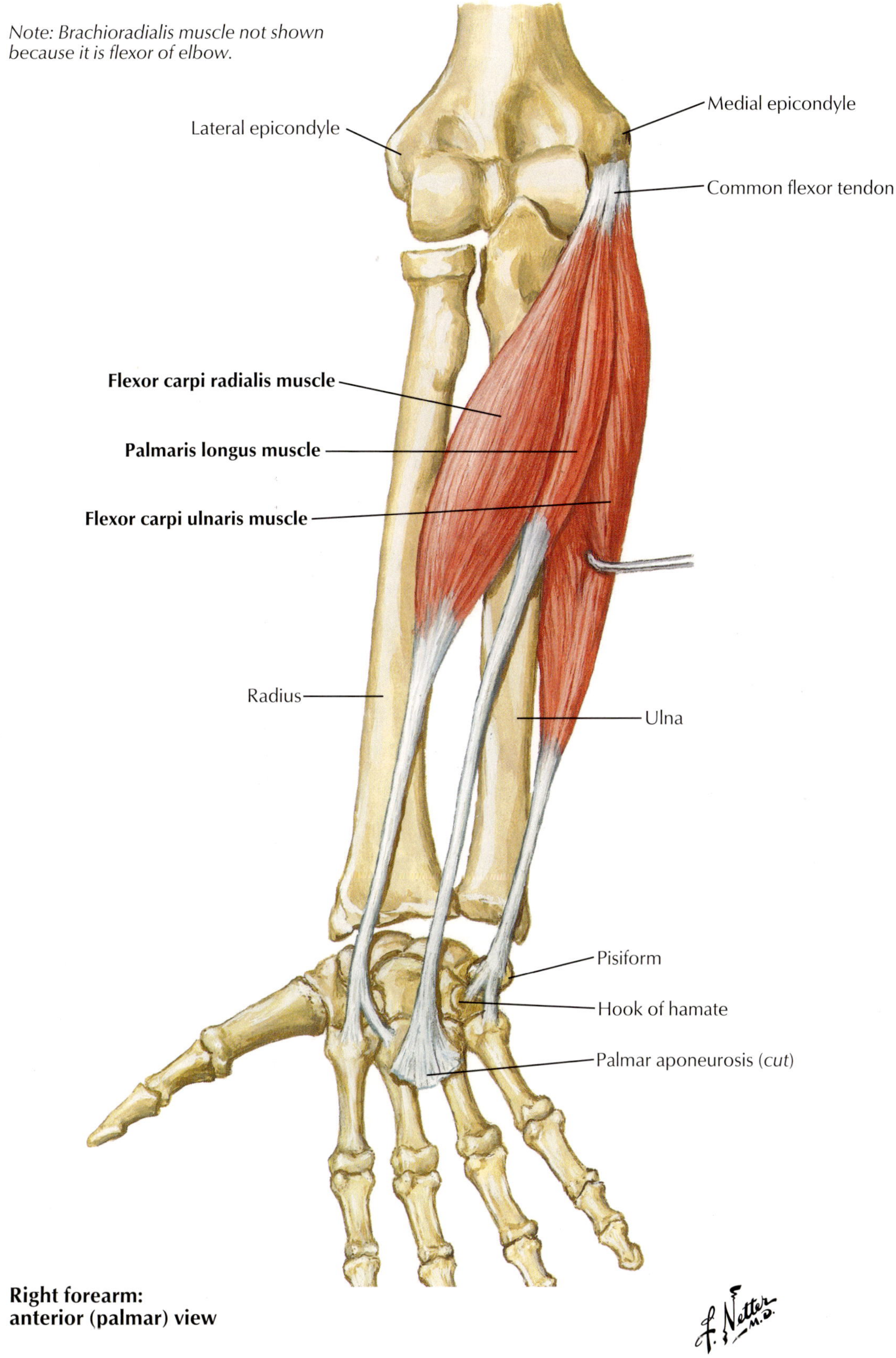

Right forearm: anterior (palmar) view

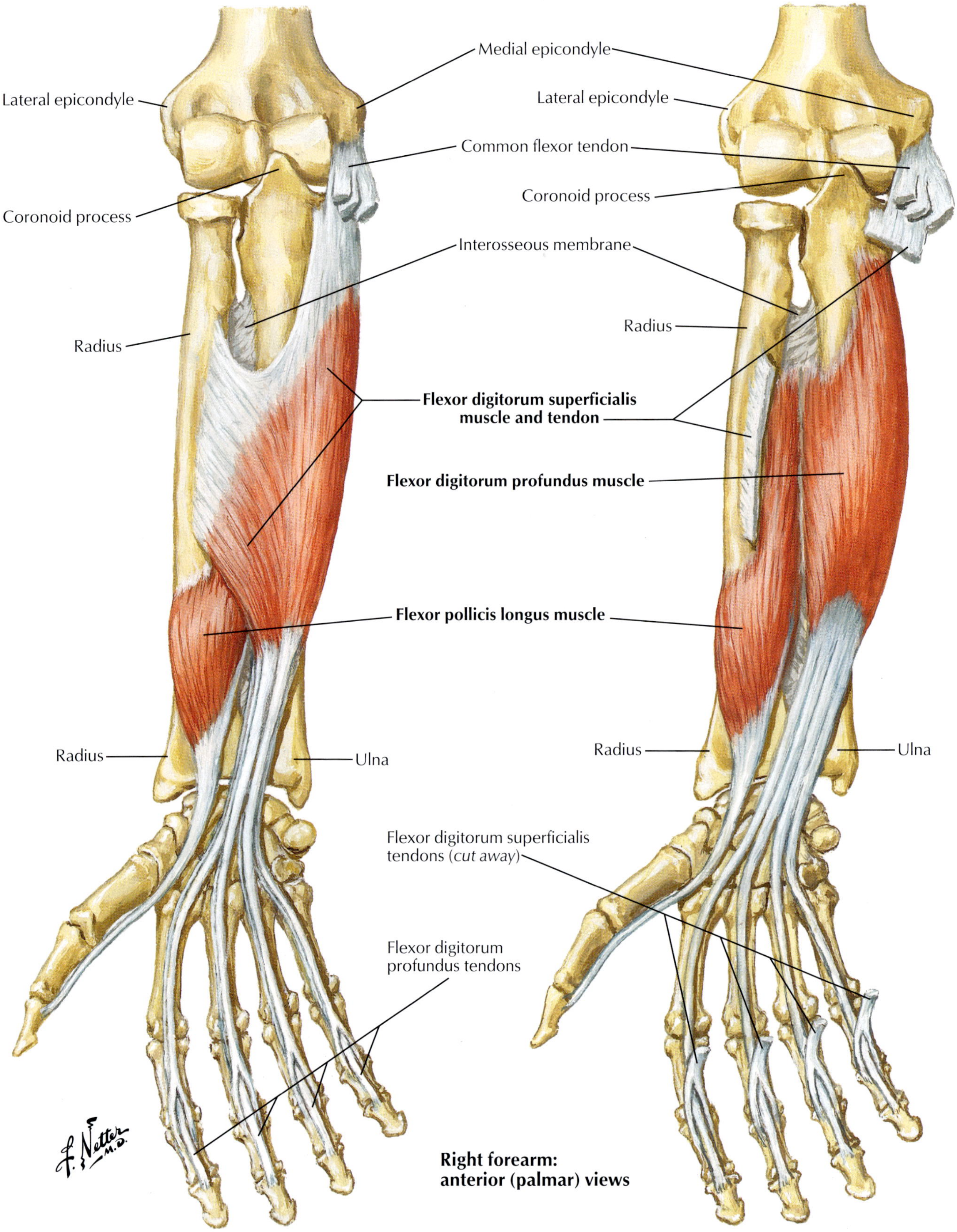

Right forearm: anterior (palmar) views

Muscles of Forearm (Superficial Layer): Posterior View

See also Plates 457, 466

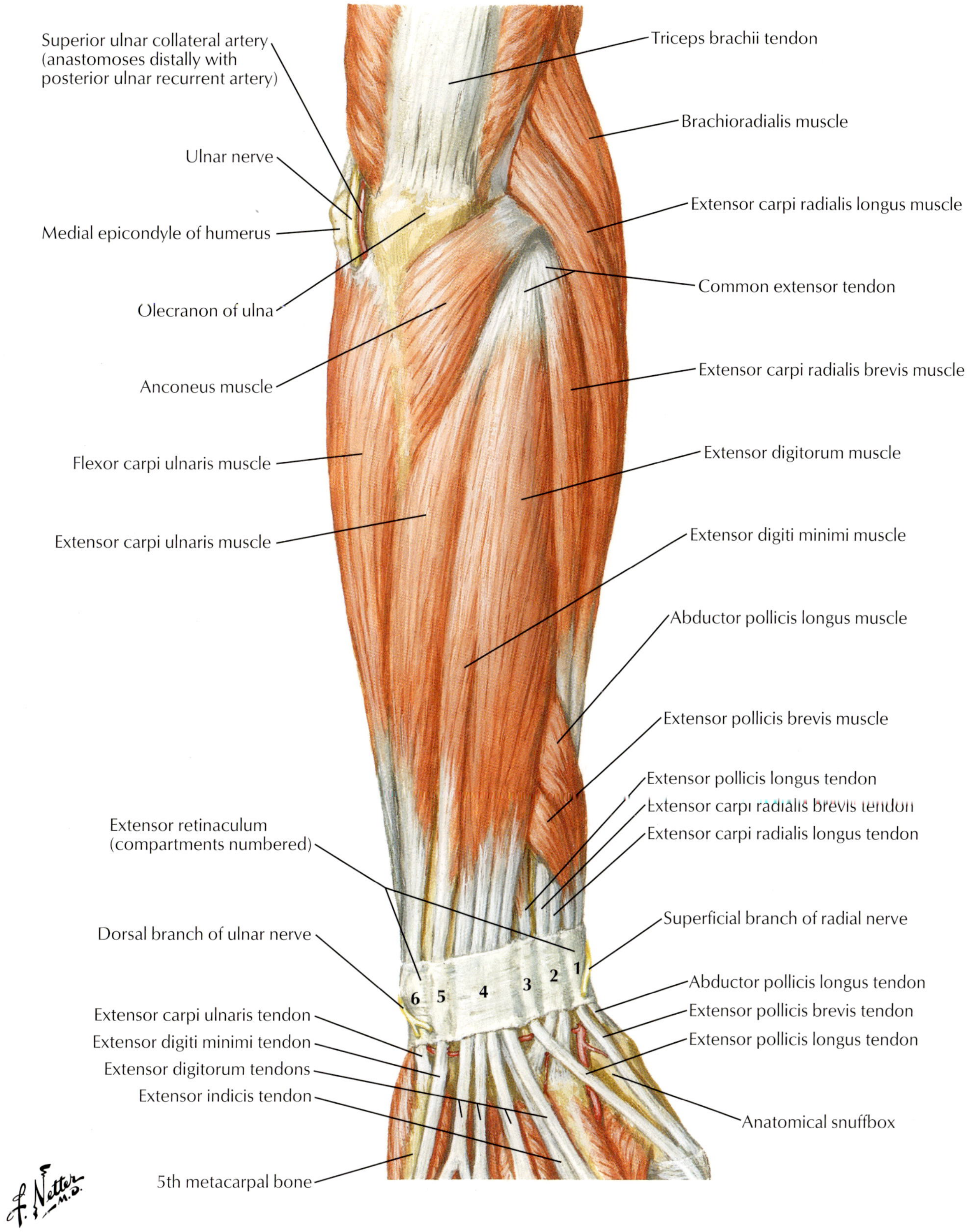

Muscles of Forearm (Deep Layer): Posterior View

See also **Plates 402, 457**

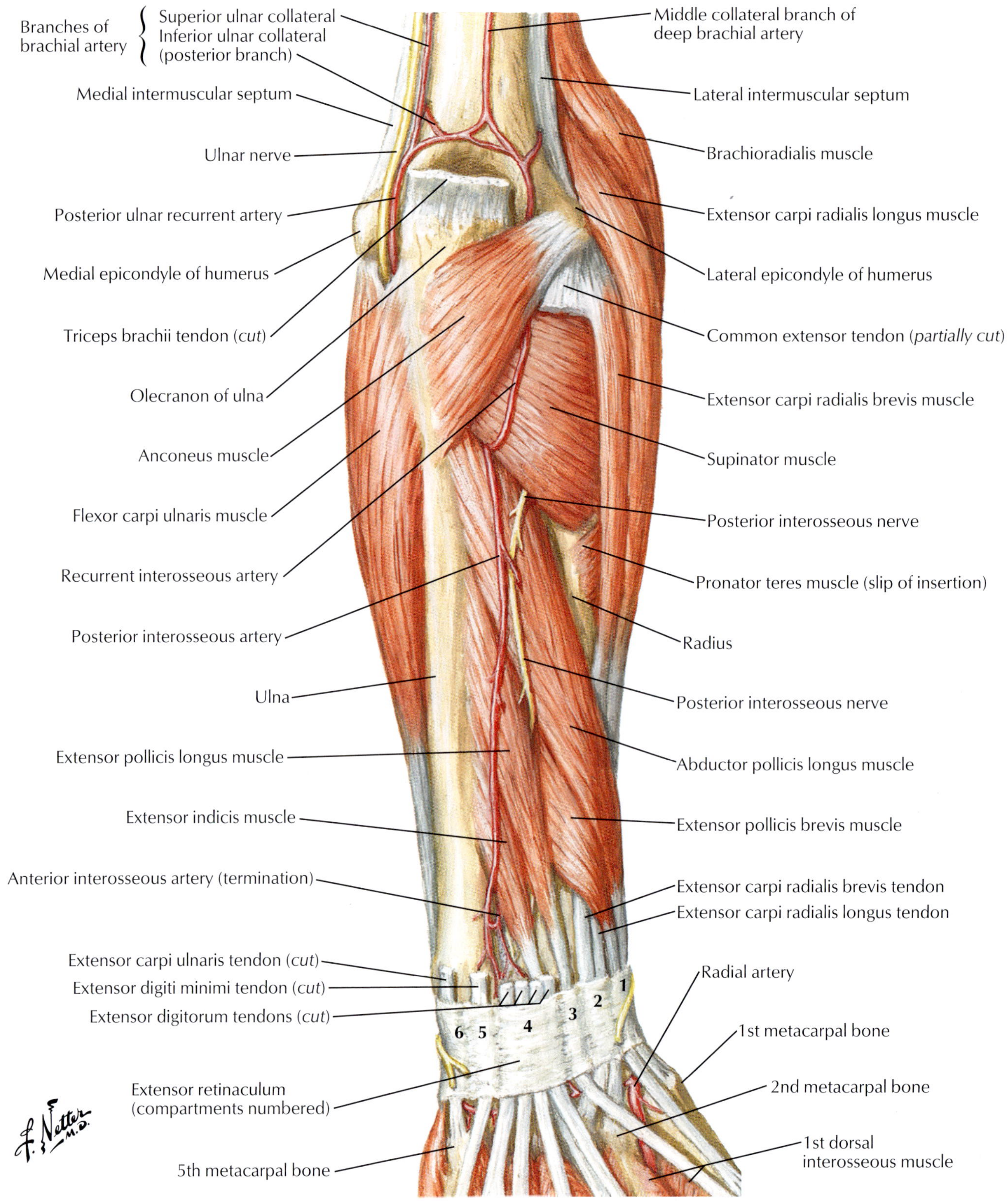

Muscles of Forearm (Superficial Layer): Anterior View

See also Plates 463, 464

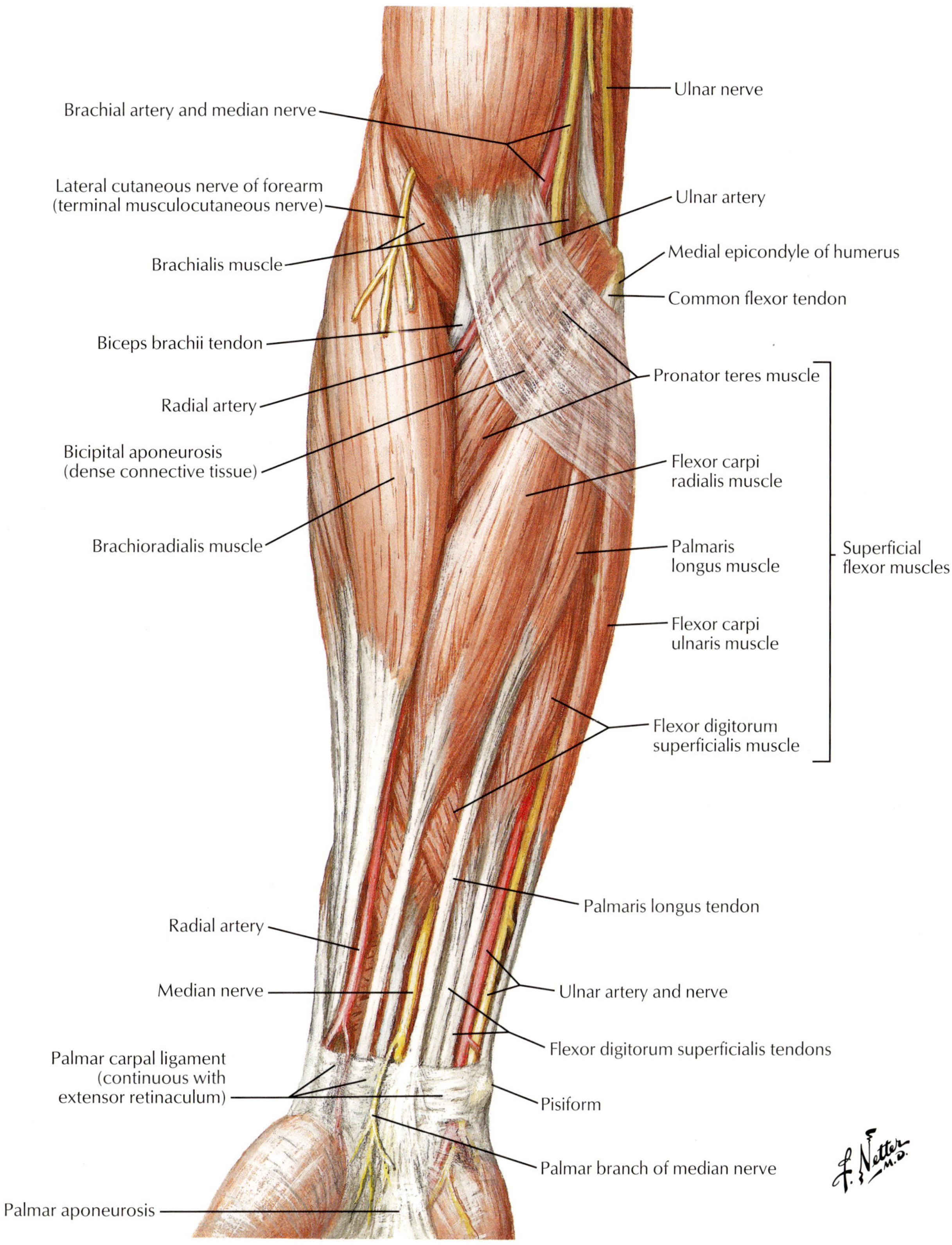

Muscles of Forearm (Intermediate Layer): Anterior View

See also **Plates 420, 463, 464**

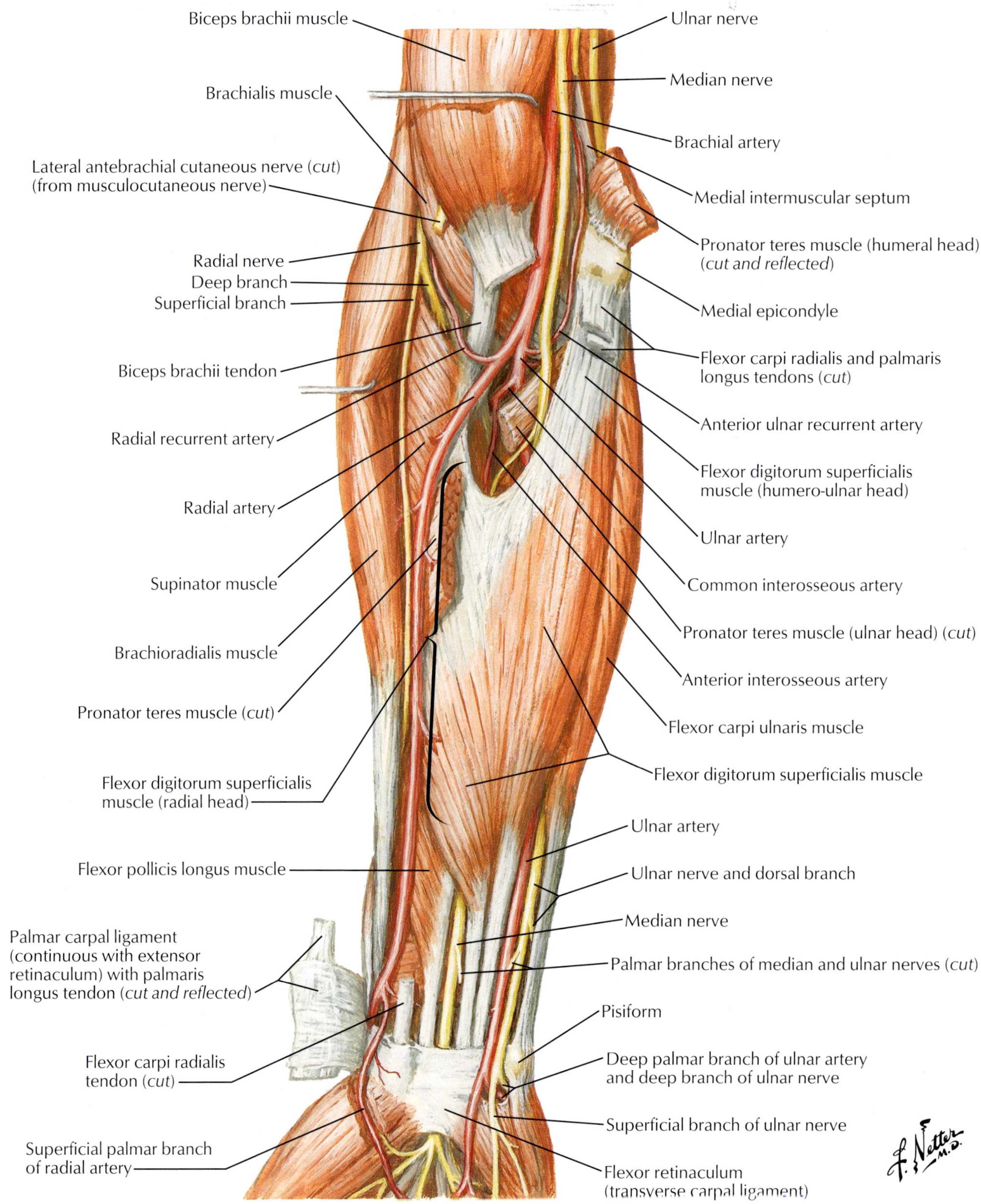

Muscles of Forearm (Deep Layer): Anterior View

See also Plates 426, 464

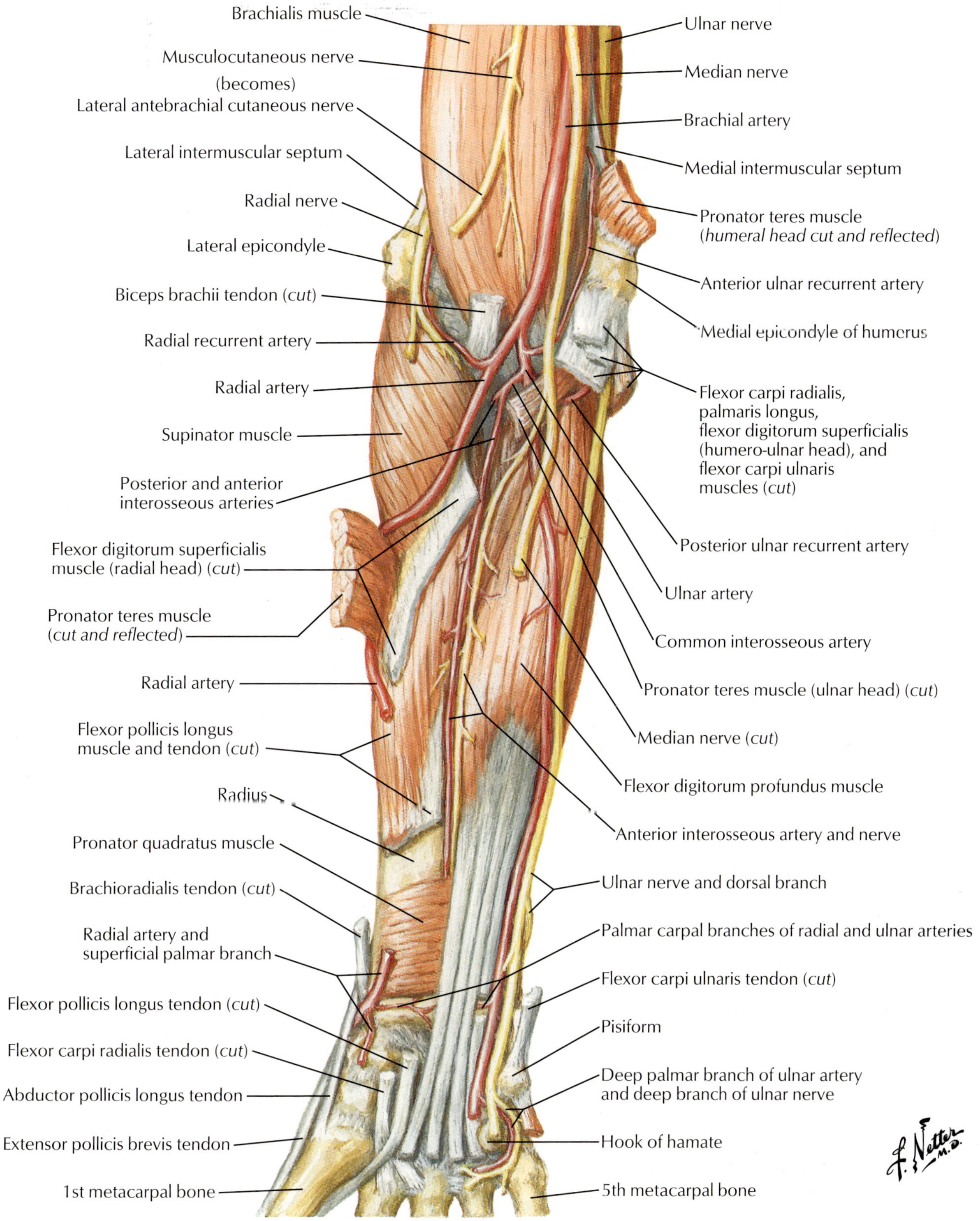

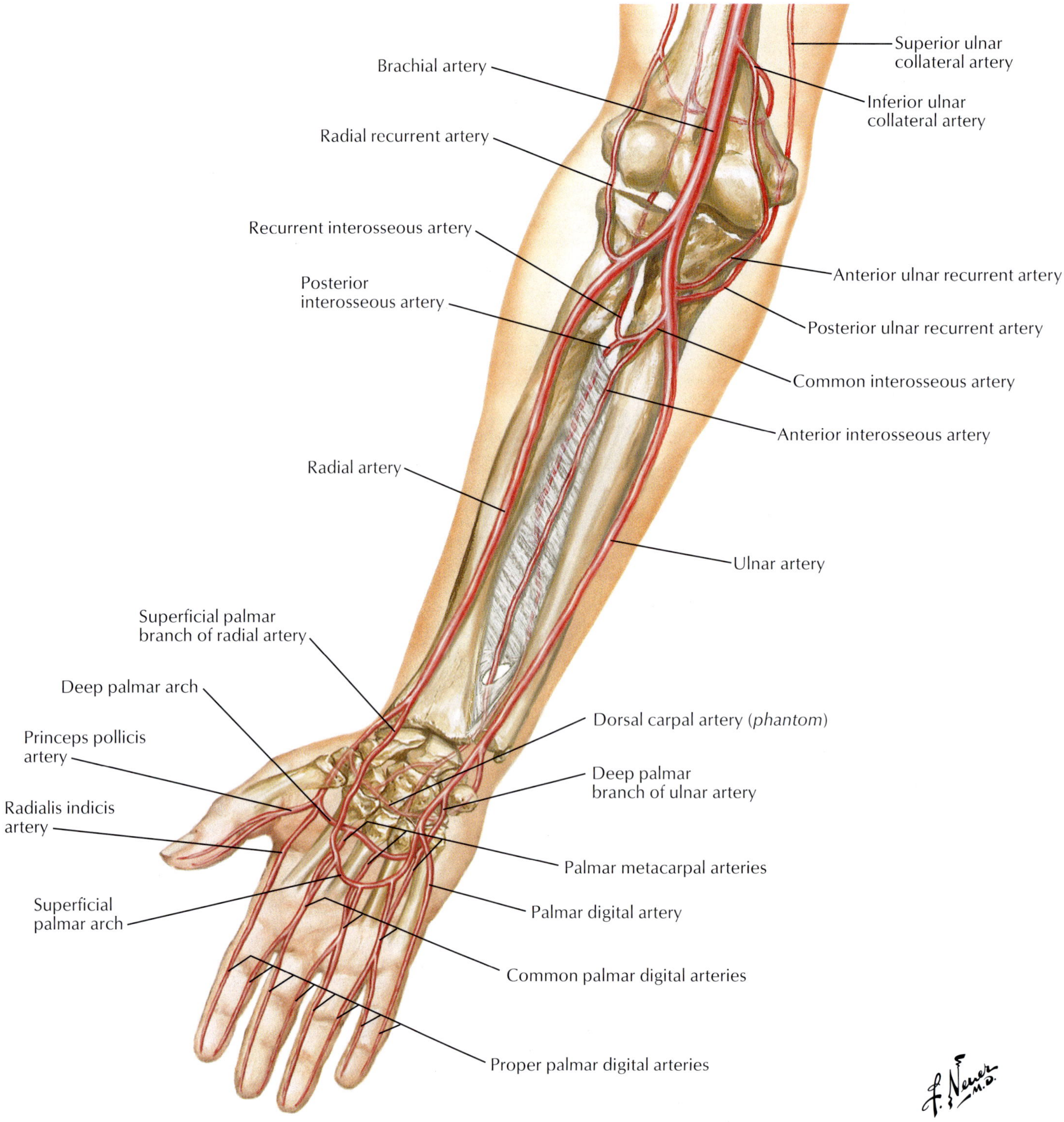
Brachial artery
Radial recurrent artery
Recurrent interosseous artery
Posterior interosseous artery
Radial artery
Superficial palmar branch of radial artery
Deep palmar arch
Princeps pollicis artery
Radialis indicis artery
Superficial palmar arch
Superior ulnar collateral artery
Inferior ulnar collateral artery
Anterior ulnar recurrent artery
Posterior ulnar recurrent artery
Common interosseous artery
Anterior interosseous artery
Ulnar artery
Dorsal carpal artery (*phantom*)
Deep palmar branch of ulnar artery
Palmar metacarpal arteries
Palmar digital artery
Common palmar digital arteries
Proper palmar digital arteries

Forearm: Serial Cross Sections, Anterior View

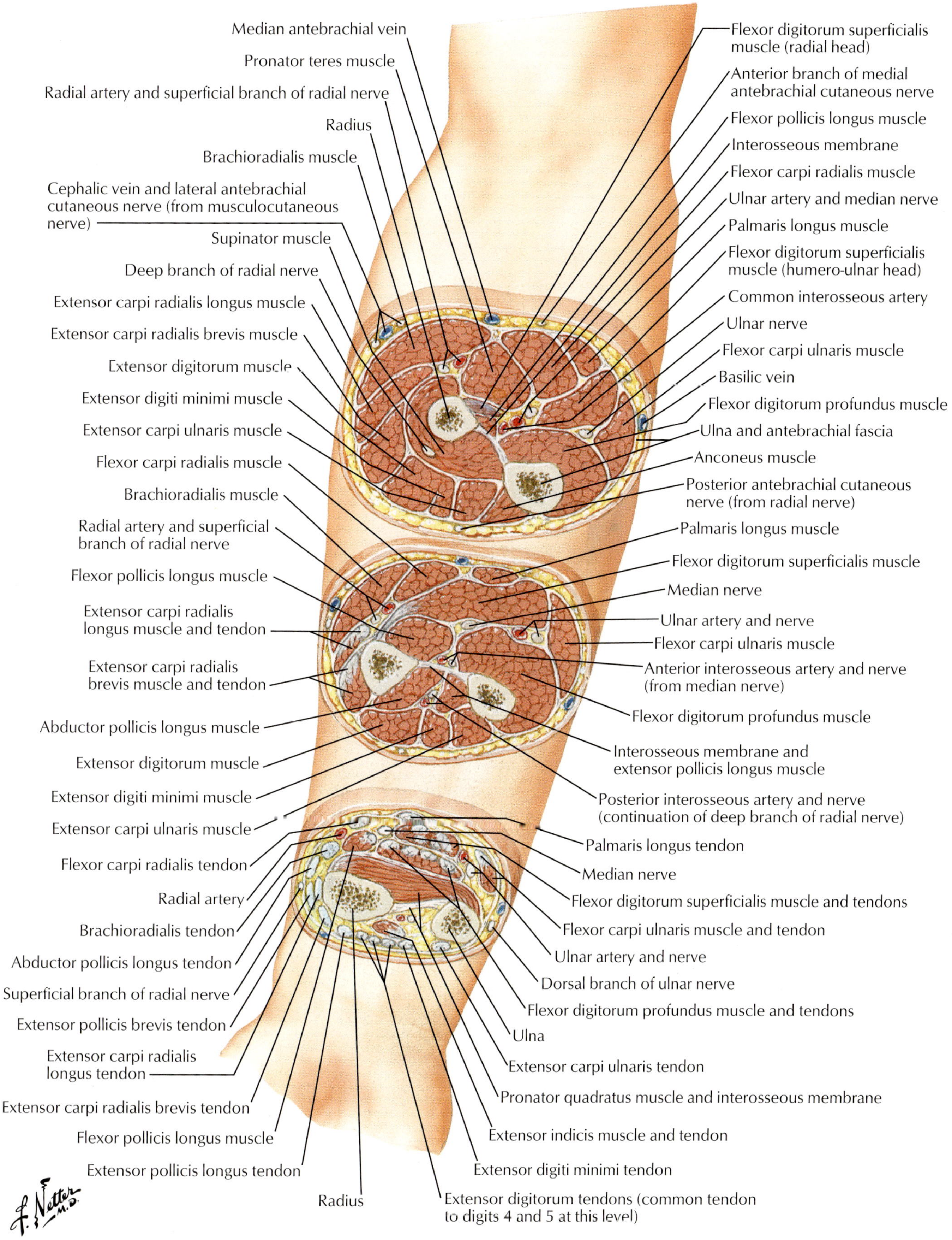

Attachments of Muscles of Forearm: Anterior View

See also Plate 422

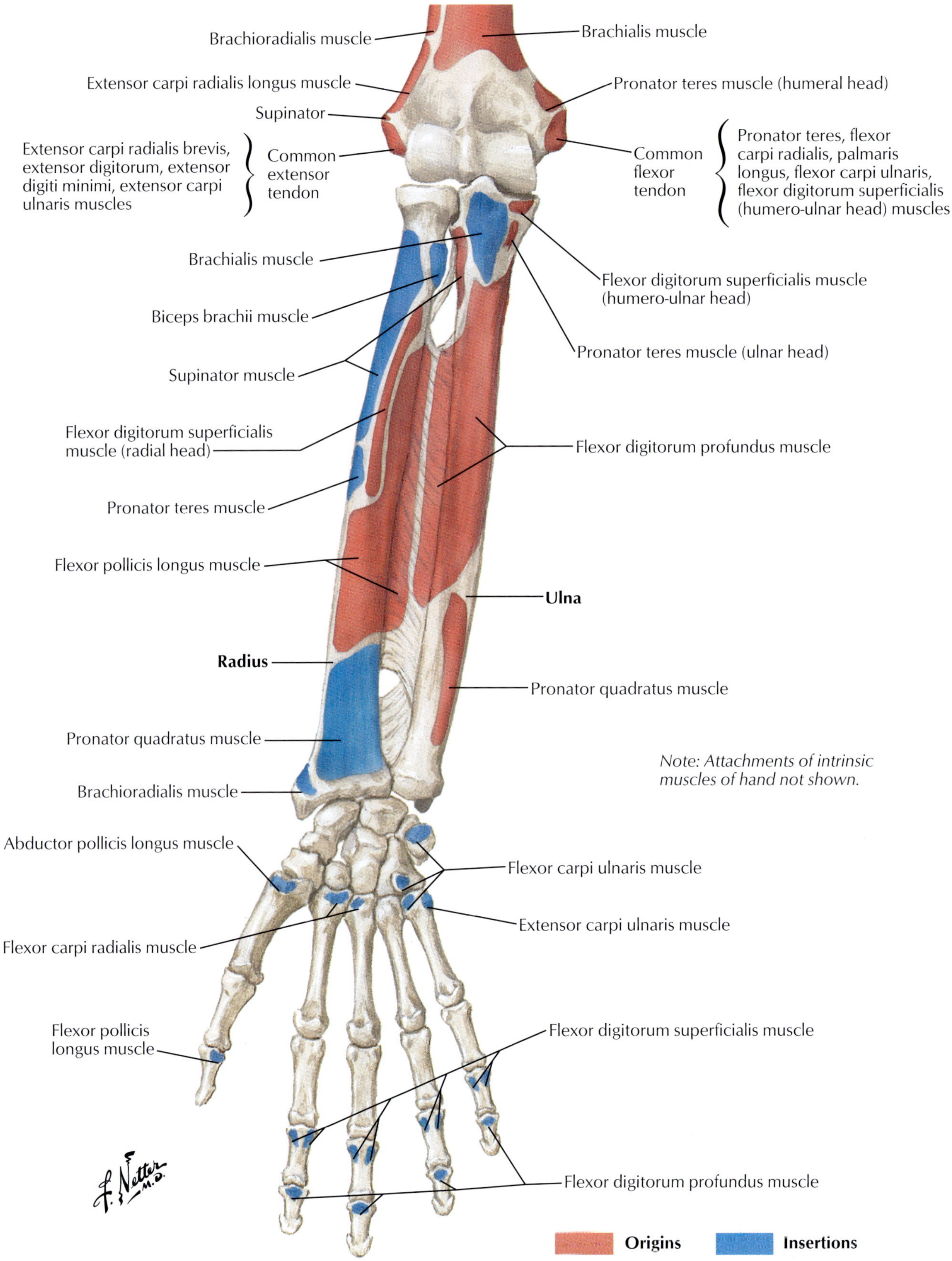

Attachments of Muscles of Forearm: Posterior View

See also Plate 427

Note: Attachments of intrinsic muscles of hand not shown.

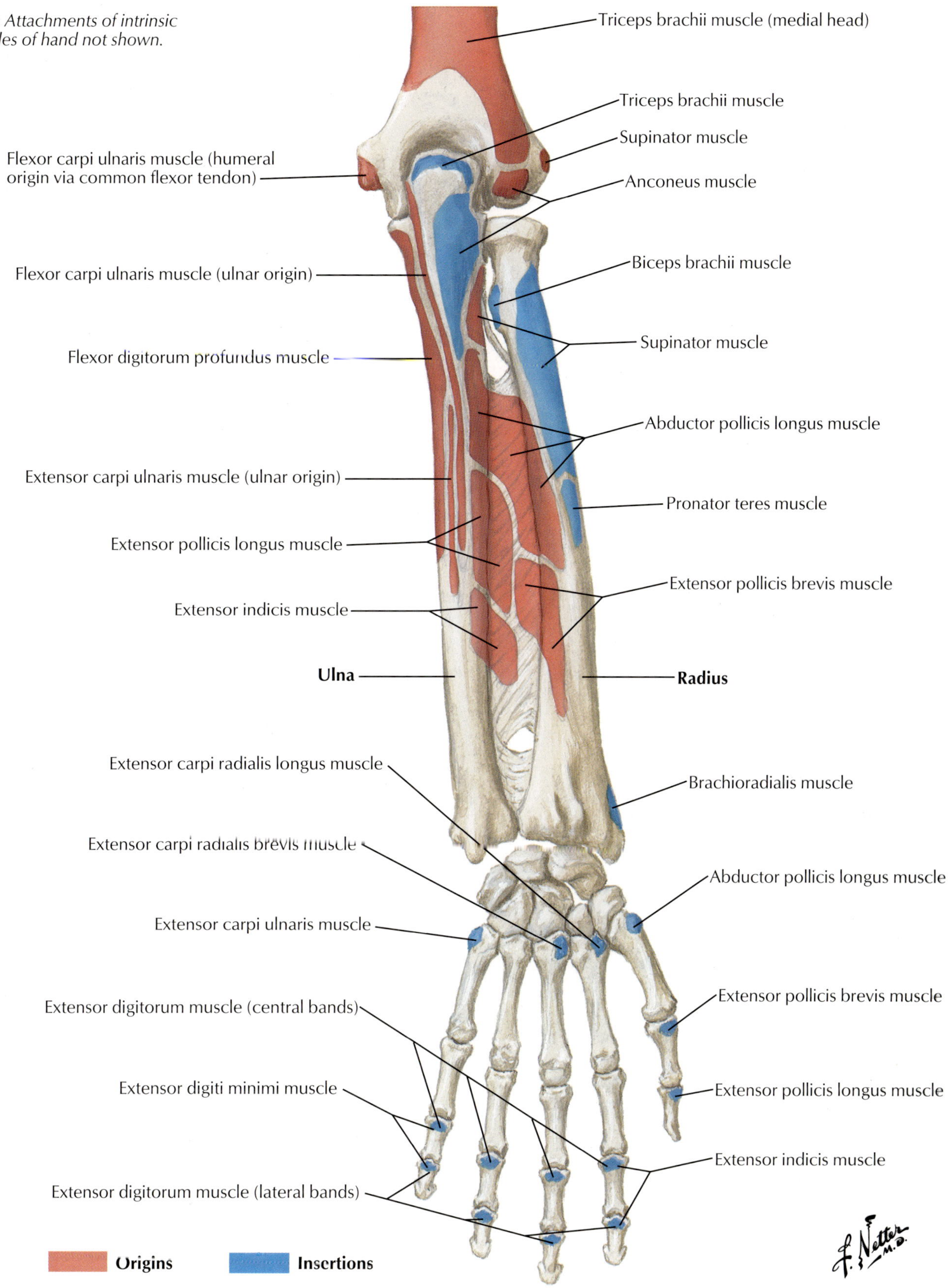

Carpal Bones

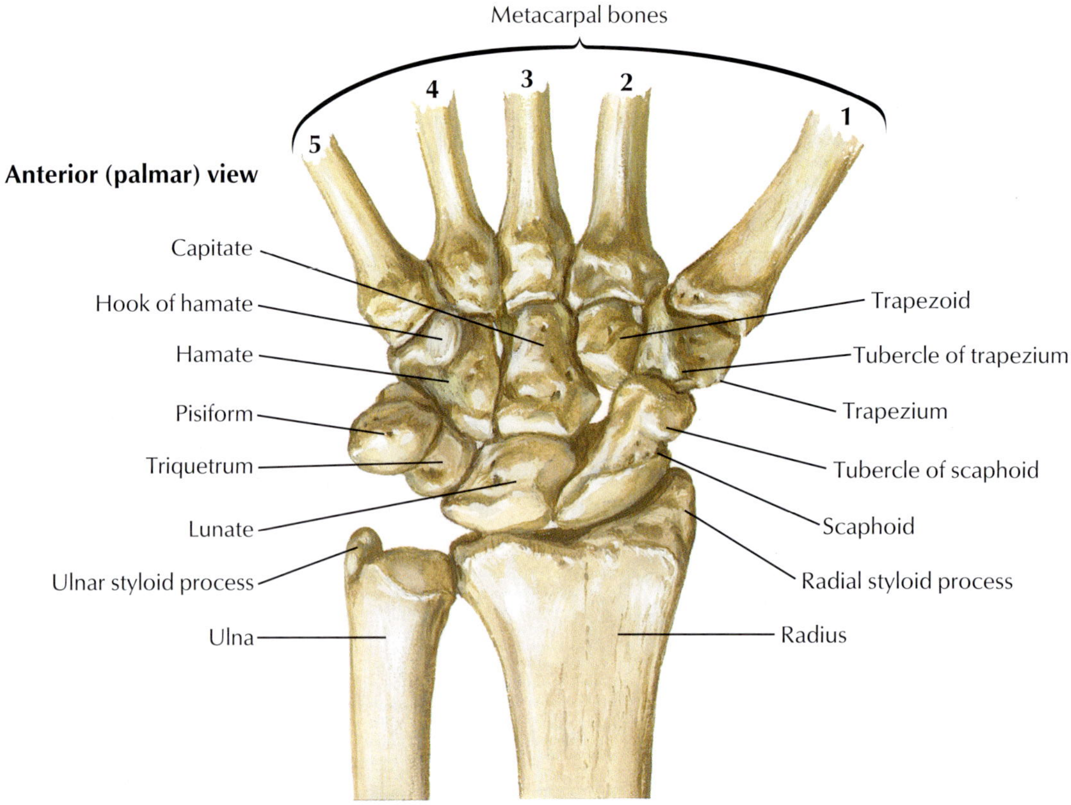

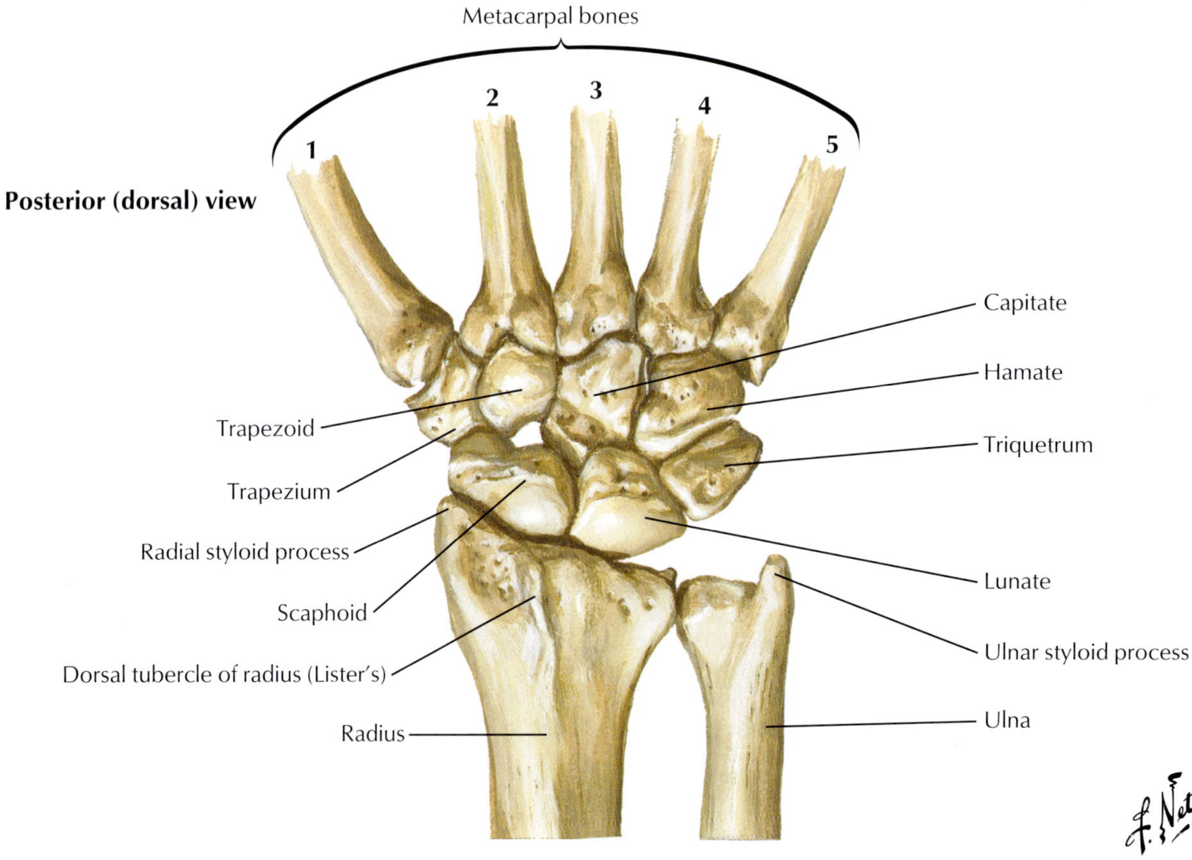

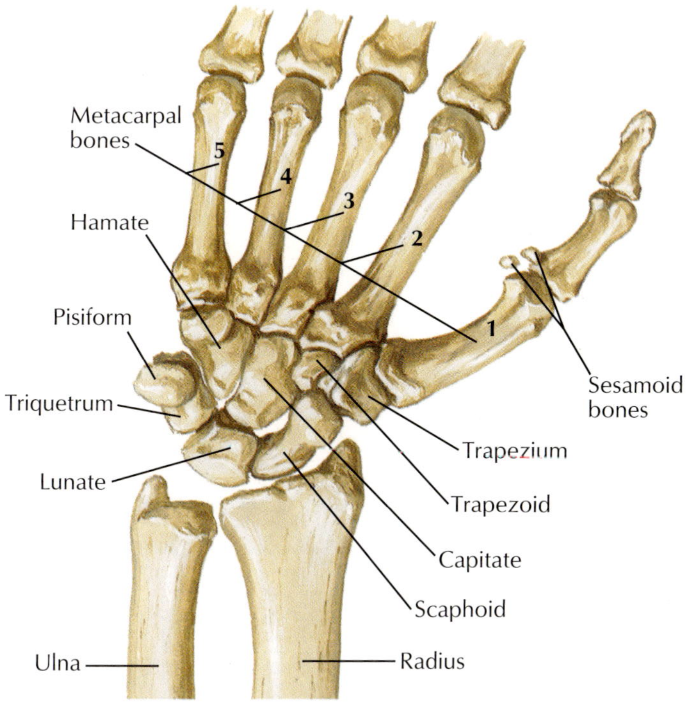

Position of carpal bones with hand in abduction: anterior (palmar) view

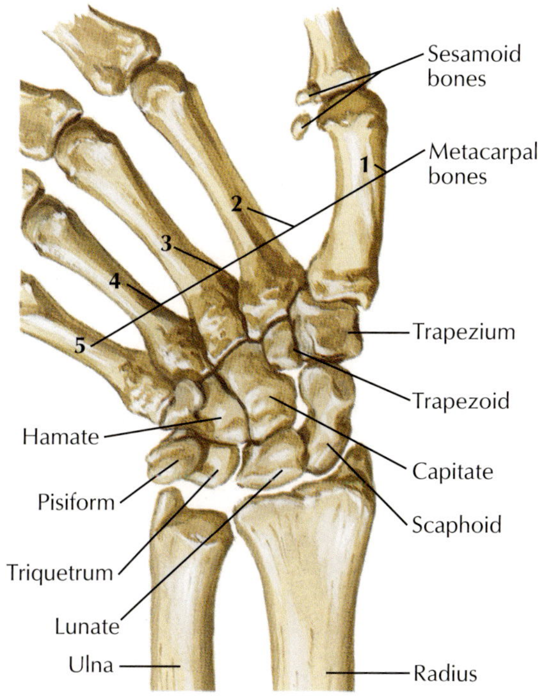

Position of carpal bones with hand in adduction: anterior (palmar) view

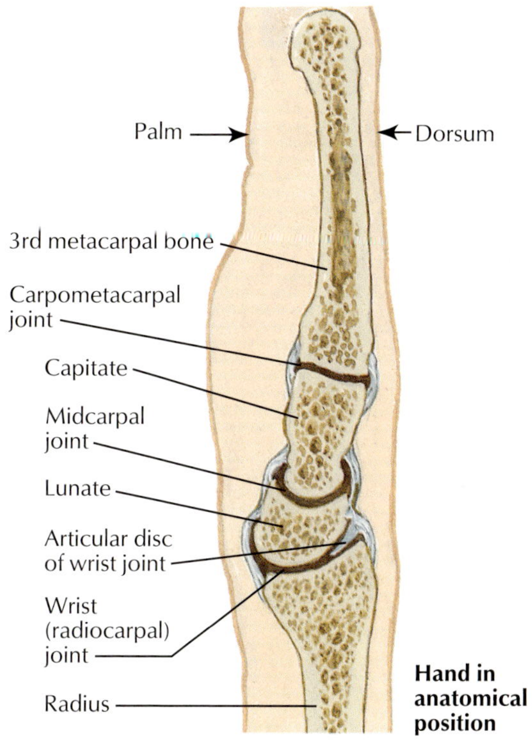

Hand in anatomical position

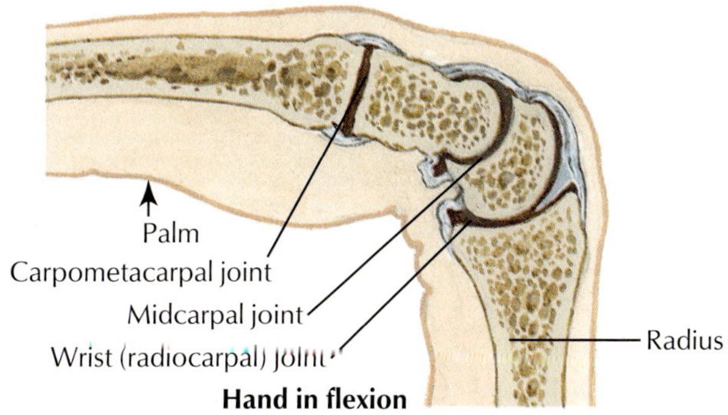

Hand in flexion

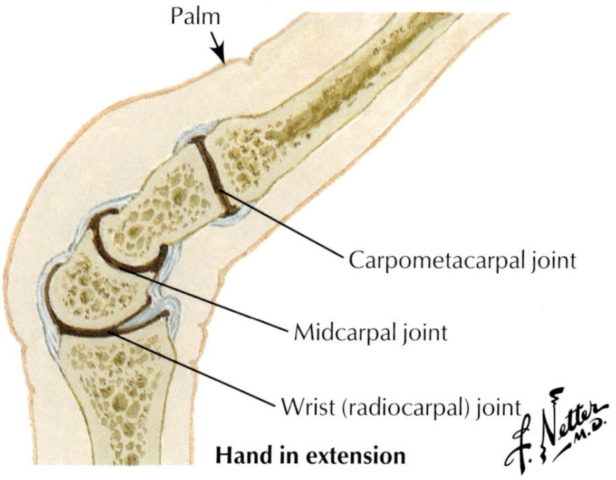

Hand in extension

Sagittal sections through wrist and middle finger

Carpal tunnel: palmar view

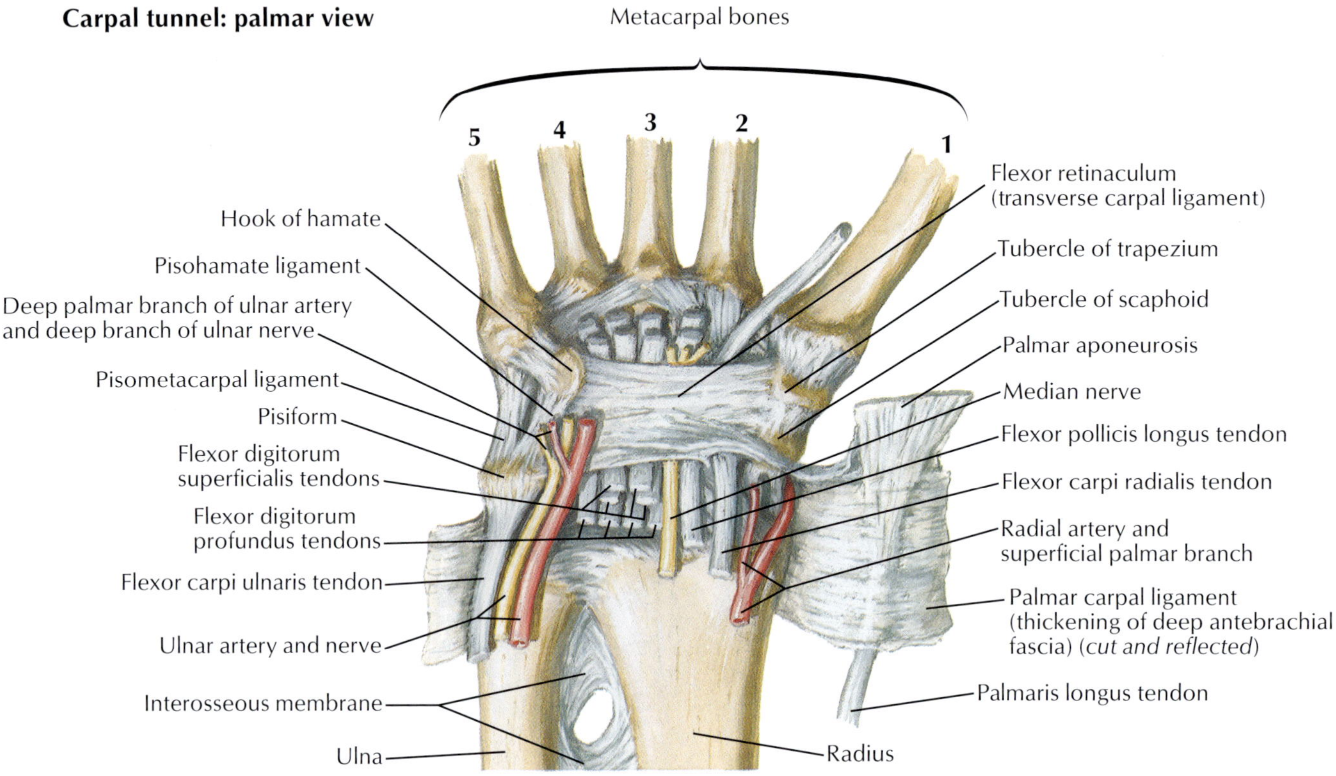

Flexor retinaculum removed: palmar view

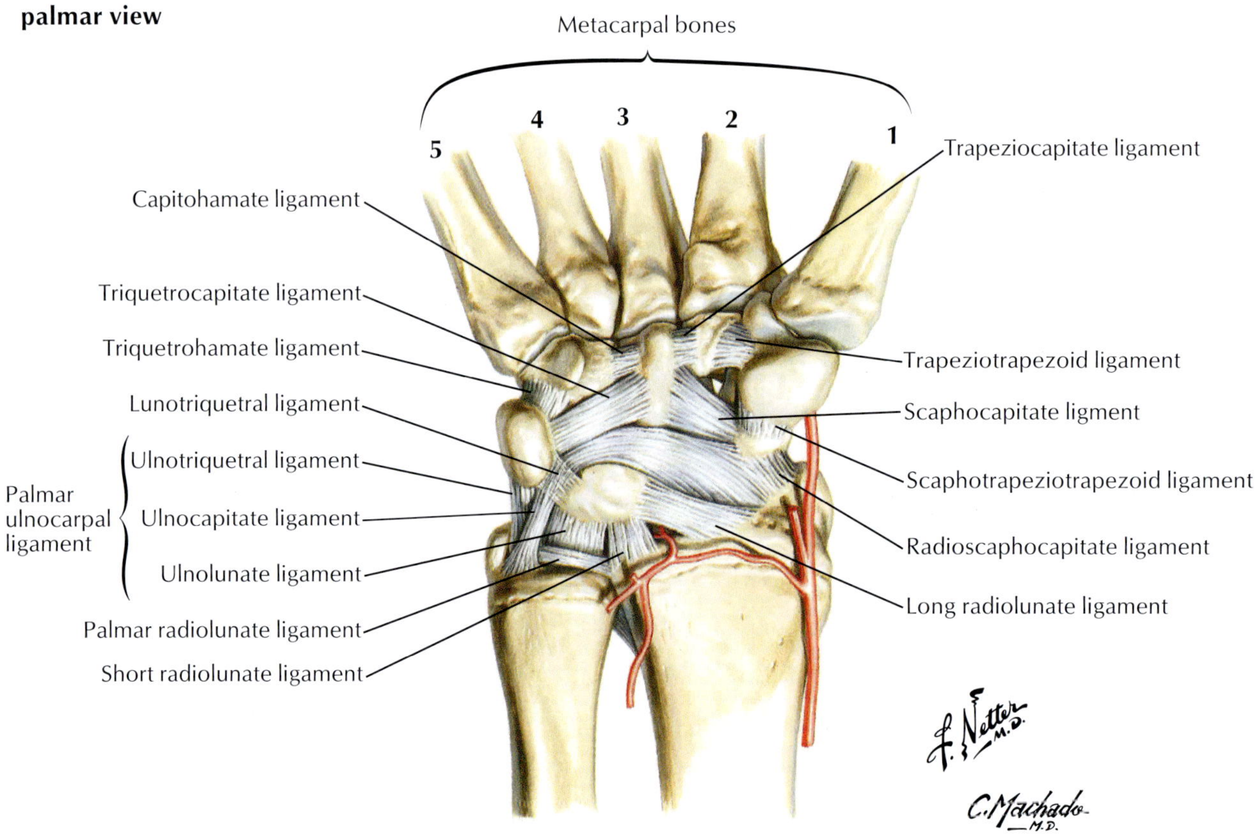

See also Plate 425

Posterior (dorsal) view

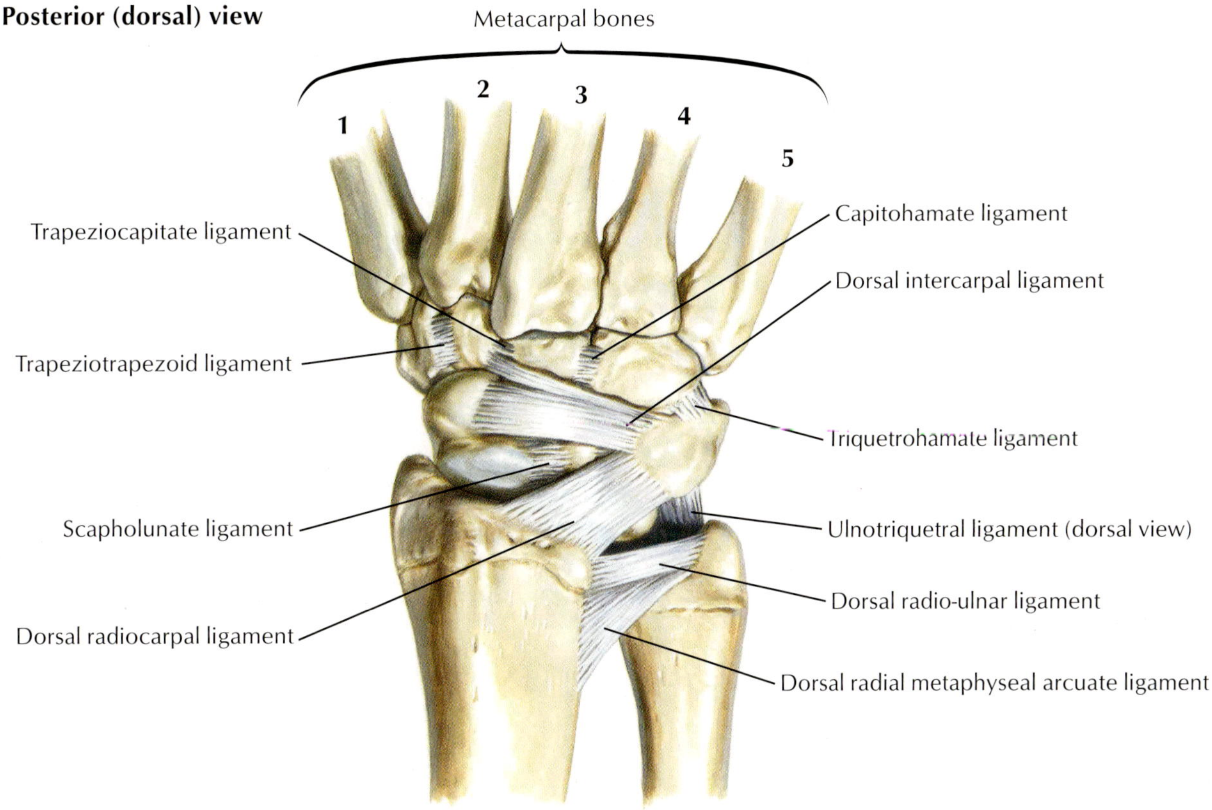

Coronal section: dorsal view

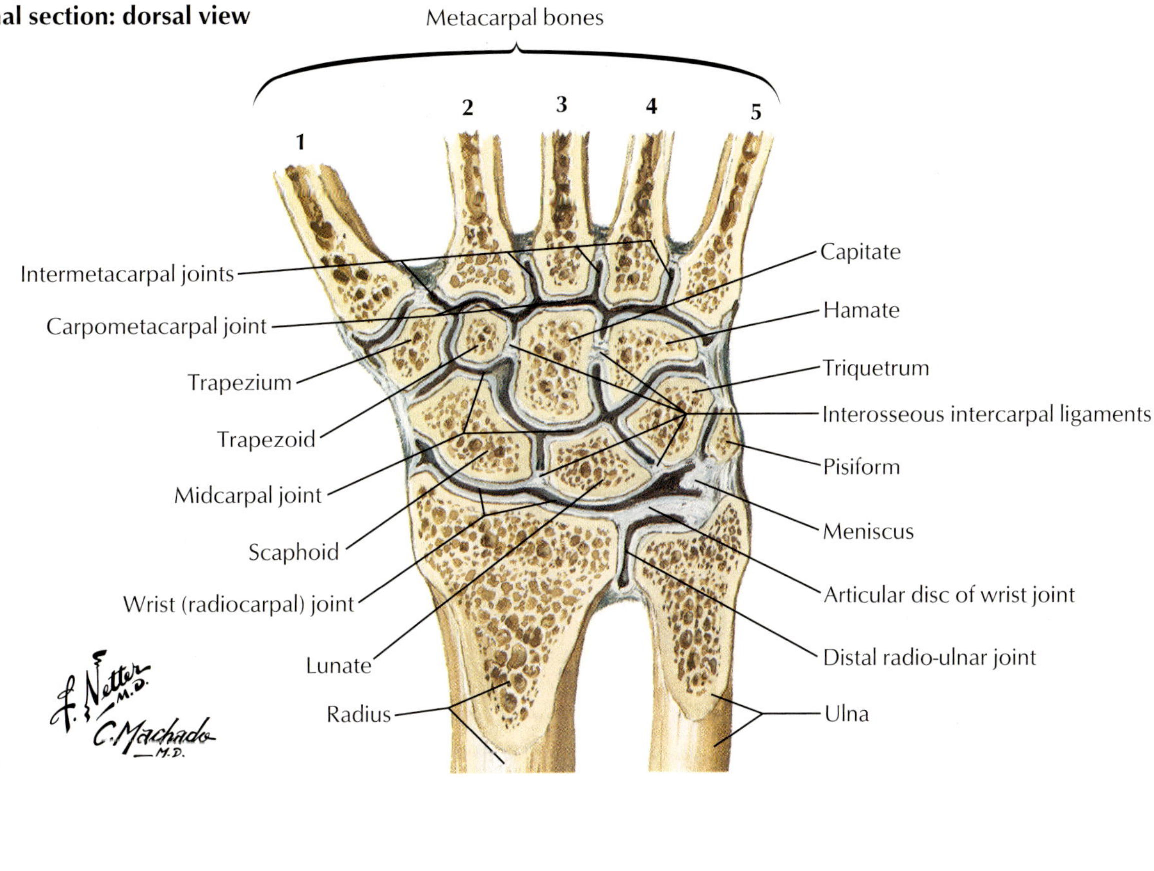

Bones of Wrist and Hand

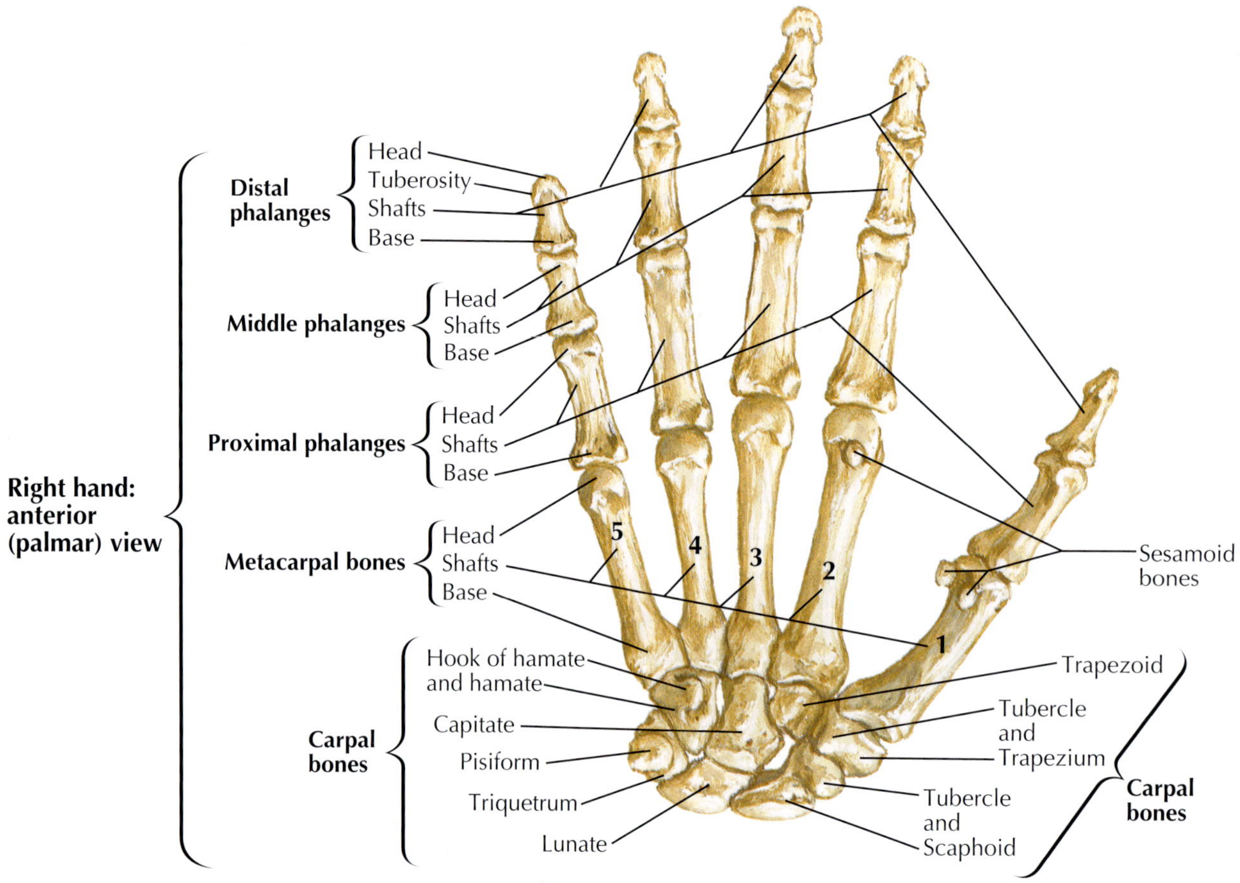

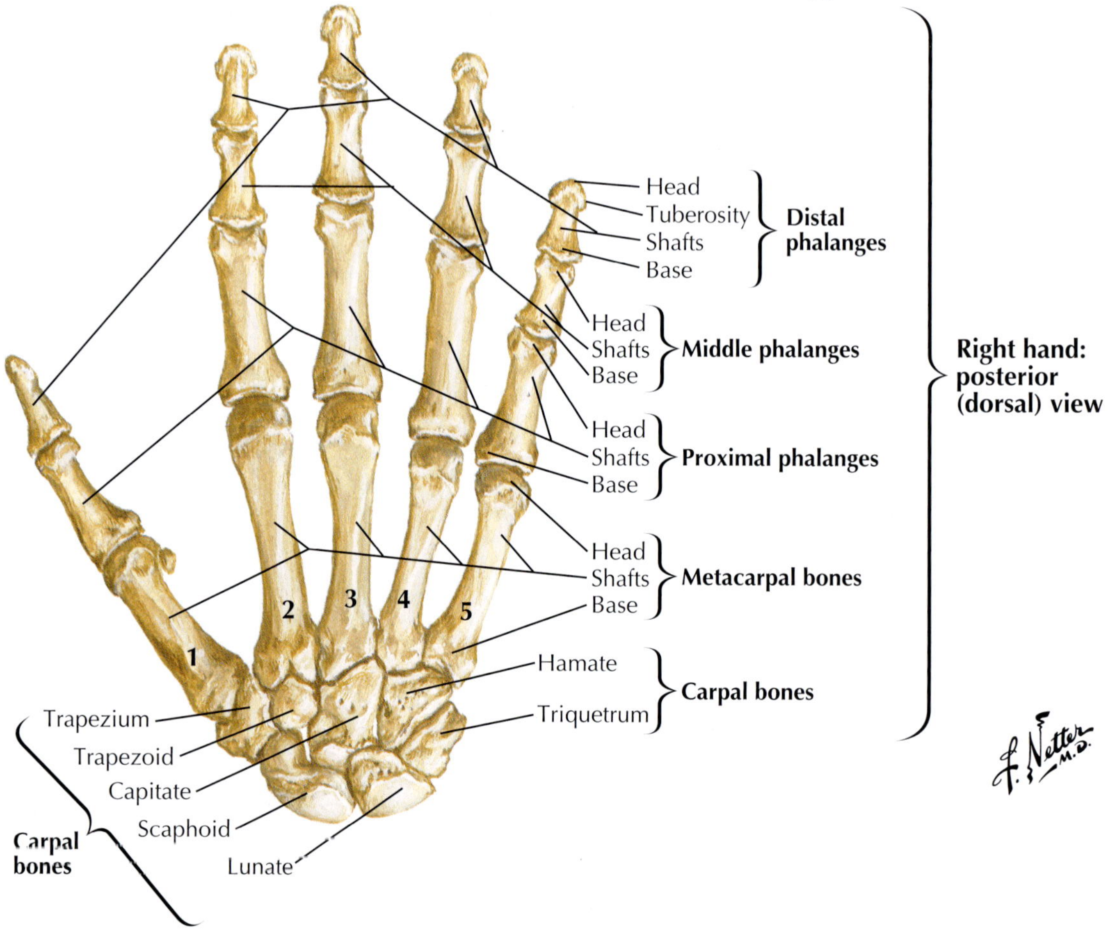

See also Plate 456

Anteroposterior view

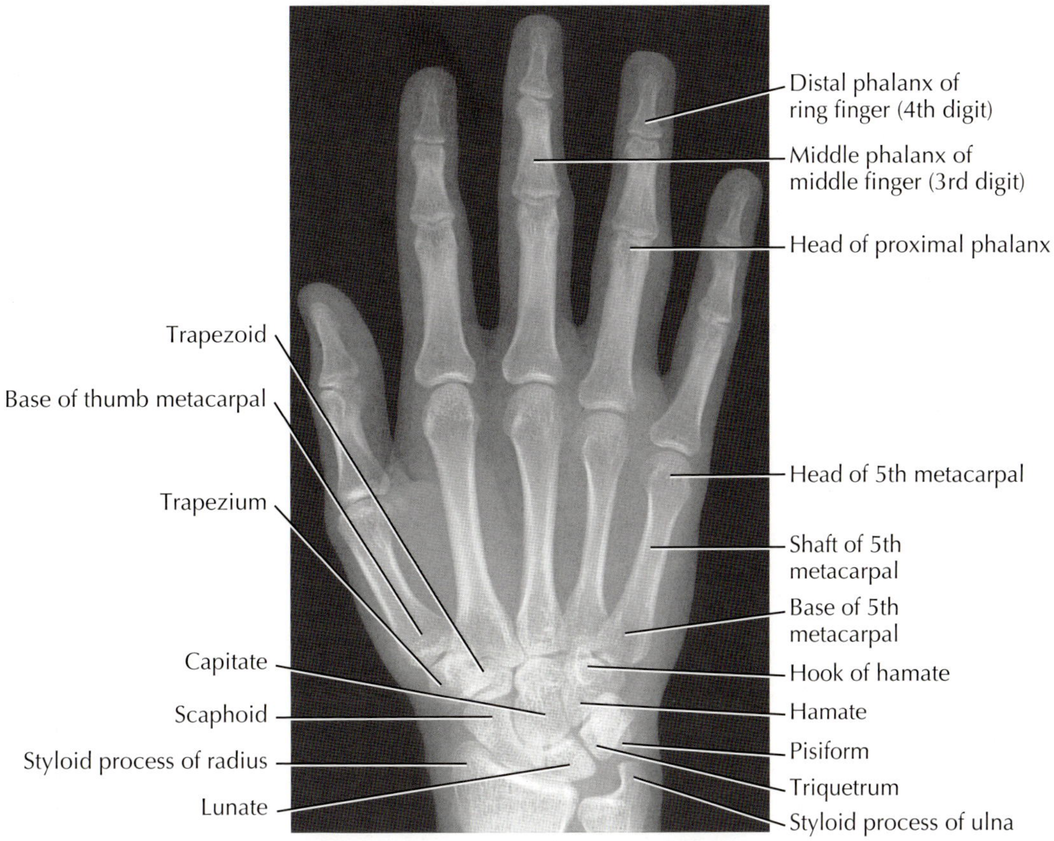

Lateral view

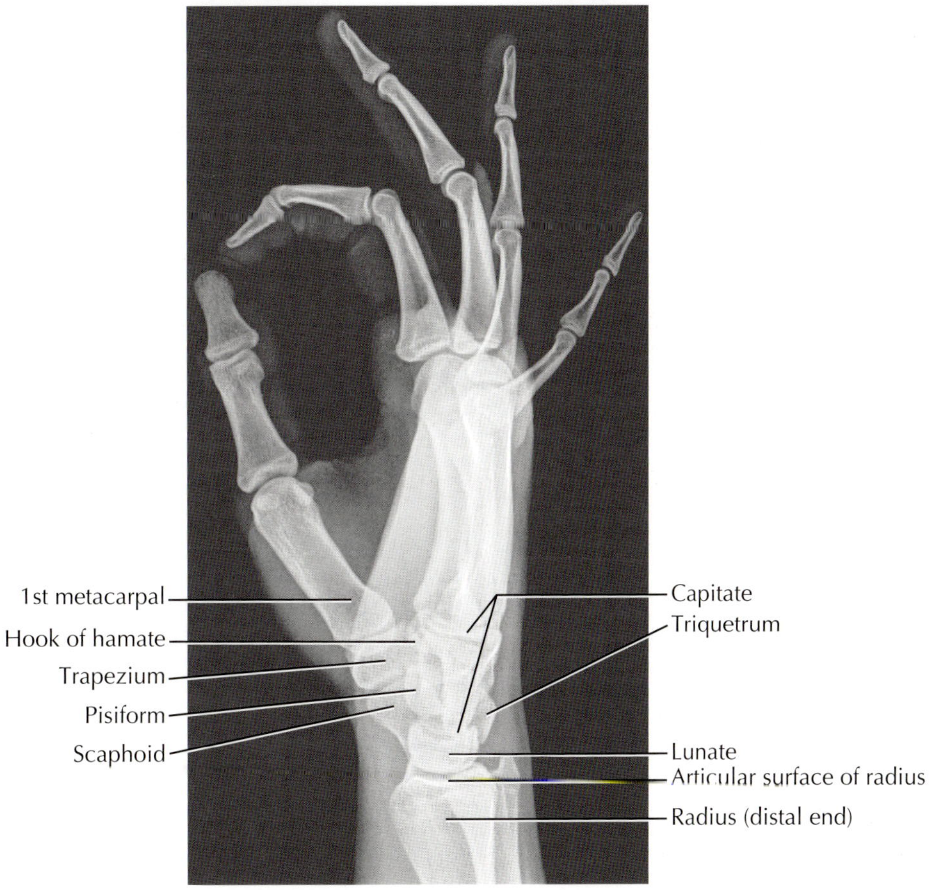

Metacarpophalangeal and Interphalangeal Ligaments

See also **Plates 448, 451**

Anterior (palmar) view

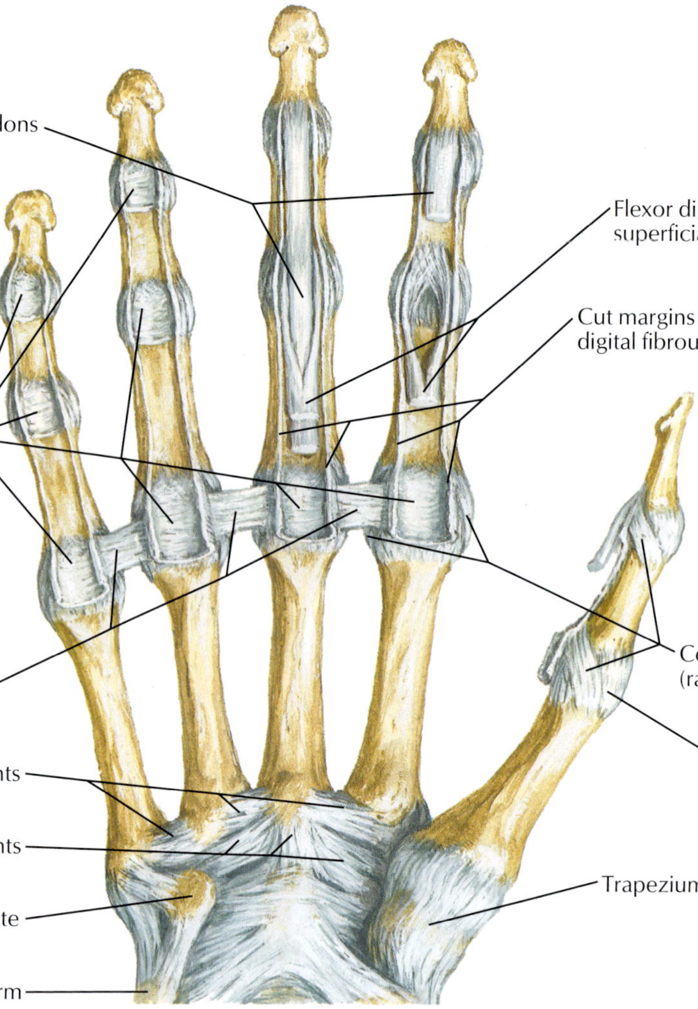

In extension: medial view

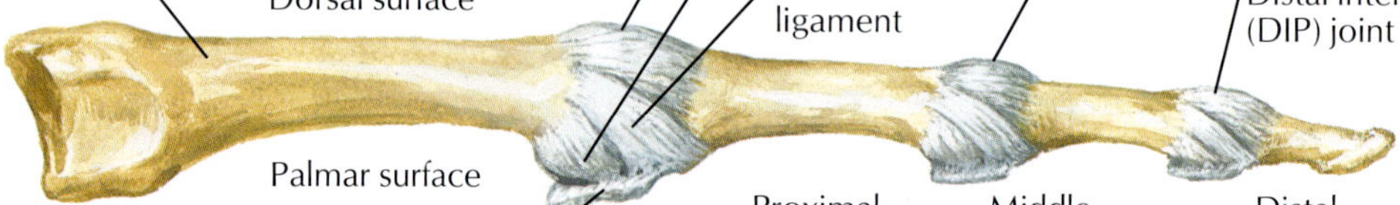

In flexion: medial view

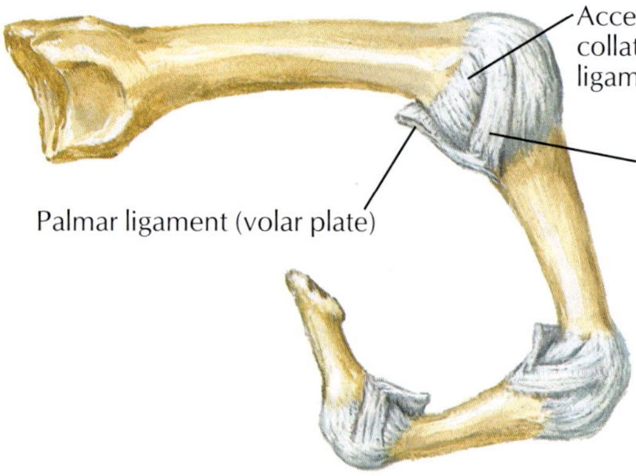

Note: Ligaments of metacarpophalangeal and interphalangeal joints are similar.

Anterior (palmar) views

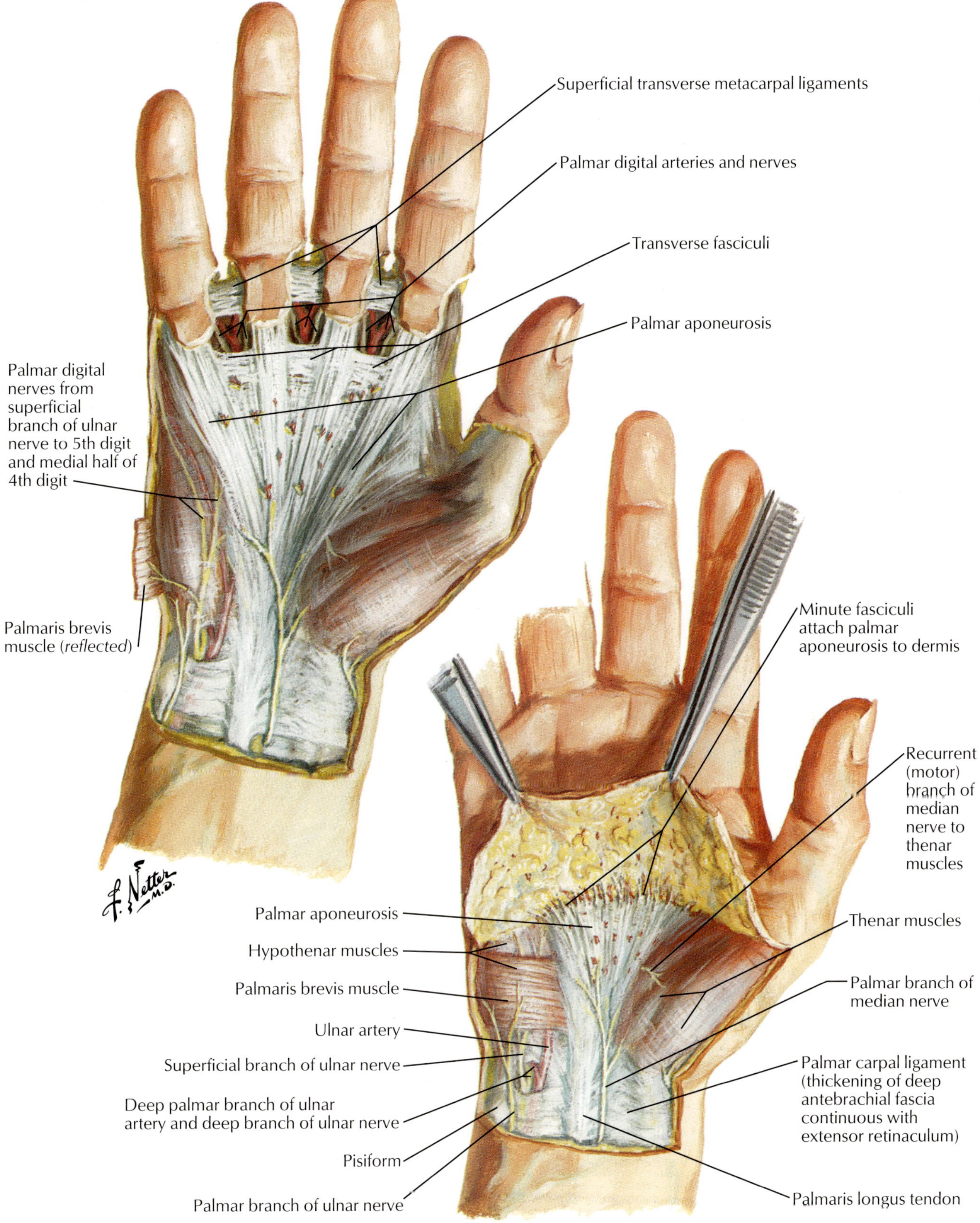

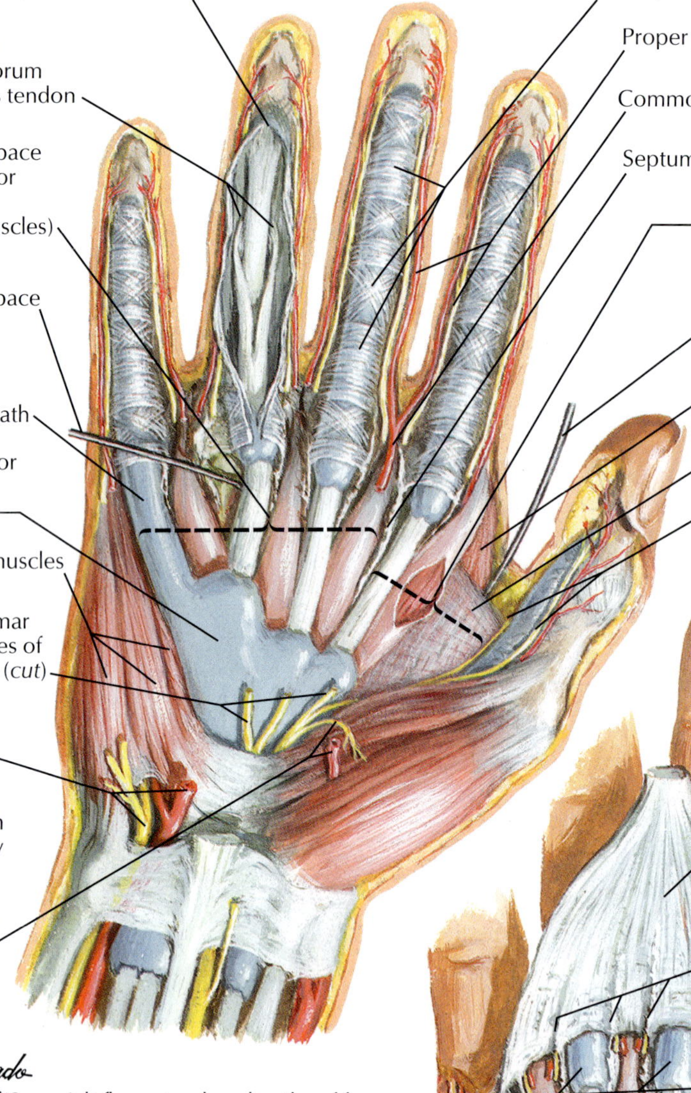

Anterior (palmar) views

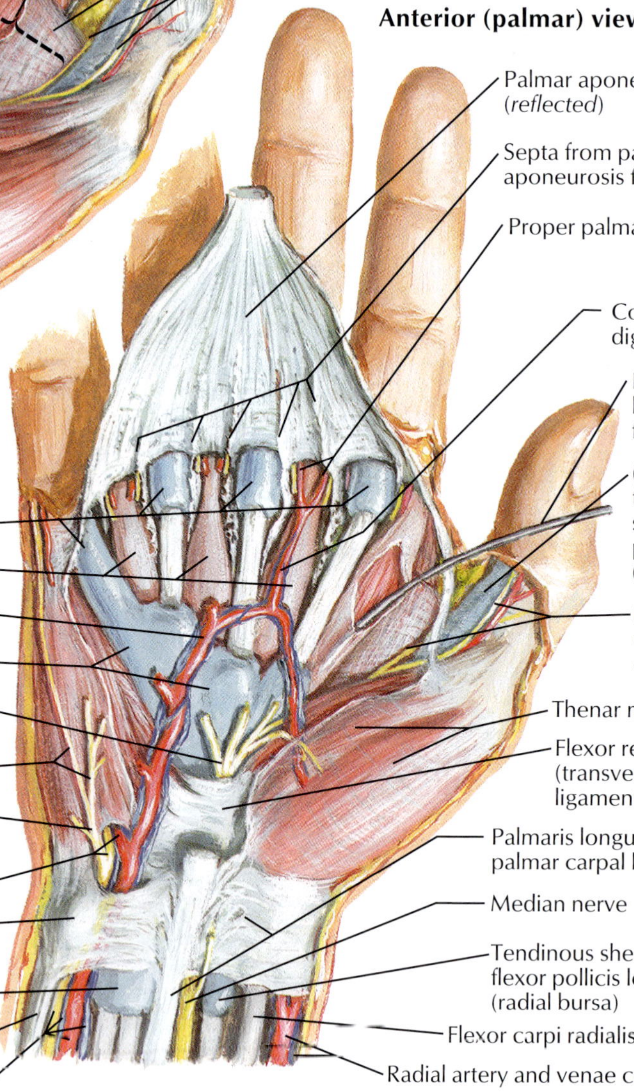

Lumbrical Muscles and Bursae, Spaces, and Sheaths: Schema

See also Plate 445

Common variation

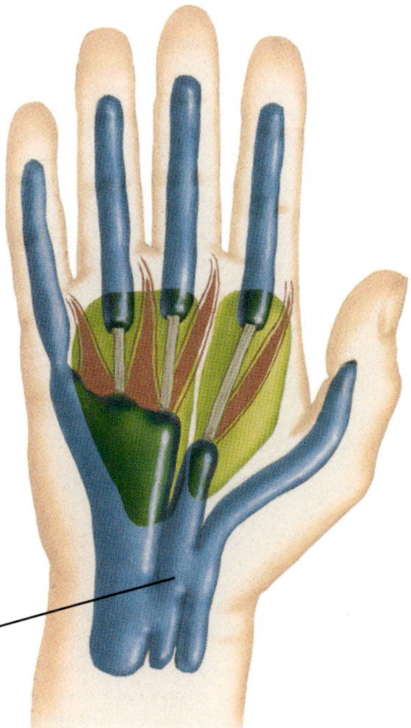

Usual arrangement

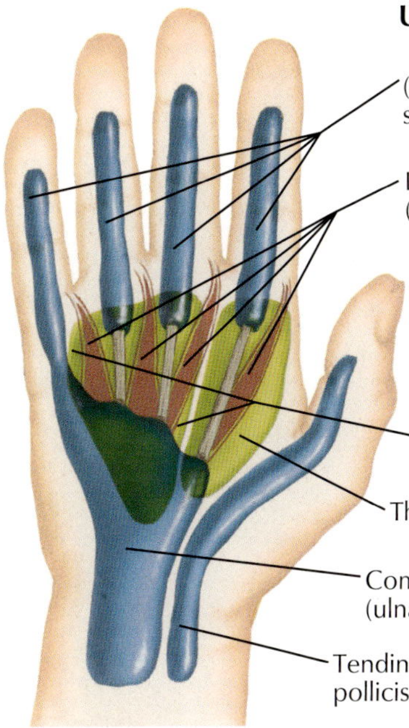

Lumbrical muscles: schema

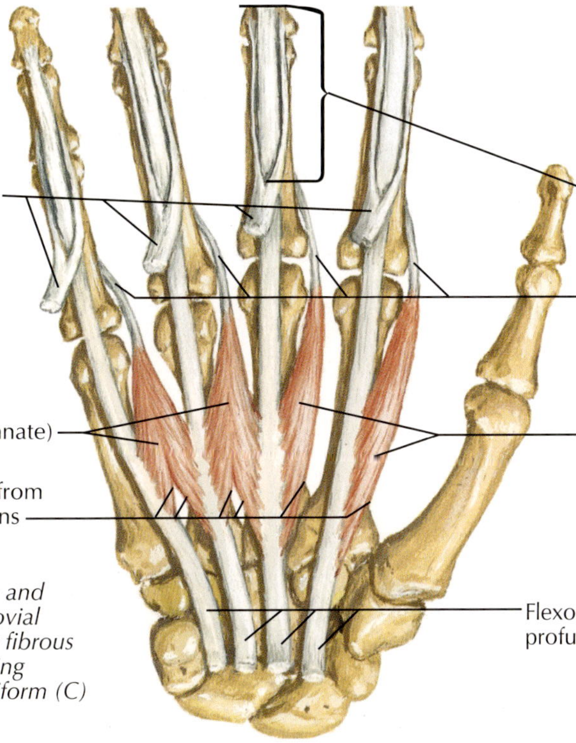

Note: Flexor digitorum superficialis and profundus tendons encased in synovial sheaths are bound to phalanges by fibrous digital sheaths made up of alternating strong anular (A) and weaker cruciform (C) parts (pulleys).

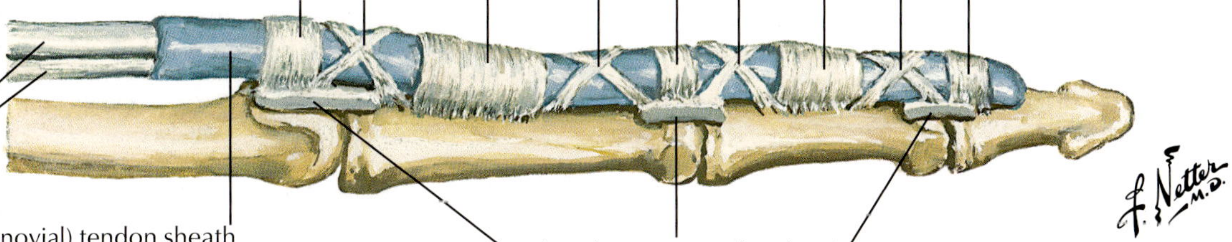

See also Plates 459, 460

Palmar view

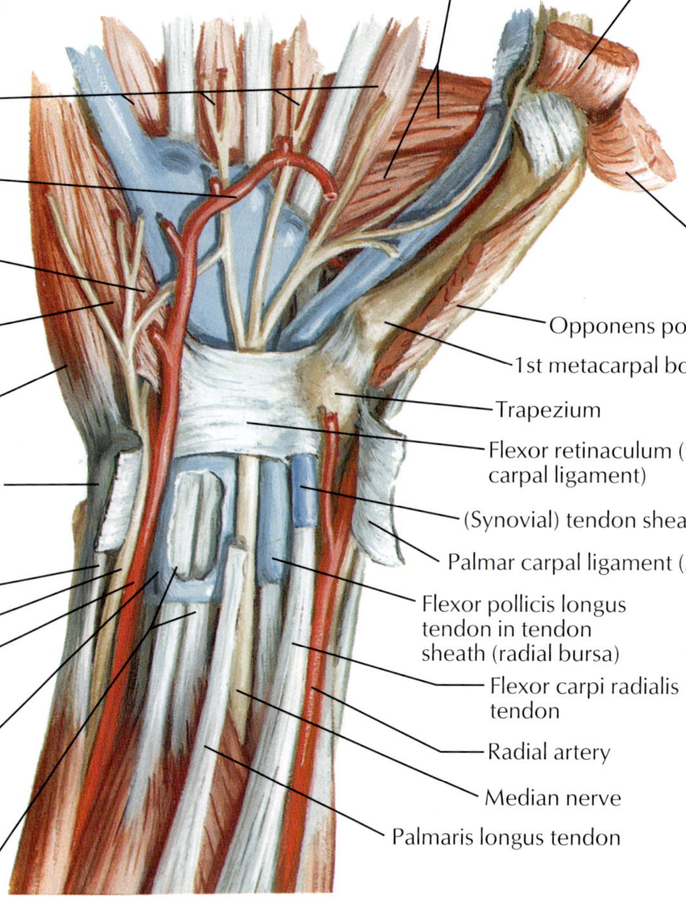

Cross section of wrist demonstrating carpal tunnel

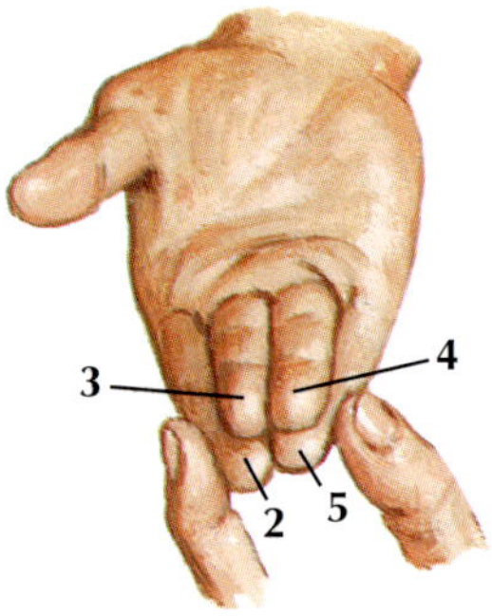

Simple method of demonstrating arrangement of flexor digitorum superficialis tendons within carpal tunnel

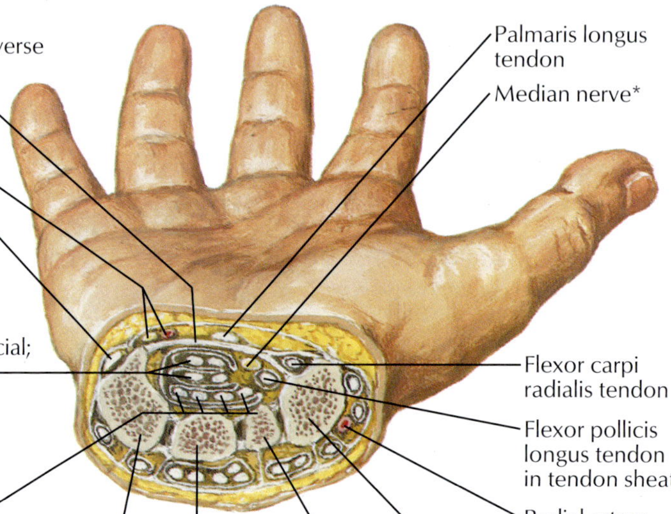

*Contents of carpal tunnel

Bursae, Spaces, and Tendon Sheaths of Hand

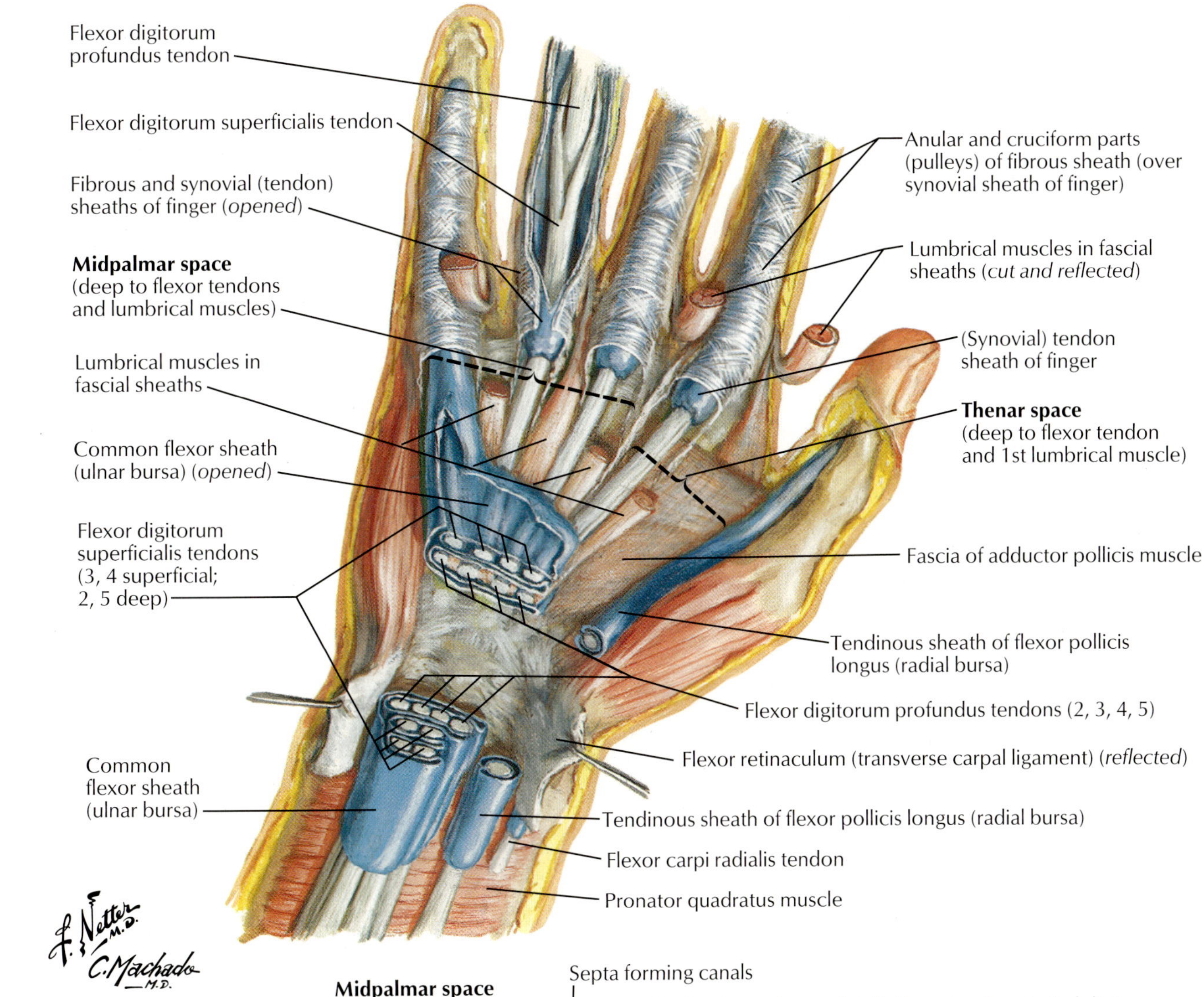

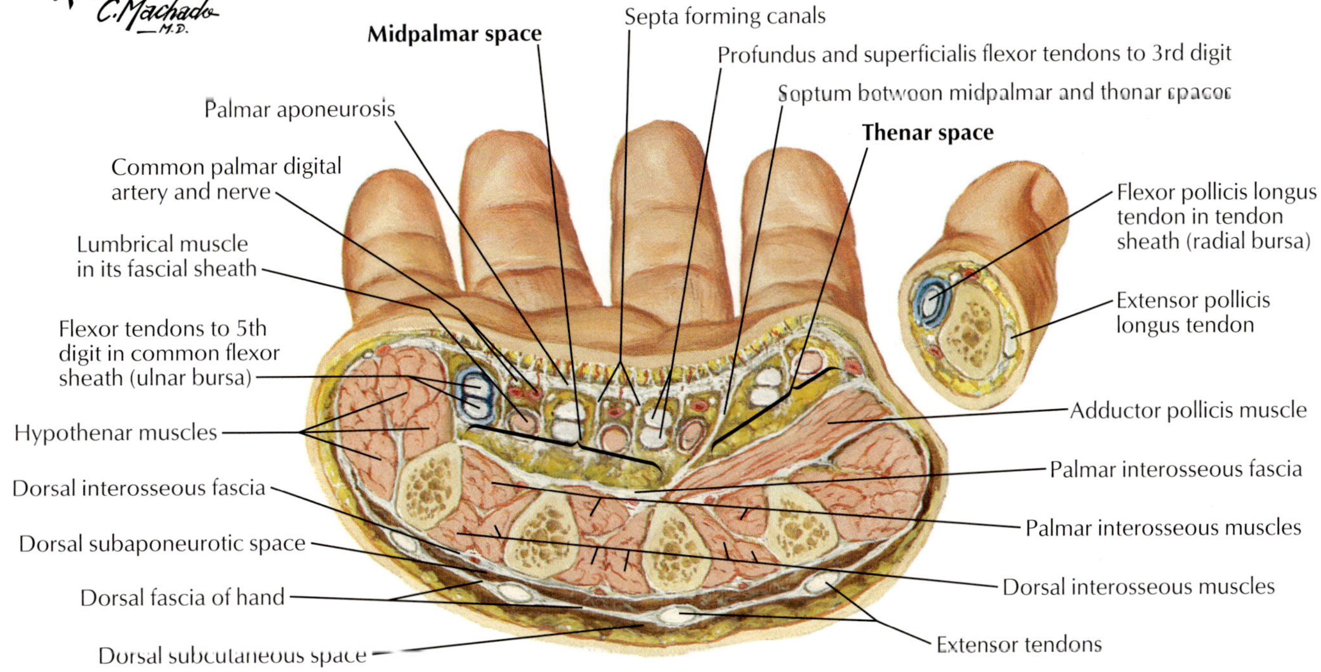

Flexor and Extensor Tendons in Fingers

See also Plate 445

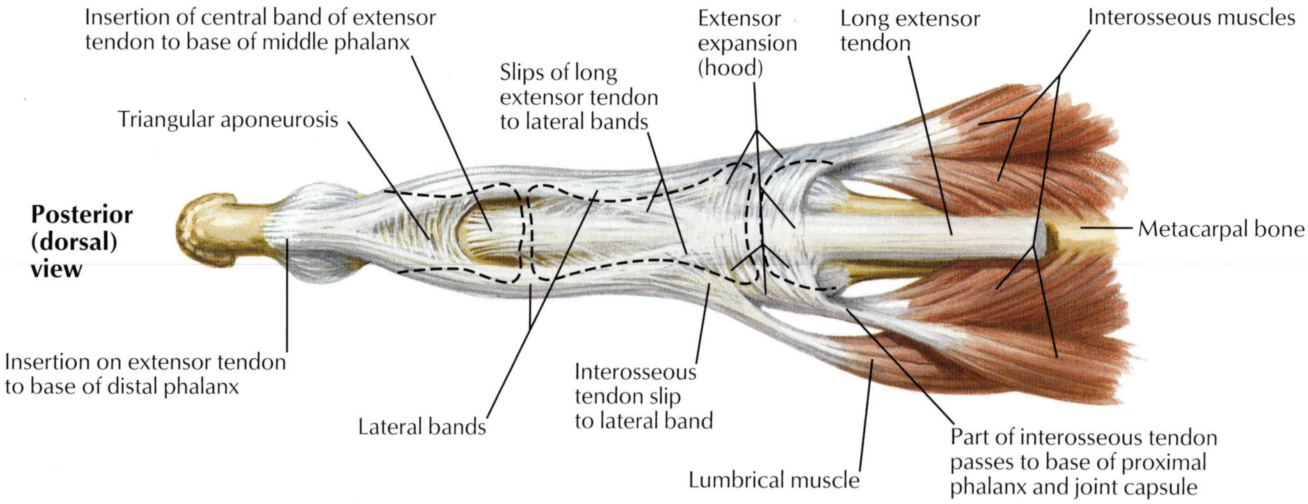

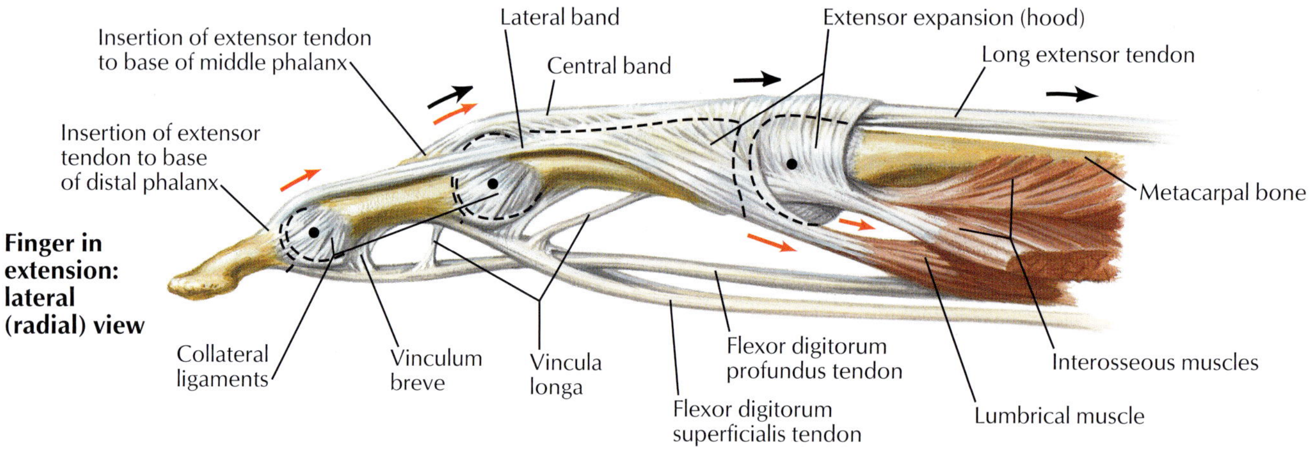

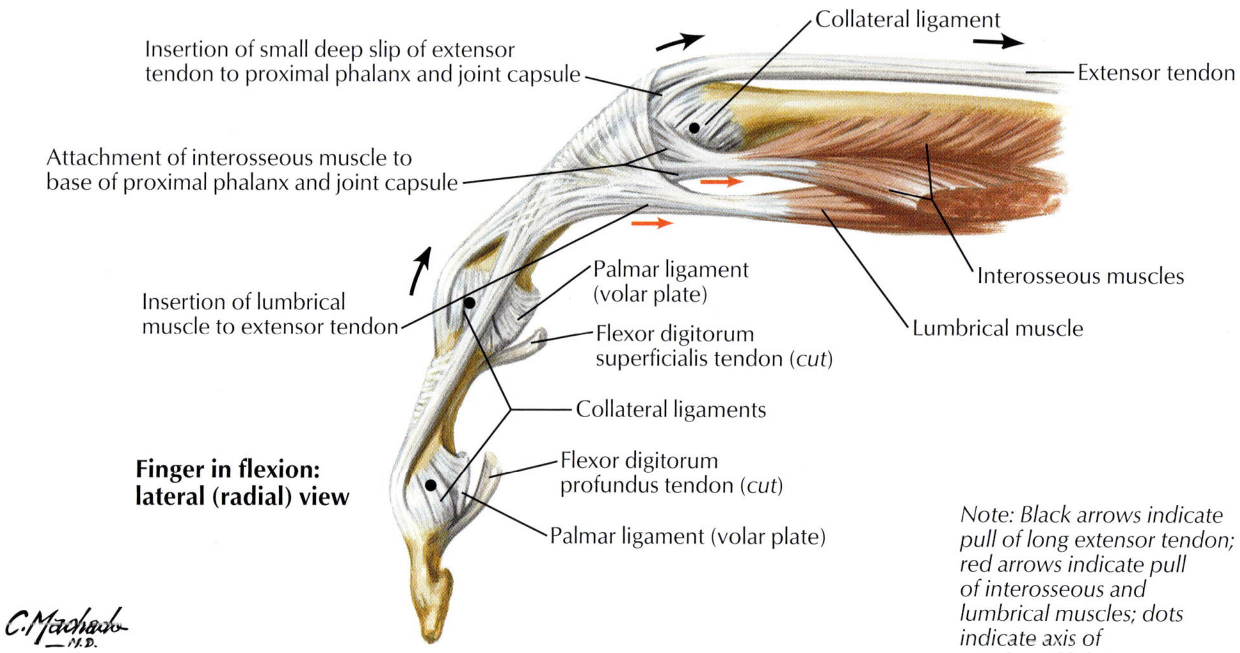

Note: Black arrows indicate pull of long extensor tendon; red arrows indicate pull of interosseous and lumbrical muscles; dots indicate axis of rotation of joints.

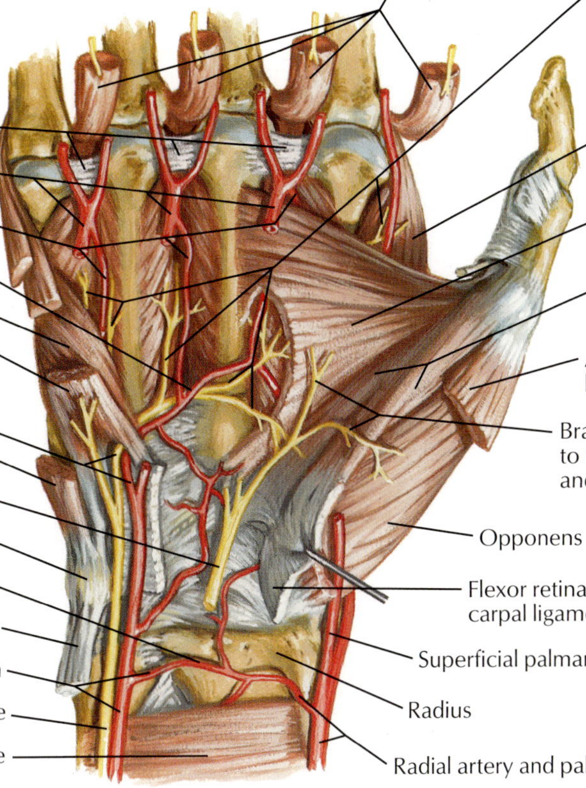

Anterior (palmar) view

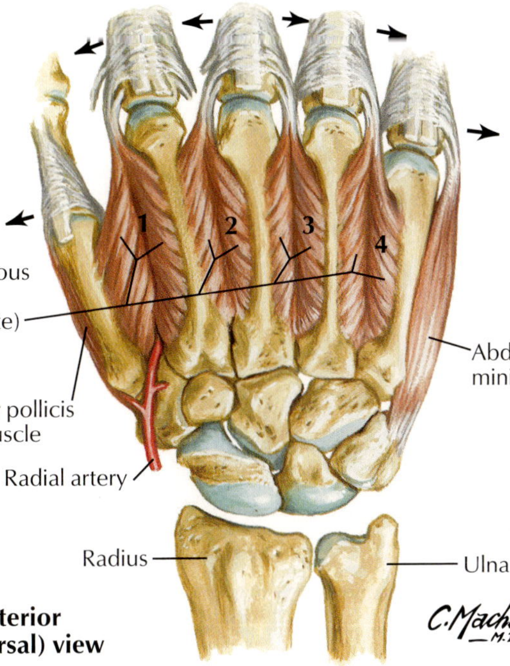

Posterior (dorsal) view

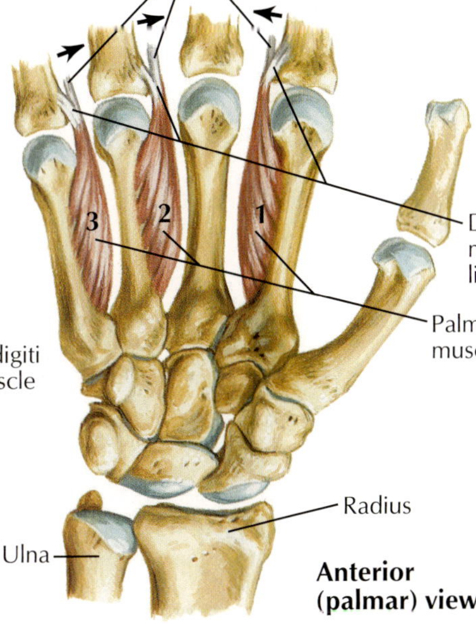

Anterior (palmar) view

Note: Arrows indicate action of muscles.

See also Plate 420

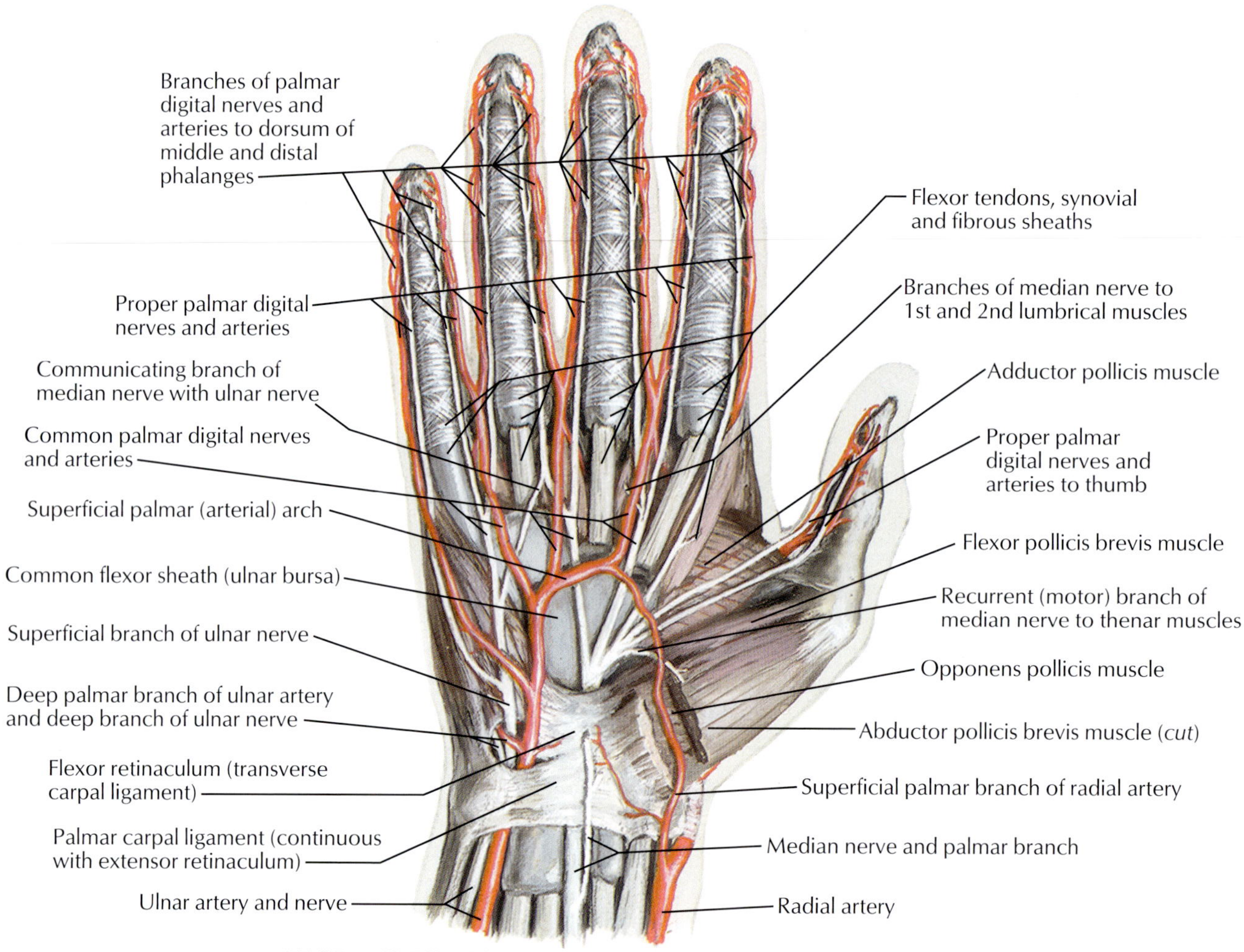

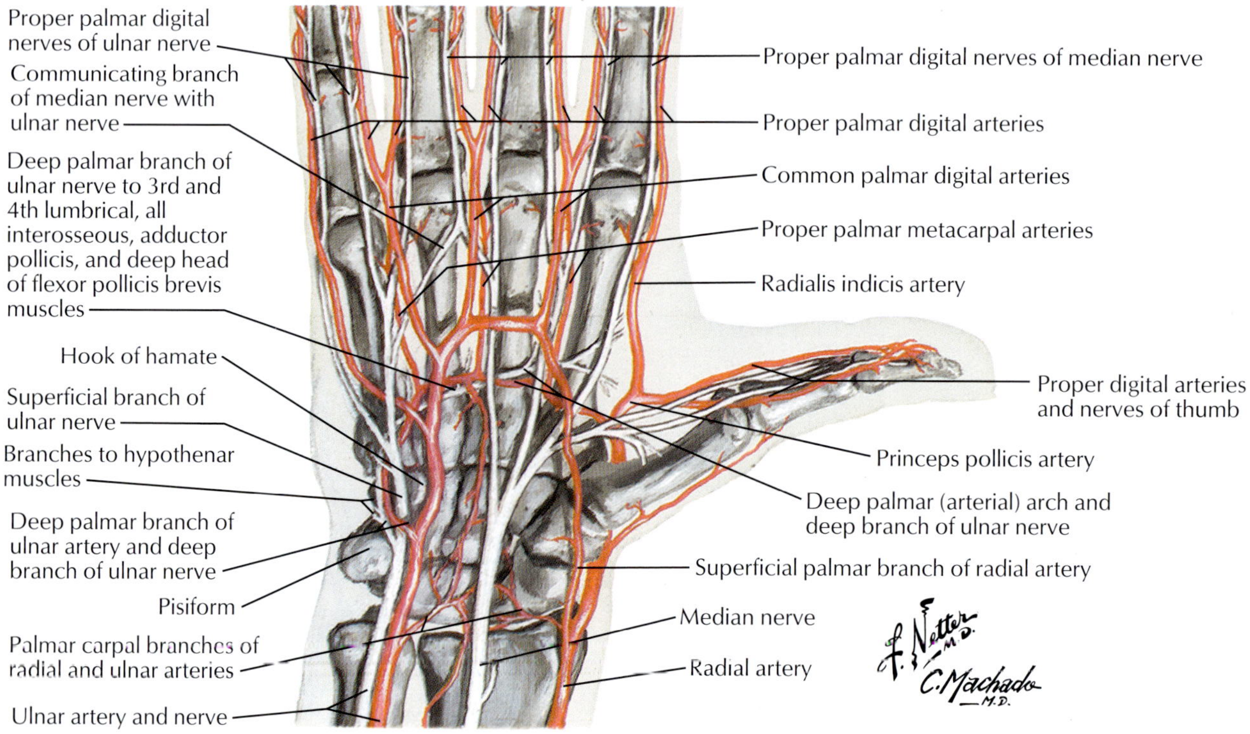

Wrist and Hand: Superficial Radial Dissection

See also Plate 466

Lateral (radial) view

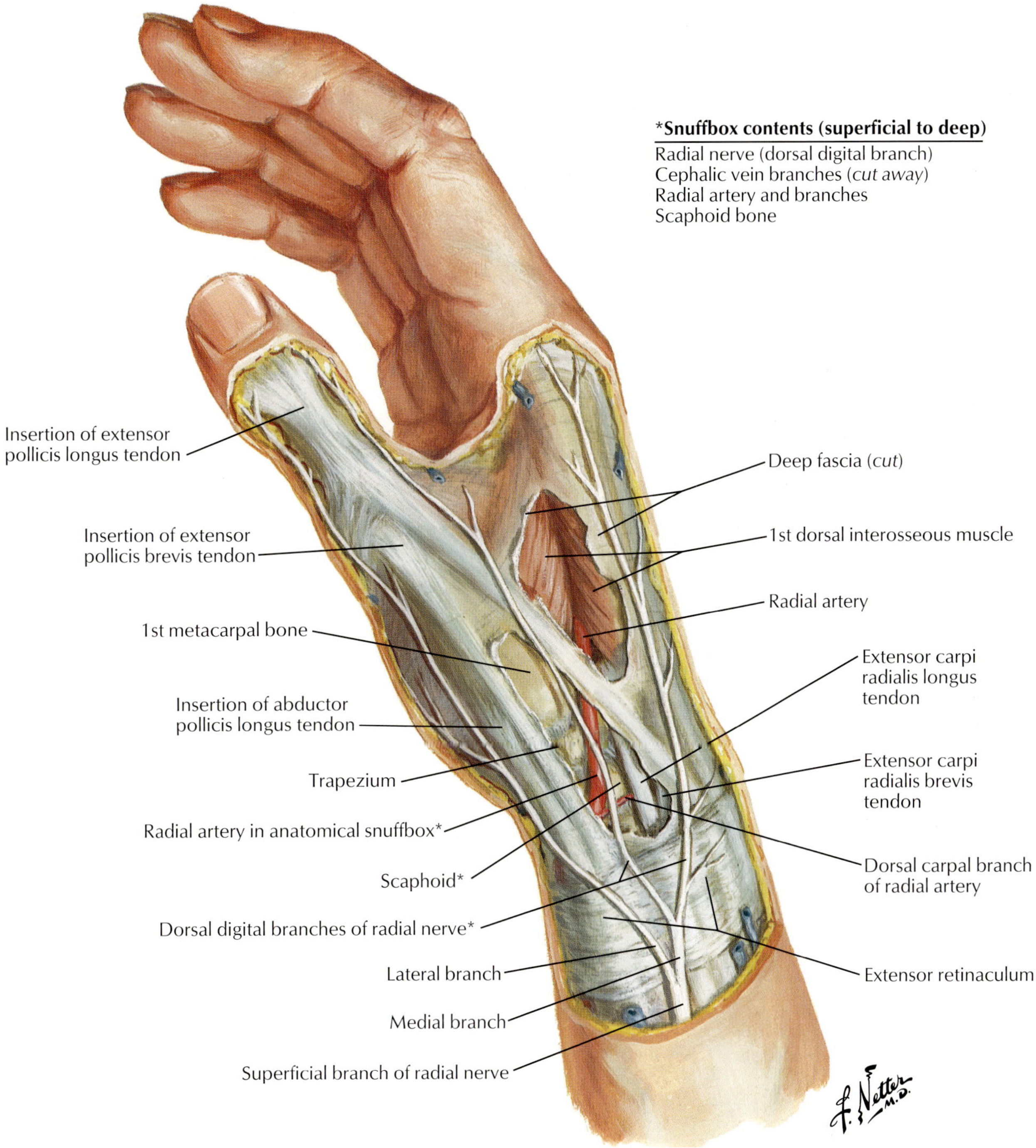

***Snuffbox contents (superficial to deep)**

Radial nerve (dorsal digital branch)
Cephalic vein branches (*cut away*)
Radial artery and branches
Scaphoid bone

See also Plates 402, 403

Posterior (dorsal) view

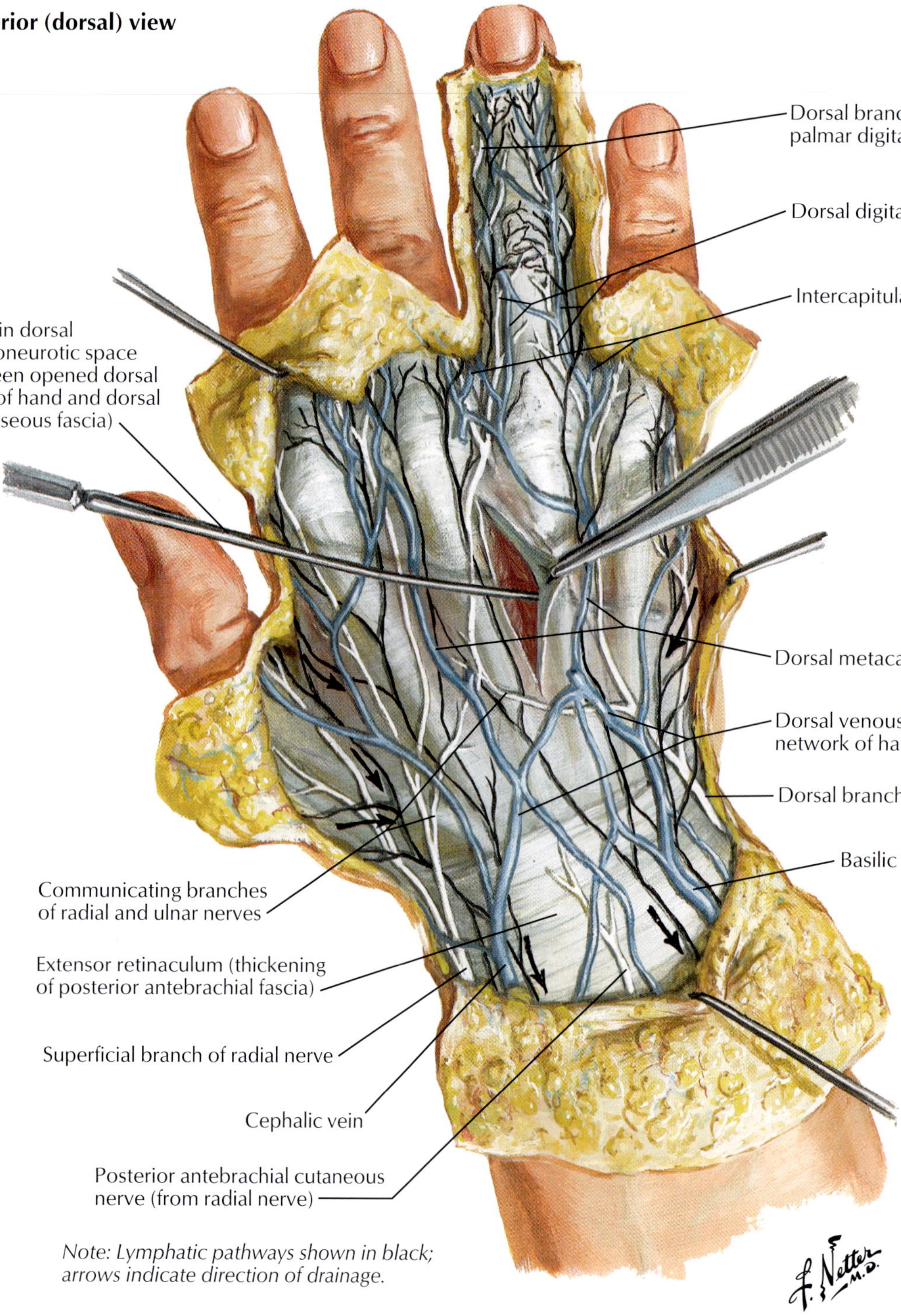

Note: Lymphatic pathways shown in black; arrows indicate direction of drainage.

Wrist and Hand: Deep Dorsal Dissection

See also Plate 445

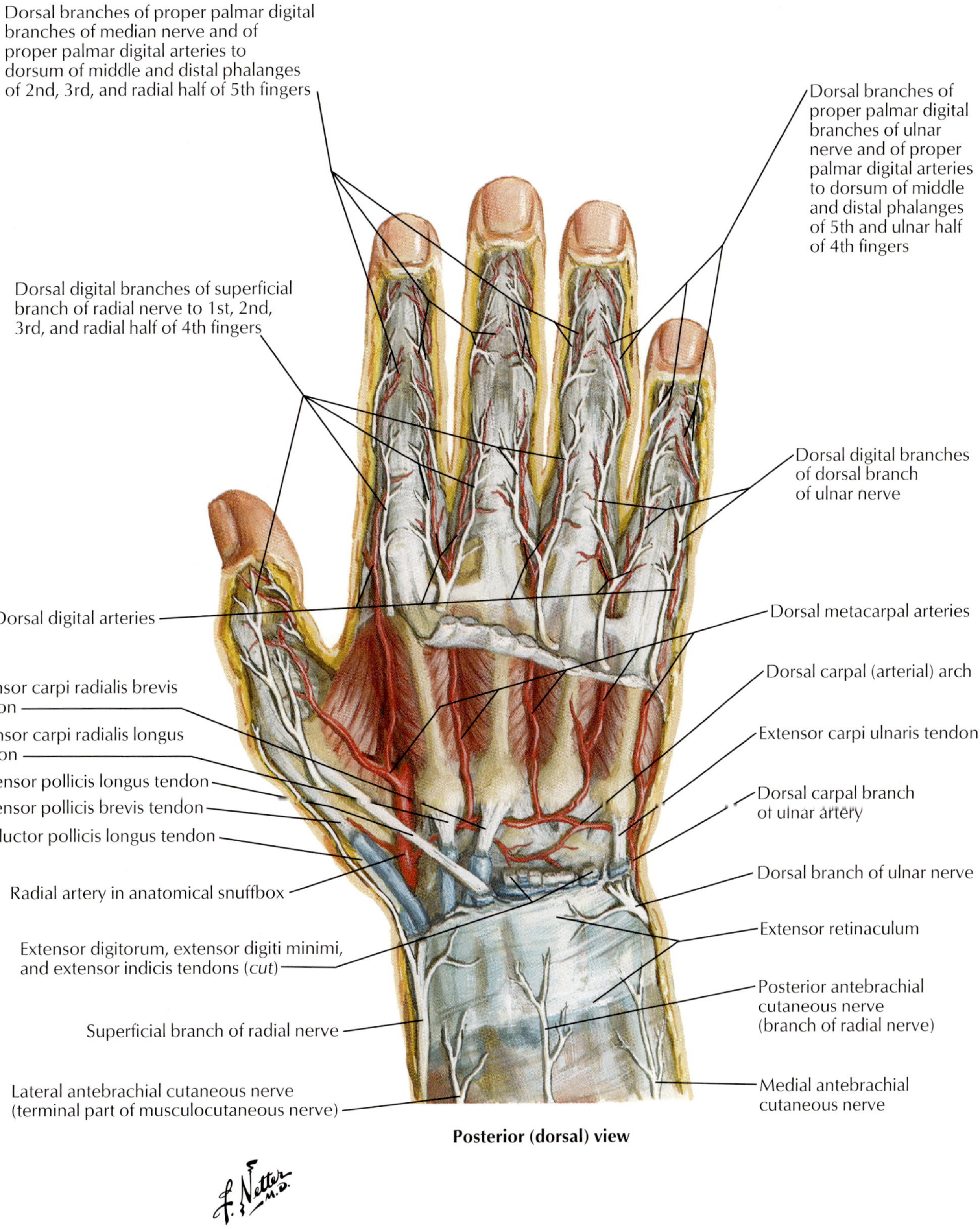

Posterior (dorsal) view

See also Plates 430, 431

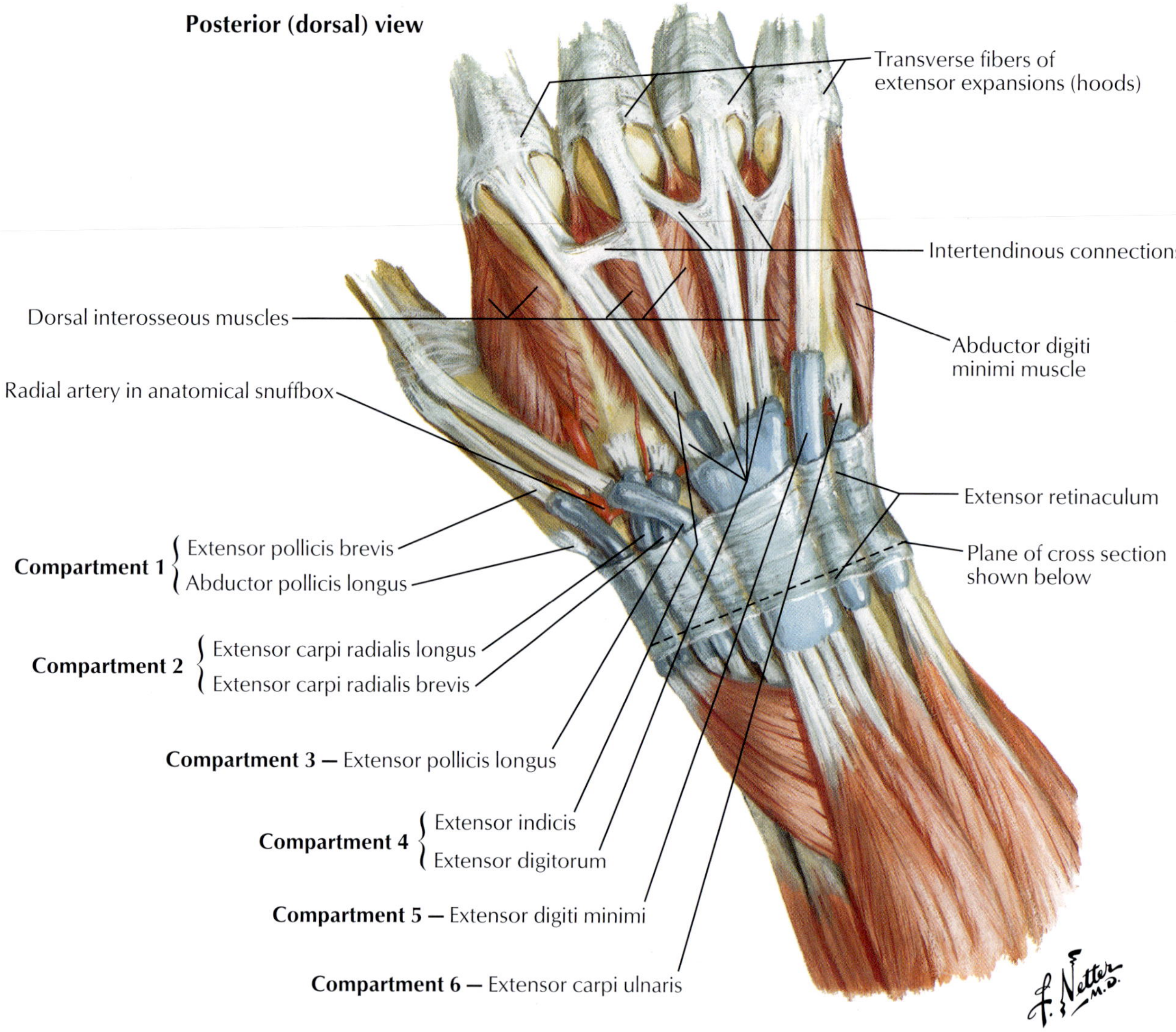

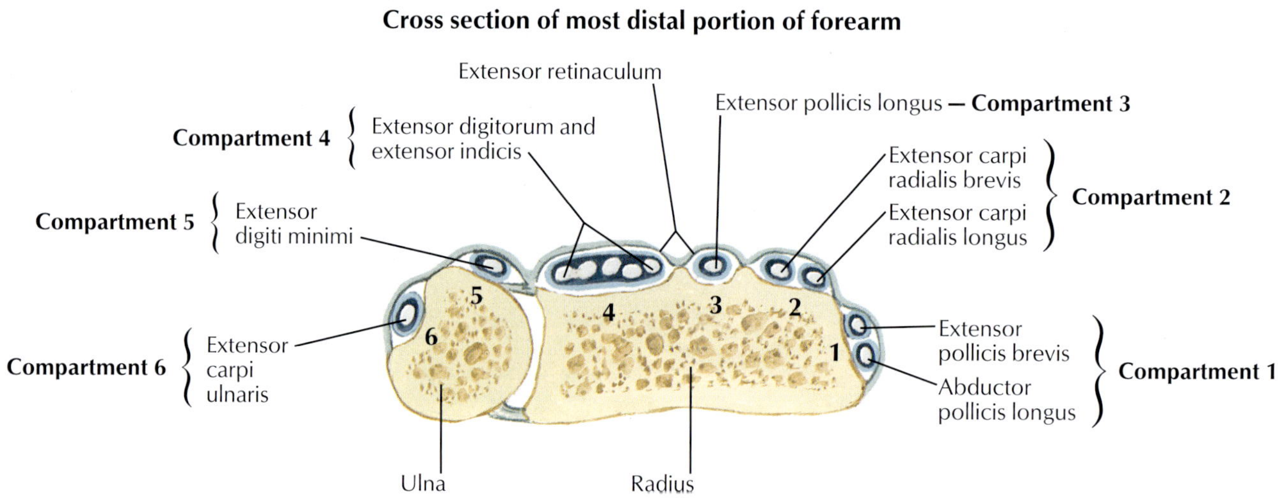

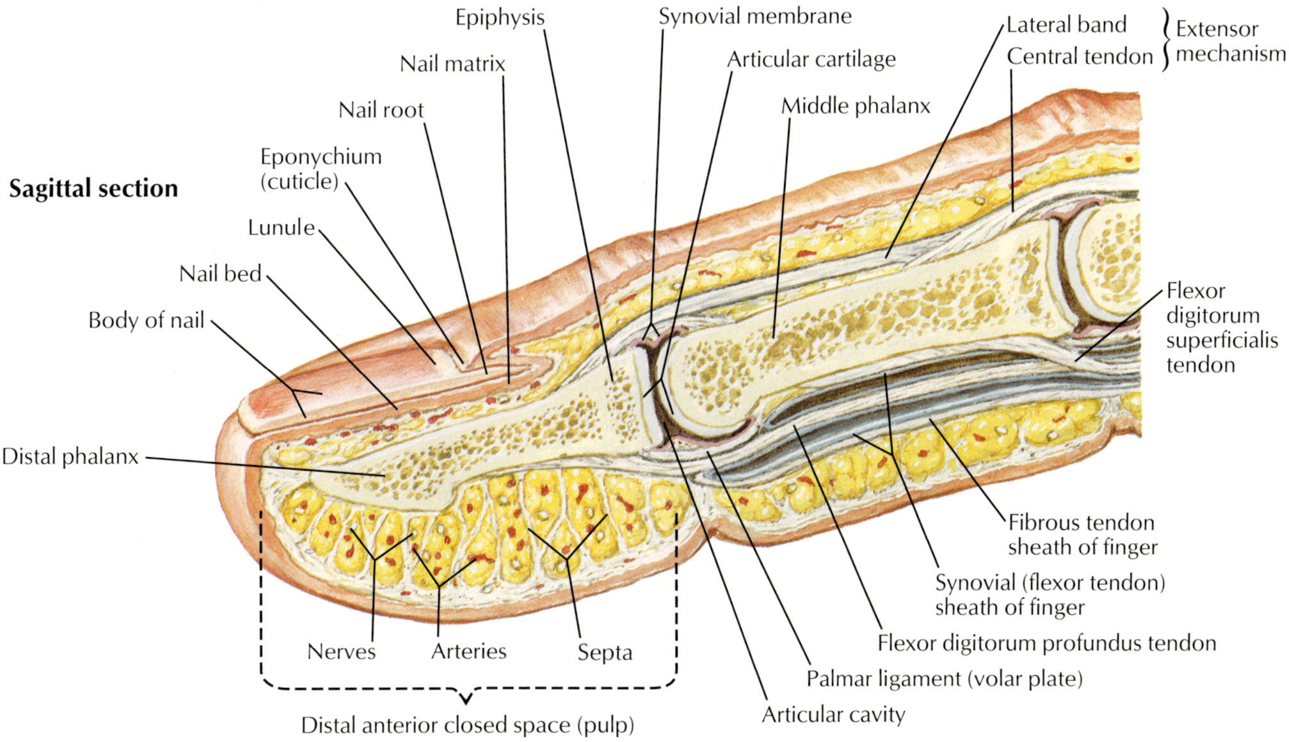

Sagittal section

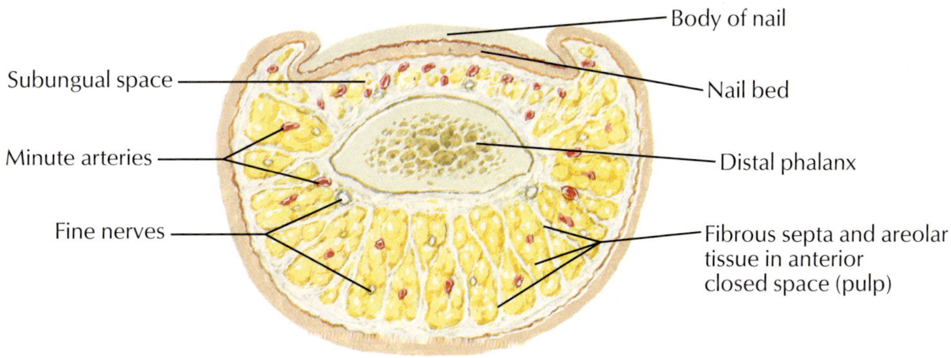

Cross section through distal phalanx

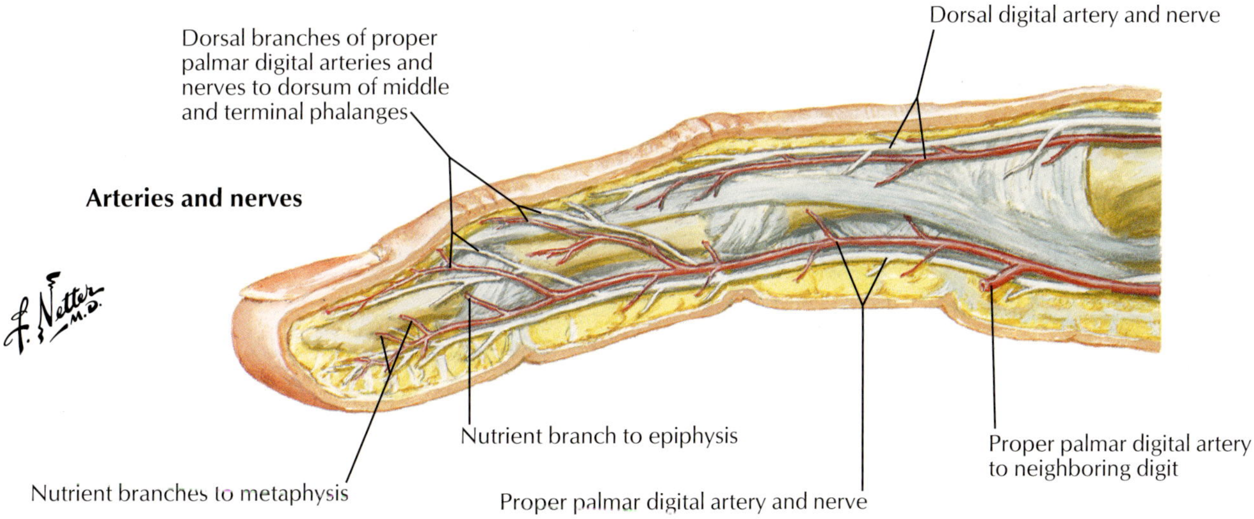

Arteries and nerves

Cutaneous Innervation of Wrist and Hand

See also **Plates 400, 449**

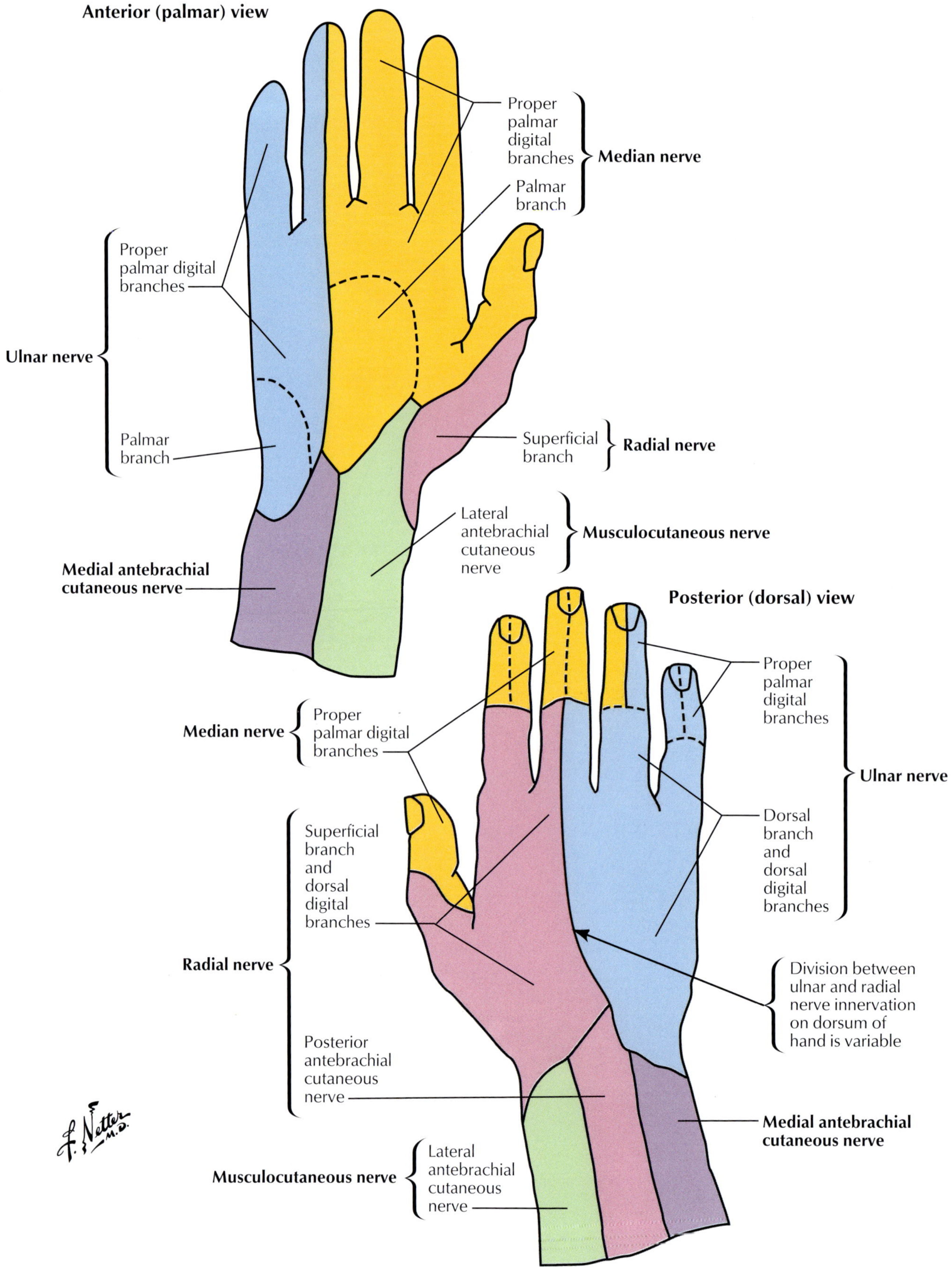

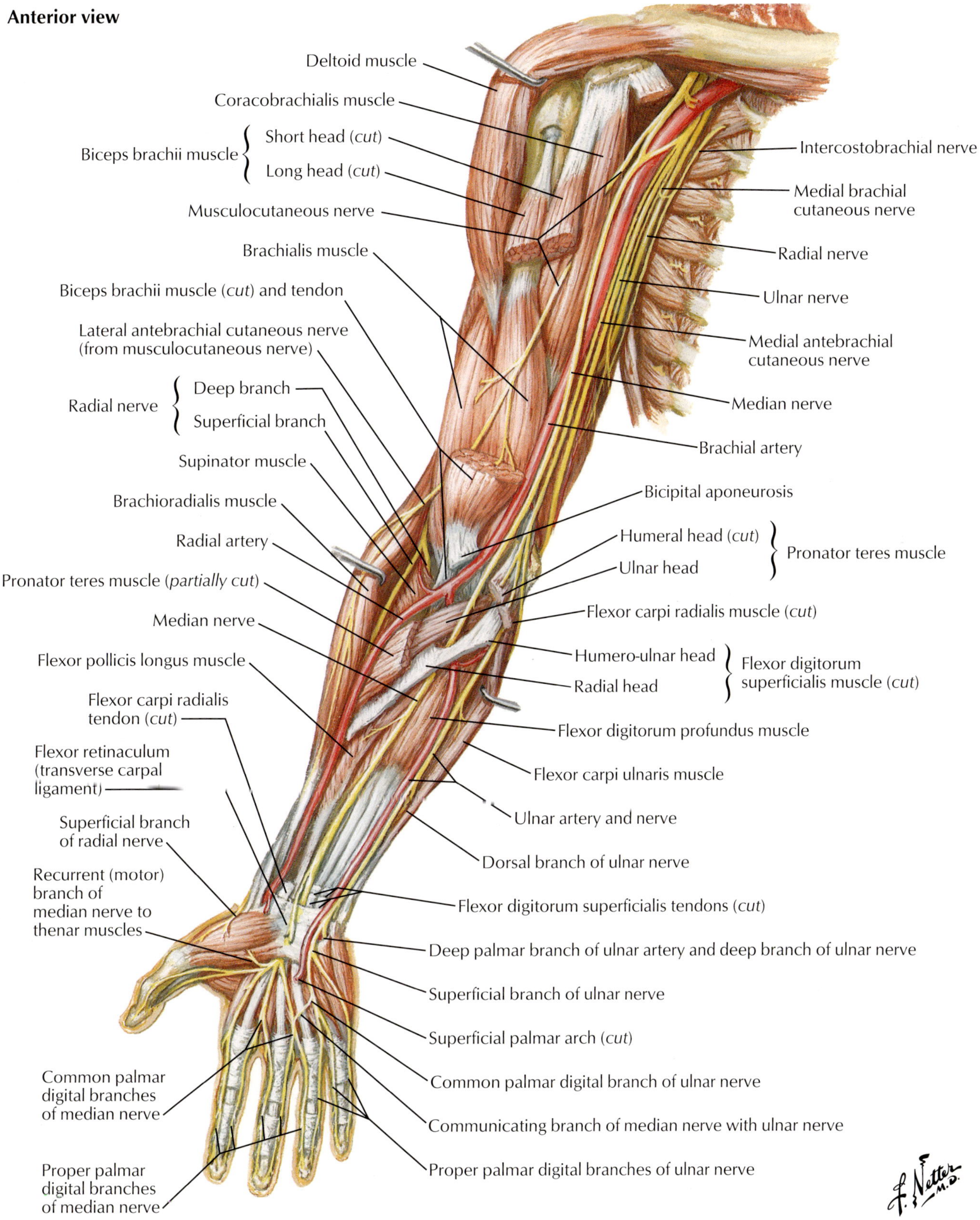
Anterior view
Deltoid muscle
Coracobrachialis muscle
Biceps brachii muscle
Short head (cut)
Long head (cut)
Musculocutaneous nerve
Brachialis muscle
Biceps brachii muscle (cut) and tendon
Lateral antebrachial cutaneous nerve (from musculocutaneous nerve)
Radial nerve
Deep branch
Superficial branch
Supinator muscle
Brachioradialis muscle
Radial artery
Pronator teres muscle (partially cut)
Median nerve
Flexor pollicis longus muscle
Flexor carpi radialis tendon (cut)
Flexor retinaculum (transverse carpal ligament)
Superficial branch of radial nerve
Recurrent (motor) branch of median nerve to thenar muscles
Common palmar digital branches of median nerve
Proper palmar digital branches of median nerve
Intercostobrachial nerve
Medial brachial cutaneous nerve
Radial nerve
Ulnar nerve
Medial antebrachial cutaneous nerve
Median nerve
Brachial artery
Bicipital aponeurosis
Humeral head (cut)
Ulnar head
Pronator teres muscle
Flexor carpi radialis muscle (cut)
Humero-ulnar head
Radial head
Flexor digitorum superficialis muscle (cut)
Flexor digitorum profundus muscle
Flexor carpi ulnaris muscle
Ulnar artery and nerve
Dorsal branch of ulnar nerve
Flexor digitorum superficialis tendons (cut)
Deep palmar branch of ulnar artery and deep branch of ulnar nerve
Superficial branch of ulnar nerve
Superficial palmar arch (cut)
Common palmar digital branch of ulnar nerve
Communicating branch of median nerve with ulnar nerve
Proper palmar digital branches of ulnar nerve
F. Netter M.D.

See also Plates 400, 410, 416

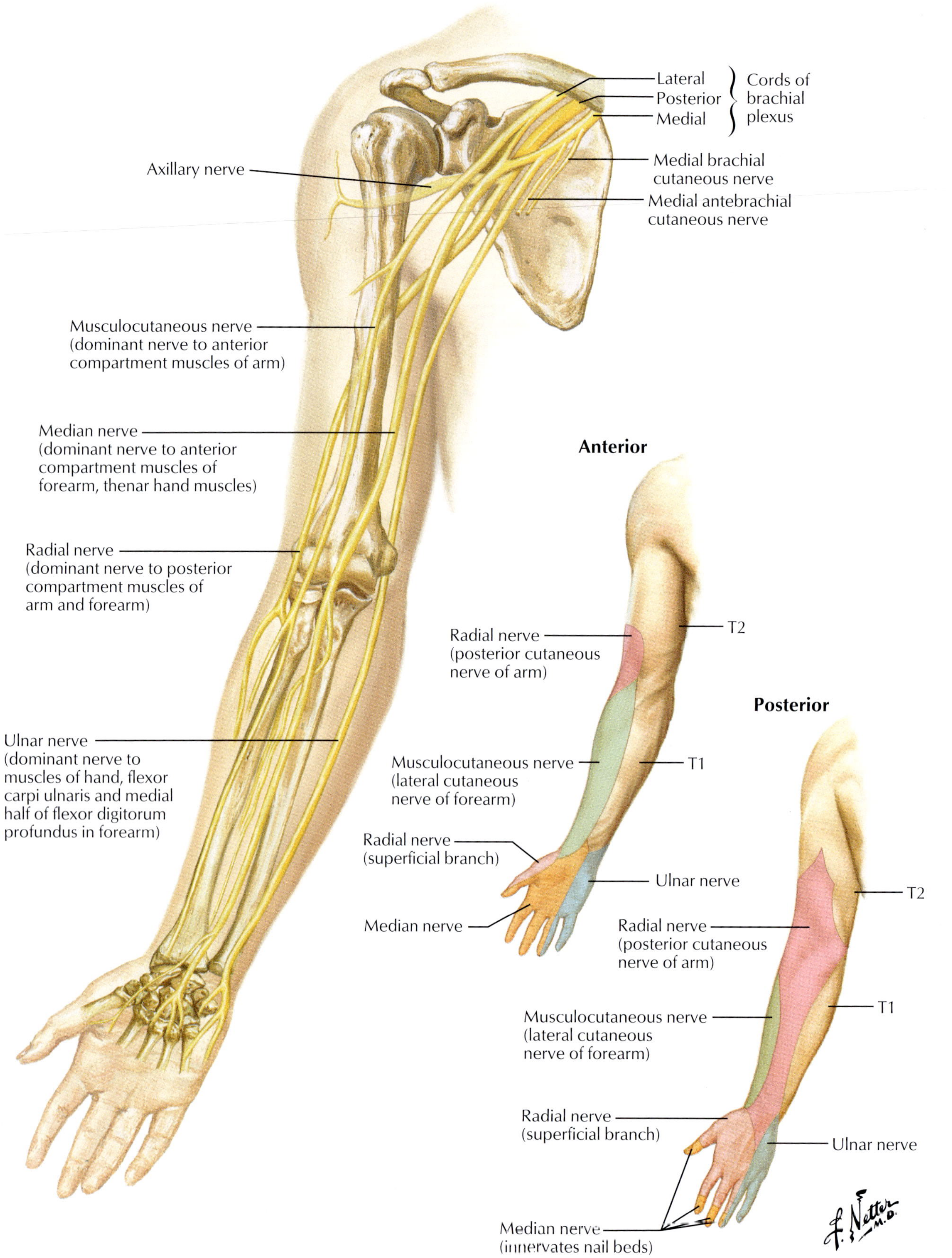

See also Plate 417

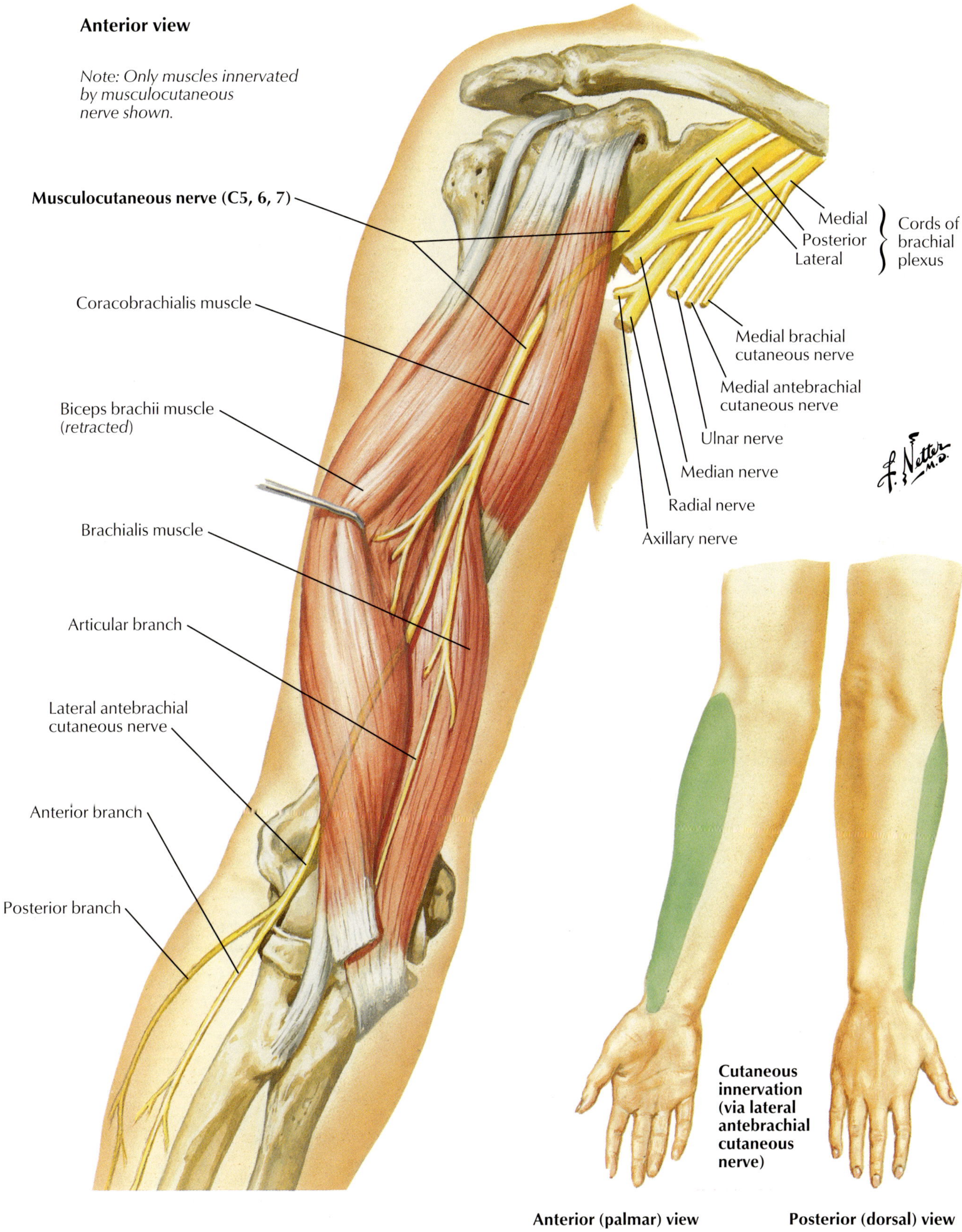

Median Nerve

See also Plates 400, 432, 433

Anterior view

Note: Only muscles innervated by median nerve shown.

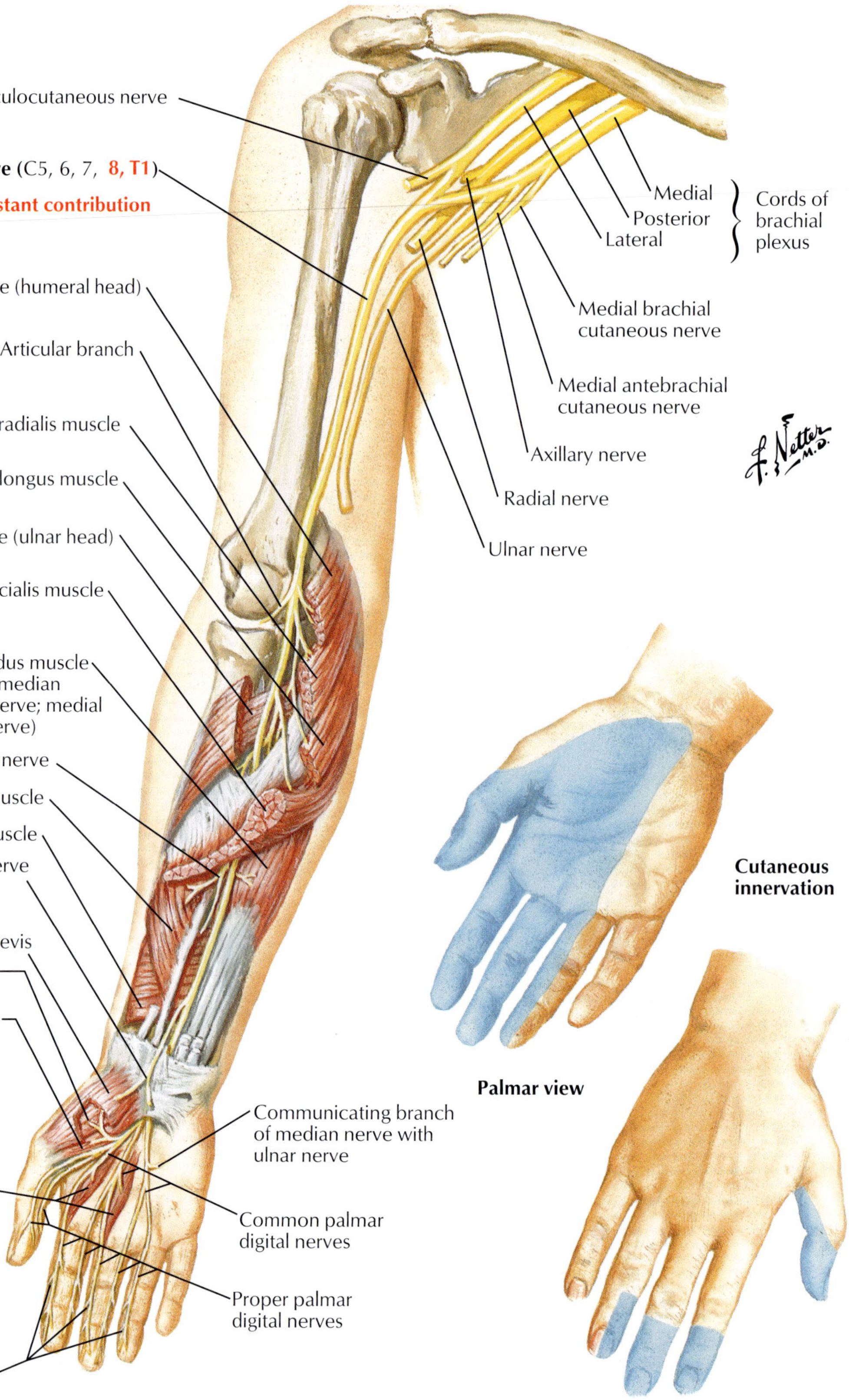

Cutaneous innervation

Palmar view

Posterior (dorsal) view

Ulnar Nerve

See also Plates 432, 434

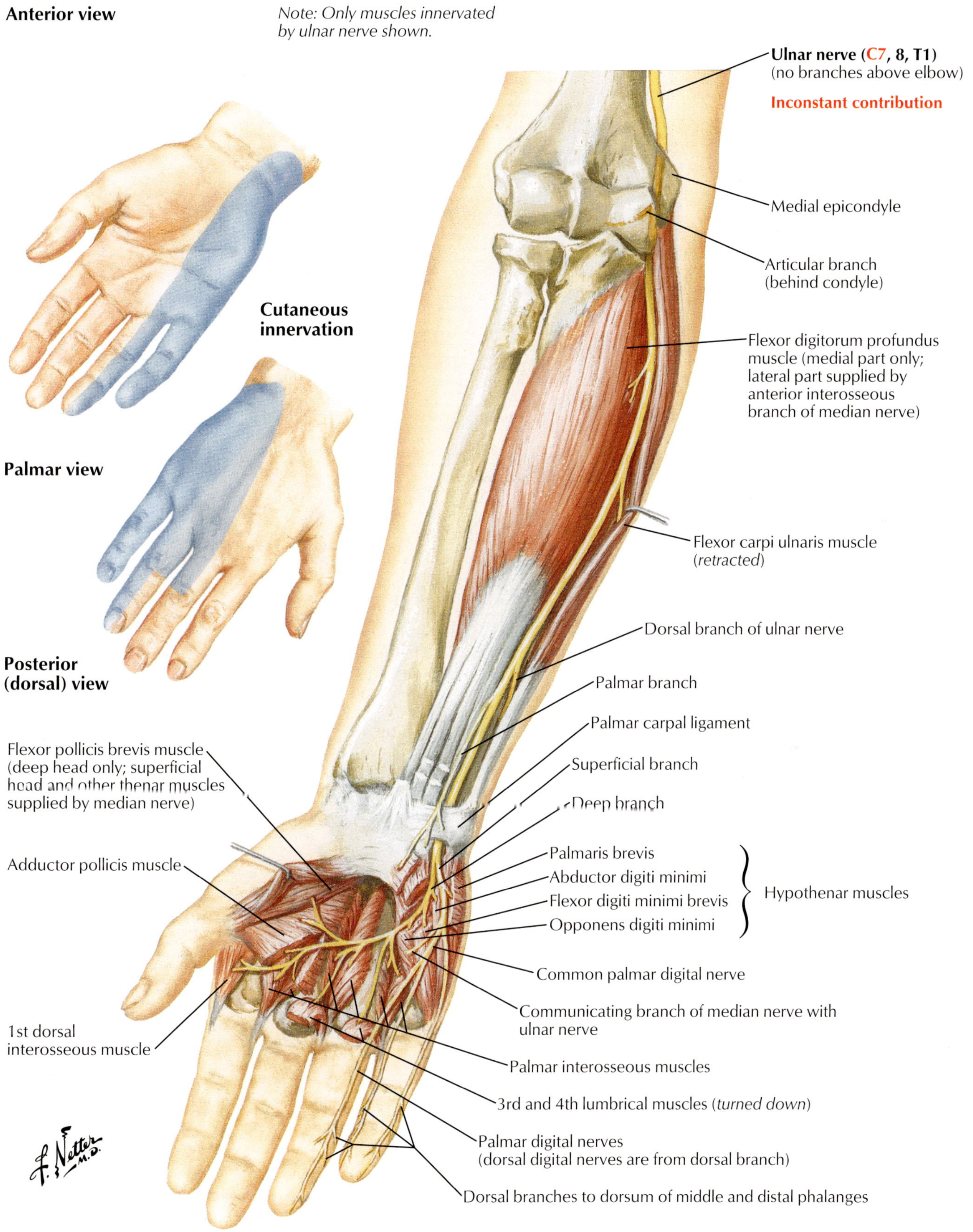

Radial Nerve in Arm and Nerves of Posterior Shoulder

See also Plates 413, 418

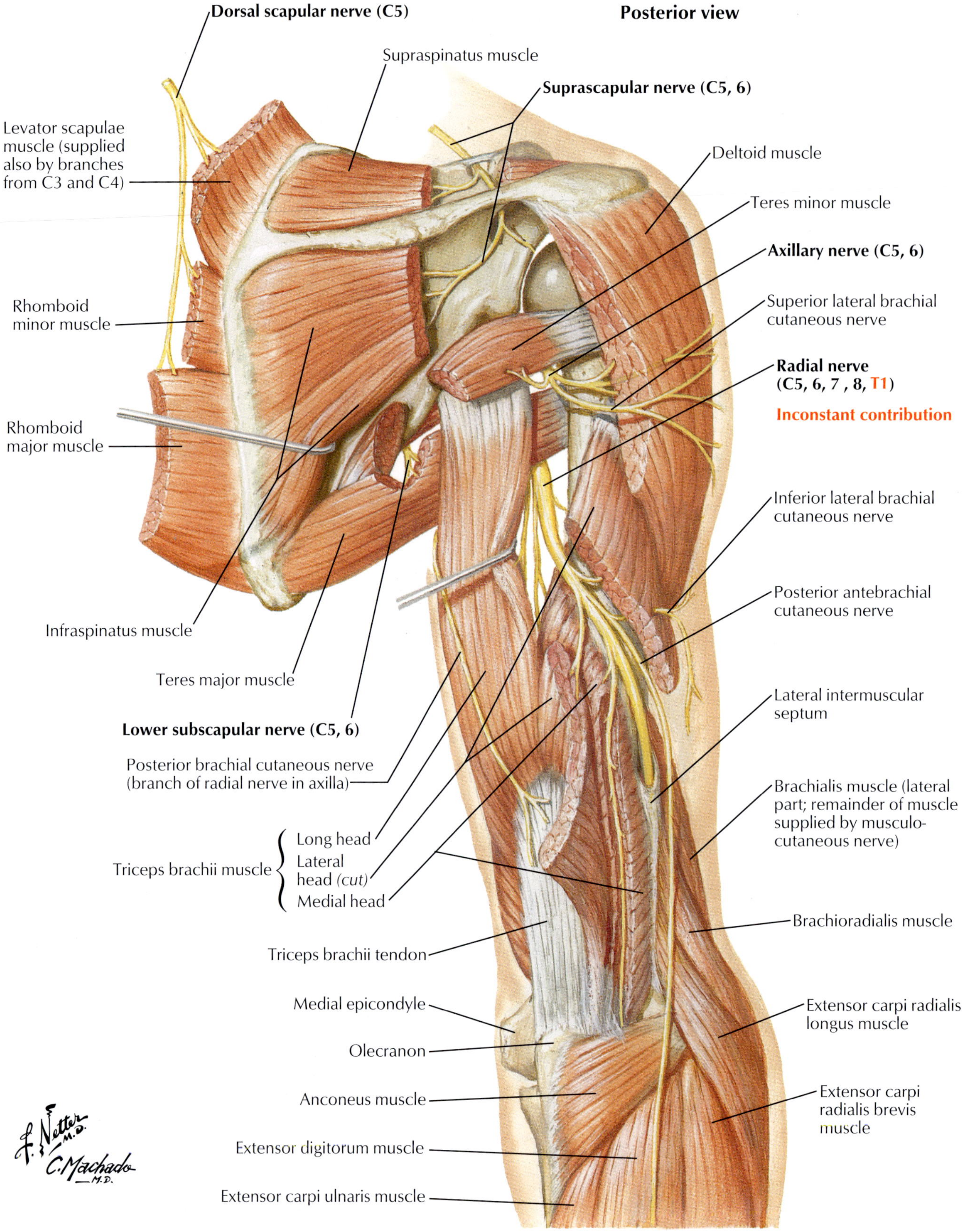

Radial Nerve in Forearm

See also Plates 430, 454

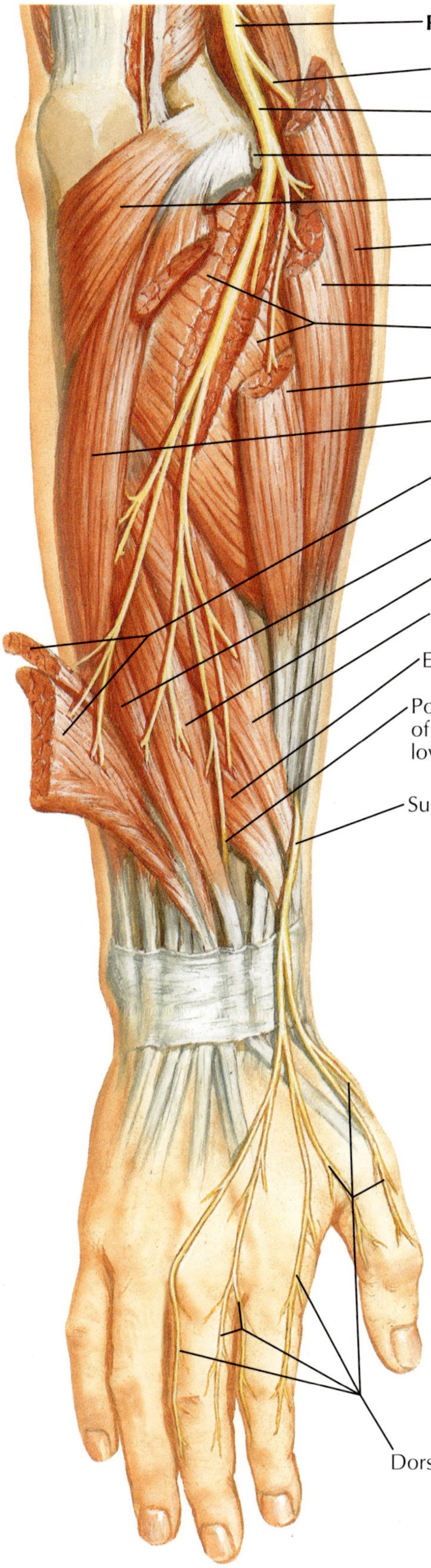

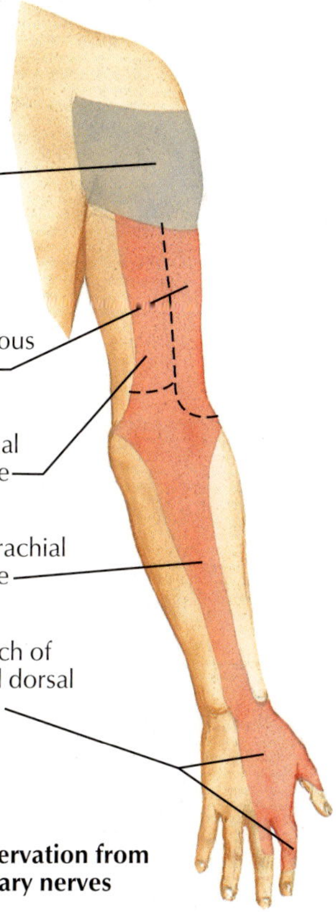

Cutaneous innervation from radial and axillary nerves

Shoulder MRI, CT Scan, and Arthrogram

See also Plate 408

MRI

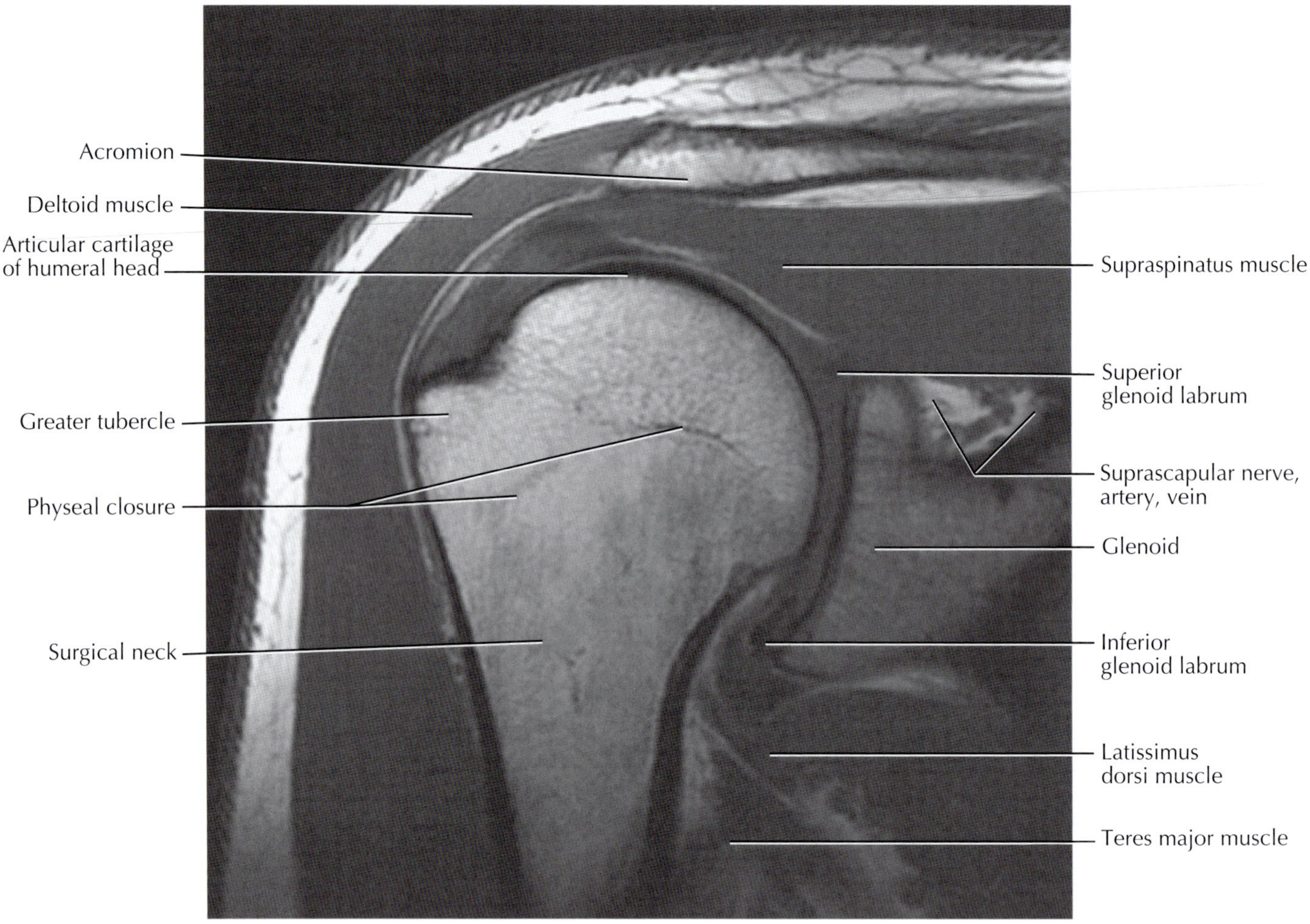

CT

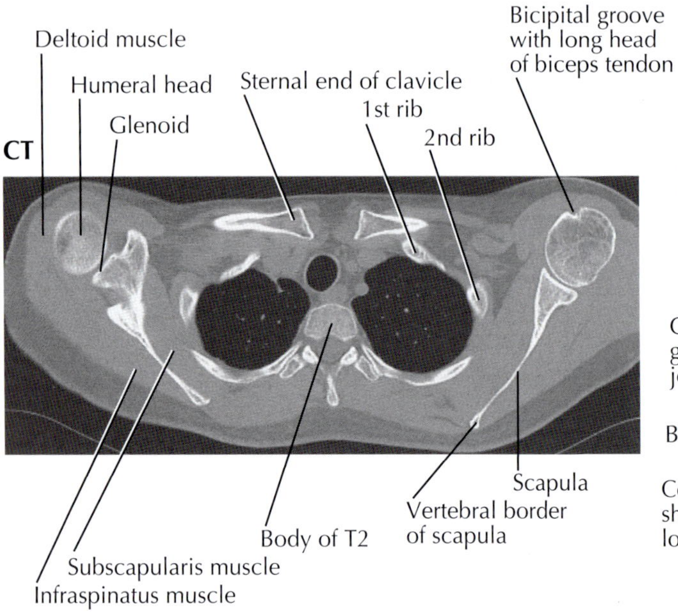

Arthrogram: glenohumeral joint

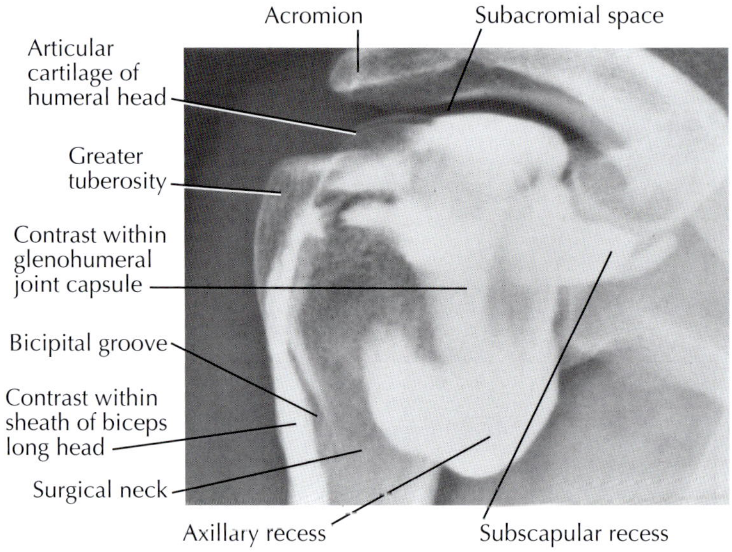

MUSCLE	PROXIMAL ATTACHMENT (ORIGIN)	DISTAL ATTACHMENT (INSERTION)	INNERVATION	MAIN ACTIONS	BLOOD SUPPLY	MUSCLE GROUP
Abductor digiti minimi	Pisiform bone and tendon of flexor carpi ulnaris	Medial side of base of proximal phalanx of little finger (5th digit)	Ulnar nerve (deep branch)	Abducts little finger	Deep palmar branch of ulnar artery	Hand
Abductor pollicis brevis	Flexor retinaculum, tubercles of scaphoid and trapezium	Lateral side of base of proximal phalanx of thumb	Median nerve (recurrent branch)	Abducts thumb	Superficial palmar branch of radial artery	Hand
Abductor pollicis longus	Posterior surface of ulna, radius, and interosseous membrane	Base of 1st metacarpal	Radial nerve (posterior interosseous)	Abducts and extends thumb at carpometacarpal joint	Posterior interosseous artery	Posterior forearm
Adductor pollicis	*Oblique head*: bases of 2nd and 3rd metacarpals and capitate and adjacent bones *Transverse head:* anterior surface of 3rd metacarpal	Medial side of base of proximal phalanx of thumb	Ulnar nerve (deep branch)	Adducts thumb	Deep palmar arch	Hand
Anconeus	Posterior surface of lateral epicondyle of humerus	Lateral surface of olecranon and posterior proximal ulna	Radial nerve (C5–T1)	Assists triceps in extending elbow, abducts ulna in pronation	Deep brachial artery	Arm
Biceps brachii	*Long head:* supraglenoid tubercle of scapula *Short head:* tip of coracoid process of scapula	Radial tuberosity, fascia of forearm via bicipital aponeurosis	Musculocutaneous nerve (C5,C6)	Flexes and supinates forearm at elbow	Muscular branches of brachial artery	Arm
Brachialis	Distal half of anterior surface of humerus	Coronoid process and tuberosity of ulna	Musculocutaneous nerve and radial nerve (C7)	Flexes forearm at elbow	Radial recurrent artery, muscular branches of brachial artery	Arm
Brachioradialis	Proximal 2/3 of lateral supracondylar ridge of humerus	Lateral side of distal end of radius	Radial nerve	Weak flexion of forearm when forearm is midpronated	Radial recurrent artery	Posterior forearm
Coracobrachialis	Tip of coracoid process of scapula	Middle third of medial surface of humerus	Musculocutaneous nerve	Flexes and adducts arm at shoulder	Muscular branches of brachial artery	Arm
Deltoid	Lateral third of anterior clavicle, lateral acromion, inferior edge of spine of scapula	Deltoid tuberosity of humerus	Axillary nerve	*Clavicular part*: flexes and medially rotates arm *Acromial part:* abducts arm beyond initial 15 degrees done by supraspinatus *Spinal part:* extends and laterally rotates arm	Posterior circumflex humeral artery, deltoid branch of thoraco-acromial artery	Shoulder
Dorsal interosseous muscles	Adjacent sides of two metacarpal bones	Base of proximal phalanges, extensor expansion of digits 2–4	Ulnar nerve (deep branch)	Abduct digits from axial line of hand (3rd digit); flex digits at metacarpophalangeal joint and extend interphalangeal joints	Deep palmar arch	Hand
Extensor carpi radialis brevis	Lateral epicondyle of humerus	Dorsal base of 3rd metacarpal and slip to 2nd metacarpal	Radial nerve (deep branch)	Extends and abducts hand at wrist	Radial artery, radial recurrent artery	Posterior forearm
Extensor carpi radialis longus	Distal third of lateral supracondylar ridge of humerus	Dorsal base of 2nd metacarpal and slip to 3rd metacarpal	Radial nerve	Extends and abducts hand at wrist	Radial artery, radial recurrent artery	Posterior forearm

Variations in spinal nerve contributions to the innervation of muscles, their arterial supply, their attachments, and their actions are common themes in human anatomy. Therefore, expect differences between texts and realize that anatomical variation is normal.

MUSCLE	PROXIMAL ATTACHMENT (ORIGIN)	DISTAL ATTACHMENT (INSERTION)	INNERVATION	MAIN ACTIONS	BLOOD SUPPLY	MUSCLE GROUP
Extensor carpi ulnaris	Lateral epicondyle of humerus and posterior border of ulna	Dorsal base of 5th metacarpal	Radial nerve (posterior interosseous)	Extends and adducts hand at wrist	Posterior interosseous artery	Posterior forearm
Extensor digiti minimi	Lateral epicondyle of humerus	Extensor expansion of 5th digit	Radial nerve (posterior interosseous)	Extends 5th digit	Posterior interosseous artery	Posterior forearm
Extensor digitorum	Lateral epicondyle of humerus	Extensor expansions of medial four digits	Radial nerve (posterior interosseous)	Extends medial four digits, assists in wrist extension	Posterior interosseous artery	Posterior forearm
Extensor indicis	Posterior surface of ulna and interosseous membrane	Extensor expansion of 2nd digit	Radial nerve (posterior interosseous)	Extends 2nd digit and helps extend hand at wrist	Posterior interosseous artery	Posterior forearm
Extensor pollicis brevis	Posterior surface of radius and interosseous membrane	Dorsal base of proximal phalanx of thumb	Radial nerve (posterior interosseous)	Extends proximal phalanx of thumb at carpometacarpal joint	Posterior interosseous artery	Posterior forearm
Extensor pollicis longus	Posterior surface of middle third of ulna, interosseous membrane	Dorsal base of distal phalanx of thumb	Radial nerve (posterior interosseous)	Extends distal phalanx of thumb at interphalangeal and metacarpophalangeal joints	Posterior interosseous artery	Posterior forearm
Flexor carpi radialis	Medial epicondyle of humerus	Base of 2nd metacarpal	Median nerve	Flexes and abducts hand at wrist	Radial artery	Anterior forearm
Flexor carpi ulnaris	*Humeral head:* medial epicondyle of humerus *Ulnar head:* olecranon and posterior border of ulna	Pisiform bone, hook of hamate, base of 5th metacarpal	Ulnar nerve	Flexes and adducts hand at wrist	Posterior ulnar recurrent artery	Anterior forearm
Flexor digiti minimi brevis	Flexor retinaculum and hook of hamate bone	Medial side of base of proximal phalanx of little finger	Ulnar nerve (deep branch)	Flexes proximal phalanx of little finger	Deep palmar branch of ulnar artery	Hand
Flexor digitorum profundus	Medial and anterior surface of proximal 3/4 of ulna and interosseous membrane	Palmar base of distal phalanges of medial four digits	*Medial part:* ulnar nerve *Lateral part:* median nerve	Flexes distal phalanges of medial four digits, assists with flexion of hand at wrist	Anterior interosseous artery, muscular branches of ulnar artery	Anterior forearm
Flexor digitorum superficialis	*Humero-ulnar head:* medial epicondyle of humerus and coronoid process of ulna *Radial head:* superior half of anterior radius	Bodies of middle phalanges of medial four digits	Median nerve	Flexes middle and proximal phalanges of medial four digits, flexes hand at wrist	Ulnar and radial arteries	Anterior forearm
Flexor pollicis brevis	Flexor retinaculum and tubercle of trapezium	Lateral side of base of proximal phalanx of thumb	Median nerve (recurrent branch)	Flexes proximal phalanx of thumb	Superficial palmar branch of radial artery	Hand
Flexor pollicis longus	Anterior surface of radius and interosseous membrane	Palmar base of distal phalanx of thumb	Median nerve (anterior interosseous)	Flexes phalanges of thumb	Anterior interosseous artery	Anterior forearm
Infraspinatus	Infraspinous fossa of scapula and deep fascia	Middle facet of greater tubercle of humerus	Suprascapular nerve	Lateral rotation of arm (with teres minor)	Suprascapular artery	Shoulder

MUSCLE	PROXIMAL ATTACHMENT (ORIGIN)	DISTAL ATTACHMENT (INSERTION)	INNERVATION	MAIN ACTIONS	BLOOD SUPPLY	MUSCLE GROUP
Latissimus dorsi	Spinous processes of T7–L5 vertebrae, thoracolumbar fascia, iliac crest, last 3 ribs	Intertubercular sulcus of humerus	Thoracodorsal nerve	Extends, adducts, and medially rotates humerus at shoulder	Thoracodorsal artery, dorsal perforating branches of 9th, 10th, and 11th posterior intercostal, subcostal, and first three lumbar arteries	Shoulder
Levator scapulae	Posterior tubercles of transverse processes of C1–C4	Medial border of scapula from superior angle to spine	Ventral rami of C3–C4 and dorsal scapular nerve	Elevates scapula medially, inferiorly rotates glenoid cavity	Dorsal scapular artery, transverse cervical artery, ascending cervical artery	Superficial back
Lumbrical, first and second	Lateral two tendons of flexor digitorum profundus	Lateral sides of extensor expansion of digits 2 and 3	Median nerve (digital branches)	Extend digits at interphalangeal joints, flex metacarpophalangeal joints	Superficial and deep palmar arches	Hand
Lumbrical, third and fourth	Medial three tendons of flexor digitorum profundus	Lateral sides of extensor expansion of digits 4 and 5	Ulnar nerve (deep branch)	Extend digits at interphalangeal joints, flex metacarpophalangeal joints	Superficial and deep palmar arches	Hand
Opponens digiti minimi	Flexor retinaculum and hook of hamate bone	Palmar surface of 5th metacarpal	Ulnar nerve (deep branch)	Draws 5th metacarpal anteriorly and rotates it to face thumb	Deep palmar branch of ulnar artery	Hand
Opponens pollicis	Flexor retinaculum and tubercle of trapezium	Lateral side of 1st metacarpal	Median nerve (recurrent branch)	Draws 1st metacarpal forward and rotates it medially	Superficial palmar branch of radial artery	Hand
Palmar interosseous muscles	Sides of metacarpals 2, 4, and 5	Bases of proximal phalanx and extensor expansion of digits 2, 4, and 5	Ulnar nerve (deep branch)	Adducts digits toward axial line of hand (3rd digit); flexes digits at metacarpophalngeal joint and extends interphalangeal joints	Deep palmar arch	Hand
Palmaris brevis	Palmar aponeurosis and flexor retinaculum	Skin of medial border of palm	Superficial palmar branch of ulnar nerve	Deepens hollow of hand, assists grip	Superficial palmar arch	Hand
Palmaris longus	Medial epicondyle of humerus	Distal half of flexor retinaculum and palmar aponeurosis	Median nerve	Flexes hand at wrist and tenses palmar aponeurosis	Posterior ulnar recurrent artery	Anterior forearm
Pectoralis major	Sternal half of clavicle, sternum to 7th rib, cartilages of true ribs, aponeurosis of external oblique muscle	Lateral lip of intertubercular sulcus of humerus	Medial and lateral pectoral nerves	Flexes and adducts arm, rotates arm medially	Pectoral branch of thoraco-acromial artery, perforating branches of internal thoracic artery	Pectoral region/ axilla
Pectoralis minor	Outer surface of upper margin of ribs 3–5	Coracoid process of scapula	Medial pectoral nerve	Lowers lateral angle of scapula and protracts scapula	Pectoral branch of thoraco-acromial and intercostal lateral thoracic arteries	Pectoral region/ axilla
Pronator quadratus	Distal fourth of anterior ulna	Distal fourth of anterior radius	Median nerve (anterior interosseous)	Pronates forearm	Anterior interosseous artery	Anterior forearm
Pronator teres	Two heads: medial epicondyle of humerus and coronoid process of ulna	Midway along lateral surface of radius	Median nerve	Pronates forearm and assists with elbow flexion	Anterior ulnar recurrent artery	Anterior forearm

MUSCLE	PROXIMAL ATTACHMENT (ORIGIN)	DISTAL ATTACHMENT (INSERTION)	INNERVATION	MAIN ACTIONS	BLOOD SUPPLY	MUSCLE GROUP
Rhomboid major	Spinous processes of T2–T5 vertebrae	Medial border of scapula below base of spine of scapula	Dorsal scapular nerve	Fixes scapula to thoracic wall and retracts and rotates it to depress glenoid cavity	Dorsal scapular OR deep branch of transverse cervical artery, dorsal perforating branches of the upper five or six posterior intercostal arteries artery	Superficial back
Rhomboid minor	Ligamentum nuchae, spines of C7 and T1 vertebrae	Medial border of scapula at spine of scapula	Dorsal scapular nerve	Fixes scapula to thoracic wall and retracts and rotates it to depress glenoid cavity	Dorsal scapular artery OR deep branch of transverse cervical artery, dorsal perforating branches of the upper five or six posterior intercostal arteries	Superficial back
Serratus anterior	Lateral surfaces of upper 8–9 ribs	Costal surface of medial border of scapula	Long thoracic nerve	Protracts and rotates scapula and holds it against thoracic wall	Lateral thoracic artery	Shoulder
Subclavius	Upper border of 1st rib and its cartilage	Inferior surface of middle third of clavicle	Nerve to subclavius	Anchors and depresses clavicle	Clavicular branch of thoraco-acromial artery	Shoulder
Subscapularis	Subscapular fossa	Lesser tubercle of humerus	Upper and lower subscapular nerves	Medially rotates arm at shoulder and adducts it, helps hold humeral head in glenoid cavity	Subscapular artery, lateral thoracic artery	Shoulder
Supinator	Lateral epicondyle of humerus, supinator crest of ulna	Lateral, posterior, and anterior surfaces of proximal third of radius	Radial nerve (deep branch)	Supinates forearm	Radial recurrent artery, posterior interosseous arteries	Posterior forearm
Supraspinatus	Supraspinous fossa of scapula and deep fascia	Superior facet of greater tubercle of humerus	Suprascapular nerve	Initiates arm abduction, acts with rotator cuff muscles	Suprascapular artery	Shoulder
Teres major	Posterior surface of inferior angle of scapula	Medial lip of intertubercular sulcus of humerus	Lower subscapular nerve	Adducts and medially rotates arm	Circumflex scapular artery	Shoulder
Teres minor	Upper 2/3 of posterior surface of lateral border of scapula	Inferior facet of greater tubercle of humerus	Axillary nerve	Laterally rotates arm	Circumflex scapular artery	Shoulder
Trapezius	Superior nuchal line, external occipital protuberance, nuchal ligament, spinous processes of C7–T12	Lateral third of clavicle, acromion, and spine of scapula	Accessory nerve (cranial nerve XI)	Elevates, retracts, and rotates scapula; lower fibers depress scapula	Transverse cervical artery, dorsal perforating branches of posterior intercostal arteries	Superficial back
Triceps brachii	*Long head:* infraglenoid tubercle of scapula *Lateral head:* upper half of posterior humerus *Medial head:* distal 2/3 of medial and posterior humerus	Posterior surface of olecranon process of ulna	Radial nerve	Extends forearm at elbow; long head stabilizes head of abducted humerus and extends and adducts arm at shoulder	Branch of profunda brachii artery	Arm

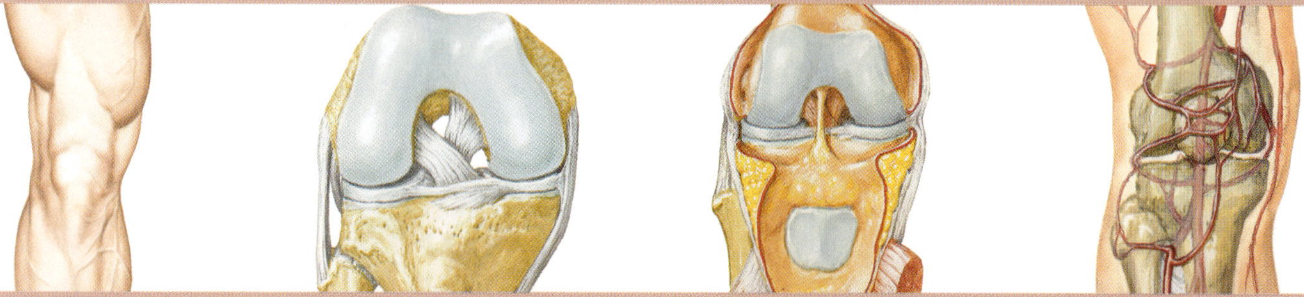

7 LOWER LIMB

Topographic Anatomy
Plate 468

468 Lower Limb: Surface Anatomy

Cutaneous Anatomy
Plates 469–472

469 Dermatomes of Lower Limb

470 Superficial Nerves and Veins of Lower Limb: Anterior View

471 Superficial Nerves and Veins of Lower Limb: Posterior View

472 Lymph Vessels and Nodes of Lower Limb

Hip and Thigh
Plates 473–492

473 Hip (Coxal) Bone

474 Hip Joint

475 Hip Joint: Anteroposterior Radiograph

476 Femur

477 Bony Attachments of Muscles of Hip and Thigh: Anterior View

478 Bony Attachments of Muscles of Hip and Thigh: Posterior View

479 Muscles of Thigh: Anterior Views

480 Muscles of Thigh: Anterior Views (continued)

481 Muscles of Hip and Thigh: Lateral View

482 Muscles of Hip and Thigh: Posterior Views

483 Psoas and Iliacus Muscles

484 Lumbosacral and Coccygeal Plexuses
485 Lumbar Plexus
486 Sacral and Coccygeal Plexuses
487 Arteries and Nerves of Thigh: Anterior Views
488 Arteries and Nerves of Thigh: Anterior Views (continued)
489 Arteries and Nerves of Thigh: Posterior View
490 Nerves of Hip and Buttock
491 Arteries of Femoral Head and Neck
492 Thigh: Serial Cross Sections

Knee

Plates 493–499

493 Knee: Medial and Lateral Views
494 Knee: Anterior Views
495 Knee: Interior
496 Knee: Cruciate and Collateral Ligaments
497 Knee: Anteroposterior Radiograph and Posterior View
498 Knee: Posterior and Sagittal Views
499 Arteries of Thigh and Knee: Schema

Leg

Plates 500–510

500 Tibia and Fibula
501 Tibia and Fibula (continued)
502 Attachments of Muscles of Leg
503 Muscles of Leg (Superficial Dissection): Posterior View
504 Muscles of Leg (Intermediate Dissection): Posterior View
505 Muscles of Leg (Deep Dissection): Posterior View
506 Muscles of Leg: Lateral View
507 Muscles of Leg (Superficial Dissection): Anterior View
508 Muscles of Leg (Deep Dissection): Anterior View
509 Arteries of Knee, Leg, and Foot
510 Leg: Cross Sections and Fascial Compartments

Ankle and Foot

Plates 511–524

511 Bones of Foot
512 Bones of Foot (continued)
513 Calcaneus
514 Ligaments and Tendons of Ankle
515 Ligaments and Tendons of Foot: Plantar View
516 Tendon Sheaths of Ankle
517 Muscles of Dorsum of Foot: Superficial Dissection
518 Dorsum of Foot: Deep Dissection
519 Sole of Foot: Superficial Dissection
520 Muscles of Sole of Foot: First Layer
521 Muscles of Sole of Foot: Second Layer
522 Muscles of Sole of Foot: Third Layer
523 Interosseous Muscles and Deep Arteries of Foot
524 Interosseous Muscles of Foot

Neurovasculature

Plates 525–529

525 Femoral Nerve and Lateral Cutaneous Nerve of Thigh
526 Obturator Nerve
527 Sciatic Nerve and Posterior Cutaneous Nerve of Thigh
528 Tibial Nerve
529 Common Fibular (Peroneal) Nerve

Regional Scans

Plates 530–531

530 Hip Radiograph, Arthrogram, and MRI
531 Ankle: Radiographs

Muscle Tables

See also Plates 470, 471

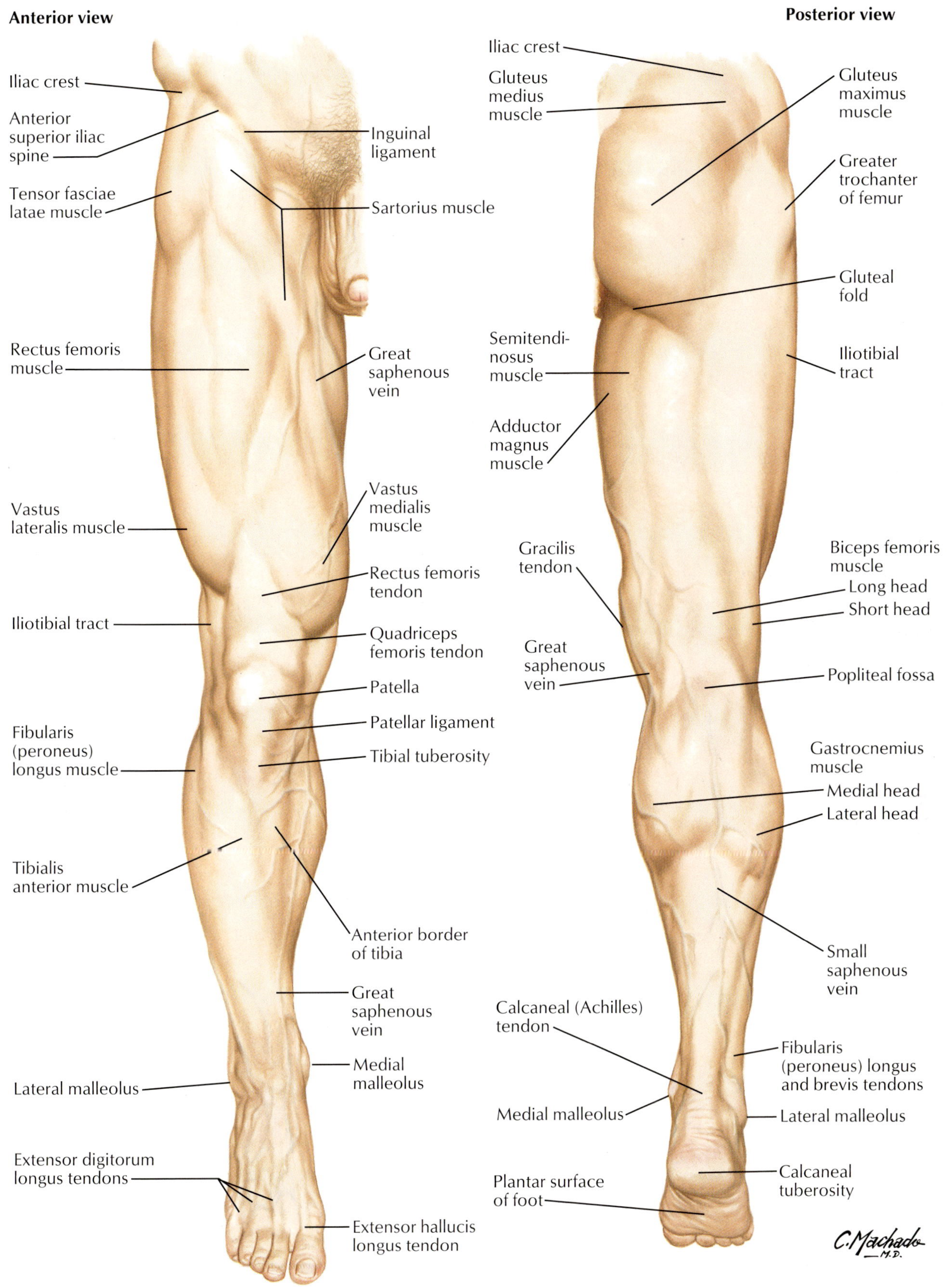

See also Plate 162

Schematic demarcation of dermatomes (according to Keegan and Garrett) shown as distinct segments. There is actually considerable overlap between any two adjacent dermatomes.

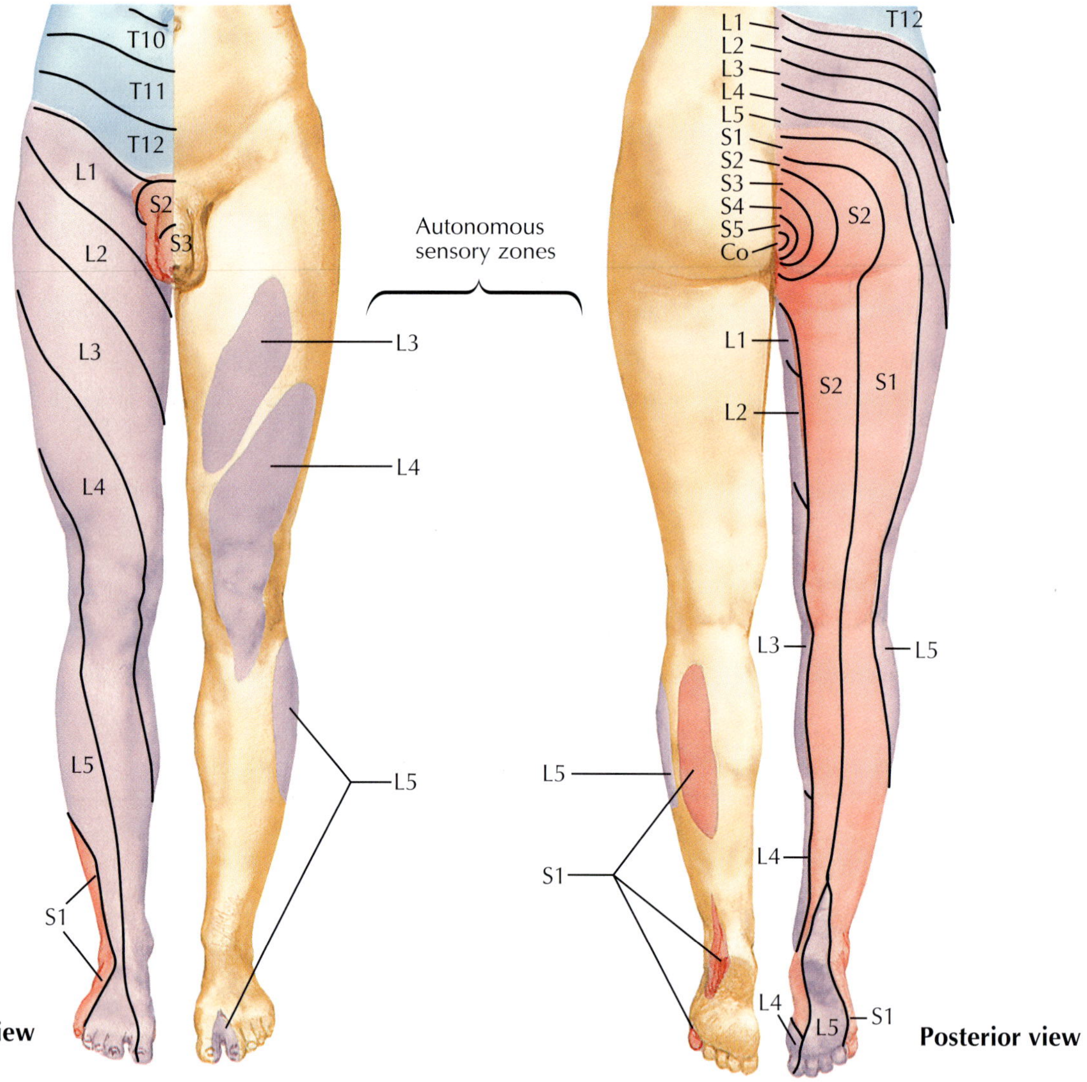

Anterior view

Segmental innervation of lower limb movements

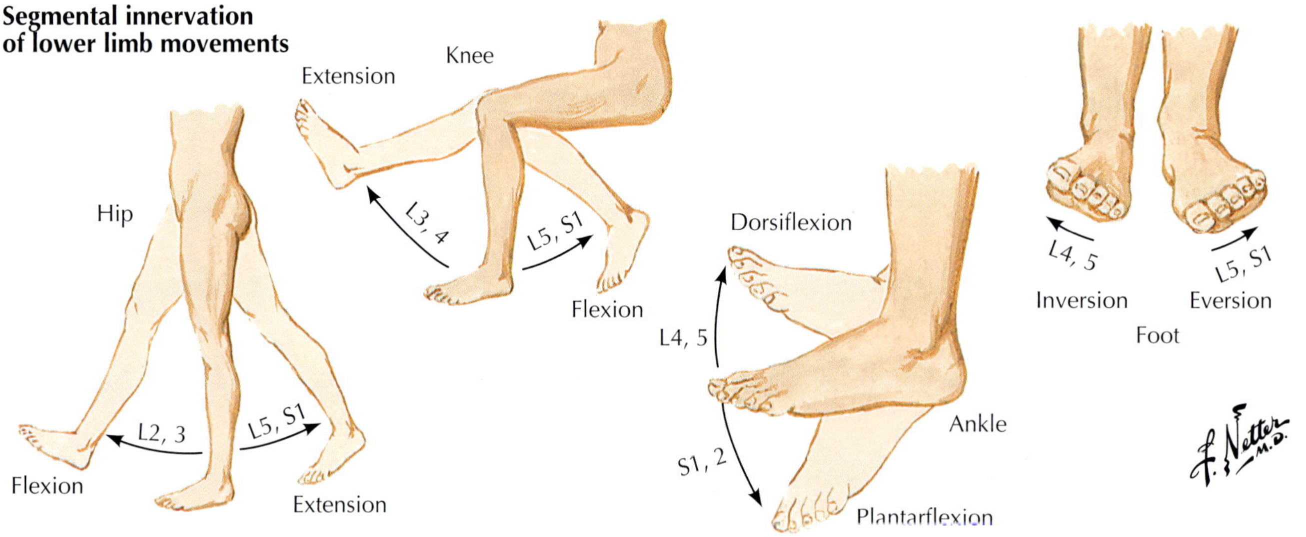

Superficial Nerves and Veins of Lower Limb: Anterior View

See also Plates 525, 526, 529

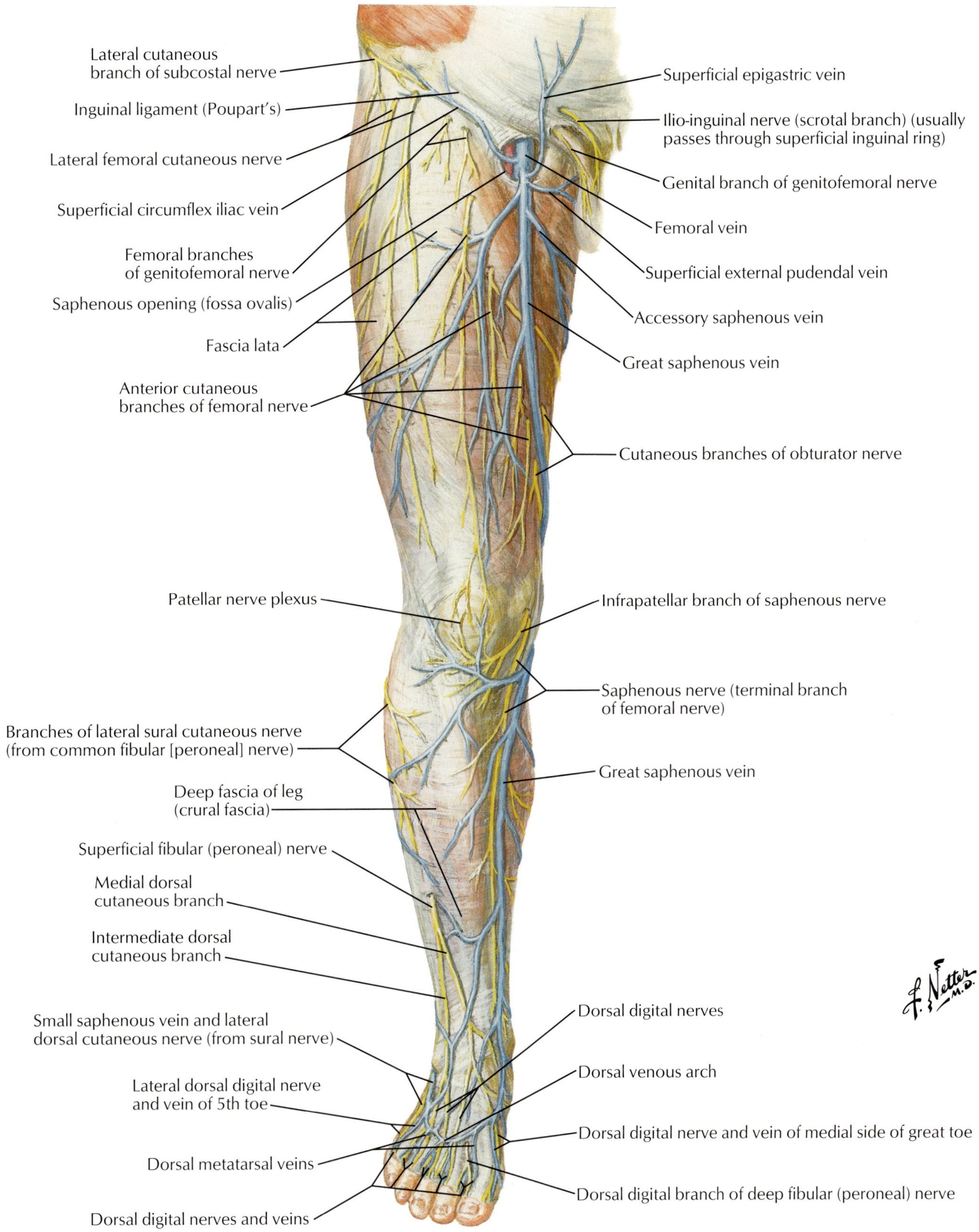

Superficial Nerves and Veins of Lower Limb: Posterior View

See also Plates 527, 528

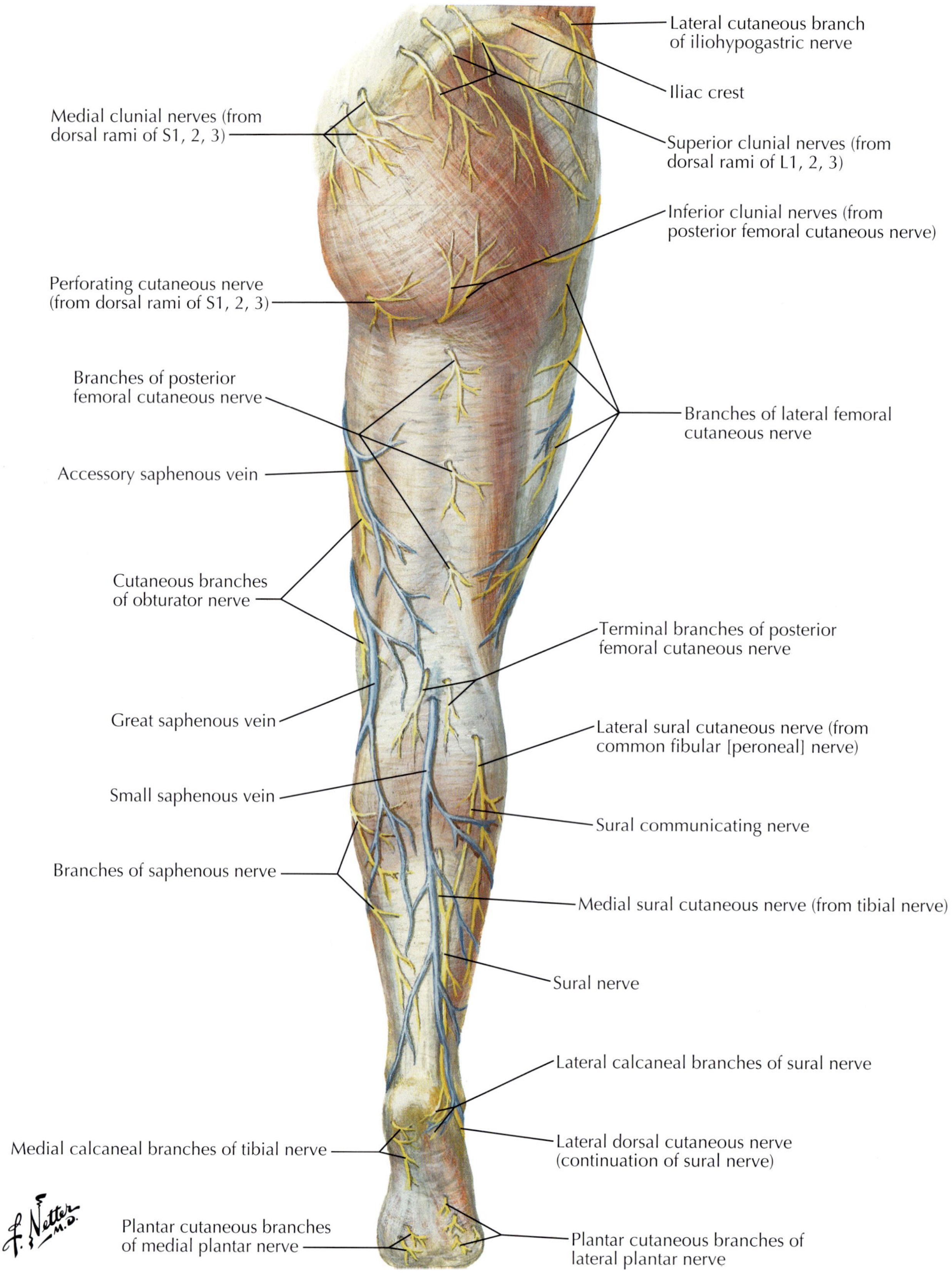

Lymph Vessels and Nodes of Lower Limb

See also Plates 385, 386

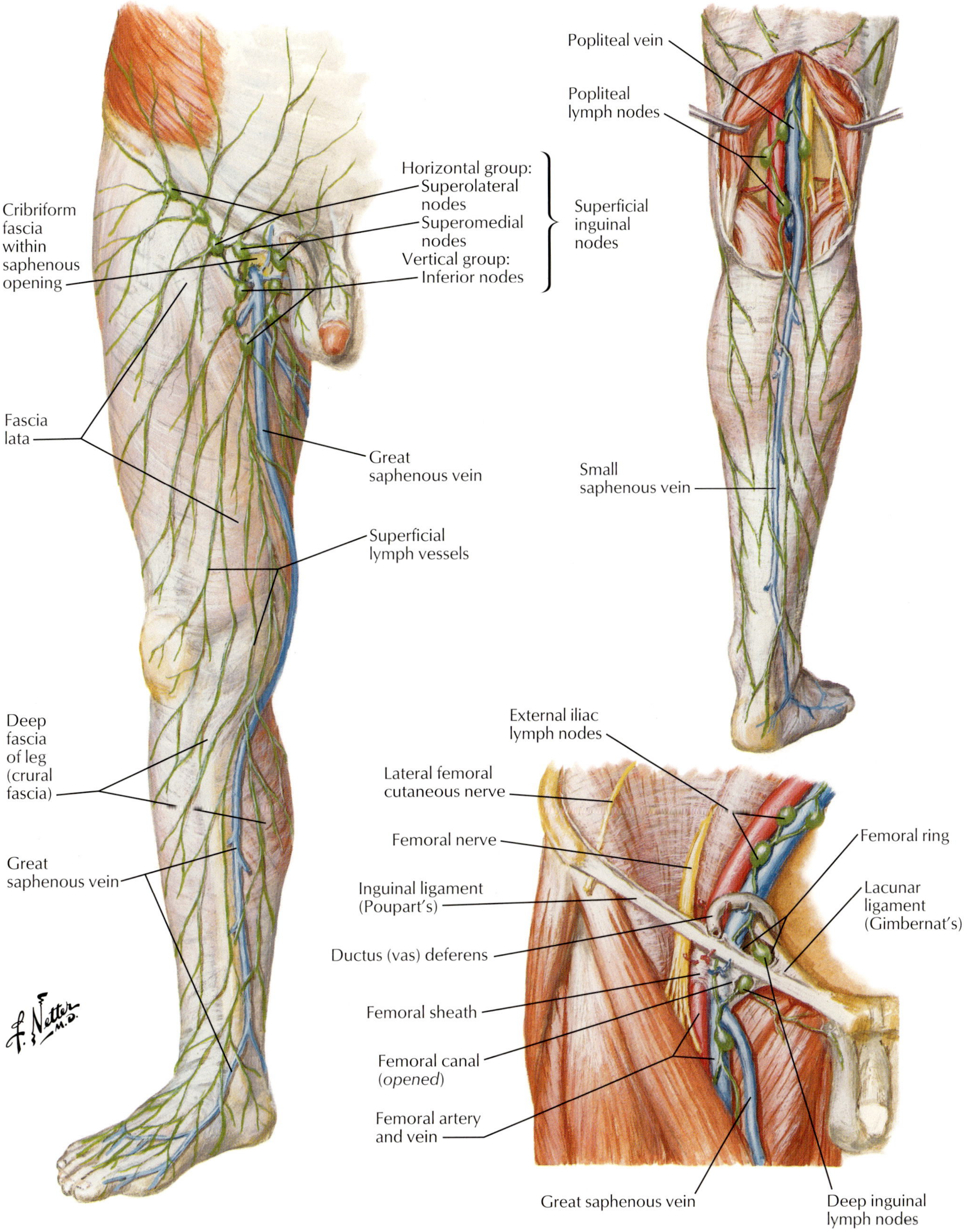

See also Plates 243, 333, 334

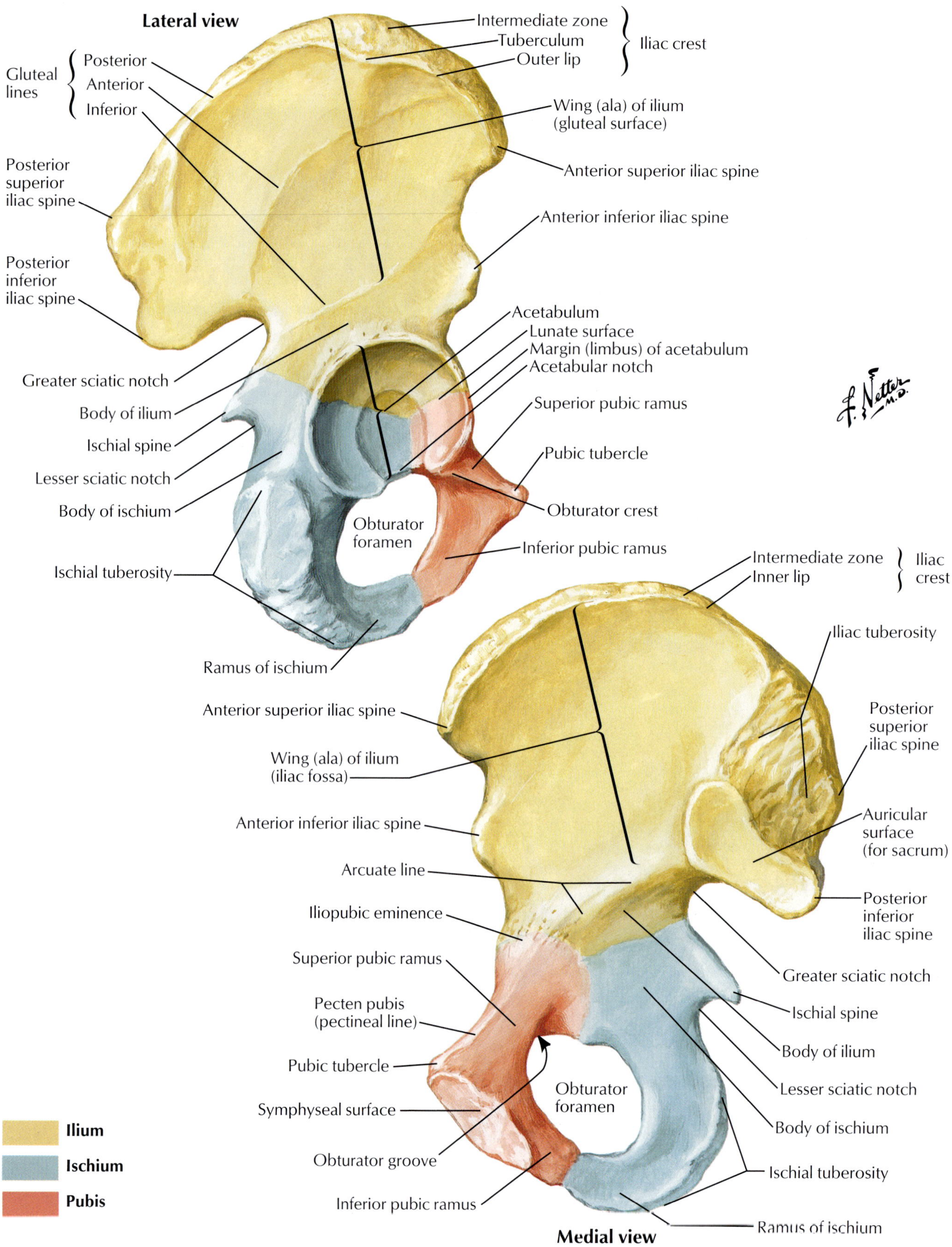

See also Plates 330, 334

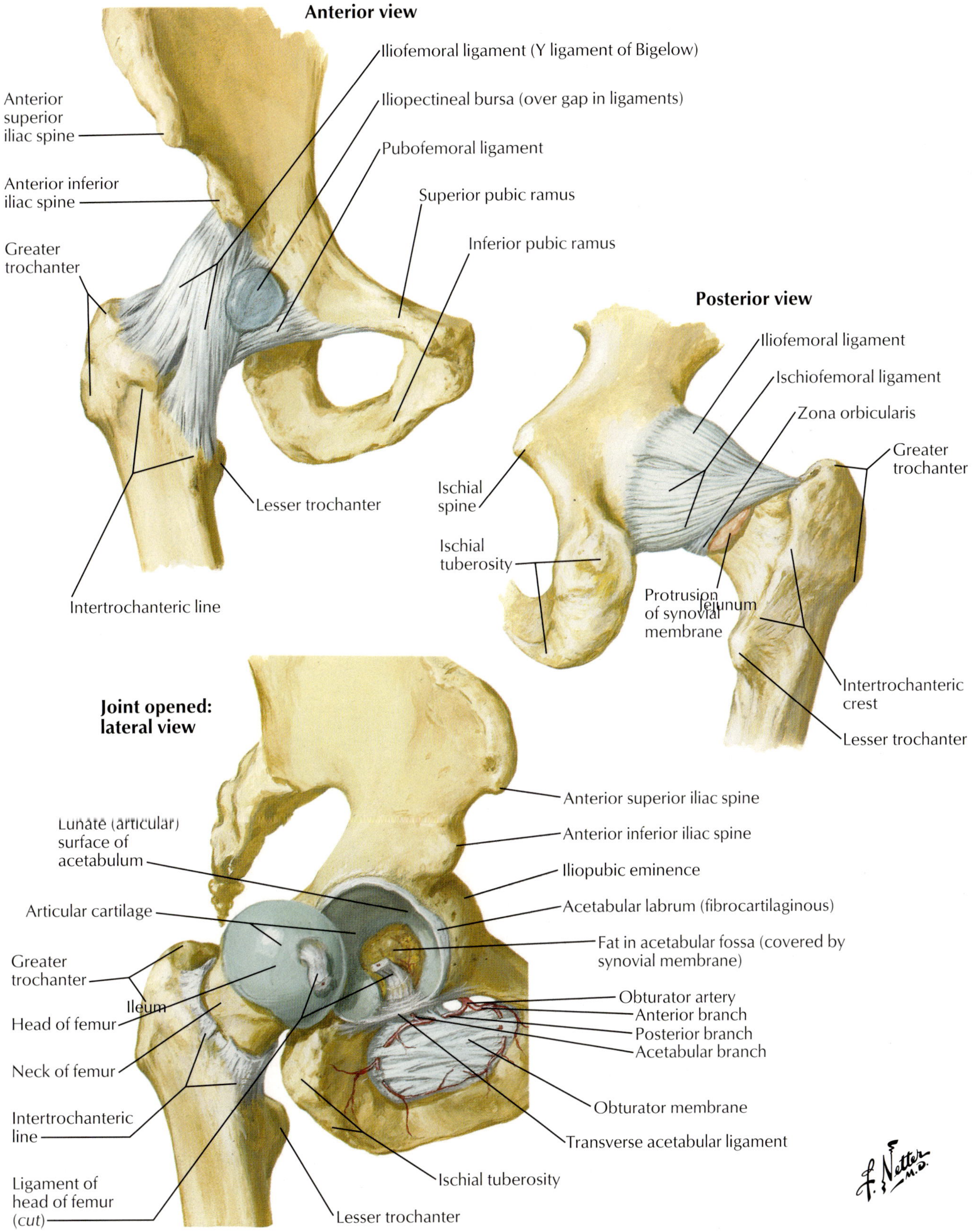

See also Plates 331, 474, 478

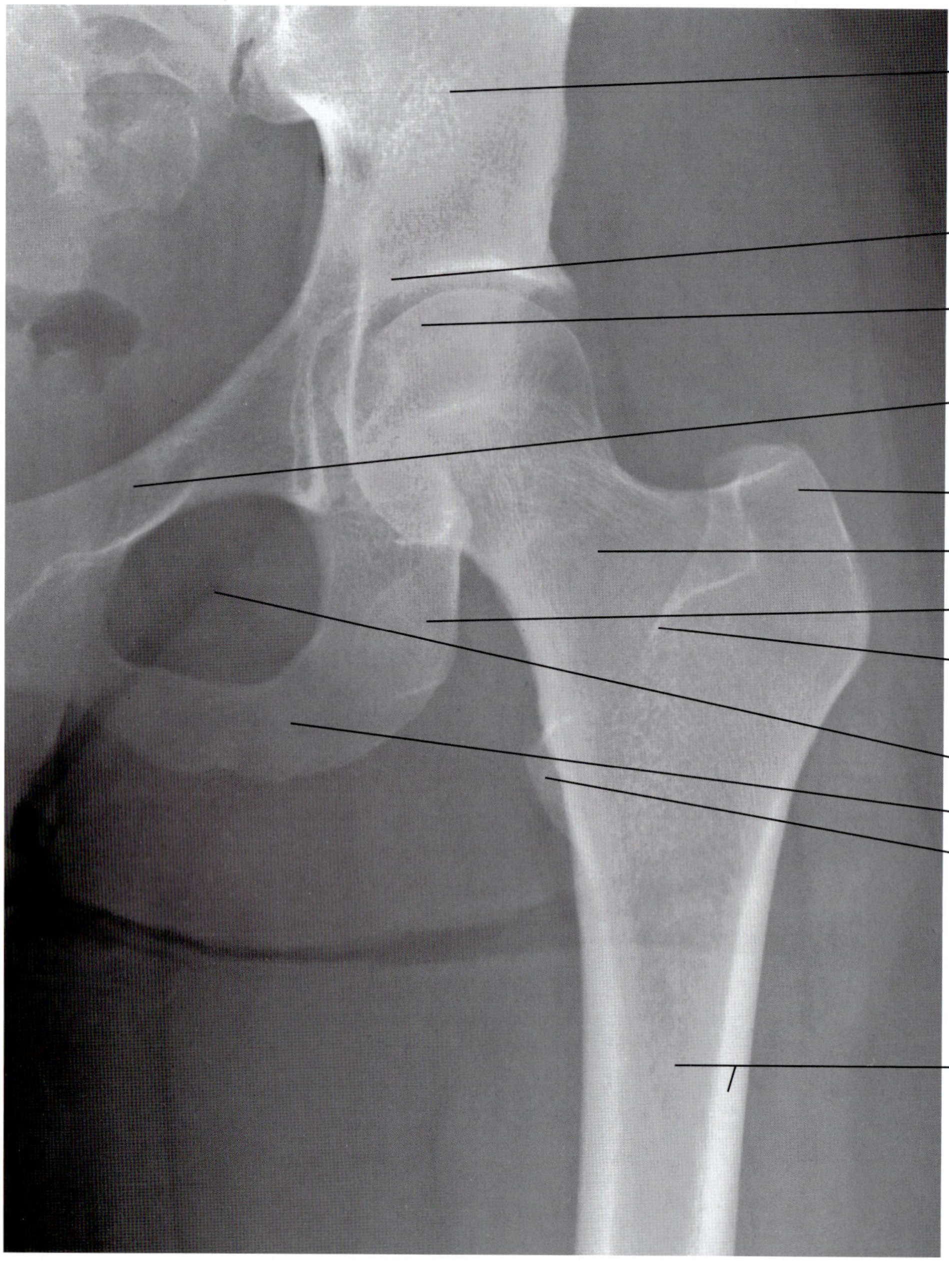

See also Plate 491

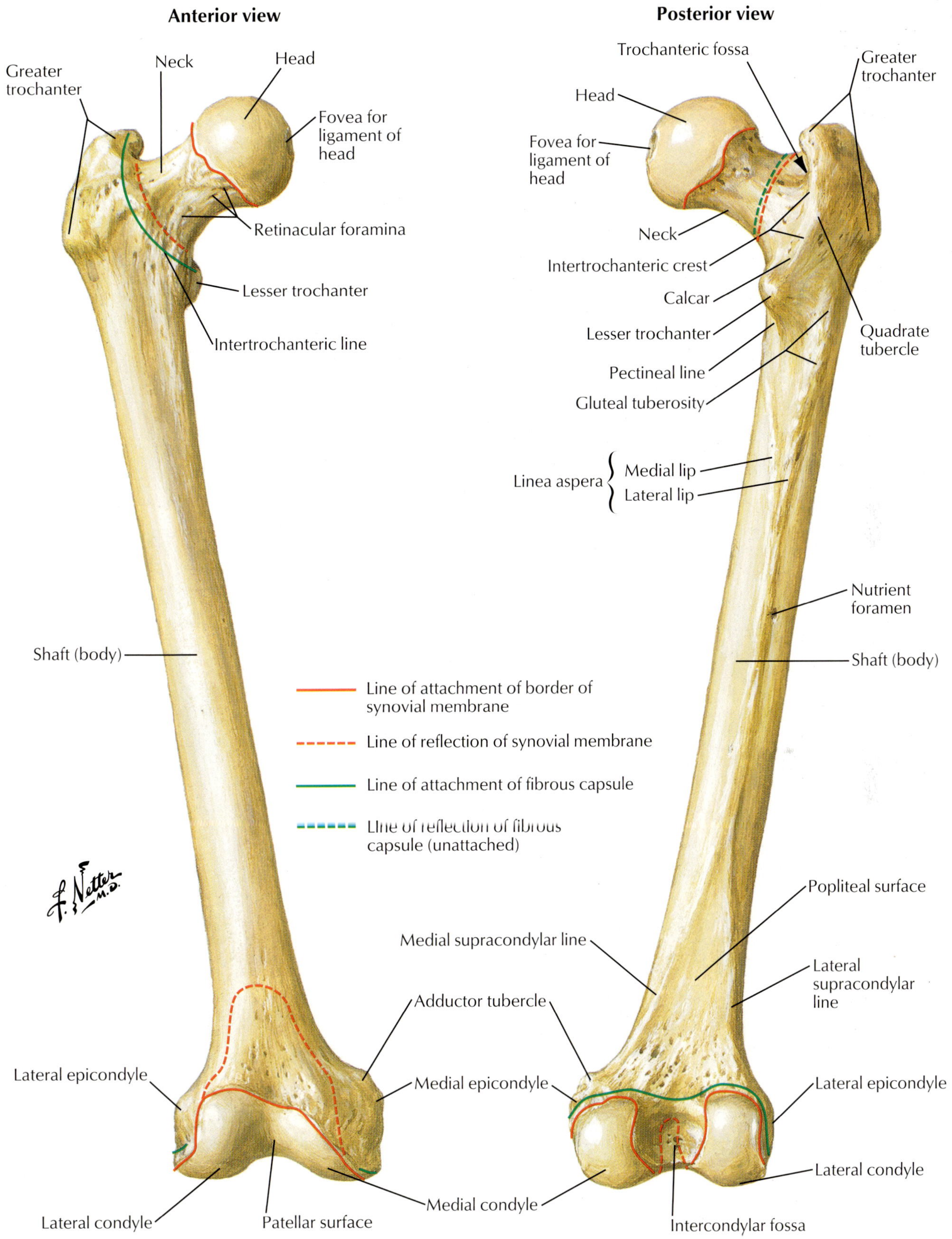

Bony Attachments of Muscles of Hip and Thigh: Anterior View

See also Plate 530

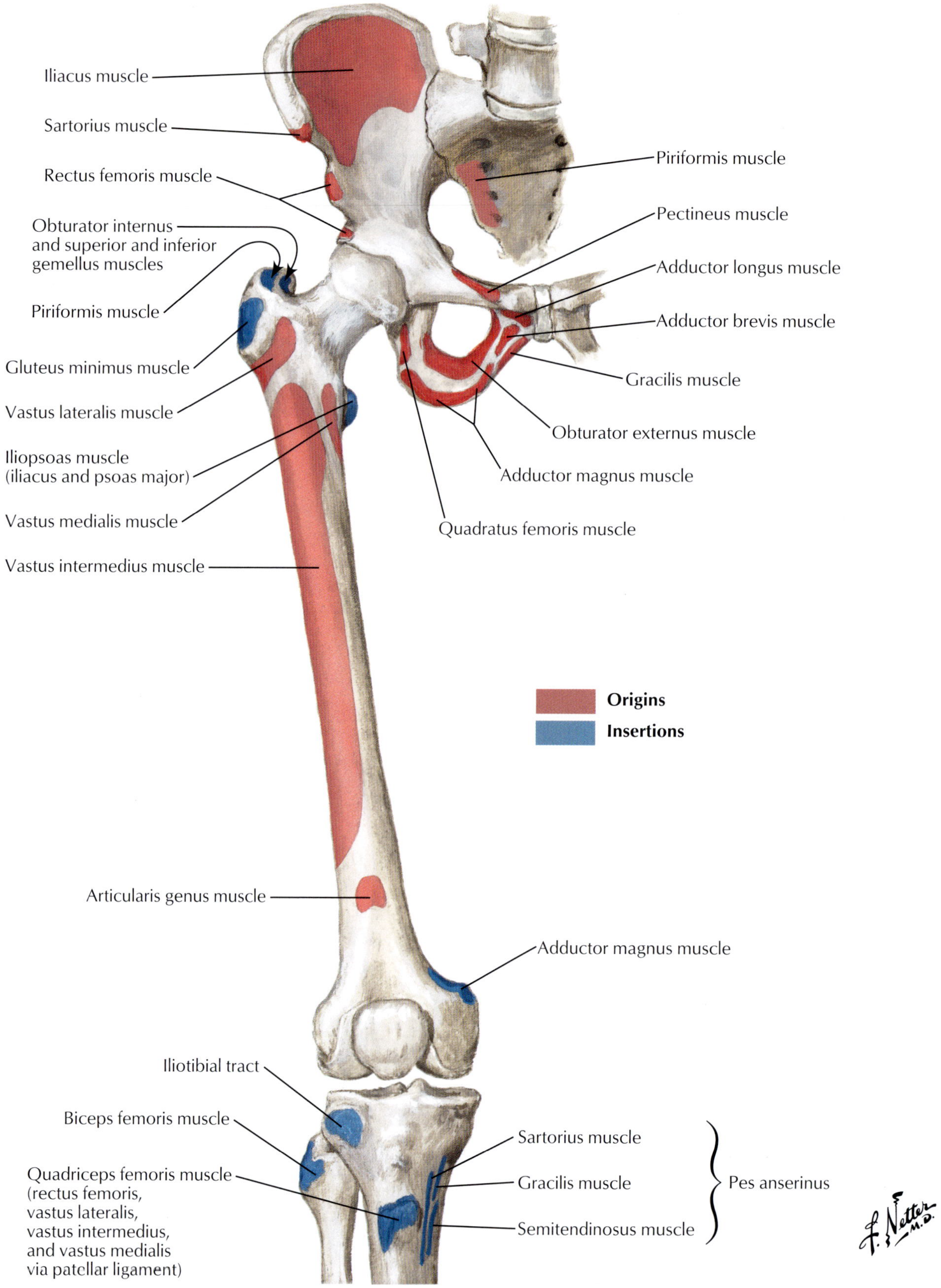

Bony Attachments of Muscles of Hip and Thigh: Posterior View

See also Plate 475

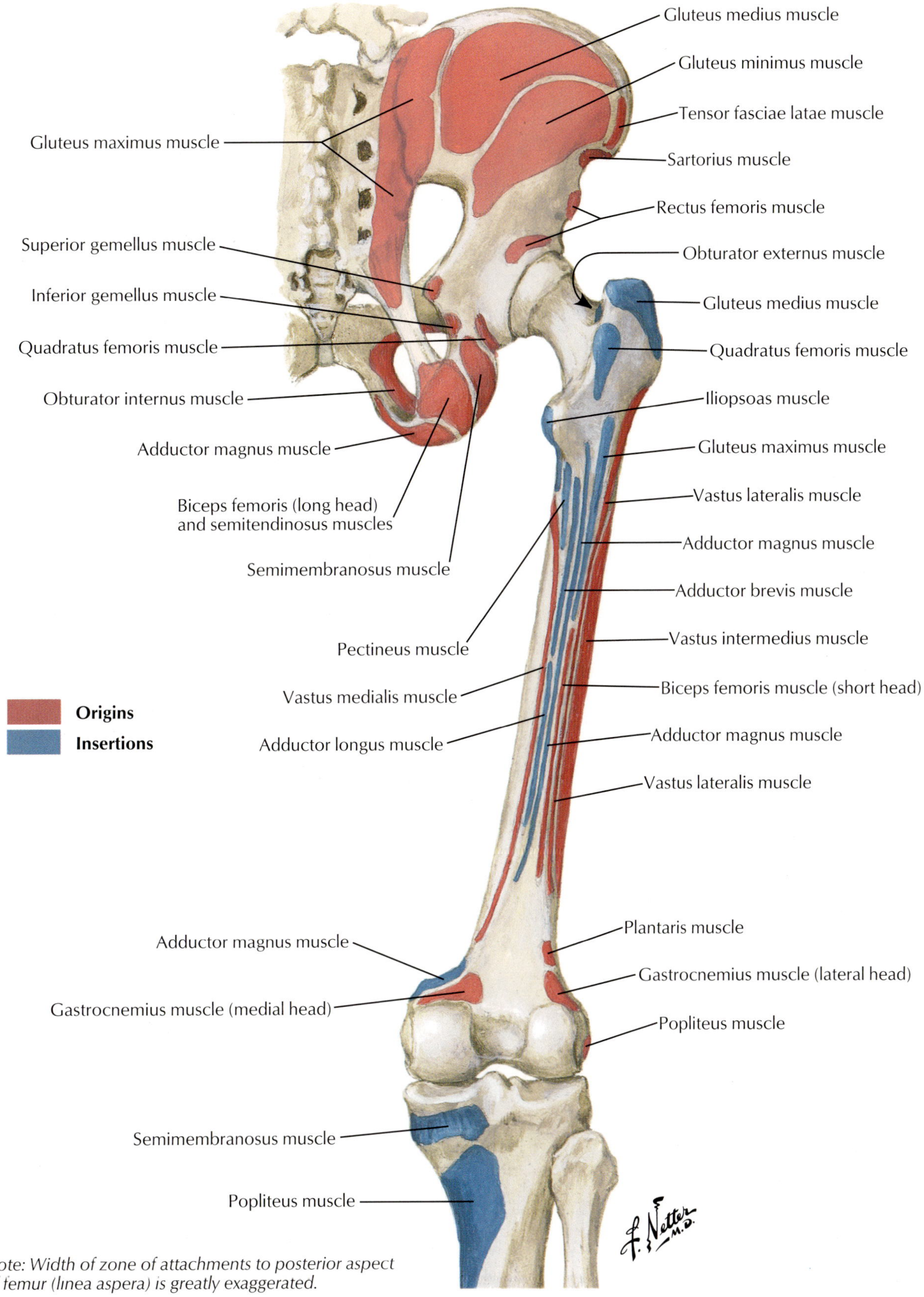

Note: Width of zone of attachments to posterior aspect of femur (linea aspera) is greatly exaggerated.

Muscles of Thigh: Anterior Views

See also **Plate 258**

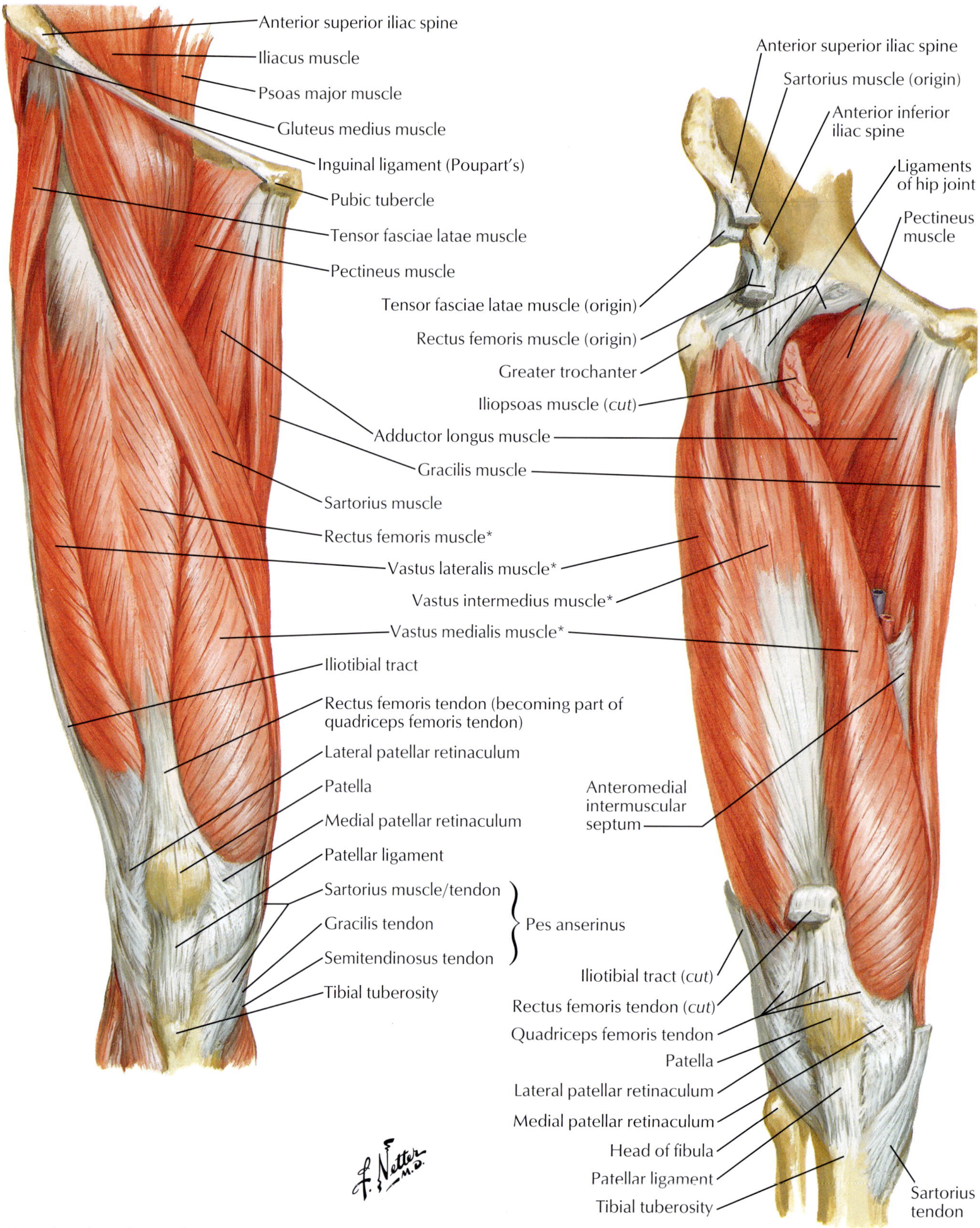

*Muscles of quadriceps femoris

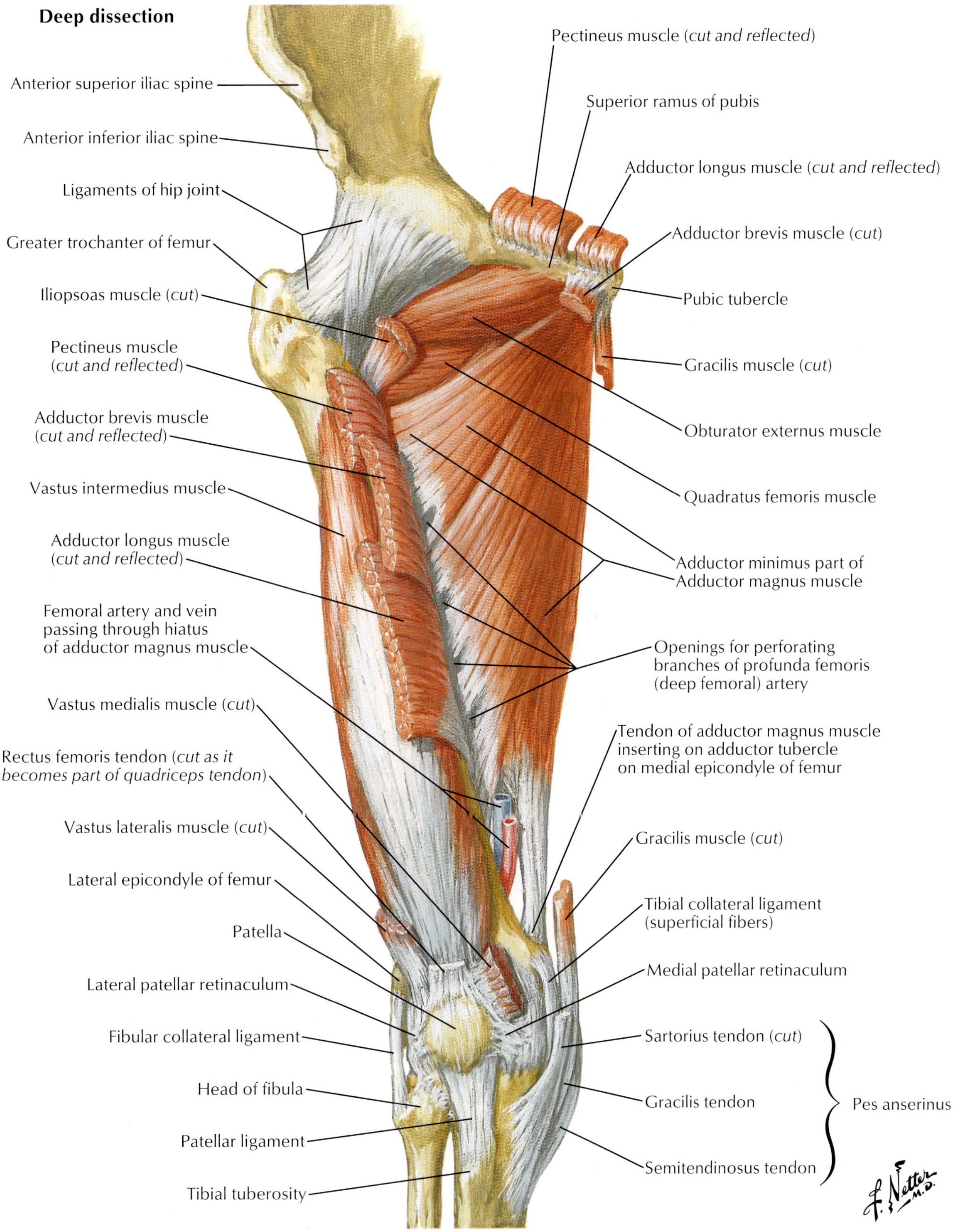
Deep dissection
Anterior superior iliac spine
Anterior inferior iliac spine
Ligaments of hip joint
Greater trochanter of femur
Iliopsoas muscle (cut)
Pectineus muscle (cut and reflected)
Adductor brevis muscle (cut and reflected)
Vastus intermedius muscle
Adductor longus muscle (cut and reflected)
Femoral artery and vein passing through hiatus of adductor magnus muscle
Vastus medialis muscle (cut)
Rectus femoris tendon (cut as it becomes part of quadriceps tendon)
Vastus lateralis muscle (cut)
Lateral epicondyle of femur
Patella
Lateral patellar retinaculum
Fibular collateral ligament
Head of fibula
Patellar ligament
Tibial tuberosity
Pectineus muscle (cut and reflected)
Superior ramus of pubis
Adductor longus muscle (cut and reflected)
Adductor brevis muscle (cut)
Pubic tubercle
Gracilis muscle (cut)
Obturator externus muscle
Quadratus femoris muscle
Adductor minimus part of Adductor magnus muscle
Openings for perforating branches of profunda femoris (deep femoral) artery
Tendon of adductor magnus muscle inserting on adductor tubercle on medial epicondyle of femur
Gracilis muscle (cut)
Tibial collateral ligament (superficial fibers)
Medial patellar retinaculum
Sartorius tendon (cut)
Gracilis tendon
Semitendinosus tendon
Pes anserinus
F. Netter M.D.

See also Plate 468

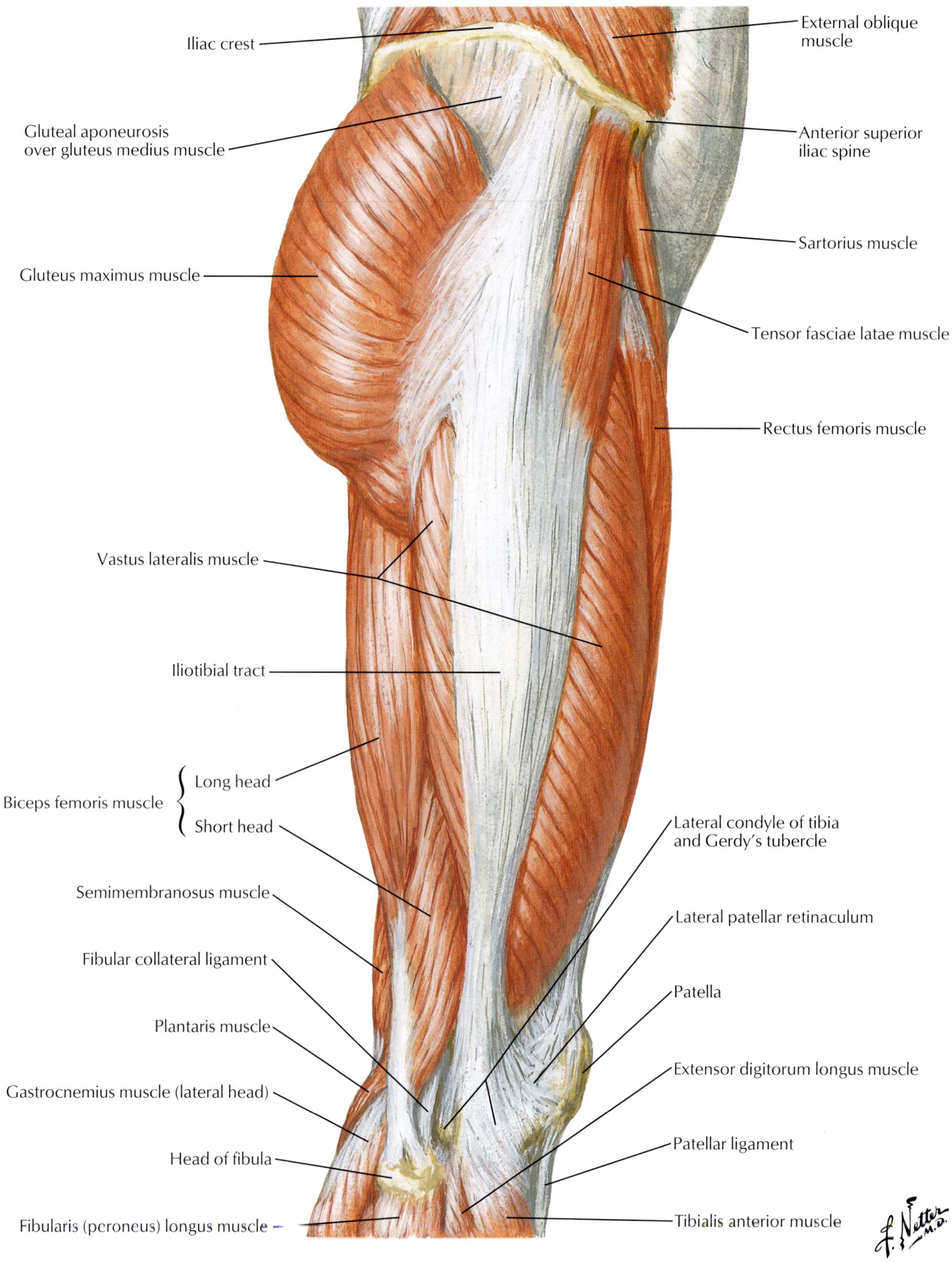

Muscles of Hip and Thigh: Posterior Views

See also **Plates 338, 339, 488**

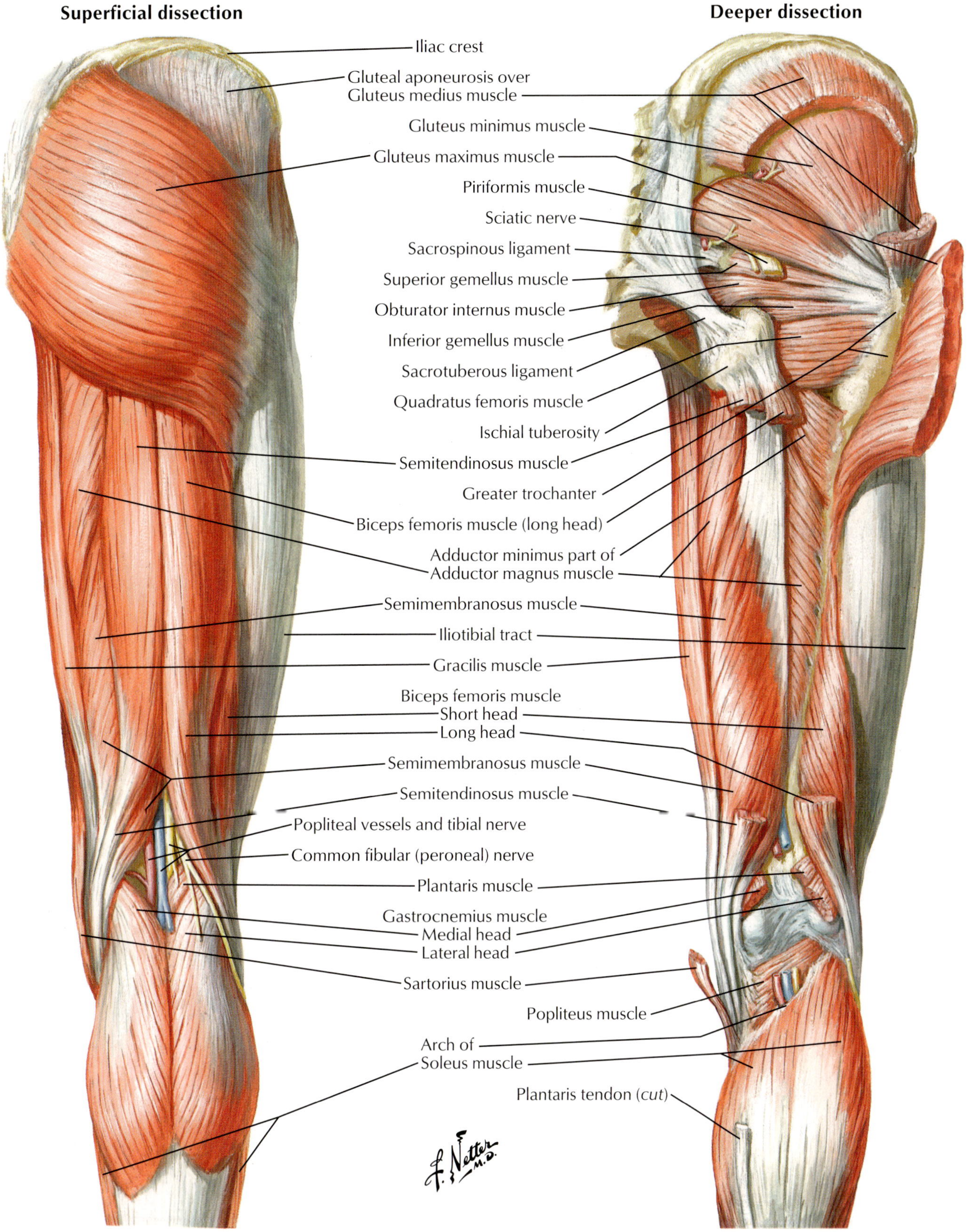

Psoas and Iliacus Muscles

See also **Plates 253, 258, 262**

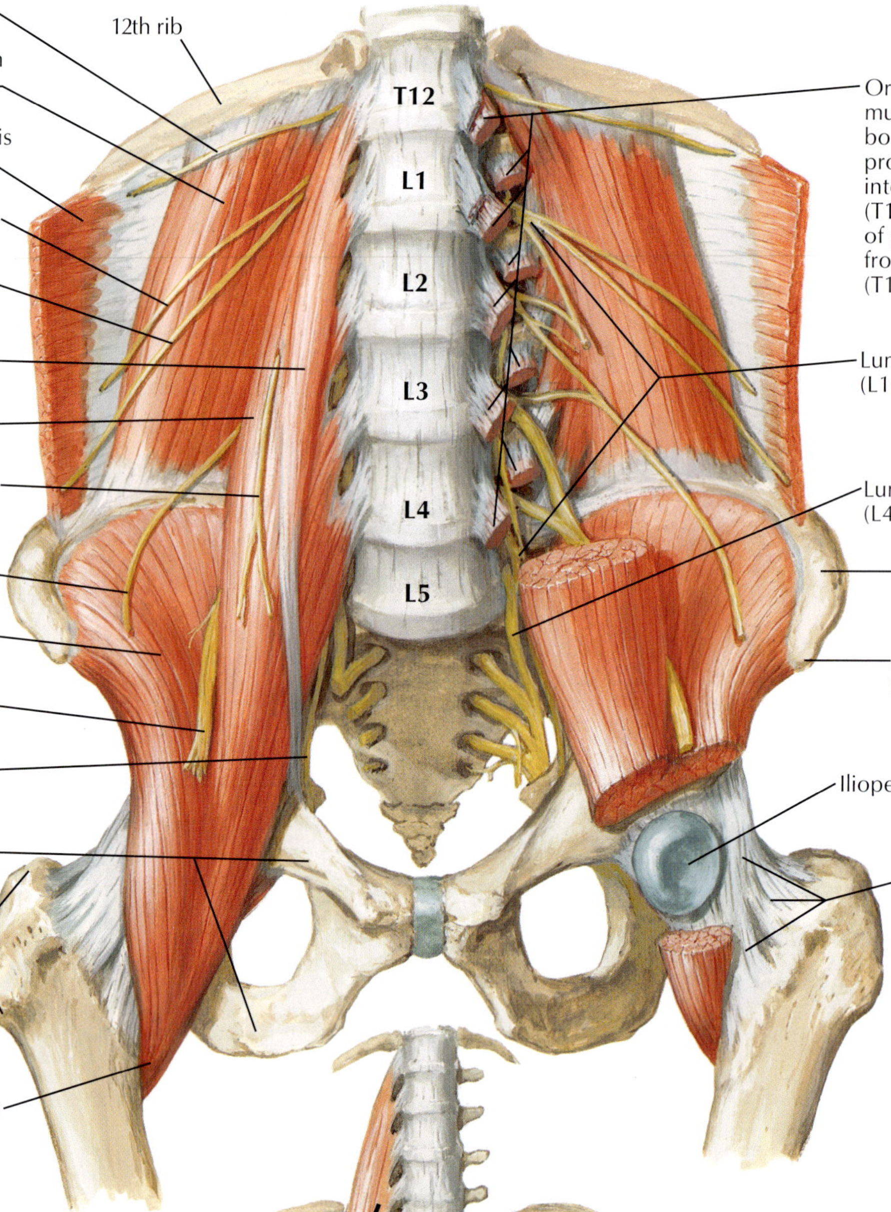

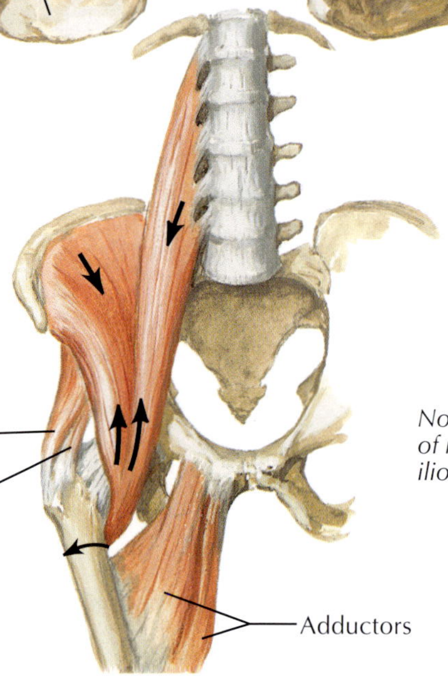

Note: Arrows indicate direction of action of muscles (iliacus/psoas superiorly, iliopsoas inferiorly).

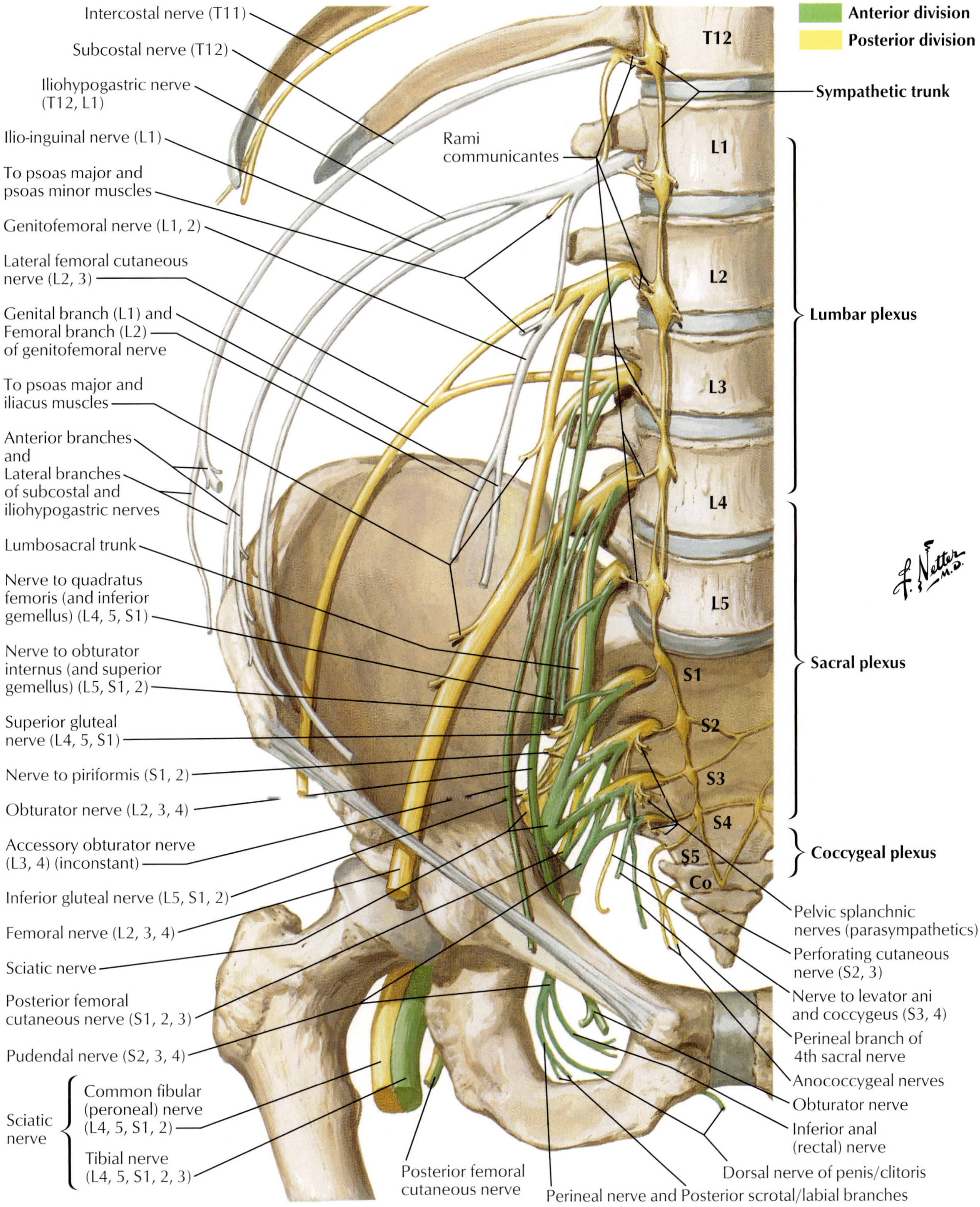

Anterior division
Posterior division
Intercostal nerve (T11)
Subcostal nerve (T12)
Iliohypogastric nerve (T12, L1)
Ilio-inguinal nerve (L1)
To psoas major and psoas minor muscles
Genitofemoral nerve (L1, 2)
Lateral femoral cutaneous nerve (L2, 3)
Genital branch (L1) and Femoral branch (L2) of genitofemoral nerve
To psoas major and iliacus muscles
Anterior branches and Lateral branches of subcostal and iliohypogastric nerves
Lumbosacral trunk
Nerve to quadratus femoris (and inferior gemellus) (L4, 5, S1)
Nerve to obturator internus (and superior gemellus) (L5, S1, 2)
Superior gluteal nerve (L4, 5, S1)
Nerve to piriformis (S1, 2)
Obturator nerve (L2, 3, 4)
Accessory obturator nerve (L3, 4) (inconstant)
Inferior gluteal nerve (L5, S1, 2)
Femoral nerve (L2, 3, 4)
Sciatic nerve
Posterior femoral cutaneous nerve (S1, 2, 3)
Pudendal nerve (S2, 3, 4)
Sciatic nerve
Common fibular (peroneal) nerve (L4, 5, S1, 2)
Tibial nerve (L4, 5, S1, 2, 3)
Posterior femoral cutaneous nerve
Rami communicantes
T12
L1
L2
L3
L4
L5
S1
S2
S3
S4
S5
Co
Sympathetic trunk
Lumbar plexus
Sacral plexus
Coccygeal plexus
F. Netter M.D.
Pelvic splanchnic nerves (parasympathetics)
Perforating cutaneous nerve (S2, 3)
Nerve to levator ani and coccygeus (S3, 4)
Perineal branch of 4th sacral nerve
Anococcygeal nerves
Obturator nerve
Inferior anal (rectal) nerve
Dorsal nerve of penis/clitoris
Perineal nerve and Posterior scrotal/labial branches

See also Plate 262

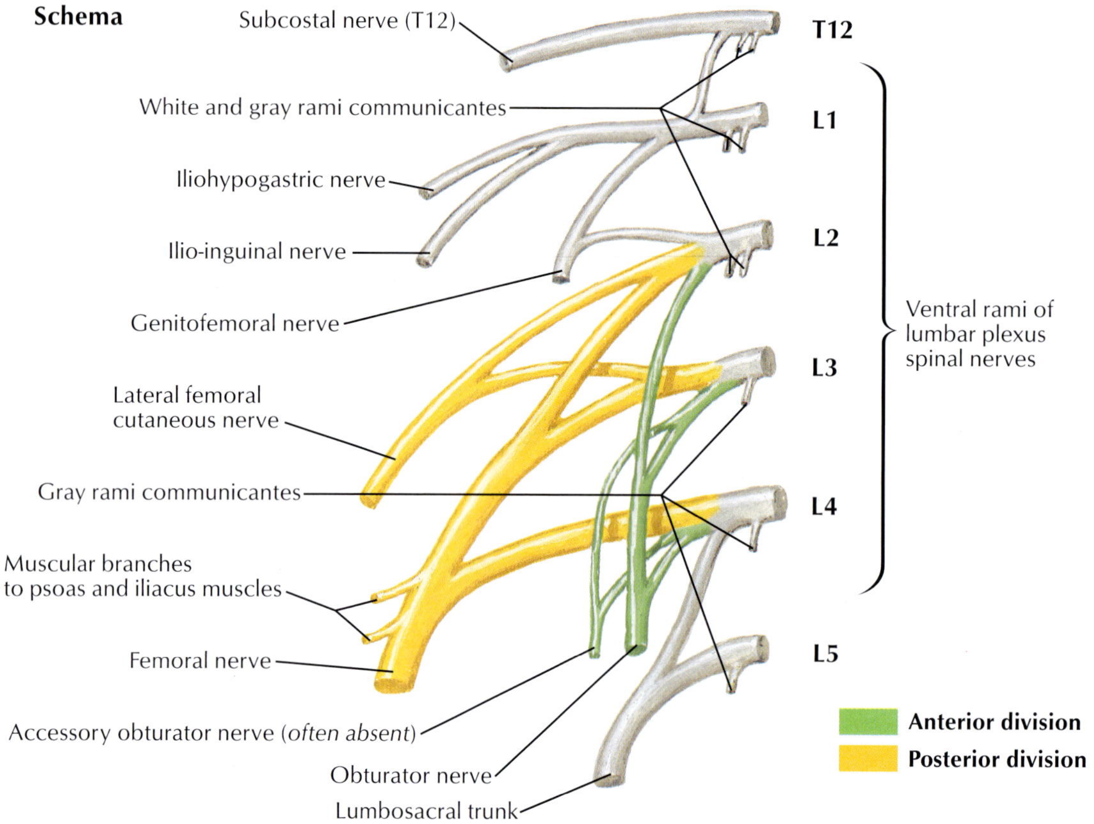

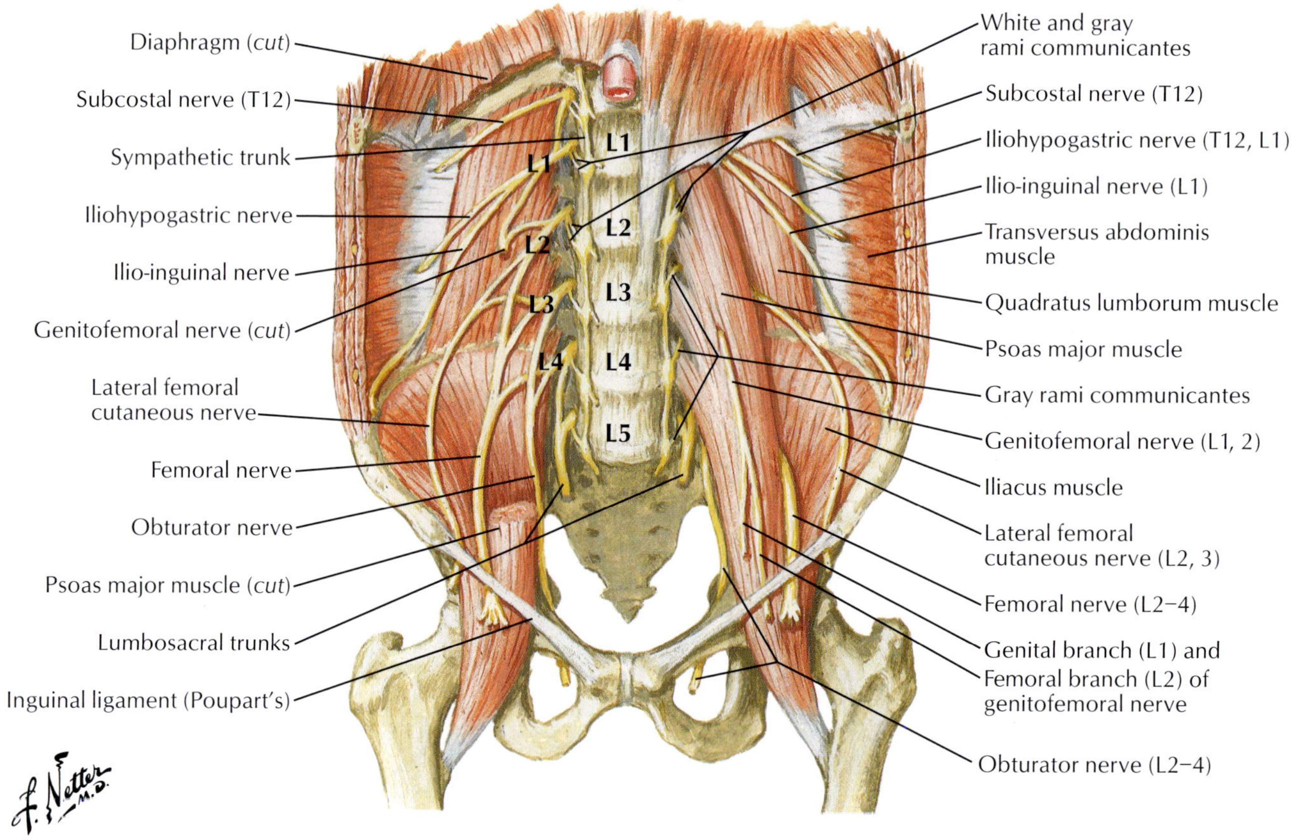

Sacral and Coccygeal Plexuses

See also Plate 262

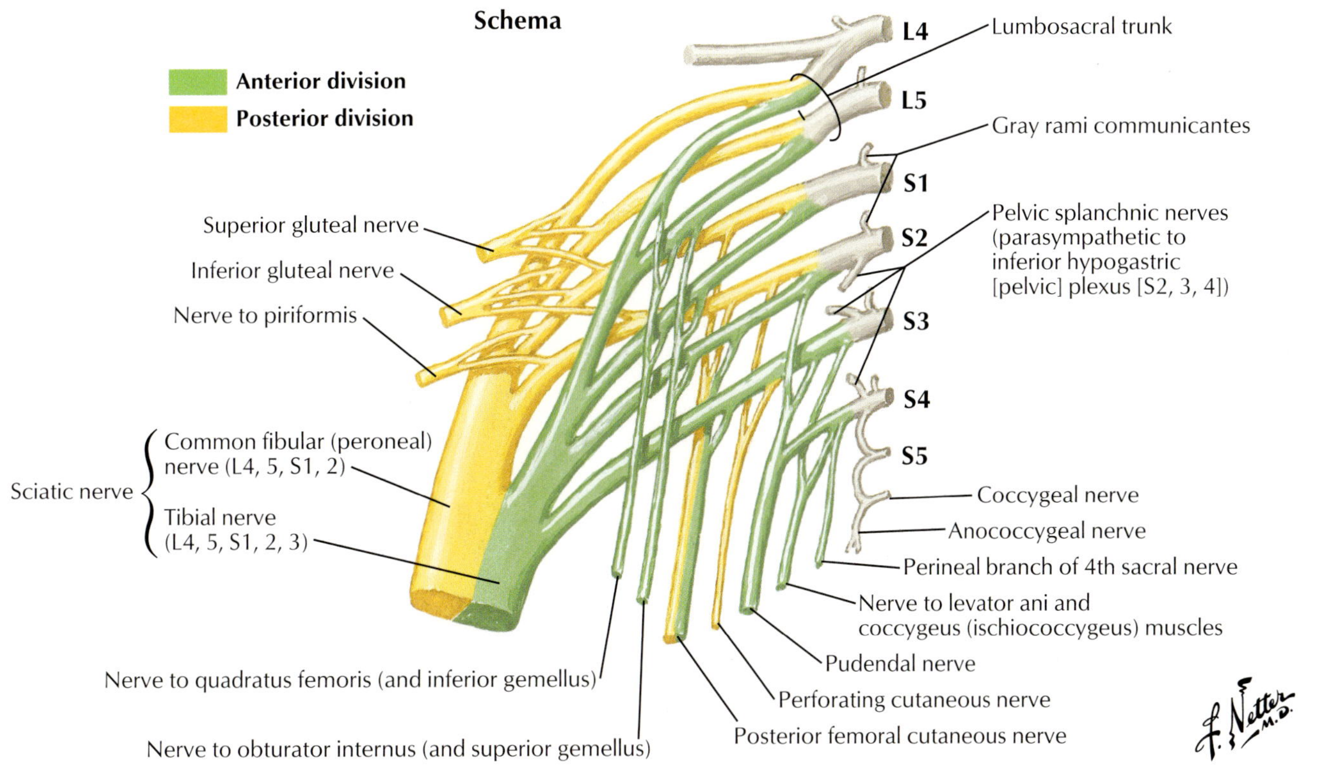

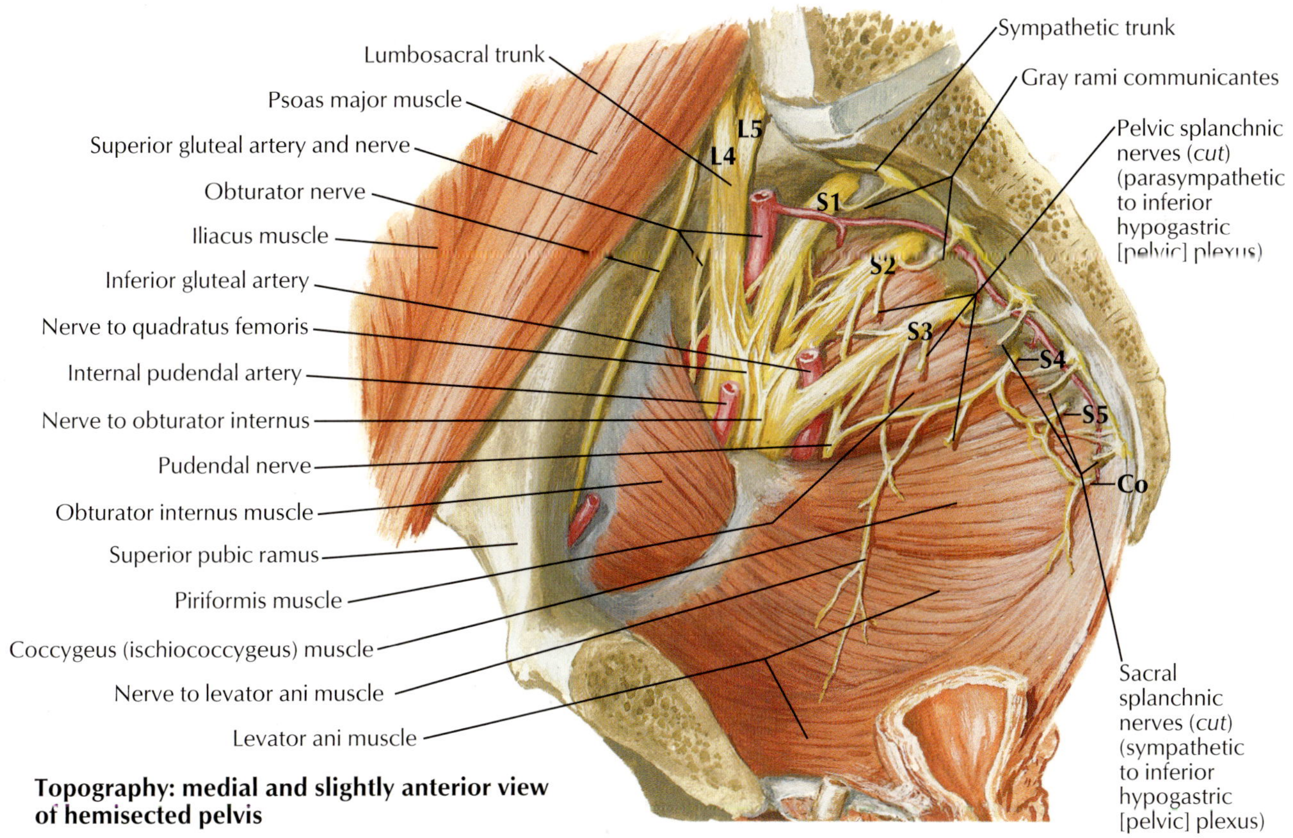

Topography: medial and slightly anterior view of hemisected pelvis

Arteries and Nerves of Thigh: Anterior Views

See also Plate 525

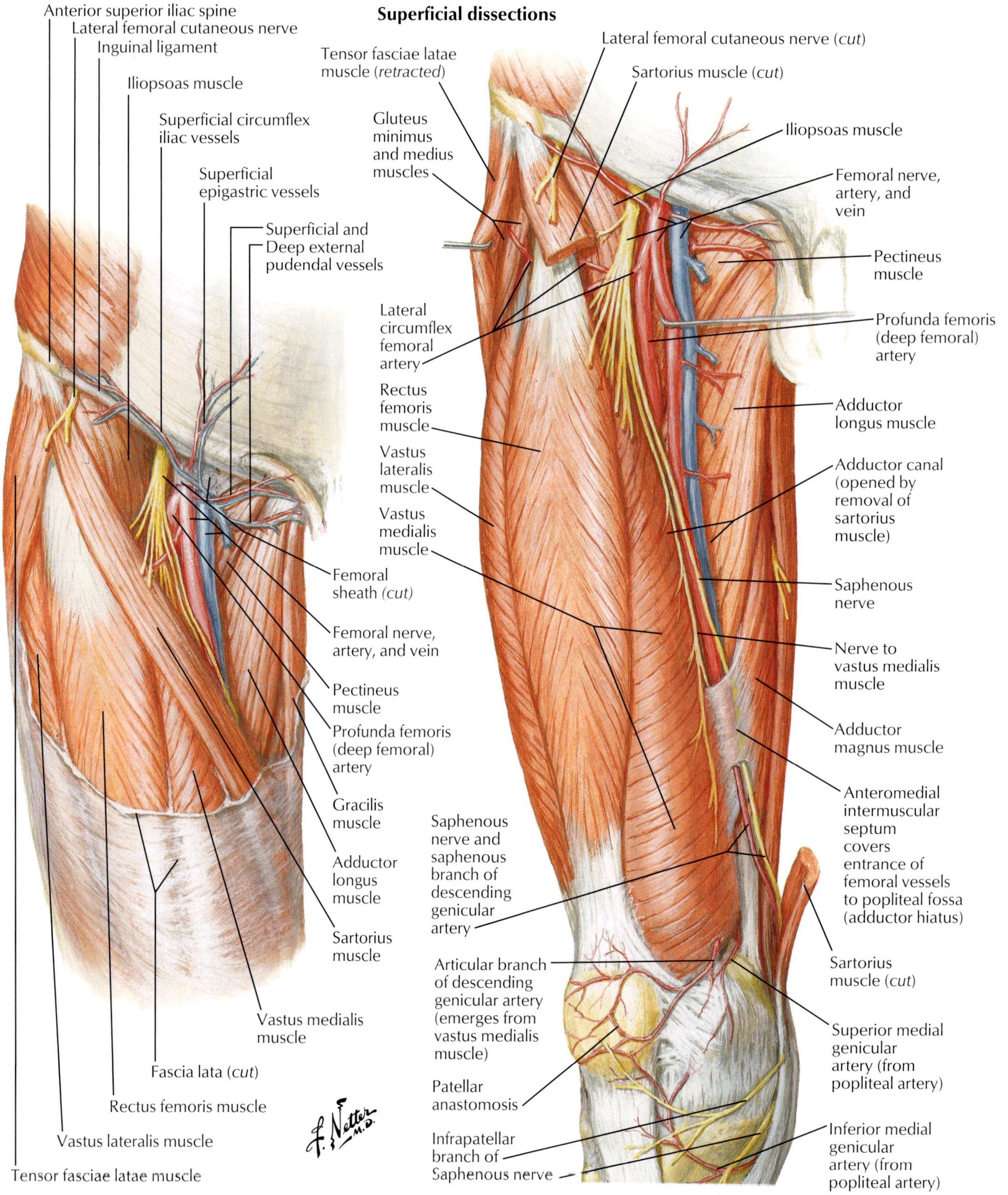

Arteries and Nerves of Thigh: Anterior Views (continued)

See also **Plates 525, 526**

Deep dissection

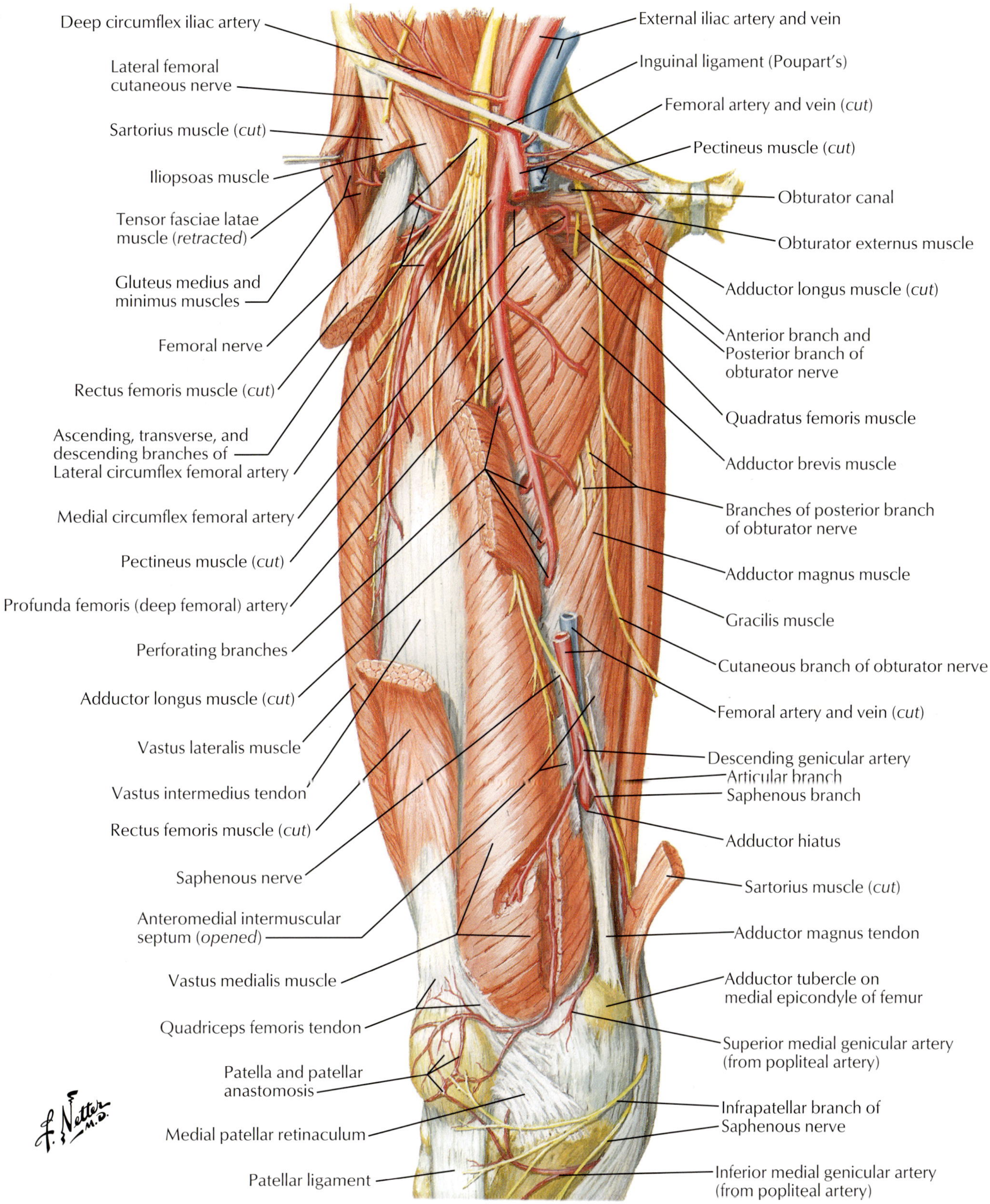

See also Plate 527

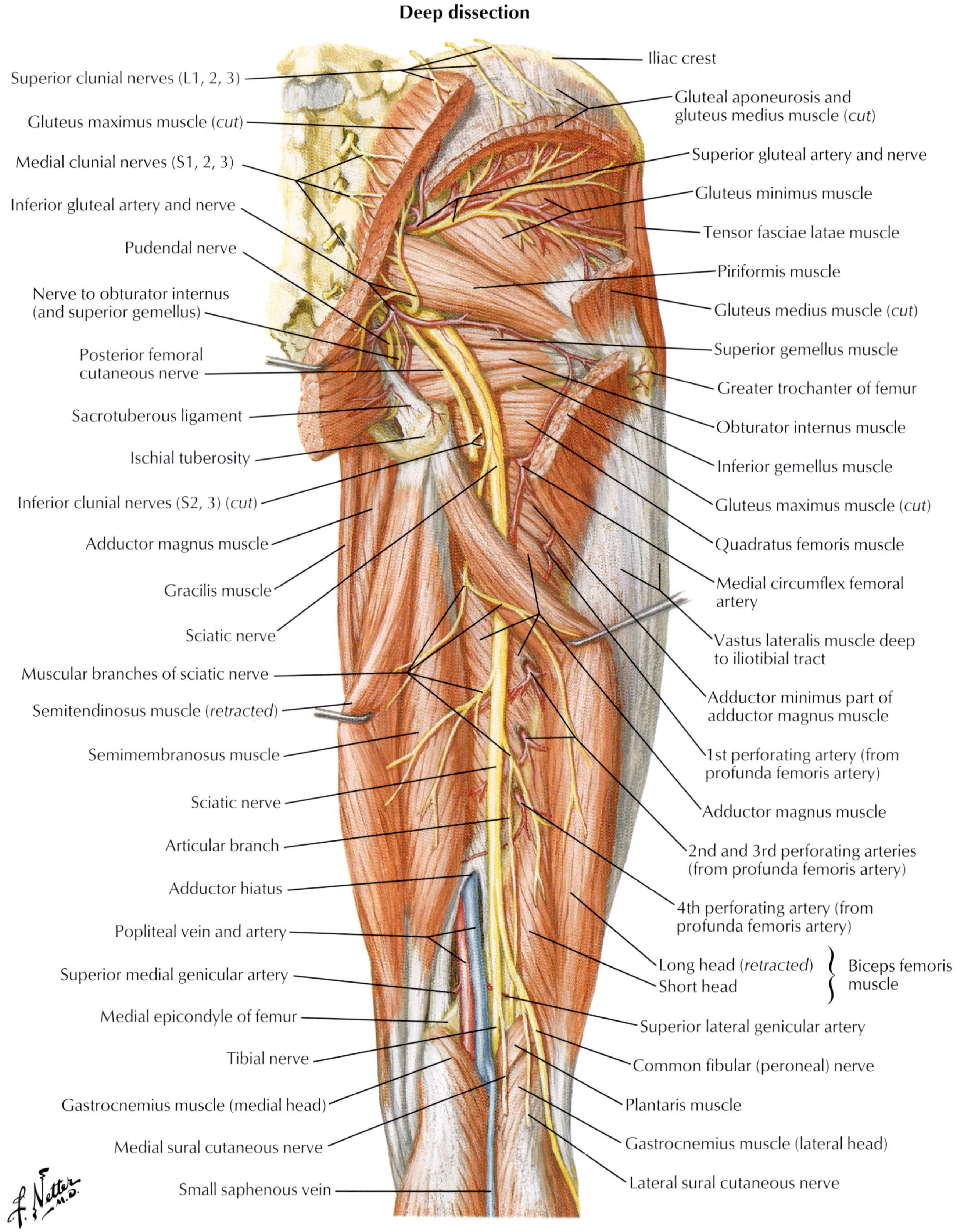

Nerves of Hip and Buttock

See also Plate 333

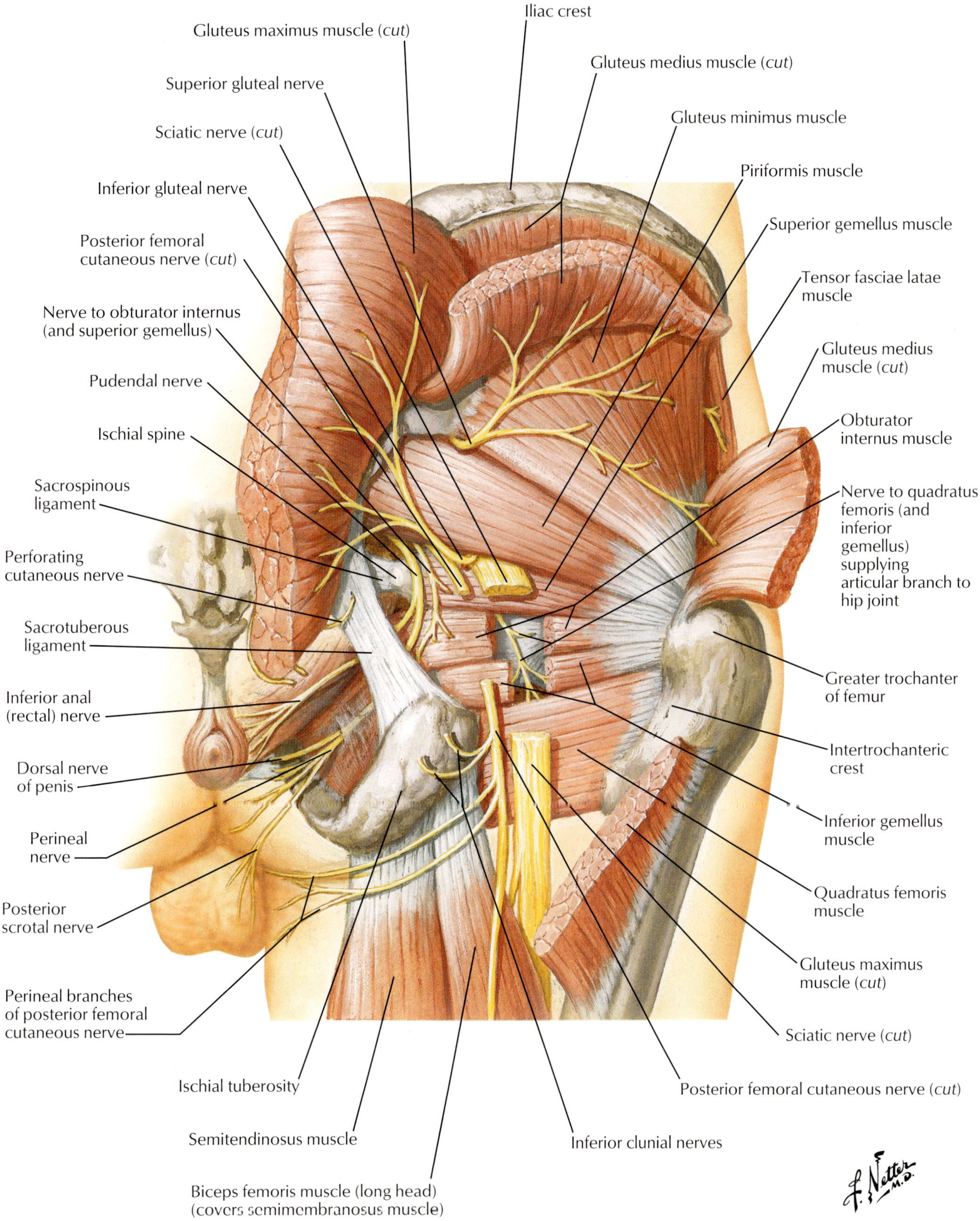

Arteries of Femoral Head and Neck

See also **Plates 499, 530**

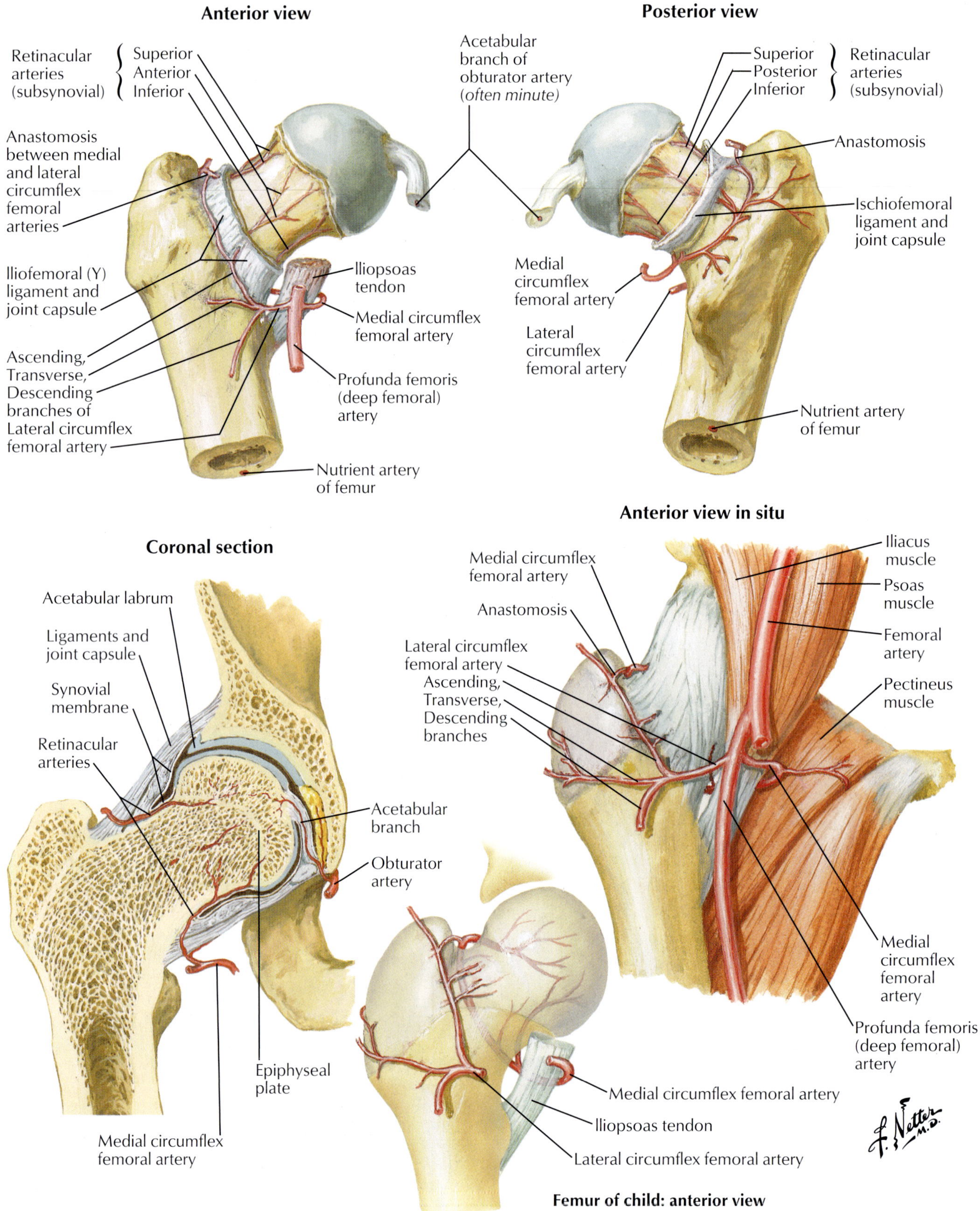

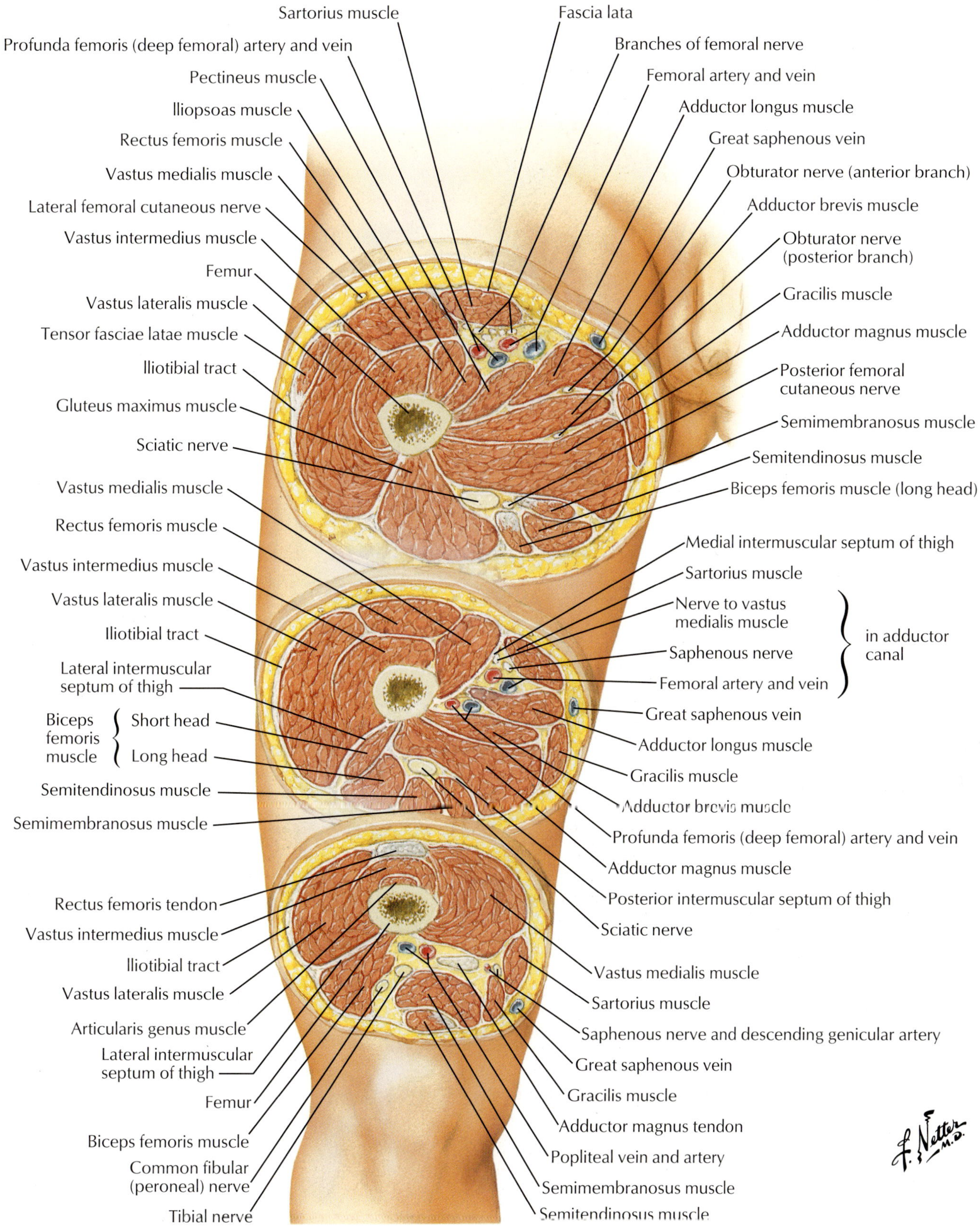
Sartorius muscle
Fascia lata
Profunda femoris (deep femoral) artery and vein
Branches of femoral nerve
Pectineus muscle
Femoral artery and vein
Iliopsoas muscle
Adductor longus muscle
Rectus femoris muscle
Great saphenous vein
Vastus medialis muscle
Obturator nerve (anterior branch)
Lateral femoral cutaneous nerve
Adductor brevis muscle
Vastus intermedius muscle
Obturator nerve (posterior branch)
Femur
Gracilis muscle
Vastus lateralis muscle
Adductor magnus muscle
Tensor fasciae latae muscle
Posterior femoral cutaneous nerve
Iliotibial tract
Semimembranosus muscle
Gluteus maximus muscle
Semitendinosus muscle
Sciatic nerve
Biceps femoris muscle (long head)
Vastus medialis muscle
Medial intermuscular septum of thigh
Rectus femoris muscle
Sartorius muscle
Vastus intermedius muscle
Nerve to vastus medialis muscle
Vastus lateralis muscle
Saphenous nerve
Iliotibial tract
Femoral artery and vein
in adductor canal
Lateral intermuscular septum of thigh
Great saphenous vein
Biceps femoris muscle
Short head
Long head
Adductor longus muscle
Gracilis muscle
Semitendinosus muscle
Adductor brevis muscle
Semimembranosus muscle
Profunda femoris (deep femoral) artery and vein
Adductor magnus muscle
Posterior intermuscular septum of thigh
Rectus femoris tendon
Sciatic nerve
Vastus intermedius muscle
Iliotibial tract
Vastus medialis muscle
Vastus lateralis muscle
Sartorius muscle
Articularis genus muscle
Saphenous nerve and descending genicular artery
Lateral intermuscular septum of thigh
Great saphenous vein
Gracilis muscle
Femur
Adductor magnus tendon
Biceps femoris muscle
Popliteal vein and artery
Common fibular (peroneal) nerve
Semimembranosus muscle
Tibial nerve
Semitendinosus muscle
F. Netter M.D.

Medial view

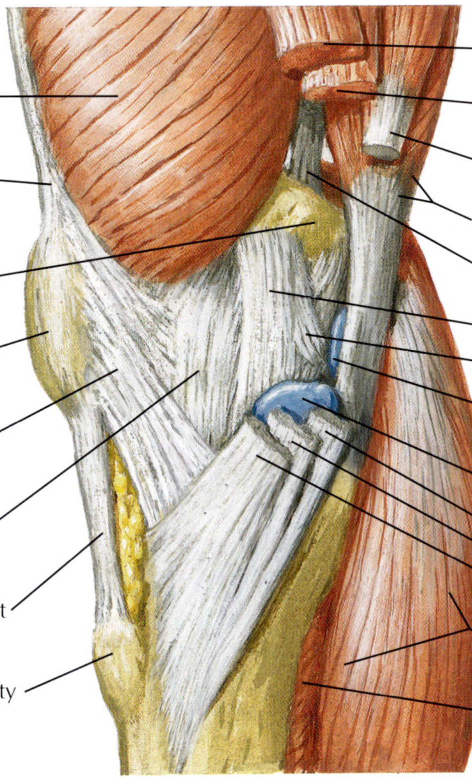

Lateral view

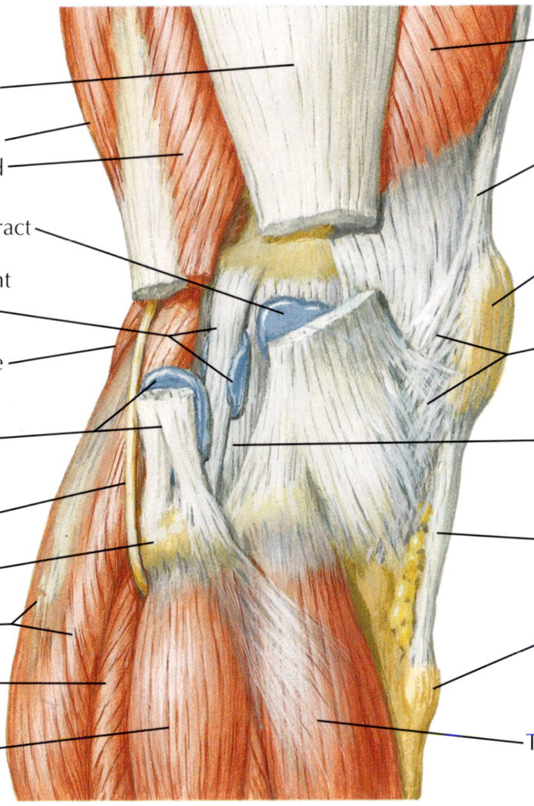

Right knee in extension

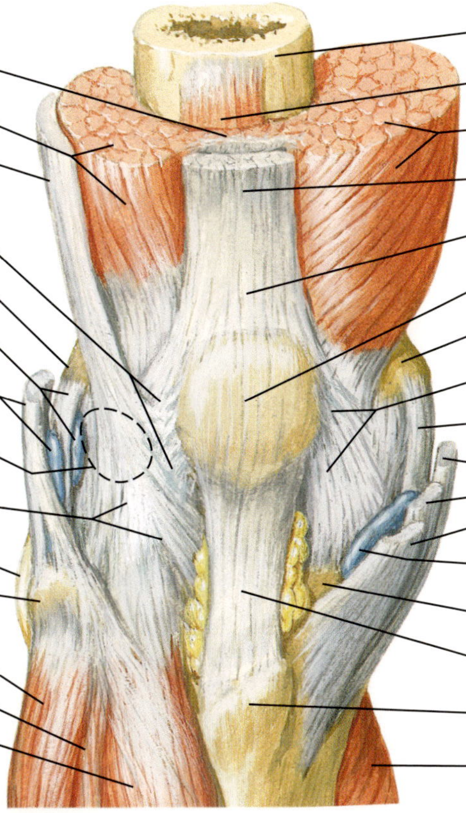

Joint opened, knee slightly in flexion

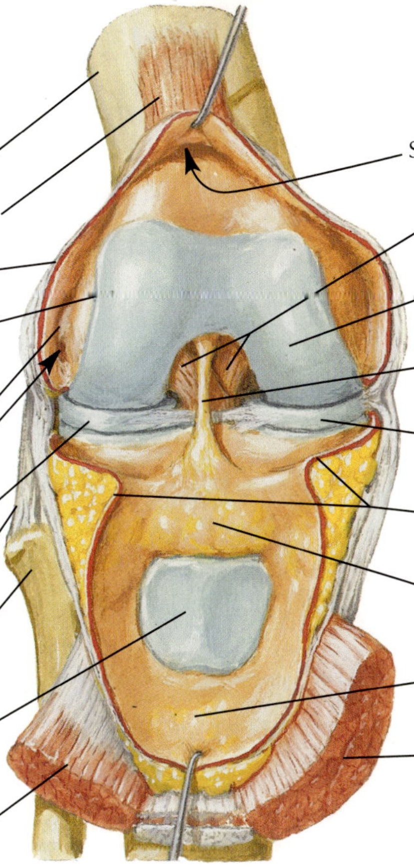

Knee: Interior

See also **Plate 501**

Inferior view

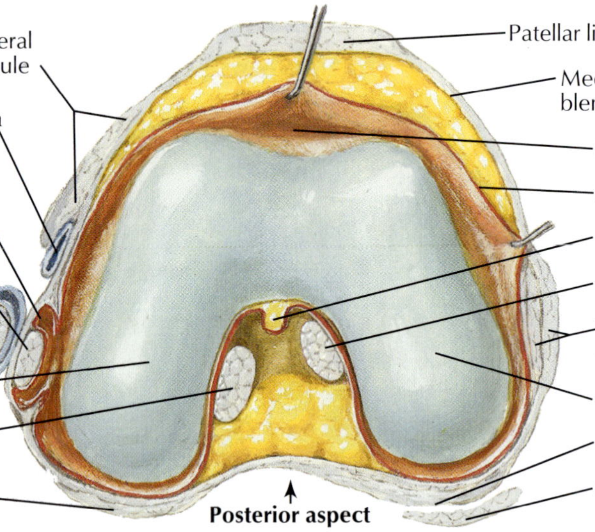

Superior view

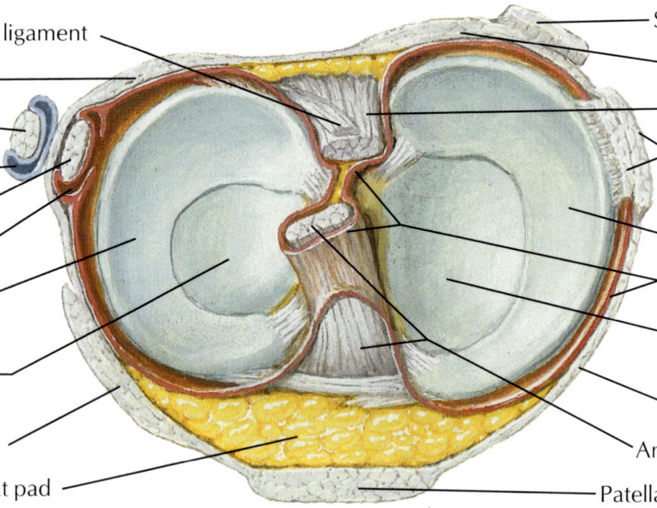

Superior view: ligaments and cartilage removed

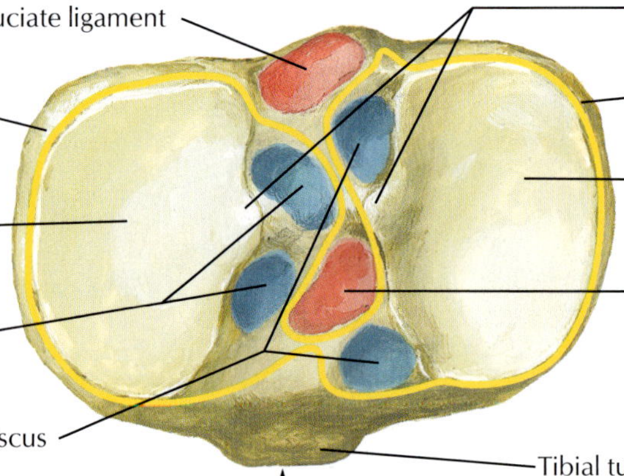

Right knee in flexion: anterior view

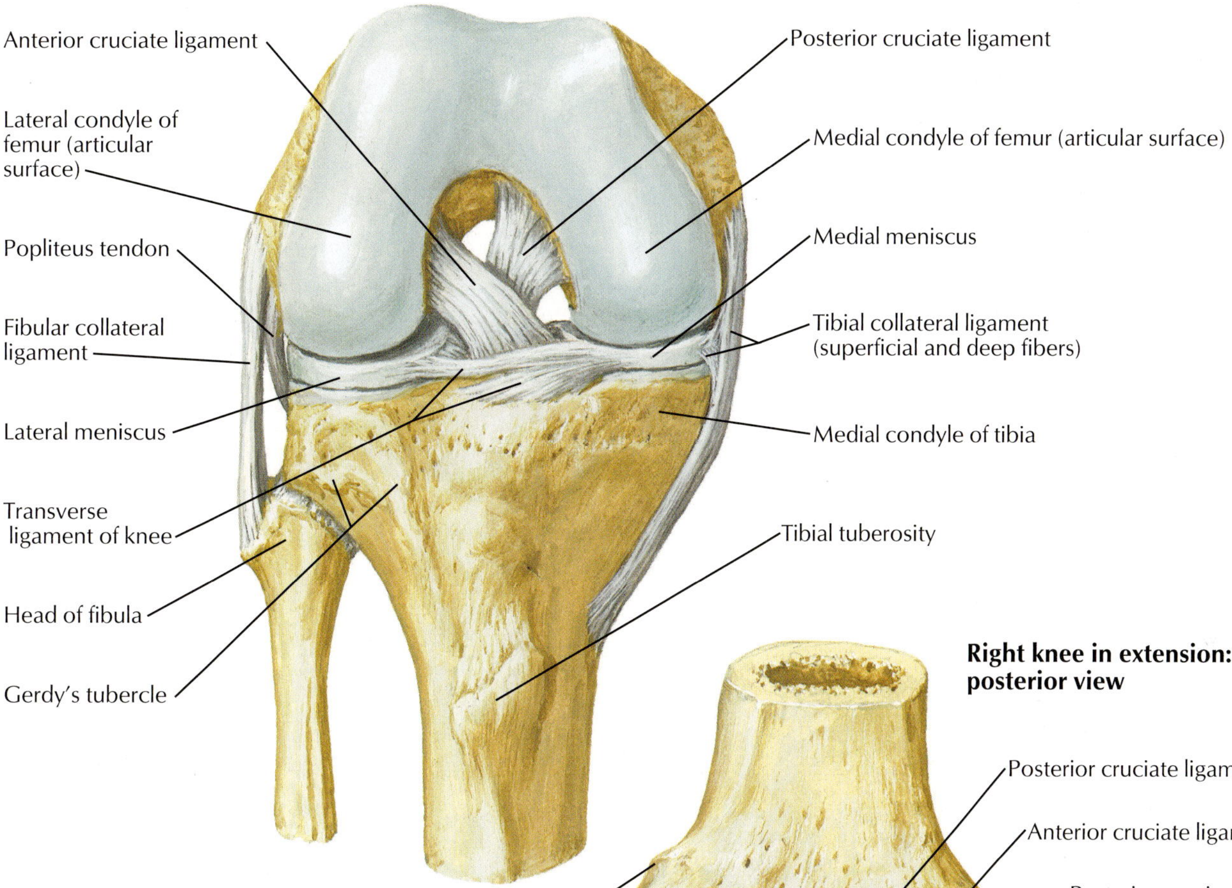

Right knee in extension: posterior view

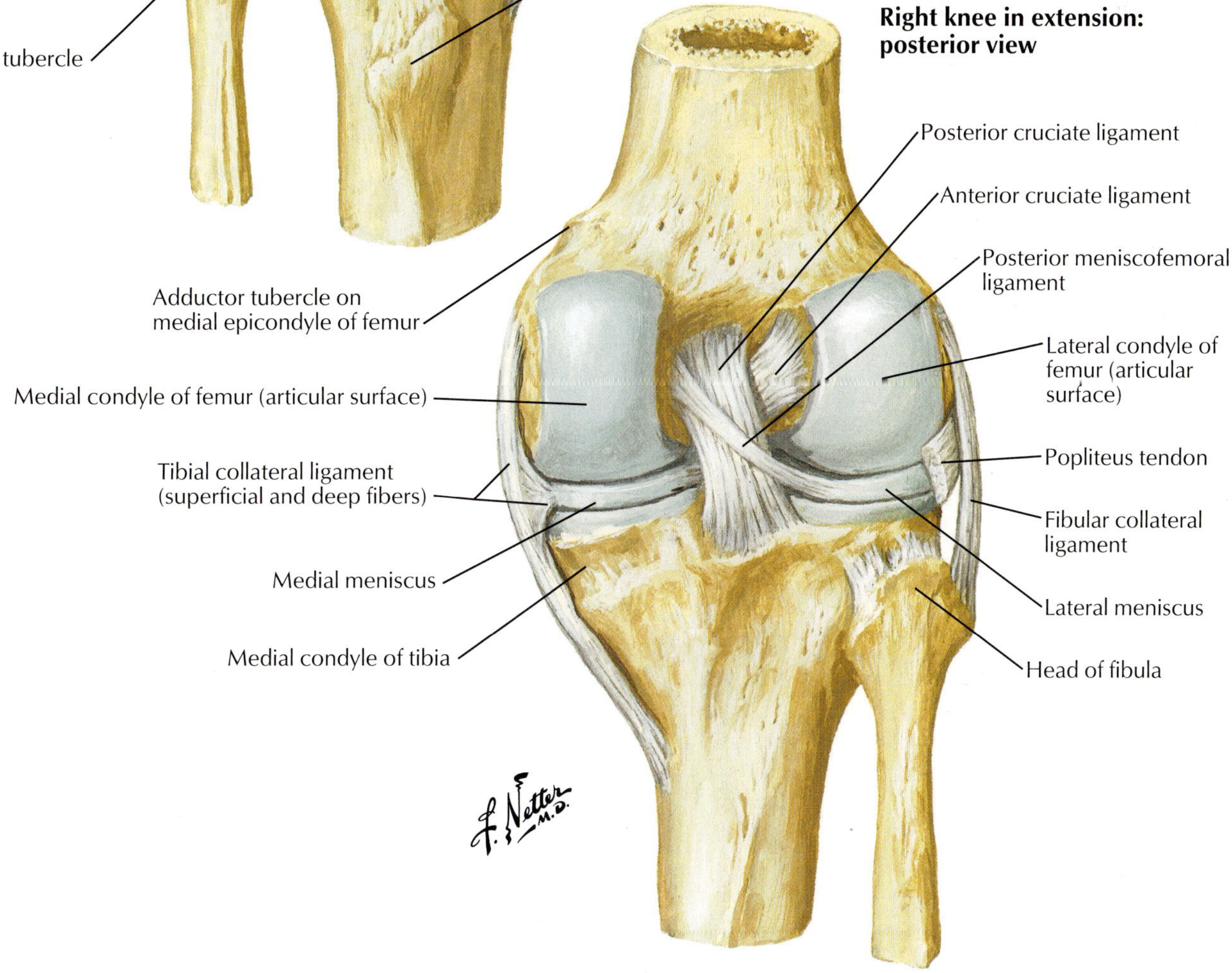

Knee: Anteroposterior Radiograph and Posterior View

See also **Plate 494**

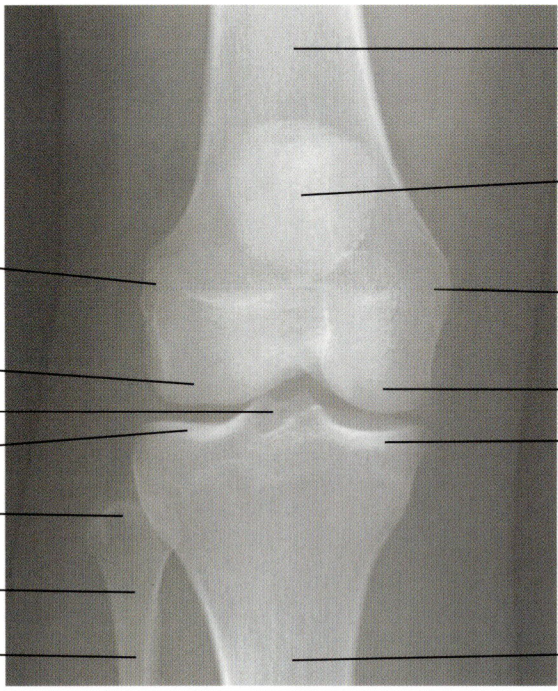

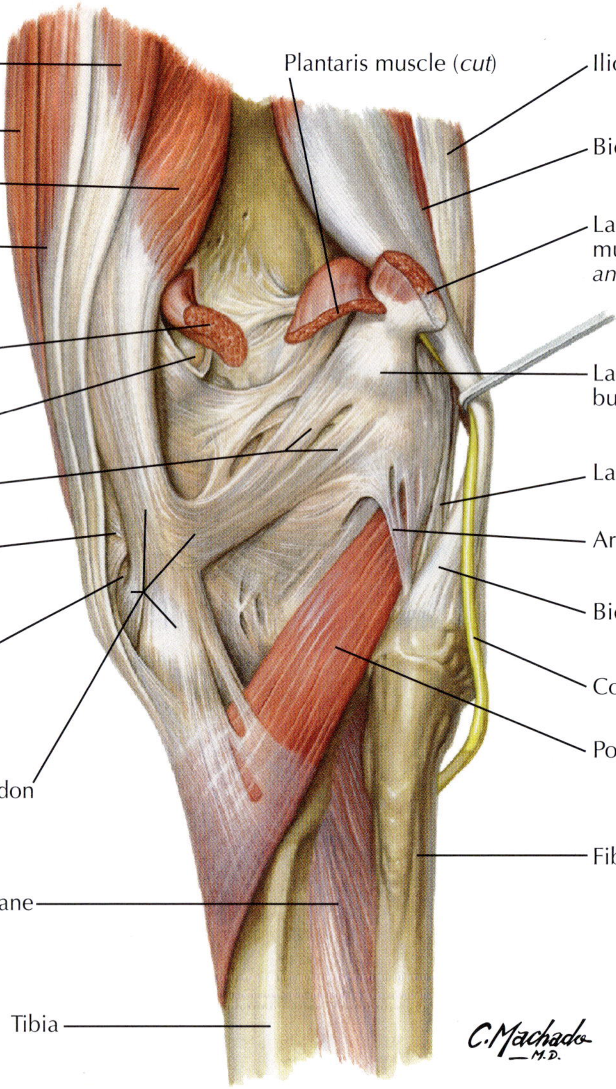

Right knee: posterior view

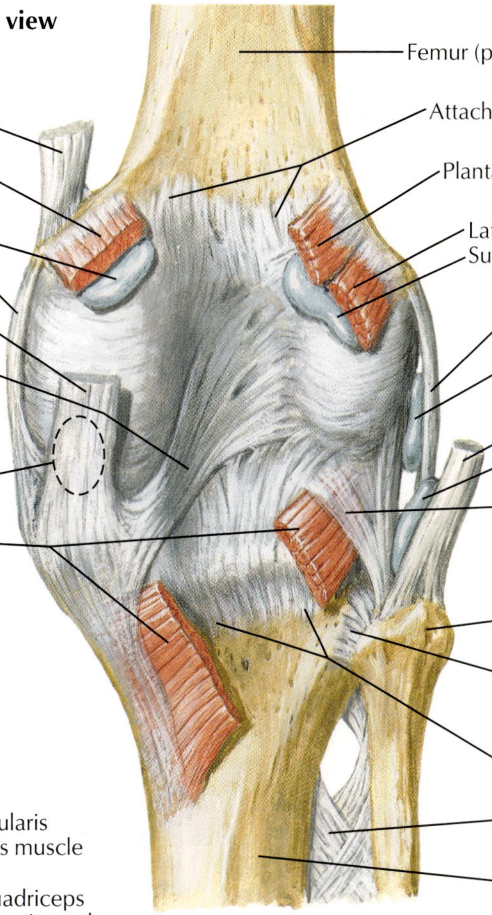

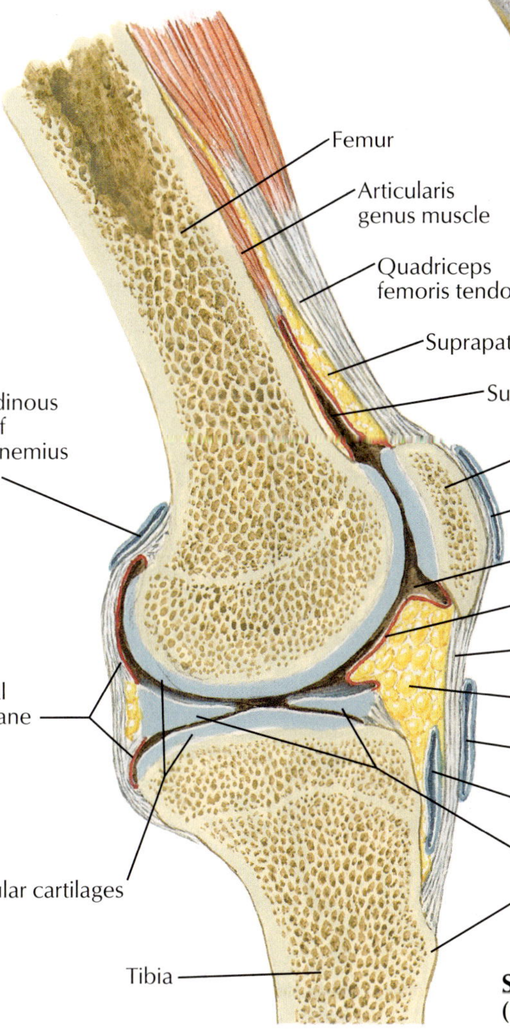

Sagittal section (lateral to midline of knee)

See also Plates 491, 508, 509, 518

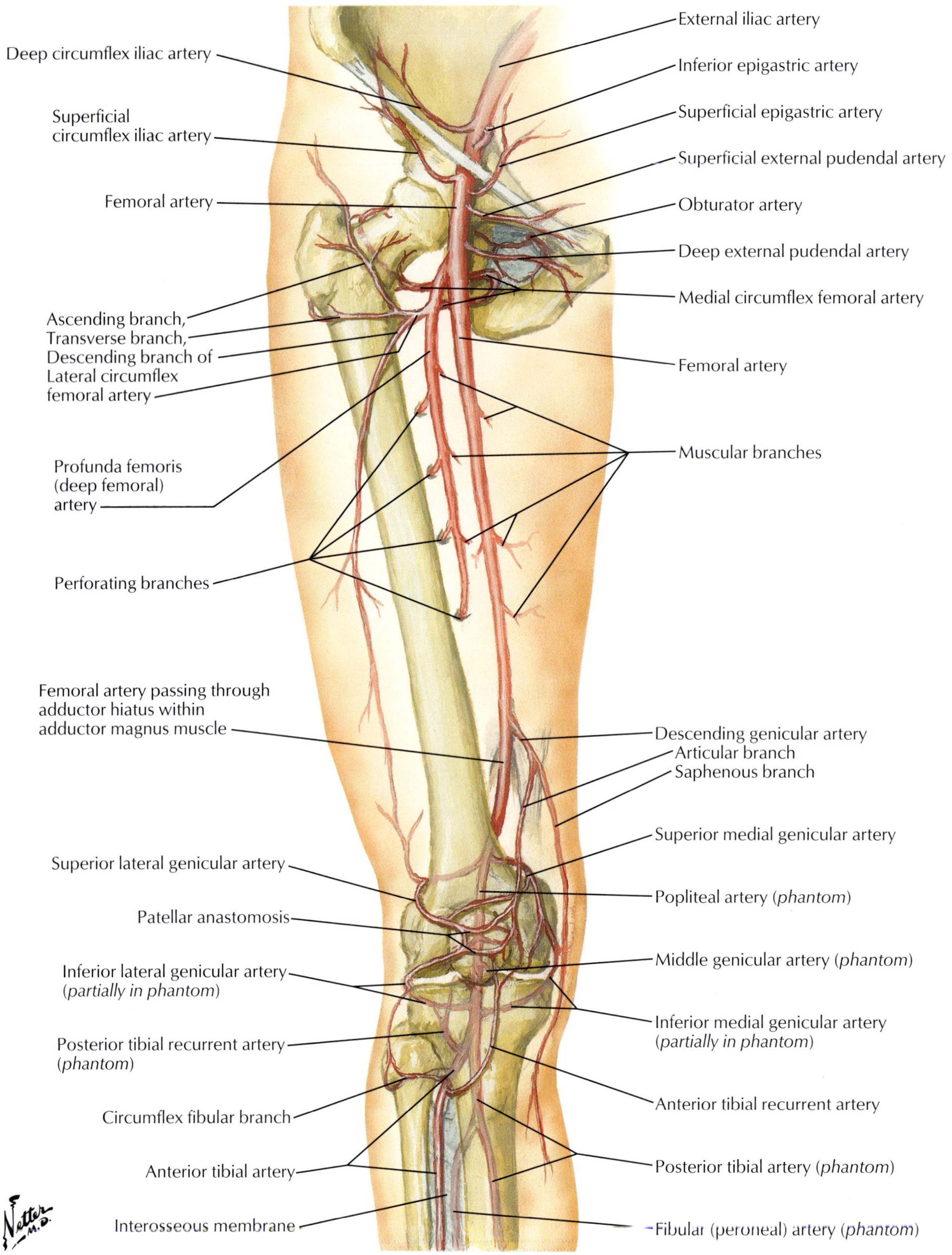

Bones of right leg

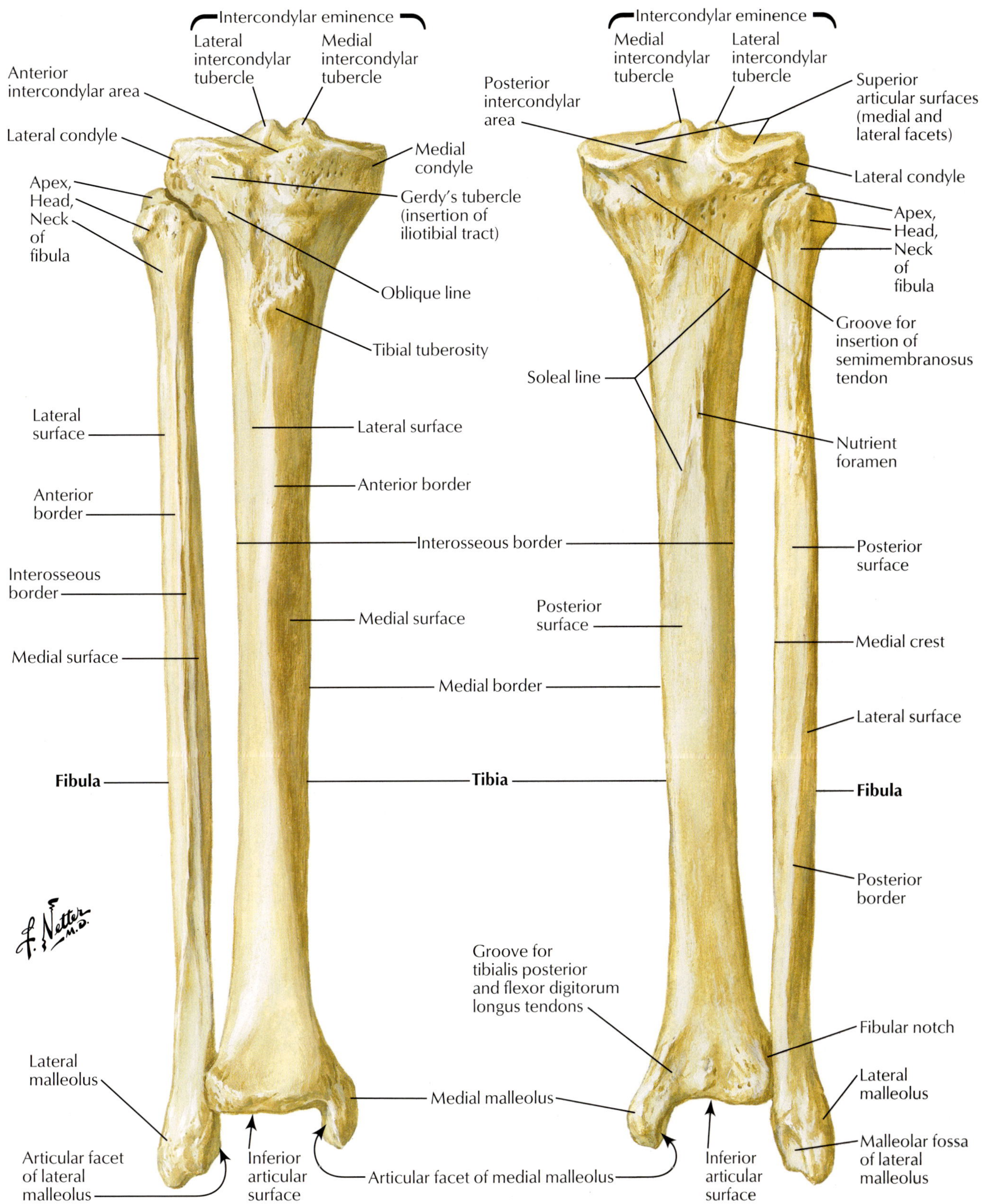

See also Plate 495

Anterior view with ligament attachments

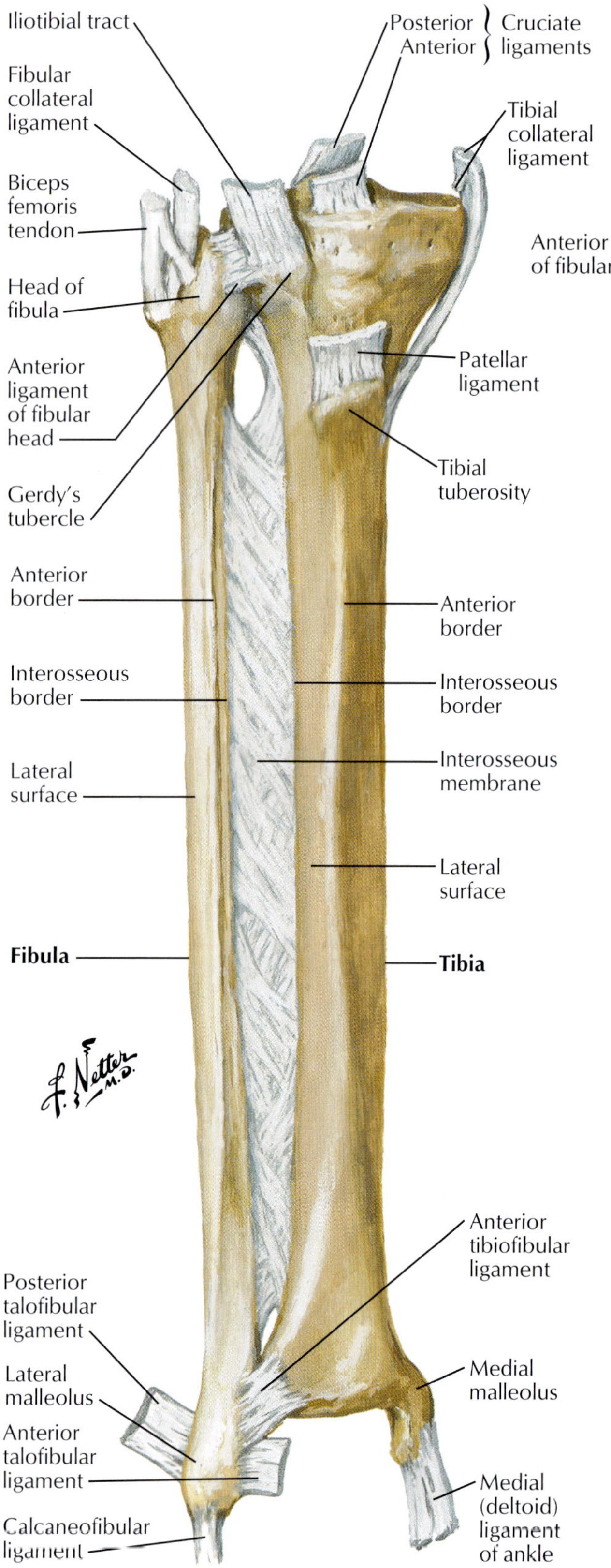

Superior view

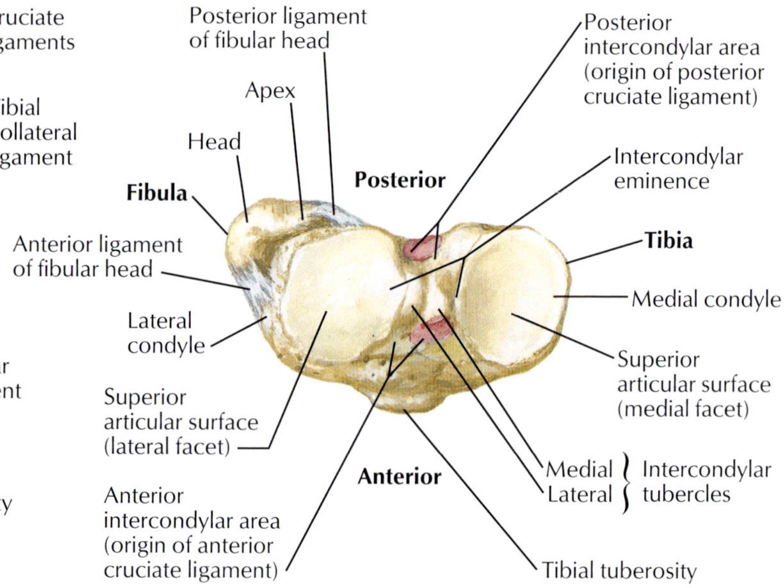

Cross section

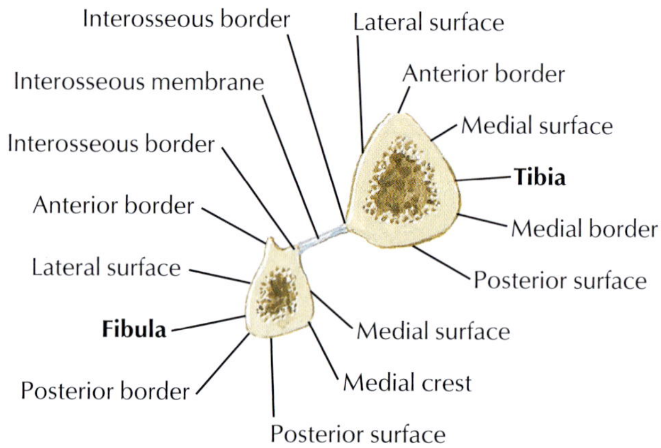

Inferior view

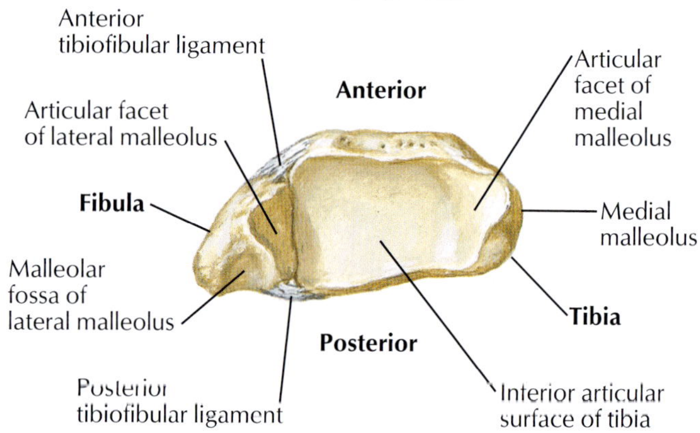

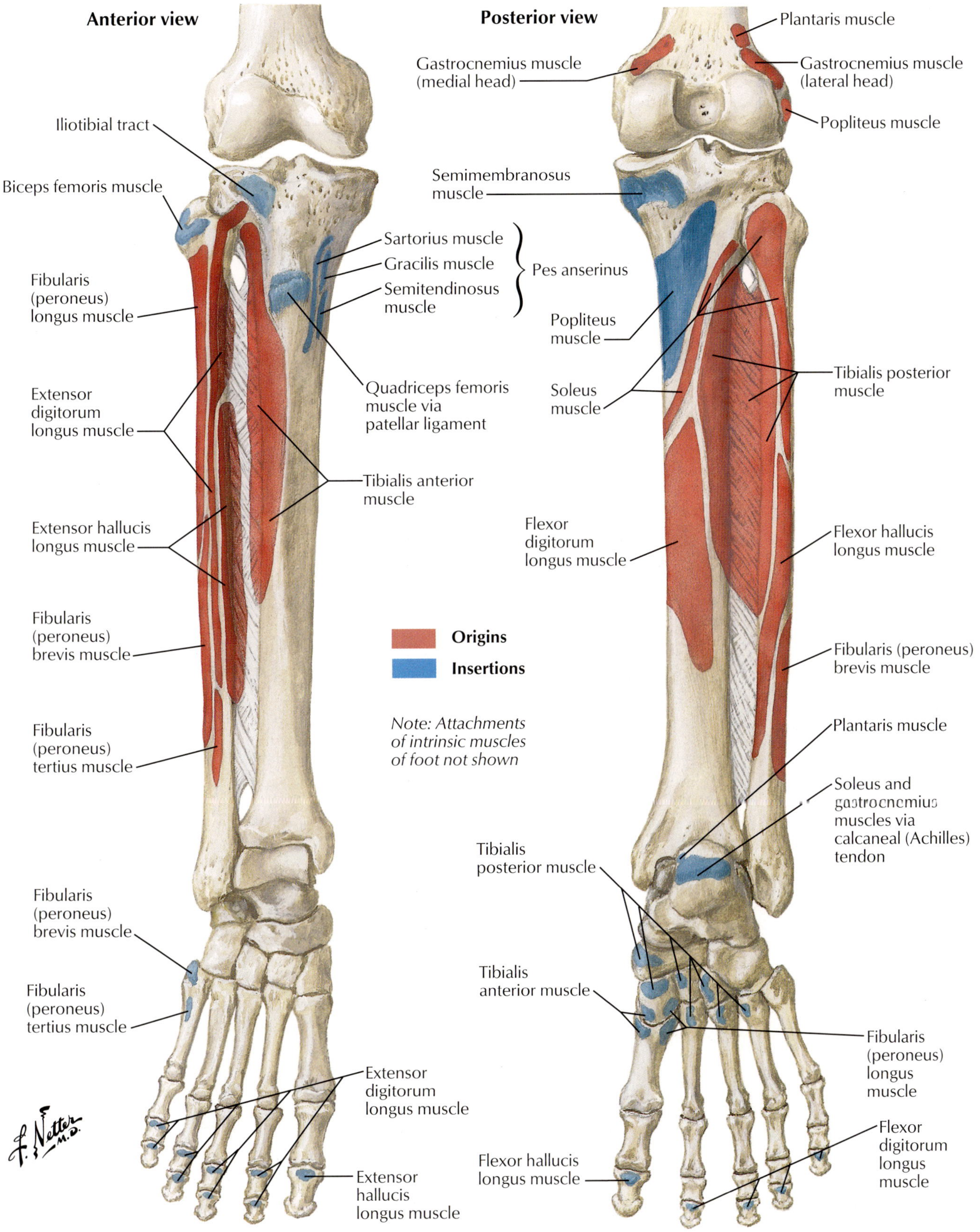
Anterior view
Iliotibial tract
Biceps femoris muscle
Fibularis (peroneus) longus muscle
Extensor digitorum longus muscle
Extensor hallucis longus muscle
Fibularis (peroneus) brevis muscle
Fibularis (peroneus) tertius muscle
Fibularis (peroneus) brevis muscle
Fibularis (peroneus) tertius muscle
Sartorius muscle
Gracilis muscle
Semitendinosus muscle
Pes anserinus
Quadriceps femoris muscle via patellar ligament
Tibialis anterior muscle
Extensor digitorum longus muscle
Extensor hallucis longus muscle
Origins
Insertions
Note: Attachments of intrinsic muscles of foot not shown
Posterior view
Gastrocnemius muscle (medial head)
Semimembranosus muscle
Popliteus muscle
Soleus muscle
Flexor digitorum longus muscle
Tibialis posterior muscle
Tibialis anterior muscle
Flexor hallucis longus muscle
Plantaris muscle
Gastrocnemius muscle (lateral head)
Popliteus muscle
Tibialis posterior muscle
Flexor hallucis longus muscle
Fibularis (peroneus) brevis muscle
Plantaris muscle
Soleus and gastrocnemius muscles via calcaneal (Achilles) tendon
Fibularis (peroneus) longus muscle
Flexor digitorum longus muscle

Muscles of Leg (Superficial Dissection): Posterior View

See also Plate 528

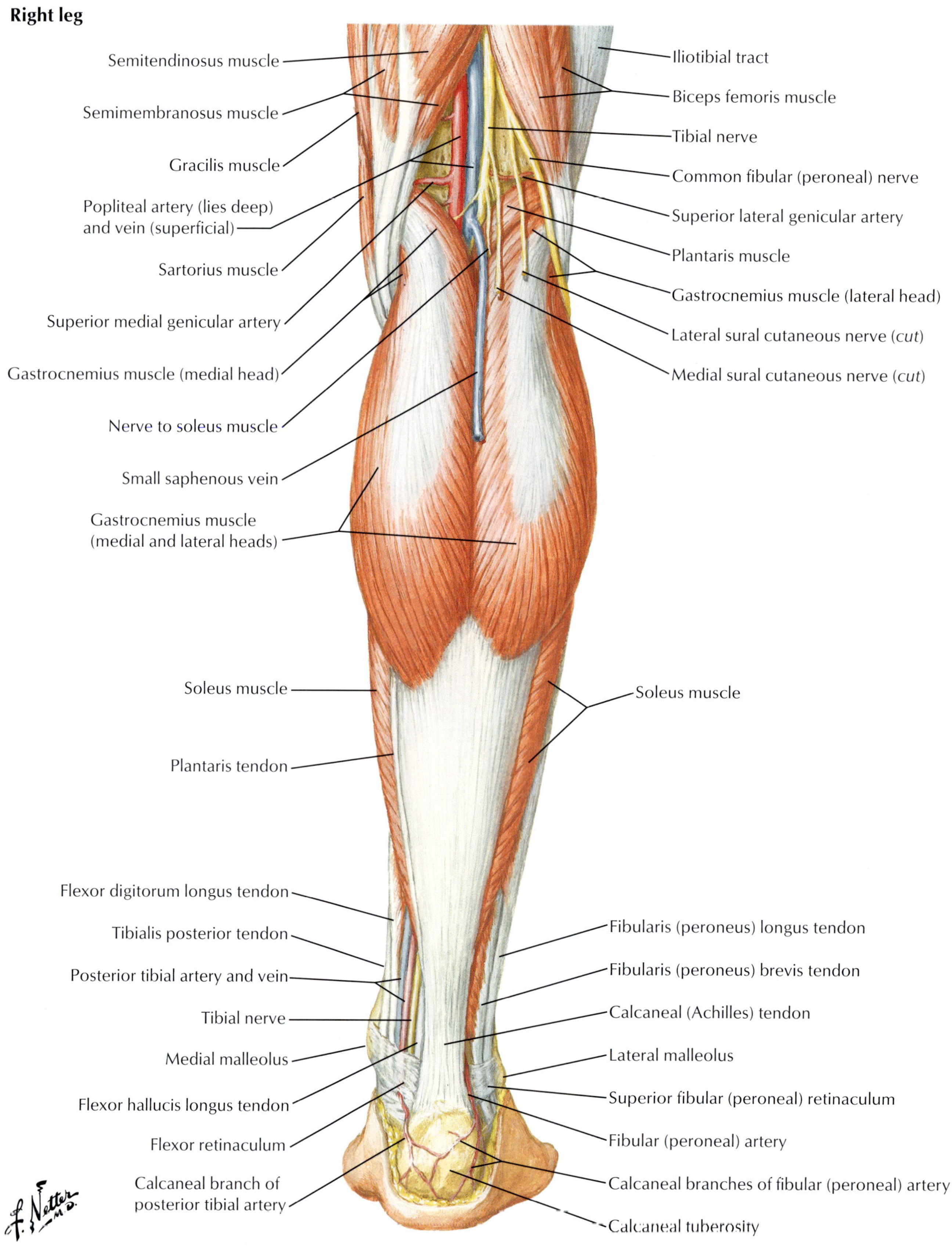

Muscles of Leg (Intermediate Dissection): Posterior View

See also Plate 528

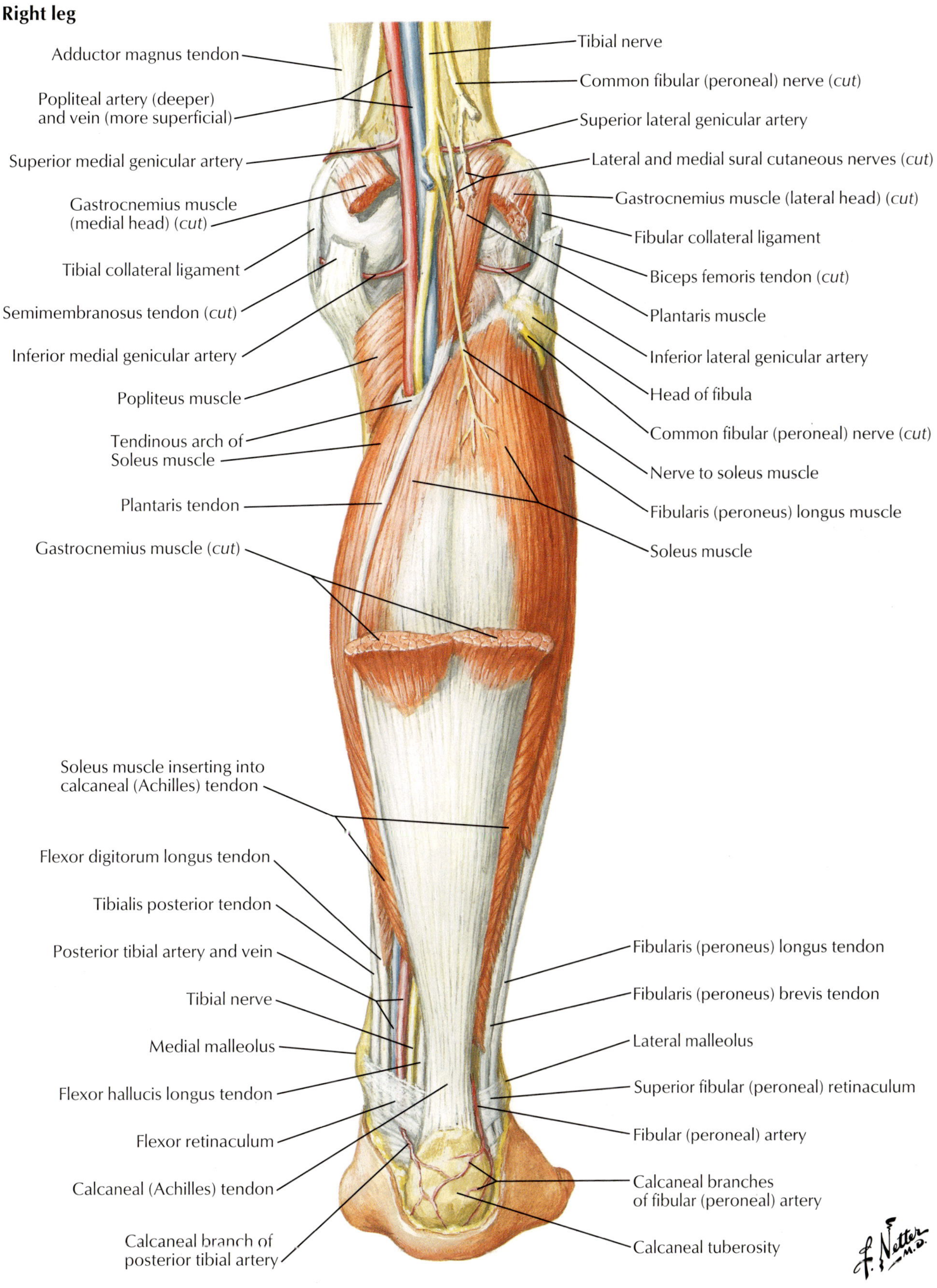

See also Plate 528

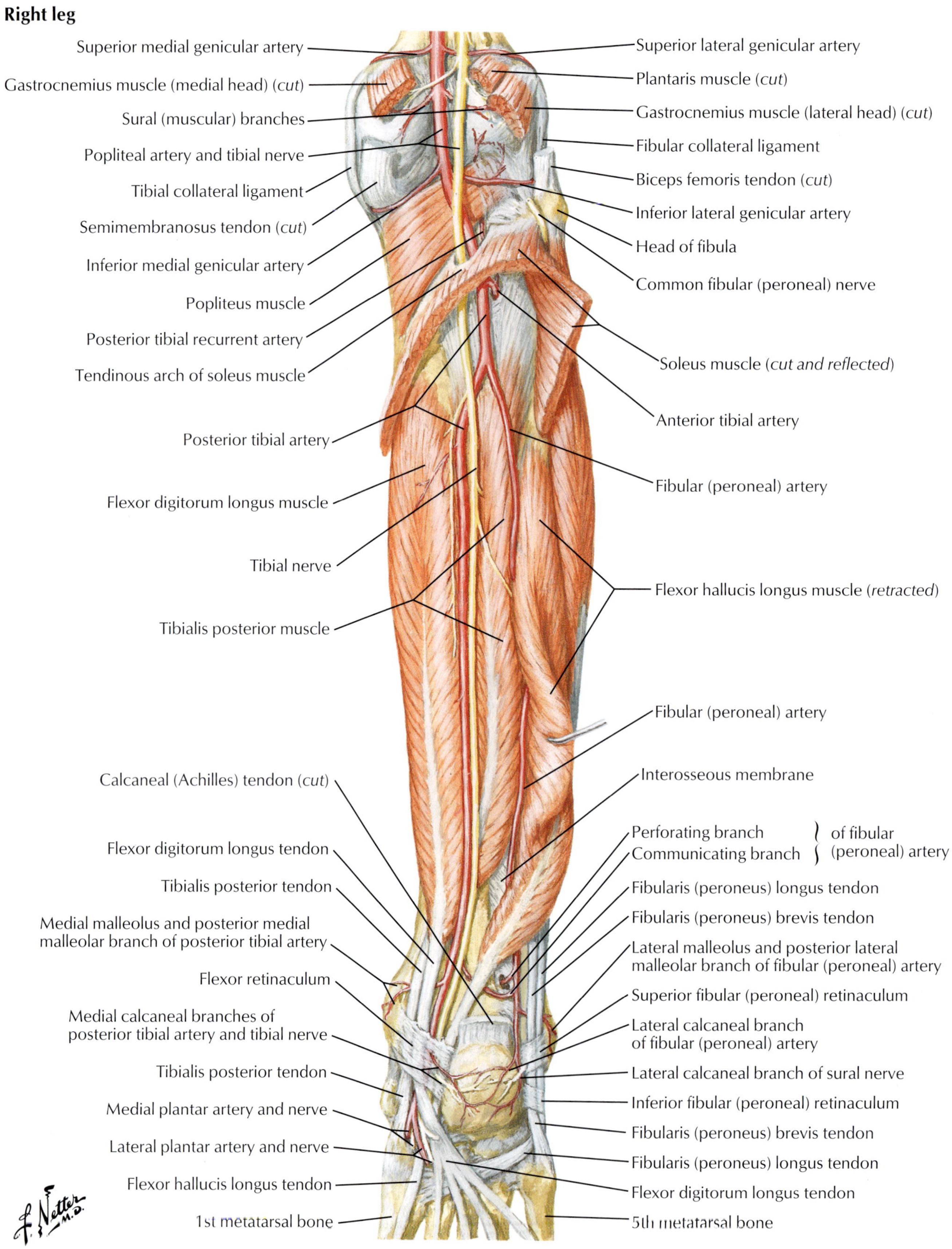

Muscles of Leg: Lateral View

See also Plates 516, 529

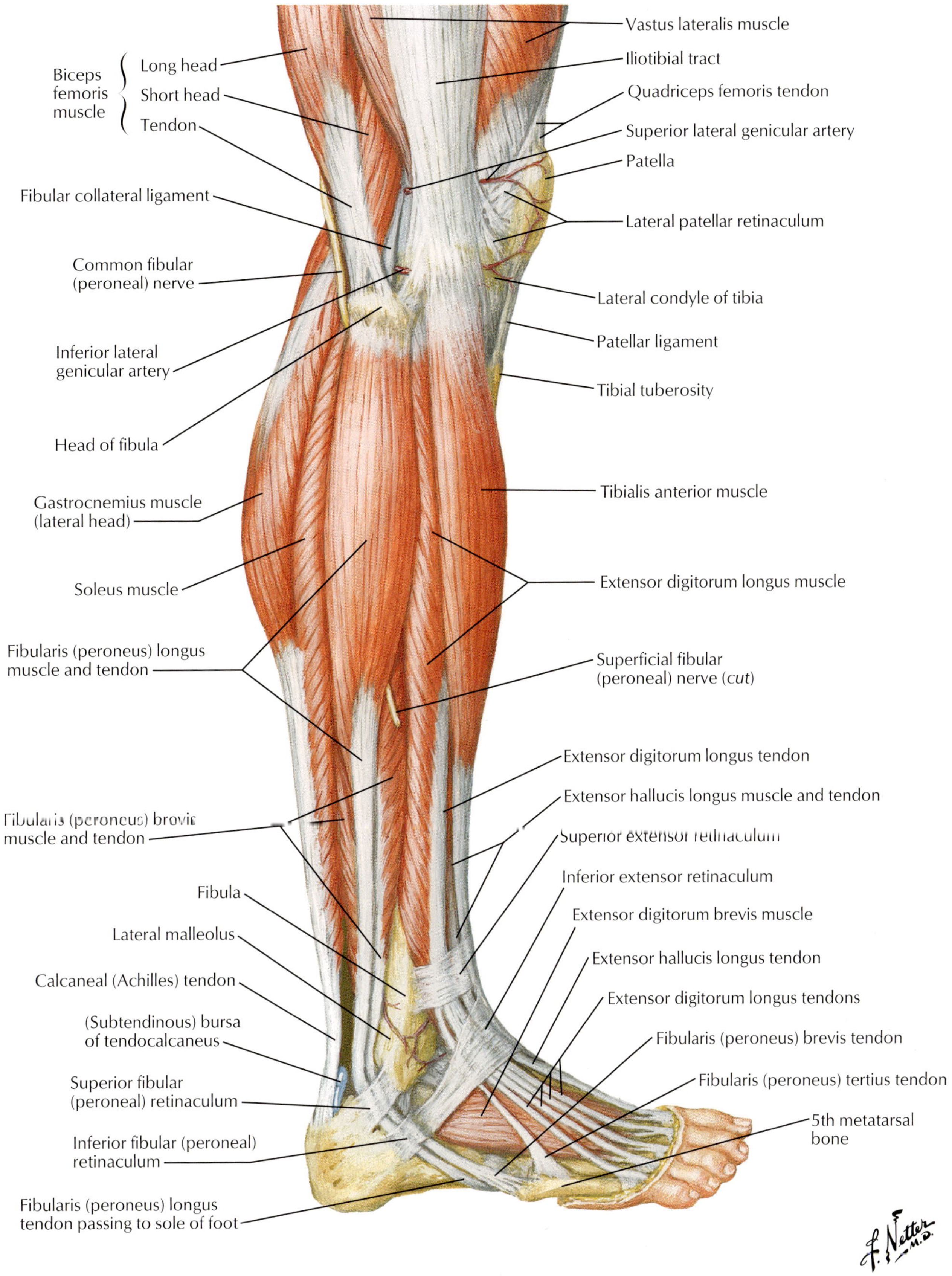

See also Plate 529

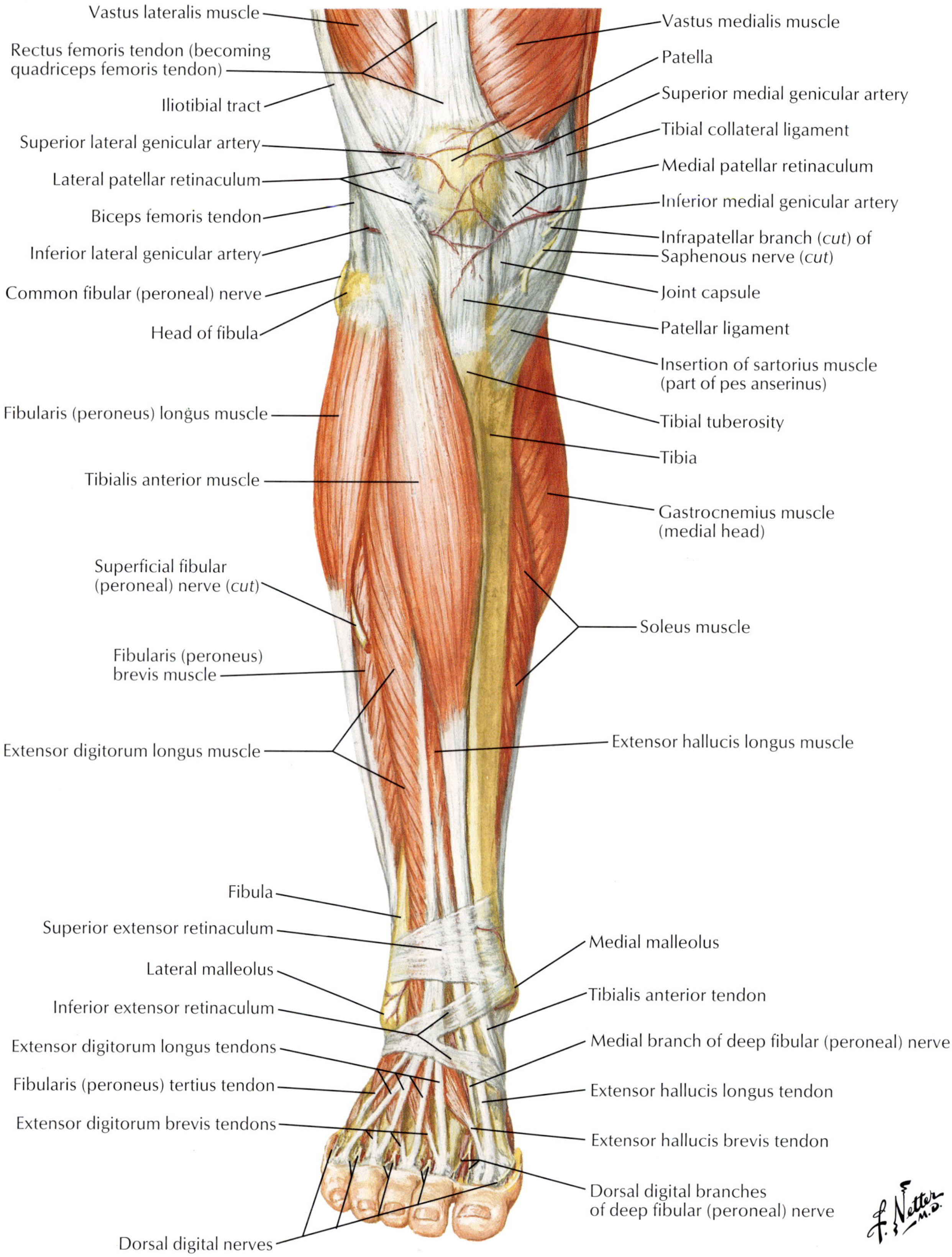

Muscles of Leg (Deep Dissection): Anterior View

See also **Plates 499, 523, 529**

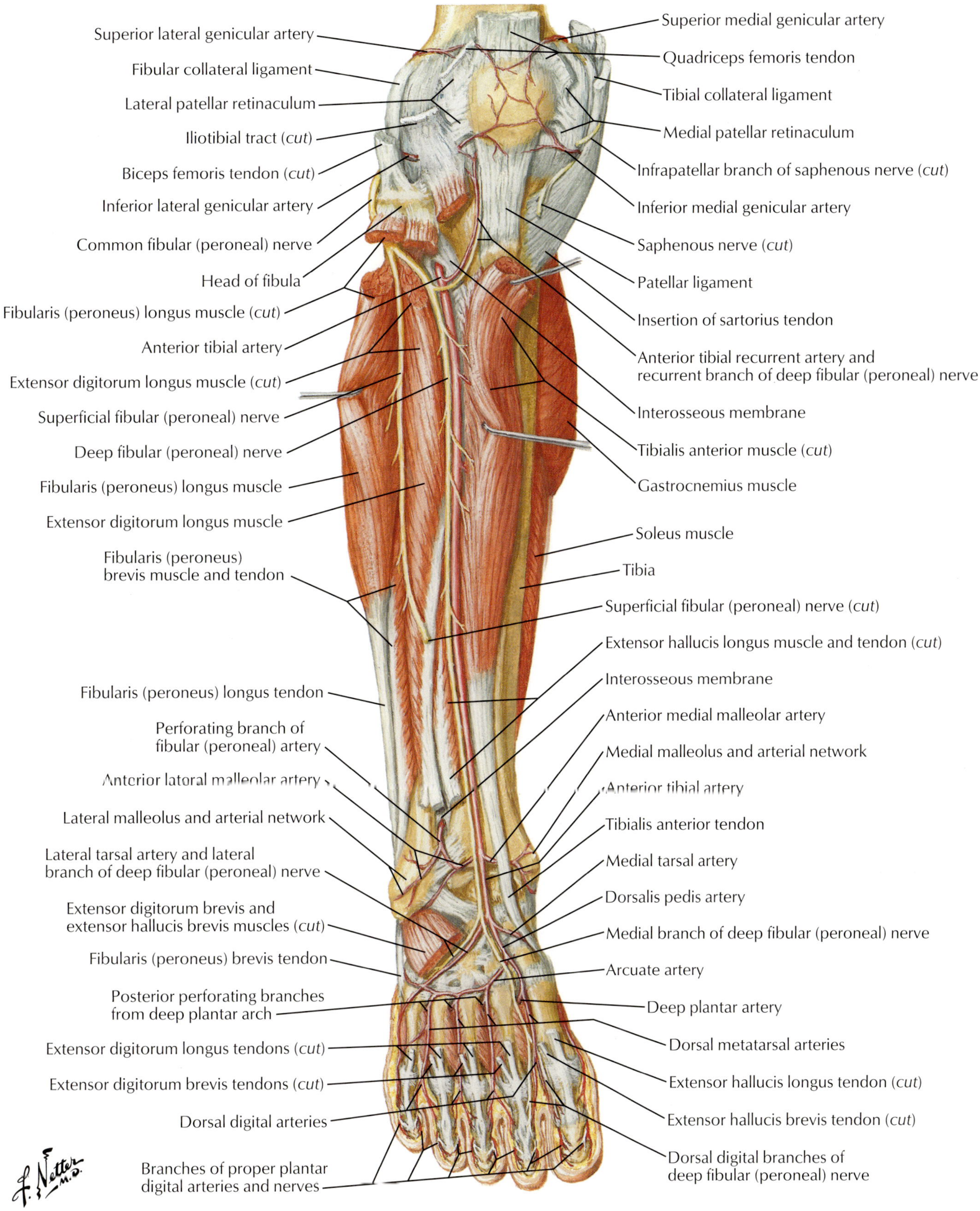

Arteries of Knee, Leg, and Foot

See also **Plate 531**

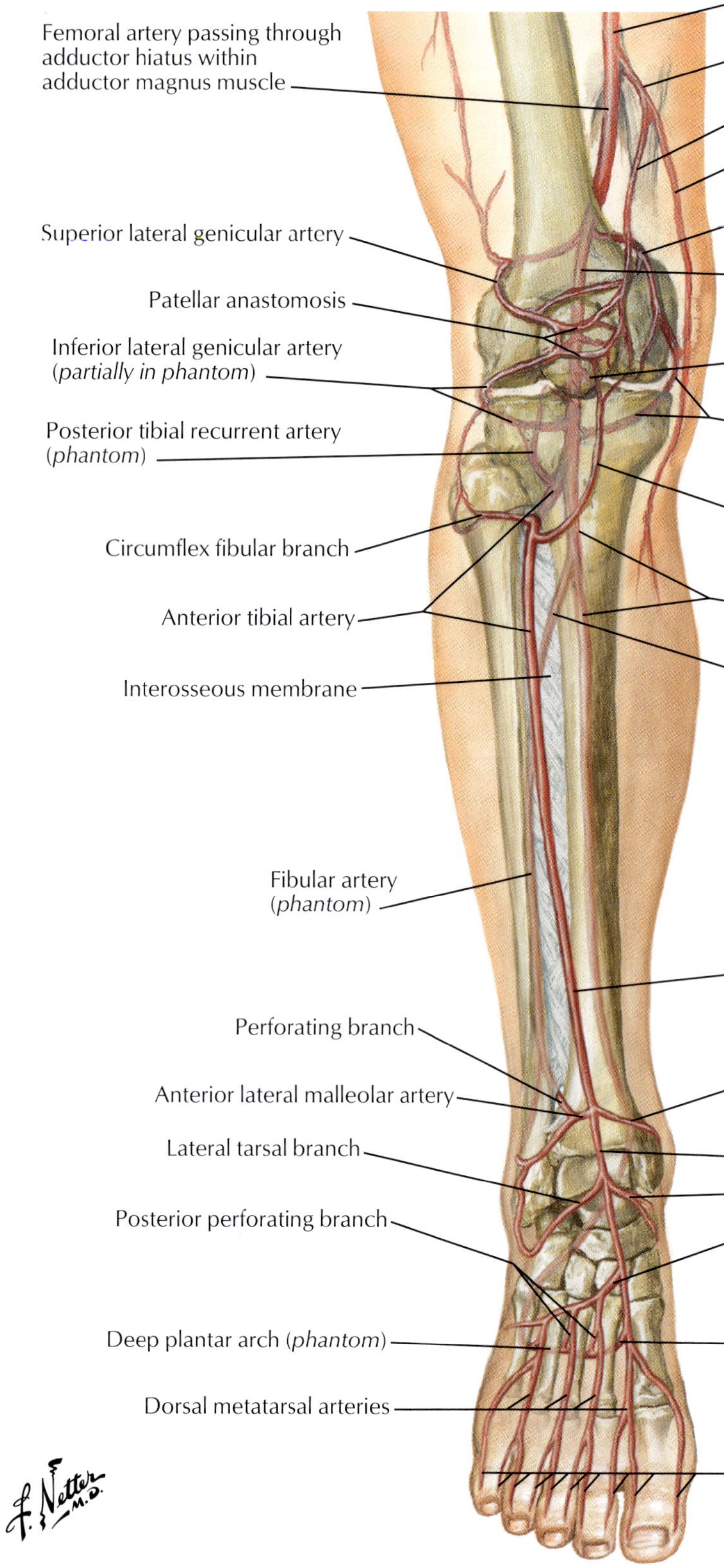

Leg: Cross Sections and Fascial Compartments

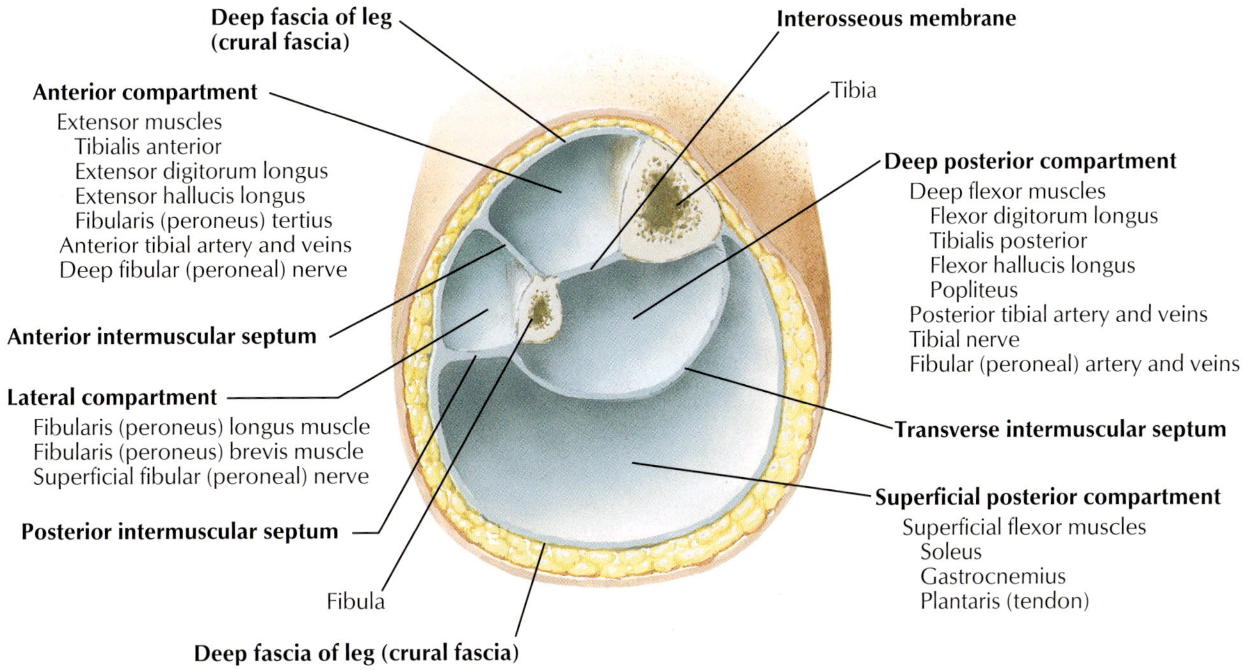

Cross section just above middle of leg

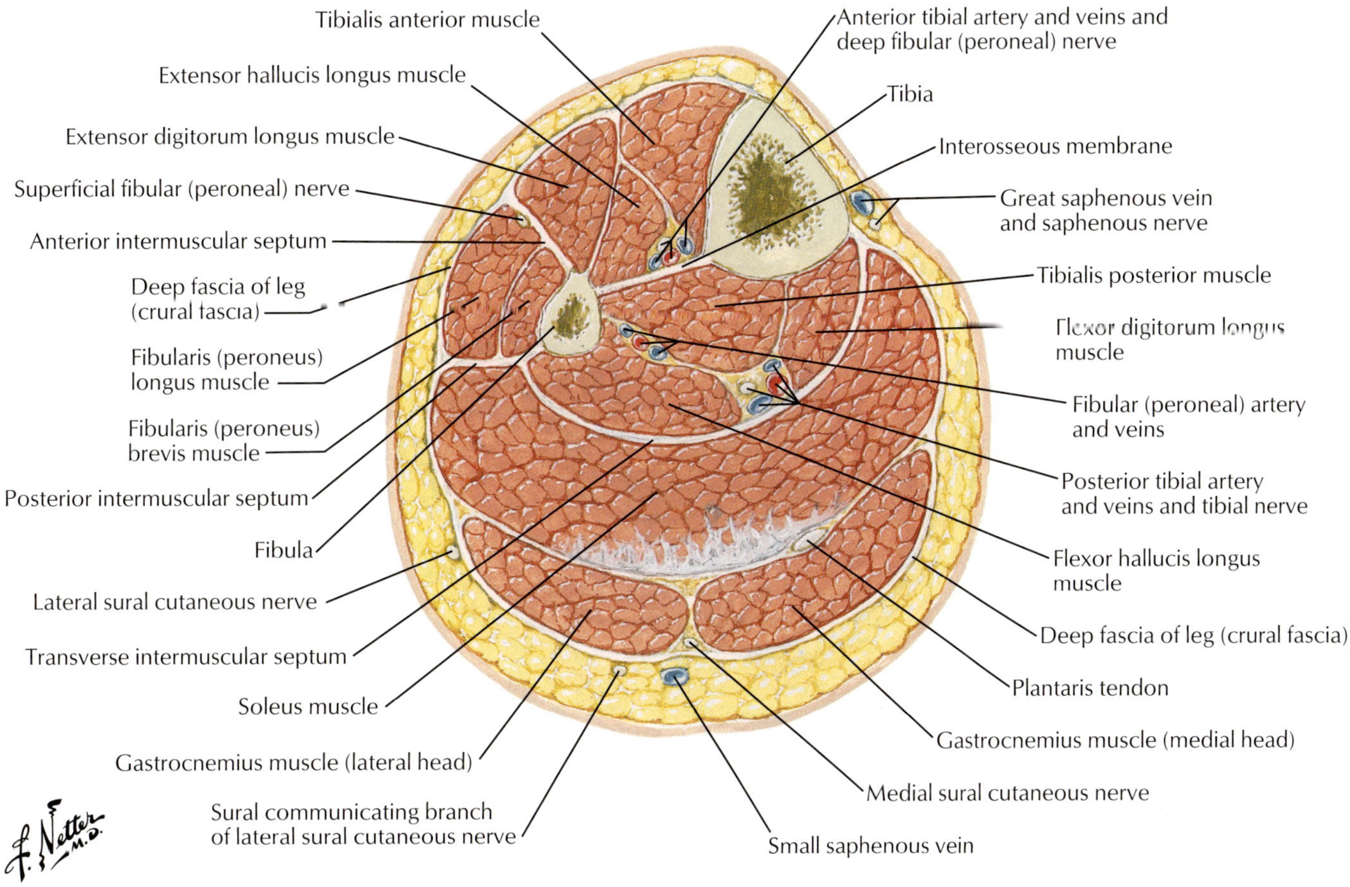

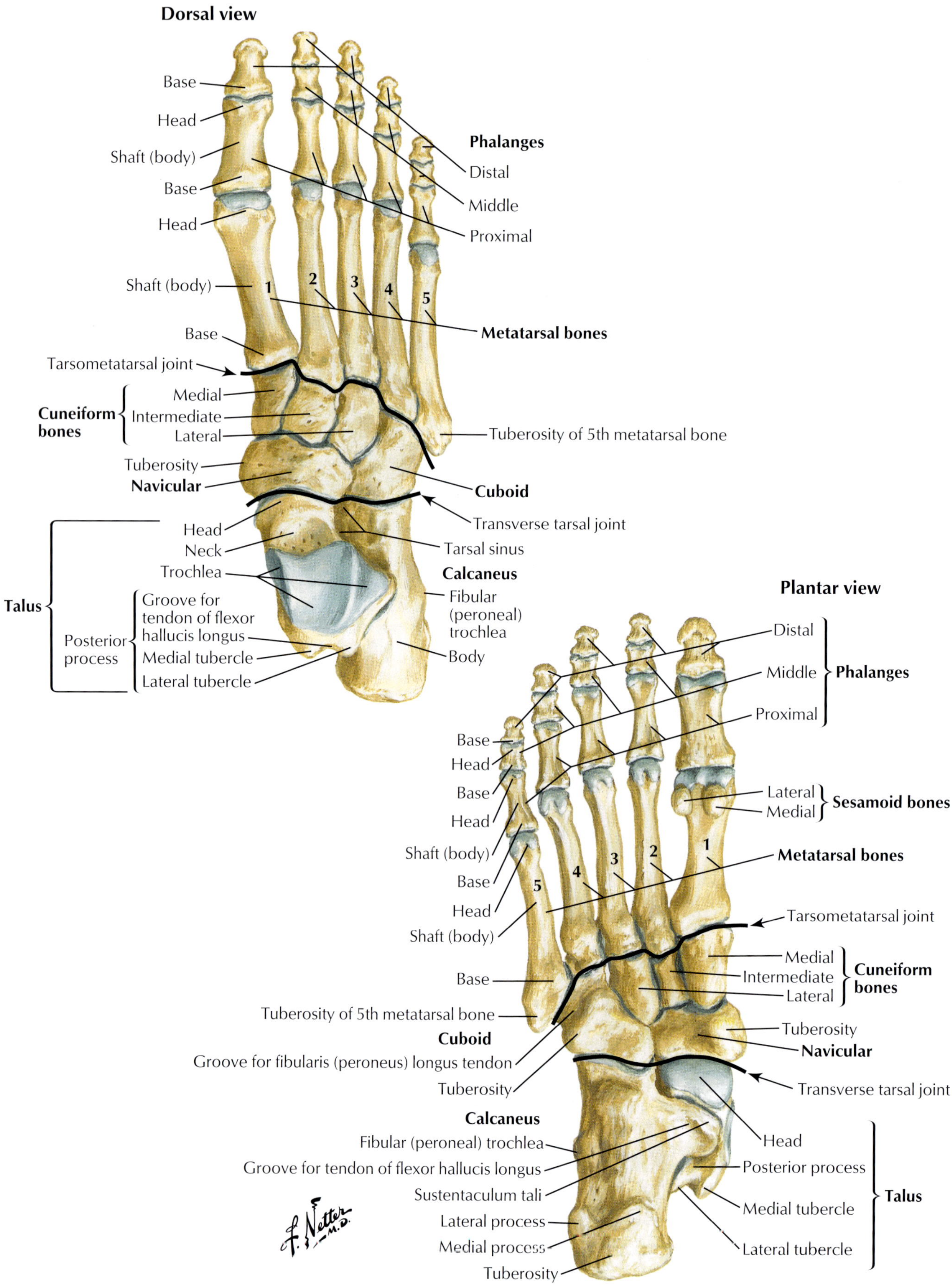
Dorsal view
Base
Head
Shaft (body)
Base
Head
Shaft (body)
Base
Tarsometatarsal joint
Cuneiform bones
Medial
Intermediate
Lateral
Tuberosity
Navicular
Phalanges
Distal
Middle
Proximal
1
2
3
4
5
Metatarsal bones
Tuberosity of 5th metatarsal bone
Cuboid
Transverse tarsal joint
Tarsal sinus
Calcaneus
Fibular (peroneal) trochlea
Body
Talus
Head
Neck
Trochlea
Posterior process
Groove for tendon of flexor hallucis longus
Medial tubercle
Lateral tubercle
Plantar view
Distal
Middle
Proximal
Phalanges
Base
Head
Base
Head
Shaft (body)
Base
Head
Shaft (body)
Base
Tuberosity of 5th metatarsal bone
Cuboid
Groove for fibularis (peroneus) longus tendon
Tuberosity
Lateral
Medial
Sesamoid bones
Metatarsal bones
Tarsometatarsal joint
Medial
Intermediate
Lateral
Cuneiform bones
Tuberosity
Navicular
Transverse tarsal joint
Calcaneus
Fibular (peroneal) trochlea
Groove for tendon of flexor hallucis longus
Sustentaculum tali
Lateral process
Medial process
Tuberosity
Head
Posterior process
Medial tubercle
Lateral tubercle
Talus

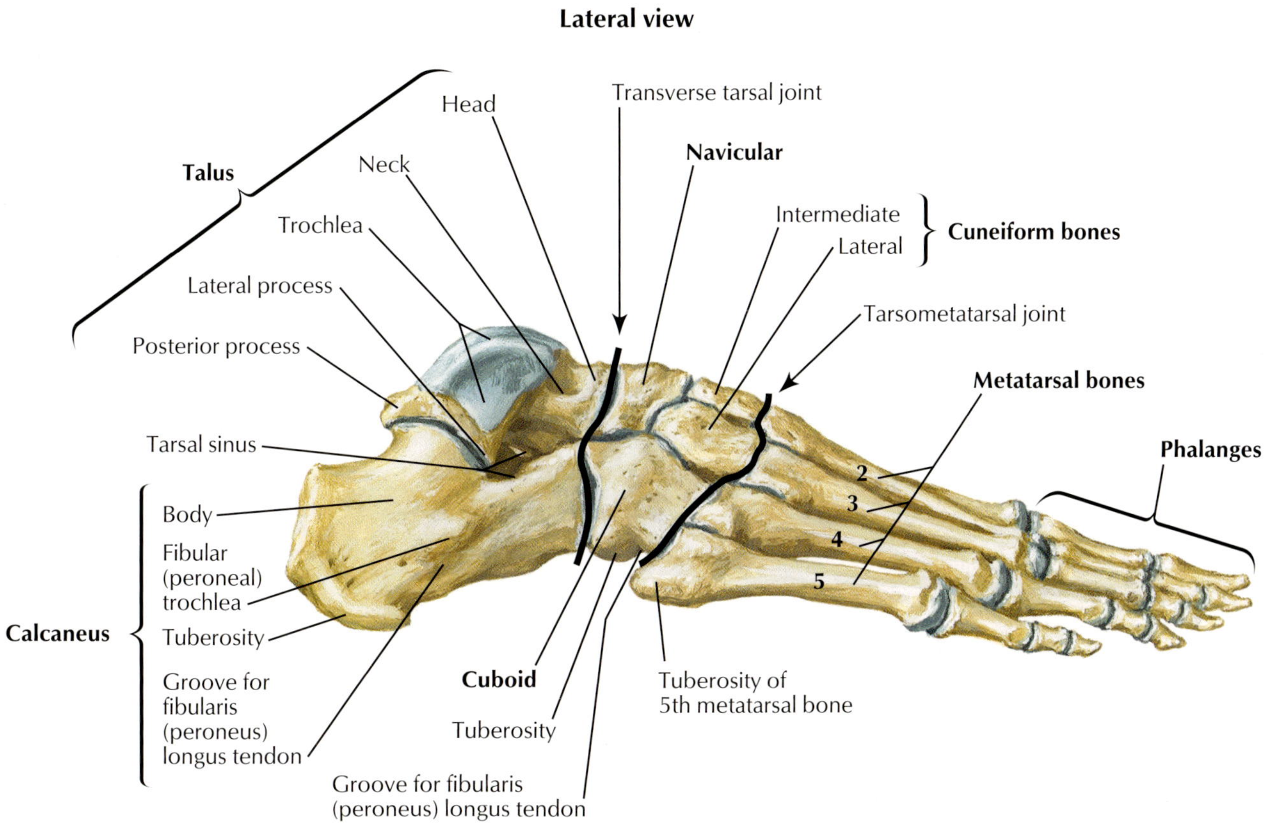
Lateral view
Talus
Head
Neck
Trochlea
Lateral process
Posterior process
Transverse tarsal joint
Navicular
Intermediate
Lateral
Cuneiform bones
Tarsometatarsal joint
Metatarsal bones
2
3
4
5
Phalanges
Tarsal sinus
Calcaneus
Body
Fibular (peroneal) trochlea
Tuberosity
Groove for fibularis (peroneus) longus tendon
Cuboid
Tuberosity
Groove for fibularis (peroneus) longus tendon
Tuberosity of 5th metatarsal bone

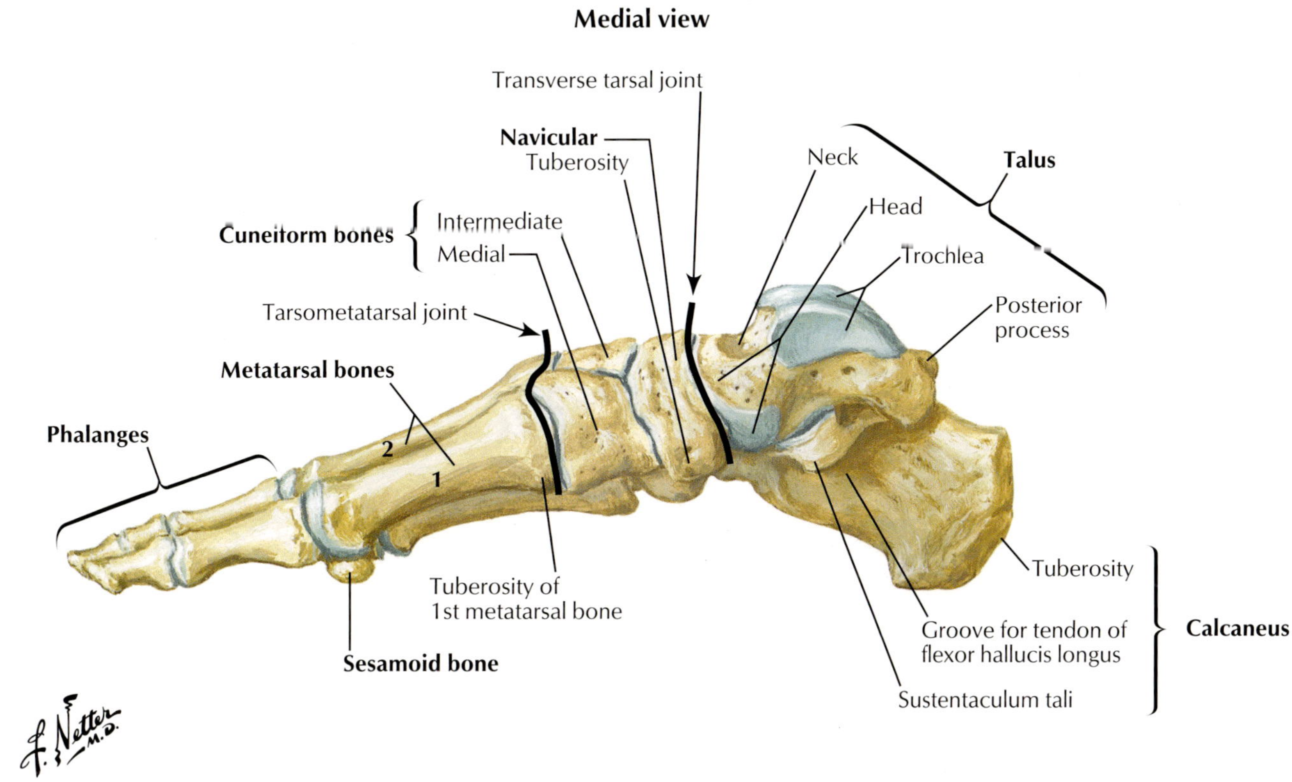
Medial view
Transverse tarsal joint
Navicular
Tuberosity
Cuneiform bones
Intermediate
Medial
Tarsometatarsal joint
Metatarsal bones
2
1
Phalanges
Neck
Talus
Head
Trochlea
Posterior process
Tuberosity
Calcaneus
Groove for tendon of flexor hallucis longus
Sustentaculum tali
Tuberosity of 1st metatarsal bone
Sesamoid bone
F. Netter M.D.

Calcaneus

See also Plate 531

Right foot

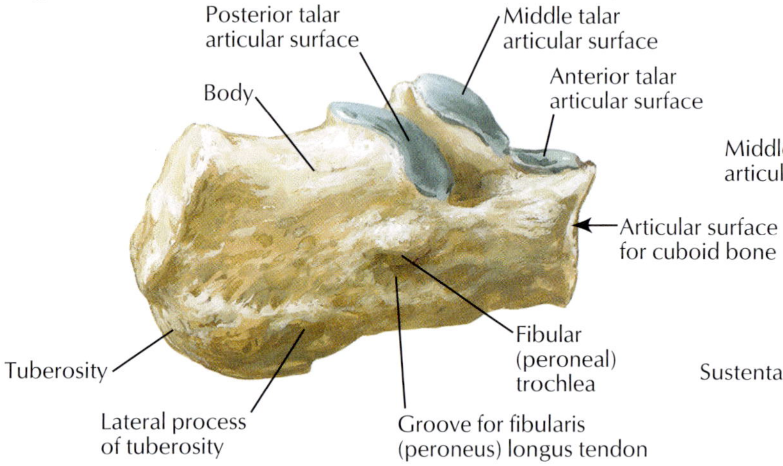

Lateral view

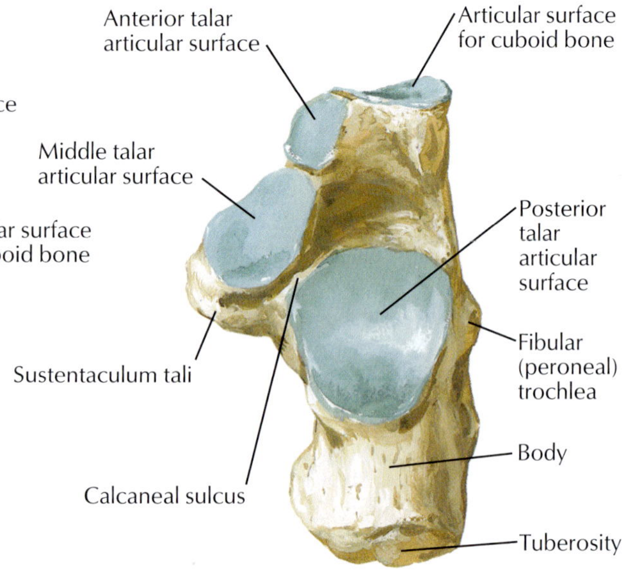

Superior view

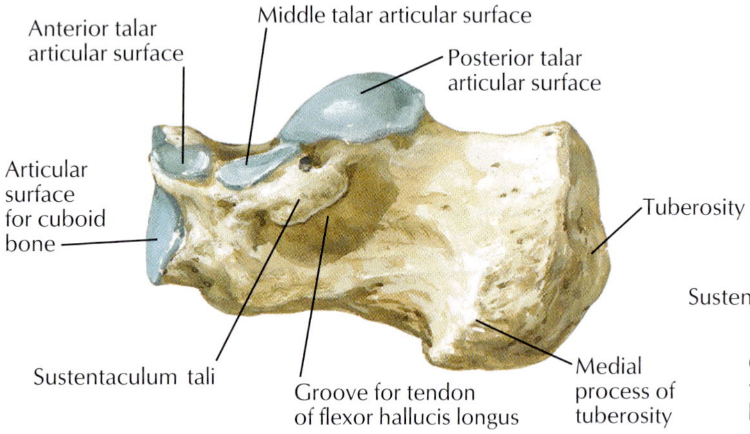

Medial view

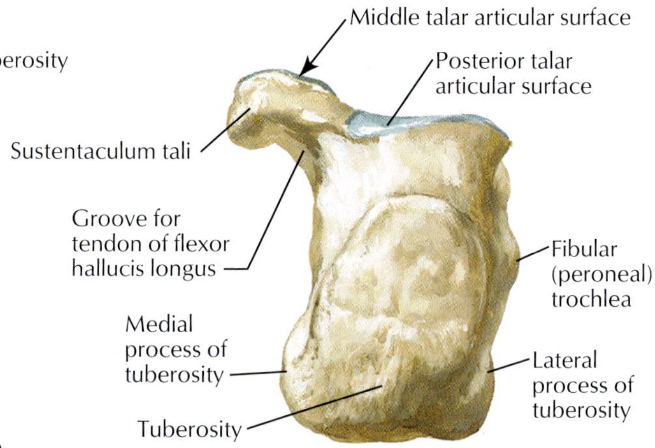

Posterior view

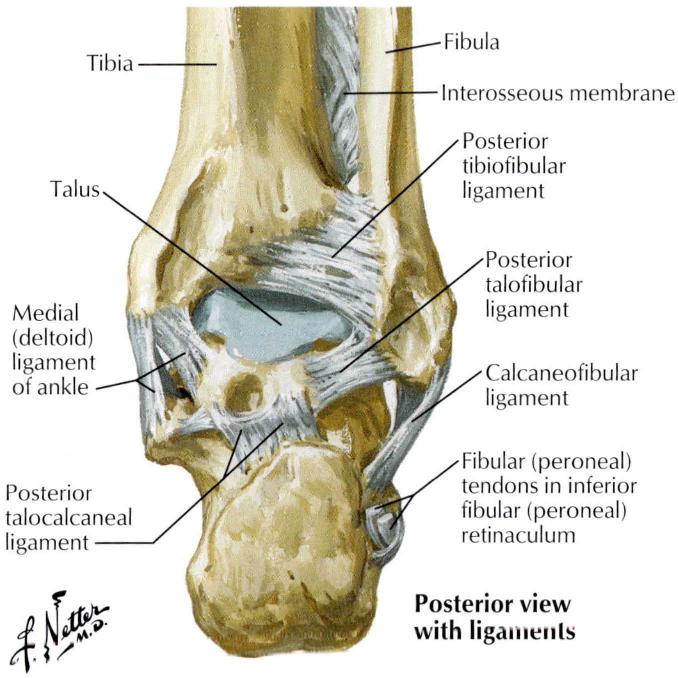

Posterior view with ligaments

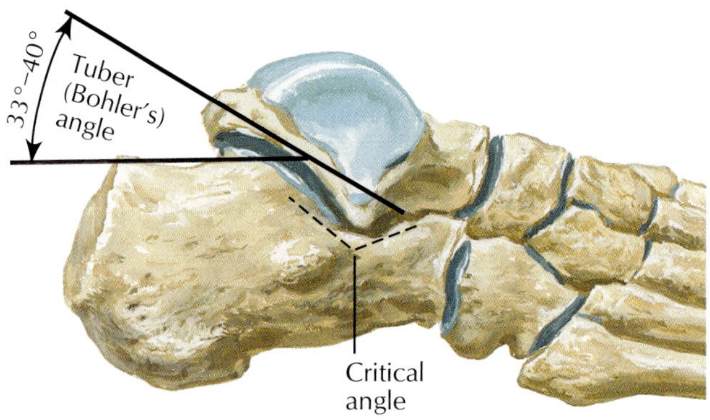

Functional relations of calcaneus

Ligaments and Tendons of Ankle

See also Plate 531

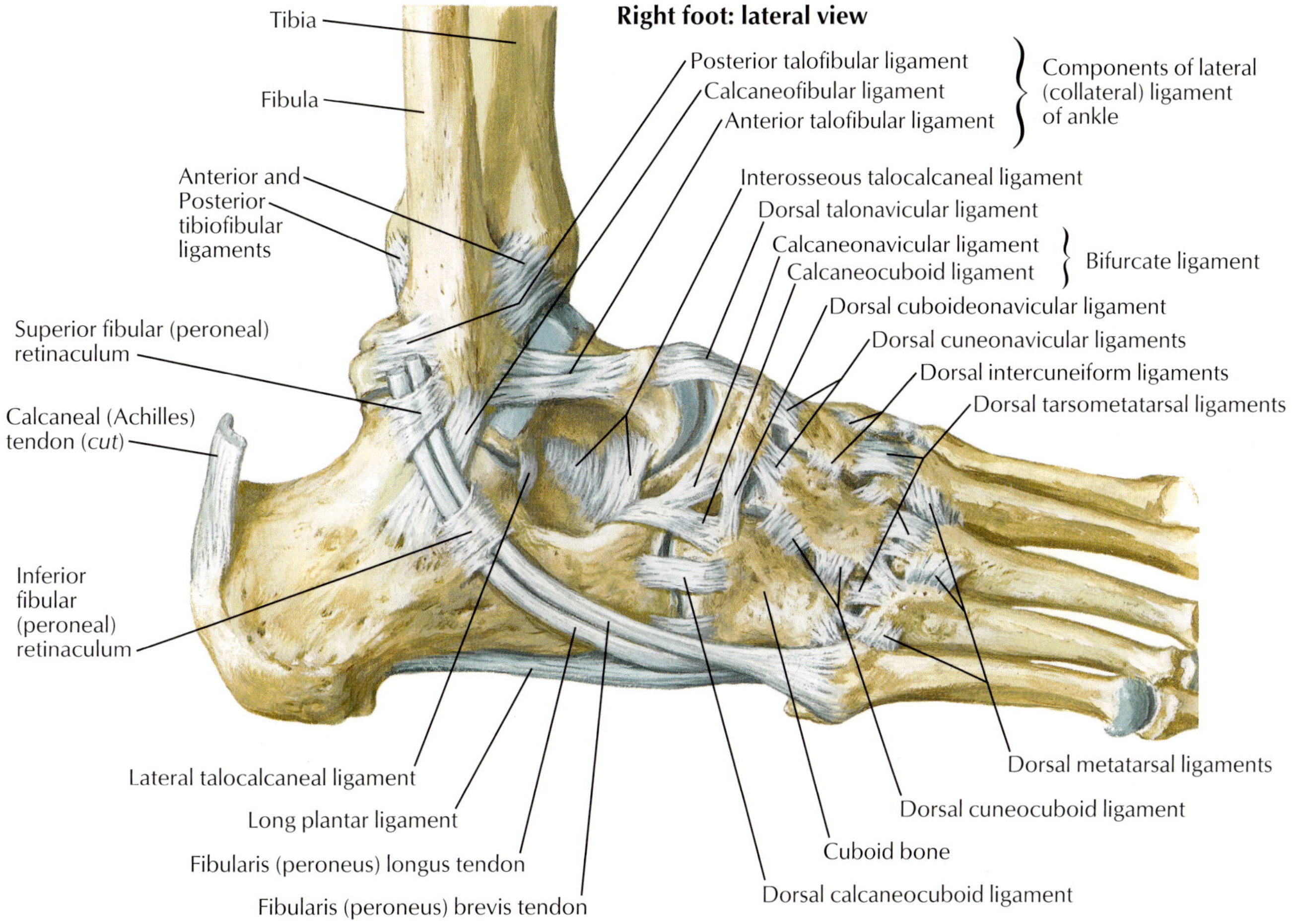

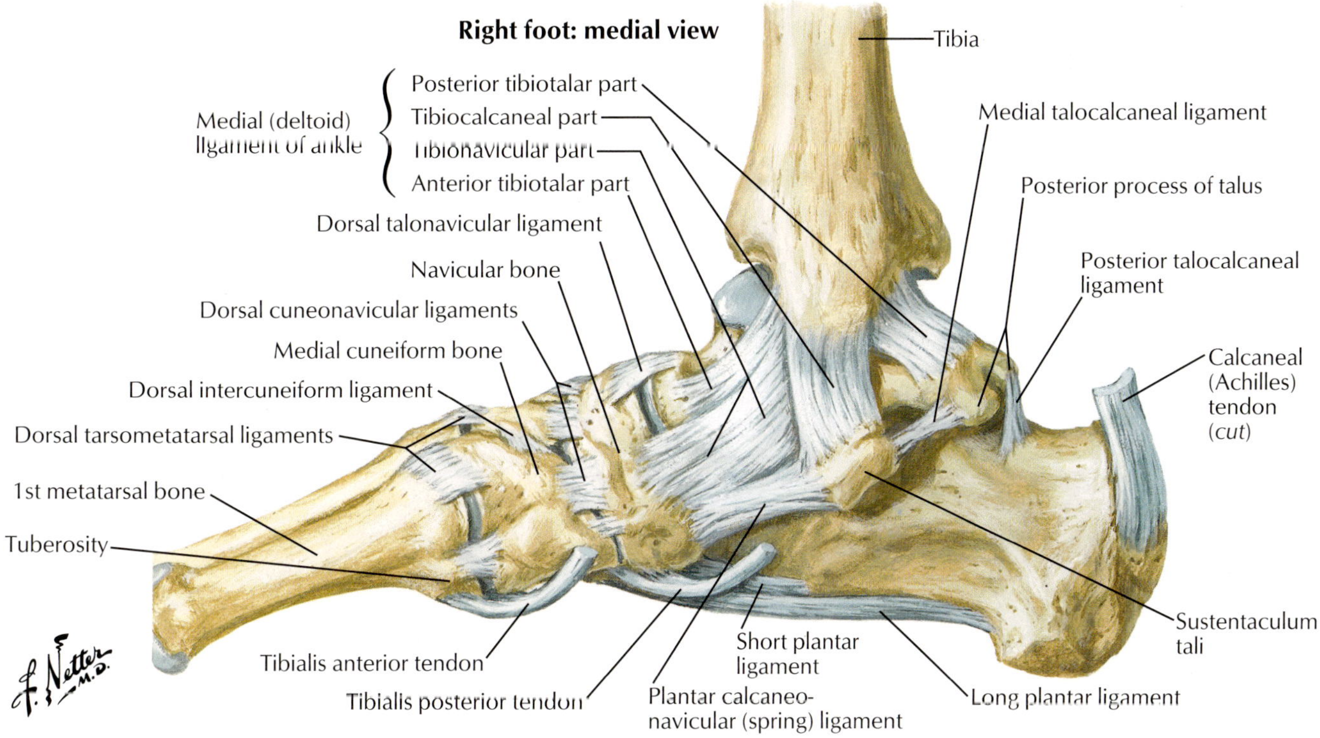

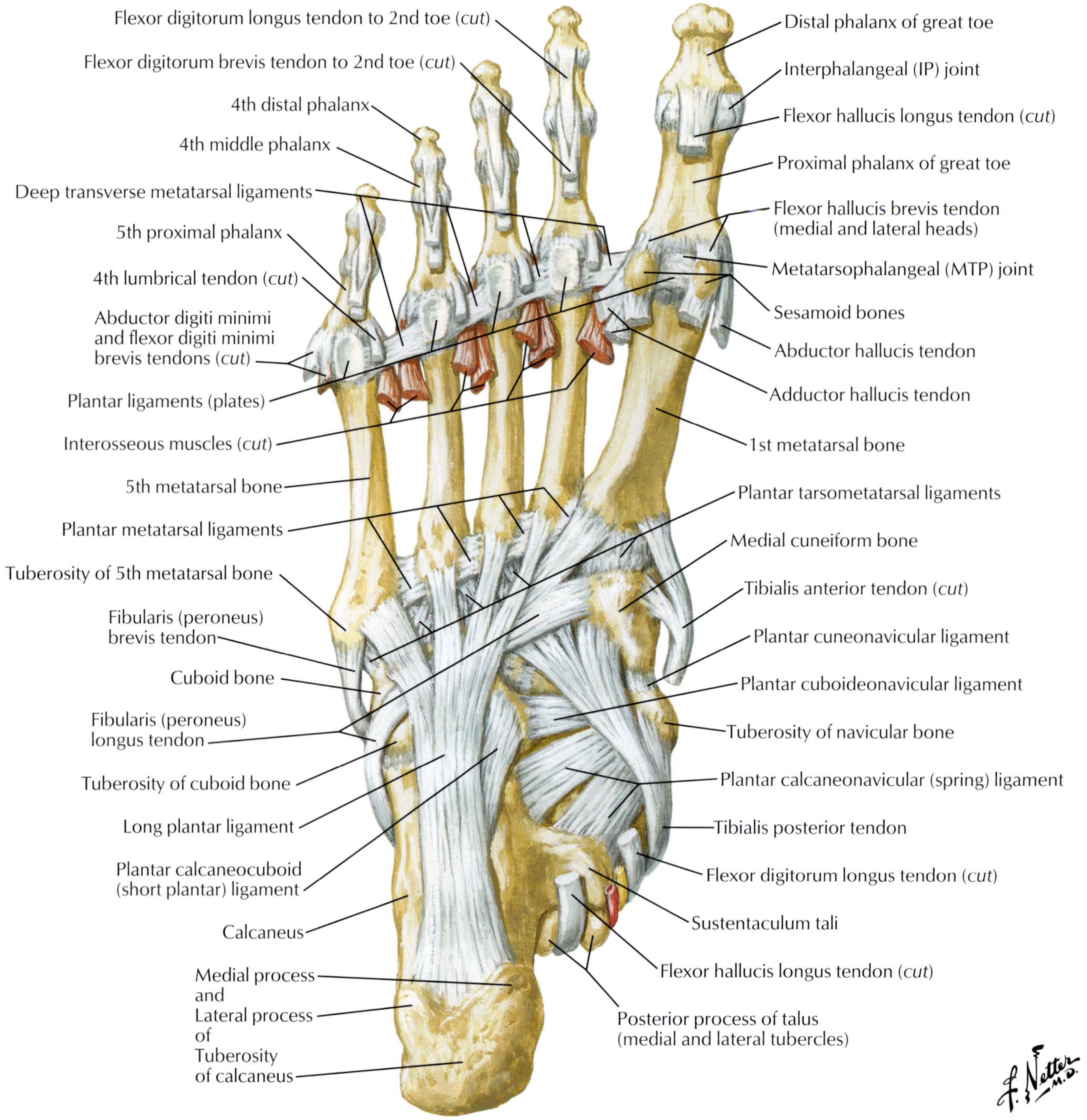

Capsules and ligaments of metatarsophalangeal and interphalangeal joints: lateral view

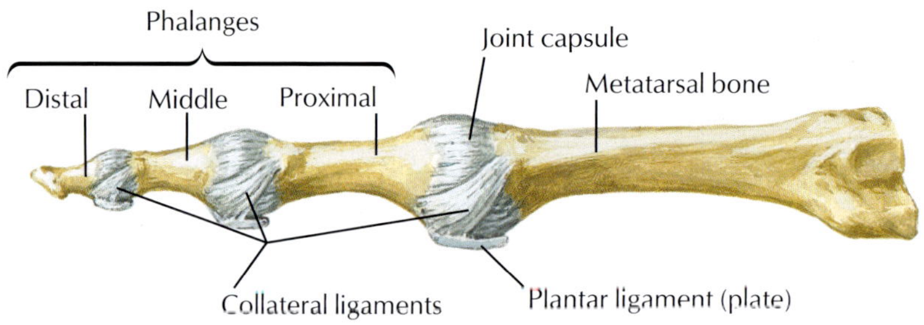

See also Plate 506

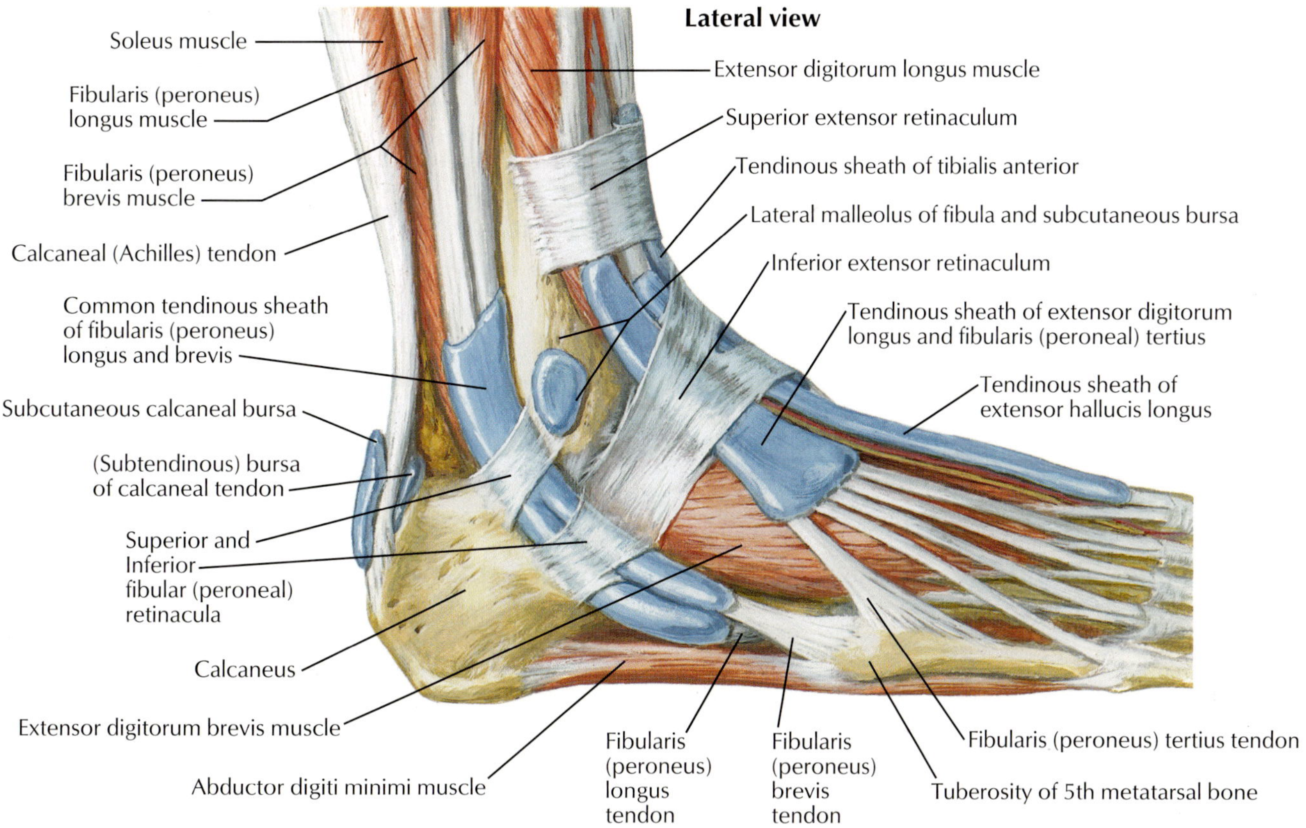

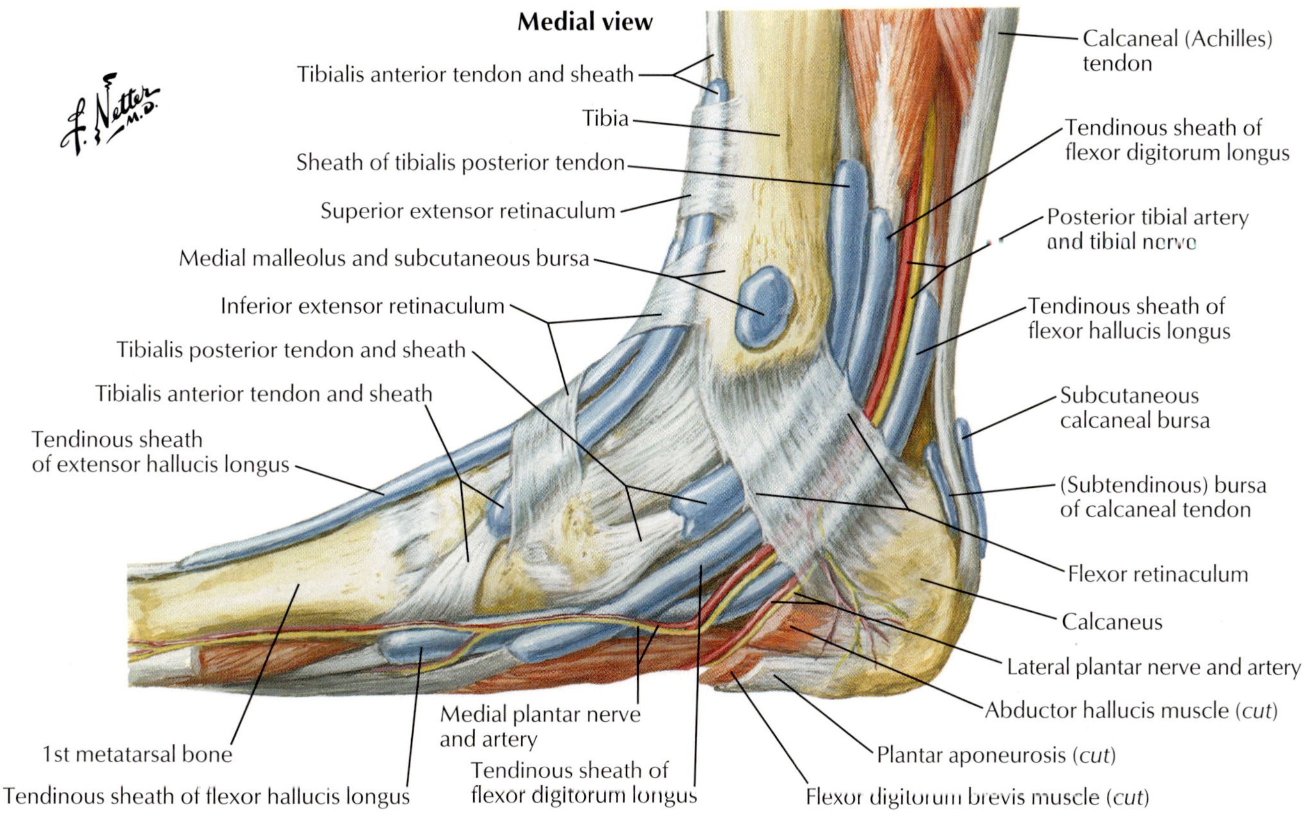

See also Plate 529

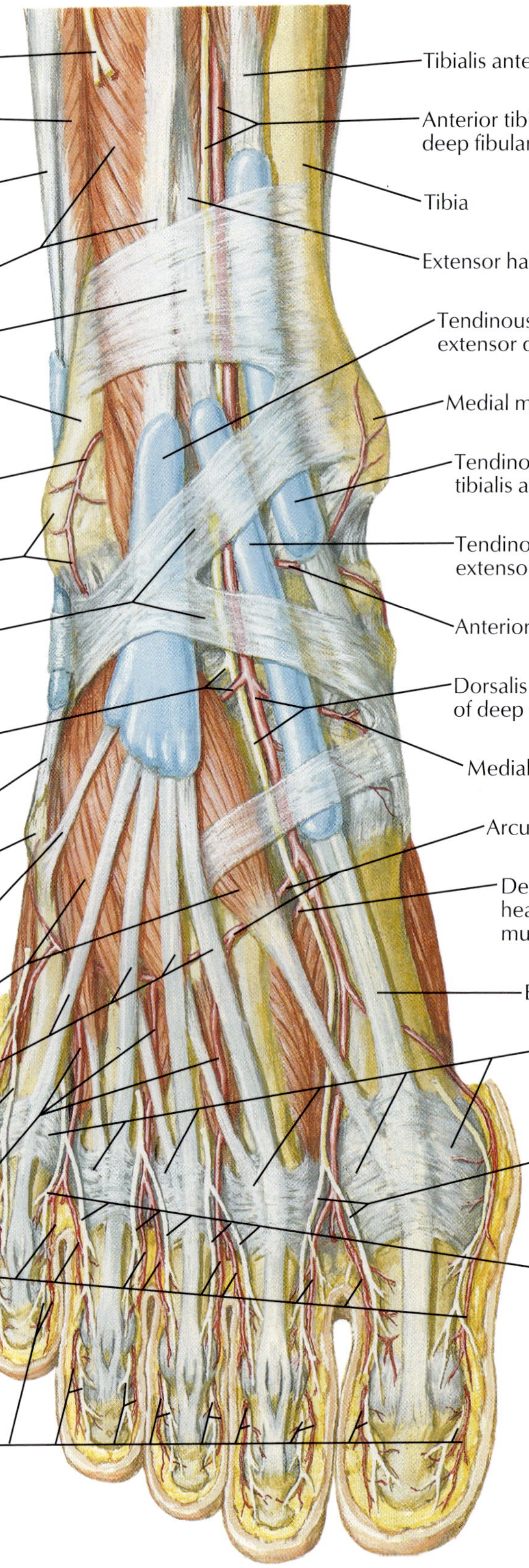

Dorsum of Foot: Deep Dissection

See also Plates 509, 523

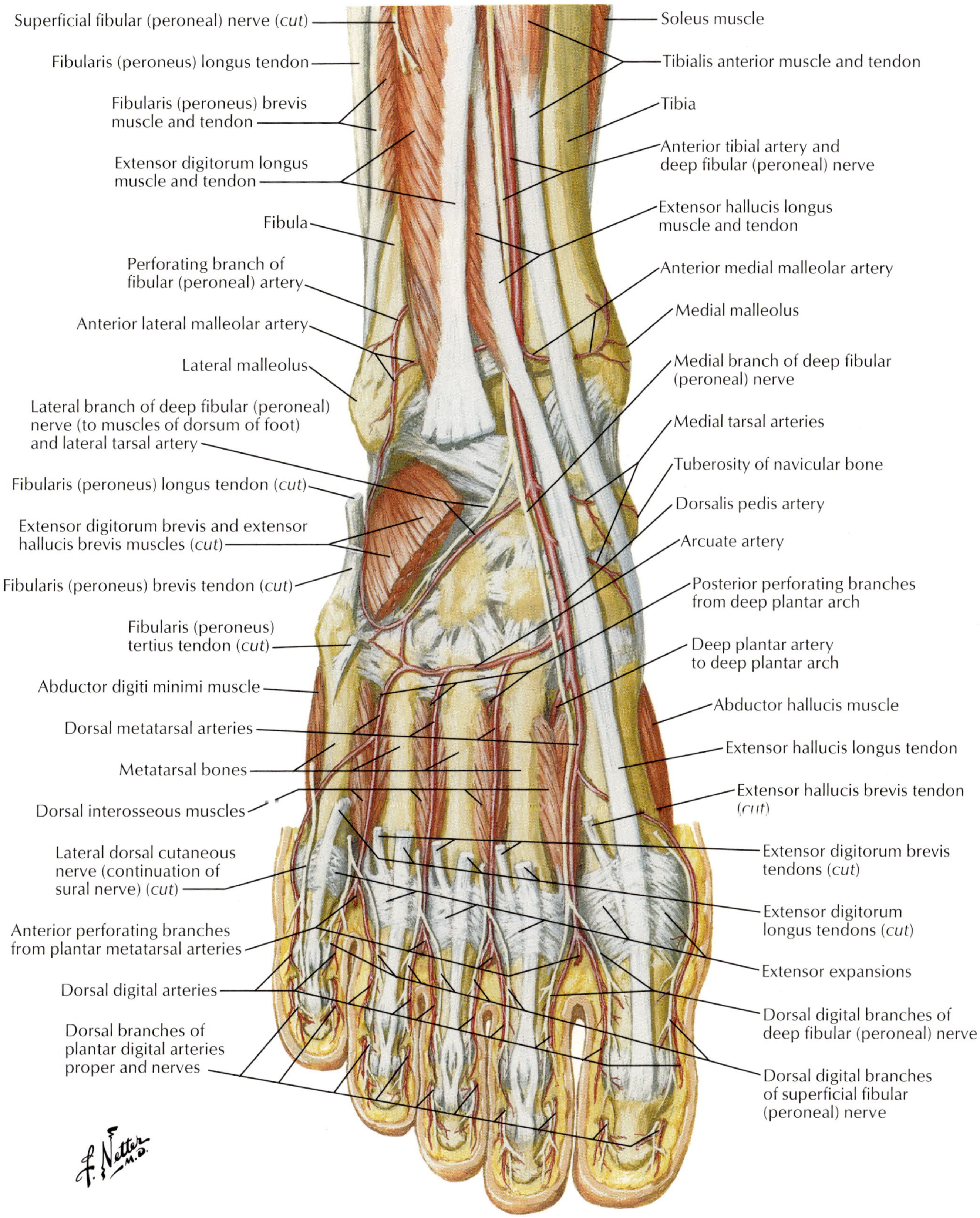

Sole of Foot: Superficial Dissection

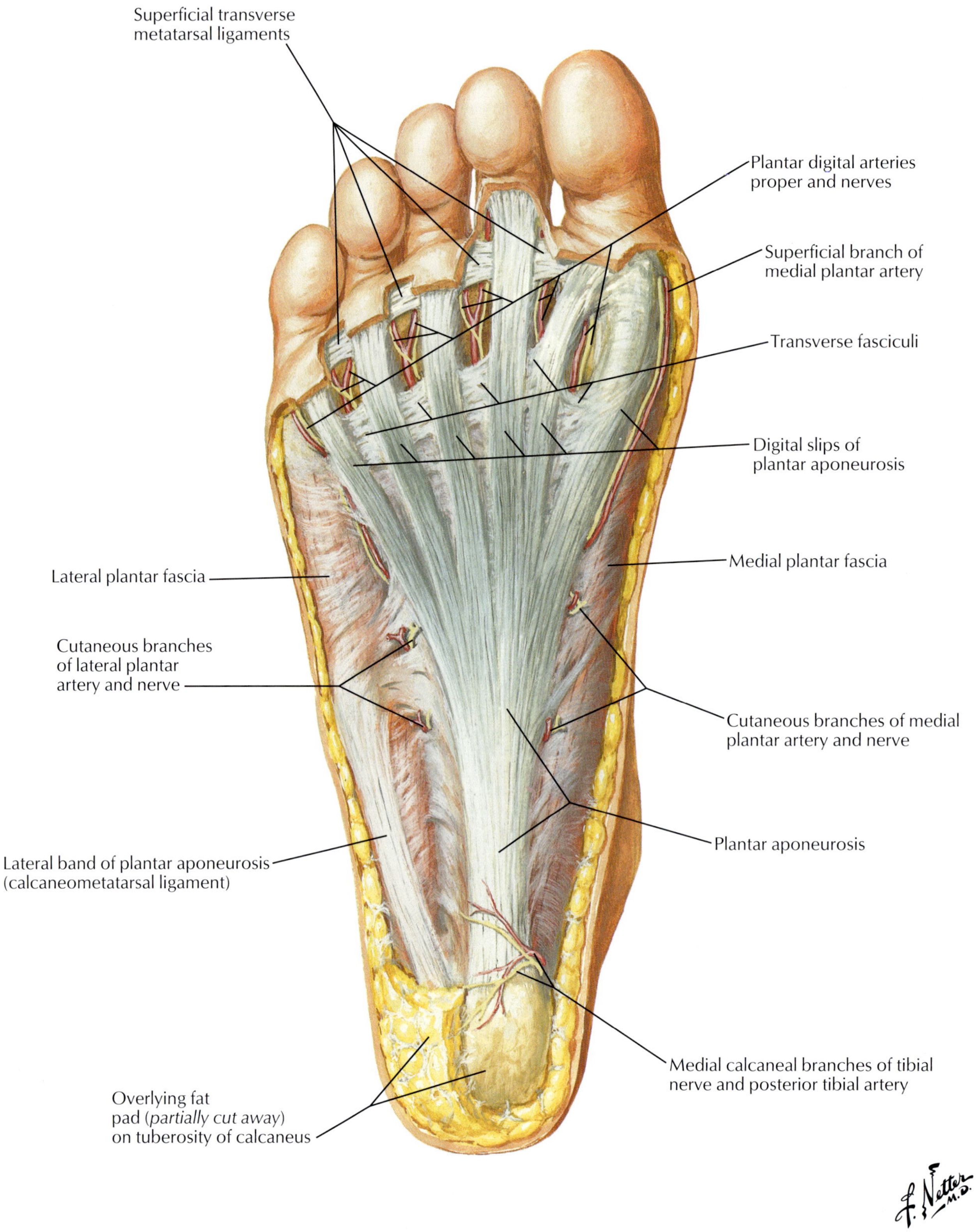

Muscles of Sole of Foot: First Layer

See also **Plate 528**

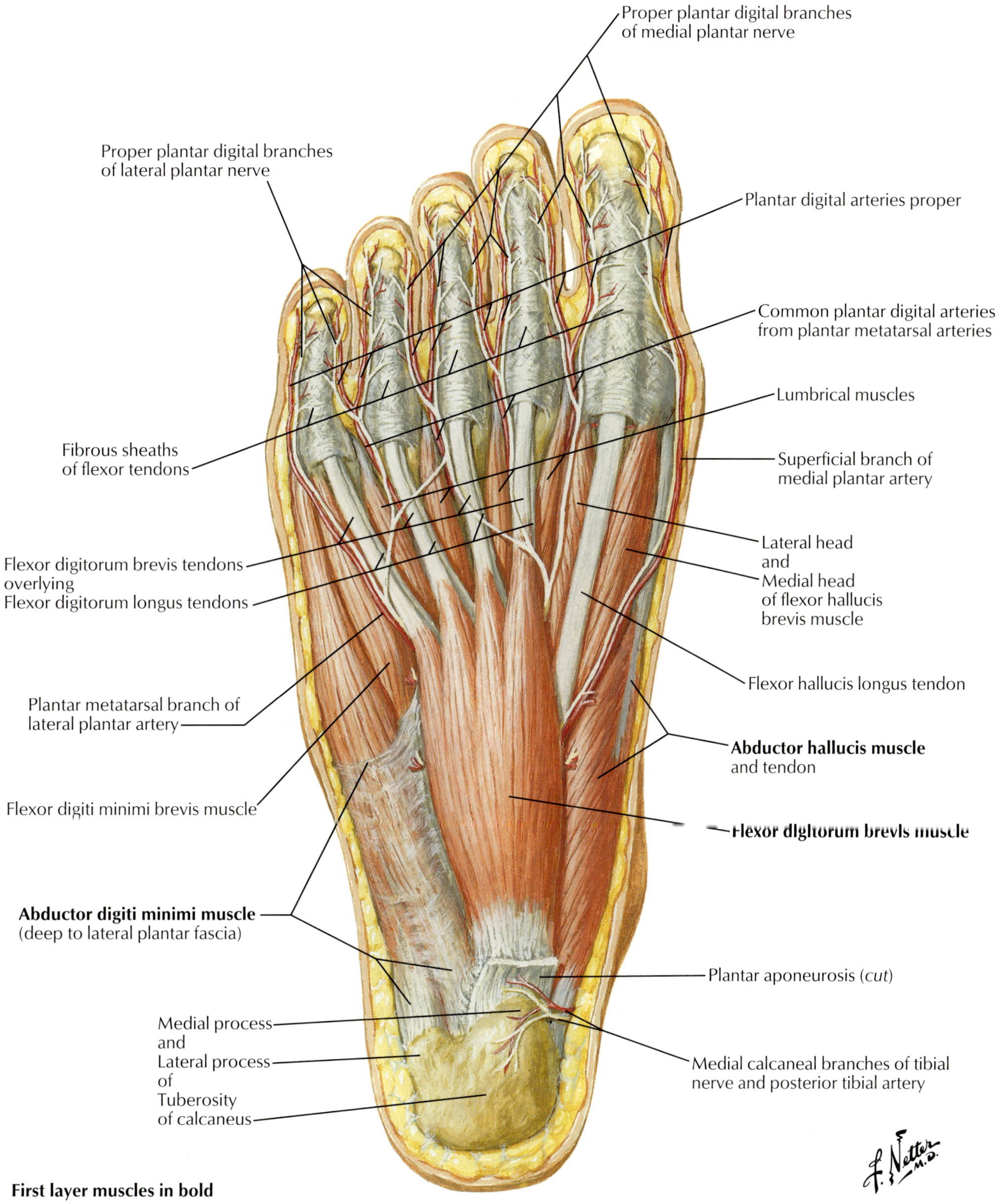

First layer muscles in bold

Muscles of Sole of Foot: Second Layer

See also Plate 528

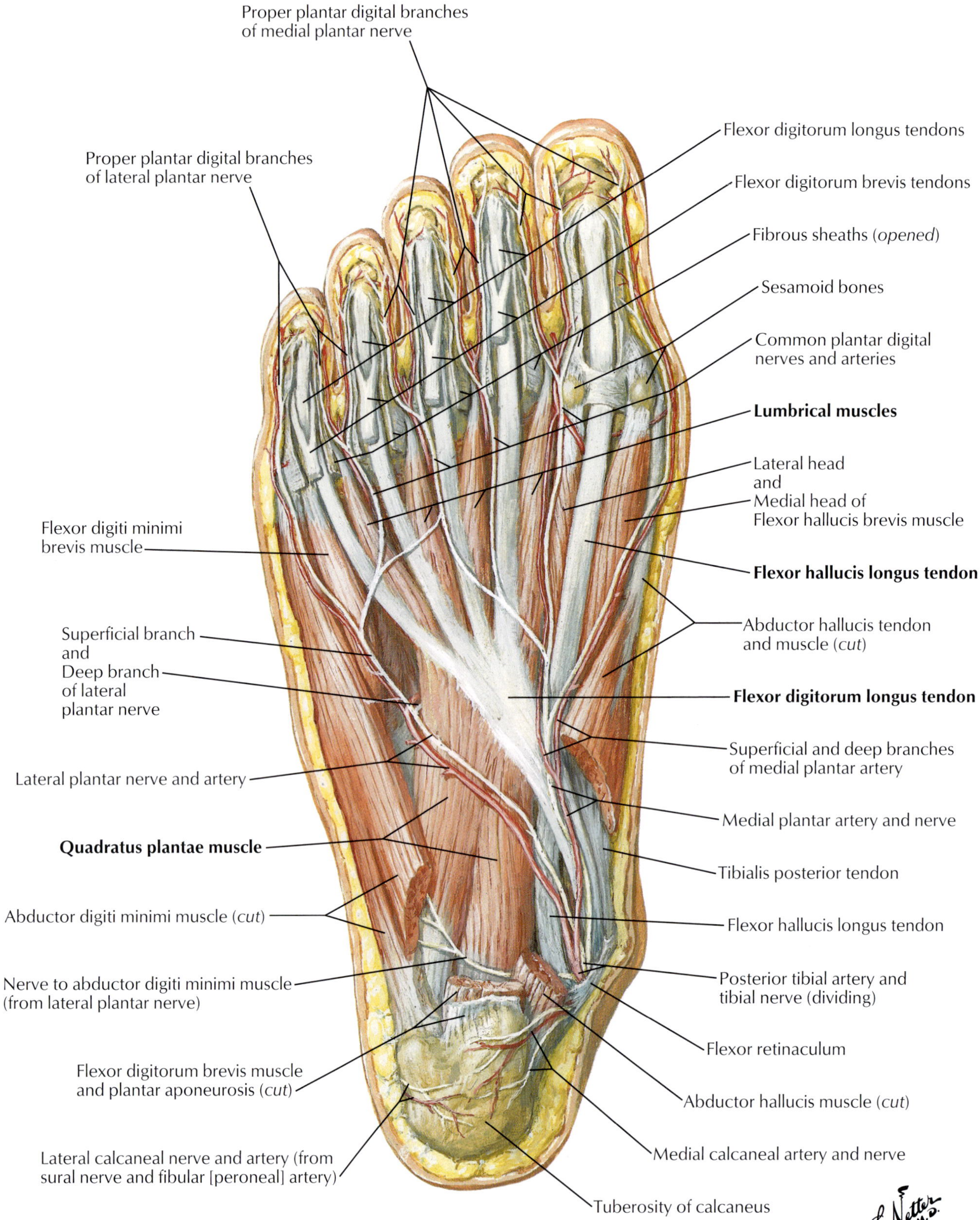

Second layer tendons and muscles in bold

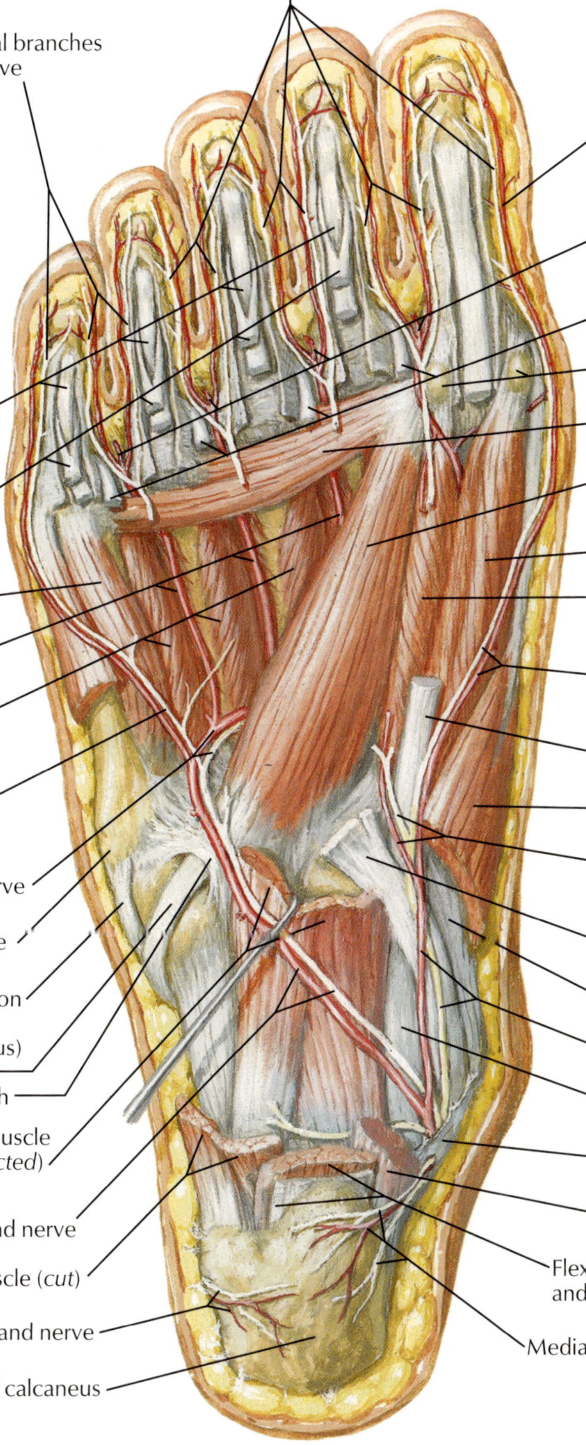

Third layer muscles in bold

Interosseous Muscles and Deep Arteries of Foot

See also Plates 508, 518

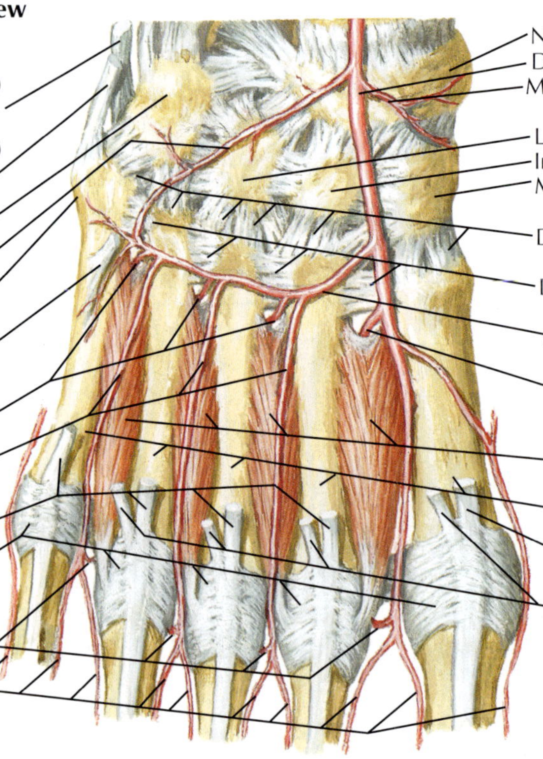

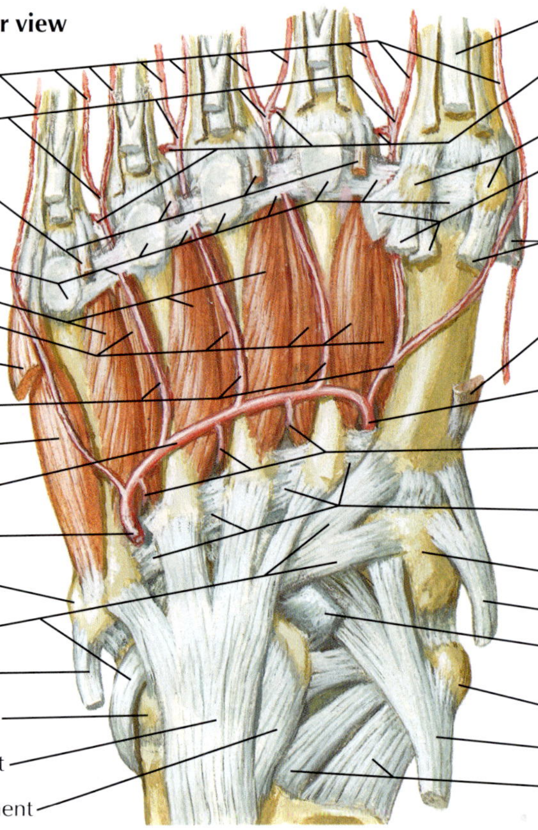

Fourth layer muscles in bold

Interosseous Muscles of Foot

See also Plate 452

Dorsal view

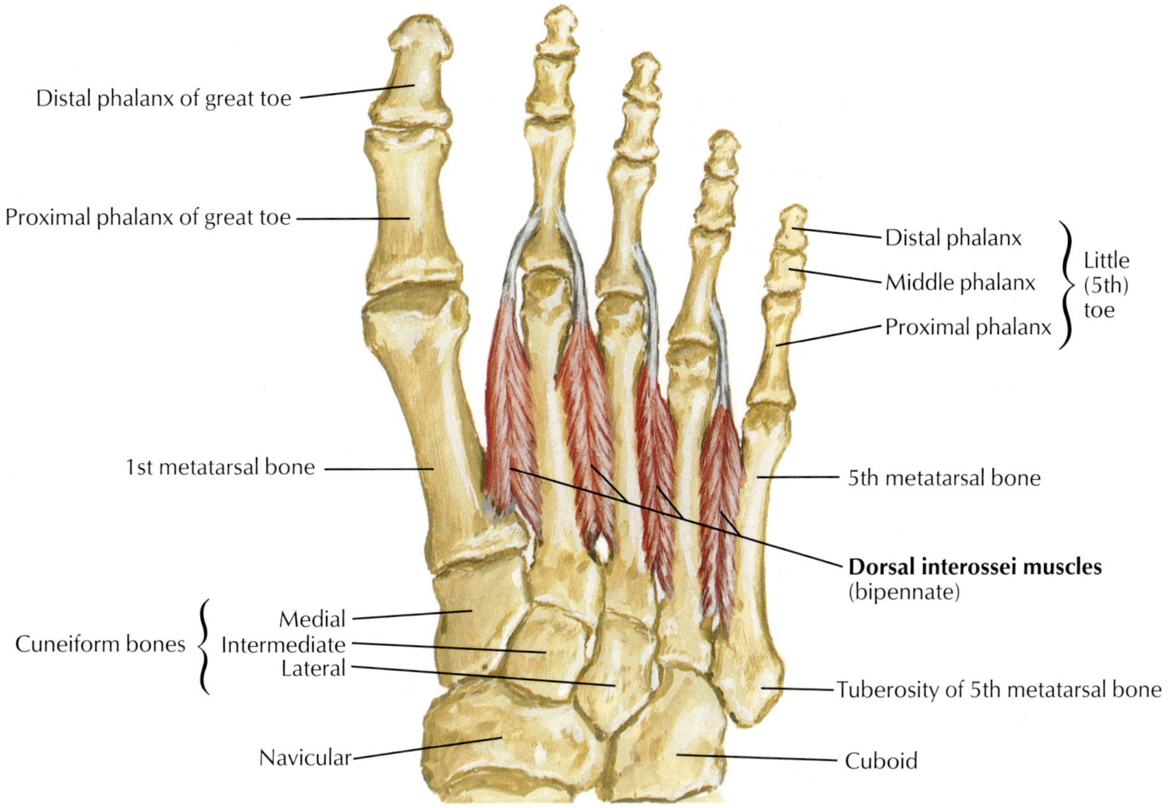

Plantar view

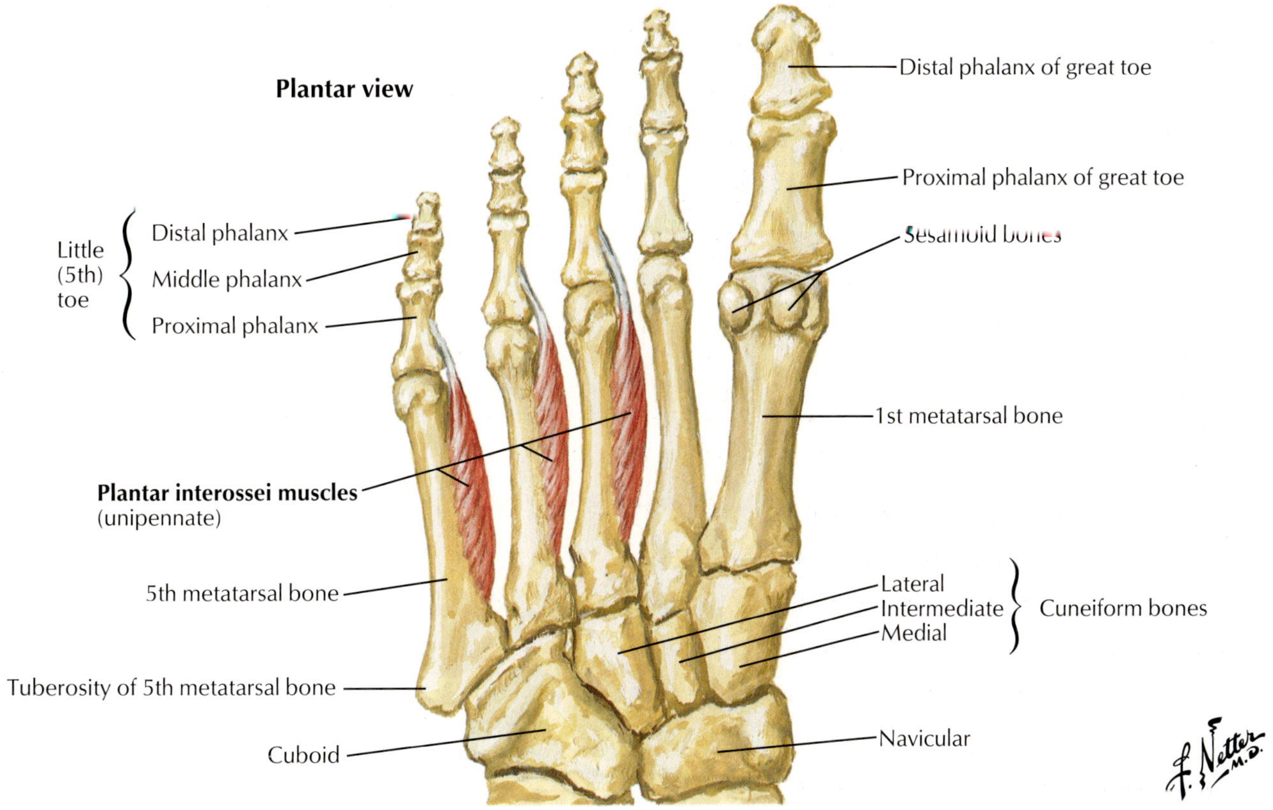

Femoral Nerve and Lateral Cutaneous Nerve of Thigh

See also Plates 262, 487, 488

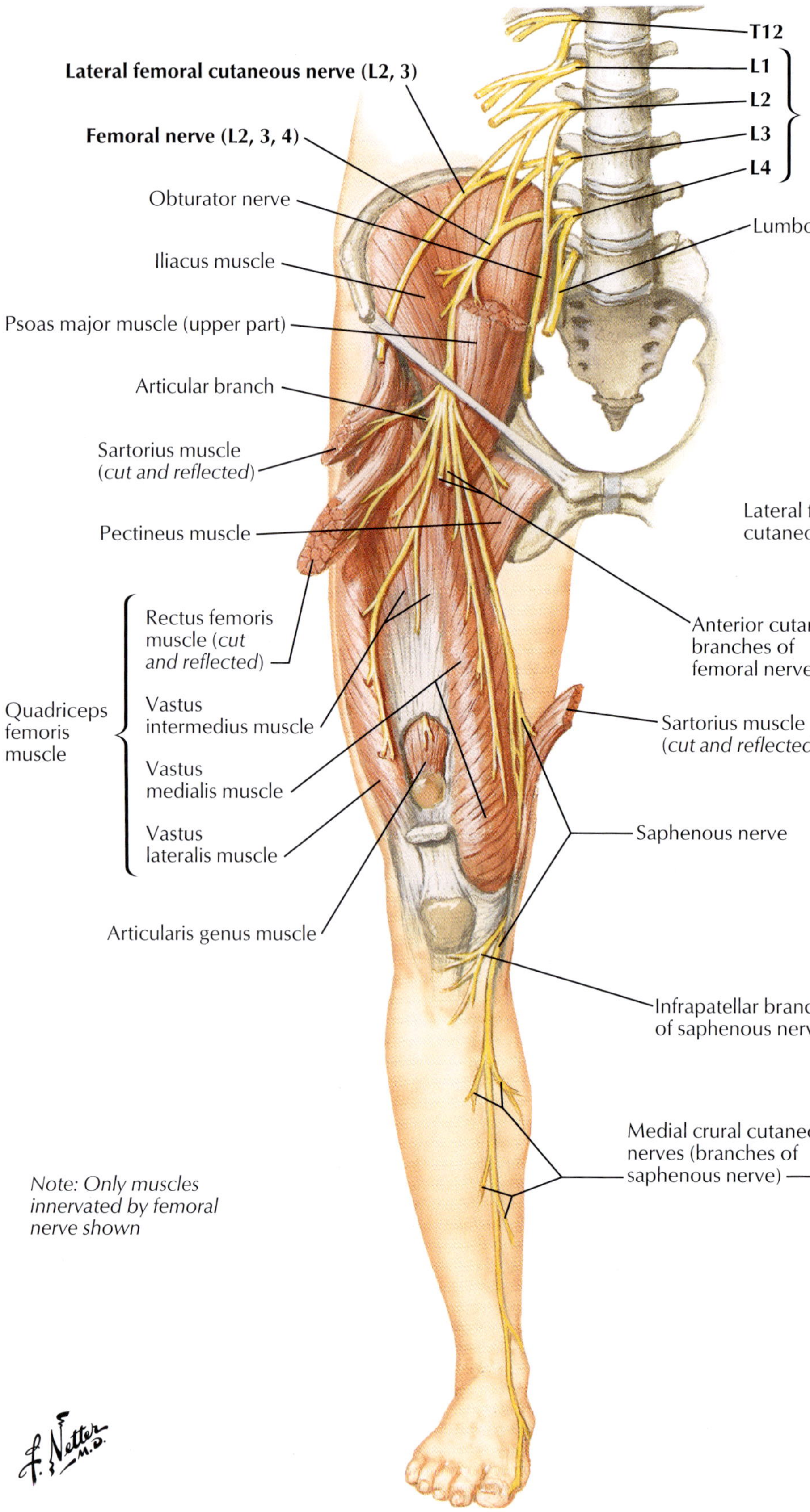

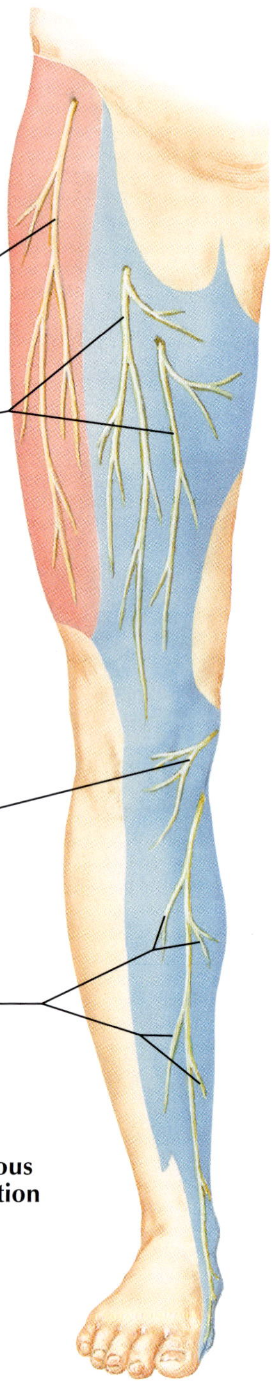

See also Plate 488

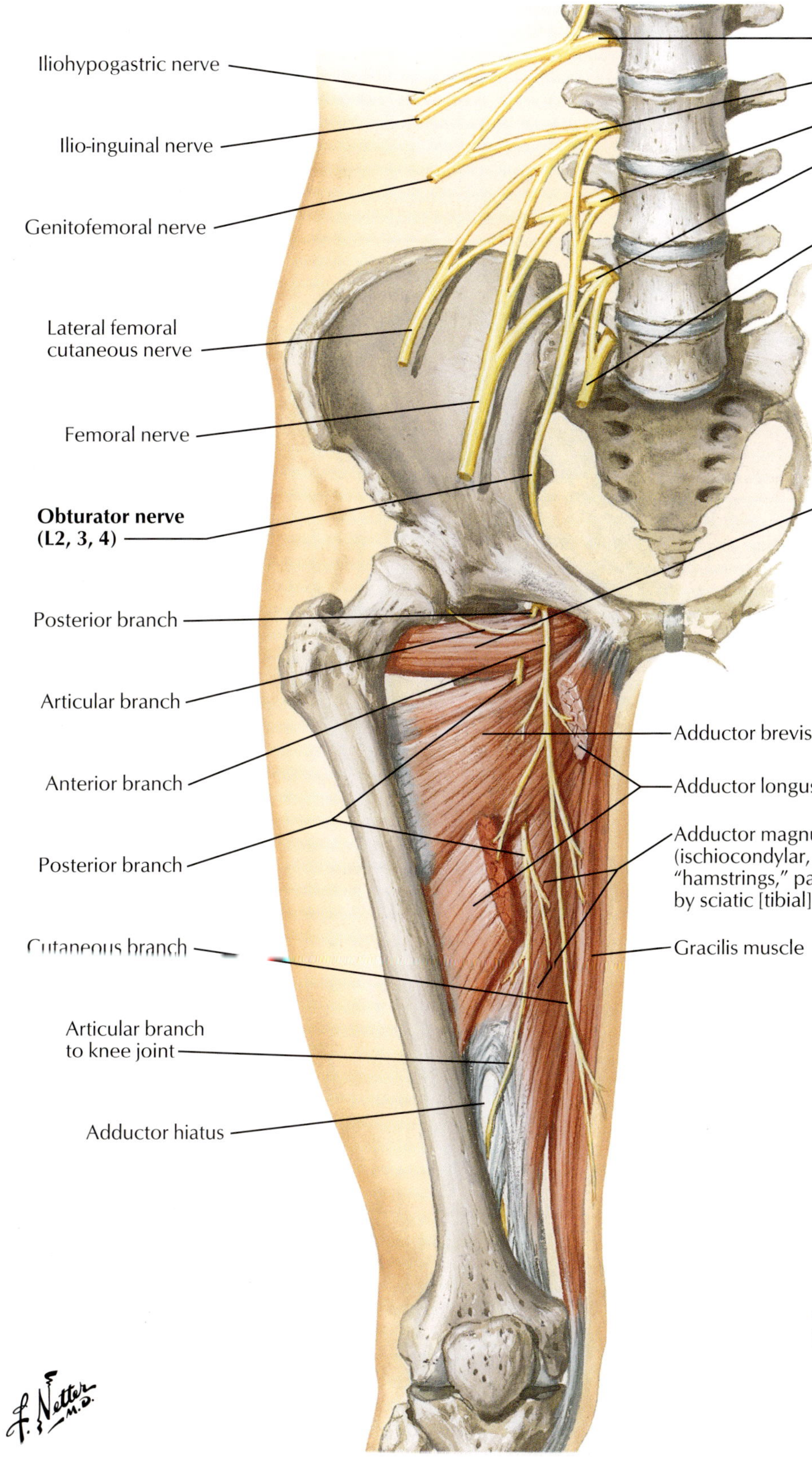

Note: Only muscles innervated by obturator nerve shown

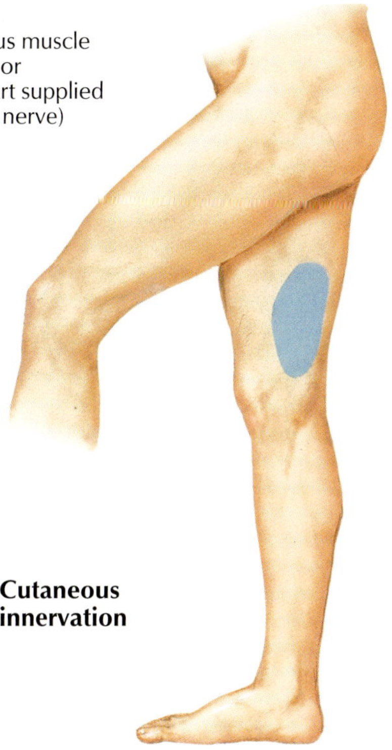

Cutaneous innervation

See also Plate 489

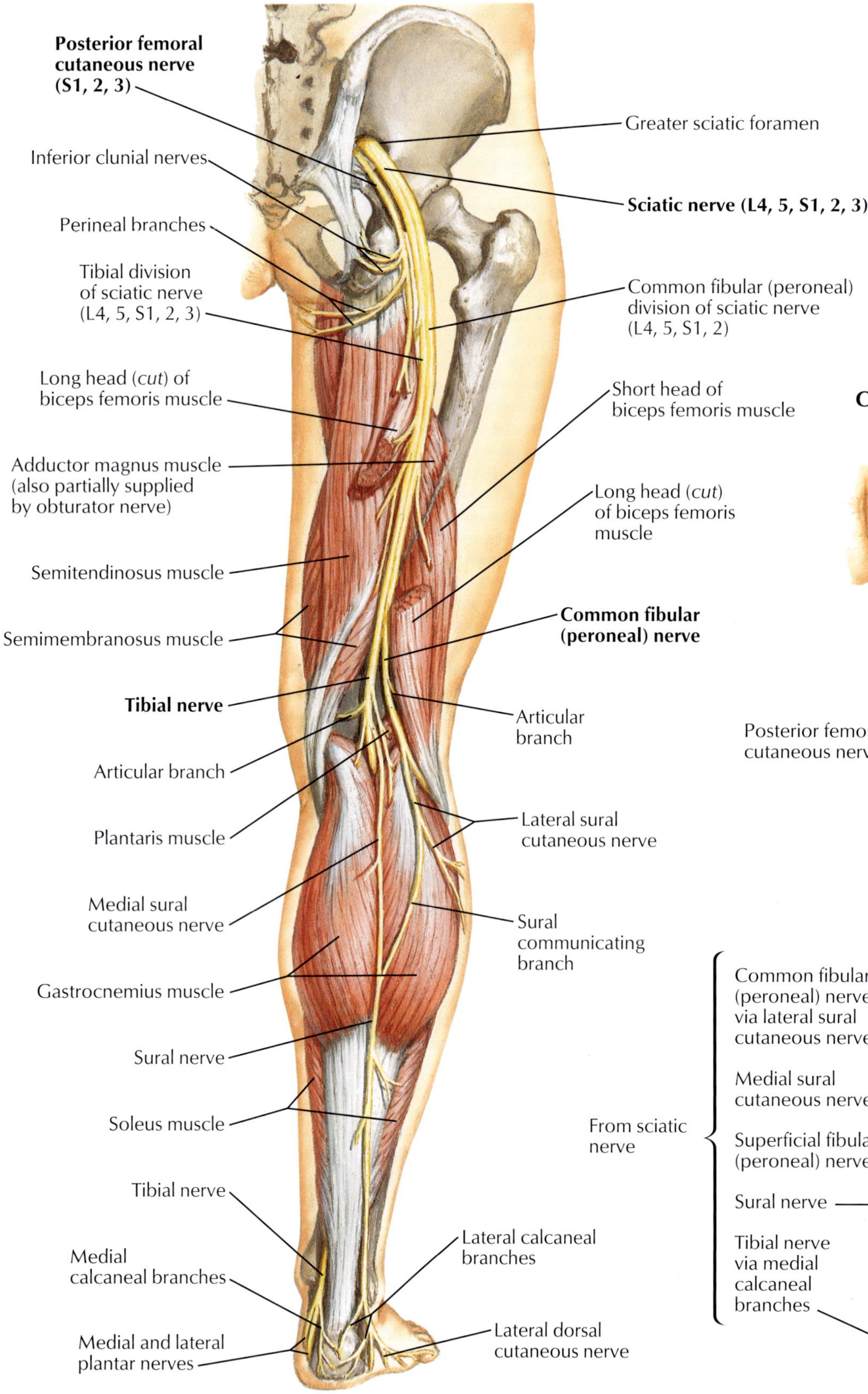

Cutaneous innervation

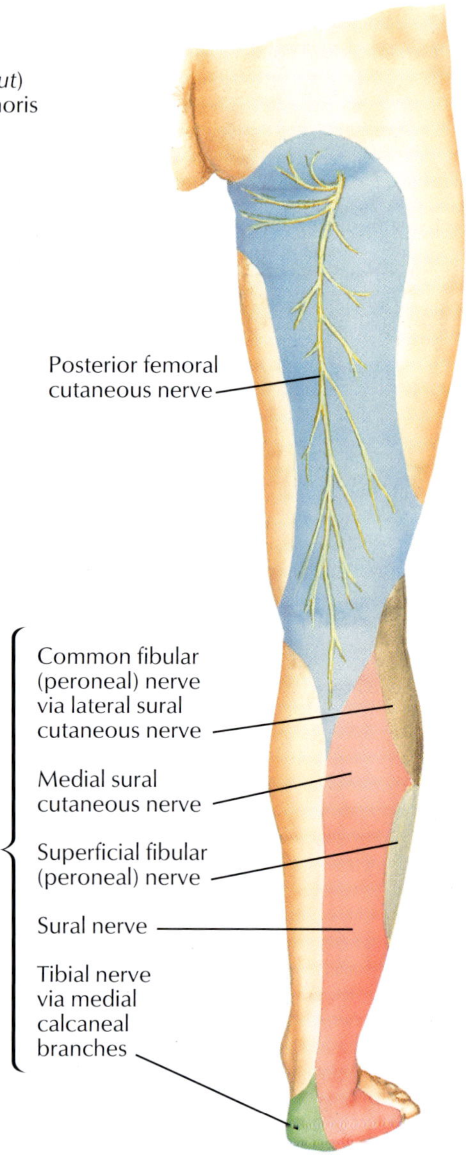

See also Plates 503, 520, 521

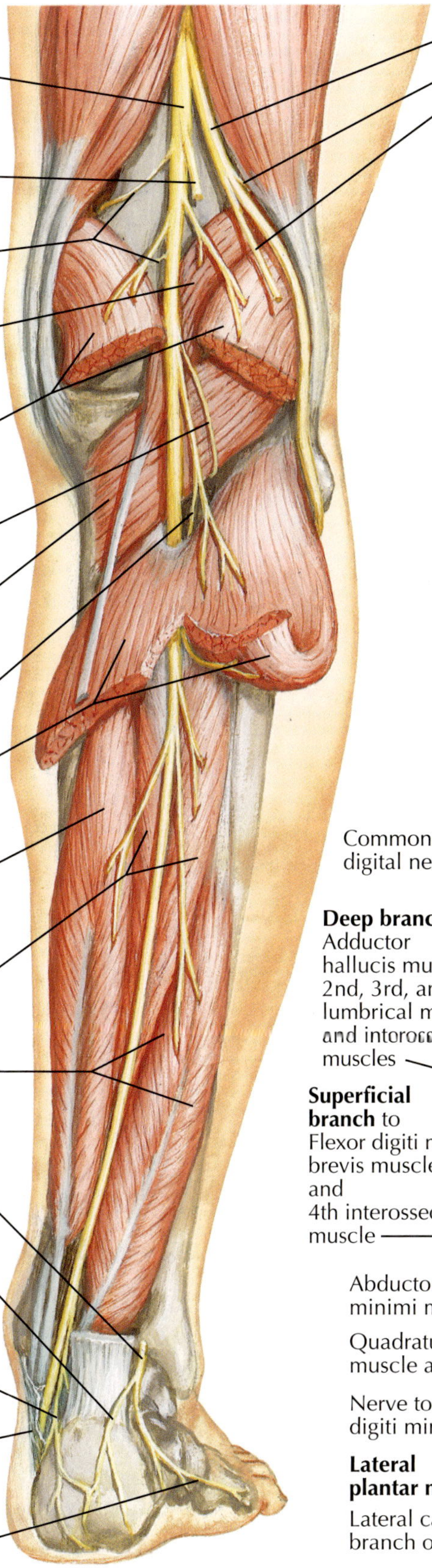

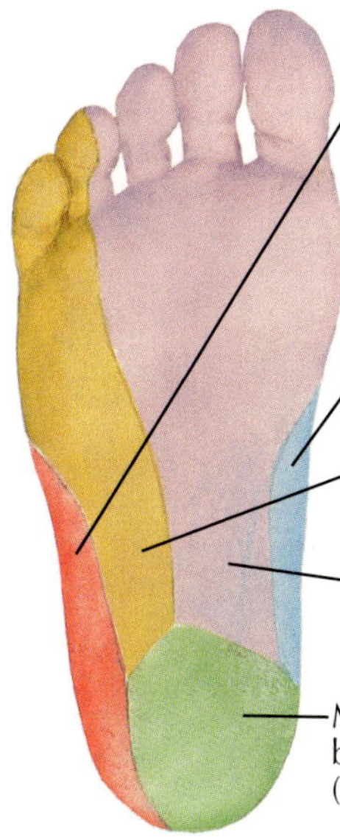

Cutaneous innervation of sole

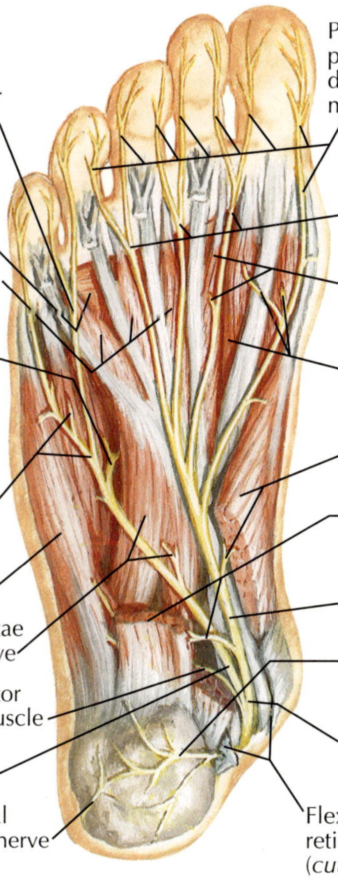

Note: Articular branches not shown

Common Fibular (Peroneal) Nerve

See also **Plates 506, 508, 516**

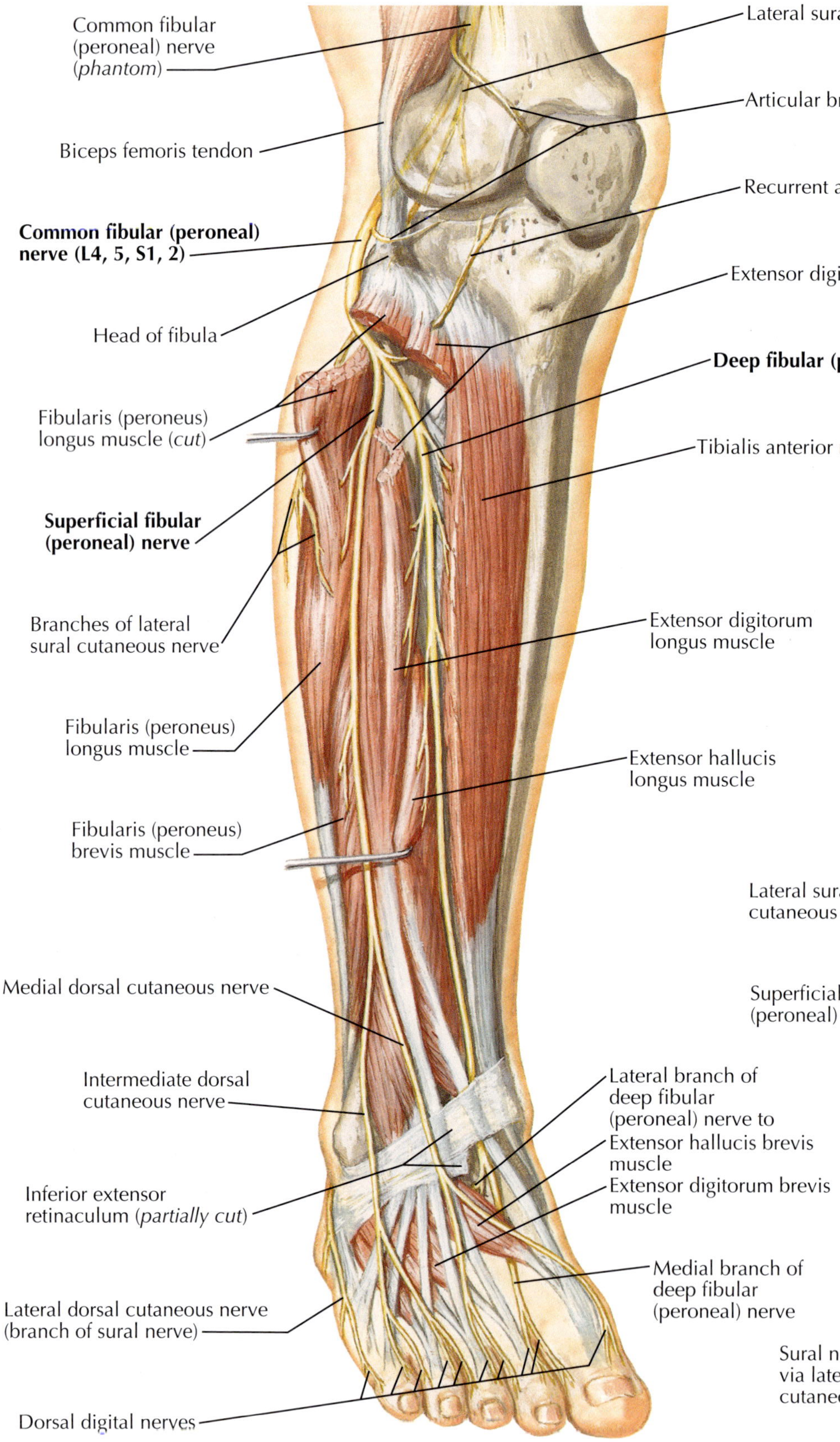

Cutaneous innervation

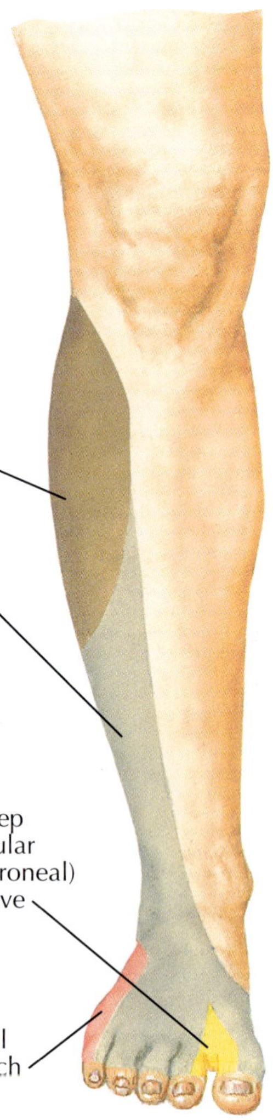

See also **Plates 330, 477, 491**

Radiograph

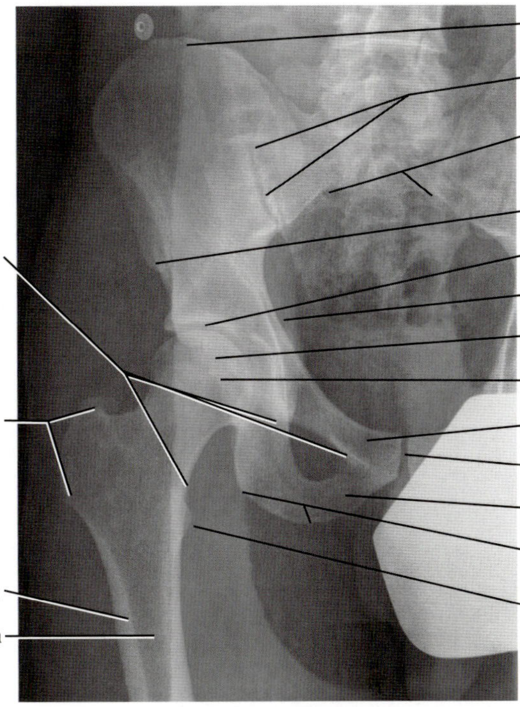

Arthrogram of hip

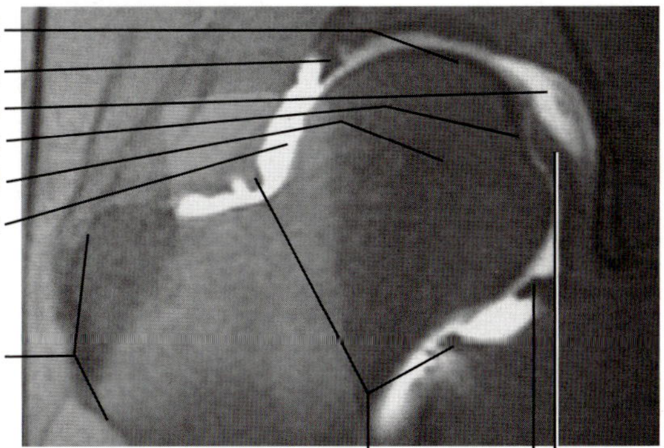

MRI

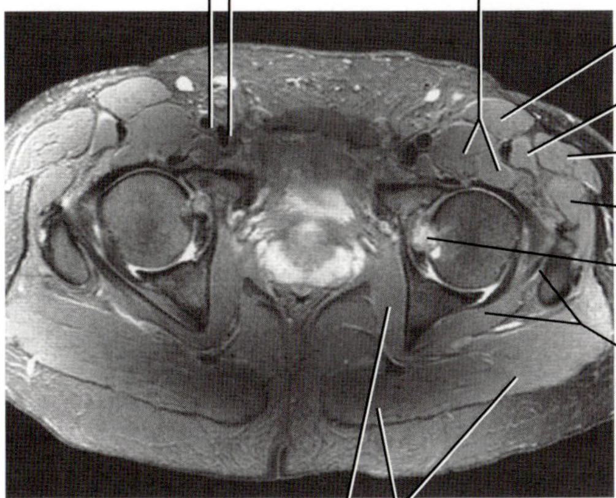

See also Plates 506, 513, 514

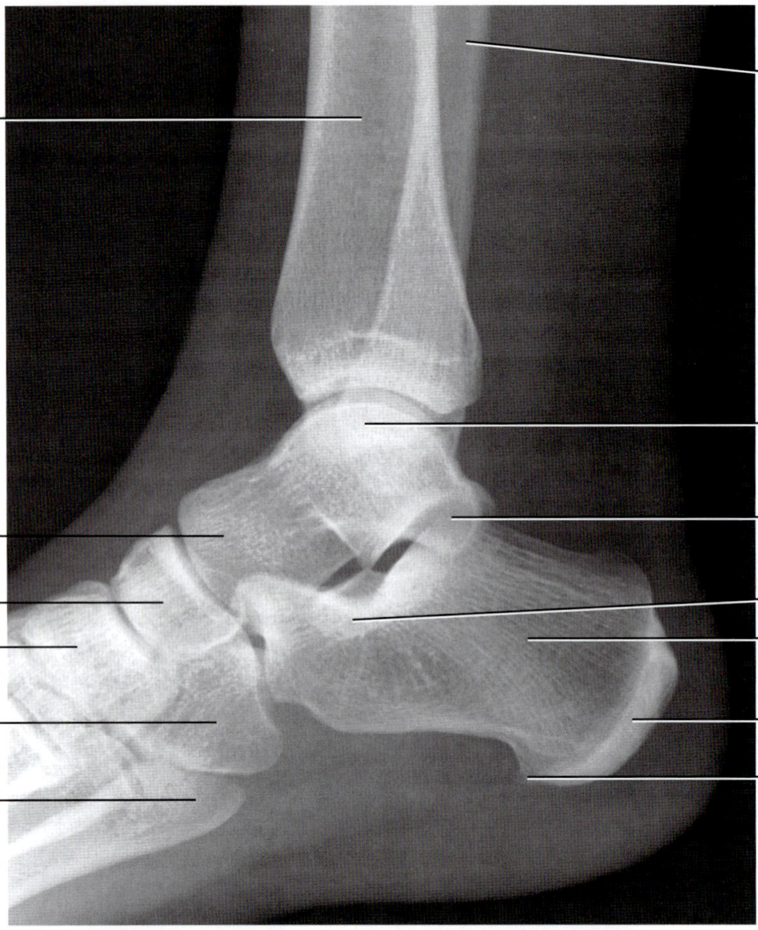

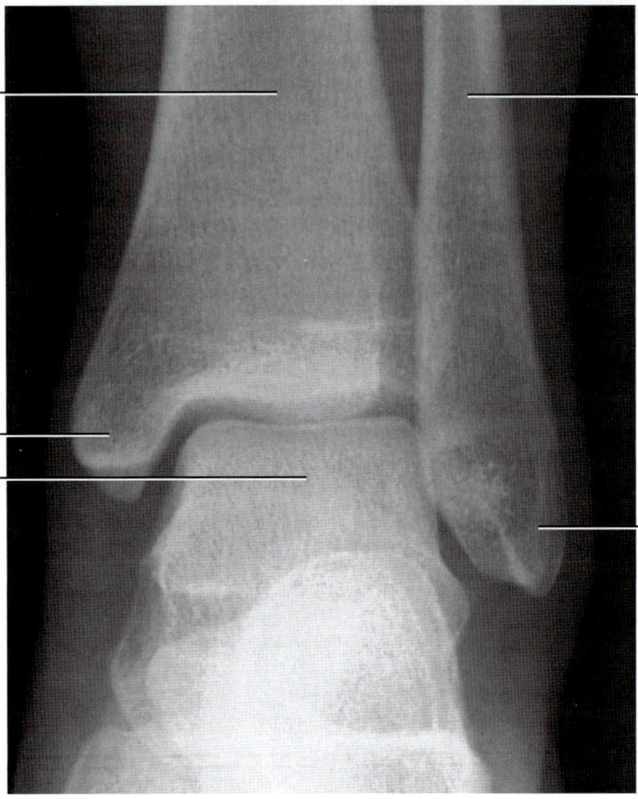

MUSCLE	PROXIMAL ATTACHMENT (ORIGIN)	DISTAL ATTACHMENT (INSERTION)	INNERVATION	MAIN ACTIONS	BLOOD SUPPLY	MUSCLE GROUP
Abductor digiti minimi	Medial and lateral tubercles of tuberosity of calcaneus, plantar aponeurosis, and intermuscular septum	Lateral side of base of proximal phalanx of 5th digit	Lateral plantar nerve	Abducts and flexes 5th digit	Medial-lateral plantar artery, plantar metatarsal and plantar digital arteries to 5th digit	Foot
Abductor hallucis	Medial tubercle of tuberosity of calcaneus, flexor retinaculum, and plantar aponeurosis	Medial side of base of proximal phalanx of 1st digit	Medial plantar nerve	Abducts and flexes 1st digit	Medial plantar and 1st plantar metatarsal arteries	Foot
Adductor brevis	Body and inferior pubic ramus	Pectineal line and proximal part of linea aspera of femur	Obturator nerve	Adducts thigh at hip, weak hip flexor	Profunda femoris, medial circumflex femoral, and obturator arteries	Medial thigh
Adductor hallucis	*Oblique head:* bases of 2nd through 4th metatarsals *Transverse head:* ligaments of metatarsophalangeal joints of digits 3-5	Tendons of both heads lateral to side of base of proximal phalanx of 1st digit	Deep branch of lateral plantar nerve	Adducts 1st digit, maintains transverse arch of foot	Medial and lateral plantar arteries and plantar arch, plantar metatarsal arteries	Foot
Adductor longus	Body of pubis inferior to pubic crest	Middle third of linea aspera of femur	Obturator nerve (anterior division)	Adducts thigh at hip	Profunda femoris and medial circumflex femoral arteries	Medial thigh
Adductor magnus	Inferior pubic ramus, ramus of ischium *Hamstring part*: ischial tuberosity	Gluteal tuberosity, linea aspera, medial supracondylar line *Hamstring part:* adductor tubercle of femur	*Adductor part:* obturator nerve *Hamstring part:* sciatic nerve (tibial division)	*Adductor part:* adducts and flexes thigh *Hamstring part:* extends thigh	Femoral, profunda femoris, and obturator arteries	Medial thigh
Articularis genus	Distal femur on anterior surface	Suprapatellar bursa	Femoral nerve	Pulls suprapatellar bursa superiorly with extension of knee	Femoral artery	Anterior thigh
Biceps femoris	*Long head:* ischial tuberosity *Short head:* Linea aspera and lateral supracondylar line of femur	Lateral side of head of fibula	*Long head:* sciatic nerve (tibial division) (L5 S2) *Short head:* sciatic nerve (common fibular division)	Flexes and laterally rotates leg, extends thigh at hip	Perforating branches of profunda femoris, inferior gluteal, and medial circumflex femoral arteries	Posterior thigh
Dorsal interossei (four muscles)	Adjacent sides of 1st through 5th metatarsals	*1st:* medial side of proximal phalanx of 2nd digit *2nd through 4th*: lateral sides of digits 2–4	Lateral plantar nerve	Abduct 2nd through 4th toes, flex metatarsophalangeal joints, and extend phalanges	Arcuate artery, dorsal and plantar metatarsal arteries	Foot
Extensor digitorum brevis and extensor hallucis brevis	Superolateral surface of calcaneus, lateral talocalcaneal ligament, cruciate crural ligament	First tendon into dorsal surface of base of proximal phalanx of great toe; other 3 tendons into lateral sides of tendons of extensor digitorum longus to digits 2-4	Deep fibular nerve	Aids the extensor digitorum longus in extending of 4 medial digits at the metatarsophalangeal and interphalangeal joints	Dorsalis pedis, lateral tarsal, arcuate, and fibular arteries	Foot

Variations in spinal nerve contributions to the innervation of muscles, their arterial supply, their attachments, and their actions are common themes in human anatomy. Therefore, expect differences between texts and realize that anatomical variation is normal.

MUSCLE	PROXIMAL ATTACHMENT (ORIGIN)	DISTAL ATTACHMENT (INSERTION)	INNERVATION	MAIN ACTIONS	BLOOD SUPPLY	MUSCLE GROUP
Extensor digitorum longus	Lateral condyle of tibia, proximal 3/4 of anterior surface of interosseous membrane and fibula	Middle and distal phalanges of lateral four digits	Deep fibular nerve	Extends lateral four digits and dorsiflexes foot at ankle	Anterior tibial artery	Anterior leg
Extensor hallucis longus	Middle part of anterior surface of fibula and interosseous membrane	Dorsal aspect of base of distal phalanx of great toe	Deep fibular nerve	Extends great toe, dorsiflexes foot at ankle	Anterior tibial artery	Anterior leg
Fibularis peroneus brevis	Distal 2/3 of lateral surface of fibula	Dorsal surface of tuberosity on lateral side of 5th metatarsal	Superficial fibular nerve	Everts foot and weakly plantarflexes foot at ankle	Anterior tibial and fibular arteries	Lateral leg
Fibularis peroneus longus	Head and proximal 2/3 of lateral fibula	Plantar base of 1st metatarsal and medial cuneiform	Superficial fibular nerve	Everts foot and weakly plantarflexes foot at ankle	Anterior tibial and fibular arteries	Lateral leg
Fibularis peroneus tertius	Distal third of anterior surface of fibula and interosseous membrane	Dorsum of base of 5th metatarsal	Deep fibular nerve	Dorsiflexes foot at ankle and aids in eversion of foot	Anterior tibial artery	Anterior leg
Flexor digiti minimi brevis	Base of 5th metatarsal	Lateral base of proximal phalanx of 5th digit	Superficial branch of lateral plantar nerve	Flexes proximal phalanx of 5th digit	Lateral plantar artery, plantar digital artery to 5th digit, arcuate artery	Foot
Flexor digitorum brevis	Medial tubercle of tuberosity of calcaneus, plantar aponeurosis, and intermuscular septum	Both sides of middle phalanges of lateral four digits	Medial plantar nerve	Flexes 2nd through 5th digits	Medial and lateral plantar arteries and plantar arch, plantar metatarsal and plantar digital arteries	Foot
Flexor digitorum longus	Medial part of posterior tibia inferior to soleal line	Plantar bases of distal phalanges of lateral four digits	Tibial nerve	Flexes lateral four digits and plantarflexes foot at ankle; supports longitudinal arches of foot	Posterior tibial artery	Posterior leg
Flexor hallucis brevis	Plantar surfaces of cuboid and lateral cuneiform	Both sides of base of proximal phalanx of 1st digit	Medial plantar nerve	Flexes proximal phalanx of 1st digit	Medial plantar artery, first plantar metatarsal artery	Foot
Flexor hallucis longus	Distal 2/3 of posterior fibula and interosseous membrane	Base of distal phalanx of great toe (hallux)	Tibial nerve	Flexes all joints of great toe, weakly plantarflexes foot at ankle	Fibular artery	Posterior leg
Gastrocnemius	*Lateral head:* lateral aspect of lateral condyle of femur *Medial head:* popliteal surface above medial condyle of femur	Posterior aspect of calcaneus via calcaneal tendon	Tibial nerve	Plantarflexes foot at ankle joint, assists in flexion of knee joint, raises heel during walking	Popliteal and posterior tibial arteries	Posterior leg
Gluteus maximus	Ilium posterior to posterior gluteal line, dorsal surface of sacrum and coccyx, sacrotuberous ligament	Most fibers end in iliotibial tract that inserts into lateral condyle of tibia; some fibers insert into gluteal tuberosity of femur	Inferior gluteal nerve	Extends flexed thigh, assists in lateral rotation, and abducts thigh	Inferior gluteal arteries mainly, and superior gluteal arteries occasionally	Gluteal region

MUSCLE	PROXIMAL ATTACHMENT (ORIGIN)	DISTAL ATTACHMENT (INSERTION)	INNERVATION	MAIN ACTIONS	BLOOD SUPPLY	MUSCLE GROUP
Gluteus medius	Lateral surface of ilium between anterior and posterior gluteal lines	Lateral surface of greater trochanter of femur	Superior gluteal nerve	Abducts and medially rotates thigh at hips; steadies pelvis on leg when opposite leg is raised	Superior gluteal artery	Gluteal region
Gluteus minimus	Lateral surface of ilium between anterior and inferior gluteal lines	Anterior surface of greater trochanter of femur	Superior gluteal nerve	Abducts and medially rotates thigh at hips; steadies pelvis on leg when opposite leg is raised	Main trunk and deep branch of superior gluteal artery	Gluteal region
Gracilis	Body and inferior ramus of pubis	Superior part of medial surface of tibia	Obturator nerve	Adducts thigh, flexes and medially rotates leg	Profunda femoris artery, medial circumflex femoral artery	Medial thigh
Iliacus (Iliopsoas)	Superior 2/3 of iliac fossa, iliac crest, ala of sacrum, anterior sacro-iliac ligaments	Lesser trochanter of femur and shaft inferior to it, to psoas major tendon	Femoral nerve	Flexes thigh at hips and stabilizes hip joint, acts with psoas major	Iliac branches of iliolumbar artery	Anterior thigh
Inferior gamellus	Ischial tuberosity	Medial surface of greater trochanter of femur	Nerve to quadratus femoris	Laterally rotates extended thigh at the hip	Medial circumflex femoral artery	Gluteal region
Lumbricals	Tendons of flexor digitorum longus	Medial side of dorsal digital expansions of lateral 4 digits	*Medial one:* medial plantar nerve *Lateral three*: lateral plantar nerve	Flexes proximal phalanges at MTP joint, extends phalanges at PIP and DIP joints	Lateral plantar artery and plantar metatarsal arteries	Foot
Obturator externus	Margins of obturator foramen, obturator membrane	Trochanteric fossa of femur	Obturator nerve	Laterally rotates thigh, stabilizes head of femur in acetabulum	Medial circumflex femoral artery, obturator artery	Medial thigh
Obturator internus	Pelvic surface of obturator membrane and surrounding bone	Medial surface of greater trochanter of femur	Nerve to obturator internus	Laterally rotates extended thigh, abducts flexed thigh at hip	Internal pudendal and obturator arteries	Gluteal region
Pectineus	Superior ramus of pubis	Pectineal line of femur	Femoral nerve and sometimes obturator nerve	Adducts and flexes thigh at hip	Medial circumflex femoral artery, obturator artery	Medial thigh
Piriformis	Anterior surface of sacral segments 2–4, sacrotuberous ligament	Superior border of greater trochanter of femur	Ventral rami of L5, S1, S2	Laterally rotates extended thigh, abducts flexed thigh at hip	Superior and inferior gluteal arteries, internal pudendal artery	Gluteal region
Plantar interossei (three muscles)	Bases and medial sides of 3rd through 5th metatarsals	Medial sides of bases of proximal phalanges of 3rd through 5th digits	Lateral plantar nerve	Adduct digits (3-5) and flex metatarsophalangeal joint and extend phalanges	Lateral plantar artery and plantar arch, plantar metatarsal and plantar digital arteries	Foot
Plantaris	Inferior end of lateral supracondylar line of femur and oblique popliteal ligament	Posterior aspect of calcaneus via calcaneal tendon	Tibial nerve	Weakly assists gastrocnemius	Popliteal artery	Posterior leg
Popliteus	Lateral aspect of lateral condyle of femur, lateral meniscus	Posterior tibia superior to soleal line	Tibial nerve (L4–S1)	Weakly flexes knee and unlocks it by rotating femur on fixed tibia	Inferior medial and lateral genicular arteries	Posterior leg
Psoas major (Iliopsoas)	Transverse processes of lumbar vertebrae, sides of bodies of T12–L5 vertebrae, intervening intervertebral discs	Lesser trochanter of femur	Ventral rami of first lumbar nerve	Acting superiorly with iliacus, flexes hip; acting inferiorly, flexes vertebral column laterally; used to balance trunk in sitting position; acting inferiorly with iliacus, flexes trunk	Lumbar branches of iliolumbar artery	Anterior thigh
Quadratus femoris	Lateral margin of ischial tuberosity	Quadrate tubercle on intertrochanteric crest of femur	Nerve to quadratus femoris	Laterally rotates thigh at hip	Medial circumflex femoral artery	Gluteal region

MUSCLE	PROXIMAL ATTACHMENT (ORIGIN)	DISTAL ATTACHMENT (INSERTION)	INNERVATION	MAIN ACTIONS	BLOOD SUPPLY	MUSCLE GROUP
Quadratus plantae	Medial and lateral sides of plantar surface of calcaneus	Posterolateral edge of flexor digitorum longus tendon	Lateral plantar nerve	Corrects for oblique pull of flexor digitorum longus tendon, thus assists in flexion of toes	Medial and lateral plantar arteries and deep plantar arterial arch	Foot
Rectus femoris (quadriceps)	Anterior inferior iliac spine and ilium superior to acetabulum	Base of patella and to tibial tuberosity via patellar ligament	Femoral nerve	Extends leg at knee joint and flexes thigh at hip joint	Profunda femoris and lateral circumflex femoral arteries	Anterior thigh
Sartorius	Anterior superior iliac spine and superior part of notch below it	Superior part of medial surface of tibia	Femoral nerve	Abducts, laterally rotates, and flexes thigh; flexes knee joint	Femoral artery	Anterior thigh
Semimembranosus	Ischial tuberosity	Posterior part of medial condyle of tibia	Sciatic nerve (tibial division)	Flexes leg, extends thigh	Perforating branch of profunda femoris and medial circumflex femoral arteries	Posterior thigh
Semitendinosus	Ischial tuberosity	Superior part of medial surface of tibia	Sciatic nerve (tibial division)	Flexes leg, extends thigh	Perforating branch of profunda femoris and medial circumflex femoral arteries	Posterior thigh
Soleus	Posterior aspect of head of fibula, proximal 1/4 of posterior surface of fibula, soleal line of tibia	Posterior aspect of calcaneus via calcaneal tendon	Tibial nerve	Plantarflexes foot at ankle, stabilizes leg over foot	Popliteal, posterior tibial, and fibular arteries	Posterior leg
Superior gemellus	Outer surface of ischial spine	Medial surface of greater trochanter of femur	Nerve to obturator internus	Laterally rotates extended thigh at the hip	Inferior gluteal and internal pudendal arteries	Gluteal region
Tensor fasciae latae	Anterior superior iliac spine and anterior part of iliac crest	Iliotibial tract that attaches to lateral condyle of tibia	Superior gluteal nerve	Abducts, medially rotates, and flexes thigh at hip; helps to keep knee extended	Ascending branch of lateral circumflex femoral artery	Gluteal region
Tibialis anterior	Lateral condyle, proximal half of lateral tibia, interosseous membrane	Medial plantar surfaces of medial cuneiform and base of 1st metatarsal	Deep fibular nerve	Dorsiflexes foot at ankle and inverts foot	Anterior tibial artery	Anterior leg
Tibialis posterior	Posterior tibia below soleal line, interosseous membrane, proximal half of posterior fibula	Tuberosity of navicular bone, all cuneiforms, cuboid, and bases of 2nd through 4th metatarsals	Tibial nerve	Plantarflexes foot at ankle and inverts foot	Fibular artery	Posterior leg
Vastus intermedius (quadriceps)	Anterior and lateral surfaces of body of femur	Base of patella and to tibial tuberosity via patellar ligament	Femoral nerve	Extends leg at knee joint	Lateral circumflex femoral and profunda femoris arteries	Anterior thigh
Vastus lateralis (quadriceps)	Greater trochanter, lateral lip of linea aspera of femur	Base of patella and to tibial tuberosity via patellar ligament	Femoral nerve	Extends leg at knee joint	Lateral circumflex femoral and profunda femoris arteries	Anterior thigh
Vastus medialis (quadriceps)	Intertrochanteric line, medial lip of linea aspera of femur	Base of patella and to tibial tuberosity via patellar ligament	Femoral nerve	Extends leg at knee joint	Femoral and profunda femoris arteries	Anterior thigh

References

Plates 8, 36-38, 43-45

Lang J. Clinical Anatomy of the Nose, Nasal Cavity, and Paranasal Sinuses. Thieme Medical Publishers, New York, 1989.

Plates 19-21

Baccetti T, Franchi L, McNamara J Jr. The cervical vertebral maturation (CVM) method for the assessment of optimal treatment timing in dentofacial orthopedics. Semin Orthod 2005;11:119-29.

Roman PS. Skeletal maturation determined by cervical vertebrae development. Eur J Orthod 2002;24:303-11.

Plate 23

Tubbs RS, Kelly DR, Humphrey ER, et al. The tectorial membrane: anatomical, biomechanical, and histological analysis. Clin Anat 2007;20:382-6.

Plates 25, 27-29, 48, 49, 58, 67, 70

Noden DM, Francis-West P. The differentiation and morphogenesis of craniofacial muscles. Dev Dyn 2006;235: 1194-218.

Plates 32, 34, 126-132

Tubbs RS, Salter EG, Oakes WJ. Anatomic landmarks for nerves of the neck: a vade mecum for neurosurgeons. Neurosurgery 2005;56:256-60.

Plate 48

Benninger B, Lee BI. Clinical importance of morphology and nomenclature of distal attachment of temporalis tendon. J Maxillofac Surg 2012;70:557-61.

Plates 50, 58

Benninger B, Kloenne J, Horn JL. Clinical anatomy of the lingual nerve and identification with ultrasonography. Br J Oral Maxillofac Surg 2013;51:541-4.

Plates 57, 62

Benninger B, Andrew K, Carter B. Clinical measurements of hard palate and implications for subepithelial connective tissue grafts with suggestions for palatal nomenclature. J Oral Maxillofac Surg 2012;70:149-53.

Plates 65, 95, 96

Kierner AC, Mayer R, v Kirschlhofer K. Do the tensor tympani and tensor veli palatini muscles of man form a functional unit? A histochemical investigation of their putative connections. Hear Res 2002;165:48-52.

Plates 74, 75

Benninger B, Barrett R. A head and neck lymph node classification using an anatomical grid system while maintaining clinical relevance. J Oral Maxillofac Surg 2011;69: 2670-3.

Plates 80-82

Ludlow CL. Central nervous system control of the laryngeal muscles in humans. Respir Physiol Neurobiol 2005;147: 205-22.

Plates 102-116

Rhoton AL. Cranial Anatomy and Surgical Approaches. Congress of Neurological Surgeons, Schaumburg, IL, 2003.

Plates 105, 141

Tubbs RS, Hansasuta A, Loukas M, et al. Branches of the petrous and cavernous segments of the internal carotid artery. Clin Anat 2007;20:596-601.

Plates 117-119, 125

Schrott-Fischer A, Kammen-Jolly K, Scholtz AW, et al. Patterns of GABA-like immunoreactivity in efferent fibers of the human cochlea. Hear Res 2002;174:75-85.

Plates 160, 175

Tubbs RS, Loukas M, Slappy JB, et al. Clinical anatomy of the C1 dorsal root, ganglion, and ramus: a review and anatomical study. Clin Anat 2007;20:624-7.

Plate 162

Lee MWL, McPhee RW, Stringer MD. An evidence-based approach to human dermatomes. Clin Anat 2008;21: 363-73.

Plates 162, 399, 469, 513

Forester O. The dermatomes in man. Brain 1933; 56:1-39.

Garrett FD. The segmental distribution of the cutaneous nerves in the limbs of man. Anat Rec 1948;102:409-37.

Keegan JJ. Dermatome hypalgesia with posterolateral herniation of lower cervical intervertebral disc. J Neurosurg 1947;4:115-39.

Plate 168

Turnball IM. Bloody supply of the spinal cord. In Vinken PJ, Bruyn GW (eds). Handbook of Clinical Neurology, XII. Amsterdam, 1972, pp 478-91.

Plate 169

Stringer MD, Restieaux M, Fisher AL, Crosado B. The vertebral venous plexuses: the internal veins are muscular and external veins have valves. Clin Anat 2012;25:609-18.

Plates 174, 175

Tubbs RS, Mortazavi MM, Loukas M, et al. Anatomical study of the third occipital nerve and its potential role in occipital headache/neck pain following midline dissections of the craniocervical junction. J Neurosurg Spine 2011; 15:71-5.

Plates 179-181

Hassiotou F, Geddes D. Anatomy of the human mammary gland: current status of knowledge. Clin Anat 2013;26: 29-48.

Plates 197, 198

Jackson CL, Huber JF. Correlated applied anatomy of the bronchial tree and lungs with a system of nomenclature. Dis Chest 1943;9:319-26.

Plate 200
Ikeda S, Ono Y, Miyazawa S, et al. Flexible bronchofiberscope. Otolaryngology (Tokyo) 1970;42:855.

Plate 215
Angelini, P, Velasco JA, Flamm S. Coronary anomalies: incidence, pathophysiology, and clinical relevance. Circulation 2002;105:2449-54.

Plates 215, 216
Chiu IS, Anderson RH. Can we better understand the known variations in coronary arterial anatomy? Ann Thorac Surg 2012;94:1751-60.

Plate 222
James TN. The internodal pathways of the human heart. Prog Cardiovasc Dis 2001;43:495-535.

Plates 222-224
Hildreth V, Anderson RH, Henderson DJ. Autonomic innervation of the developing heart: origins and function. Clin Anat 2009;22:36-46.

Plate 236
Ang HJ, Gill YC, Lee WJ, et al. Anatomy of thoracic splanchnic nerves for surgical resection. Clin Anat 2008;21:171-7.

Plate 279
Elias H. Morphology of the Liver. New York, Academic Press, 1969.

MacSween RNM, Anthony PP, Scheuer PJ, et al (eds). Pathology of the Liver. London, Churchill Livingstone, 2002.

Robinson PJ. MRI of the Liver: A Practical Guide. New York, Taylor & Francis, 2006.

Plates 283, 284
Odze RD. Surgical Pathology of the GI Tract, Liver, Biliary Tract, and Pancreas. Philadelphia, Saunders, 2004.

Plate 305
Thomas MD. In The Ciba Collection of Medical Illustrations, vol 3, part II. Summit, NJ, CIBA, p 78.

Plates 321, 344, 362, 374, 392
Stormont TJ, Cahill DR, King BF, Myers RP. Fascias of the male external genitalia and perineum. Clin Anat 1994;7: 115-24.

Plates 335, 340, 346, 350, 355, 356
Oelrich TM. The striated urogenital sphincter muscle in the female. Anat Rec 1983;205:223-32.

Plates 339, 344
Myers RP, Goellner JR, Cahill DR. Prostate shape, external striated urethral sphincter, and radical prostatectomy: the apical dissection. J Urol 1987;138:543-50.

Plates 339, 344, 361, 362
Oelrich TM. The urethral sphincter muscle in the male. Am J Anat 1980;158:229-46.

Plate 381
Flocks RH, Kerr HD, Elkins HB, et al. Treatment of carcinoma of the prostate by interstitial radiation with radio-active gold (Au 198): A preliminary report. J Urol 1952;68:510-22.

Plate 399
Keegan JJ, Garrett FD. The segmental distribution of the cutaneous nerves in the limbs of man. Anat Rec 1948;102:409.

Plate 469
Keegan JJ. Neurological interpretation of dermatome hypalgesia with herniation of the lumbar intervertebral disc. J Bone Joint Surg Am 1944;26:238-48.

Last RJ. Innervation of the limbs. J Bone Joint Surg Br 1949;31:452.

Index

References are to plate numbers. In most cases, structures are listed under singular nouns

A

Abdomen
autonomic nerves and ganglia of, 297
axial CT images of, 322–323
bony framework of, 243
left lower quadrant, 244
left upper quadrant, 244
regions and planes of, 244
right lower quadrant, 244
right upper quadrant, 244
Scarpa's layer of, 245
subcutaneous tissue of, 245
surface anatomy of, 242
ureters in, 313
Abdominal aorta, 176, 192, 229, 259, 264, 267–268, 271, 283–284, 303, 308, 310, 314–315, 320–321, 341–342, 345, 376, 378–381, 390
arteriogram of, 285
axial CT images of, 323
transverse section of, 326–328
Abdominal ostium, 352
Abdominal viscera, 263
Abdominal wall
anterior
arteries of, 251
deep dissection of, 247
intermediate dissection of, 246
internal view of, 249
nerves of, 253
superficial dissection of, 245
veins of, 252
paramedian section of, 321
posterior
arteries of, 259
internal view of, 258
lymph vessels and nodes of, 261
nerves of, 262
peritoneum of, 268
veins of, 260
posterolateral, 250
Abdominis muscle
rectus, 242, 246, 249
transversus, 7, 172–173, 176, 247, 249, 483, 485
tendon of origin of, 172–173, 176
Abducent nerve (VI), 13, 55, 85–86, 88, 105, 115, 118, 122
distribution of, 119
lateral rectus muscle and, 122
schema of, 122
Abducent nucleus, 117–118, 122
Abductor digiti minimi muscle, 449, 452, 457, 464, 467, 516, 518, 520–523, 528, 531
nerve to, 521
Abductor digiti minimi tendon, 515
Abductor hallucis muscle, 516, 518, 520–523, 528, 531
Abductor hallucis tendon, 515, 520–521
Abductor pollicis brevis muscle, 427, 430, 449, 452–453, 463, 467
Abductor pollicis longus muscle, 427, 430–431, 436–438, 466–467
radial area for, 425
Abductor pollicis longus tendon, 430, 434, 436, 454, 456–457
Aberrant ductule, 368
Accessory hemi-azygos vein, 189, 204, 228, 234, 240
Accessory nerve (XI), 32–34, 42, 55, 71, 74–75, 105, 115, 117–118, 128, 130, 174
cranial root of, 128
distribution of, 119
inferior, 13
in jugular fossa, 12
schema of, 128
spinal roots of, 13, 128
in foramen magnum, 12
Accessory nucleus, 117–118
oculomotor, 117–118, 122, 133
Accessory process, 155
Acetabular fossa, 396, 474, 530
Acetabular labrum, 334, 474, 491, 530
Acetabular ligament, transverse, 334, 474
Acetabular margin, 333–334, 338
Acetabular notch, 334, 473
Acetabulum, 334, 473
lunate surface of, 396, 473–474
margin of, 473
radiograph of, 331, 475
Achilles tendon, 468, 502–506, 514, 516
Acinus, 201
Acoustic meatus
external, 6, 10, 15, 94–95, 98
internal, 8, 13, 94, 124–125
Acoustic opening, internal, 99
Acromial anastomosis, 414
Acromial angle, 405–406
Acromial plexus, 414
Acromioclavicular joint, 408, 411
Acromioclavicular joint capsule, 408
Acromioclavicular joint space, 407
Acromion, 29, 185, 398, 408–409, 411, 413–415, 417, 467
of scapula, 183, 405–407
Adamkiewicz, artery of, 167
Adductor brevis muscle, 477–478, 480, 488, 492, 526, 531
Adductor canal, 487, 492
Adductor hallucis muscle, 522–523, 528, 531
Adductor hallucis tendon, 515
Adductor hiatus, 488–489, 499, 509, 526
Adductor longus muscle, 396, 477–480, 487–488, 492, 526, 531
Adductor magnus muscle, 468, 477–478, 480, 482, 487–489, 492, 499, 509, 526–527, 531
adductor minimus part of, 480, 482, 489
Adductor magnus tendon, 492–493, 498, 504
Adductor pollicis muscle, 447, 449–450, 453, 464, 467
fascia of, 450
Adductor tubercle, 476, 488, 496
Adenohypophysis, 141, 148–149
Adenoid, 36
Aditus (laryngeal inlet), 64, 66, 69
Adnexa, 352
Afferent fibers, 117–118, 122–126, 128–130, 133
of autonomic reflex pathways, 304
of kidneys and upper ureters, 318
of liver and biliary tract, 306
from olfactory bulb, 120
of pancreas, 307
of reproductive organs, 393–394
of tracheobronchial tree, 207
of urinary bladder and lower ureter, 395
Agger nasi, 36–37
Aggregate lymphoid nodules (Peyer's patches), 272, 275
Airway, intrapulmonary
schema of, 201
structure of, 201
subdivisions of, 201
Ala, 10, 157
of ilium, 243, 330, 334, 338, 473
of nose, 1
of sacrum, radiograph of, 331
Alar cartilage
major, 37–38, 42
lateral crus, 35
medial crus, 35, 38
minor, 35
Alar fascia, 26
Alar fibrofatty tissue, 35, 37
Alar folds, 494
Alar ligaments, 23
posterior, 23
Alcock's, pudendal canal, 291, 370, 376, 380, 382–383, 389, 391
Alveolar artery
inferior, 40, 47, 51, 58, 73
lingual branch of, 72
mental branch of, 51, 72
mylohyoid branch of, 18, 72
superior
anterior, 51, 54
dental branches of, 54
middle, 51, 54
posterior, 51, 54, 72
Alveolar ducts, 201
opening of, 201
Alveolar foramen, 6
Alveolar nerve (V_2)
inferior, 18, 47, 49–51, 58, 61, 71, 123, 132, 135
superior, 61
anterior, 52, 71
dental branches of, 54
gingival branches of, 54
middle, 52, 54, 71
nasal branch of, 18
posterior, 52–54, 71
Alveolar periosteum, 63
Alveolar pores (of Kohn), 201
Alveolar process, 4, 6, 8, 16, 37
of maxilla, 43
Alveolar recess, 43
Alveolar sacs, 201
Alveolar vein
inferior, 47, 73
posterior superior, 73
Alveolar wall
capillary bed within, 202
capillary plexuses within, 202
Alveoli, 201
Alveus, of hippocampus, 113
Amacrine cells, 121
Ampulla
of ductus deferens, 362
of ear, 94, 98
anterior, 97
lateral, 97
posterior, 97
of fallopian tube, 352–353
of rectum, 346
of semicircular ducts
lateral, 125
posterior, 125
superior, 125
Amygdaloid body, 111, 113, 120, 136

Anal canal, 371
arteries of, male, 376
longitudinal muscle of, 338–339
muscularis mucosae of, 371–372
veins of, female, 377
Anal columns, 371
Anal crypt, 371
Anal glands, 371
Anal (rectal) nerves
branch of, 357
inferior, 388–389, 391–392, 484, 490
Anal pit, 366
Anal sinus, 371
Anal sphincter muscle
external, 276, 303, 321, 335, 340, 346, 355–356, 359–360, 370, 376, 382, 397
attachment of, 337
deep, 344, 369, 371–374
perineal views of, 373
subcutaneous, 344, 369, 371–374
superficial, 344, 369, 371–374
internal, 370–372
Anal triangle, 358
Anal tubercle, 366
Anal valve, 371
Anal verge, 371
Anastomosis
in arteries to brain, 139
internal to external carotid artery, 138
paravertebral, 168
prevertebral, 168
Anastomotic loops, 287, 290
to anterior spinal artery, 167
of ileal arteries, 272
of jejunal arteries, 272
to posterior spinal artery, 167
Anastomotic vein
inferior (of Labbé), 103, 146
superior (of Trolard), 103
Anatomical snuffbox, 398, 430, 454, 456–457
Anconeus muscle, 406, 418, 430–431, 436, 438, 465–467
nerve to, 418
Angle of mandible, 1, 15, 17, 66
Angular artery, 3, 35, 51, 72, 87, 139
Angular gyrus, 106
branch to, 142–143
Angular notch, 269
Angular vein, 3, 73, 87
Ankle
dorsiflexion of, 469
ligaments of, 514
medial ligament of, 501
plantarflexion of, 469
radiographs of, 531
tendon sheaths of, 516
tendons of, 514
Anococcygeal body (ligament), 337, 355–356, 360, 373–374
Anococcygeal nerve, 389, 391, 484, 486
Anocutaneous line, 370–372
Anoderm, 371
Anorectal hiatus, 338
Anorectal junction
circular muscle layer of, 339
conjoined longitudinal muscle of, 339
Anorectal line, 371
Anorectal musculature, 372
Ansa cervicalis, 31, 129–130
inferior root of, 32, 34, 71, 76, 129–130
superior root of, 32, 34, 71, 76, 129–130
Ansa of Galen, 82
Ansa pectoralis, 415
Ansa subclavia, 131, 206, 223–224, 236
Anserine bursa, 493–494
Antebrachial cutaneous nerves
lateral, 400–401
branches of, 401
medial, 400
branches of, 401
posterior, 400–401
Antebrachial fascia, 436
deep, 441
Antebrachial vein, median, 401–402, 436
Anterior chamber of eye, 83, 89–92
endothelium of, 90
Anterolateral central (lenticulostriate) arteries, 138, 140–142, 144
Anteromedial central (perforating) arteries, 141
Antihelix, 1, 95
crura of, 95
Antitragus, 1, 95
Anular ligament of radius, 424
Anular (intercartilaginous) ligaments, 199
Anulus fibrosus, 21, 155, 159
collagen lamellae of, 159
Anus, 337, 340, 354, 358, 360, 366, 373
Aorta, 26, 204, 216–217, 226, 258, 306, 309, 320
abdominal, 176, 192, 229, 259, 264, 267–268, 271, 283–284, 303, 308, 310, 314–315, 320–321, 341–342, 345, 376, 378–381, 390
arteriogram of, 285
axial CT images of, 323
transverse section of, 326–328
ascending, 139, 212, 214, 217, 220–222, 237, 240
coronal section of, 214
axial CT images of, 322
thoracic (descending), 139, 168, 188, 191, 213, 228–229, 233, 237, 240–241
lung groove for, 196
transverse section of, 324–325
ureteric branch from, 314
Aortic arch, 76–77, 139, 193, 203, 207–212, 218, 222, 228–230, 233, 239
lung groove for, 196
Aortic arch lymph node of ligamentum arteriosum, 205
Aortic heart valve, 210, 214, 218–222
left semilunar cusp of, 218–222
posterior semilunar cusp of, 218–222
right semilunar cusp of, 218–222
Aortic hiatus, 192
Aortic lymph nodes, lateral, 261, 316, 384
Aortic plexus, 300
Aortic sinus, 210, 220
Aorticorenal ganglion, 163, 262, 297, 299–303, 317–319, 387, 392–393, 395
left, 388, 394
Apical collecting vessels, 75
Apical foramina, 63
Apical ligament, of dens, 23, 64–65
Appendicular artery, 273, 287–288, 301–302
Appendicular lymph nodes, 296
Appendicular plexus, 301–302
Appendicular vein, 291–292
Appendix, 127, 275
of epididymis, 365, 367
fibrous, of liver, 277
omental (epiploic), 265
of testis, 365, 367
vermiform, 265, 273–276
orifice of, 274
vesicular, 352, 367
Arachnoid, 101, 103, 110
dura mater interface with, 103
superior cerebral veins penetrating, 103
Arachnoid granulations, 101–103, 110
granular foveolae for, 9
Arachnoid mater, 165–166
Arcuate arteries, 312, 517–518, 523
lymph vessels along, 316
Arcuate eminence, 11, 94
Arcuate ligament
dorsal radial metaphyseal, 442
lateral, 192, 258
medial, 192, 258
median, 192, 258
Arcuate line, 243, 247, 249, 251, 255, 330, 334–335, 338, 473
of ilium, 336
Arcuate (infundibular) nucleus, 148
Arcus tendineus fasciae pelvis, 351
Areola, 179
Areolar glands (of Montgomery), 179
Areolar tissue, 245, 344
loose, 103
Areolar venous plexus, 252
Arm
arteries of, 420
cutaneous nerves of, 401
muscles of
anterior view of, 417
posterior view of, 418
radial nerve in, 465
serial cross sections of, 421
superficial veins of, 401
Arrector pili muscles, innervation to, 163
Arteriae rectae, 288, 305
Arterial arch, deep plantar, 522
Arterial circle of iris
major, 90, 92–93
minor, 90, 92–93
Arterial rete, marginal, 96
Arteries. *See also specific arteries*
of abdominal wall
anterior, 251
posterior, 259
of anal canal, male, 376
of arm, 420
of brain, 137
frontal section of, 142
frontal view of, 142
inferior view of, 140
lateral view, 143
medial view, 143
schema of, 139
of duodenum, 284, 286
of esophagus, 233
of eye, intrinsic, 92
of face, 3
of femoral head and neck, 491
of foot, 509
deep, 523
of forearm, 435
of hand, 453
of head of pancreas, 286
of hypothalamus and hypophysis, 149
intrarenal, 312
of iris, 93
of knee, 499, 509
of large intestine, 288
of leg, 509
of liver, 283–284
of mallear stria, 96
of mammary gland, 180
to meninges, 137
of nasal cavity, 40
of oral and pharyngeal regions, 72
of orbit and eyelids, 87
of pancreas, 284
of pelvic organs, female, 378
of pelvis
female, 380
male, 381

Arteries *(Continued)*
of perineum, 382
male, 383
of posterior cranial fossa, 144
of proximal forearm, 420
of rectum, male, 376
of scalp, 3
of small intestine, 287
of spinal cord
intrinsic distribution of, 168
schema of, 167
of spleen, 283–284
of stomach, 283
of suprarenal glands, 320
of testis, 379
of thigh, 499
anterior view, 487–488
posterior view, 489
of upper limb, 460
of ureters, 314
of urinary bladder, 314
of uterus, 382
of wrist, 449
Arteriole
macular
inferior, 92
superior, 92
nasal retinal
inferior, 92
superior, 92
temporal retinal
inferior, 92
superior, 92
Artery of Adamkiewicz, 167
Articular cartilage, 424, 458, 467, 474, 498, 530
Articular cavities, 184, 458, 498
of sternoclavicular joint, 404
Articular disc, 184
inferior, 18
of sternoclavicular joint, 404
of temporomandibular joint, 48–49
of wrist joint, 439, 442
Articular facet
cervical
anterior, 19
inferior, 20
superior, 19–20
of dens, posterior, 23
for sacrum, 155, 157
thoracic
inferior, 154
superior, 154
for vertebral body
inferior, 184
superior, 184
transverse process of, 184
Articular nerve, recurrent, 529
Articular process
cervical
inferior, 20–21
superior, 20–21
lumbar
inferior, 155–156, 158–159
superior, 155, 158–159
sacral, superior, 157
thoracic
inferior, 154
superior, 154
Articular tubercle, 6, 10, 49
inferior, 18
Articularis genus muscle, 477, 492, 494, 498, 525, 531
Ary-epiglottic fold, 66–67, 80
Arytenoid cartilage, 79
muscular process of, 79–80
vocal process of, 79–80
Arytenoid muscle
oblique, 67, 69, 80, 82, 151
action of, 81
ary-epiglottic part of, 80, 82
transverse, 64, 67, 69, 80, 82, 151
action of, 81
Ascending aorta, 139, 212, 214, 217, 220–222, 237, 240
coronal section of, 214
Ascending connections, 224
Asterion, 6
Atlanto-axial joint
lateral, 22
capsule of, 22–23
median, 23
Atlanto-axial ligament, 23
Atlanto-occipital joint, capsule of, 22–23
Atlanto-occipital ligament, anterior, 23
Atlanto-occipital membrane
anterior, 22, 64–65
posterior, 22
Atlas (C1), 15, 22–23, 160
anterior view of, 21, 153
arch of
anterior, 7, 19, 21, 64
posterior, 19, 151, 175
articular facet for
anterior, 19
superior, 19
dens of, articular facet for, 19
groove for vertebral artery, 19
inferior view of, 19
lateral mass of, 19
lateral view of, 153
posterior view of, 153
spinal nerves relation to, 161
superior articular surface of lateral mass for occipital condyle, 19
superior view of, 19
transverse foramen of, 19
transverse ligament of, 23
transverse process of, 19, 22, 30, 173
tubercle of
anterior, 19, 21, 23
posterior, 19, 172–173
vertebral foramen of, 19
Atrioventricular (AV) bundle (of His), 222
Atrioventricular (AV) node, 222
Atrium, 221
left, 211–213, 218, 220–221, 241
oblique vein of (of Marshall), 211–212, 215, 218
right, 209–214, 217, 220–221, 227, 241
Auditory (pharyngotympanic, eustachian) tube. *See* Pharyngotympanic (auditory, eustachian) tube
Auerbach's plexus, 305
Auricle, 94, 99
concha of, 95
lobule of, 95
Auricle (atrial appendage)
left, 209, 211–212, 215–216, 218, 221–222
right, 209, 211, 217, 221
Auricular artery
anterior, 3
deep, 51, 72, 96
posterior, 3, 34, 51, 72, 96, 102, 137, 139, 175
Auricular cartilage, 42
Auricular muscles, nerve branches to, 124
Auricular nerve
anterior, 123
branches to muscles, 124
Auricular nerve *(Continued)*
great, 2, 31–33, 130, 174–175
posterior, 24, 50, 124
occipital branch of, 124
Auricular surface, 473
of sacrum, 157–158
Auricular tubercle (of Darwin), 95
Auricular vein, posterior, 3, 32, 73
Auricularis muscle
anterior, 25, 151
innervation of, 119
posterior, 25, 151
superior, 25, 151
Auriculotemporal nerve, 2, 18, 46, 49–51, 71–72, 123, 126, 135
Auscultation
of heart, 210
precordial areas of, 210
Auscultatory triangle, 152, 241, 250
Autonomic nerves
of abdomen, 297
of biliary tract, 306
of duodenum, 298–300
in head, 132
of kidneys, 317–318
of large intestine, 302–303
of liver, 306
of lower limb, 469
in neck, 131
of pancreas, 307
of small intestine, 301, 303
of stomach, 298–300
of suprarenal glands, 319
in thorax, 206
of ureters, 317–318
of urinary bladder, 317
Autonomic reflex pathways, 304
Axilla, 178
anterior view, 415
posterior wall of, 410
suspensory ligament of, 412
Axillary artery, 180, 186, 195, 214, 251, 412, 414–415, 419
acromial branch of, 420
clavicular branch of, 420
deltoid branch of, 420
left, 190
right, 190
Axillary fascia, 412
Axillary fold
anterior, 178
posterior, 178
Axillary fossa, 238–240
Axillary lymph node, 412
anterior, 181–182
apical, 181–182
central, 181–182
lateral, 181–182, 403
posterior, 181–182
Axillary nerve, 400, 410–411, 413, 415–416, 418, 461–463, 465–466
branches of, 410
superior lateral brachial cutaneous nerve from, 174, 400–401
Axillary recess, 408, 467
Axillary tail (of Spence), 180
Axillary vein, 186, 195, 214, 252, 403, 412
intercostal tributaries to, 252
Axis (C2), 15, 22–23, 47, 160
anterior view of, 19, 21, 153
body of, 19, 22
dens of, 7, 19, 21, 64
inferior articular facet for, 19
interarticular part of, 19
lateral view of, 153
pedicle of, 19

Axis (C2) *(Continued)*
  posterior view of, 153
  posterosuperior view of, 19
  spinal nerves relation to, 161
  spinous process of, 171, 173
  transverse process of, 19
    posterior tubercle, 30
Azygos vein, 189, 191, 203–204, 206, 213, 227, 229, 234, 237, 239–241
  lung groove for, 196
  transverse section of, 324

B

Back
  lumbar region of, 176
  muscles of
    deep layers, 173
    intermediate layers, 172
    superficial layers, 171
  nerves of, 174
  surface anatomy of, 152
Bartholin's gland
  greater, 356–357, 367, 382
    primordium of, 367
  opening of, 354
Basal collecting vessels, 75
Basal nuclei, 111
Basal vein (of Rosenthal), 145–147
Basilar artery, 137, 139–142, 144, 167
  imaging of, 150–151
Basilar membrane, 98
Basilic vein, 398, 401–403, 415, 421, 436, 455
  median, 402
Basivertebral vein, 169
Batson, vertebral venous plexus of, 104, 166, 169
Bertin, renal column of, 311
Biceps brachii muscle, 178, 239–240, 398, 405, 409–410, 412–413, 415, 417, 419, 421, 432–434, 437–438, 460, 462, 467
Biceps brachii tendon, 238–239, 408, 411, 413, 417, 424
Biceps femoris muscle, 468, 477–478, 481–482, 489–490, 492–493, 497, 502–503, 506, 527, 531
Biceps femoris tendon, 333, 493–494, 497–498, 501, 504–505, 507–508, 529
Bicipital aponeurosis, 402, 417, 419, 432, 460
Bifid spinous process, 20
Bifurcate ligament, 514
Bile canaliculi, 279
Bile ducts, 127, 267–268, 271–272, 277–279, 281, 283–284, 286
  extrahepatic, 280
  innervation of, 163–164
  sphincter of, 280
  transverse section of, 325–326
Biliary tract, autonomic nerves of, 306
Bipolar cells, 121
Biventer lobule, 114
Bladder. *See* Urinary bladder
Bladder-prostate junction, 396
Blood vessels. *See* Vessels
Bloodless fold of Treves, 273
Bohler's angle, 513
Bones
  of elbow, 422
  of foot, 511–512
  of forearm, 425
  of hand, 443
  of nasal cavity, 45
  of paranasal sinuses, 45
  of pelvis, 333–334
  around teeth, 63
  of thorax, 183
  of wrist, 439, 443
Bony labyrinths, 97–98
  orientation of, 99
Bony spicule, 20
Brachial artery, 180, 414–415, 417, 419–421, 432–435, 460
  branches of, 431
  middle collateral branch of, 431
  muscular branch of, 419
  in situ, 419
Brachial cutaneous nerves
  inferior lateral, 400–401
  medial, 253, 400–401
  posterior, 400–401
  superior lateral, 174, 400–401
Brachial fascia, 412, 421
Brachial plexus, 1, 29–32, 71, 160, 180, 186, 190, 195, 203, 208, 225, 227–229, 412–413, 415
  anterior divisions of, 416
  communication to, 130
  cords of, 461–463
    lateral, 416, 419, 461–463
    medial, 416, 419, 461–463
    posterior, 416, 461–463
  inferior trunks of, 71, 410, 416
  lateral cord of, 214
  middle trunks of, 71, 410, 416
  posterior divisions of, 416
  roots of, 416
  schema of, 416
  superior trunks of, 71, 410, 416
  terminal branches of, 416
Brachial veins, 415, 421
Brachialis muscle, 405–406, 415, 417, 419, 421, 432–434, 437, 460, 462, 465, 467
  insertion of, 424
Brachiocephalic trunk, 33, 76–78, 137, 139, 187, 190, 203, 208–211, 214, 229, 233, 238
Brachiocephalic vein, 73, 76, 187, 205
  left, 77, 170, 189, 203, 208–209, 214, 227–229, 234, 238
  lung groove for, 196
  right, 77, 170, 189, 203, 208–209, 227, 234, 238
Brachioradialis muscle, 398, 405, 417–419, 421, 430–433, 436–438, 460, 465
Brachioradialis tendon, 434, 436
Brachium
  of inferior colliculus, 112
  of superior colliculus, 112
Brain, 43
  arteries of, 137
    frontal section of, 142
    frontal view of, 142
    inferior view of, 140
    lateral view, 143
    medial view, 143
    schema of, 139
  veins of
    deep, 146
    subependymal, 147
  ventricles of, 109
Brainstem
  cranial nerve nuclei in, 117–118
  median sagittal section of, 116
  posterior view of, 116
Breast
  lymphatic drainage of, 182
  pathway to/from opposite, 181
  suspensory ligament of, 179
Bregma, 9
Bridging veins, 101, 103–104, 110
  imaging of, 150
Broad ligament, 313, 340–342, 350, 367
  anterior lamina of, 353
  mesometrium of, 352
Broad ligament *(Continued)*
  mesosalpinx of, 342, 352
  mesovarium of, 352
  posterior lamina of, 353
Bronchi, 201
  cartilages of, 201
  extrapulmonary, 199
  inferior lobar, 199–200
    anterior basal, 200
    anteromedial basal, 200
    lateral basal, 200
    medial basal, 200
    posterior basal, 200
  innervation of, 119, 163–164
  intermediate, 196
  intrapulmonary, 199
  large intrasegmental, 201
  lingular, 199–200
    inferior, 200
    superior, 200
  main
    left, 196, 199–200, 203–204, 213, 228–231, 237, 240
    right, 199–200, 204, 213, 227, 229, 237, 240
  major, 199
  middle lobar, 199–200
    lateral, 200
    medial, 200
  nomenclature of, schema of, 200
  right, 210
  segmental, 201
  small intrasegmental, 201
  superior, 200
  superior division, 199–200
    anterior, 200
    apicoposterior, 200
  superior lobar (eparterial), 199–200
    anterior, 200
    apical, 200
    posterior, 200
    right, 196, 203
Bronchial artery, 202, 204
  esophageal branch of, 204, 233
  left, 196, 228
    inferior, 204, 233
    superior, 204, 233
  right, 196, 204, 227, 233
Bronchial veins, 204
  left, 204
  right, 204
Bronchioles, 201
  respiratory, 201–202
  terminal, 201–202
    elastic fibers of, 201
    smooth muscle of, 201
Bronchomediastinal lymphatic trunk, 205
Bronchopulmonary (hilar) lymph nodes, 196, 205, 227–228
Bronchopulmonary segments, 197–198
  anterior, 197–198
  anterior basal, 197–198
  anteromedial basal, 197–198
  apical, 197–198
  apicoposterior, 197–198
  inferior lingular, 197–198
  lateral, 197–198
  lateral basal, 197–198
  medial, 197–198
  medial basal, 197–198
  posterior, 197–198
  posterior basal, 197–198
  superior, 197–198
  superior lingular, 197–198
Buccal artery, 51, 72
Buccal nerve (V_3), 2, 50–51, 61, 71, 123
Buccinator crest, of mandible, 70
Buccinator lymph nodes, 74

Buccinator muscle, 25, 43, 46–50, 57, 65, 70, 72, 124, 151
Buccopharyngeal fascia, 26, 47, 64–65
Bulb
of penis, 360–361, 363
artery of, 361, 383
of vestibule, 350, 356–357, 382
artery of, 350, 357, 382
Bulb of vestibule, 348
Bulbar conjunctiva, 83, 85, 89–90, 92
Bulbospongiosus muscle, 321, 344, 348, 350, 355–357, 359, 361, 373–374, 382–383, 395, 397
Bulbo-urethral duct, opening of, 362–363
Bulbo-urethral (Cowper's) gland, 249, 321, 344, 348, 361–363, 367
duct of, 361
primordium of, 367
Bulging septum, 36
Bundle
left, 222
right, 222
Bundle of His, 222
Burns, suprasternal space of, 26–27, 64
Buttock, nerves of, 490

C

Calcaneal artery
lateral, 521–522
medial, 521–522
Calcaneal bursa, subcutaneous, 516
Calcaneal nerve
lateral, 521–522
medial, 521–522
Calcaneal sulcus, 513
Calcaneal (Achilles) tendon, 468, 502–506, 514, 516
Calcaneal tuberosity, 468, 503–504
Calcaneocuboid ligament, 514, 523
dorsal, 514
Calcaneofibular ligament, 501, 513–514
Calcaneonavicular ligament, 514
Calcaneus bone, 511–513, 515–516, 531
tuberosity of, 515, 519–522, 531
Calcar avis, 112–113
Calcarine sulcus, 106–108, 112, 121
Callosomarginal artery, 142–143
Calot's triangle, 280, 284
Calvaria, 103
inferior view of, 9
superior view of, 9
Calyces
major, 311
transverse section of, 327
minor, 311
Camper chiasm, 448
Camper's (fatty) layer, 245, 321, 344, 355, 358
Canal of Schlemm, 89–90, 92–93
Canine teeth, 62–63
Capillary plexus, of infundibular process, 149
Capitate, 439, 442–443, 449
radiographs of, 444
Capitohamate ligament, 441–442
Capitulum, 405, 422–423
Capsular ligaments, 408
Cardiac impression, 196
Cardiac nerves
cervical, 206, 225, 236
inferior, 223–224
middle, 223–224
superior, 223
thoracic, 190, 206, 225, 236
Cardiac notch, 232, 269
of left lung, 195
Cardiac orifice, 270
Cardiac plexus, 127, 206, 223–224, 236
branches to, 206
Cardiac veins, 215
anterior, 215
great, 215
middle, 211, 215
small, 215
Cardinal (transverse cervical or Mackenrodt's) ligament, 342–343, 350–351
Carinal lymph nodes, inferior, 205
Caroticotympanic artery, 96, 138
Caroticotympanic nerve, 96, 124, 126
Carotid artery, 34
common, 3, 26, 30–31, 33–34, 55, 71–73, 76–78, 126, 129, 131–132, 134–135, 137, 139, 187, 195, 207, 229, 233
left, 170, 190, 203, 208–211, 214, 238
right, 170, 190, 203, 210
external, 3, 27–28, 31, 34, 46–47, 51, 54–55, 59, 71–73, 76–78, 96, 102, 126, 131–132, 134–135, 137, 139
indirect branch of, 138
internal to, 138
schema of, 34
internal, 3, 13, 34, 42, 47, 49, 53, 55, 71–72, 76–78, 87–88, 96, 100, 102, 124, 126, 129, 131–135, 137, 139–142
caroticotympanic branch of, 139
in carotid canal, 12
cavernous segment of, 105, 138
cerebral part of, 138
cervical part of, 138
to external, 138
imaging of, 150
left, 143–144
meningeal branch of, 138
meningohypophyseal trunk of, 102
nerve plexus and, 122
in petrous part of temporal bone, 138
petrous parts of, 138
right, 143
Carotid autonomic plexus, 12
Carotid body, 34, 126, 131, 137, 207
Carotid canal, 10, 12, 100
greater, 13
Carotid groove, 11
Carotid nerve
external, 163
internal, 53, 55, 131–132, 134, 163, 225
Carotid plexus
common, 131–132
external, 131–132, 134, 163
internal, 13, 53, 88, 96, 124, 132–133, 163
Carotid sheath, 26–27
Carotid sinus, 126, 131–132, 137, 207
Carotid sinus nerve (of Hering), 71, 126, 131
Carotid tubercle (of Chassaignac), 21–22
Carpal arch, dorsal, 456
Carpal artery, dorsal, 435
Carpal bones, 439, 443
Carpal ligament, transverse, 433, 441, 447, 449
Carpometacarpal joint, 439, 442
Carpometacarpal ligaments, palmar, 445
Cartilage
of pharyngotympanic (auditory, eustachian) tube, 42
of larynx, 79
thyroid, 1
Cartilage end plate, 159
Cauda equina, 160–161, 166, 176
transverse section of, 327
Caudal mesonephric tubules, 367
residua of, 367
Caudate nucleus, 111, 142
anterior vein of, 146–147
body of, 109, 111
head of, 111–113, 144, 146
imaging of, 151
posterior vein of, 146
terminal, 147
tail of, 109, 111, 113
transverse veins of, 146–147
Caudate process, 277
Caval opening, 192, 258
Cave of Retzius, 247, 321
Cavernous nerves, of penis, 388, 394
Cavernous plexus, 122
Cavernous sinus, 87, 105, 137, 141
efferent hypophyseal vein to, 149
emissary vein communicating with, 73
inferior, artery to, 138
Cavum septum pellucidum, 101
Cecal artery, 302
anterior, 273, 287–288
posterior, 273, 287–288
Cecal folds, 273, 341, 345
Cecal plexus, 302
Cecal vein
anterior, 291–292
posterior, 291–292
Cecum, 127, 263, 265, 273, 275–276, 341, 345
vascular fold of, 273
Celiac ganglion, 163–164, 236, 262, 297–304, 306–307, 317–319, 387–388, 392–395
Celiac lymph nodes, 235, 261, 293–295
Celiac plexus, 127, 236, 298–299, 301–302, 317–319, 388, 393
Celiac trunk, 192, 226, 229, 233, 259, 264, 268, 271, 281, 283–284, 286–287, 300, 303, 307–308, 310, 321, 388
arteriogram of, 285
axial CT images of, 322
transverse section of, 325–326
Cement of teeth, 63
Central arteries
anterolateral, 138, 140–142, 144
anteromedial, 141
posteromedial, 141
Central canal, of spinal cord, 109–110, 116, 118
Central collecting vessels, 75
Central lobule, 114, 116
Central sulcal arteries, 142–143
Central sulcus
of insula, 100
of Rolando, 106–107
Central tendon, of diaphragm, 191–192
Central vein, 278–279
Cephalic vein, 178, 185–186, 214, 252, 398, 401–403, 409, 412, 415, 421, 436, 455
accessory, 401–402
median, 402
Cerebellar artery
inferior
anterior, 137, 139–142, 144, 167
choroidal branch of, 144
posterior, 137, 139–140, 142, 144, 167
tonsillar branch of, 144
superior, 137, 139–142, 144, 167
lateral branch of, 144
vermian branch of, 144
Cerebellar hemispheric veins, inferior, 145
Cerebellar notch
anterior, 114
posterior, 114
Cerebellar nuclei
dentate, 114
emboliform, 114
fastigial, 114
globose, 114

Cerebellar peduncles
inferior, 114–116, 125, 145
middle, 114–116, 145
superior, 114–116, 145
decussation of, 114
Cerebellar vein
precentral, 145
superior, 145
Cerebellomedullary cistern, vein of, 145
Cerebellum, 99, 107, 112, 114, 147
anterior lobe of, 114
biventer lobule of, 114
central lobule of, 114
dentate nucleus of, 116
flocculonodular lobe of, 114
flocculus of, 114–115
fourth ventricle and, 114, 116
horizontal fissure of, 114
imaging of, 151
medullary velum of
inferior, 114
superior, 114
posterior lobe of, 114
posterolateral (dorsolateral) fissure of, 114
postlunate fissure of, 114
primary fissure of, 114
quadrangular lobule of, 114
retrotonsillar fissure of, 114
secondary (postpyramidal) fissure of, 114
semilunar lobule
inferior, 114
superior, 114
simple lobule of, 114
tonsil of, 114, 116
vermis of, 114
central lobule of, 114, 116
culmen of, 114, 116
declive of, 114, 116
folium of, 114, 116
lingula of, 114, 116
nodule of, 114, 116
pyramid of, 114, 116
tuber of, 114, 116
uvula of, 114, 116
Cerebral aqueduct, 107–110, 116, 118, 147–148
imaging of, 151
Cerebral arterial circle (of Willis), 140–141
Cerebral arteries, 103
anterior, 137–142, 144, 146
branches of, 142
cingular branches of, 143
imaging of, 150–151
left, 143
medial frontal branches of, 142–143
right, 143
terminal branches of, 143
middle, 137–142, 144
imaging of, 150
left, 143
occipitotemporal branches of, 143
temporal branches of, 142–143
terminal branches of, 143
posterior, 137–142, 144, 167
calcarine branch to, 143–144
dorsal branch of, 143–144
imaging of, 150
parieto-occipital branch to, 143–144
right, 143
temporal branches of, 143–144
terminal branches of, 143
Cerebral crus, 108, 114–115, 140, 146
Cerebral fissure, longitudinal, 108, 144, 146
imaging of, 151
Cerebral hemisphere, 103
Cerebral peduncle, 107, 116
Cerebral sulcus, lateral, 142
Cerebral veins, 101
anterior, 145–146
great (of Galen), 104–105, 107, 116, 145–147
imaging of, 150
inferior, 103, 105, 146
internal, 101, 109, 112, 145–147
imaging of, 150
middle
deep, 101, 145–147
superficial, 101, 103, 105, 146
superficial, 103
superior, 103
opening of, 102
Cerebrospinal fluid, circulation of, 110
Cerebrum
frontal lobe of, 106
frontal pole of, 106, 108
inferior margin of, 108
occipital lobe of, 106
occipital pole of, 106
parietal lobe of, 106
temporal lobe of, 106, 142
temporal pole of, 106, 108
Cervical artery
ascending, 33, 71–72, 76–78, 139, 167, 414
deep, 137, 139, 167
superficial, 76–77, 139, 174
transverse, 32–33, 78, 414–415
Cervical canal, 352
Cervical cardiac nerves, 206, 225, 236
inferior, 223–224
middle, 223–224
superior, 223
Cervical fascia, 185
deep
investing layer of, 409
superficial layer of, 64
investing layer of, 25–27
pretracheal layer of, 27
prevertebral layer of, 26
superficial layer of, 26
Cervical ganglion
middle, 71, 129, 223–224, 236
superior, 53, 55, 163, 223–224, 236
Cervical ligament, transverse, 342–343, 350–351
Cervical lordosis, 153
Cervical lymph nodes
anterior deep, 74
anterior superficial, 74
deep inferior, 205, 235
deep lateral, 75
inferior deep lateral, 74
posterior lateral superficial, 74
superior deep lateral, 74
superior lateral superficial, 74
transverse chain, 74
Cervical muscles, deep, 26
Cervical nerve, transverse, 2, 31–32, 130
Cervical (cupula, dome of) parietal pleura, 193–194, 227–228
Cervical plexus, 174–175
ansa cervicalis of, 129
branches from, 2
schema of, 33, 130
Cervical spinal nerves
C1, 128, 160
dorsal ramus of, 175
dorsal roots of, 115
ventral ramus of, 71, 129
vertebrae relation to, 161
C2, 128
dermatome of, 162
dorsal ramus of, 174–175
ventral ramus of, 32, 71, 129, 174
vertebrae relation to, 161
Cervical spinal nerves *(Continued)*
C3, 128
dermatome of, 162
dorsal ramus of, 174–175
ventral ramus of, 32, 129, 174, 190
vertebrae relation to, 161
C4, 128
dermatome of, 162
dorsal ramus of, 174–175
ventral ramus of, 71, 190
vertebrae relation to, 161
C5
dermatome of, 162
dorsal ramus of, 174–175
ventral ramus of, 32, 190
vertebrae relation to, 161
C6
dorsal ramus of, 174–175
transverse process of, 137
vertebrae relation to, 161
C7
dorsal ramus of, 174
vertebrae relation to, 161
C8, 160
dorsal ramus of, 174
vertebrae relation to, 161
dorsal rami of, 2, 22
enlargement of, 161
groove for, 20–21
Cervical sympathetic cardiac nerve
inferior, 131
middle, 131
superior, 131–132
Cervical sympathetic ganglion
middle, 33, 131
superior, 47, 126, 129, 131–134, 207
Cervical sympathetic trunk, 132, 236
Cervical sympathetic trunk ganglion, 225
Cervical triangle, posterior, 26
Cervical vein, deep
left, 170
right, 170
Cervical vertebrae
anterior view of, 21
anulus fibrosus of, 21
arteries of, 167
body of, 20–21, 156
C1 (*See* Atlas (C1))
C2 (*See* Axis (C2))
C3, 15, 19
bifid spinous process of, 20
costal lamella, 20
foramen transversarium of, 20
inferior articular facet for, 19–20
inferior articular process for, 21
inferior aspect of, 20
intervertebral foramen for, 21
lamina of, 20
pedicle of, 20
spinal nerves relation to, 161
transverse process of, 20, 30
vertebral body of, 20
vertebral foramen of, 20
C4, 19
anterior view of, 20
articular surface of, 20
body of, 20
foramen transversarium of, 20
inferior articular facet, 20
inferior articular process of, 20
lamina of, 20
spinal nerve groove, 20
spinal nerves relation to, 161
spinous process of, 20
superior articular facet, 20
superior articular process of, 20–21

Cervical vertebrae *(Continued)*
superior aspect of, 20
transverse process of, 20
uncinate process of, 20
C5, spinal nerves relation to, 161
C6
anterior tubercle of, 22
spinal nerves relation to, 161
C7, 15, 26, 160
anterior view of, 20, 153
articular surface of, 20
body of, 20
bony spicule of, 20
costal lamella of, 20
foramen transversarium of, 20
lamina of, 20
lateral view of, 153
pedicle of, 20
posterior view of, 153
spinal nerves relation to, 161
spinous process of, 20, 22, 152, 171–173, 409
superior articular process and facet of, 20
transverse process of, 20, 30
uncinate process of, 20
vertebral foramen of, 20
intervertebral disc of, 21–22
nucleus pulposus of, 21
transverse process of, 21
uncinate processes of, 21
uncovertebral joints, 21
upper, 19
Cervicofacial division, 24
Cervicothoracic (stellate) ganglion, 131, 206, 223–224, 236
Cervix, 351, 393
of uterus, 340, 342–343, 350, 352
Chassaignac, carotid tubercle of, 21–22
Check ligament, 85
Chest scans, axial CT images, 237
Chiasmatic cistern, 110
Choanae, 10, 16, 36, 38, 49, 57, 66–67, 100
Chorda tympani, 96
Chorda tympani nerve, 12, 50, 61, 71, 95, 123–125, 132, 134–136
Chordae tendineae, 217–218, 220
Choroid, 89, 91–92
Choroid plexus, 112–113, 116
of fourth ventricle, 107, 110, 115–116, 146
of lateral ventricle, 101, 109–111, 140, 144, 146
of third ventricle, 107, 109–110, 144
Choroid vein, superior, 146–147
Choroidal artery
anterior, 138, 140–142, 144
posterior lateral, 144
posterior medial, 140, 144
Choroidal veins, superior, 101
Ciliary arteries
anterior, 92–93
recurrent branch of, 93
posterior, 87
long, 92–93
short, 92–93
Ciliary body, 89–92
blood vessels of, 92
orbiculus ciliaris of, 91
Ciliary ganglion, 52, 55, 88, 122–123, 132–133, 164
nasociliary (sensory) root of, 88, 122–123, 132–133
oculomotor (parasympathetic) root of, 88, 122, 132–133
schema of, 133
sympathetic root of, 88, 122, 132–133
Ciliary muscle, 89–90, 122, 133, 151
circular fibers of, 90
innervation of, 119
meridional fibers of, 90
Ciliary nerves
long, 52, 88, 122–123, 132–133
short, 52, 88, 122–123, 132–133
Ciliary processes, 89–91
Ciliary vein, anterior, 90, 92–93
veins draining into, 93
Cingulate gyrus, 107
isthmus of, 107–108
Cingulate sulcus, 107
Circular esophageal muscle, 65, 67, 69, 231–232
in V-shaped area of Laimer, 69, 77
Circular fibers, 90
Circular folds (valves of Kerckring), 272, 280
Circular intramuscular plexus, 305
Circular muscle, 305
of anorectal junction, 339
of colon, 274
of duodenum, 270, 280
of ileum, 272, 274
of jejunum, 272
of rectum, 371–372
of stomach, 232, 270
of vermiform appendix, 275
Circular sulcus, 106
Circulation, prenatal and postnatal, 226
Cistern
chiasmatic, 110
of corpus callosum, 110
interpeduncular, 110
prepontine, 110
quadrigeminal, 110
Cisterna chyli, 261, 295, 297, 316
Claustrum, 111
Clavicle, 1, 25, 27–29, 31, 178–179, 183–187, 193–195, 210, 214, 227–228, 238, 398, 404–405, 408–412, 414–415
acromial end of, 404
acromial facet of, 404
anteroposterior radiograph of, 407
conoid tubercle, 404
shaft of, 404
sternal end of, 404, 467
sternal facet of, 404
subclavian groove, 404
trapezoid line of, 404
Clavicular head, 27, 29
of sternocleidomastoid muscle, 1
Clavipectoral fasciae, 185, 412
Cleft of Luschka, 21
Clinoid process
anterior, 8, 11
posterior, 11
Clitoris, 356, 373
body of, 340, 366
crus of, 340, 348, 350, 356–357
deep artery of, 357, 382
dorsal artery of, 357, 382
dorsal nerve of, 357, 391–392, 484
dorsal vein of, deep, 335–337, 340, 343, 346, 357
frenulum of, 354
glans of, 354, 366
prepuce of, 354
suspensory ligament of, 355–357
Clivus, 11, 23
Clunial nerves
inferior, 174, 389, 391, 471, 489–490, 527
medial, 471, 489
middle, 174
superior, 174, 250, 471, 489
Coccygeal cornu, 157
Coccygeal ligament, 160
Coccygeal nerve, 160–161, 486
Coccygeal plexus, 484, 486
Coccygeus (ischiococcygeus) muscle, 258, 335–339, 380, 388–390, 397, 486
nerve to, 484, 486
Coccyx, 157–158, 160–161, 243, 330, 333–336, 356, 369
anterior view of, 153
lateral view of, 153
measurements of, 332
posterior view of, 153
radiography of, 156
tip of, 337, 339, 358, 360, 373, 396
transverse process of, 157
Cochlea, 55, 94, 97, 99
helicotrema of, 94, 98
modiolus of, 98
osseous, 98
scala tympani of, 94
scala vestibuli of, 94
section through turn of, 98
Cochlear aqueduct, 98
Cochlear cupula, 97
Cochlear duct, 94, 97–99
Cochlear (spiral) ganglion, 125
Cochlear nerve, 94, 97–99, 119, 125
Cochlear nuclei
anterior, 117–118, 125
posterior, 117–118, 125
Cochlear recess, 97
Colic artery
ascending branch of, 288, 376
descending branch of, 265, 268, 288, 376
left, 259, 288, 297, 302, 313, 376
middle, 281, 284, 287–288, 301–302, 321
right, 287–288, 302, 313
Colic flexure
left (splenic), 263–266, 269, 271, 276, 278, 281, 302, 320
axial CT images of, 322
right (hepatic), 263, 265–266, 269, 271, 276, 278, 281, 315
transverse section of, 325
Colic impression, 277, 282
Colic lymph nodes
left, 296
middle, 296
right, 296
Colic plexus
left, 297, 302
middle, 301–302
right, 302
Colic vein
left, 291–292
middle, 281, 290, 292
right, 290–292
Collagen lamellae, of anulus fibrosus, 159
Collar of Helvetius, 232
Collateral artery
middle, 418, 420–421
radial, 418, 420–421
ulnar
inferior, 419–420, 431, 435
superior, 419–421, 430–431, 435
Collateral eminence, 112
Collateral ligaments, 445, 451, 496
accessory, 445
fibular, 480–481, 493–496, 498, 501, 504–506, 508
of foot, 515
lateral, 497
radial, 424
tibial, 480, 493–498, 501, 504–505, 507–508
ulnar, 424
Collateral sulcus, 107–108
Collateral trigone, 112

Colles' fascia, 344, 348, 350, 355–361, 369, 373–374, 382–383, 389
superficial, 359
Colliculus
facial, 116
inferior, 107, 112, 115–116
brachia of, 115
brachium of, 112
left, 145
seminal, 348
superior, 107–108, 112, 115–117, 133, 144
brachia of, 115
brachium of, 112
left, 145
Colon
ascending, 127, 265, 268, 271, 276, 309, 341, 345
transverse section of, 326–328
circular muscle of, 274
descending, 265, 271, 276, 302, 315, 341, 345
axial CT images of, 322–323
innervation of, 163–164
transverse section of, 325–328
innervation of, 163
radiography of, 156
sigmoid, 263, 265, 276, 302, 341–342, 345, 369–372, 390
innervation of, 163–164
transverse, 263–265, 267, 271, 276, 281–282, 290, 321
axial CT images of, 322–323
transverse section of, 325–328
tributary from, 291
Commissure
anterior, 107, 116, 120, 147–148
of fornix, 113
habenular, 107, 112, 116
of labia majora
anterior, 354
posterior, 354
of lips, 1
posterior, 107, 112, 116, 366
Common bony limbs, 97–98
Common membranous limbs, 97–98
Common tendinous ring (of Zinn), 85–86, 88, 122
Common trunk, 46, 73
Common-extensor tendon, 406
Communicating artery
anterior, 137–143
imaging of, 150
posterior, 105, 137–144
imaging of, 150
Communicating nerve, sural, 471
Communicating vein, 31, 170
Compressor urethrae muscle, 335, 350, 356–357, 382, 397
growth of, 347
Concha
of auricle, 95
inferior, 16
Conducting system, of heart, 222
Condylar canal, 10, 13
Condylar fossa, 10
Condylar process, of mandible, 15, 17
head of, 6
Condyles
of femur
lateral, 476, 494–497
medial, 476, 494–497
of mandible, 7
occipital, 8, 10–11, 16
of tibia
lateral, 481, 497, 500–501, 506
medial, 494, 496–497, 500–501
Cone of light, 95
Cones, 121
Conjoined longitudinal muscle, 370–372
Conjoint tendon, 246, 249, 255–256
Conjunctiva, 93
Conjunctival artery, posterior, 93
Conjunctival fornix
inferior, 83
superior, 83
Conjunctival vein, posterior, 93
Conjunctival vessels, 92
Connective tissue
of skull, 103
subserous, 305
Conoid ligament, 404, 408, 411
Conoid tubercle, 404
Conus arteriosus, 209, 217–219
Conus elasticus, 80, 82
Conus medullaris, 156, 160–161
transverse section of, 327
Cooper's ligament, 179, 246–247, 249, 255, 257–258
Coraco-acromial ligament, 408, 411, 413, 417
Coracobrachialis muscle, 239–240, 405, 410, 412–413, 415, 417, 419, 421, 460, 462, 467
Coracobrachialis tendon, 410, 413
Coracoclavicular ligament, 408, 411
Coracohumeral ligament, 408
Coracoid process, 185–186, 405–408, 410–415, 417, 419
of scapula, 183
Cornea, 83, 85, 89–90, 92–93
Corneal limbus, 83
Corneoscleral junction, 83
Corniculate cartilage, 79
Corniculate tubercle, 66–67, 80
Coronal sulcus, 366
Coronal suture, 4–9, 14
Coronary arteries, 215, 221
imaging of, 216
left, 215–216, 220
anterior interventricular branch of (left anterior descending artery), 215–216
circumflex branch of, 215–216, 219
interventricular branch of, 209
interventricular septal branches of, 215–216
left (obtuse) marginal branch of, 215–216
posterior left ventricular branch of, 215
posterolateral branches of, 216
right, 209, 211, 215–216, 219–220
atrial branch of, 215
AV nodal branch of, 216, 219
interventricular septal branches of, 215
posterior interventricular branch of (posterior descending artery), 211, 215–216, 219
right (acute) marginal branch of, 215–216
SA nodal branch of, 215–216
Coronary ligament, 277, 321
hepatorenal portion of, 277
of liver, 268
Coronary sinus, 211–213, 215, 218, 241
opening of, 214, 217, 220
valve (thebesian) of, 217
Coronary sulcus, 209, 211
Coronoid fossa, 405, 422
Coronoid process
of mandible, 6–7, 15, 17, 42
temporalis muscle insertion to, 6
of ulna, 422, 425, 429
radiographs of, 423
Corpora cavernosa, of penis, 360
Corpora quadrigemina, 108
Corpus albicans, 352
Corpus callosum, 107, 109, 112, 142, 144
cistern of, 110
dorsal vein of, 145, 147
genu of, 107–108, 111, 113, 147
imaging of, 151
imaging of, 151
posterior cerebral artery to, 143
rostrum of, 107, 142, 146
splenium of, 107–108, 111, 113, 116, 144–147
imaging of, 151
sulcus of, 107
trunk of, 107, 142
Corpus cavernosum, 344, 359, 361, 363
tunica albuginea of, 359, 363
Corpus luteum, 352
Corpus spongiosum, 344, 348, 359–361, 363
tunica albuginea of, 359, 363
Corpus striatum, 111, 142
Corrugator cutis ani muscle, 371–372
Corrugator supercilii muscle, 25, 124, 151
Corti
spiral ganglion of, 98
spiral organ of, 94, 98
Cortical lymph vessels, 316
Cortical radiate (interlobular) arteries, 312
lymph vessels along, 316
Costal cartilages, 183–184, 243, 404
fifth, 191, 213
first, 193, 238
second, 240
seventh, 195
sixth, 409
transverse section of, 324
Costal facet, 154
inferior, 154, 184
superior, 154, 184
transverse, 154, 184
Costal groove, 184
Costal impressions, 277
Costal lamella, 20
Costocervical trunk, 33, 137, 139, 170
Costochondral joints, 184
Costoclavicular ligament, 184, 404, 412
impression for, 404
Costocoracoid ligament, 412
Costocoracoid membrane, 412
Costodiaphragmatic recess, 193–195, 210, 214, 227–228, 309, 315
transverse section of, 324
Costomediastinal space, 195
Costotransverse joint, 238
Costotransverse ligament, 184
lateral, 184
superior, 184
Costoxiphoid ligament, 184
Cough receptors, 207
Cowper's gland, 249, 321, 344, 348, 361–363, 367
duct of, 361
primordium of, 367
Cranial base
foramina and canals of
inferior view of, 12
superior view of, 13
inferior view of, 10
nerves of, 55
superior view of, 11
vessels of, 55
Cranial fossa
anterior, 11
middle, 11
posterior, 11
arteries of, 144
veins of, 145
Cranial imaging, 150–151

- **Cranial mesonephric (Gartner's) duct**, 367
- **Cranial mesonephric tubules**, 367
- **Cranial nerves**
  - motor and sensory distribution of, 119
  - nuclei of, in brainstem, 117–118
- **Cranial root**
  - of accessory nerve, 128
  - of vagus nerve, 127
- **Craniocervical ligaments**
  - external, 22
  - internal, 23
- **Cremaster fascia**, 247, 365, 368
  - on spermatic cord, 256
- **Cremaster muscle**, 247, 256, 365, 397
  - lateral origin, 246, 255
  - medial origin, 246, 255
  - on spermatic cord, 253, 256
- **Cremasteric arteries**, 251, 256–257, 379
- **Cremasteric veins**, 256, 379
- **Cribriform fascia**
  - over saphenous opening, 252
  - within saphenous opening, 472
- **Cribriform plate**, 8, 11, 36–39, 120
  - foramina of, 13
- **Crico-arytenoid muscle**
  - lateral, 80, 82, 151
    - action of, 81
  - posterior, 67, 69, 80, 82, 151
    - action of, 81
- **Crico-esophageal tendon**, 69
- **Cricoid cartilage**, 15, 27–28, 64, 69–70, 76, 79–80, 82, 193, 203, 230–231
  - arch of, 79
  - arytenoid articular surface of, 79
  - lamina of, 79–80
    - prominence over, 66
- **Cricopharyngeus muscle**, 65, 67, 69–70, 77–78, 82, 230
- **Cricothyroid artery**, 72, 76
- **Cricothyroid joint**, 79, 81
- **Cricothyroid ligament**, 76, 79
  - median, 28, 70, 76, 79, 199
- **Cricothyroid muscle**, 28, 70, 76, 80, 82, 127, 151
  - action of, 81
  - oblique part, 80
  - straight part, 80
- **Crista galli**, 5, 8, 11, 38
- **Crista terminalis**, 217, 222
- **Crown of tooth**, 63
- **Cruciate ligaments**, 23, 494, 496
  - anterior, 495–496, 501
    - attachment of, 495
  - posterior, 495–496, 501
    - attachment of, 495
- **Crura**
  - of antihelix, 95
  - cerebral, 108, 114–115, 140, 146
  - of clitoris, 340, 348, 350, 356–357
  - of diaphragm, 176, 315
    - left, 229, 264
    - right, 229, 258, 264
    - transverse section of, 324–327
  - of fornix, 107, 111, 113, 144
  - of penis, 348, 359–361, 363
- **Crural artery**
  - anterior, 96
  - posterior, 96
- **Crural fascia**, 470, 510
- **Crux of helix**, 95
- **Crypts of Lieberkühn**, 275
- **Cubital fossa**, 398
- **Cubital lymph nodes**, 403
- **Cubital vein, median**, 398, 401, 403
- **Cuboid bones**, 511–512, 514, 523–524, 531
  - articular surface for, 513
  - tuberosity of, 515, 523
- **Cuboideonavicular ligament**
  - dorsal, 514
  - plantar, 515
- **Culmen**, 114, 116
- **Cuneate fasciculus**, 115–116
- **Cuneate tubercle**, 115–116
- **Cuneiform bones**, 511–512, 523–524, 531
  - intermediate, 523–524
  - lateral, 523–524
  - medial, 514–515, 523–524
- **Cuneiform tubercle**, 66–67, 80
- **Cuneocuboid ligament, dorsal**, 514
- **Cuneonavicular ligaments**
  - dorsal, 514
  - plantar, 515
- **Cuneus**, 107
  - apex of, 108
- **Cupula of pleura**, 76
  - parietal, 193–194, 227–228
- **Cuspid teeth**. *See* Canine teeth
- **Cutaneous nerves**
  - antebrachial
    - lateral, 400–402, 417, 421, 433–434, 436, 456, 459–460, 462
    - medial, 400–402, 415–416, 419, 421, 436, 456, 459–463
    - posterior, 400–402, 418, 421, 436, 455–456, 459, 465–466
  - of arm, 401
  - brachial
    - anterior, 410
    - inferior lateral, 400–401, 418, 465–466
    - medial, 253, 400–401, 415–416, 419, 421, 460–463
    - posterior, 401, 410, 418, 465–466
    - from posterior, 400
    - superior lateral, 174, 400–401, 410, 413, 418, 465–466
  - dorsal
    - intermediate, 529
    - lateral, 470–471, 517–518, 527–529
    - medial, 529
  - femoral
    - lateral, 253, 257, 262, 308, 387, 470–472, 483–485, 487–488, 492
    - posterior, 160, 174, 389, 391, 471, 484, 486, 489–490, 492, 527
  - of forearm, 402, 461–462
  - of hand, 459, 463–464
  - of head, 2
  - lateral
    - of forearm, 402
    - of thigh, 525
  - medial crural, 525
  - of neck, 2, 31
  - perforating, 389, 391, 471, 484, 486, 490
  - of shoulder, 401
  - sural
    - lateral, 470–471, 489, 503–504, 510, 527–529
    - medial, 471, 489, 503–504, 510, 527–528
  - of wrist, 459
- **Cuticle**, 458
- **Cystic artery**, 283–284
- **Cystic duct**, 277, 280, 283–284
- **Cystic lymph nodes**, 294
- **Cystohepatic (Calot's) triangle**, 280, 284

D

- **Dartos fascia**, 245, 344, 358–360, 365, 368, 373, 383
- **Darwin, auricular tubercle of**, 95
- **Deciduous teeth**, 62
- **Declive**, 114, 116
- **Deep artery**
  - of clitoris, 357, 382
  - of penis, 359, 363, 383
- **Deep cervical lymph nodes, inferior**, 205, 235
- **Deep fascia, of leg**, 470, 510
- **Deep (Buck's) fascia, of penis**, 245–247, 321, 344, 358–361, 365, 373–374, 381, 383
  - intercavernous septum of, 359–360, 363
- **Deltoid muscle**, 27, 29, 152, 171, 174, 178, 214, 238–240, 398, 404–406, 408–410, 412–413, 415, 417–419, 421, 460, 465, 467
- **Deltoid tuberosity**, 405–406
- **Deltopectoral groove**, 398
- **Deltopectoral lymph node**, 403
- **Deltopectoral triangle**, 409
- **Denonvilliers' fascia**, 321, 339, 344, 362, 369, 374
- **Dens**
  - apical ligament of, 23, 64–65
  - of atlas, 19
  - of axis, 7, 19, 21, 64
  - posterior articular facet of, 23
- **Dental plexus, inferior**, 123
- **Dental pulp**, 63
- **Dentate gyrus**, 107, 109, 112–113, 120
- **Dentate line**, 371
- **Dentate nucleus, of cerebellum**, 116
- **Denticulate ligament**, 165–166
- **Dentinal tubules of teeth**, 63
- **Dentine of teeth**, 63
- **Depressor anguli oris muscle**, 25, 48, 124
- **Depressor labii inferioris muscle**, 25, 48, 124, 151
- **Depressor septi nasi muscle**, 25, 35, 124, 151
- **Dermatomes**
  - levels of, 162
  - of lower limb, 469
  - schematic demarcation of, 162
  - of upper limb, 399
- **Descemet's membrane**, 90
- **Descending artery**
  - anterior, 215–216
  - posterior, 211, 215–216, 219
- **Descending pathway**, 133
- **Diagonal conjugate**, 332
- **Diaphragm**, 187, 195, 203, 206, 208, 210, 214, 227–230, 232–234, 241, 249, 251, 258, 260, 266–267, 269, 277, 282, 306, 308–309, 315, 321, 328, 388, 485
  - abdominal surface of, 192
  - central tendon of, 191–192, 258
  - costal origin of, slips of, 187
  - costal part of, 192
  - crura of, 176, 315
    - left, 192, 229, 264
    - right, 192, 229, 258, 264
    - transverse section of, 324–327
  - dome of
    - left, 193–194
    - right, 193–194
  - lumbar part of, 192
  - pelvic, 369
    - female, 335–337, 340
    - inferior fascia of, 355–356, 360, 370
    - interior fascia of, 372
    - male, 338–339, 344
    - superior fascia of, 343, 346, 355, 370, 372
  - sternal part of, 187, 192
  - thoracic surface of, 191
  - transverse section of, 324
- **Diaphragmatic constriction**, 230
- **Diaphragmatic fascia**, 315
- **Diaphragmatic ligament**, 367
- **Digastric fossa**, 17
- **Digastric muscle**, 27, 151
  - anterior belly of, 28–29, 31, 34, 43, 46, 50, 58, 70
    - innervation of, 119
  - mastoid notch for, 10

Digastric muscle *(Continued)*
phantom, 34
posterior belly of, 27–29, 34, 46–47, 50–51, 58–59, 67, 70, 75, 124
innervation of, 119
nerve to, 24
Digastric tendon, intermediate, 47, 59
fibrous loop for, 27–28, 58–59
Digital artery
dorsal, 456, 458, 508–509, 517, 523
palmar, 435
common, 435
proper, 435
proper, 453
Digital fibrous sheaths, 445
Digital nerves, dorsal, 402, 458, 466, 470, 507, 529
Digital veins, dorsal, 402, 470
Digits
extensors of, 427
flexors of, 429
Dilator pupillae muscle, 90, 122, 133, 151
Diploë, 9
Diploic veins, 101, 103
frontal, 101
occipital, 101
temporal
anterior, 101
posterior, 101
Direct vein, lateral, 146–147
Distal interphalangeal (DIP) joint, 398, 445
Distributing vein, 279
Dome of pleura, parietal, 193–194, 227–228
Dorsal artery
of clitoris, 357, 382
of penis, 359, 361, 383
deep, 379, 383
Dorsal nerve
of clitoris, 357, 391–392, 484
of penis, 359, 361, 383, 387–389, 394, 484, 490
Dorsal nucleus, of vagus nerve, 117
posterior, 118
Dorsal rami, 254
of cervical spinal nerves, 2, 22–24
of lumbar spinal nerves, 158, 174
of sacral spinal nerves, 174
of spinal nerves, 165–166
of thoracic spinal nerves, 174, 177, 250
Dorsal root ganglion, 129, 133, 166, 177, 188, 254, 300, 303–304, 306–307, 318, 395
Dorsal rootlets, of spinal nerves, 160
Dorsal vein
of clitoris, deep, 335–337, 340, 343, 346, 357
of corpus callosum, 145, 147
of penis
deep, 245, 339, 344, 359, 361, 379, 381
superficial, 245, 252, 329, 359, 381
Dorsal venous network, 402, 455
Dorsiflexion, of ankle, 469
Dorsum of foot, 518
Douglas, recto-uterine pouch of, 340, 342, 352, 369
Duct system, of liver, 278
Ductus arteriosus, 226
Ductus (vas) deferens, 249, 255–257, 259, 313, 344–345, 348, 362, 364–365, 367–369, 387, 394, 472
ampulla of, 362
artery to, 251, 259, 365, 376, 379, 381
inferior, 381
Ductus reuniens, 98
Ductus venosus, 226
Duodenal flexure
inferior, 272
superior, 272
Duodenal fold
inferior, 264, 271
superior, 264
Duodenal fossa
inferior, 264, 271
superior, 264
Duodenal impression, 277
Duodenal muscle fibers, 280
Duodenal papilla
major (of Vater), 272, 280
minor, 272, 280
Duodenojejunal flexure, 264, 271–272, 281, 315, 320
Duodenojejunal junction, 176
Duodenum, 127, 267–269, 271, 277–278, 281, 308, 313, 315, 320
arteries of, 284, 286
ascending part of, 264, 271–272
autonomic nerves of, 298–300
descending part of, 176, 264, 266, 271–272, 280
transverse section of, 326
inferior part of, 264, 271–272, 321
mucosa and musculature of, 272
in situ, 271
superior part of, 270–272
transverse section of, 325
suspensory muscle of, 264
transverse section of, 327
veins of, 289
Dura mater, 38, 95, 98, 102–103, 110, 120
arachnoid interface with, 103
endosteal layer, 103
meningeal layer, 101, 103
periosteal layer, 101
skull interface with, 101, 103
spinal, 160, 165–166, 170, 176
posterior intercostal artery branch to, 168
superior cerebral veins penetrating, 103
Dural sac, termination of, 160–161
Dural venous sinuses
sagittal section of, 104
superior view of, 105

E

Ear
ampulla of, 94, 98
bony and membranous labyrinths of, 97–98
orientation of, 99
external, 95
innervation of, 119
tympanic cavity of, 96
vestibule of, 94, 97–98
Edinger-Westphal nucleus, 117–118, 122, 133
Efferent ductules, 367–368
Efferent fibers, 117–118, 122–124, 126, 128–130
of autonomic reflex pathways, 304
to olfactory bulb, 120
Ejaculatory duct
beginning of, 362
opening of, 362–363, 367, 396
Elbow
bones of, 422
ligaments of, 424
radiographs of, 423
Elliptical recess, 97
Emissary vein, 13, 73, 101, 103
condylar, 170
mastoid, 3, 101, 170
in mastoid foramen, 12
occipital, 101
parietal, 3, 101
parietal foramen for, 9
to superior sagittal sinus, 13
Enamel of teeth, 63
Endolymphatic duct, 13, 97–99
Endolymphatic sac, 98
Endometrium, 352
Endopelvic fascia, female, 343
Enteric plexus, 304
Ependyma, 109
Epicolic lymph nodes, 296
Epicondyles
of femur
lateral, 476, 480, 497
medial, 476, 488–489, 493–494, 496–497
of humerus
lateral, 405–406, 417–418, 422–424, 426, 428–429, 431, 434, 466
medial, 405–406, 417–419, 422–424, 426–434, 464–465
Epicranial aponeurosis, 3, 25, 103, 175
Epicranius muscle, occipital belly of, 151
Epididymal duct, 368
Epididymis, 364, 368, 394
appendix of, 365, 367
body of, 365, 368
head of, 365, 368
sinus of, 368
tail of, 368
Epidural hematoma, site of, 101, 103
Epidural space, fat in, 166
Epigastric artery
inferior, 245, 247, 249, 251, 255–257, 259, 268, 314, 341, 343, 345, 376, 378–379, 381, 499
cremasteric branch of, 247, 249, 259
pubic branch of, 247, 249, 255, 259, 343, 345
transverse section of, 328
superficial, 186, 208, 245, 247, 251, 259, 487, 499
superior, 185, 187–188, 247, 251
Epigastric lymph nodes, inferior, 261
Epigastric region, 244
Epigastric veins
inferior, 245, 247, 249, 252, 255–257, 260, 268, 341, 345, 378–379, 381
pubic branch of, 255
transverse section of, 328
superficial, 186, 242, 245, 252, 260, 329, 470, 487
superior, 187, 189, 247, 252
Epiglottis, 15, 60, 64, 66–69, 78–80, 82, 136, 230
Epiphysis, 458
nutrient branches to, 458
Episcleral artery, 92
Episcleral space, 85, 89
Episcleral vein, 92–93
segment of, 93
Epithelial tag, 366
Epithelium, gingival, 63
Epitympanic recess, 94–95
Eponychium, 458
Epoöphoron, 352, 367
Erector spinae muscles, 152, 171–173, 176–177, 188, 238, 254, 309
transverse section of, 324, 328
Esophageal artery, 204
Esophageal hiatus, 192, 264
Esophageal impression, 277
Esophageal mucosa, 69, 232
Esophageal muscles, 64, 199
circular, 65, 67, 69
in V-shaped area of Laimer, 69, 77
longitudinal, 65, 67, 69, 77
attachment of, 69
cricoid attachment of, 65, 67
Esophageal plexus, 127, 203, 206, 213, 227–229, 234, 236, 300
nerve branches to, 236
sympathetic branch to, 206

Esophageal prominence, 212
Esophageal sphincter, inferior, 230
Esophageal submucosa, 69, 232
Esophageal veins, 292
Esophagogastric junction, 214, 232
  transverse section of, 324
Esophagus, 26, 64, 66, 70, 78, 80, 127, 191, 203–204, 213–214, 227–228, 232–234, 236, 238–241, 258, 260, 264, 268, 302, 308, 310, 321
  abdominal part of, 230, 233, 269
  arteries of, 233
  inferior phrenic artery recurrent branch to, 259
  longitudinal muscle of, 270
  lung area for
    left, 196
    right, 196
  lung groove for
    left, 196
    right, 196
  lymph vessels and nodes of, 235
  musculature of, 231
  nerves of, 236
  in situ, 229
  topography and constrictions of, 230
  veins of, 234
  zone of sparse muscle fibers, 69–70
Ethmoidal air cells, 43–44, 85
  anterior
    of newborn, 45
    openings of, 36–37
  middle
    of newborn, 45
    openings of, 36–37
  posterior
    of newborn, 45
    opening of, 36–37
Ethmoidal artery
  anterior, 13, 87
    anterior lateral nasal branch of, 40
    anterior meningeal branch of, 102
    anterior septal branch of, 40
    external nasal branch of, 40
  posterior, 13, 87, 102
    septal and lateral nasal branches of, 40
Ethmoidal bone, 4, 6, 8, 11
  anterior ethmoidal foramen of, 14
  cribriform plate of, 8, 11, 36–38, 120
  crista galli of, 8, 11, 38
  nasal concha of
    highest, 37
    middle, 4, 8, 37
    superior, 8, 37
  orbital plate of, 4, 6, 14
  perpendicular plate of, 4, 8, 38
  uncinate process of, 36–37, 44
    of newborn, 45
Ethmoidal bulla, 36–37
Ethmoidal foramen
  anterior, 4, 13–14
  posterior, 4, 13
Ethmoidal nerve (V_1)
  anterior, 13, 52, 88, 122–123
    external nasal branches of, 2, 39, 41, 52, 123
    internal nasal branches of, 123
    lateral internal nasal branch of, 39, 41
    medial internal nasal branch of, 39, 41
  posterior, 13, 52, 88, 122–123
Ethmoidal process, of inferior nasal concha, 37
Ethmoidal vein
  anterior, 13
  posterior, 13
Eustachian tube. *See* Pharyngotympanic (auditory, eustachian) tube
Eversion, of foot, 469
Extension
  of hip, 469
  of knee, 469, 494
Extensor carpi radialis brevis muscle, 398, 418, 427, 430–431, 436–438, 465–467
Extensor carpi radialis brevis tendon, 430–431, 436, 454, 456–457
Extensor carpi radialis longus muscle, 398, 405, 418, 421, 427, 430–431, 436–438, 465–467
  groove for, 425
Extensor carpi radialis longus tendon, 430–431, 436, 454, 456–457
Extensor carpi ulnaris muscle, 398, 427, 430, 436–438, 465–467
Extensor carpi ulnaris tendon, 430–431, 436, 456–457
Extensor digiti minimi muscles, 427, 430, 436–438, 466–467
Extensor digiti minimi tendon, 427, 430–431, 456–457
Extensor digitorum brevis muscle, 506, 508, 516–518, 529, 531
Extensor digitorum brevis tendon, 507–508, 518, 523
Extensor digitorum longus muscle, 506–508, 510, 516–518, 529, 531
Extensor digitorum longus tendon, 468, 481, 494, 502, 506–508, 517–518, 523
  tendinous sheath of, 517
Extensor digitorum muscle, 418, 427, 430, 436–438, 465–467
Extensor digitorum tendon, 398, 427, 430–431, 436, 456–457
Extensor expansion system, 448, 451–452, 457, 517–518, 523
Extensor hallucis brevis muscle, 508, 517–518, 529, 531
Extensor hallucis brevis tendon, 507–508, 518, 523
Extensor hallucis longus muscle, 506–508, 510, 518, 529, 531
Extensor hallucis longus tendon, 468, 502, 506–508, 517–518, 523
  tendinous sheath of, 516–517
Extensor indicis muscle, 427, 431, 436, 438, 466–467
Extensor indicis tendon, 398, 430, 436, 456–457
Extensor pollicis brevis muscle, 431, 438, 466–467
  radial area for, 425
Extensor pollicis brevis tendon, 430, 434, 436, 454, 456–457
Extensor pollicis longus muscle, 431, 436, 438, 466–467
  radial area for, 425
Extensor pollicis longus tendon, 398, 430, 450, 454, 456–457
Extensor retinaculum, 402, 430–433, 454–457
  inferior, 506–507, 516–517, 529
  superior, 506–507, 516–517
Extensor tendons, 450–451
  common, 405, 427, 430–431, 437
  in fingers, 451
  long, 451
  at wrist, 457
External capsule, 111
External jugular vein, 1
External occipital protuberance (inion), 6, 8, 10, 16, 152
External os, 352
Extrahepatic bile ducts, 280
Extraperitoneal fascia, 7, 176, 245, 256–257, 390
Extraperitoneal space, 370
Extreme capsule, 111
Eye
  anterior chamber of, 83, 89–92
    endothelium of, 90
  innervation of, 119, 163–164
  intrinsic arteries and veins of, 92
  posterior chamber of, 83, 89–92
  vascular supply of, 93
Eye muscle, extrinsic, 86, 92
Eyeball, 43, 89
  fascia of, 85
  fascial sheath of, 85, 89
Eyelashes (cilia), 83
Eyelids, 83
  arteries and veins of, 87
  tarsus of, 85

F

Face
  arterial supply sources of, 3
  muscles of, 124
    innervation of, 119
  superficial arteries and veins of, 3
Facial artery, 3, 31, 34–35, 42, 46–47, 51, 72–73, 77, 87, 132, 134, 137, 139
  inferior labial branch of, 35
  lateral nasal branch of, alar branches of, 3
  superior labial branch of, 35
    nasal septal branch of, 40
  tonsillar branch of, 68
  transverse, 3, 34–35, 46, 72, 87
Facial canal, 125
  prominence of, 95
Facial colliculus, 116
Facial expression muscles, 25, 47
Facial lymph nodes, 74
Facial nerve (VII), 13, 34, 42, 47, 50–51, 53, 55, 71, 94, 96, 99, 105, 115, 118, 123–124, 132, 135–136
  branches of, 24, 46, 164
  buccal branches of, 24
  cervical branch of, 24
  communication to, 126
  distribution of, 119
  geniculum of, 50, 53, 99, 117, 125–126, 132
  intermediate nerve (of Wrisberg), 61, 105, 115, 124–125, 132, 134, 136
    distribution of, 119
  internal genu of, 118
  marginal mandibular branch of, 24, 31
  motor nucleus of, 124–125
  schema of, 124
  stylomastoid foramen and, 12, 24
  temporal branches of, 24
  trunk of, 24
  zygomatic branches of, 24
Facial (intermediate) nerve (VIII), chorda tympani of, 12
Facial nucleus, 117–118
Facial plexus, 132
Facial vein, 3, 31–32, 42, 46–47, 59, 73, 87
  common, 3, 32
  common trunk for, 46, 59, 73
  deep, 3, 73, 87
  transverse, 3, 73
Falciform ligament, 7, 249, 263, 268–269, 277
  of liver, 251, 292
Fallopian tube. *See* Uterine (fallopian) tube
False cords. *See* Ventricular folds
False pelvis, 334, 341
False ribs, 183
Falx cerebelli, 104, 145
Falx cerebri, 38, 43, 103–105, 142, 145
Fascia
  of hand, 450
  of legs, 510
  of orbit and eyeball, 85

Fascia lata, 245–246, 385, 470, 472, 487, 492
Scarpa's layer attachment to, 245
of thigh, 350, 355, 358–359
Fascial ligaments, of uterus, 351
Fascial sheath, 85, 89, 450
Fasciculus
cuneate, 115–116
gracile, 115–116
longitudinal
dorsal, 148
medial, 114, 116
mammillothalamic, 107
Fat tissue, 179, 397
Fauces, 68
Femoral artery, 247, 251, 256, 259, 358, 379, 385, 396–397, 472, 480, 487–488, 492, 499, 509, 530
deep, 397
in femoral sheath, 257
lateral circumflex, 487–488, 491, 499
medial circumflex, 488–489, 491, 499
muscular branches of, 499
opening for, 258
perforating branches of, 499
Femoral canal, 472
lymph nodes in, 257
Femoral cutaneous nerves
lateral, 253, 257, 262, 308, 387, 525–526
posterior, 160, 174, 389, 527
perineal branch of, 391, 527
Femoral nerve, 160, 249, 255, 262, 385, 387, 396–397, 472, 483–485, 487–488, 525–526
anterior cutaneous branches of, 387, 470, 525
branches of, 492
deep to iliopsoas fascia, 257
of thigh, 525
Femoral ring, 255, 257, 341, 343, 345, 472
Femoral sheath, 246–247, 249, 257, 472, 487
femoral vessels in, 257
Femoral vein, 246–247, 252, 256, 260, 358, 379, 385, 396–397, 470, 472, 480, 487–488, 492, 530
in femoral sheath, 257
opening for, 258
Femur, 476, 492, 494, 498
adductor tubercle of, 476
condyles of
lateral, 476, 494–497
medial, 476, 494–497
epicondyles of
lateral, 476, 480, 497
medial, 476, 488–489, 493–494, 496–497
gluteal tuberosity, 476
head of, 396, 474–476, 530
arteries of, 491
ligament of, 474, 476
radiograph of, 331
intercondylar fossa of, 476
intertrochanteric crest of, 476
intertrochanteric line of, 476
lateral supracondylar line of, 476
ligaments of, 491
linea aspera of, 476
neck of, 396–397, 474–476
arteries of, 491
nutrient artery of, 491
nutrient foramen of, 476
patellar surface of, 476
pectineal line of, 476
popliteal surface of, 476, 498
quadrate tubercle of, 476
radiograph of, 331, 475, 497, 530
retinacular foramina of, 476
shaft of, 476
Femur *(Continued)*
trochanter of, 475
greater, 152, 243, 330, 468, 474, 476, 479–480, 483, 489–490, 530
lesser, 243, 258, 330, 474–476, 530
radiograph of, 331
trochanteric fossa of, 476
Fibroelastic membranes, of esophagus, 231
Fibromuscular stroma, 362
Fibrous appendix, of liver, 277
Fibrous capsule, 282, 315
Fibrous pericardium, 195, 208, 212, 227–228
Fibrous septum, 372
transverse, 371–373
Fibrous sheath, 450, 453, 458, 521
Fibrous tendon, 458
Fibrous trabecula, 148
Fibrous trigone
left, 219
right, 219
Fibula, 497, 500–501, 506–507, 513–514, 517–518
anterior border of, 500–501
anterior ligament of, 501
apex of, 500–501
head of, 479–481, 493–494, 496–498, 500–501, 504–508, 529
anterior ligament of, 501
posterior ligament of, 498
interosseous border of, 500–501
interosseous membrane of, 501
lateral malleolus of, 468, 500–501, 503–508, 517–518, 531
lateral surface of, 500–501
medial surface of, 500
neck of, 497, 500
posterior ligament of, 501
radiographs of, 497, 531
Fibula bursa, lateral malleolus of, 516
Fibular artery, 499, 503–505, 509–510, 521
calcaneal branches of, 503–505
communicating branch of, 505
perforating branch of, 505, 508, 517–518
posterior lateral malleolar branch of, 505
Fibular nerve, 529
common, 482, 484, 486, 489, 492–494, 497, 503–508, 527–529
articular branch of, 527–529
sural communicating branch of, 527
deep, 508, 510, 517–518, 529
dorsal digital branch of, 470, 507–508, 517–518
lateral branch of, 508, 517–518, 529
medial branch of, 507–508, 517–518, 529
recurrent branch of, 508
superficial, 470, 506–508, 510, 517–518, 527, 529
dorsal digital branches of, 517–518
intermediate dorsal cutaneous branch of, 470
medial dorsal cutaneous branch of, 470
Fibular notch, 500
Fibular retinaculum
inferior, 505–506, 514, 516
superior, 503–506, 514, 516
Fibular veins, 510
Fibularis (peroneus) brevis muscle, 506–508, 510, 516–518, 529, 531
Fibularis brevis tendon, 468, 502–506, 508, 514–518, 522–523
common tendinous sheath of, 516
Fibularis (peroneus) longus muscle, 468, 481, 493–494, 502–504, 506–508, 510, 516, 529, 531
Fibularis longus tendon, 468, 504–506, 508, 514–518, 522–523
common tendinous sheath of, 516
Fibularis (peroneus) tertius muscle, 502, 531
Fibularis tertius tendon, 506–507, 516–518, 523
Filiform papillae, 60
Filum terminale externum, 160, 166
Fimbriae, 111
of fallopian tube, 352–353
of hippocampus, 107, 109, 112–113, 120
Fimbriated fold, 56
Fingers, 458
anterior closed space of, 458
areolar tissue in, 458
arteries of, 458
articular cavity of, 458
cross section through, 458
dorsum of, lymph vessels passing to, 403
in extension, 451
extensor tendons in, 451
fibrous septa in, 458
fibrous tendon sheath of, 458
fine nerves of, 458
in flexion, 451
flexor tendons in, 451
minute arteries of, 458
nerves of, 458
posterior view of, 451
subungual space of, 458
tendon sheaths of, 448
Flank
left, 244
right, 244
Flexion
of hip, 469
of knee, 469
Flexor carpi radialis muscle, 417, 419, 428, 432, 434, 436–437, 460, 463, 467
Flexor carpi radialis tendon, 398, 433–434, 436, 441, 447, 449–450, 460
Flexor carpi ulnaris muscle, 398, 418, 430–434, 436–438, 460, 464, 467
Flexor carpi ulnaris tendon, 398, 434, 436, 441, 447, 449, 452
Flexor digiti minimi brevis muscle, 449, 452, 464, 467, 520–523, 528, 531
Flexor digiti minimi brevis tendon, 515
Flexor digitorum brevis muscle, 516, 520–522, 528, 531
Flexor digitorum brevis tendon, 515, 520–522
Flexor digitorum longus muscle, 502, 505, 510, 528, 531
Flexor digitorum longus tendon, 503–505, 515, 520–522
tendinous sheath of, 516
Flexor digitorum profundus muscle, 429, 434, 436–438, 460, 463–464, 467
Flexor digitorum profundus tendon, 429, 436, 445, 447–451, 458
Flexor digitorum superficialis muscles, 429, 432–434, 436–437, 460, 463, 467
Flexor digitorum superficialis tendons, 398, 405, 429, 432, 436, 441, 445, 447–451, 458, 460
Flexor hallucis brevis muscle, 520–523, 528, 531
Flexor hallucis brevis tendon, 523
Flexor hallucis longus muscle, 502, 505, 510, 528, 531
Flexor hallucis longus tendon, 503–505, 515, 520–523
groove for, 513
tendinous sheath of, 516
Flexor muscles, superficial, 432
Flexor pollicis brevis muscle, 449, 452–453, 463–464, 467

Flexor pollicis longus muscle, 405, 429, 433–434, 436–437, 447, 460, 463, 467
tendinous sheath of, 448, 450
Flexor pollicis longus tendon, 434, 436, 441, 449–450
Flexor retinaculum, 433, 441, 447, 449–450, 452–453, 460, 503–505, 516, 521–522, 528
Flexor sheath, common, 447–450, 453
Flexor tendon, 450, 453
common, 405–406, 428–429, 432, 437–438
fibrous sheaths of, 520
in fingers, 451
at wrist, 449
Flexor tendon sheath, 447
Floating ribs, 183
Flocculonodular lobe, 114
Flocculus, 114–115
Folds of iris, 90
Foliate papillae, 60, 136
Folium, 114, 116
Follicle (graafian), 352
Fontanelle
anterior, 14
posterior, 14
Foot
arteries of, 509
bones of, 511–512
deep arteries, 523
dorsum of, 518
muscles of, 517
eversion of, 469
interosseous muscles of, 523–524
inversion of, 469
ligaments of, 515
muscles of sole of
first layer, 520
second layer, 521
third layer, 522
plantar surface of, 468
sole of, 519
tendons of, 515
Foramen
interventricular (of Monro), 107, 109–110, 112, 116, 146–147
of Luschka, 109–110
of Magendie, 109–110, 116, 118
Foramen cecum, 11, 13, 60, 64
Foramen lacerum, 10, 13, 100
recurrent artery of, 138
Foramen magnum, 8, 10, 12–13, 100, 128
Foramen ovale, 6, 10, 12–13, 16, 49–50, 100, 226
branch to, 138
valve of, 218
Foramen rotundum, 5, 13, 52
branch to, 138
maxillary nerve entering, 53
Foramen spinosum, 10, 13, 16, 50, 100
accessory, 12
branch to, 138
Foramen transversarium, 20–21
bony spicule dividing, 20
septated, 20
Forearm
arteries of, 435
bones of, 425
cutaneous nerves of, 402, 461–462
muscles of
attachments of, 437–438
deep layer, 431, 434
extensors of wrist and digits, 427
flexors of digits, 429
flexors of wrist, 428
intermediate layer, 433
rotators of radius, 426
superficial layer, 430, 432
Forearm *(Continued)*
proximal, arteries of, 420
radial nerve in, 466
serial cross sections of, 436
superficial veins of, 402
Fornix, 107, 113, 148
anterior, 351
body of, 107, 109, 113, 116
columns of, 107, 111–113, 146
commissure of, 113
conjunctival
inferior, 83
superior, 83
crus of, 107, 111, 113, 144
imaging of, 151
vaginal, 352
anterior, 340
posterior, 340
Fossa ovalis, 214, 217, 226, 470
limbus of, 217
Fovea, inferior, 116
Fovea capitis, 530
Fovea centralis in macula, 89, 92
Free taenia, 265, 273–274, 276, 369, 372
Frenulum, 274
artery to, 59
of clitoris, 354
of labia minora, 354
of lower lip, 56
of penis, 360
of tongue, 46, 56
of upper lip, 56
Frontal artery, 3
polar, 142–143
Frontal bone, 1, 4, 6, 8–11, 35, 37, 83–84
foramen cecum of, 11
frontal crest of, 11
glabella of, 4, 6
groove for anterior meningeal vessels, 11
groove for superior sagittal sinus of, 11
growth of, 45
lateral view of, 14
nasal spine of, 37–38
of newborn, 14
orbital surface, 4
sinus of, 8, 37–38
squamous part of, 14, 37–38
superior surface of orbital part, 11
superior view of, 14
supra-orbital notch of, 4, 6
Frontal crest, 9, 11
Frontal gyrus
inferior
opercular part of, 106
orbital part of, 106
triangular part of, 106
medial, 107
middle, 106
superior, 106
Frontal (anterior) horn, 109
Frontal lobe, 106
Frontal nerve, 13, 52, 85, 88, 122–123, 132
Frontal operculum, 106
Frontal pole, 106, 108
Frontal sinus, 7, 36–38, 43–44, 64
growth of, 45
Frontal sulcus
inferior, 106
superior, 106
Frontal (metopic) suture, 14
Frontal vein, 3
Frontobasal artery
lateral, 140, 142–143
medial, 138, 140, 142–143
Frontonasal canal
infundibulum leading to, 37
opening of, 37
Frontonasal duct, 36
opening of, 44
Fundiform ligament, 245, 255, 344
Fundus
of gallbladder, axial CT images of, 323
of stomach, 230, 232, 269–270
transverse section of, 324
of urinary bladder, 344, 346, 348
of uterus, 340, 342, 346, 352
sagittal CT images of, 375
Fungiform papilla, 60, 136
Funiculus, lateral, 116

G

Galen, great cerebral veins of, 104–105, 107, 116, 145–147
imaging of, 150
Gallaudet's fascia, 344, 348, 350, 355–356, 359–361, 369
Gallbladder, 127, 193, 263, 266, 269, 277–278, 280–281, 284
axial CT images of, 322
fundus of, axial CT images of, 323
innervation of, 163–164
transverse section of, 325
Ganglion, of trigeminal nerve, 117–118, 132
Ganglion cells, 121
Gartner's duct, 367
Gasserian ganglion, 105, 117–118
Gastric artery
left, 233, 259, 266, 268, 283–284, 297–300, 388
arteriogram of, 285
esophageal branch of, 233, 236, 283
right, 272, 280, 283–284, 298–300
arteriogram of, 285
short, 268, 282–284, 300
Gastric canal, longitudinal folds of, 270
Gastric folds (rugae), 232, 270
transverse section of, 324
Gastric impression, 277, 282
Gastric lymph nodes, 235, 293–294
Gastric plexus, 388
left, 297–299
right, 298–299
Gastric veins
left, 234, 289–292
esophageal tributary of, 289
right, 234, 289–290, 292
short, 234, [illegible]
Gastrocnemius muscle, 478, 481, 489, 493–494, 502–508, 510, 527–528, 531
lateral head of, 468, 482, 497–498, 503
lateral subtendinous bursa of, 498
medial head of, 468, 482, 497–498, 503
Gastrocolic ligament, 266
anterior layers of, 266
posterior layers of, 266
Gastroduodenal artery, 272, 280, 283–284, 286–287, 300–301, 306
arteriogram of, 285
plexus on, 299
Gastroduodenal plexus, 301, 306
Gastro-omental (gastro-epiploic) artery, 268, 282
anastomosis of, 266
left, 283–284, 289, 292, 300
plexus on, 298–299
right, 266, 283–284, 286–287, 289, 292, 300
Gastro-omental (gastro-epiploic) lymph nodes, 293
Gastro-omental (gastro-epiploic) vein, 268, 282
left, 234
right, 234, 289, 291
Gastropancreatic fold, 266

Gastrophrenic ligament, 266, 268, 308
Gastrosplenic (gastrolienal) ligament, 266–267, 282
Gemellus muscle, 530
inferior, 396–397, 477–478, 482, 489–490, 531
nerve to, 490
superior, 477–478, 482, 489–490, 531
nerve to, 484, 489
Genial tubercle, 58
Genicular artery
descending, 487–488, 492, 499, 509
inferior
lateral, 499, 504–509
medial, 488, 499, 504–505, 507–509
middle, 499, 509
superior
lateral, 489, 499, 503–509
medial, 487–489, 499, 503–505, 507–509
Geniculate body
lateral, 108, 111–112, 115–117, 121, 133, 140, 144–146
medial, 108, 111–112, 115–116, 140, 144–146
Geniculate ganglion, 50, 53, 96, 99, 117, 124–126, 132, 136
Geniculate nucleus, dorsal lateral
left, 121
right, 121
Geniculum, of facial nerve, 50, 53, 99, 117, 125–126, 132
Genioglossus muscle, 43, 47, 59, 64, 129, 151
superior mental spine for origin of, 58
Geniohyoid fascia, 26
Geniohyoid muscle, 26, 43, 58–59, 64, 129–130, 151
communication with cervical plexus, 33
Genital cord, 367
Genital tubercle
anal pit of, 366
anal tubercle of, 366
epithelial tag of, 366
glans area of, 366
lateral part of, 366
urogenital fold of, 366
Genitalia
external
female, 354
homologues of, 366
innervation of, 163–164
male, 358–359
internal, homologues of, 367
lymph vessels and nodes of
female, 384
male, 386
nerves of
female, 391
male, 387
Genitofemoral nerve, 257, 262, 308, 313, 387, 483, 485, 526
femoral branches of, 253, 257, 262, 387, 470, 484–485
genital branch of, 253, 255–257, 262, 365, 387, 470, 484–485
nerves to, 484
transverse section of, 328
Genu
of corpus callosum, 107–108, 111, 113, 147
imaging of, 151
internal, of facial nerve, 118
of internal capsule, 111
Gerdy's tubercle, 481, 494, 496, 500–501
Gerota's fascia. *See* Renal (Gerota's) fascia
GI tract, innervation of, 119
Gimbernat's (lacunar) ligament, 246–247, 249, 255, 257–258, 472
Gingiva, lamina propria of, 63
Gingival epithelium, 63
Gingival groove, 63
Glabella, 1, 4, 6
Gland lobules, 179
Gland orifices, 280
Glans, of clitoris, 354, 366
Glans penis, 329, 344, 360, 363, 366
corona of, 360
neck of, 360
Glenohumeral joint, 408, 467
capsule of, 418
Glenohumeral ligament
inferior, 408
middle, 408
superior, 408
Glenoid cavity, of scapula, 183, 405, 407–408, 467
Glenoid labrum, 408, 467
Globus pallidus, 109, 111
Glomerulus, 120
Glossoepiglottic fold
lateral, 60
median, 60
Glossoepiglottic ligament, median, 80
Glossopharyngeal nerve (IX), 34, 42, 55, 61, 71–72, 105, 115, 117–118, 124, 126–127, 131–132, 134–136, 207
branch of, 164
carotid branch of, 34, 127, 132
in carotid sheath, 47
carotid sinus branch (of Hering), 71, 126, 131
distribution of, 119
inferior, 13
inferior (petrosal) ganglion of, 55, 96, 126, 135–136, 207
in jugular fossa, 12
lesser petrosal nerve from, 123
lingual branches of, 61, 126
pharyngeal branches of, 126
schema of, 126
superior ganglion of, 126
tonsillar branches of, 61, 68, 71, 126
tympanic branch of, 12
Gluteal aponeurosis, 309, 481–482, 489
over gluteus medius muscle, 250
Gluteal artery
inferior, 259, 314, 376, 380–381, 486, 489
superior, 259, 314, 376, 380–381, 486, 489
Gluteal fold, 152, 468
Gluteal lines
anterior, 334, 473
inferior, 334, 473
posterior, 334, 473
Gluteal nerves
inferior, 160, 484, 486, 489–490
superior, 160, 484, 486, 489–490
Gluteal vein, superior, 260, 291
Gluteus maximus muscle, 152, 171, 174, 250, 309, 339, 356, 359–360, 373–374, 388–389, 391, 396, 468, 478, 481–482, 489–490, 492, 530–531
Gluteus medius muscle, 152, 309, 396–397, 468, 478–479, 482–483, 487–490, 530–531
gluteal aponeurosis over, 250
Gluteus minimus muscle, 477, 482–483, 487–490, 531
Gluteus minimus tendon, 396
Gonads, 364, 367
Graafian follicle, 352
Gracile fasciculus, 115–116
Gracile tubercle, 115–116
Gracilis muscle, 477, 480, 482, 487–489, 492–493, 497, 502–503, 526, 531
Gracilis tendon, 468, 477, 479–480, 493–494
Granular foveolae, 9, 101, 103
Granule cell, 120
Gray matter
imaging of, 151
intermediolateral nucleus of, preganglionic sympathetic cell bodies in, 53, 133–135
lateral horn of, 165–166, 319
of spinal nerves, 165
Gray rami communicantes, 131, 133–135, 163, 166, 177, 188, 206, 224–225, 227–228, 236, 254, 262, 297, 300, 303–304, 317–318, 388, 390, 393–395, 485–486
of spinal nerves, 165
to and from sympathetic trunk, 165
Great auricular nerve, 2
Great cardiac vein, 215
Great cerebral veins (of Galen), 104–105, 107, 116, 145–147
imaging of, 150
Great toe
dorsal digital nerve and vein of, 470
phalanx of, 515, 524
Great vessels
pericardium at site of reflection from, 209
of superior mediastinum, 203
Greater occipital nerve, 2
Groin
left, 244
right, 244
Gubernaculum, 364, 367
Gyrus
angular, 106
branch to, 142–143
cingulate, 107
isthmus of, 107
dentate, 107, 109, 113, 120
frontal
inferior, 106
medial, 107
middle, 106
superior, 106
lingual, 107
long, 106
occipitotemporal
lateral, 107–108
medial, 107–108
orbital, 108
parahippocampal, 107–109, 120
postcentral, 106
precentral, 106
straight, 108
subcallosal, 107
supramarginal, 106
temporal
inferior, 106, 108
middle, 106
superior, 106

H

Habenula, 111
Habenular commissure, 107, 112, 116
Habenular trigone, 112, 116
Hair cells
inner, 98
outer, 98
Hamate, 440, 442–443, 449
hook of, 428, 434, 439, 441, 443–445, 453
radiographs of, 444
Hand
arteries of, 453
bones of, 443
bursae of, 450
cutaneous nerves of, 459, 463–464
deep dorsal dissection of, 456
dorsum of, lymph vessels passing to, 403
fascia of, 450
intrinsic muscles of, 452
nerves of, 453

Hand *(Continued)*
palmar dissections
deeper, 447
superficial, 446
radiographs of, 444
spaces of, 450
superficial dorsal dissection of, 455
superficial radial dissection of, 454
tendon sheaths of, 450
Handle of malleus, 95–96
Hard palate, 64, 68
Hasner's valve, 84
Haustra, 273, 276
Head
autonomic nerves in, 132
bony framework of, 15
cutaneous nerves of, 2
lymph vessels and nodes of, 74
of malleus, 95
skin of, 103
surface anatomy of, 1
Heart, 127, 230
anterior exposure of, 209
apex of, 209, 211, 241
base and diaphragmatic surface of, 211
conducting system of, 222
coronal section of, 214
diaphragmatic surface of, 215
fibrous skeleton of, 219–220
inferior border (acute margin) of, 209
innervation of, 119, 163–164
left border (obtuse margin) of, 193, 209
nerves of, 223–224
radiography of, 156
radiology and auscultation of, 210
right border of, 193
in situ, 208
sternocostal surface of, 215
Heart valves, 219–220
aortic, 210, 214, 218–222
mitral, 210, 213–214, 218–222, 241
pulmonary, 217, 219, 222
pulmonic, 210
tricuspid, 210, 213–214, 217, 219–222, 241
Helicotrema, 94, 97–98
Helix, 1, 95
crux of, 95
Hemi-azygos vein, 189, 191, 213, 234
accessory, 189, 204, 228, 234, 240
Hepatic artery, 278, 280, 283–284
branch of, 279
common, 259, 266, 272, 280–281, 283–284, 286–287, 297, 300, 306
arteriogram of, 285
intermediate, 284
proper, 267–268, 271–272, 277–278, 280–281, 283–284, 286, 300, 321
arteriogram of, 285
transverse section of, 325
Hepatic ducts, 280
common, 277–278, 280–281, 284
Hepatic lymph nodes, 293–294
Hepatic plexus, 298–299, 301, 306
common, 297
pyloric branch from, 127
vagal branch from, 298
vagal branch to, 236
Hepatic portal veins, 214, 226, 234, 267, 271–272, 277–278, 281, 283–284, 289–291, 294, 321
tributaries of, 292
Hepatic veins, 226, 234, 260, 268, 277–278
Hepatoduodenal ligament, 266–267, 269, 278
transverse section of, 325
Hepatogastric ligaments, 267, 269, 278
Hepatopancreatic ampulla (of Vater), 280
sphincter of, 280, 306
Hering-Breuer reflex, 207
Hesselbach's inguinal triangle, 249, 255
transversalis fascia within, 255
Heubner, recurrent artery of, 138, 140–143
Hilar lymph nodes, 196, 205, 227–228
Hilum, 196, 282, 311
of lungs
left, 209
right, 209
Hip
arthrogram of, 530
extension of, 469
flexion of, 469
magnetic resonance imaging of, 530
muscles of
attachments of, 477–478
lateral view, 481
posterior views, 482
nerves of, 490
radiograph of, 530
Hip (coxal) bone, 473
Hip joint, 474
anteroposterior radiograph, 475
articular branch to, 490
ligaments of, 479–480
Hippocampal sulcus, 113
Hippocampus, 111–113
alveus of, 113
fimbria of, 107, 109, 112–113, 120
Hook of hamate, 428, 434, 439, 441, 443, 445, 453
radiographs of, 444
Horizontal cells, 121
Horizontal fissure, 114
of lungs, right, 193–196
Horizontal plate, 8, 10, 16, 36–38, 57, 62, 100
Humeral artery
anterior circumflex, 413–415, 417, 419–420
posterior circumflex, 413–415, 418–420
Humeral ligament, transverse, 408
Humeral lymph nodes, 181–182
Humeral vein, posterior circumflex, superficial branches of, 401
Humerus, 419, 421, 429
anatomical neck of, 405–407
anterior view of, 405
anteroposterior radiograph of, 407
capitulum of, 405, 422–423
coronoid fossa of, 405, 422
deltoid tuberosity of, 405–406
epicondyles of
lateral, 405–406, 417–418, 422–424, 426, 428–429, 431, 434, 466
medial, 405–406, 417–419, 422–424, 426–434, 464–465
greater tubercle of, 405–407, 413, 417, 467
crest of, 405
head of, 405–407, 467
intertubercular sulcus, 405
lateral supracondylar ridge, 405–406
lesser tubercle of, 405–407, 417
crest of, 405
medial supracondylar ridge, 405–406, 422
olecranon fossa of, 406, 422–423
posterior view of, 406
radial fossa of, 405
radial groove of, 406
shaft of, 238–240
surgical neck of, 238, 405–407, 467
trochlea of, 405–406, 422–423
ulnar nerve groove, 406, 422
Hyaloid canal, 89
Hydatid of Morgagni, 352
Hymenal caruncle, 350, 354
Hyo-epiglottic ligament, 64, 79
Hyoglossus muscle, 28–29, 34, 58–59, 68, 70, 73, 129, 151
origin of, 58
Hyoid bone, 15, 27–29, 31, 34, 46–47, 59, 64, 67, 70, 76, 78–79, 82
body of, 15, 58
greater horn of, 15, 58, 70
prominence caused by, 66
tip of, 67, 77
lesser horn of, 15, 58
Hypochondriac region
left, 244
right, 244
Hypochondrium
left, 244
right, 244
Hypogastric nerves, 297, 302–303, 317–318, 387–388, 392–395
left, 390
right, 390
Hypogastric plexus, 486
inferior, 163, 297, 302–303, 317–318, 387–388, 390, 392–395
superior, 163, 297, 302–303, 317–318, 341, 345, 387, 390, 392–395
Hypogastric region, 244
Hypogastric (neurovascular) sheath, 343
Hypoglossal canal, 8, 10, 12, 129
Hypoglossal nerve (XII), 33–34, 42, 47, 50, 55, 59, 71–73, 75, 105, 115, 118, 129–130
in carotid sheath, 47
distribution of, 119
in hypoglossal canal, 12
meningeal branch of, 129
schema of, 129
vena comitans of, 47, 59, 73
Hypoglossal nucleus, 117–118, 129
Hypoglossal trigone, 116
Hypoglossus muscle, 47
Hypophyseal artery
inferior, 138, 141, 149
superior, 138, 141, 149
Hypophyseal fossa, 7
of newborn, 45
Hypophyseal portal veins
long, 141, 149
primary plexus of, 149
secondary plexus of, 149
short, 149
Hypophyseal veins, efferent, 141, 149
Hypophysis, 105, 107–108, 148
arteries and veins of, 149
in sella turcica, 36
Hypothalamic area, lateral, 136
Hypothalamic artery, 141
Hypothalamic sulcus, 107, 116, 148
Hypothalamic vessels, 149
Hypothalamohypophyseal tract, 148
Hypothalamus, 109, 148, 303
arteries and veins of, 149
principal nuclei of, 148
arcuate (infundibular), 148
dorsomedial, 148
mammillary body, 148
paraventricular, 148
posterior, 148
supra-optic, 148
ventromedial, 148
Hypothenar eminence, 398
Hypothenar muscles, 446–447, 450, 453, 464
Hysterosalpingogram, of uterus, 353

I

Ileal arteries, 287–288, 290
anastomotic loops of, 272
Ileal orifice, 276

Ileal papilla, 274
Ileal vein, 290–291
Ileocecal fold (bloodless fold of Treves), 273
Ileocecal junction, fibers around, 274
Ileocecal lips, 274
Ileocecal recess
inferior, 273
superior, 273
Ileocecal region, 273–274
Ileocolic artery, 273, 287–288, 301–302, 313
Ileocolic lymph nodes, 296
Ileocolic plexus, 301–302
Ileocolic vein, 290–292
Ileum, 263, 272, 276, 290, 295
fibers to, 274
terminal part of, 265, 273–274, 341
transverse section of, 327–328
Iliac artery
common, 259, 265, 268, 297, 308, 313–314, 376, 378–381, 390
ureteric branch from, 314
deep circumflex, 249, 257, 343, 381, 488, 499
ascending branch of, 251, 259
external, 249, 255–257, 259, 268, 273, 291, 297, 308, 313, 340–345, 350, 353, 370, 376, 378–381, 390, 488, 499
internal, 259, 288, 297, 308, 313–314, 343, 376, 378–381, 390
superficial circumflex, 245, 247, 251, 259, 487, 499
Iliac crest, 152, 158, 171–174, 242–243, 250, 308–309, 315, 329–330, 333, 468, 471, 481–483, 489–490, 530
inner lip of, 243, 330, 334, 473
intermediate zone of, 243, 330, 334, 473
outer lip of, 243, 330, 334, 473
tuberculum of, 243, 330, 473
Iliac fascia, 257, 343
Iliac fossa, 333–334, 341
Iliac lymph nodes
common, 261, 296, 316, 384, 386
external, 261, 296, 316, 386, 472
lateral, 384
medial, 384
internal, 261, 296, 316, 384, 386
Iliac plexus
common, 297, 390
external, 297, 390
internal, 297, 390
Iliac spine
anterior
inferior, 243, 258, 330, 333–334, 338, 473–474, 479–480
superior, 242–243, 245–246, 255–256, 258, 329–330, 333–334, 355, 358, 468, 473–474, 479–481, 483, 487
posterior
inferior, 158, 334, 473
superior, 152, 158, 333–334, 473
Iliac tubercle, 333–334
Iliac tuberosity, 330, 473
Iliac vein
common, 260, 265, 379, 381, 390
deep circumflex, 249, 257, 260, 343
tributaries to, 252
external, 249, 255–257, 260, 273, 291, 340–345, 350, 353, 370, 377, 379, 381, 488
internal, 260, 343, 377, 379, 381
superficial circumflex, 242, 245, 252, 260, 329, 470, 487
Iliacus fascia, 370
Iliacus muscle, 255, 258, 308, 328, 343, 370, 396–397, 477, 479, 483, 485–486, 491, 525, 530–531
nerves to, 484–485
Iliococcygeus muscle, 335–339, 350, 373
Iliocostalis cervicis muscles, 172
Iliocostalis lumborum muscles, 172
Iliocostalis muscles, 172
Iliocostalis thoracis muscles, 172
Iliofemoral ligament, 474, 483, 491
Iliohypogastric nerve, 160, 174, 262, 308–309, 387, 392, 483–485, 526
anterior branch of, 253
cutaneous branches of
anterior, 253, 262, 387
lateral, 250, 253, 471
transverse section of, 328
Ilio-inguinal nerve, 160, 253, 256, 262, 308–309, 387, 391–392, 470, 483–485, 526
anterior scrotal branch of, 253
scrotal branches of, anterior, 262
transverse section of, 328
Iliolumbar artery, 259, 314, 380–381
Iliolumbar ligament, 158, 309, 333
Iliolumbar vein, 260
Iliopectineal bursa, 474, 483
Iliopectineal line, 370
Iliopsoas fascia, 257, 487
Iliopsoas muscle, 249, 396–397, 477–480, 487–488, 492
Iliopsoas tendon, 491
Iliopubic eminence, 243, 330, 333–334, 338, 473–474
Iliopubic tract, 255, 341, 343, 345
Iliotibial tract, 468, 477, 479, 481–482, 489, 492–495, 497, 501–503, 506–508
Ilium
arcuate line of, 336
body of, 334, 473
radiography of, 156, 331
wing of, 243, 330, 334, 338, 473
Incisive canal, 8, 36–39, 41, 64
anastomosis in, 40, 51, 54
communication through, 41
Incisive fossa, 10, 12, 16, 57, 62
Incisive papilla, 57
Incisor teeth, 62–63, 230
Incus, 94–95, 98, 125
lenticular process of, 95
long limb of, 95
short limb of, 95
Inferior ganglion
of glossopharyngeal nerve, 55, 96, 126, 135–136, 207
of vagus nerve, 55, 127–129, 136, 207
Inferolateral trunk, 138
Infradiaphragmatic fascia, 232
Infraglenoid tubercle, 405–406
Infraglottic region, 82
Infrahyoid artery, 76
Infrahyoid fascia, 26–27
Infrahyoid muscles, 28
fascia of, 26, 412
Inframammary lymph nodes, 182
Infra-orbital artery, 3, 35, 51, 54, 72, 83, 87
Infra-orbital canal, infra-orbital nerve entering, 52
Infra-orbital foramen, 4, 6, 35
of newborn, 14
Infra-orbital groove, 4
Infra-orbital margin, 1
Infra-orbital nerve (V_2), 2, 35, 52–55, 71, 83, 85, 122–123
entering infra-orbital canal, 52
internal nasal branches of, 41
superior alveolar branches of, 123
Infra-orbital recess, 43
Infra-orbital vein, 3, 73
Infrapatellar bursa
deep, 498
subcutaneous, 498
Infrapatellar fat pads, 494–495, 498
Infrapatellar synovial fold, 494–495
Infraspinatus fascia, 171, 174, 409
Infraspinatus muscle, 152, 171, 177, 188, 238–240, 406, 409, 411–414, 418, 465, 467
Infraspinatus tendon, 408, 411, 413, 418
Infraspinous fascia, 250
Infraspinous fossa, 406
of scapula, 183
Infratemporal crest, 6
Infratemporal fossa, 6, 16
Infratrochlear nerve, 2, 35, 83, 88
from nasociliary nerve, 52
Infundibular nucleus, 148
Infundibular process, 148
capillary plexus of, 149
Infundibular recess, 109
Infundibular stem, 148
Infundibulum, 115, 141, 148
of fallopian tube, 352–353
leading to frontonasal canal, 37
Inguinal canal, 256–257
Inguinal falx, 246–247, 249, 255–256
Inguinal fold, 367
Inguinal hernia, 255
Inguinal ligament (Poupart's), 242, 245–247, 255–258, 329, 336, 355, 358–359, 385, 468, 470, 472, 479, 485, 488
reflected, 246–247, 255
Inguinal lymph node
deep, 384–386, 472
highest, 261, 384–386
superficial, 261, 296, 384–386, 472
Inguinal region
dissections of, 255
left, 244
right, 244
Inguinal ring
deep, 245, 249, 255–256, 341–343, 345, 364
lateral crus, 255
medial crus, 255
superficial, 245, 255–256, 355, 359, 364–365
Inguinal triangle (Hesselbach's), 249, 255
transversalis fascia within, 255
Inion, 6, 8, 10, 16, 152
Inlet venule, 279
Inner hair cell, 98
Insula (island of Reil), 106, 111, 142
central sulcus of, 106
circular sulcus of, 106
limen of, 106
long gyrus of, 106
short gyri of, 106
Interalveolar septa, 17
Interarytenoid notch, 66
Interatrial septum, 217, 241
Intercalated lymph nodes, 74–75
Intercapitular veins, 402
Intercarpal ligament, dorsal, 442
Intercartilaginous ligaments, 199
Intercavernous septum, of deep fascia of penis, 359–360, 363
Intercavernous sinuses
anterior, 104–105
posterior, 104–105
Interchondral joints, 184
Interclavicular ligament, 184, 404
Intercondylar eminence, 495, 497, 500–501
Intercondylar fossa, 476
Intercostal artery, 188
anterior, 187–188, 251
collateral branches of, 187
lower, anastomoses with, 251
posterior, 167–168, 185–186, 188, 227–228
branch to vertebral body and dura mater, 168
dorsal branch of, 168, 188
lateral cutaneous branch of, 188

Intercostal artery *(Continued)*
lateral mammary branches of lateral cutaneous branches of, 180
right, 188
spinal branch of, 168, 188
third right, 204, 233
supreme, 137, 139
Intercostal lymph nodes, 235
Intercostal membrane
external, 177, 185–186, 188, 254, 413
internal, 177, 188, 227–228, 254, 413
Intercostal muscles, 179, 195, 214, 238–240
external, 173, 177, 185–186, 188, 227–228, 241, 246, 251, 254, 413
innermost, 177, 187–188, 227–228, 241, 251, 254
internal, 177, 185–188, 241, 251, 254
Intercostal nerves, 160, 179, 186–188, 225, 227–228, 484
anterior branch of, 177, 254
cutaneous branches of
anterior, 177, 185, 187–188, 253, 413
anterior branch of lateral, 188
lateral, 174, 177, 185–186, 188, 253, 413
posterior, 177
dorsal ramus of, 177
eighth, 206
first, 224, 416
lateral branch of, 177
lower, 190
medial branch of, 177
posterior branch of, 177, 413
sixth, 206
third, 236
ventral ramus of, 177
Intercostal veins
anterior, 187, 189
collateral branches of, 187
internal, 252
posterior, 189, 227–228, 234
superior
left, 228, 234
right, 189, 227, 234
tributaries to axillary vein, 252
Intercostal vessels, 179
Intercostobrachial nerve, 186, 253, 400–401, 413, 415, 460
Intercrural fibers, 245, 255–256
Intercuneiform ligaments, dorsal, 514
Interdigitating fibers, of levator veli palatini muscle, 57
Interfoveolar ligament, 249
Interglobular spaces of teeth, 63
Intergluteal (natal) cleft, 152
Interlobar arteries, 312
lymph vessels along, 316
Interlobar lymph vessels, 205
Intermaxillary suture, 10, 35
Intermediate bursa, 448
Intermediate nerve (of Wrisberg), 61, 105, 115, 124–125, 132, 134, 136
distribution of, 119
Intermediolateral cell column, 304, 319
Intermediolateral nucleus, of gray matter, preganglionic sympathetic cell bodies in, 53, 133–135
Intermesenteric (para-aortic) plexus, 262, 297, 301–303, 317–318, 388, 390, 392–395
renal branches from, 317
transverse section of, 328
upper ureteric branches from, 317
Intermetacarpal joints, 442
Intermuscular septum
anterior, 510
anteromedial, 479, 487–488
lateral, 417–418, 421, 431, 434, 465, 492
medial, 417–419, 421, 431, 433–434, 492
transverse, 510
Intermuscular stroma, 305
Internal capsule, 109, 142
anterior limb of, 111
cleft for, 111
genu of, 111
posterior limb of, 111
retrolenticular part of, 111
Internal os, 352
Interosseous artery
anterior, 420, 431, 433–436
common, 420, 433–436
posterior, 431, 434–436
recurrent, 420, 431, 435
Interosseous fascia, dorsal, 450
Interosseous intercarpal ligaments, 442
Interosseous membrane, 425, 429, 436, 441, 497–499, 505, 508–510
Interosseous muscles, 451, 515, 523
attachment of, 451
dorsal, 447, 450, 452, 454, 457, 464, 467, 518, 523, 531
first, 431
of foot, 523–524
palmar, 450, 452, 464, 467
plantar, 522, 531
Interosseous nerve
anterior, 434, 436, 463
of leg, 528
posterior, 431, 436, 466
Interosseous talocalcaneal ligament, 514
Interosseous tendon, 451
Interpectoral (Rotter's) lymph nodes, 181–182
Interpeduncular cistern, 110
Interpeduncular fossa, posterior perforated substance in, 108
Interphalangeal (IP) joint, 515
Interphalangeal ligaments, 445
Interproximal spaces of teeth, 63
Intersigmoid recess, 265, 313
Intersphincteric groove, 370–372
Interspinalis cervical muscle, 173, 177
Interspinalis lumbar muscle, 173, 177
Interspinalis thoracic muscle, 177
Interspinous ligament, 158–159
Interspinous plane, 244
Interthalamic adhesion, 107, 109, 111–112, 116, 147–148
Intertragic notch, 95
Intertransversarii muscles, 173, 177
Intertransverse ligament, 184
Intertrochanteric crest, 474–476, 490
Intertrochanteric line, 474
Intertubercular plane, 244
Intertubercular sulcus, 405
Intertubercular tendon sheath, 408, 413, 417
Interureteric crest, 348
Interventricular artery, anterior, diagonal branch of, 215
Interventricular foramen (of Monro), 107, 109–110, 112, 116, 146–147
Interventricular septum, 221, 241
membranous part of, 217
muscular part of, 213, 217–218, 220–222
Interventricular sulcus
anterior, 209, 241
posterior, 211–212
Intervertebral discs, 158–159
cervical, 21–22
lumbar, 155
radiography of, 156
lumbosacral, 192, 334
thoracic, 191, 239–240
transverse section of, 326–328
Intervertebral foramen, 21, 154–155, 157–159
dorsal root of, 177
Intervertebral vein, 169
Intestinal glands, 305
Intestinal lymphatic trunk, 295
Intestinal trunk, 261
Intestines, 226. *See also* Large intestine; Small intestine
innervation of, 163–164
intrinsic autonomic plexuses of, 305
mesenteric relations of, 264–265
Intra-articular ligament, of head of rib, 184
Intraarticular sternocostal ligament, 184
Intraculminate vein, 145
Intralaminar nuclei, 112
Intralobular arteriole, 279
Intralobular bile ductule, 279
Intramuscular plexus
circular, 305
longitudinal, 305
Intraparietal lobule, 106
Intrapulmonary airways
schema of, 201
structure of, 201
subdivisions of, 201
Intrapulmonary blood circulation, schema of, 202
Intrapulmonary lymph nodes, 205
Intrarenal arteries, 312
Intrinsic autonomic plexuses, of intestines, 305
Intrinsic muscles, 60, 129
Inversion, of foot, 469
Investing fascia, 344, 348, 350, 355–356, 359–361, 369
Iridocorneal angle, 89–90, 92
trabecular meshwork and spaces of, 90
Iris, 83, 89, 91–92
arteries and veins of, 93
folds of, 90
major arterial circle of, 90, 92–93
minor arterial circle of, 90, 92–93
Irritant receptors, 207
Ischial spine, 158, 243, 258, 330, 333–338, 376, 389, 473–474, 490, 530
measurements of, 332
radiograph of, 331
Ischial tuberosity, 158, 243, 330, 333–334, 337, 339, 355–356, 358–361, 370, 373, 473–475, 482, 489–490, 530
measurements of, 332
Ischio-anal fossa, 356, 359–360, 370, 373
anterior recess of, 249, 348, 350, 374
communication in, 374
fat body of, 355, 358, 370, 396
posterior recess of, 374
pus in, 374
transverse fibrous septum of, 370, 372
Ischiocavernosus muscle, 340, 348, 350, 355–357, 359–361, 369, 373, 382–383, 397
Ischiococcygeus muscle, 258, 335–337
Ischiofemoral ligament, 474, 491
Ischiopubic ramus, 333–334, 339, 344, 350, 355–356, 358, 360–362, 373
Ischium, 397, 475
body of, 473
radiograph of, 331
ramus of, 473
Island of Reil. *See* Insula
Isthmus
of cingulate gyrus, 107–108
of fallopian tube, 352
of thyroid gland, 76
of uterus, 352

Longitudinal muscle *(Continued)*
of ileum, 272, 274
inferior, 47, 151
of jejunum, 272
outer, of stomach, 232, 270
of rectum, 371–372
superior, 47, 151
of vermiform appendix, 275
Longitudinal pharyngeal muscles, 65, 67, 69
Longus capitis muscle, 29–30, 42, 47, 151
communication with cervical plexus, 33
nerves to, 130
Longus colli muscle, 26, 30, 151, 229
communication with cervical plexus, 33
innervation of, 416
nerves to, 130
Loop of Heiss, 347
Lower limb
dermatomes of, 469
lymph vessels and nodes of, 472
movements of, 469
superficial nerves of, 470–471
superficial veins of, 470–471
surface anatomy, 468
Lumbar artery, 167, 259
anastomoses with, 251
Lumbar cistern, 156
Lumbar ganglion, 297
first, 163
Lumbar lordosis, 153
Lumbar lymph nodes, 261, 384
Lumbar lymph trunks, 316
Lumbar lymphatic trunk, 295
Lumbar plexus, 160, 225, 483–485, 525–526
muscular branches from, 262
Lumbar region, 176
left, 244
right, 244
vertebral ligaments, 159
Lumbar spinal nerves, 176
dorsal and ventral roots of, 166
enlargement of, 161
L1, 160
dermatome of, 162
dorsal ramus of, 174
posterior rami of, 250
spinous process of, 176
ventral ramus of, 174, 388
vertebrae relation to, 161
L2
dermatome of, 162
dorsal ramus of, 174
ganglion of, 390
posterior rami of, 250
ventral ramus of, 158
vertebrae relation to, 161
L3
dermatome of, 162
dorsal ramus of, 174
posterior rami of, 250
ventral ramus of, 393
vertebrae relation to, 161
L4, 158
dermatome of, 162
vertebrae relation to, 161
L5, 160, 390
dermatome of, 162
dorsal ramus of, 158
ventral ramus of, 388
vertebrae relation to, 161
ventral ramus of, 485
Lumbar triangle (of Petit), 152, 250
internal oblique muscle in, 171
Lumbar trunk
left, 261
right, 261
Lumbar trunk ganglion
lower, 225
upper, 225
Lumbar veins, 310
ascending, 260, 310
right, 260
Lumbar vertebrae, 155, 243
arteries of, 167
articulated, lateral view of, 155
body of, 155, 159
L1, 160
body of, 158, 267
spinal nerve relation to, 161
L2
body of, 176
spinal nerve relation to, 161
superior view of, 155
L3
body of, 341, 345
posterior view of, 155
spinal nerve relation to, 161
L4
body of, 334
posterior view of, 155
spinal nerve relation to, 161
L5, 160
body of, 156, 158, 334
radiograph of, 331
sagittal CT images of, 375
spinal nerve relation to, 161
radiography of, 156
section through, 166
spinous process of, transverse section of, 328
transverse processes of, 243, 330
Lumbocostal ligament, 309
Lumbocostal triangle, 192
Lumbocostal trigone, 258
Lumbosacral intervertebral discs, 334
transverse process of, 192
Lumbosacral plexus, 262, 317, 484
Lumbosacral region, vertebral ligaments, 158
Lumbosacral trunks, 262, 317, 388, 483–486, 525–526
Lumbrical muscles, 448–452, 463–464, 467, 520–521, 523, 528, 531
tendons of, 522
Lumbrical tendon, 448, 515
Lumen, 305
Lunate bone, 439, 442–443
radiographs of, 444
Lunate sulcus, 106
Lunate (articular) surface, 334
Lungs, 179, 315
apex of, 193
innervation of, 119, 163–164
left, 196, 208, 212, 214, 238–240
anterior border of, 196
apex of, 194, 196
bronchopulmonary segments of, 197–198
cardiac impression of, 196
cardiac notch of, 193, 195
diaphragmatic surface of, 196
esophagus area of, 196
hilum of, 209
inferior border of, 193–194, 196
inferior lobe of, 195–198, 324
lymph vessels and nodes of, 205
oblique fissure of, 193–194, 196, 239
root of, 190
superior lobe of, 195–198, 213, 237
trachea area of, 196
lymph nodes of, 205
lymph vessels of, 205
lymphatic drainage routes of, 205
medial views of, 196
Lungs *(Continued)*
radiography of, 156
right, 196, 208, 210, 214, 238–240
anterior border of, 196
apex of, 196
bronchopulmonary segments of, 197–198
cardiac impression of, 196
diaphragmatic surface of, 196
esophagus area of, 196
hilum of, 209
horizontal fissure of, 193–196
inferior border of, 193–194, 196
inferior lobe of, 195–198, 324
lymph vessels and nodes of, 205
middle lobe of, 195–198, 213
oblique fissure of, 193–196
root of, 190
superior lobe of, 195–198, 237
trachea area of, 196
in situ, anterior view of, 195
topography of
anterior view of, 193
posterior view of, 194
Lunotriquetral ligament, 441
Lunula, 220
Lunule, 458
Luschka
cleft of, 21
foramen of, 109–110
prerectal muscle fibers of, 339
Lutea, 89
Lymph follicles, 60
Lymph nodes
of abdominal wall, posterior, 261
of esophagus, 235
in femoral canal, 257
of genitalia
female, 384
male, 386
of head and neck, 74
of kidneys, 316
of large intestine, 296
of lower limb, 472
of lung, 205
of mammary gland, 181
of pancreas, 294
of pelvis
female, 384
male, 386
of perineum, female, 385
of pharynx and tongue, 75
of small intestine, 295
of stomach, 293
transverse section of, 328, 397
of upper limb, 403
of urinary bladder, 316
Lymph vessels
of abdominal wall, posterior, 261
cortical, 316
of esophagus, 235
of genitalia
female, 384
male, 386
of head and neck, 74
of kidneys, 316
of large intestine, 296
of lower limb, 472
of lung, 205
of mammary gland, 181
medullary, 316
of pancreas, 294
of pelvis
female, 384
male, 386
of perineum, female, 385
of pharynx and tongue, 75
of small intestine, 295

Lymph vessels *(Continued)*
of stomach, 293
of upper limb, 403
of urinary bladder, 316
Lymphatic drainage, of breast, 182
Lymphatic drainage routes, of lungs, 205
Lymphatic duct, right, 182, 295
Lymphatic trunk
intestinal, 295
lumbar, 295

M

Mackenrodt's ligament, 342–343, 350–351
Macula, fovea centralis in, 89, 92
Macular arteriole
inferior, 92
superior, 92
Macular venule
inferior, 92
superior, 92
Macular zone, 121
Macule, 92
Magendie, foramen of, 109–110, 116, 118
Mallear fold
anterior, 95
posterior, 95
Mallear stria, arteries of, 96
Malleolar artery
anterior lateral, 508–509, 517–518
anterior medial, 508–509, 517–518
Malleolus
lateral, 468, 500–501, 503–508, 517–518, 531
medial, 468, 500–501, 503–505, 507–508, 516–518, 531
Malleus, 94–95, 98
anterior ligament of, 95
handle of, 95–96
head of, 95, 125
lateral process of, 95
superior ligament of, 95
Mammary gland
anterolateral dissection, 179
arteries of, 180
lymph nodes of, 181
lymph vessels of, 181
sagittal section of, 179
Mammillary body, 107–109, 113, 115, 148
Mammillary process, 155
Mammillothalamic fasciculus, 107
Mammillothalamic tract (of Vicq d'Azyr), 148
Mandible, 4, 6, 15, 26, 64
of aged person, 17
alveolar part of, 17
angle of, 1, 15, 17, 66
base of, 17
body of, 4, 6, 15, 17, 29, 43
buccinator crest of, 70
condylar process of, 15, 17
head of, 6
condyle of, 7
coronoid process of, 6–7, 15, 17, 42
digastric fossa of, 17
head of, 17
interalveolar septa of, 17
lingula of, 17
mandibular foramen of, 17
mandibular notch of, 6, 17
mental foramen of, 4, 6, 17
mental protuberance of, 1, 4, 17
mental spines of, 17
mental tubercle of, 4
mylohyoid groove of, 17
mylohyoid line of, 17
neck of, 17, 42
oblique line of, 6, 17, 70
pterygoid fovea of, 17
Mandible *(Continued)*
ramus of, 4–6, 15, 17, 24, 29, 47
temporalis muscle insertion to, 6
retromolar fossa of, 17
sublingual fossa of, 17
submandibular fossa of, 17
Mandibular canal, 47
Mandibular foramen, 17, 58
inferior alveolar nerve entering, 50
Mandibular fossa, 6, 10, 14, 100
inferior, 18
Mandibular lymph nodes, 74
Mandibular nerves (V_2), 88, 105, 122–123, 126, 132, 134–136
meningeal branch of, 88
Mandibular nerves (V_3), 2, 12–13, 18, 50, 71
anterior division of, 50
articular branch of, 123
lateral view of, 50
medial view of, 50
meningeal branch of, 12–13, 50, 123
motor root of, 50
parotid branches of, 123
posterior division of, 50
sensory root of, 50
superficial temporal branches of, 123
Mandibular notch, 6, 15, 17
Mandibular periosteum, 63
Manubriosternal joint, 184
Manubriosternal junction, 240
Manubriosternal synchondrosis, 404
Manubrium of sternum, 26–27, 29, 64, 183–184, 187, 195, 238–239, 404
Marginal artery, 288, 302, 376
left (obtuse), 215
right, 216
Marginal collecting vessels, 75
Marginal plexus, 302
Marginal sulcus, 107
Masseter muscle, 24, 27, 29, 42, 46–48, 151
deep part of, 48
insertion of, 6
superficial part of, 48
Masseteric artery, 6, 49, 51, 72
Masseteric fascia, 25
Masseteric nerve (V_3), 6, 49–51, 71, 123
Mastication, muscles involved in, 48–49
innervation of, 119
Mastoid air cells, 7, 42, 55, 96
Mastoid angle, 11
Mastoid antrum, 90
Mastoid canaliculus, 10, 12
Mastoid emissary vein, 3
in mastoid foramen, 12
Mastoid foramen, 10, 12–13, 16
Mastoid lymph nodes, 74
Mastoid notch, 10
Mastoid process, 6, 10, 15–16, 24, 27, 29–30, 58–59, 100, 173
Maxilla, 4, 6, 8, 10
alveolar process of, 4, 6, 8, 16, 37, 43
anterior nasal spine of, 4, 6, 8, 37
frontal process of, 4, 6, 35, 37, 83
incisive canal of, 8, 37–38
incisive fossa of, 10
infra-orbital foramen of, 4, 6
infratemporal surface of, 6
intermaxillary suture of, 10
nasal crest of, 38
nasal spine of, anterior, 35, 38
nasal surface of, 8
of newborn, 14, 45
orbital surface of, 4
palatine process of, 7 8, 10, 16, 36–38, 57, 62, 100
tuberosity of, 6, 16
zygomatic process of, 4, 10
Maxillary artery, 18, 34, 40, 49–51, 54–55, 71–72, 96, 102, 132, 134–135, 137, 139
posterior lateral nasal branch of, 51
Maxillary bone, 42
Maxillary nerve (V_2), 13, 39, 50, 52, 54–55, 71, 88, 105, 122–123, 132, 134–136
entering foramen rotundum, 53
meningeal branch of, 88, 123
nasal branches of
nasopalatine, 123
posterior inferior lateral, 39, 54
posterior superior, 53
posterior superior lateral, 39, 41, 54, 123
posterior superior medial, 123
pharyngeal branch of, 39, 123
Maxillary nerves (V_2), 2
Maxillary ostium, 55
Maxillary periosteum, 63
Maxillary plexus, 132
Maxillary sinus, 5, 7, 42, 44, 53, 55, 86
growth of, 45
middle, 43
of newborn, 45
opening of, 36–37, 43–44
postsynaptic fibers to, 53
recesses of, 43
transverse section of, 42
wall of, 54
Maxillary veins, 73, 87
McBurney's point, 275
Medial eminence, 116
Medial ligament, of ankle, 514
Median aperture, 109–110, 116, 118
of fourth ventricle, 147
Median nerve, 400, 415–417, 419, 421, 432–434, 436, 441, 447, 449, 452–453, 459–463
articular branch of, 463
communicating branch of, 453, 460, 463–464
digital branch, 400
palmar branch of, 400, 402, 432–433, 446, 453, 459, 463
palmar digital branches of, 400, 456, 459
common, 447, 460
proper, 460
recurrent branch of, 446–447, 453, 460
Median nuclei, 112
Median raphe
of levator ani muscle, 337
levator plate, 336
between mylohyoid muscles, 58
Median sulcus, 60
dorsal, 116
Mediastinal lymph nodes, 238
posterior, 235
Mediastinal nodes, anterior, pathway to, 181
Mediastinal pleurae, 191, 209
Mediastinum
anterior, 191
lung area for, 196
cross section of, 213
lateral view of
left, 228
right, 227
superior, great vessels of, 203
Mediastinum testis, 368
Medulla oblongata, 13, 42, 53, 107, 116, 125, 135, 164, 224, 303, 318
in foramen magnum, 12
lower part of, 136
nuclear layer of, 114
Medullary artery, segmental, 167–168
Medullary lamina
external, 112
internal, 112

Medullary lymph vessels, 316
Medullary vein
anteromedian, 145
segmental, 169
anterior, 169
posterior, 169
Medullary velum
inferior, 107, 114, 116
superior, 107, 114–116
Meibomian (tarsal) glands, 83
Meissner's plexus, 305
Membranous labyrinths, 97–98
orientation of, 99
Membranous septum
atrioventricular part of, 213, 217–222
interventricular part of, 213, 218–222
Meningeal arteries, 102
accessory, 12–13, 51, 96, 102
anterior, 87
dorsal, 138
middle, 13, 18, 49–51, 71–72, 96, 101–103, 105, 132, 137–139
branches of, 103
frontal branches of, 102
left, 137
parietal branches of, 102
posterior, 3, 13
in mastoid foramen, 12
Meningeal nerve, 13
Meningeal plexus, middle, 132
Meningeal sheath, 85–86, 93
Meningeal vein, middle, 13, 101, 103
Meningeal vessels
anterior, groove for, 11
middle, 12
groove for, 11
grooves for branches of, 8–9
posterior, groove for, 11
Meninges, 13, 101, 103
arteries to, 137
Meningohypophyseal trunk, 102, 138
cavernous sinus branches of, 102
meningeal branches of, 102
tentorial branches of, 102, 138
Meniscofemoral ligament, posterior, 495–496
Meniscus, 442
lateral, 494–496, 498
attachment of horns of, 495
medial, 494–496
attachment of horns of, 495
Mental foramen, 4, 6, 17
Mental nerve, 2, 50, 71, 123
Mental protuberance, 1, 4, 17
Mental vein, 73
Mentalis muscle, 25, 48, 124, 151
Meridional fibers, 90
Mesencephalic nucleus, of trigeminal nerve, 117–118, 123, 136
Mesencephalic vein
lateral, 145
posterior, 147
Mesenteric artery
inferior, 259, 264, 271, 288, 297, 302, 308, 310, 313–314, 376, 378–379, 388
superior, 176, 226, 259, 264, 268, 271–273, 281, 284, 286–288, 290, 294, 298–301, 307–308, 310, 313–315, 321, 388
arteriogram of, 285
axial CT images of, 322–323
transverse section of, 327–328
Mesenteric ganglia, 297
celiac, 127
inferior, 163, 297, 302–303, 317, 387–388, 392–395
superior, 127, 163–164, 262, 299–304, 307, 317–319, 387–388, 392–395
Mesenteric lymph nodes
inferior, 261, 296
superior, 261, 293–296
Mesenteric plexus
inferior, 297, 302, 388
superior, 297–299, 301, 307, 388
Mesenteric vein
inferior, 234, 264, 281, 289, 291–292, 294, 377
superior, 176, 234, 268, 271–272, 281, 287, 289–292, 294, 315
transverse section of, 326–328
Mesentericoparietal recess (fossa), 264
Mesentery, 176, 265, 272, 321
peritoneal layers of, 305
root of, 268, 271, 281, 313, 341, 345
transverse section of, 328
Meso-appendix, 273, 275, 301
Mesocolic taenia, 273–274, 276
Mesocolon
sigmoid, 265, 268, 276, 288, 308, 313, 369
transverse, 263–268, 271, 276, 281, 288, 290, 308, 321
attachment of, 281–282
Mesometrium, of broad ligament, 352
Mesonephric (wolffian) duct, 364, 367
Mesonephric tubules, 367
caudal, 367
residua of, 367
cranial, 367
Mesosalpinx
of broad ligament, 342, 352
laminae of, 353
Mesovarium, 350
of broad ligament, 352
laminae of, 353
Metacarpal arteries
dorsal, 456
palmar, 435, 452
Metacarpal bones, 439–443, 445, 451
fifth, 430–431, 434
first, 431, 434, 449, 454
radiographs of, 444
second, 431
Metacarpal ligaments
deep transverse, 445, 452
palmar, 445
superficial transverse, 402, 446
Metacarpal veins, dorsal, 455
Metacarpophalangeal joint, 445
Metacarpophalangeal ligaments, 445
Metaphysis, nutrient branches to, 458
Metatarsal arteries, dorsal, 509, 517–518, 523
Metatarsal bones, 511–512, 515, 523–524
fifth, 505–506
first, 505, 514
tuberosity of, 516–517, 522–523, 531
Metatarsal ligaments
deep transverse, 515, 523
dorsal, 514, 523
superficial transverse, 519
Metatarsal veins, dorsal, 470
Metatarsophalangeal (MTP) joint, 515
Midbrain, imaging of, 151
Midcarpal joint, 439, 442
Midclavicular line
left, 244
right, 244
Midline groove, 60
Midpalmar space, 447–448, 450
Minute fasciculi, 446
Mitral cell, 120
Mitral heart valve, 210, 213–214, 218–222
anterior cusp of, 213, 218–221
commissural cusp of, 219–220
leaflet of, 241
left fibrous ring of, 219
posterior cusp of, 213, 218–221
Mixed fibers, 117–118
Modiolus, 25
of cochlea, 98
Molar minor salivary glands, 57
Molar teeth, 62–63
growth of, 45
Monocular fields, 121
Monro, interventricular foramen of, 107, 109–110, 112, 116, 146–147
Mons pubis, 354
Morgagni
hydatid of, 352
urethral lacunae of, 363
Motor nucleus
of facial nerve, 124–125
of trigeminal nerve, 117–118, 123, 136
Mucosa, 305
of duodenum, 272
esophageal, 69, 232
of ileum, 272
of large intestine, 276
olfactory, 120
distribution of, 39
of stomach, 270
Mucous glands, 60
crypt of, 60
duct of, 60
innervation of, 164
Müllerian duct, 367
Müller's (tarsal) muscle, superior, 83
Multifidus lumborum muscles, 173
Multifidus muscles, 176–177
Multifidus thoracis muscles, 173
Muscles
anorectal, 372
of arm
anterior view of, 417
posterior view of, 418
of back
deep layers, 173
intermediate layers, 172
superficial layers, 171
of dorsum of foot, 517
of duodenum, 272
of esophagus, 231
of eye, extrinsic, 86
of face, 124
facial expression, 25, 47
innervation of, 119
of forearm
attachments of, 437–438
deep layer, 431, 434
extensors of wrist and digits, 427
flexors of digits, 429
flexors of wrist, 428
intermediate layer, 433
rotators of radius, 426
superficial layer, 430, 432
of hand, 452
of hip
attachments of, 477–478
lateral view, 481
posterior views, 482
of large intestine, 276
of larynx, 80
action of intrinsic, 81
of leg
attachments of, 502
deep dissection, 505, 508
intermediate dissection, 504
lateral view of, 506
superficial dissection, 503, 507

Muscles *(Continued)*
in mastication, 48–49
innervation of, 119
of neck
anterior view of, 27
infrahyoid and suprahyoid, 28
lateral view of, 29
scalene and prevertebral, 30
of pharynx
lateral view of, 70
partially opened posterior view of, 67
sagittal section, 65
of rotator cuff, 411
of shoulder, 409
of soft palate, 65
of sole of foot
first layer, 520
second layer, 521
third layer, 522
of thigh, 479–480
attachments of, 477–478
lateral view, 481
posterior views, 482
of tongue, 60, 129
inferior longitudinal, 129
superior longitudinal, 129
transverse, 129
vertical, 129
Muscular artery, 92–93
Muscular vein, 92
Muscularis mucosae, 305, 371
of anal canal, 371–372
of rectum, 372
Musculocutaneous nerve, 415–417, 419, 421, 433–434, 436, 459–463
anterior branch of, 462
articular branch of, 462
posterior branch of, 462
terminal part of, 400–401, 432
Musculofascial extensions
to urethra, 337
to vagina, 337
Musculophrenic arteries, 186–187, 195, 208, 251
Musculophrenic vein, 186–187, 252
Myelencephalon, 303
Myenteric (Auerbach's) plexus, 305
Mylohyoid artery, 51
mylohyoid nerve to, 51, 58
Mylohyoid groove, 17
Mylohyoid line, 17
Mylohyoid muscle, 27–29, 31, 34, 43, 46–47, 50, 58–59, 64, 70, 151
innervation of, 119
median raphe between, 58
nerve to, 49–50, 58, 123
Mylohyoid nerve, 18, 47, 51, 71
to mylohyoid artery, 51
Myometrium, 352

N

Nail bed, 458
Nail body, 458
Nail matrix, 458
Nail root, 458
Nares, 1
anterior, 1
Nasal aperture, posterior, 16, 38
Nasal artery
dorsal, 3, 35, 51, 72, 83, 87, 139
external, 35
lateral, 35
Nasal bone, 1, 4, 6, 8, 35, 37–38
of newborn, 14, 45
Nasal cartilage, accessory, 35
Nasal cavity, 43, 84–85
arteries of, 40
autonomic innervation of, 53
bones of, 45
floor of, 36
growth of, 45
innervation of, 119
lateral wall of, 36–37, 40–41
medial wall of, 38
nerves of, 39, 41
postsynaptic fibers to, 53
Nasal concha
highest, 37
of newborn, 45
inferior, 4–5, 8, 36–37, 42–44, 66, 84
ethmoidal process of, 37
growth of, 45
middle, 4, 8, 36–37, 43–44, 84
growth of, 45
of newborn, 45
superior, 8, 36–37
of newborn, 45
Nasal crest, 38
Nasal meatus
inferior, 36, 43, 84
middle, 36, 43
atrium of, 36
of newborn, 45
opening into, 44
superior, 36
of newborn, 45
Nasal nerve
external, 35
lateral
inferior, 132
posterior, 132
superior, 132
posterior, 134
Nasal retinal arteriole
inferior, 92
superior, 92
Nasal retinal venule
inferior, 92
superior, 92
Nasal septal cartilage, 35
lateral process of, 35, 37–38
Nasal septum, 5, 16, 38, 40–41, 43, 64, 66
bony, 8
growth of, 45
nerves of, 39
schematic hinge of, 40–41
Nasal slit, 13
Nasal spine, 37–38
anterior, 4, 6, 8, 37–38
posterior, 10, 37–38
Nasal vein
dorsal, 3
external, 73
Nasal vestibule, 36, 38, 42
Nasal wall, lateral view of, 8
Nasalis muscle, 124, 151
alar part of, 25, 35
transverse part of, 25, 35
Nasion, 4
Nasociliary nerve (V_1), 13, 52, 85, 88, 122–123, 132–133
Nasofrontal vein, 3, 73, 87
Nasolabial lymph nodes, 74
Nasolabial sulcus, 1
Nasolacrimal canal, opening of, 37
Nasolacrimal duct, 84
of newborn, 45
opening of, 36, 84
Nasolacrimal foramen, of newborn, 45
Nasopalatine nerve (V_2), 39, 41, 53, 61
greater palatine nerves communication with, 54
groove for, 38
Nasopalatine nerve (V_2) *(Continued)*
in incisive fossa, 12
septal branch of, 54
Nasopalatine vessels, groove for, 38
Nasopharynx, 64, 66, 94, 105
airway to, 36
Navicular bone, 511–512, 514, 523–524, 531
tuberosity of, 515, 518, 523
Navicular fossa, 344, 363
Neck
autonomic nerves in, 131
bony framework of, 15
cutaneous nerves of, 2, 31
fascial layers of, 26
lymph vessels and nodes of, 74
muscles of
anterior view of, 27
infrahyoid and suprahyoid, 28
lateral view of, 29
scalene and prevertebral, 30
nerves of, 32–33
of scapula, 183
skin of, 26
subcutaneous tissue of, 26
superficial veins of, 31
surface anatomy of, 1
triangle of, 175
posterior, 171, 185
vessels of, 32–33
Nerves. *See also specific nerves*
of abdominal wall
anterior, 253
posterior, 262
of back, 174
of buttock, 490
of esophagus, 236
of external genitalia
female, 391
male, 387
of hand, 453
of head, 2
of heart, 223–224
of hip, 490
of larynx, 82
of lower ureter, 395
of nasal cavity, 39, 41
of neck, 2, 32–33
of oral and pharyngeal regions, 71
of orbit, 88
of pelvic viscera
female, 390
male, 388
of perineum
female, 391
male, 389
of reproductive organs
female, 393
male, 394
of shoulder, 465
of teeth, 63
of thigh
anterior view, 487–488
posterior view, 489
of upper limb, 400, 460–461
of urinary bladder, 395
of wrist, 449
Nervus intermedius, 96
Neurohypophysis, 141, 148–149
Neurovascular compartment, 421
Neurovascular sheath, 343
Newborn, skull of, 14
Nipple, 178–179, 329
Node of Cloquet or Rosenmüller, 261
Nodule, of inferior vermis, 114, 116
Nose, 35
ala of, 1
innervation of, 164
transverse section of, 42

Nostril, 1
Nuchal line
inferior, 10, 16
superior, 10, 16, 171–173
Nucleus ambiguus, 117–118, 126–128
Nucleus of lens, 90–91
Nucleus pulposus, 21, 155, 159
Nutrient artery, of femur, 491
Nutrient foramen, of femur, 476

O

Obex, 116
Oblique fissure, of lungs
left, 193–194, 196, 239
right, 193–196
Oblique muscle
external, 7, 171–172, 174, 176, 178–179, 185, 188, 242, 245–247, 249–251, 253–256, 258, 309, 328–329, 341, 345, 409–410, 481
aponeurosis of, 7, 245–247, 253, 255, 257, 355, 359
aponeurotic part of, 7, 245–247, 253, 255, 257
deep fascia over, 358
muscular part of, 245
transverse section of, 326, 328
inferior, 85–86, 122, 151
internal, 7, 171–172, 176, 185, 246–247, 249–251, 255–256, 258, 309, 328, 341, 345
aponeurosis of, 7, 247, 253
aponeurotic part of, 7, 247, 253
in lumbar triangle (of Petit), 171
tendon of origin of, 176
transverse section of, 328
superior, 85–86, 88, 122, 151
innervation of, 119
Oblique vein, of left atrium, 211
Obliquus capitis inferior muscle, 172, 175, 177
Obliquus capitis superior muscle, 172–173, 175, 177
Obturator anastomotic artery, 345
Obturator artery, 249, 255, 259, 313–314, 342–343, 376, 378, 380–381, 388, 396, 491, 499
accessory, 255, 257, 376, 380
acetabular branch of, 474, 491
anterior branch of, 474
posterior branch of, 474
right, 381
Obturator canal, 334–336, 338, 342–343, 346, 380, 488
Obturator crest, 334, 473
Obturator externus muscle, 397, 477–478, 480, 488, 526, 531
Obturator fascia, 335–336, 338, 342, 346, 350, 356, 370, 380
Obturator foramen, 243, 330, 473, 475
radiograph of, 331
Obturator groove, 473
Obturator internus muscle, 249, 258, 335–339, 343, 346, 348, 350, 361, 370, 376, 380, 389, 396–397, 477–478, 482, 486, 489–490, 530–531
nerve to, 484, 486, 489–490
transverse section of, 397
Obturator internus tendon, 337, 530
Obturator lymph nodes, 384
Obturator membrane, 334, 350, 474
Obturator nerves, 249, 262, 313, 378, 388, 390, 483–486, 525–526
accessory, 262, 484 485
anterior branch of, 488, 492, 526
articular branch of, 526
Obturator nerves *(Continued)*
cutaneous branches of, 471, 488, 526
posterior branch of, 488, 492, 526
branches of, 488
Obturator vein, 249, 255, 260, 291, 377, 396
accessory, 255, 257
right, 381
Occipital artery, 3, 34, 72–73, 102, 137, 139, 175
descending branch of, 34, 175
groove for, 10
mastoid branch of, 102, 137
medial, 143
meningeal branch of, 3
sternocleidomastoid branch of, 34, 72
Occipital bone, 6, 8–11, 22, 160
basilar part of, 8, 10–11, 22, 30, 36–38, 57, 65–68
clivus, 11
condylar canal and fossa of, 10
foramen magnum of, 8, 10
groove for inferior petrosal sinus, 8, 11
groove for occipital sinus, 11
groove for posterior meningeal vessels, 11
groove for superior sagittal sinus, 11
groove for transverse sinus, 11
hypoglossal canal of, 8, 10
jugular foramen of, 8
jugular process of, 30
lateral view of, 14
of newborn, 14
nuchal line of
inferior, 10
superior, 10
occipital crest of
external, 10
internal, 11
occipital protuberance of
external, 8, 10
internal, 11
pharyngeal tubercle of, 10, 64
superior view of, 14
transverse sinus of, groove for, 8
Occipital condyle, 8, 10–11, 16, 30, 100, 129
lateral mass for, 19
superior articular surface for, 19
Occipital crest
external, 10, 16
internal, 11
Occipital groove, 10
Occipital horn, 109–113, 144, 147
Occipital lobe, 106
projection on, 121
Occipital lymph nodes, 74
Occipital nerve
greater, 2, 130, 174–175
lesser, 2, 32–33, 130, 174–175
third, 2, 174–175
Occipital pole, 106
Occipital protuberance
external (inion), 6, 8, 10, 16, 152
internal, 11
Occipital sinus, 104, 145
groove for, 11
Occipital sulcus, transverse, 106
Occipital vein, 3, 73
internal, 147
Occipitalis muscle, 175
innervation of, 119
Occipitofrontalis muscle
frontal belly of, 25, 35, 124, 151
occipital belly of, 25, 124, 175
Occipitomastoid suture, 16
Occipitotemporal gyrus
lateral, 107–108
medial, 107–108
Occipitotemporal sulcus, 107–108
Oculomotor nerve (III), 55, 86, 88, 105, 115, 117–118, 122, 132, 145
branch of, 164
distribution of, 119
inferior branch of, 85, 88, 122
schema of, 122
superior branch of, 13, 85, 88, 122
Oculomotor nucleus, 117–118, 122
accessory, 117–118, 122, 133
Odontoblast layer of teeth, 63
Olecranon, of ulna, 418, 422, 425, 427, 430–431, 465
radiographs of, 423
Olecranon bursa, subcutaneous, 424
Olecranon fossa, 406, 422
radiographs of, 423
Olfactory bulb, 39, 43, 108, 120
afferent fibers from, 120
cells of, 120
efferent fibers to, 120
Olfactory cells, 120
Olfactory mucosa, 120
distribution of, 39
Olfactory nerves (I), 13, 39, 41
distribution of, 119
fibers of, 120
schema of, 120
Olfactory nucleus, anterior, 120
Olfactory stria
lateral, 120
medial, 120
Olfactory sulcus, 108
Olfactory tract, 39, 107–108, 115, 120
lateral nucleus, 120
Olfactory trigone, 120
Olfactory tubercle, 120
Olivary complex, inferior, 118
Olive, 115
Omental (epiploic) appendices, 265, 276
transverse section of, 328
Omental bursa
cross section of, 267
lesser sac, 267, 321
stomach reflected, 266
superior recess of, 266, 268, 277, 321
Omental (epiploic) foramen (of Winslow), 266–267, 269, 278, 321
Omental taenia, 273, 276
Omental (epiploic) veins, 234
Omentum
greater, 262, 265, 267, 269, 276, 278, 321
transverse section of, 327–328
lesser, 267–269, 278, 299, 321
anterior layer of, 280, 298
posterior layer of, 298
right free margin of, 271–272, 281
Omohyoid muscle, 26, 28, 31, 58, 151, 185, 195, 405, 409, 412, 415
fascia of, 185
inferior belly of, 1, 27–29, 32, 129–130
communication with cervical plexus, 33
nerves to, 71
phantom, 34
superior belly of, 27–29, 31, 129–130
communication with cervical plexus, 33
nerves to, 71
Operculum
frontal, 106
orbital, 106
parietal, 106
Ophthalmic artery, 13, 51, 55, 72, 85, 87, 133, 137–139, 141, 144
continuation of, 87
inferior, 87
muscular branch of, 87
supra-orbital branch of, 72
supratrochlear branch of, 72
zygomatic branches of, 87

Ophthalmic nerve (V_1), 2, 50, 52, 55, 88, 105, 122–123, 132–136
  frontal branch of, 13
  lacrimal branch of, 13
  nasociliary branch of, 13
  tentorial branch of, 88, 123
Ophthalmic vein
  inferior, 93
  superior, 13, 73, 85, 87, 93, 105
Opponens digiti minimi muscle, 449, 452, 464, 467
Opponens pollicis muscle, 449, 452–453, 463, 467
Optic canal, 4, 8, 13, 85
Optic chiasm, 43, 105, 107–108, 115, 121, 138, 141–142, 146–148
Optic disc, 85, 92
Optic nerve (II), 13, 43, 55, 85, 88–89, 92, 105, 107–108, 133, 144–145
  distribution of, 119
  internal sheath of, vessels of, 93
  left, 138
  meningeal sheath of, 86, 93
  right, 138
  schema of, 121
Optic radiation, 121
Optic tract, 108–109, 113, 115, 121, 140, 145
Ora serrata, 89, 91–92
Oral cavity, 38, 43, 64
  afferent innervation of, 61
  floor of, 58
  inspection of, 56
  roof of, 57
Oral region
  arteries of, 72
  nerves of, 71
  veins of, 73
Orbicularis oculi muscle, 124, 151
  orbital part of, 25
  palpebral part of, 25, 83
Orbicularis oris muscle, 6, 25, 35, 47–48, 124, 151
Orbiculus ciliaris, 91
Orbit, 44
  arteries and veins of, 87
  fascia of, 85
  frontal and slightly lateral view of, 4
  growth of, 45
  medial wall of, 43
  nerves of, 88
  surface of, 4
Orbital fat, 43
Orbital fat body, 85
Orbital fissure
  inferior, 4, 6, 16, 85
  superior, 4–5, 13, 85
    branch to, 138
Orbital gyri, 108
Orbital muscles, 43
Orbital operculum, 106
Orbital plate, of newborn, 14
Orbital process, of palatine bone, 4, 37
Orbital septum, 83
Orbital sulci, 108
Orbitofrontal artery
  lateral, 140, 142–143
  medial, 138, 140, 142–143
Oropharynx, 26, 64, 66, 68, 230
Os
  external, 352
  internal, 352
Osseous cochlea, 98
Osseous spiral lamina, 97–98
Osteomeatal unit, 36, 44
Otic capsule, 97–98
Otic ganglion, 18, 49–50, 96, 123–124, 126, 132, 134–136, 164
  schema of, 135
Outer hair cells, 98
Oval (vestibular) window, 14, 97
  stapes in, 98
    base of, 94
Ovarian arteries, 313–314, 341–343, 378, 382, 390, 393
  tubal branches of, 382
  ureteric branch from, 314
Ovarian plexus, 390, 393
Ovarian veins, 260, 313, 341–343, 378, 382
  tubal branches of, 382
Ovary, 313, 340–342, 350, 352, 367, 378, 390, 393
  corpus albicans of, 352
  corpus luteum of, 352
  follicle (graafian) of, 352
  ligament of, 340–342, 350–352, 367
  right, 353
  suspensory ligament of, 340–343, 352–353, 367, 378

P

Palate
  growth of, 45
  hard, 64, 68
  innervation of, 119, 164
  postsynaptic fibers to, 53
  soft, 36, 38, 56, 64, 66, 68
    innervation of, 119
    muscles of, 65
Palatine aponeurosis, 57, 65
Palatine artery
  ascending, 51, 68, 72
    tonsillar branches of, 51, 68
  descending, 54–55, 72
  greater, 40, 51, 54–55, 57
    sphenopalatine artery anastomosis with, 54
  lesser, 40, 51, 54–55, 68
    tonsillar branch of, 68
Palatine bone, 8, 10, 37
  horizontal plate of, 8, 10, 16, 36–38, 57, 62, 100
  nasal crest of, 38
  nasal spine of, posterior, 10, 38
  of newborn, 14, 45
  orbital process of, 4, 37
  palatine foramen of
    greater, 10, 12, 37–38
    lesser, 10, 12, 37–38
  perpendicular plate of, 8, 37–38
  posterior nasal spine of, 37
  pyramidal process of, 10, 14, 16
  sphenoidal process of, 37
Palatine folds, transverse, 57
Palatine foramen
  greater, 10, 12, 37–38, 40, 57, 62
  lesser, 10, 12, 37–38, 40, 57, 62
Palatine glands, 57, 64, 68
Palatine nerves (V_2)
  descending, 134
  greater, 39, 41, 53–55, 57, 61, 71, 123, 132, 134
    in greater palatine foramen, 12
    nasopalatine nerve communication with, 54
    posterior inferior lateral nasal branch of, 41
  lesser, 39, 41, 53–55, 61, 71, 123, 132, 134
    in lesser palatine foramen, 12
Palatine process, 7–8, 10, 16
  of maxilla, 36–38, 57, 62, 100
Palatine raphe, 57
Palatine tonsil, 47, 56–57, 60, 64, 66, 68
Palatine vein, 73
  external, 73
Palatine vessels, 12
Palatoglossal arch, 47, 56, 60, 68
Palatoglossus muscle, 47, 57, 59–60, 68, 127, 151
Palatomaxillary suture, 10
Palatopharyngeal arch, 47, 56, 60, 66, 68
Palatopharyngeal sphincter, 65
Palatopharyngeus muscle, 47, 57, 59–60, 65, 67–69, 127, 151
Palmar aponeurosis, 402, 428, 432, 441, 446–447, 450
Palmar arch
  deep, 435, 452
  superficial, 435, 449, 453
Palmar carpal arterial arch, 452
Palmar carpal ligament, 402, 432–433, 441, 446–447, 449, 453, 464
Palmar crease, proximal, 398
Palmar digital arteries, 435, 446, 453, 456
  common, 435, 447, 450, 452–453
  proper, 435, 447, 458
Palmar digital nerves, 402, 446–447, 453, 464
  common, 450, 463–464
  proper, 447, 453, 458, 463
Palmar digital veins, 402
Palmar ligaments, 445, 448, 451, 458
Palmar metacarpal arteries, 435
  proper, 453
Palmar radiolunate ligament, 441
Palmar ulnocarpal ligament, 441
Palmaris brevis muscle, 446, 464, 467
Palmaris carpi ulnaris muscle, 428
Palmaris longus muscle, 428, 432, 434, 436, 463, 467
Palmaris longus tendon, 398, 433, 436, 441, 446–447, 449
Palmate folds, 352
Palpebral arterial arches
  inferior, 87
  superior, 87
Palpebral artery
  lateral, 87
    inferior, 87
    superior, 87
  medial, 87
    inferior, 87
    superior, 87
Palpebral conjunctiva, 83, 85
  inferior, 83
  superior, 83
Palpebral ligament
  lateral, 83, 85
  medial, 83, 85
Pampiniform venous plexus, 252, 365, 379, 381
Pancreas, 127, 176, 267–268, 281, 320–321
  autonomic nerves of, 307
  axial CT images of, 322
  body of, 266, 281
    axial CT images of, 322
  head of, 266, 271–272, 281
    arteries of, 286
    axial CT images of, 323
  innervation of, 163–164
  lymph vessels and nodes of, 294
  neck of, 281
  in situ, 281
  tail of, 266, 281–282, 308
    artery to, 284
  transverse section of, 325
  uncinate process of, 281
    transverse section of, 327

Pancreatic arteries, 284
anastomotic branch of, 284
dorsal, 283–284, 286–287
greater, 284, 286
inferior, 284, 286–287
Pancreatic duct, 280
accessory (of Santorini), 272, 281
main (of Wirsung), 272, 280–281
Pancreatic lymph nodes, 294
right superior, 293
Pancreatic notch, 281
Pancreatic veins, 289, 291
great, 289
Pancreaticoduodenal artery
anterior inferior, 284, 286, 300
plexus on, 298–299
anterior superior, 266, 283–284, 286–287, 300
plexus on, 298–299
inferior, 284, 286–288, 301
posterior inferior, 284, 286, 300
plexus on, 299
posterior superior, 283–284, 286–287, 300
plexus on, 299
Pancreaticoduodenal lymph nodes, 294
Pancreaticoduodenal plexus, inferior, 301
Pancreaticoduodenal vein
anterior inferior, 289, 291–292
anterior superior, 289, 291–292
posterior inferior, 289, 291
posterior superior, 289, 292
Papilla, 63
fibers to, 274
filiform, 60
foliate, 60, 136
fungiform, 60, 136
ileal, 274
incisive, 57
keratinized tip of, 60
lacrimal
inferior, 83–84
superior, 83–84
parotid, 56
renal, 311
vallate, 60, 136
Papillary muscle, 213, 241
anterior, 217–218, 220–222
posterior, 217–218, 220–222
Paracentral artery, 142–143
Paracentral lobule, 107
Paracentral sulcus, 107
Paracolic gutter
left, 265, 341, 345
transverse section of, 328
right, 265, 273, 341, 345
transverse section of, 328
Paracolic lymph nodes, 296
Paradidymis, 367
Paraduodenal fossa, 264
Parahippocampal gyrus, 107–109, 120
Paramedian arteries, posteromedial, 141
Paramesonephric (müllerian) duct, 367
Paranasal sinuses
bones of, 45
changes with age of, 45
coronal section, 43
horizontal section, 43
innervation of, 164
lateral dissection, 44
sagittal section, 44
Pararectal fossa, 341–342, 345, 370
Pararenal fat, 176, 315
transverse section of, 327
Parasternal lymph nodes, 181–182
Parasympathetic fibers, 122–124, 126, 133, 135
of autonomic reflex pathways, 304
of kidneys and upper ureters, 318
Parasympathetic fibers *(Continued)*
of liver and biliary tract, 306
of pancreas, 307
of reproductive organs, 393–394
of tracheobronchial tree, 207
of urinary bladder and lower ureter, 395
Parasympathetic nervous system, schema of, 164
Parathyroid gland, 78
inferior, 77–78
superior, 77–78
Paratracheal lymph nodes, 235
left, 205
right, 205
Para-umbilical veins, 249, 292
in round ligament of liver, 252
tributaries of, 252
Para-urethral (Skene's) ducts, 367
openings of, 354
primordium of, 367
Paravertebral anastomoses, 168
Paravesical endopelvic fascia, 348
Paravesical fossa, 342
Paravesical pouch, 350
Parietal artery, 3
anterior, 142–143
posterior, 142–143
Parietal bone, 4, 6, 8–11
groove for middle meningeal vessels, 11
lateral view of, 14
mastoid angle, 11
of newborn, 14
superior view of, 14
tuber of, 14
Parietal emissary vein, 3
Parietal foramen, 9
Parietal lobe, 106
Parietal lobule, inferior
angular gyrus of, 106
supramarginal gyrus of, 106
Parietal lymph nodes, posterior, 235
Parietal operculum, 106
Parietal peritoneum, 257, 265, 267–268, 321, 341, 344–346, 348
diaphragmatic part of, 306
transverse section of, 328
Parietal pleurae, 208
cervical (cupula, dome of), 193–194, 227–228
costal part of, 190–191, 195, 203, 208, 227–229
left border of, 194
right border of, 194
diaphragmatic part of, 190–191, 195, 203, 208, 229
mediastinal part of, 190–191, 195, 203, 208–209, 212–213, 227–229
Parietal vein, 3
Parieto-occipital sulcus, 106–107
Parolfactory area, 107
Paroöphoron, 367
Parotid duct (of Stensen), 24, 46, 48–49, 72
opening of, 56
Parotid fascia, 25
Parotid gland, 24, 27, 29, 31, 42, 46–47, 66, 94, 126, 135
accessory, 46
bed of, 47
innervation of, 163–164
Parotid lymph nodes
deep, 74
superficial, 74
Parotid papilla, 56
Parotid space, 34
Pars distalis, 148
Pars flaccida, 95
Pars interarticularis, 155
Pars intermedia, 148
Pars tensa, 95
Pars tuberalis, 148
Parturition, neuropathways in, 392
Passavant's ridge, 65
Patella, 468, 479–481, 488, 493–494, 498, 506–507
radiograph of, 497
Patellar anastomosis, 487–488, 499, 509
Patellar capsule, 495
Patellar ligament, 468, 479–481, 488, 493–495, 498, 501–502, 506–508
Patellar nerve plexus, 470
Patellar retinaculum, 495
lateral, 479–481, 493–494, 506–508
medial, 479–480, 488, 493–495, 507–508
Pecten, 371
Pecten pubis, 243, 330, 334, 338, 473
Pectinate ligament, 90
Pectinate line, 371
Pectinate muscles, 217
Pectineal fascia, 247
Pectineal ligament (Cooper's), 246–247, 249, 255, 257–258
Pectineal line, 243, 330, 334, 473
Pectineus muscle, 396–397, 477–480, 487–488, 491–492, 525, 531
Pectoral fasciae, 179, 412
Pectoral lymph nodes, 181–182
Pectoral nerve
lateral, 185, 412, 415–416
medial, 185, 412, 415–416
Pectoralis major muscle, 27, 29, 31, 179, 182, 185–186, 188, 195, 213–214, 238–242, 245–246, 398, 405, 409–410, 412, 415, 417, 419, 421, 467
abdominal part of, 409
clavicular head of, 178, 214, 409
fascia of, 412
pectoral fascia and, 179, 412
sternal head of, 178
sternocostal head of, 214, 409
Pectoralis major tendon, 419, 421
Pectoralis minor muscle, 182, 185–186, 195, 214, 238–241, 405, 410, 412–413, 415, 417, 419, 467
fascia of, 185, 412
Pectoralis minor tendon, 410, 415
Pedicle
cervical, 20
lumbar, 155–156, 158–159
thoracic, 154
Pedis artery, dorsal, 508, 517–518, 523
Peduncles
cerebellar
inferior, 114–116, 125, 145
middle, 114–116, 145
superior, 114–116, 145
cerebral, 107, 116
Pelvic brim, 350
sacral part of, 157
Pelvic diaphragm, 369
female, 335–337, 340
inferior fascia of, 355–356, 360, 370, 383
interior fascia of, 372
male, 338–339, 344
superior fascia of, 343, 346, 355, 370, 372
Pelvic fascia, tendinous arch of, 343, 346, 348
Pelvic inlet, radiograph of, 331
Pelvic ligaments, 353
Pelvic organs, arteries and veins of, female, 378
Pelvic outlet
anteroposterior diameter of, 332
transverse diameter of, 332
Pelvic viscera
female, 340, 342
male, 344

Pelvic viscera *(Continued)*
nerves of
female, 390
male, 388
Pelvis
bones of, 333–334
bony framework of, 330
false, 334, 341
female, 397
arteries of, 380
contents of, 341
diaphragm, 335–337, 340
lymph vessels and nodes of, 384
measurements of, 332
radiograph of, 331
viscera of, 340, 342
ligaments of, 333–334
linea terminalis of, 343, 345
male
arteries of, 381
bladder-prostate junction, 396
contents of, 345
diaphragm, 338–339
lymph vessels and nodes of, 386
measurements of, 332
radiograph of, 331
veins of, 381
viscera of, 344
sagittal CT images of, 375
surface anatomy of, 329
true, 334
ureters in, 313
Penis, 360
body (shaft) of, 329, 366
bulb of, 360–361, 363
artery of, 361, 383
cavernous nerves of, 388, 394
corpus cavernosum of, 359–360, 363
corpus spongiosum of, 359, 363
crus of, 348, 359–361, 363
deep artery of, 359, 363, 383
deep (Buck's) fascia of, 245–247, 321, 344, 358–361, 365, 373–374, 381, 383
intercavernous septum of, 359–360, 363
dorsal artery of, 359, 361, 383
deep, 379, 383
dorsal nerve of, 359, 361, 383, 387–389, 394, 484, 490
dorsal vein of
deep, 245, 339, 344, 359, 361, 379, 381
hiatus for, 338
superficial, 245, 252, 329, 359, 381
frenulum of, 360
fundiform ligament of, 245, 255, 344
glans, 329, 344, 360, 363, 366
corona of, 360
neck of, 360
lateral superficial vein of, 359
raphe of, 366
sagittal CT images of, 375
skin of, 358–360, 365
superficial fascia of, 245–247, 344, 358–360, 365
suspensory ligament of, 246, 344
transverse section through, 359
tunica albuginea of, 359, 363
Perforated substance
anterior, 108, 115, 120
male, 343
posterior, 108, 115
Perforating arteries, 489
anteromedial, 141
posteromedial, 141
Perforating cutaneous nerve, 389, 391
Perforating radiate (capsular) arteries, 312
Perforating veins, 401–402
anterior, 189
Peri-anal skin, 371–372
Peri-anal space, 370–371, 374
Peri-anal tissues, 366
Pericallosal artery, 142–143
posterior, 144
Pericardiacophrenic artery, 187, 203, 208–209, 213, 227, 251
left, 190–191, 228
right, 190–191
Pericardiacophrenic vein, 187, 203, 208–209, 213, 227
left, 191, 228
right, 191
Pericardiacophrenic vessels, 212
Pericardial cavity, 213
Pericardial reflection, 211, 217–218
Pericardial sac, 212
Pericardial sinus
oblique, 212–213, 241
transverse, 209, 212, 217–218
Pericardium, 26, 191, 203, 208–209, 212, 229–230
bare area of, 193
diaphragmatic part of, 212
fibrous, 195, 208, 212, 227–228
at site of reflection from great vessels, 209
sternocostal part of, 212
Perichoroidal space, 89–90
Pericranium, 103
Periglandular plexus, 305
Periglomerular cell, 120
Perimuscular rectal venous plexus, 291, 377
Perineal artery, 350, 357, 381–383
transverse, 383
Perineal body, 339, 344, 346, 355–356, 360–362, 369, 373, 383
growth of, 347
Perineal compartment, superficial, 374
Perineal fascia
deep, 344, 348, 350, 355–356, 359–361, 369, 374
superficial, 344, 348, 350, 355, 357–361, 369, 373–374, 382–383, 389
transverse, deep, 362, 369
Perineal flexure, 396
Perineal ligament, transverse, 336, 343–344, 346, 355, 361, 383
anterior thickening of, 338
Perineal lymph vessels, 386
Perineal membrane, 249, 258, 321, 335, 339–340, 344, 346, 348, 350, 355–357, 359–362, 373–374, 382–383, 389
anterior thickening of, 343–344, 346
superior aspect of, 381
Perineal muscle
deep, fascia of, 336
transverse
deep, 249, 321, 335, 340, 344, 356–357, 361–362, 369, 374, 382, 397
superficial, 321, 335, 355–357, 359–361, 369, 373–374, 382–383, 397
Perineal nerve, 357, 370, 388–389, 391, 484, 490
deep branches of, 357, 389, 391
superficial branches of, 357, 389, 391
Perineal raphe, 354, 366
Perineal space
female
deep, 357
superficial, 357
male, 361
superficial, 344, 350, 355–356, 359–361, 382–383
inferior fascia of, 344
Perineal vein, 383
Perineopelvic spaces, 374
Perineum
arteries of, 382
male, 383
female, 340, 354
deep perineum and, 356
interdigitating fibers of, 337
superficial dissection of, 355
lymph vessels and nodes of, female, 385
male, 344
deeper dissection, 359
superficial dissection, 358
nerves of
female, 391
male, 389
surface anatomy of, 329
veins of, 382
male, 383
Periodontium, 63
Periorbita, 85
Periosteum
alveolar, 63
mandibular, 63
maxillary, 63
Periportal arteriole, 279
Periportal bile ductule, 279
Periportal space, 279
Perirenal fat, 176, 315
transverse section of, 327
Perisinusoidal spaces, 279
Peritoneal fold, 266, 345
Peritoneal layers, of mesentery, 305
Peritoneal reflection, 369
Peritoneum, 7, 176, 232, 249, 256, 276, 301, 308, 315, 320, 340, 355, 378. *See also specific peritoneums*
inferior extent of, 393–394
of pararectal fossa, 370
of pelvic viscera, 390
of posterior abdominal wall, 268
Peritoneum reflection, 371
Peri-ureteric loops, 317
Perivascular fibrous capsule, 278
Permanent teeth, 62–63
Perpendicular plate, 8, 37–38
Pes anserinus, 477, 479–480, 493–494, 502
Pes hippocampi, 112–113
Petit, lumbar triangle of, 152, 250
internal oblique muscle in, 171
Petropharyngeus muscle, 67
Petrosal artery, superficial, 96
descending branch of, 96
Petrosal nerve
deep, 39, 53, 124, 126, 132, 134
greater, 13, 39, 53, 55, 61, 88, 96, 124–126, 132, 134, 136
in foramen lacerum, 12
groove for, 11, 99
hiatus for, 13
lesser, 12–13, 50, 88, 95–96, 123–124, 126, 135
groove for, 11
hiatus for, 13
Petrosal sinus
inferior, 13, 104–105
groove for, 8, 11
superior, 55, 99, 104–105, 145
groove for, 8, 11
Petrosal vein, 105, 145
Petrosquamous fissure, 14
Petrotympanic fissure, 10, 12
Peyer's patches, 272, 275
Phalanges
foot, 511–512
distal, 511, 515, 524
middle, 511, 515, 524
proximal, 511, 515, 524

Phalanges *(Continued)*
hand, 445
distal, 443–444, 458
middle, 443–444, 458
proximal, 443–444
Pharyngeal aponeurosis, 65, 67, 69
Pharyngeal artery, 51
artery of, 54
ascending, 34, 51, 55, 72, 96, 137, 139
meningeal branches of, 13, 102, 137
pharyngeal branch of, 68
tonsillar branch of, 68
Pharyngeal constrictor muscle, 64, 82
inferior, 29, 65, 67, 69–70, 77–78, 82, 127, 151, 231
cricopharyngeus part of, 69, 230–231
middle, 29, 59, 65, 67–70, 77, 127, 151
superior, 47, 49, 51, 57, 59, 65, 67–70, 72, 77, 127, 151
glossopharyngeal part of, 59, 65
Pharyngeal muscles, longitudinal, 65, 67, 69
Pharyngeal nerve, 134
Pharyngeal plexus, 61, 71, 126–127, 131–132
Pharyngeal raphe, 36, 64–65, 67–68, 77, 231
Pharyngeal recess, 36, 42, 66, 68
Pharyngeal region
arteries of, 72
nerves of, 71
veins of, 73
Pharyngeal tonsil, 36, 38, 64, 66–68
imaging of, 151
Pharyngeal tubercle, 10, 38, 64–65, 67–68
basilar part of, 22
Pharyngobasilar fascia, 57, 59, 65, 67, 70, 75
Pharyngo-epiglottic fold, 67, 69
fibers to, 65
Pharyngo-esophageal constriction, 230
Pharyngo-esophageal junction, 69
Pharyngotympanic (auditory, eustachian) tube, 94–96, 98, 100, 127
cartilage of, 42, 49, 57, 65, 67–68, 100
lateral lamina of, 100
medial lamina of, 100
groove for, 10
opening of, 36
pharyngeal opening of, 64, 66, 68, 126
Pharynx
afferent innervation of, 61
innervation of, 119
lymph vessels and nodes of, 75
median section of, 64
muscles of
lateral view of, 70
partially opened posterior view of, 67
sagittal section, 65
opened posterior view of, 66
posterior view of, 77
posterior wall of, 56
zone of sparse muscle fibers, 69, 77
Philtrum, 1, 56
Phrenic arteries, inferior, 229, 233, 236, 259, 283, 297–298, 320, 388
anterior branch of left, 192
lateral branch of left, 192
left, 192, 266, 268, 284, 299, 310, 319–320
recurrent branch of, 259, 283
right, 192, 284, 299, 310, 319
Phrenic ganglion, 192, 299
Phrenic lymph nodes
inferior, 261
pathway to, 181
juxta-esophageal, 235
superior, 235
Phrenic nerve, 26, 30–33, 71–72, 76, 130–131, 186–187, 190, 195, 203, 208–209, 213, 223, 227–229, 238, 251, 297, 319, 413, 415–416
afferent fibers, 190
efferent fibers, 190
left, 190–192, 212, 228
anterior branch of, 192
pericardial branch of, 190
phrenico-abdominal branches of, 190
right, 190–191, 212, 239, 306, 319
anterior branch of, 192
Phrenic plexus, inferior, 297–298, 388
left, 299, 319
right, 299, 319
Phrenic veins, inferior, 260, 310
Phrenicocolic ligament, 266, 268
Phrenico-esophageal ligament, 232
Physeal closure, 467
Pia mater, 101, 103, 109, 166
overlying spinal cord, 165
Pial arterial plexus, 168
Pial plexus, 167
peripheral branches from, 168
Pial venous plexus, 169
Pigment cells, 121
Pigment epithelium, 90
Pillar (rod) cells, 98
Pineal body, 107, 111–112, 115–116
Pineal gland, imaging of, 151
Pineal recess, 109
Piriform fossa, 66, 80, 230
Piriform lobe, 120
Piriformis muscle, 258, 335–338, 380, 388–389, 397, 477, 482, 486, 489–490, 531
nerve to, 484, 486
Pisiform bone, 428, 432–434, 439–443, 445–447, 449, 452
radiographs of, 444
Pisohamate ligament, 441
Pisometacarpal ligament, 441
Pituitary gland, 36, 105, 107–108, 148
adenohypophysis (anterior lobe) of, 141, 148–149
cleft of, 148
imaging of, 151
neurohypophysis (posterior lobe) of, 141, 148–149
Pituitary stalk, 115, 141, 148
Plantar aponeurosis, 516, 519–522
Plantar arch, deep, 509, 523
posterior perforating branches from, 508–509, 518
Plantar artery
deep, 508–509, 517, 523
lateral, 505, 516, 519, 522–523
plantar metatarsal branch of, 520
medial, 516, 519, 521–522
deep branches of, 521–522
proper plantar digital branch of, 522
superficial branch of, 520–521
Plantar calcaneocuboid ligament, 515
Plantar calcaneonavicular ligament, 514–515, 523
Plantar digital arteries, 519–521, 523
branches of, 508, 517–518
Plantar digital nerves, 519, 521, 528
branches of, 508
Plantar fascia
lateral, 519
medial, 519
Plantar ligaments, 515, 523
of foot, 515
long, 514–515, 523
short, 514
Plantar metatarsal arteries, 520, 522–523
perforating branches from, 518
Plantar metatarsal ligaments, 515, 523
Plantar nerve
lateral, 505, 516, 519, 521–522, 527–528
plantar cutaneous branches of, 471
plantar digital branches of, 520–522
superficial branch of, 522
medial, 516, 519, 521–522, 527–528
deep branches of, 522
plantar cutaneous branches of, 471
plantar digital branches of, 520–521
Plantar surface, of foot, 468
Plantarflexion, of ankle, 469
Plantaris muscle, 478, 481–482, 489, 493, 498, 502–505, 527–528, 531
Plantaris tendon, 482, 503–504, 510
Platysma muscle, 25–27, 31, 124, 151
Pleurae, 166, 196, 309
mediastinal, 191, 209
parietal, 208
cervical (cupula, dome of), 193–194, 227–228
costal part of, 190–191, 194–195, 203, 208, 227–229
diaphragmatic part of, 190–191, 195, 203, 208, 229
mediastinal part of, 190–191, 195, 203, 208–209, 212–213, 227–229
visceral, 202
Pleural cavity, 213
costodiaphragmatic recess of, 193–195, 227–228
costomediastinal recess of, 193
left, 191
right, 191
Pleural reflection, 193–195
Plica semilunaris, 83–84
Pons, 107, 115–116, 135–136
imaging of, 151
Pontine arteries, 140–142, 144
Pontine taste area, 136
Pontine vein
lateral, 145
transverse, 145
Pontomesencephalic vein, anterior, 145
Popliteal artery, 482, 487, 489, 492, 499, 503–505, 509
Popliteal fossa, 468, 487
Popliteal ligament
arcuate, 495, 497–498
oblique, 495, 497–498
Popliteal lymph nodes, 472
Popliteal tendon, origin of, 494
Popliteal vein, 472, 482, 489, 492, 503–504
Popliteus muscle, 478, 482, 497–498, 502, 504–505, 528, 531
nerve to, 528
Popliteus tendon, 495–496
Porta hepatis, 277
Portacaval anastomoses, 292
Portal arteriole, 279
Portal space, limiting plate of, 279
Portal triad, 267, 271, 278, 281
transverse section of, 325
Portal veins, 278
axial CT images of, 322–323
branch of, 279
hepatic, 214, 226, 234, 267, 271–272, 277–278, 281, 283–284, 289–291, 294, 321
tributaries of, 292
long hypophyseal, 141, 149
short hypophyseal, 149
transverse section of, 325
Postanal space
deep, 374
superficial, 374
Postcaval lymph nodes, 316
Postcentral gyrus, 106

Postcentral sulcal arteries, 142
Postcentral sulcus, 106, 143
Posterior chamber of eye, 83, 89–92
Posterolateral (dorsolateral) fissure, 114
Posteromedial central (paramedian) arteries, 141
Posteromedial central (perforating) arteries, 141
Postganglionic fibers, 53, 133, 135
  of autonomic reflex pathways, 304
  of kidneys and upper ureters, 318
  of liver and biliary tract, 306
  of pancreas, 307
  of reproductive organs, 393–394
  of urinary bladder and lower ureter, 395
Postlunate fissure, 114
Postnatal circulation, 226
Potential spaces, female, 343
Poupart's, Inguinal ligament, 242, 245–247, 255–258, 329, 336, 355, 358–359, 385, 468, 470, 472, 479, 485, 488
  reflected, 255
Pre-aortic lymph nodes, 296, 384, 386
Precaval lymph nodes, 316
Prececal lymph nodes, 296
Precentral cerebellar vein, 145
Precentral gyrus, 106
Precentral sulcal arteries, 142–143
Prechiasmatic groove, 11
Precordial areas, of auscultation, 210
Preculminate vein, 145
Precuneal artery, 143
Precuneus, 107
Prefrontal artery, 140, 142
Prefrontal sulcal arteries, 143
Preganglionic fibers, 53, 133, 135
  of autonomic reflex pathways, 304
  of kidneys and upper ureters, 318
  of liver and biliary tract, 306
  of pancreas, 307
  of reproductive organs, 393–394
  of urinary bladder and lower ureter, 395
Preganglionic sympathetic cell bodies, 53, 133–135
Premammillary artery, 141
Premolar teeth, 62–63
Prenatal circulation, 226
Preoccipital notch, 106
Prepatellar bursa, subcutaneous, 498
Prepontine cistern, 110
Prepuce, 344, 366
  of clitoris, 354
Preputial (Tyson's) gland, opening of, 360
Prepyloric vein, 289, 291
Prerectal muscle fibers (of Luschka), 339
Pre-rolandic arteries, 142–143
Presacral fascia, 343, 374
Presacral space, 343, 374
Pretracheal fascia, 26, 64
  visceral layer of, 199
Pretracheal lymph nodes, 76
Prevertebral anastomoses, 168
Prevertebral fascia, 26, 47, 64–65
Prevertebral muscles, 30
Prevesical fascia, umbilical, 344
Prevesical lymph nodes, lateral, 316
Prevesical plexus, 386
Prevesical space, 374
Primary fissure, 114
Primary teeth, 62
Princeps pollicis artery, 435, 453
Procerus muscle, 25, 35, 124, 151
Processus vaginalis, 364
Profunda brachii artery, 415, 418–421
  superior lateral, 413
Profunda femoris artery, 487–489, 491–492, 499
  perforating branches of, 480, 488
Profunda femoris vein, 492
Promontorial (middle sacral) lymph nodes, 316, 384, 386
Promontory, 94
  sacral, 157, 330, 333–334, 336, 340, 342, 345, 390
    measurements of, 332
  with tympanic plexus, 95
Pronator quadratus muscle, 426, 434, 436–437, 450, 452, 463, 467
Pronator teres muscle, 405, 417, 419, 426, 431–434, 436–438, 460, 463, 467
Proprioceptive fibers, 123
Prostate, 249, 321, 339, 344, 348, 361–363, 367, 369
  apex of, 362
  base of, 362
  capsule of, 348
  central zone of, 362
  fibromuscular stroma of, 362
  innervation of, 163–164
  lymphatic drainage from, 386
  peripheral zone of, 362
  primordium of, 367
  transitional zone of, 362
Prostate gland, 396
Prostatic ducts, openings of, 362–363
Prostatic plexus, 317, 388, 394–395
Prostatic sinus, 362–363
Prostatic urethra, 348, 363
Prostatic utricle, 362–363, 367
Prostatic venous plexus, 381
Proximal interphalangeal (PIP) joint, 398, 445
Psoas fascia, 176, 315
Psoas major muscle, 176, 192, 255, 258–260, 262, 271, 308–309, 315, 328, 341, 343, 345, 378, 479, 483, 485–486, 525, 530–531
  nerves to, 484–485
  origin of, 483
  transverse section of, 327–328
Psoas minor muscle, 258, 328, 341, 345, 483
  nerves to, 484–485
  origin of, 483
Psoas muscles, 491
Pterion, 6
Pterygoid artery, 51
  lateral, 51
  medial, 51
Pterygoid canal, 54
  artery of, 51, 54–55, 96, 138
  nerve (vidian) of, 39, 41, 52–53, 55, 96, 123–124, 126, 132, 134, 136
Pterygoid fossa
  inferolateral view of, 16
  posterior view of, 16
Pterygoid fovea, 17
Pterygoid hamulus, 6, 10, 16, 37, 49–50, 57, 65, 68, 70, 100
  of newborn, 45
Pterygoid muscle
  lateral, 6, 42, 49–51, 151
  medial, 24, 42, 47, 49–51, 57, 67, 71, 151
Pterygoid nerve (V_3)
  lateral, 50, 71, 123
  medial, 49–50, 71, 123
Pterygoid plate
  lateral, 15–16, 42, 49, 70, 100
  medial, 16, 49, 57, 65, 68, 100
    hamulus of, 15
    right, 55
Pterygoid plexus, 73, 87
  deep facial vein from, 3
Pterygoid process
  hamulus of, 6, 10, 16, 37
  lateral plate of, 6, 8, 10, 16, 37–38
Pterygoid process *(Continued)*
  medial plate of, 6, 8, 10, 16, 37–38
    of newborn, 45
  pterygoid fossa of, 10
  scaphoid fossa of, 10
Pterygomandibular raphe, 15, 47, 49, 51, 57, 65, 68, 70
Pterygomaxillary fissure, 6
Pterygopalatine fossa, 6, 54
  nasal branches in, 53
  pterygopalatine ganglion in, 53
Pterygopalatine ganglion, 39, 41, 52, 54–55, 61, 71, 122–124, 126, 132, 134, 136, 164
  ganglionic branches to, 52
  pharyngeal branch of, 61
  in pterygopalatine fossa, 53
  schema of, 134
Pubic arch, 243, 330
  measurements of, 332
Pubic bone, 321, 335–336, 361
  growth of, 347
  sagittal CT images of, 375
  transverse section of, 397
Pubic crest, 255, 338
Pubic ligament, inferior, 243, 330, 336–339, 343–344, 346, 355, 361
Pubic ramus, 530
  inferior, 243, 330, 337, 340, 348, 473–474, 483
  superior, 243, 330, 333–334, 338, 340, 344, 360, 473–474, 480, 483, 486
    radiograph of, 331
Pubic symphysis, 242–243, 255–256, 258, 329–330, 333, 336–340, 343–344, 346, 355, 357–358, 361, 380, 397, 530
  measurements of, 332
  radiograph of, 331
  superior portion of, 396
Pubic tubercle, 242–243, 246–247, 256, 258, 329–330, 333–334, 338–339, 355, 360, 473, 479–480
Pubic vein, 260
Pubis, 244
  body of, 396
  radiograph of, 331, 475
  symphyseal surface of, 390
Pubocervical fascia
  horizontal portion of, 351
  vertical portion of, 351
Pubococcygeus muscle, 335–339, 350, 373
Pubofemoral ligament, 474
Puboprostatic ligament
  lateral, 346
  medial, 346
Puborectalis muscle, 321, 335, 337–339, 373, 397
  left, 335
Pubovesical ligament
  lateral, 343, 346
  medial, 343, 346
Pudendal artery, 370
  external
    deep, 251, 259, 379, 487, 499
    superficial, 245, 251, 259, 379, 487, 499
  internal, 259, 314, 357, 361, 376, 380–383, 396–397, 486
    perineal branch of, 361
Pudendal canal (Alcock's), 291, 370, 376, 380, 382–383, 389, 391
Pudendal cleft, 354
Pudendal nerve, 160, 262, 303, 370, 383, 388–397, 484, 486, 489–490
Pudendal vein, 370
  external, 252, 260
    deep, 379, 487
    superficial, 245, 379, 470, 487
  internal, 260, 291, 377, 383, 396–397

Pudendum, 354
Pulmonary arteries, 202
left, 196, 203, 210–211, 218, 226, 228, 240
right, 196, 203, 209, 211, 217–218, 226–227, 240
Pulmonary heart valve, 217, 219, 222
anterior semilunar cusp of, 217, 219
left semilunar cusp of, 217, 219
right semilunar cusp of, 217, 219
Pulmonary ligament, 195–196, 205, 227–228
Pulmonary (intrapulmonary) lymph nodes, 205
Pulmonary plexus, 127, 207, 236
anterior, 206
branches to, 206
posterior, 206
Pulmonary trunk, 203, 209–210, 212, 217, 221–222, 226, 237, 240
bifurcation of, 214
Pulmonary veins, 202
inferior
left, 196, 211, 213
right, 196, 211, 213, 217, 241
left, 203, 212, 218, 221, 226, 228
right, 203, 212, 218, 222, 226–227
septum of, 202
superior
left, 196, 209, 211, 218
right, 196, 209, 211, 217, 221
Pulmonic heart valve, 210
Pulvinar, 111–112
left, 145
right, 145
of thalamus, 108, 112, 115–116, 140, 146
Pupil, 83
Purkinje fibers
of left bundle, 222
of right bundle, 222
Putamen, 109, 111
Pyloric antrum, 269
Pyloric canal, 269
transverse section of, 325
Pyloric lymph nodes, 294
Pyloric orifice, 272
Pyloric sphincter, 270
Pyloric zone, 270
Pylorus, 269–271
transverse section of, 325
Pyramid, cerebellar, 115
decussation of, 115–116
of inferior vermis, 114, 116
Pyramidal eminence, 96
Pyramidal lobe, of thyroid gland, 76
Pyramidal process, 10, 14, 16
Pyramidalis muscle, 246, 256, 328

Q

Quadrangular lobule, 114
Quadrangular space, 413–414
Quadrate ligament, 424
Quadrate tubercle, 476
Quadratus femoris muscle, 477–478, 480, 482, 488–490, 531
nerve to, 484, 486, 490
Quadratus lumborum fascia, 176, 192, 258–260, 262, 308, 315, 328, 341, 345
transverse section of, 328
Quadratus lumborum muscle, 173, 176, 309, 483, 485
Quadratus plantae muscle, 521–522, 528, 531
Quadratus plantae nerve, 528
Quadriceps femoris muscle, 502, 525
Quadriceps femoris tendon, 460, 477, 488, 493–494, 498, 506–508
Quadrigeminal cistern, 110
imaging of, 151

R

Radial artery, 419–420, 431–436, 441, 447, 449, 452–454, 456–457, 460
dorsal carpal branch of, 454
palmar branch of, 433, 453
superficial, 434–435, 441, 447, 452–453
palmar carpal branches of, 434, 452
Radial collateral artery, 418, 420–421
Radial collateral ligament, 424
Radial fossa, 405, 422
Radial groove, 406
Radial longitudinal crease, 398
Radial metaphyseal arcuate ligament, dorsal, 442
Radial nerve, 400, 410, 413, 415–416, 418, 421, 433–434, 454, 459–463, 465
in arm, 465
communicating branches of, 455
deep branch of, 433, 436, 460, 466
dorsal digital branches, 400, 454, 459, 466
in forearm, 466
inferior lateral brachial cutaneous nerve from, 400–401
lateral branch of, 454
medial branch of, 454
posterior antebrachial cutaneous nerve from, 400–401, 459
posterior brachial cutaneous nerve from, 400–401
superficial branch of, 400, 402, 430, 433, 436, 454–456, 459–460, 466
Radial notch, of ulna, 422, 425
Radial recurrent artery, 419–420, 433–435
Radial tuberosity, 417, 422, 425
radiograph of, 423
Radialis indicis artery, 435, 453
Radiate ligament, of head of rib, 184
Radiate sternocostal ligament, 184, 404
Radicular artery
anterior, 167–168
posterior, 168
Radicular vein, segmental, 169
anterior, 169
posterior, 169
Radiocarpal joint, 439, 442
articular disc of, 439, 442
Radiocarpal ligament, dorsal, 442
Radiology, of heart, 210
Radiolunate ligament
long, 441
palmar, 441
short, 441
Radioscaphocapitate ligament, 441
Radio-ulnar joint, distal, 442
Radio-ulnar ligament, dorsal, 442
Radius, 422, 426–429, 431, 434, 436–439, 441–442, 452
anterior border of, 425
anterior surface of, 425
dorsal (Lister's) tubercle of, 425
head of, 417, 422–423, 425
interosseous border of, 425
interosseous membrane of, 425, 429
neck of, 422–423, 425
posterior border of, 425
posterior surface of, 425
radiograph of, 423
rotators of, 426
styloid process of, 425, 439
radiographs of, 444
Rathke's pouch, 45
Rectal artery
inferior, 288, 376, 380–383
middle, 259, 288, 302, 313, 343, 376, 378, 380–381
Rectal artery *(Continued)*
superior, 259, 268, 288, 297, 302–303, 313, 376, 378
branch of, 288
Rectal fascia, 342–343, 355, 362, 369–372, 374
Rectal lymph nodes
middle, 296
superior, 296
Rectal nerves
inferior, 303, 388–389, 391–392, 484, 490
superior, 303
Rectal plexus, 302–303, 317, 388, 390
communication between, 377
external, 377
internal, 377
middle, 302
superior, 297, 302
Rectal vein
inferior, 292, 377
right, 291
middle, 260, 291–292, 377
right, 291
superior, 268, 291–292, 377
Rectal venous plexus, 260
external, 291, 371–372
internal, 371–372
perimuscular, 291
Rectocervical spaces, 342
Rectococcygeus muscle, 258
Rectoprostatic (Denonvilliers') fascia, 321, 339, 344, 362, 369, 374
Rectosigmoid arteries, 376
Rectosigmoid junction, 276, 369, 371–372
Recto-urethralis superior muscle, 339
Recto-uterine fold, 342
Recto-uterine ligament, 342
Recto-uterine pouch (of Douglas), 340, 342, 352, 369
Rectovaginal spaces, 342–343
Rectovesical fascia, 362, 374
Rectovesical pouch, 321, 344–345, 369
Rectovesical space, 374
Rectum, 258, 265, 268, 276, 308, 321, 335–337, 340–341, 343–346, 362, 371, 378, 390
ampulla of, 346
arteries of, male, 376
circular muscle layer of, 371–372
innervation of, 163–164
longitudinal muscle layer of, 371–372
muscularis mucosae of, 372
radiography of, 156
sagittal CT images of, 375
in situ, 369
transverse folds of, 371
transverse section of, 397
veins of, female, 377
Rectus abdominis muscle, 7, 178, 185–186, 188, 242, 246–247, 249, 251, 253–256, 321, 328–329, 341, 343–345, 355
axial CT images of, 322
sagittal CT images of, 375
transverse section of, 324, 328
Rectus capitis muscle
anterior, 30, 42, 75, 151
communication with cervical plexus, 33
nerves to, 130
lateral, 30, 151
communication with cervical plexus, 33
nerves to, 130
posterior
major, 172–173, 175, 177
minor, 172–173, 175, 177
Rectus femoris muscle, 396–397, 468, 477, 479, 481, 487–488, 492, 525, 530–531
Rectus femoris tendon, 468, 479–480, 494, 507

Rectus muscle
  inferior, 85–86, 122, 151
    branches to, 88
  lateral, 85–86, 88, 151
    abducent nerve and, 122
    check ligament of, 85
    innervation of, 119
    tendon of, 89
  medial, 85–86, 88, 122, 151
    branches to, 88
    check ligament of, 85
    tendon of, 89
  superior, 85–86, 88, 122, 151
    tendon of, 93
Rectus sheath, 186, 245–246
  anterior layer of, 7, 185, 245–246, 253, 255, 344, 355
  cross section of, 7
  posterior layer of, 7, 247, 251, 253, 255
  transverse section of, 328
Recurrent artery
  of foramen lacerum, 138
  of Heubner, 138, 140–143
  radial, 419–420, 433–435
  tibial
    anterior, 499, 508–509
    posterior, 499, 505, 509
  ulnar
    anterior, 420, 433–435
    posterior, 420, 431, 434–435
Recurrent interosseous artery, 435
Recurrent process, 120
Red nucleus, 108, 117–118
  imaging of, 151
Reissner's membrane, 98
Renal artery, 297, 311–312, 314, 318, 321, 378–379, 395
  anterior branch of, 312
  capsular branches of, 312
  left, 259, 302, 308, 310, 315, 320, 388
    arteriogram of, 285
    transverse section of, 327
    ureteric branch of, 310
  pelvic branch of, 312
  perirenal branches of, 312
  posterior branch of, 312
  right, 259, 300, 308, 310
    ureteric branch of, 310
  in situ, 310
  ureteric branch of, 312, 314
Renal capsule, 311
Renal column (of Bertin), 311
Renal (Gerota's) fascia, 315, 320
  anterior layer, 176, 315
  posterior layer, 176, 315
  transverse section of, 327
Renal ganglion, 317–319, 394
Renal impression, 277, 282
Renal papilla, 311
Renal parenchyma, 311
Renal pelvis, 311
  transverse section of, 327
Renal plexus, 297, 317–319, 395
  left, 302, 388
Renal segments, 312
Renal sinus, 311
  fat in, 311
Renal vein, 311, 314, 321, 378–379
  left, 234, 260, 308, 310, 315, 320
    axial CT images of, 323
    transverse section of, 327
  right, 234, 260, 308, 310
    axial CT images of, 323
    transverse section of, 327
  in situ, 310
Reproductive organs, innervation of
  female, 393
  male, 394
Respiratory bronchioles, 201–202
Rete testis, 368
Reticular nucleus, 112
Retina, 92
  ciliary part of, 89–91
  nonpigmented and pigmented regions of, 93
  optic part of, 89, 91
  pigment epithelium of, 90
  structure of, 121
Retinacular arteries, 491
Retinal arteriole
  nasal
    inferior, 92
    superior, 92
  temporal
    inferior, 92
    superior, 92
Retinal artery, 92
  central, 87, 89, 92–93
Retinal vein, 92
  central, 89, 92–93
Retinal venule
  nasal
    inferior, 92
    superior, 92
  temporal
    inferior, 92
    superior, 92
Retrobulbar fat, 85
Retrocecal recess, 265, 273
Retromandibular vein, 3, 31–32, 42, 46–47, 59, 87
  anterior branch, 32, 46, 73
    common trunk for, 46, 73
  common trunk for, 59
  posterior branch, 32, 46, 73
Retromolar fossa, 17
Retropharyngeal lymph nodes, 75
Retropharyngeal space, 26, 47, 64–65
Retropubic space, 321, 343, 346, 374
  areolar tissue in, 344
  fat in, 247, 339
  vesical venous plexus in, 344
Retropubic venous plexus, 346
Retrotonsillar fissure, 114
Retrotonsillar vein
  of cerebellomedullary cistern, 145
  superior, 145
Retzius, retropubic space of, 247, 321, 346, 371
Rhinal sulcus, 107–108
Rhomboid fossa, of fourth ventricle, 115
Rhomboid major muscle, 171, 174, 177, 188, 238–240, 250, 406, 409, 465, 467
Rhomboid minor muscle, 171, 177, 406, 409, 465, 467
Ribs, 210, 237, 239–240
  angle of, 183–184
  associated joints and, 184
  body of, 183
  costal groove of, 184
  eighth, 183–184, 213
  eleventh, 183, 309
  false, 183
  fifth, 183–184, 210
  first, 15, 21, 30, 76, 160, 183–184, 189, 193–194, 208, 210, 227–229, 238, 404, 415, 467
    lung groove for, 196
  floating, 183
  fourth, 183–184
  head of, 183–184
    intra-articular ligament of, 184
    radiate ligament of, 184
  neck of, 183–184
  ninth, 183, 282
  second, 179, 183–184, 404, 467
Ribs *(Continued)*
  seventh, 154, 183–184, 241
  sixth, 179, 183–184
    posterior view of, 184
  tenth, 183
  third, 183–184, 210
  true, 183
  tubercle of, 183–184
  twelfth, 160, 171, 183, 192, 243, 309, 315
    radiography of, 156
Right bundle, 222
  Purkinje fibers of, 222
  subendocardial branches of, 222
Risorius muscle, 25, 124, 151
Rod cells, 98, 121
Rolandic arteries, 142–143
Rolando, central sulcus of, 106–107
Root canal, 63
Rosenthal, basal vein of, 145–147
Rostrum, of corpus callosum, 107, 142, 146
Rotator cuff, muscles of, 411
Rotatores cervicis muscles, 173, 177
  brevis, 173
  longus, 173
Rotatores thoracis muscles, 173, 177
  brevis, 173
  longus, 173
Rotter's lymph nodes, 181–182
Round ligament
  of liver, 249, 269, 277–278, 292, 313
    transverse section of, 328
  para-umbilical veins in, 252
  of uterus, 260, 340–342, 350–351, 353, 355, 367, 378, 382
    terminal part of, 350
Round (cochlear) window, 14, 94, 97–98
  fossa of, 95

S

SA node. *See* Sinu-atrial node
Saccule, 94, 97–98, 125
Sacral artery
  lateral, 167, 259, 314, 380–381
    spinal branches of, 167
  median, 259, 288, 314, 342–343, 376, 378, 380–381
Sacral canal, 157, 338
Sacral cornu, 157
Sacral crest
  intermediate, 157
  lateral, 157
  median, 157, 334–335
Sacral foramina, 530
  anterior, 157, 333, 338
  posterior, 157, 333
  radiograph of, 331
Sacral ganglion, first, 163, 297
Sacral hiatus, 157
Sacral kyphosis, 153
Sacral lymph nodes, 384, 386
  lateral, 261
  middle, 261, 386
Sacral nerve, perineal branch of, 486
Sacral plexus, 160, 225, 318, 388, 393–395, 484, 486
  right, 302
Sacral promontory, 157, 330, 333–334, 336, 340, 342, 345, 390
  measurements of, 332
Sacral spinal cord, 303
Sacral spinal nerves
  dorsal and ventral roots of, 166
  S1, 160
    dermatome of, 162
    dorsal ramus of, 174
    ventral ramus of, 388, 392

Sacral spinal nerves *(Continued)*
S2
dermatome of, 162
dorsal ramus of, 174
S3
dermatome of, 162
dorsal ramus of, 174
S4, dermatome of, 162
S5, 160
dermatome of, 162
Sacral splanchnic nerves, 163
Sacral tuberosity, 157
Sacral vein
lateral, 260
median, 260, 291, 342, 378, 381
Sacral vertebrae
anterior view of, 153
lateral view of, 153
posterior view of, 153
S1, radiography of, 156
Sacrococcygeal ligaments
anterior, 333, 336, 338, 343–344
lateral, 158, 333–334
posterior, 158, 334
deep, 333
superficial, 333
Sacrogenital fold, 268, 345, 370
Sacro-iliac joint, 338, 530
measurements of, 332
radiograph of, 331
Sacro-iliac ligaments
anterior, 333
posterior, 158, 333–334
Sacrospinous ligament, 158, 333–335, 337, 339, 388, 482, 490
Sacrotuberous ligament, 158, 333–335, 337, 339, 356, 374, 380, 388–389, 391, 396, 482, 489–490
Sacro-uterine ligament, 342
Sacrum, 152, 158, 160–161, 243, 330, 337–338
ala of, radiograph of, 331
anterior view of, 153
apex of, 157
arteries of, 167
articular facet for, 155
auricular surface of, 158
base of, 157
lateral view of, 153
posterior view of, 153
radiography of, 156, 331
sagittal CT images of, 375
Sagittal sinus
inferior, 101, 104–105, 145–147
superior, 101–105, 107, 110, 146
emissary vein to, 13
groove for, 9, 11
imaging of, 150–151
superior cerebral veins entering, 103
Sagittal suture, 5, 9, 14
Salivary glands, 46–47. *See also* Sublingual glands; Submandibular glands
lingual minor, 56
molar minor, 57
Salivatory nucleus
inferior, 117–118, 126, 135
superior, 53, 117–118, 124, 134
Salpingopharyngeal fold, 66, 68
Salpingopharyngeus muscle, 65, 67–68, 127, 151
Santorini, accessory pancreatic duct of, 272, 281
Saphenous nerve, 487–488, 492, 508, 525, 528
branches of, 471
infrapatellar branch of, 470, 487–488, 507–508, 525
Saphenous opening, 246, 252, 355, 358, 470
cribriform fascia over, 252
Falciform margin of, 257
Saphenous vein, 487
accessory, 470–471
great, 245–246, 252, 260, 358, 397, 468, 470–472, 492, 510
small, 468, 470–472, 489, 503, 510
Sartorius muscle, 396–397, 468, 477, 479, 481–482, 487–488, 492–493, 497, 502–503, 507, 525, 530–531
Sartorius tendon, 479–480, 493–494, 508
Scala tympani, 94, 97–98
Scala vestibuli, 94, 97–98
Scalene lymph nodes, inferior, 205
Scalene muscle, 27–28, 30
anterior, 26, 29–33, 71–73, 76, 151, 186–187, 190, 195, 203, 208, 214, 227–229, 413–415
slips of origin of, 30
communication with cervical plexus, 33
innervation of, 416
middle, 26, 29–30, 32, 71–73, 151, 186, 413
nerves to, 130
posterior, 26, 29–30, 151, 186, 229, 413
slips of origin of, 30
Scalp
skin of, 3, 25, 103
subcutaneous tissue of, 25
superficial arteries and veins of, 3
Scaphocapitate ligament, 441
Scaphoid bone, 439, 442–443, 454
radiographs of, 444
tubercle of, 439, 441, 443
Scaphoid fossa, 95, 100
Scapholunate ligament, 442
Scaphotrapeziotrapezoid ligament, 441
Scapula, 177, 188, 210, 238–240, 413, 467
acromial angle of, 405–406
acromion of, 183, 405–407
anastomoses around, 414
anterior view of, 405
body of, 412
circumflex scapular vessel groove, 406
coracoid process of, 183, 405–407
glenoid cavity of, 183, 405, 407–408, 467
inferior angle of, 152, 241, 405–406
infraglenoid tubercle of, 405–406
infraspinous fossa of, 183, 406
lateral border of, 405–407
medial border of, 152, 405–406
neck of, 183, 405–406
posterior view of, 406
spine of, 152, 171, 174, 183, 194, 406–407, 409, 411–414
subscapular fossa of, 183, 405
superior angle of, 405–406
superior border of, 405–406, 411
supraglenoid tubercle of, 405
suprascapular notch of, 183, 405–406
supraspinous fossa of, 183, 406
vertebral border of, 467
Scapular artery
circumflex, 413–415, 417, 420
groove for, 406
dorsal, 32–33, 170, 414–415
Scapular ligament, superior transverse, 408, 410–411, 413–414
Scapular nerve, dorsal, 415–416, 465
Scapular vein, circumflex, groove for, 406
Scapulohumeral dissection, 413
Scapulothoracic dissection, 413
Scarpa, vestibular ganglion of, 97
Scarpa's layer, 245, 321, 344, 358–359
fascia lata attachment of, 245
Schlemm, canal of, 89–90, 92–93
Schwalbe's line, 90
Sciatic foramen
greater, 158, 333–335, 527
lesser, 158, 333–334
Sciatic nerve, 160, 397, 482, 484, 489–490, 492, 527
articular branch of, 489
common fibular division of, 527
left, 396
muscular branches of, 489
right, 396
Sciatic notch
greater, 243, 330, 473
lesser, 243, 330, 473
Sclera, 83, 85, 89–93
lamina cribrosa of, 89
Scleral spur, 89–90
Scleral venous sinus, 89–90, 92–93
veins draining, 93
Scrotal arteries, posterior, 381, 383
Scrotal fascia, superficial, 373
Scrotal ligament (gubernaculum), 367
Scrotal nerve
anterior, 387
posterior, 388–389, 490
Scrotal veins, anterior, 252
Scrotum, 329, 364, 366
contents of, 365
sagittal CT images of, 375
septum of, 344, 365, 368, 373, 383
skin of, 365, 368
superficial fascia of, 245–247, 344, 358, 365, 383
Sebaceous glands, 83
Secondary (postpyramidal) fissure, 114
Segmental artery
inferior, 312
anterior, 312
posterior, 312
superior, 312
anterior, 312
Segmental bronchus, 201
Sella turcica, 7–8, 11, 38, 64
dorsum sellae of, 11
hypophyseal fossa of, 11
hypophysis in, 36
posterior clinoid process of, 11
tuberculum sellae of, 11
Semicircular canals
anterior, 55, 97–98
plane of, 99
lateral, 97–99
prominence of, 94
posterior, 97–98
plane of, 99
Semicircular ducts, 94
anterior, 97–99
lateral, 97–99
ampulla of, 125
posterior, 97–99
ampulla of, 125
superior, ampulla of, 125
Semilunar fold, 68, 276
Semilunar ganglion. *See* Trigeminal ganglion
Semilunar hiatus, 36–37, 44
of newborn, 45
Semilunar lobule
inferior, 114
superior, 114
Semimembranosus bursa, 493, 498, 502–503, 527
Semimembranosus muscle, 478, 481–482, 489–490, 492–493, 497–498, 531
bursa of, 497
Semimembranosus tendon, 493, 495, 497–498, 504–505
groove for, 500
Seminal colliculus, 348, 362

Seminal vesicles, 249, 344–345, 362, 367, 369
Seminiferous tubules, 368
Semispinalis capitis muscle, 171–173, 175, 177
Semispinalis cervicis muscle, 173, 175, 177
Semispinalis thoracis muscle, 173, 177
Semitendinosus muscle, 468, 477–478, 482, 489–490, 492–493, 497, 502–503, 527, 531
Semitendinosus tendon, 479–480, 493–494
Sensory cortex, 136
Septa forming canals, 450
Septal area, 120
Septal cartilage, 35, 38
Septal nasal cartilage. *See* Nasal septal cartilage
Septal nuclei, 120
Septal papillary muscle, 217, 220–221
Septomarginal trabecula (moderator band), 217, 221–222
Septum
- bulging, 36
- fibrous, 372
  - transverse, 371–373
- nasal, 5
- of pulmonary veins, 202
- of scrotum, 344, 365, 368, 373, 383

Septum pellucidum, 107, 109, 111–113, 142, 144, 146, 148
- anterior vein of, 146–147
- posterior veins of, 147

Serosa (visceral peritoneum), 272, 275, 282, 305
Serous glands of von Ebner, 60
Serratus fascia, anterior, 412
Serratus muscle
- anterior, 171, 177–179, 188, 214, 238–242, 245–246, 250, 253–254, 329, 398, 405, 409–410, 413, 415, 467
  - digitations of, 185–186
  - transverse section of, 324
- posterior
  - inferior, 171–172, 176–177, 241, 250, 309
  - superior, 171–172, 177, 241

Sesamoid bone
- foot, 511, 515, 521–523
- hand, 439, 443

Shenton's line, 530
Short radiolunate ligament, 441
Shoulder
- anteroposterior radiograph of, 407
- arthrogram of, 467
- computed tomography of, 467
- cutaneous nerves of, 401
- glenohumeral joint, 408
- joint capsule of, 413
- magnetic resonance imaging of, 467
- muscles of, 409
- nerves of, 465
- superficial veins of, 401

Sigmoid artery, 259, 268, 288, 302, 376
Sigmoid colon, 263, 265, 276, 302, 341–342, 345, 369–372, 390
- innervation of, 163–164

Sigmoid lymph nodes, 296
Sigmoid mesocolon, 265, 268, 276, 288, 308, 313, 369
Sigmoid plexus, 302
Sigmoid sinus, 55, 99, 104–105
- groove for, 8, 11
- imaging of, 150
- inferior, 13

Sigmoid vein, 268, 291–292, 377
Sinu-atrial (SA) nodal artery, 222
Sinu-atrial (SA) node, 215, 222
Sinuses, 44. *See also specific sinuses*
- confluence of, 99, 104–105, 146
- of newborn, 45

Sinusoids, 278–279
Skene's ducts, 367
- openings of, 354

Skin
- of neck, 26
- of penis, 358–360, 365
- peri-anal, 371–372
- of scalp, 3, 25, 103
- of scrotum, 365, 368

Skull
- anterior view of, 4
- anteroposterior radiograph of, 5
- base of, 66
- connective tissue of, 103
- dura mater interface with, 101, 103
- lateral radiograph of, 7
- lateral view of, 6
- midsagittal section of, 8
- of newborn, 14
- nuchal line of, superior, 171–173

Small intestine, 127, 263, 321
- arteries of, 287
- autonomic nerves of, 301, 303
- innervation of, 163–164
- lymph vessels and nodes of, 295
- transverse section of, 328
- veins of, 290

Soft palate, 36, 38, 56, 64, 66, 68
- innervation of, 119
- muscles of, 65

Sole
- of foot, 519
  - cutaneous innervation of, 528
- muscles of
  - first layer, 520
  - second layer, 521
  - third layer, 522

Soleus muscle, 482, 493, 502–508, 510, 516, 518, 527–528, 531
- arch of, 482
- nerve to, 503–504
- tendinous arch of, 504–505

Solitary lymphoid nodules, 272
Solitary tract nucleus, 117–118, 124, 126–127, 224, 318
- rostral part of, 136

Somatic efferent fibers, of urinary bladder and lower ureter, 395
Sound reception, pathway of, 94
Spaces
- of hand, 450
- of Retzius, 346
- triangular, 413

Spermatic cord, 249, 256, 359–360, 383, 396
- artery to ductus deferens in, 251
- cremaster fascia on, 256
- cremaster muscle on, 253, 256
- external spermatic fascia on, 245, 253, 255–256
- internal spermatic fascia on, 257
- testicular vessels in, 379

Spermatic fascia
- external, 246–247, 256, 344, 358–360, 365, 368, 383
  - of spermatic cord, 245, 253, 255–256
- internal, 245, 247, 256, 365, 368
  - on spermatic cord, 257

Spheno-ethmoidal recess, 36–37
Sphenoidal bone, 4, 6, 8, 10–11, 15, 42
- anterior clinoid process, 8, 11
- body of, 8, 11, 38
  - jugum, 11
  - prechiasmatic groove, 11
  - sella turcica, 11
- carotid groove of, 11

Sphenoidal bone *(Continued)*
- clivus of, 11
- crest of, 38
- foramen ovale of, 10
- foramen spinosum of, 10
- greater wing of, 4, 6–8, 10–11
  - groove for middle meningeal vessels, 11
  - orbital surface of, 4
- infratemporal crest of, 6
- lesser wing of, 4–5, 8, 11
- of newborn, 45
- optic canal of, 8
- pterygoid hamulus of, 6, 10, 16, 37
- pterygoid process of, 10
  - hamulus of, 6, 10, 16, 37
  - lateral plate of, 6, 8, 10, 16, 37–38
  - medial plate of, 6, 8, 10, 16, 37–38
  - pterygoid fossa of, 10
  - scaphoid fossa of, 10
- sella turcica of, 8, 11
  - dorsum sellae, 11
  - hypophyseal fossa, 11
  - posterior clinoid process, 11
  - tuberculum sellae, 11
- sphenoidal sinus of, 8, 37–38
- spine of, 10, 16, 100

Sphenoidal concha, of newborn, 45
Sphenoidal emissary foramen (of Vesalius) (inconstant), 13
Sphenoidal fontanelle, of newborn, 14
Sphenoidal process, of palatine bone, 37
Sphenoidal sinus, 8, 36–38, 43–44, 55, 64, 68, 85, 105, 138
- of newborn, 45
- opening of, 8, 36–37, 44

Sphenomandibular ligament, 18, 49, 51
- inferior, 18

Spheno-occipital synchondrosis, 64
Sphenopalatine artery, 40, 51, 54, 72
- posterior lateral nasal branches of, 40, 54
- posterior septal branch of, 40
- posterior septal branches of, 40, 51
  - greater palatine artery anastomosis with, 54

Sphenopalatine foramen, 6, 8, 16, 37, 40–41, 51
- opening of, 37

Sphenopalatine vessels, in incisive fossa, 12
Sphenoparietal sinus, 104–105
- superficial middle cerebral vein draining to, 146

Spherical recess, 97
Sphincter pupillae muscle, 90, 122, 133, 151
- innervation of, 119

Sphincter urethrae muscle, 335, 339–340, 346, 348, 355–356, 374, 395, 397
- growth of, 347

Sphincter urethrovaginalis muscle, 346, 350, 355–357, 397
Spinal artery
- anterior, 139–140, 142, 144, 167–168
  - anastomotic loops to, 167
  - spinal segmental medullary branches of, 139
- posterior, 140, 142, 167–168
  - anastomotic loops to, 167
  - left, 144, 168
  - right, 168

Spinal cord, 53, 238–239, 319
- arteries of
  - intrinsic distribution of, 168
  - schema of, 167
- central canal of, 109–110, 116, 118
- descending tracts in, 207
- dorsal horn of, 165
- gray matter of, 165–166

Spinal cord *(Continued)*
imaging of, 151
lateral horn of, 165–166, 319
lumbar part of, 395
pia mater overlying, 165
radiography of, 156
sacral, 303, 395
in situ, 160
termination of, 161
thoracic part of, 133, 207, 304, 306–307
thoracolumbar, 303
veins of, 169
ventral horn of, 165
white matter of, 165
Spinal dura mater, 160, 165–166, 170, 176
posterior intercostal artery branch to, 168
Spinal ganglion, dorsal root of, 165, 188
Spinal membranes, 165
Spinal meninges, 304
Spinal nerve roots, 300
posterior view of, 165
vertebrae relation to, 161
Spinal nerve trunk, 254
Spinal nerves, 26, 166, 177, 225, 304. *See also* Cervical spinal nerves; Lumbar spinal nerves; Sacral spinal nerves; Thoracic spinal nerves
dorsal ramus of, 165–166
lateral branch of, 166
medial branch of, 166
dorsal root of, 165–166, 188, 304, 395
dorsal rootlets of, 160, 165
groove for, 20–21
origin of, 166
cross section of, 166
recurrent (meningeal) branches of, 166
ventral ramus of, 165–166
ventral root of, 165–166, 188, 304, 395
ventral rootlets of, 165
Spinal perivascular plexus, 304
Spinal sensory ganglion, 300, 303–304, 318, 395
Spinal vein
anterior, 145, 169
posterior, 145, 169
Spinalis cervicis muscle, 172
Spinalis muscle, 172
Spinalis thoracis muscle, 172
Spino-umbilical line, 275
Spinous process, 237
cervical, 20, 22, 152, 171–173, 409
lumbar, 155–156, 158–159, 176
transverse section of, 328
thoracic, 154, 156, 171–172, 174, 194, 409
Spiral ganglion of Corti, 98
Spiral lamina
hamulus of, 97
osseous, 97–98
Spiral ligament, 98
Spiral organ of Corti, 94, 98
Splanchnic nerves
greater, 163, 192, 206, 227–228, 236, 254, 262, 297–304, 306–307, 317, 319, 387–388, 392–394
left, 191, 213, 236
right, 191, 236
least, 163, 192, 206, 262, 297, 299–304, 317–319, 387–388, 392–394
lesser, 163, 192, 206, 254, 262, 297–304, 317–319, 387–388, 392–394
lumbar, 163, 297, 302–303, 317–319, 387–388, 390, 392–395
pelvic, 164, 302–303, 317–318, 388, 390, 392, 394–395, 484, 486
sacral, 163, 303, 317, 388, 486
thoracic, 225, 319
Spleen, 193–194, 267, 269, 278, 281–282, 320
anterior extremity of, 282
arteries of, 283–284
axial CT images of, 322–323
hilum of, 282
inferior border of, 282
posterior extremity of, 282
superior border of, 282
transverse section of, 324–326
veins of, 289
Splenic artery, 259, 268, 271, 281–284, 286–287, 297–300, 306–307, 321
arteriogram of, 285
axial CT images of, 322
splenic branches of, 283
transverse section of, 325
Splenic lymph nodes, 293–294
Splenic plexus, 297–299
Splenic red pulp, 282
Splenic trabeculae, 282
Splenic vein, 234, 267–268, 282, 287, 289–292, 320–321
axial CT images of, 322–323
transverse section of, 325–326
Splenic white pulp, 282
Splenium, of corpus callosum, 107–108, 111, 113, 116, 144–147
imaging of, 151
Splenius capitis muscle, 29, 171–172, 175, 177
Splenius cervicis muscle, 171–172, 175, 177
Splenorenal (lienorenal) ligament, 266, 268, 282, 308
Spongy urethra, 363
bulbous portion of, 348
Squamous suture, 14
Stapedius muscle, 55, 96, 151
innervation of, 119, 124
pyramidal eminence and tendon of, 95
Stapes, 95–96
base of, in oval window, 94
footplate of, 95
limbs of, 94
Stellate ganglion, 131, 206, 223–224, 236
Stellate veins, 311
Stensen, parotid duct of, 24, 48–49, 72
opening of, 56
Sternal head, 27, 29
of sternocleidomastoid muscle, 1
Sternalis muscle (inconstant), 185
Sternoclavicular joint, 193, 238, 404
Sternocleidomastoid lymph nodes, 74
Sternocleidomastoid muscle, 26–27, 29, 31–32, 34, 46–47, 75, 128, 130, 151, 171, 175, 185, 195, 404, 409–410, 415
accessory nerve to, 128
clavicular head of, 1, 178
innervation of, 119
medial margin of, 76
sternal head of, 1, 178
Sternocostal articulations
anterior view of, 184
left anterolateral view of, 184
right posterolateral view of, 184
Sternocostal joint, 404
Sternocostal triangle, 187
Sternohyoid muscle, 26–29, 31, 58, 129, 151, 185, 187, 195, 404
communication with cervical plexus, 33
fascia of, 185
nerves to, 71
Sternothyroid muscle, 26–29, 31, 82, 129–130, 151, 185, 187, 195
communication with cervical plexus, 33
fascia of, 185
nerves to, 71
Sternum, 25, 177, 188, 191, 213, 237, 241, 409
angle of, 183
body of, 178, 183, 185, 187, 189, 242–243
jugular notch of, 183
manubrium of, 26–27, 29, 64, 183–184, 187, 195, 238–239
xiphoid process of, 178, 183, 185
Stomach, 193, 214, 229, 232–233, 263, 266–267, 277–278, 280–282, 321
air in, 210
arteries of, 283
autonomic nerves of, 298–300
axial CT images of, 322
body of, 269
axial CT images of, 322
cardiac part of, 230, 232, 269–270
fundus of, 230, 232, 269–270
transverse section of, 324
gastric zone of, 270
innervation of, 163–164
lymph vessels and nodes of, 293
mucosa of, 270
pyloric part of, 269, 298
radiography of, 156
in situ, 269
transverse section of, 325
vagal branches to, 236
veins of, 289
Straight arteries, 287–288
branch of, 305
Straight gyrus, 108
Straight sinus, 99, 104–105, 110, 145–147
imaging of, 150
in tentorium cerebelli, 107
Straight veins, 290
Strap muscles, innervation of, 119
Stretch receptors, 207
Stria medullaris, 112, 116
of thalamus, 107
Stria terminalis, 109, 112–113
Striate artery, distal medial, 138, 140–143
Striatum, 111
Styloglossus muscle, 42, 47, 51, 59, 65, 70, 129, 151
Stylohyoid ligament, 15, 59, 65, 68, 70
Stylohyoid muscle, 27–29, 34, 42, 46–47, 50–51, 58–59, 67, 70, 124
innervation of, 119
nerve to, 24
Styloid process, 6, 10, 14–16, 18, 29–30, 34, 42, 58–59, 66–67, 70, 96
of radius, 425, 439
radiographs of, 444
of ulna, 425, 439
radiographs of, 444
Stylomandibular ligament, 15, 18
inferior, 18
Stylomastoid artery, 96
posterior tympanic branch of, 96
stapedial branch of, 96
Stylomastoid foramen, 10, 12, 100, 124, 126
facial nerve from, 24
Stylopharyngeus muscle, 47, 59, 65, 67–70, 126–127, 151
Subacromial bursa, 408, 417
Subacromial space, 467
Subaponeurotic space, dorsal, 450
Subarachnoid space, 89, 101, 103, 110, 166
imaging of, 151
Subcallosal (parolfactory) area, 107, 120
Subcallosal gyrus, 107
Subcapsular lymphatic plexus, 316

Subclavian artery, 30, 32–33, 71–73, 76, 78, 131, 137, 139, 167, 180, 186–187, 195, 208–209, 229, 233, 251, 413–415
left, 77, 170, 203, 211, 228, 238
lung groove for, 196
right, 77, 127, 170, 203, 227
Subclavian groove, 404
Subclavian lymph nodes, 74, 181–182
Subclavian lymphatic trunk, 205
Subclavian trunk, 74
left, 295
right, 261, 295
Subclavian vein, 30, 32–33, 73, 76, 186–187, 195, 205, 208–209, 229, 234, 252, 413, 415
left, 77, 170, 203, 228
right, 77, 170, 203, 227
Subclavius fascia, 412
Subclavius muscle, 151, 179, 185–186, 214, 227–228, 404, 410, 412, 415, 467
fascia of, 185, 412
Subclavius nerve, 416
Subcostal artery, 259
anastomoses with, 251
Subcostal muscles, 241, 254
Subcostal nerve, 160, 262, 308–309, 387, 392, 483–485
cutaneous branches of
anterior, 253
lateral, 250, 253, 262
lateral cutaneous branch of, 470
right, 308
Subcostal plane, 244
Subcostal vein, 260
Subcutaneous bursa, 516
lateral malleolus of, 516
Subcutaneous space, dorsal, 450
Subcutaneous tissue
of abdomen, 7
fatty layer of, 179, 245, 321, 344, 355, 358
membranous layer of, 321, 344, 355, 358–359
of neck, 26
of scalp, 3
Scarpa's layer, 245, 321, 344, 355, 359
Subdeltoid bursa, 408
Subdiaphragmatic lymph nodes, pathway to, 181
Subhiatal fat ring, 232
Sublime tubercle, 422
Sublingual artery, 46, 59
Sublingual caruncle, 40, 50
Sublingual ducts, openings of, 46, 56
Sublingual fold, 46, 56
Sublingual fossa, 17
Sublingual glands, 43, 47, 50, 56, 58, 124, 134
innervation of, 119, 163–164
Sublingual nerve, 50
Sublingual vein, 46, 59
Sublobular vein, 278–279
Submandibular duct (of Wharton), 46–47, 56, 58–59
openings of, 46, 56
Submandibular fossa, 17
Submandibular ganglion, 46, 50, 59, 71, 123, 132, 134, 164
schema of, 134
Submandibular glands, 1, 27, 29, 31, 46–47, 50, 58, 66, 72–73, 124, 134
innervation of, 119, 163–164
Submandibular lymph nodes, 74–75
Submental artery, 51, 72
Submental lymph nodes, 74–75
Submental vein, 31, 73
Submucosa, 305
esophageal, 69, 232
of ileum, 272
of jejunum, 272
Submucosal glands, 305
Submucosal (Meissner's) plexus, 305
Submucous space, 370–371, 374
Suboccipital nerve, 22, 175
Suboccipital triangle, 175
Subparotid lymph nodes, 74
Subpleural capillaries, 202
Subpleural lymphatic plexus, 205
Subpopliteal recess, 494–495
Subpubic angle, radiograph of, 331
Subpyloric lymph nodes, 293
Subscapular artery, 413–415, 420
Subscapular fossa, 405
of scapula, 183
Subscapular lymph nodes, 181–182
Subscapular nerve
lower, 410, 413, 415–416, 465
upper, 410, 415
Subscapular recess, 467
Subscapularis muscle, 177, 188, 238–240, 405, 408, 410–413, 417, 419, 467
Subscapularis tendon, 408, 411, 413
subtendinous bursa of, 408
Subserous connective tissue, 305
Subserous plexus, 305
Substantia nigra, 108, 118
Subtendinous bursa, 493–494, 498, 516
of gastrocnemius muscle, 497
lateral, 498
medial, 497
opening of, 408
of subscapularis, 408
Sulcal arteries
central, 142–143, 168
postcentral, 142
precentral, 142–143
prefrontal, 143
Sulcal vein, central
anterior, 169
posterior, 169
Sulcus
calcarine, 106–108, 112, 121
central
of insula, 106
of Rolando, 106–107
cingulate, 107
circular, 106
collateral, 107–108
of corpus callosum, 107
frontal
inferior, 106
superior, 106
hippocampal, 113
hypothalamic, 107, 116, 148
intertubercular, 405
lateral (of Sylvius), 108
anterior ramus of, 106
ascending ramus of, 106
posterior ramus of, 106
lunate, 106
marginal, 107
median, 60
dorsal, 116
nasolabial, 1
occipital, transverse, 106
occipitotemporal, 107–108
olfactory, 108
orbital, 108
paracentral, 107
parieto-occipital, 106–107
postcentral, 106, 143
rhinal, 107–108
temporal
inferior, 106, 108
superior, 106
terminal, 60
Sulcus terminalis cordis, 211
Superciliary arch, 1
Superficial fascia, 356, 368
of penis, 245–247, 344, 358–360, 365
of scrotum, 245–247, 344, 358, 365, 383
Superficial nerves, of lower limb, 470–471
Superficial veins
of arm, 401
of forearm, 402
lateral, 359
of lower limb, 470–471
of shoulder, 401
Superficialis flexor tendon, 450
Superior bulb, in jugular fossa, 12
Superior ganglion
of glossopharyngeal nerve, 126
of vagus nerve, 127–128
Superior lip, tubercle of, 1
Supinator muscle, 405, 426, 431, 433–434, 436–438, 460, 466–467
Supraclavicular lymph nodes, 74
Supraclavicular nerves, 31–33, 400
intermediate, 130, 400–401
lateral, 130, 400–401
medial, 130, 400–401
Supracondylar ridge
lateral, 405–406, 422
medial, 405–406, 422
Supradiaphragmatic fascia, 232
Supraduodenal artery, 283–284, 286–287
Supraglenoid tubercle, 405
Suprahyoid artery, 59, 72
Suprahyoid lymph nodes, 74
Suprahyoid muscles, 28
Supramarginal gyrus, 106
Supramastoid crest, 6
Supra-optic recess, 107, 109
Supra-opticohypophyseal tract, 148
Supra-orbital artery, 3, 35, 51, 72, 83, 87, 139
Supra-orbital nerve, 2, 35, 52, 83, 88, 123
lateral branch, 88
medial branch, 88
Supra-orbital notch, 1, 4, 6
of newborn, 14
Supra-orbital vein, 3, 73, 87
Suprapatellar bursa, 494, 498
Suprapatellar fat body, 498
Suprapatellar synovial bursa, 495
Suprapineal recess, 109
Suprapleural membrane (Sibson's fascia), 228
Suprapyloric lymph nodes, 293
Suprarenal arteries
inferior, 259, 310, 312, 320
middle, 259, 310, 320
branches of, 320
superior, 259, 310, 320
left, 192
Suprarenal glands, 271, 277, 281–282, 315, 320, 364
arteries of, 320
autonomic nerves of, 319
cross section through, 320
innervation of, 163
left, 194, 266, 308, 319
transverse section of, 325–326
right, 194, 268, 308, 319
transverse section of, 325–326
veins of, 320
Suprarenal impression, 277
Suprarenal plexus, 297, 302
Suprarenal vein, 320
inferior, right, 260
left, 234, 260, 310
right, 310

Suprascapular artery, 32–33, 76–78, 139, 413–415, 467
Infraspinous branch of, 414
Suprascapular foramen, 408, 411, 413–414
Suprascapular nerve, 413, 415–416, 465, 467
upper, 416
Suprascapular notch, 405–406, 413
of scapula, 183
Suprascapular vein, 467
Supraspinatus muscle, 171, 174, 405–406, 408–414, 418, 465, 467
Supraspinatus tendon, 408, 411, 413, 418
Supraspinous fossa, 406
of scapula, 183
Supraspinous ligament, 22, 158–159, 176, 333–334
Suprasternal space (of Burns), 26–27, 64
Supratonsillar fossa, 68
Supratrochlear artery, 3, 35, 51, 72, 83, 87, 139
Supratrochlear nerve, 2, 35, 52, 83, 88, 123
Supratrochlear vein, 3, 73, 87
Supraventricular crest, 217, 221
Supravesical fossa, 249
Sural nerve, 470–471, 521, 527–529
calcaneal branches of, 528
lateral, 471, 505, 528
medial, 528
Suspensory ligament
of axilla, 412
of breast, 179
of clitoris, 355–357
diaphragmatic, 364
of lens, 89
of ovary, 340–343, 352–353, 367, 378
of penis, 246, 344
Suspensory muscle, of duodenum, 264
Sustentaculum tali, 512–515, 531
Sutural (wormian) bone, 6, 9
Sweat glands
innervation to, 163
in peri-anal skin, 371
Sylvius, lateral sulcus of, 108
anterior ramus of, 106
ascending ramus of, 106
posterior ramus of, 106
Sympathetic cardiac nerve
cervical
inferior, 131
middle, 131
superior, 131–132
postganglionic, 133
Sympathetic cell bodies, preganglionic, 53, 133–134
Sympathetic fibers, 122–124, 133, 135
of autonomic reflex pathways, 304
of kidneys and upper ureters, 318
of liver and biliary tract, 306
of pancreas, 307
of reproductive organs, 393–394
of tracheobronchial tree, 207
of urinary bladder and lower ureter, 395
Sympathetic ganglion, 166, 177, 188, 317, 388, 394
cervical
middle, 33, 131
superior, 47, 126, 129, 131–134
Sympathetic nerves
thoracic, 131
of tracheobronchial tree, 207
Sympathetic nervous system, schema of, 163
Sympathetic plexus, 55
Sympathetic trunk, 26, 42, 53, 71–73, 126, 134–135, 188, 192, 206–207, 227–228, 236, 254, 258, 262, 303–304, 306, 317, 341, 345, 388, 390, 393–395, 485–486
cervical, 132
ganglion of, 304, 318, 387, 392–393
first thoracic, 133
ninth thoracic, 300
sixth thoracic, 300
left, 191, 213, 297, 307, 319
lumbar, 302
transverse section of, 328
in lumbosacral and coccygeal plexuses, 484
right, 191, 297, 307, 319, 390
sacral, 302
Symphyseal surface, 334, 473
of pubis, 390
Synchondrosis, of first rib, 404
Synovial cavities, 23
Synovial membrane, 408, 424, 458, 491, 494–495
attachment of, 495
of knee, 498
protrusion of, 474
Synovial sheaths, 453, 458

T

Taenia
fibers to, 274
of fourth ventricle, 116
Talar articular surface, 513
Talocalcaneal ligament, 513
lateral, 514
medial, 514
posterior, 514
Talofibular ligament
anterior, 501, 514
posterior, 501, 514
Talonavicular ligament, dorsal, 514
Talus bone, 511–513, 531
posterior process of, 514, 531
Tarsal artery
lateral, 508, 517, 523
medial, 508, 517–518, 523
Tarsal (meibomian) glands, 83
openings of, 83
Tarsal joint, 512
Tarsal (Müller's) muscle, superior, 83
Tarsometatarsal joint, 512
Tarsometatarsal ligaments
dorsal, 514, 523
plantar, 515
Tarsus
of eyelid, 85
inferior, 83
superior, 83, 86
Taste
nerves for, 61
pathways for, 136
Taste buds, 60
furrow of, 60
Tectal (quadrigeminal) plate, 107, 116
Tectorial membrane, 23, 98
deeper part of, 23
Tectospinal tract, 133
Tectum, imaging of, 151
Teeth, 62–63
apical foramina of, 63
bone around, 63
canine, 62–63
cement of, 63
crown of, 63
deciduous, 62
Teeth *(Continued)*
dental pulp, 63
dentinal tubules of, 63
dentine of, 63
enamel of, 63
incisors, 62–63, 230
interglobular spaces of, 63
interproximal spaces of, 63
molar, 62–63
growth of, 45
neck of, 63
odontoblast layer of, 63
permanent, 62–63
premolar, 62–63
primary, 62
root canals of, 63
roots of, 44, 63
unerupted, 5
Tegmen tympani, 94–95
Tela choroidea, of third ventricle, 109, 112, 146
Temporal artery
deep, 72, 101
anterior, 51
posterior, 6, 51
middle, 3, 101
polar, 143
superficial, 34–35, 42, 46, 51, 54, 71–73, 96, 101–102, 135, 137, 139
frontal branch of, 3, 87, 101
parietal branch of, 3, 101
Temporal bone, 4, 6, 8, 10–11, 15
acoustic meatus of
external, 6, 10
internal, 8
articular tubercle of, 6, 10
carotid canal of, 10
groove for posterior deep temporal artery of, 6
inferior, 6
jugular fossa for, 10
lambdoid suture, 6
mandibular fossa of, 6, 10, 14
mastoid canaliculus of, 10
mastoid foramen of, 10
mastoid notch of, 10
mastoid process of, 6, 10
of newborn, 14
occipital groove of, 10
oval window of, 14
petrosquamous fissure of, 14
petrotympanic fissure of, 10
petrous part of, 8, 10–11, 14, 99–100
accessory muscle bundle from, 67
arcuate eminence, 11
groove for greater petrosal nerve, 11
groove for lesser petrosal nerve, 11
groove for sigmoid sinus, 11
groove for superior petrosal sinus, 11
internal carotid artery in, 138
trigeminal impression, 11
round window of, 14
sigmoid sinus, groove for, 8
squamous part of, 6, 8, 11, 14
styloid process of, 6, 10, 14
stylomastoid foramen of, 10
superior petrosal sinus, groove for, 8
supramastoid crest of, 6
tympanic canaliculus of, 10
tympanic part of, 14
vestibular aqueduct, opening of, 8
zygomatic process of, 6, 10, 14
Temporal fascia, 25, 48, 50
deep layer, 48
superficial layer, 48
Temporal fossa, 6, 15

Temporal gyrus
  inferior, 106, 108
  middle, 106
  superior, 106
Temporal horn, 109, 112–113, 147
Temporal line
  inferior, 6
  superior, 6
Temporal lobe, 106, 115, 142
  imaging of, 151
Temporal nerves (V_3), deep, 50–51, 71, 123
Temporal operculum, 106
Temporal pole, 106, 108
Temporal retinal arteriole
  inferior, 92
  superior, 92
Temporal retinal venule
  inferior, 92
  superior, 92
Temporal sulcus
  inferior, 106, 108
  superior, 106
Temporal vein
  deep, 101
  middle, 3, 101
  superficial, 46, 73, 101
    frontal branch of, 3, 101
    parietal branch of, 3, 101
    tributary of, 103
Temporalis muscle, 48, 50, 101, 103, 151
  deep temporal nerves to, 123
  insertion of, 48
Temporalis tendon, 46
Temporofacial division, 24
Temporomandibular joint, 18, 49
  articular disc of, 48–49
  joint capsule of, 18
Temporomandibular ligament, lateral, 18
Tendinous arch, 70
  of levator ani muscle, 370
Tendinous intersection, 178, 242, 246, 329
Tendinous slips, 452
Tendocalcaneus bursa, 506
Tendon sheaths
  of ankle, 516
  of finger, 450
  of hand, 450
  of wrist, 449
Tendons
  of ankle, 514
  of foot, 515
Tenon's capsule, 85, 89
Tensor fasciae latae muscle, 396–397, 468, 479, 481, 487–490, 492, 530–531
Tensor tympani muscle, 50, 95–96, 151
  innervation of, 119
  tendon of, 95–96
Tensor tympani nerve, 50, 123
Tensor veli palatini muscle, 49–50, 57, 65, 68, 70, 95, 151
  innervation of, 119
  palatine aponeurosis from, 57, 65
Tensor veli palatini nerve, 50, 71, 123
Tensor veli palatini tendon, 57, 65, 68
Tentorial artery, 105
Tentorium cerebelli, 88, 104–105, 145–146
  straight sinus in, 107
Teres major muscle, 152, 171, 174, 177, 239–240, 405–406, 409–410, 412–415, 417–419, 421, 465, 467
Teres major tendon, 418
Teres minor muscle, 171, 174, 188, 238–239, 406, 409–414, 418, 465, 467
Teres minor tendon, 408, 411, 418
Terminal bronchiole, 201–202
  elastic fibers of, 201
  smooth muscle of, 201
Terminal ileum, 265, 273–274, 341, 345
Terminal sulcus, 60
Testicular arteries, 251, 255–257, 259, 268, 313, 345, 365, 379, 381, 387, 394
  left, 291, 308, 310
  right, 291, 297, 310
  in spermatic cord, 379
  transverse section of, 328
Testicular plexus, 387, 394
  right, 297
Testicular veins, 255–257, 260, 268, 313, 345, 379
  left, 291, 308, 310
  right, 291, 310
  in spermatic cord, 379
  transverse section of, 328
Testis, 321, 365, 367–368, 383, 394
  appendix of, 365, 367
  arteries of, 379
  descent of, 364
  lobules of, 368
  mediastinum, 368
  rete, 368
  septa of, 368
  tunica albuginea of, 359, 363, 368
  tunica vaginalis, 321
  veins of, 379
Thalamic veins, superior, 147
Thalamogeniculate arteries, 144
Thalamoperforating artery, 141, 144
Thalamostriate, superior, 101
Thalamostriate vein
  inferior, 145, 147
  posterior part of, 147
  superior, 109, 112, 146–147
Thalamotuberal (premammillary) artery, 141
Thalamus, 109, 111–113, 115, 146, 148, 303
  geniculate bodies of, 144
  left, 145
  nucleus of, 112
  pulvinar of, 108, 112, 115–116, 140, 146
  schematic representation of, 112
  stria medullaris of, 107
  third ventricle and, 107, 112, 116
  ventral posteromedial nucleus of, 136
Thenar eminence, 398
Thenar muscles, 446–447, 453, 460, 463
Thenar space, 447–448
Thigh
  arteries of, 499
    anterior view, 487–488
    posterior view, 489
  fascia lata of, 350, 355, 358–359
  muscles of, 479–480
    attachments of, 477–478
    lateral view, 481
    posterior views, 482
  nerves of
    anterior view, 487–488
    femoral, 525
    lateral cutaneous, 525
    posterior view, 489
  posterior cutaneous nerve of, 527
  serial cross sections of, 492
Third occipital nerve, 2
Thoracic (descending) aorta, 139, 168, 188, 191, 213, 228–229, 233, 237, 240–241
  lung groove for, 196
  transverse section of, 324–325
Thoracic aortic plexus, 236
Thoracic artery
  internal, 77, 139, 180, 186–188, 195, 203, 208–209, 213, 229, 233, 239–241, 251, 414
    anterior intercostal branches of, 186
    left, 190–191, 228
    medial mammary branches of, 180
    perforating branch of, 180, 185, 187–188, 413
    right, 190, 227
  lateral, 180, 185–186, 251, 413–415, 420
    lateral mammary branches of, 180
  superior, 186, 413–415, 420
Thoracic cardiac nerves, 206, 225, 236
Thoracic constriction, 230
Thoracic duct, 74, 186, 191, 195, 203, 205–206, 208, 213, 228–229, 234–235, 238–241, 258, 261, 295, 297, 316
  transverse section of, 324
Thoracic ganglion
  first, 163
  fourth, 223–224
  second, 224
  sixth, 206
  third, 223, 236
Thoracic intervertebral discs, 239–240
  T8, 191
  T9, 191
Thoracic nerve
  dorsal ramus of, 188
  lateral branch of, 188
  long, 180, 185–186, 253, 413, 415–416
  medial branch of, 188
Thoracic plexus, 206
Thoracic spinal cord, 134–135, 207, 303
Thoracic spinal nerves
  dorsal ramus of, 177
  dorsal root of, 134–135, 177
  T1, 133–135, 160
    dermatome of, 162
    dorsal ramus of, 174
    vertebrae relation to, 161
  T2, 134–135
    dermatome of, 162
    dorsal ramus of, 174
    vertebrae relation to, 161
  T3
    dermatome of, 162
    dorsal ramus of, 174
    vertebrae relation to, 161
  T4
    dermatome of, 162
    dorsal ramus of, 174
    vertebrae relation to, 161
  T5
    dermatome of, 162
    dorsal ramus of, 174
    vertebrae relation to, 161
  T6
    dermatome of, 162
    dorsal ramus of, 174
    vertebrae relation to, 161
  T7
    dermatome of, 162
    dorsal ramus of, 174, 250
    dorsal rootlets of, 160
    ventral ramus of, 392
    vertebrae relation to, 161
  T8
    dermatome of, 162
    dorsal ramus of, 174
    dorsal rootlets of, 160
    vertebrae relation to, 161

Thoracic spinal nerves *(Continued)*
T9
dermatome of, 162
dorsal ramus of, 174
vertebrae relation to, 161
T10, 388
dermatome of, 162
dorsal ramus of, 174
ventral ramus of, 388
vertebrae relation to, 161
T11
dermatome of, 162
dorsal ramus of, 174
ventral ramus of, 392
vertebrae relation to, 161
T12, 160
anterior ramus of, 250
dermatome of, 162
dorsal ramus of, 174
ventral ramus of, 174
vertebrae relation to, 161
typical, 177
ventral ramus of, 177, 188
ventral root of, 134–135, 177
Thoracic sympathetic nerves, 131
Thoracic sympathetic trunk, 236
Thoracic sympathetic trunk ganglion, first, 133
Thoracic trunk ganglion
lower, 225
upper, 225
Thoracic vein
internal, 77, 186–187, 189, 195, 209, 213, 239–241
left, 191
perforating branch of, 187
perforating tributaries to, 252
lateral, 252
Thoracic vertebrae, 154, 167, 227, 243
arteries of, 167
body of, 154, 166, 238, 241
radiography of, 156
section through, 166
T1, 15, 22, 160
anterior view of, 153
inferior articular facet for, 15
lateral view of, 153
posterior view of, 153
spinal nerves relation to, 161
spinous process of, 194
T2, spinal nerves relation to, 161
T3, spinal nerves relation to, 161
T4, spinal nerves relation to, 161
T5
anterior view of, 153
lateral view of, 153
posterior view of, 153
spinal nerves relation to, 161
T6
lateral view of, 154
spinal nerves relation to, 161
superior view of, 154
T7
posterior view of, 154
spinal nerves relation to, 161
T8, 213
posterior view of, 154
spinal nerves relation to, 161
T9
posterior view of, 154
spinal nerves relation to, 161
T10
body of, 324
spinal nerves relation to, 161
T11, spinal nerves relation to, 161

Thoracic vertebrae *(Continued)*
T12, 160
anterior view of, 153
lateral view of, 153–154
posterior view of, 153
spinal nerves relation to, 161
spinous process of, 152, 171–172, 174, 409
Thoracic wall
anterior, 185–186
internal view of, 187
internal, veins of, 189
Thoracoabdominal nerves, 254
cutaneous branches of, 185
Thoraco-acromial artery, 186, 412, 414–415, 420
acromial branch of, 414–415
clavicular branch of, 414–415
deltoid branch of, 409, 414–415
pectoral branch of, 185, 414–415
Thoraco-acromial vein, acromial branches of, 401
Thoracodorsal artery, 413–415, 420
Thoracodorsal nerve, 410, 413, 415–416
Thoraco-epigastric vein, 245, 252
Thoracolumbar fascia, 171, 174
anterior layer, 173, 176
middle layer, 176
posterior layer, 172–173, 176, 250, 309
transverse section of, 328
Thoracolumbar spinal cord, 303
Thorax
autonomic nerves in, 206
bony framework of, 183
coronal section of heart and ascending aorta, 214
cross section of
at T3 level, 238
at T3-4 disc level, 239
at T4-5 disc level, 240
at T7 level, 241
surface anatomy of, 178
Thumb, extensors of, 427
Thymus, 208, 227–228, 239
lung area for, 196
Thyro-arytenoid muscle, 80, 82, 151
action of, 81
thyro-epiglottic part of, 80, 82
Thyrocervical trunk, 32–34, 71–72, 76–78, 137, 139, 229, 233, 414
left, 170
right, 170
Thyro-epiglottic ligament, 79
Thyrohyoid membrane, 28, 64, 67, 69–70, 76, 78–79, 82
Thyrohyoid muscle, 27–29, 31, 58, 82, 129–130, 151
branch to, 34
communication with cervical plexus, 33
nerve to, 71, 130
Thyroid artery
inferior, 34, 72, 76–78, 137, 139, 223, 414
esophageal branch of, 233
superior, 31, 34, 72, 76–78, 137, 139
laryngeal branch of, 34
Thyroid articular surface, 80, 82
Thyroid capsule, 26
Thyroid cartilage, 1, 15, 27–28, 31, 64, 69–70, 76, 82, 193, 199, 203, 230–231
inferior horn of, 79
lamina of, 79–80
posterior border of, 67
laryngeal prominence of, 79
oblique line of, 28, 79
superior horn of, 67, 69–70, 79
prominence caused by, 66

Thyroid gland, 26, 28, 31, 33, 64, 76–78, 82, 193, 195, 203, 214
anterior view of, 76
fibrous capsule of, 78
isthmus of, 76
left lobe of, 76, 78
posterior view of, 77
pyramidal lobe of, 76
right lobe of, 76, 78
Thyroid lymph nodes, superior, 74
Thyroid notch, superior, 79
Thyroid vein
inferior, 31, 73, 76–78, 195, 208, 234
middle, 31, 73, 76, 78
superior, 31, 73, 76, 78, 82
Thyropharyngeus muscle, 69
Tibia, 497–498, 500–501, 507–508, 510, 513–514, 516–518
anterior border of, 468, 500–501
condyles of
lateral, 481, 497, 500–501, 506
medial, 494, 496–497, 500–501
fibular notch of, 500
Gerdy's tubercle of, 481, 494, 496, 500–501
intercondylar area of, 500
anterior, 501
posterior, 501
intercondylar tubercles of
lateral, 500–501
medial, 500–501
interosseous border of, 500–501
interosseous membrane of, 501
lateral surface of, 500–501
medial border of, 500
medial malleolus of, 468, 500–501, 503–505, 507–508, 516–518, 531
medial surface of, 500
nutrient foramen of, 500
oblique line of, 500
posterior intercondylar area of, 500
radiographs of, 497, 531
superior articular surface of, 495, 501
Tibial artery
anterior, 499, 505, 508–510, 517–518
circumflex fibular branch of, 499, 509
lateral tarsal branch of, 509
posterior, 499, 503–505, 509–510, 516, 520–521
calcaneal branch of, 503–504
medial calcaneal branches of, 505, 519
medial malleolar branch of, 505
Tibial nerve, 482, 484, 486, 489, 492, 503–505, 510, 521, 527–528
articular branch of, 527–528
lateral calcaneal branches of, 527
medial calcaneal branches of, 471, 519–520, 527–528
posterior, 516
Tibial tuberosity, 468, 479–480, 493–496, 498, 500–501, 506–507
Tibial vein
anterior, 510
posterior, 503–504, 510
Tibialis anterior muscle, 468, 481, 493–494, 502, 506–507, 510, 518, 529, 531
tendinous sheath of, 516
Tibialis anterior tendon, 508, 514–518, 523
tendinous sheath of, 517
Tibialis posterior muscle, 502, 505, 510, 528, 531
Tibialis posterior tendon, 503–504, 514–516, 521–523
Tibiofibular ligament
anterior, 501, 514
posterior, 514

Tongue, 38, 46–47, 59–60, 68
apex of, 60
body of, 43, 60, 64
dorsum of, 60
frenulum of, 46, 56
inferior longitudinal muscle of, 59
innervation of, 119
intrinsic muscles of, 60, 129
inferior longitudinal, 129
superior longitudinal, 129
transverse, 129
vertical, 129
lingual glands of, 60
longitudinal muscle of
inferior, 47, 151
superior, 47, 151
lymph follicles of, 60
lymph vessels and nodes of, 75
mucous glands of, 60
root of, 60, 64, 66–67, 69, 80
taste buds of, 60
transverse muscle of, 151
vertical muscle of, 151
Tonsil
of cerebellum, 114, 116
lingual, 60, 64, 68, 80
palatine, 47, 56–57, 60, 64, 66, 68
pharyngeal, 64, 66–68
imaging of, 151
Tonsillar artery, 51, 72
Torus levatorius, 66
Torus tubarius, 36, 38, 66, 68
posterior, opening of, 36
Trabecula, 149
artery of, 149
Trabeculae carneae, 217
Trabecular meshwork and spaces of iridocorneal angle, 90
Trachea, 15, 26, 28, 64, 70, 76–80, 127, 193, 195, 199–200, 203–204, 208, 210, 214, 227, 229–231, 233, 237–239
connective tissue sheath of, 199
cross section through, 199
elastic fibers of, 199
epithelium of, 199
glands of, 199
innervation of, 119, 163–164
lung area for
left, 196
right, 196
lymph vessels of, 199
nerves of, 199
small arteries of, 199
Tracheal cartilages, 199
Tracheal wall
anterior, 199
posterior, 199
mucosa of, 199
Trachealis muscle, 199
Tracheobronchial lymph nodes, 261
inferior, 235, 240
superior, 235, 239
left, 205
right, 205
Tracheobronchial (carinal) lymph nodes, inferior, 205
Tracheobronchial tree, innervation of, schema of, 207
Tracheo-esophageal groove, 70
Tragus, 1, 95
Transpyloric plane, 244
Transversalis fascia, 7, 176, 245, 249, 255–257, 259, 315, 321, 341, 343–344, 346, 355
within inguinal triangle, 255
transverse section of, 328
Transverse fasciculi, 446, 519
Transverse foramen, 19
Transverse ligament
of atlas, 23
of knee, 496
Transverse pericardial sinus, 209, 212, 217–218
Transverse process, 176, 184
cervical, 19, 22, 30, 173
anterior tubercle of, 20, 30
C6, 137
posterior tubercle of, 20, 30
of coccyx, 157
lumbar, 155–156, 158–159, 243, 330
lumbosacral, L1, 192
thoracic, 154
of vertebral body, articular facet for, 184
Transverse ridges, 157
Transverse sinus, 99, 104–105, 146
groove for, 8, 11
imaging of, 150
sigmoid sinus continuation of, 105
Transversospinalis muscle, 238
Transversus abdominis muscle, 7, 172–173, 176, 186–187, 245, 247, 249, 251, 253–256, 258, 262, 308–309, 328, 341, 345
aponeurosis of, 7, 251, 309
tendon of origin of, 172–173, 176, 250
transverse section of, 328
Transversus muscle, 151
Transversus thoracis muscle, 177, 186–188, 213, 241
Trapeziocapitate ligament, 441–442
Trapeziotrapezoid ligament, 441–442
Trapezium, 439, 442–443, 445, 449, 454
radiographs of, 444
tubercle of, 439, 441, 443
Trapezium bone, 439
Trapezius muscle, 1, 26–29, 31, 128, 130, 152, 171, 174–175, 177, 185–186, 188, 238–241, 250, 398, 404–406, 409–410, 412, 415, 467
accessory nerve to, 128
innervation of, 119
Trapezoid bone, 439, 442–443, 449
radiographs of, 444
Trapezoid ligament, 404, 408, 411
Treitz, ligament of, 264
Triangle
anal, 358
of auscultation, 241, 409
auscultatory, 152, 250
cystohepatic (Calot's), 280, 284
deltopectoral, 409
inguinal (Hesselbach's), 249, 255
transversalis fascia within, 255
lumbar (of Petit), 152, 250
internal oblique muscle in, 171
lumbocostal, 192
of neck, 175
posterior, 171, 185
sternocostal, 187
suboccipital, 175
urogenital, 358
Triangular aponeurosis, 451
Triangular fold, 68
Triangular fossa, 95
Triangular ligament
left, 268, 277
right, 268, 277
Triangular space, 413
Triceps brachii muscle, 152, 178, 405–406, 409–410, 413–415, 418–419, 421, 438, 465, 467
lateral head of, 152, 239–240, 398
long head of, 152, 238–240, 398
tendon of, 152, 398
Triceps brachii tendon, 424, 430–431, 465
Tricuspid heart valve, 210, 213–214, 219–221, 241
anterior cusp of, 213, 217, 219–221
posterior cusp of, 213, 217, 219–221
right fibrous ring of, 219, 222
septal cusp of, 213, 217, 219–221
Trigeminal (semilunar) ganglion, 50, 52, 88, 105, 133–136
Trigeminal impression, 11
Trigeminal nerve (V), 52, 55, 61, 99, 115, 123, 134–135, 145, 207
distribution of, 119
ganglion of, 117–118, 123, 132
mandibular division of, 2, 61
maxillary division of, 2, 61
mesencephalic nucleus of, 117–118, 123, 136
motor nucleus of, 117–118, 123, 132, 136
nuclei of, 123
ophthalmic division of, 2
schema of, 123
sensory root of, 115, 117–118, 123, 132
spinal nucleus of, 117–118, 123, 126–127
spinal tract of, 117–118, 123, 126–127
Trigeminal tubercle, 116
Trigonal ring, 347
Trigone
collateral, 112
habenular, 112, 116
hypoglossal, 116
olfactory, 120
of urinary bladder, 344, 346, 348, 362–363
vagal, 116
Triquetrocapitate ligament, 441
Triquetrohamate ligament, 441–442
Triquetrum bone, 439–440, 442–443
radiographs of, 444
Triticeal cartilage, 79
Trochanter of femur
greater, 152, 243, 330, 396–397, 468, 474–476, 479–480, 483, 489–490, 530
radiograph of, 331
lesser, 243, 258, 330, 474–476, 530
radiograph of, 331
Trochanteric fossa, 476
Trochlea, 86, 405–406, 422
fibular, 512–513
radiographs of, 423
of talus, 512, 531
Trochlear nerve (IV), 55, 85–86, 88, 105, 115–118, 122, 145
distribution of, 119
schema of, 122
superior, 13
Trochlear notch, of ulna, 425
Trochlear nucleus, 117–118, 122
Trolard
lateral lacuna of, 101–102
superior anastomotic vein of, 103
True cords. *See* Vocal fold
True pelvis, 334
True ribs, 183
Tubal artery, 96, 382
Tuber, of inferior vermis, 114, 116
Tuber (Bohler's) angle, 513
Tuber cinereum, 107–108, 115
median eminence of, 148
Tuberohypophyseal tract, 148
Tufted cell, 120
Tunica albuginea, 359, 363, 368
Tunica vaginalis
cavity of, 364
parietal layer of, 365, 368
testis, 321
visceral layer of, 365, 368

Turbinate, 36, 44
Tympanic artery
anterior, 51, 72, 96, 139
inferior, 55, 96
superior, 96
Tympanic canaliculus, 10, 12
Tympanic cavity, 53, 94–96, 98, 125–126
Tympanic membrane, 94–96, 98
Tympanic nerve, 55, 95
inferior, 96
of Jacobson, 124, 126, 135
Tympanic plexus, 96, 124, 126, 133, 135
promontory with, 95
tubal branch of, 126
Tyson's gland, opening of, 360

U

Ulna, 422, 426–429, 431, 436–439, 441–442, 452
anterior border of, 425
anterior surface of, 425
coronoid process of, 422, 425, 429
radiographs of, 423
interosseous border of, 425
interosseous membrane of, 425, 429
oblique cord of, 425
olecranon of, 398, 418, 422, 425, 427, 430–431, 465
radiographs of, 423
radial notch of, 422, 425
radiographs of, 423
styloid process of, 425, 439
radiographs of, 444
trochlear notch of, 425
Ulna fascia, 436
Ulnar artery, 419–420, 432–436, 441, 446–447, 449, 452–453, 460
carpal branch of, 456
deep palmar branch of, 433–435, 441, 446–447, 452–453, 460
palmar branch of, 453
palmar carpal branches of, 434, 452
Ulnar bursa, 449–450, 453
Ulnar collateral artery
inferior, 419–420, 431, 435
superior, 419–421, 430–431, 435
Ulnar collateral ligament, 424
Ulnar nerve, 400, 415–416, 418–419, 421, 430–434, 436, 441, 447, 449, 452–453, 459–464
articular branch of, 464
communicating branches of, 455
deep branch of, 434, 441, 446–447, 452–453, 460, 464
deep palmar branch of, 453
dorsal branch of, 400, 402, 430, 433–434, 436, 455–456, 459–460, 464
dorsal digital branch of, 400, 459
groove for, 406, 422
palmar branch of, 400, 402, 433, 446, 459, 464
palmar digital branch of, 400, 456, 459–460
superficial branch of, 433, 446–447, 453, 460, 464
superficial palmar arch of, 460
Ulnar recurrent artery
anterior, 420, 433–435
posterior, 420, 431, 434–435
Ulnar tuberosity, 417, 422, 425
Ulnocapitate ligament, 441
Ulnolunate ligament, 441
Ulnotriquetral ligament, 441–442
Umbilical artery, 226, 249, 259, 313, 376, 381
left, 249
occluded part of, 245, 257, 259, 268, 313, 343, 345, 378, 380–381
patent part of, 314, 378, 380–381
Umbilical fold
lateral, 249, 268, 341, 345
medial, 268, 341, 345, 378
median, 249, 268, 341, 345
right medial, 249
Umbilical ligament
medial, 226, 245, 249, 255–257, 259, 313–314, 341, 343, 345, 378, 380–381
left, 249
median, 256–257, 321, 341, 343, 345–346, 378, 381
Umbilical prevesical fascia, 249, 256, 343–344, 346
Umbilical region, 244
Umbilical vein, 226, 269
Umbilicus, 242, 249, 292, 329
sagittal CT images of, 375
Umbo, 95, 98
Uncal vein, 146
Uncinate process
cervical, 20
of ethmoidal bone, 36–37, 44
of newborn, 45
of pancreas, 281
transverse section of, 327
Uncovertebral joints, 21
Uncus, 107–108, 120
Unerupted teeth, 5
Upper limb
arteries of, 460
cutaneous innervation of, 400
dermatomes of, 399
lymph vessels and nodes of, 403
nerves of, 460–461
surface anatomy of, 398
Urachus, 249, 256–257, 268, 321, 341, 343–344, 346, 355, 378
median, 346
Ureteric fold, 341–342, 345
Ureteric orifice, 362
left, 348
right, 348
Ureteric plexus, 388
Ureteropelvic junction, transverse section of, 327
Ureters, 249, 257, 260, 265, 268, 297, 308, 311, 313–314, 340–346, 350, 352, 362, 369–370, 378–382, 388, 390, 395
in abdomen and pelvis, 313
arteries of, 314
autonomic nerves of, 317–318
in female, 313
innervation of, 395
left, 313
transverse section of, 328
in male, 313
retroperitoneal, 313
right, 313, 353
Urethra, 258, 335–337, 339–340, 346, 348, 351, 356, 359, 361–363, 367, 396
bulbous portion of, 363
floor of, 363
growth of, 347
hiatus for, 338
intermediate part of, 363
musculofascial extensions to, 337
pendulous portion of, 363
prostatic, 348, 363
roof of, 363
spongy, 363
bulbous portion of, 348
transverse section of, 397
Urethrae muscle
compressor, 335, 350, 356–357, 382, 397
growth of, 347
sphincter, 335, 339, 356, 374, 395, 397
growth of, 347
Urethral artery, 361, 383
Urethral crest, 362–363
Urethral fold, 366
Urethral glands (of Littré), 363
Urethral lacunae, of Morgagni, 363
Urethral meatus, external, 344
Urethral orifice, external, 329, 340, 354, 357, 360, 363, 366, 373
Urethral sphincter muscle
external, 249, 344, 361–363, 381
internal, 348, 362–363
Urethrovaginal sphincter muscle, 335
growth of, 347
Urinary bladder, 249, 256–257, 263, 268, 302, 308, 313, 321, 340, 342, 361–362, 364, 369, 378, 390, 395–396
apex of, 344, 346
arteries of, 314
autonomic nerves of, 317
body of, 344, 346
fascia of, 344
female, 341, 343, 348
growth of, 347
fundus of, 344, 346, 348
innervation of, 163–164, 395
lateral ligament of, 343
loop of Heiss, 347
lymph vessels and nodes of, 316
male, 344–345, 348
neck of, 344, 346, 348
orientation and supports of, 346
posterior loop of, 347
sagittal CT images of, 375
trigonal ring of, 347
trigone of, 344, 346, 348, 362–363
ureteric orifice of, 346
uvula of, 348, 362–363
Urinary bladder-prostate junction, 396
Urogenital fold, 366
Urogenital groove, 366
Urogenital hiatus, growth of, 347
Urogenital sinus, 367
Urogenital triangle, 358
Uterine artery, 313–314, 342, 350, 352–353, 378, 380, 382
branches of, 382
ovarian branches of, 353
vaginal branches of, 382
Uterine fascia, 343
Uterine ostium, 352
Uterine (fallopian) tube, 340–342, 350–352, 367, 378, 390, 393
abdominal ostium of, 352
ampulla of, 352–353
fimbriae of, 352–353
folds of, 352
infection of, 353
infundibulum of, 352–353
isthmus of, 352
uterine part of, 352
Uterine vein, 260, 342, 350, 352, 382
ovarian branches of, 353
superior, 377
Uterosacral fold, 313, 341, 370
Uterosacral ligament, 340, 343, 351–352
Uterovaginal fascia, 342, 350, 355
Uterovaginal plexus, 390, 392–393
Uterovaginal venous plexus, 260
Uterovesical pouch. *See* Vesico-uterine pouch

Uterus, 341, 346, 350, 367, 369, 378, 390, 393
adnexa and, 352
arteries of, 382
body of, 340, 342, 352
cervix of, 340, 342–343, 350, 352
fascial ligaments of, 351
fundus of, 340, 342, 346, 352
sagittal CT images of, 375
growth of, 349
hysterosalpingogram of, 353
isthmus of, 352
round ligament of, 260, 340–342, 350–351, 353, 355, 367, 378, 382
terminal part of, 350
supporting structures of, 350
veins of, 382
Utricle, 94, 97–98, 125
prostatic, 362
Uvula, 56, 66–68
of bladder, 348
of inferior vermis, 114, 116
of urinary bladder, 362–363
Uvular muscle, 57, 151

V

Vagal cardiac nerves, 131
Vagal fibers, 127
Vagal trigone, 116
Vagal trunk, 258, 297
anterior, 127, 206, 229, 236, 298–302, 306–307, 317, 319, 388
celiac branch of, 127, 298–299, 301
gastric branches of, 127, 298
hepatic branch of, 127, 298–299, 302, 306
posterior, 236, 299–302, 306–307, 317, 319, 388
celiac branch of, 127, 298–301, 388
gastric branch of, 299
Vagina, 335–337, 340, 346, 350, 352, 356, 367, 369, 373, 378, 393
growth of, 347
horizontal portion of, 351
musculofascial extensions to, 337
sagittal CT images of, 375
supporting structures of, 350
transverse section of, 397
vertical portion of, 351
vestibule of, 350, 354, 367
Vaginal artery, 313, 350, 353, 378, 380, 382
inferior, 343, 346
Vaginal fascia, 369
Vaginal fornix, 352
anterior, 340
posterior, 340
Vaginal orifice, 340, 354, 357, 366
Vaginal vein, 377
Vaginal venous plexus, 377, 397
Vaginal wall, 350–351
Vaginorectal fascial fibers, 343
Vagus nerve (X), 26, 32–34, 42, 55, 61, 71–72, 76–78, 105, 115, 117–118, 126–128, 131–132, 136, 164, 203, 206–208, 224, 229, 236, 303–304, 318
auricular branch of, 2, 12, 127
communication to, 126
in carotid sheath, 47
celiac branch of, 300
cervical cardiac branch of
inferior, 127
superior, 71–72, 127, 131–132
communicating branch of, 127
communication with cervical plexus, 33
cranial root of, 127
distribution of, 119
Vagus nerve (X) *(Continued)*
dorsal nucleus of, 117, 127, 303
posterior, 118
ganglion of
inferior, 55, 127–129, 236
superior, 127–128, 236
inferior, 13
inferior (nodose) ganglion of, 136, 207
in jugular fossa, 12
left, 77, 190, 203, 209, 223, 228, 238–239
meningeal branch of, 127
pharyngeal branch of, 126–127, 131–132, 236
posterior (dorsal) nucleus of, 224, 318
right, 77, 190, 203, 209, 223, 227, 238
schema of, 127
sympathetic trunk and, 73, 126
thoracic cardiac branch of, 127, 206, 223–224
vagal branches of, 236
Vallate papillae, 60, 136
Vallecula, 60, 68
Valves. *See* Heart valves
Valves of Houston, 371
Valves of Kerckring, 272, 280
Vas deferens, 249
Vascular fold, of cecum, 273
Vascular smooth muscle, innervation to, 163
Vascular system, of liver, 278
Vastus intermedius muscle, 477–480, 488, 492, 494, 525, 531
Vastus lateralis muscle, 397, 468, 477–481, 487, 489, 492–494, 506–507, 525, 531
Vastus medialis muscle, 468, 477–478, 480, 487–488, 492–494, 507, 525, 531
nerve to, 487, 492
Vater
hepatopancreatic ampulla of, 280
major duodenal papilla of, 272, 280
Veins. *See also specific veins*
of abdominal wall
anterior, 252
posterior, 260
of anal canal, female, 377
of brain
deep, 146
subependymal, 147
of duodenum, 289
of esophagus, 234
of eye, intrinsic, 92
of face, 3
of hypothalamus and hypophysis, 149
of internal thoracic wall, 189
of iris, 93
of large intestine, 291
of oral and pharyngeal regions, 73
of orbit and eyelids, 87
of pancreas, 289
of pelvic organs, female, 378
of pelvis, male, 381
of perineum, 382
male, 383
of posterior cranial fossa, 145
of rectum, female, 377
of scalp, 3
of small intestine, 290
of spinal cord, 169
of spleen, 289
of stomach, 289
of suprarenal glands, 320
of testis, 379
of uterus, 382
of vertebral column, 169–170
Vena cava, 380
inferior, 176, 203, 206, 211–212, 214, 217–218, 220, 222, 226–227, 229, 234, 237, 260, 266–268, 271, 277, 281, 286, 289, 308–310, 315, 320, 341, 345, 376, 378–379, 381, 390
axial CT images of, 322–323
groove for, 277
lung groove for, 196
transverse section of, 324–328
valve (eustachian) of, 217
superior, 76–77, 190, 203, 208–214, 217, 221–222, 226–227, 234, 237, 239–241
lung groove for, 196
Vena comitans, of hypoglossal nerve, 47, 59, 73
Venae comitantes, 59, 447
Venae rectae, 290
Venous arch, dorsal, 470
Venous plexus, 353
basilar, 104–105
external, 370
communication with, 377
in foramen magnum, 12
internal, 370
communication with, 377
of internal carotid artery, 55
pampiniform, 252, 365, 379, 381
prostatic, 344, 381
rectal, 260
external, 291
perimuscular, 291
vaginal, 377, 397
vertebral (of Batson), 104
internal, 166
around vertebral artery, 170
vesical, 381
Venous sinuses, dural
sagittal section of, 104
superior view of, 105
Ventral posteromedial nucleus, of thalamus, 136
Ventral rami
of cervical spinal nerves, 32, 71, 129, 174, 190
of lumbar spinal nerves, 158, 174, 388, 393, 485
of sacral spinal nerves, 388, 392
in situ, 160
of spinal nerves, 165–166
of thoracic spinal nerve, 174, 177, 388, 392
Ventricles (cardiac), 221
left, 209–214, 216, 218, 221, 237, 241
posterior vein of, 215
right coronary artery branches to back of, 216
right, 209, 211–214, 217, 221, 237, 241
Ventricles (cerebral), 109
fourth, 109, 116, 144, 147
cerebellum and, 114, 116
choroid plexus of, 107, 110, 115–116, 145
choroidal branch to, 144
imaging of, 151
lateral apertures of, 147
left lateral aperture of, 109
left lateral recess of, 109, 116
median apertures of, 109, 147
rhomboid fossa of, 115
taenia of, 116
vein of lateral recess of, 145
interventricular foramen (of Monro), 109–110
lateral, 109, 111, 113, 140, 147
central part of, 109
choroid plexus of, 101, 109–111, 140, 144, 146
frontal (anterior) horn of, 109
imaging of, 151

Ventricles (cerebral) *(Continued)*
lateral vein of, 147
medial vein of, 147
occipital (posterior) horn of, 109–113, 144, 147
temporal (inferior) horn of, 109, 112–113, 147
third, 109, 111–112, 116, 147
choroid plexus of, 107, 109–110, 144
imaging of, 151
infundibular recess of, 109
interthalamic adhesion of, 109
pineal recess of, 109
supra-optic recess of, 109
suprapineal recess of, 109
tela choroidea of, 109, 112, 146
thalamus and, 107, 112, 116
Ventricular folds, 80
Ventricular veins
hippocampal, 147
inferior, 147
Venule
macular
inferior, 92
superior, 92
nasal retinal
inferior, 92
superior, 92
temporal retinal
inferior, 92
superior, 92
Vermian artery, inferior, 144
Vermian vein
inferior, 145
superior, 145, 147
Vermiform appendix, 265, 273–276
orifice of, 274
Vermillion border, 1
Vermis
inferior
nodule of, 114, 116
pyramid of, 114, 116
tuber of, 114, 116
uvula of, 114, 116
superior, 114
central lobule of, 114, 116
culmen of, 114, 116
declive of, 114, 116
folium of, 114, 116
lingula of, 114, 116
Vertebrae, spinal nerve root relation to, 161
Vertebral arteries, 13, 22, 32–34, 71, 77–78, 131, 139–142, 167, 170, 175, 223, 233, 414
cervical part of, 137
in foramen magnum, 12
imaging of, 150–151
intracranial part of, 137
left, 144, 170
meningeal branches of, 13
anterior, 102, 137, 144
posterior, 102, 137, 144
right, 170
Vertebral artery, venous plexus around, 170
Vertebral body, 237
articular facet for
inferior, 184
superior, 184
transverse process of, 184
cervical, 20–21, 156
lumbar, 155, 159, 176, 267, 334, 341, 345
posterior intercostal artery branch to, 168
thoracic, 154, 166, 227, 238, 241, 324
Vertebral canal, 154–155
Vertebral column, 153
veins of, 169–170
Vertebral foramen, 19
cervical, 20
lumbar, 155
thoracic, 154
Vertebral ganglion, 131, 223–224
Vertebral ligaments
lumbar region, 159
lumbosacral region, 158
Vertebral notch
inferior, 154–155
superior, 154
Vertebral plexus, 131
Vertebral vein, 234
accessory, 170
anterior, 170
left, 170
right, 170
Vertebral venous plexus, 104
external, 169
anterior, 170
internal, 166, 169
anterior, 170
Vertebrocostal (lumbocostal) trigone, 258
Verticalis muscle, 151
Vesical artery
inferior, 259, 313–314, 343, 346, 376, 378, 380–381
prostatic branches of, 381
ureteric branch of, 314
superior, 249, 259, 313–314, 343, 376, 378, 380–381
ureteric branch from, 314
Vesical fascia, 342–344, 348, 355, 374
Vesical fold, transverse, 249, 341, 345, 353
Vesical lymph nodes, lateral, 316
Vesical plexus, 302, 317, 388, 390, 392, 394–395
Vesical vein, superior, 260, 377
Vesical venous plexus, 260, 348, 381
in retropubic space, 344
Vesicocervical fascial fibers, 343
Vesicocervical space, 343
Vesicosacral (sacrogenital) fold, 345
Vesico-uterine pouch, 340, 342, 346, 353, 369
Vesicovaginal space, 343
Vesicular appendix, 352, 367
Vessels
of ciliary body, 92
innervation of, 225
of neck, 32–33
of teeth, 63
Vestibular aqueduct
endolymphatic duct in, 98
internal opening of, 97
opening of, 8, 13, 99
Vestibular area, 116
Vestibular fold, 82
Vestibular fossa, 354
Vestibular ganglion (of Scarpa), 97, 125
Vestibular (Bartholin's) gland
greater, 356–357, 367, 382
primordium of, 367
opening of, 354
Vestibular (Reissner's) membrane, 98
Vestibular nerve, 94, 97, 99, 119, 125
inferior part of, 97, 99, 125
superior part of, 97, 99, 125
Vestibular nuclei, 117–118
inferior, 125
lateral, 125
medial, 125
superior, 125
Vestibule
bulb of, 348, 350, 356–357, 382
artery of, 350, 357, 382
of ear, 94, 97–98
of larynx, 82
nasal, 36, 38, 42
of vagina, 350, 354, 367
Vestibulocochlear nerve (VIII), 13, 94, 97, 99, 105, 115, 117–118, 125, 132
distribution of, 119
schema of, 125
Vestigial mesonephric tubule, 368
Vidian, 39, 41, 52–53, 55, 96, 123–124, 126, 132, 134, 136
Vincula longa, 451
Vinculum breve, 451
Viscera, paramedian section of, 321
Visceral (pre-aortic) lymph nodes, 261
Visceral peritoneum, 267, 272, 305, 374
Visceral pleura, 202
Visual pathway, 133
Vitreous body, 89
Vitreous chamber, 92
Vocal fold, 64, 80, 82
Vocal ligament, 79–80
Vocalis muscle, 80, 82, 151
action of, 81
Volar plates, 445, 448, 451, 458
Vomer, 4, 10, 38, 42
Vomeronasal organ, 36
Vorticose veins, 87, 92–93
anterior tributaries of, 93
bulb of, 93
posterior tributaries of, 93
suprachoroidal tributaries forming, 93
V-shaped area of Laimer, circular esophageal muscle in, 69, 231
Vulva, 354

W

White matter
imaging of, 151
of spinal nerves, 165
White rami communicantes, 131, 133–135, 163, 166, 177, 188, 206, 224–225, 227–228, 236, 254, 262, 297, 300, 303–304, 318, 388, 390, 393–395, 485
of spinal nerves, 165
to and from sympathetic trunk, 165
Willis, cerebral arterial circle of, 140–141
Winslow, omental (epiploic) foramen of, 266–267, 269, 321
Wirsung, pancreatic duct of, 272, 280–281
Wolffian duct, 364, 367
Wormian bone, 6, 9
Wrisberg, intermediate nerve of, 61, 105, 115, 124–125, 132, 134, 136
distribution of, 119
Wrist
arteries of, 449
bones of, 443
cutaneous nerves of, 459
deep dorsal dissection of, 456
extensor tendons at, 457
extensors of, 427
flexor tendons at, 449
flexors of, 428
ligaments of, 441–442
movements of, 440
nerves of, 449
palmar dissections
deeper, 447
superficial, 446
radiographs of, 444
superficial dorsal dissection of, 455
superficial radial dissection of, 454

Wrist (radiocarpal) joint, 439, 442
articular disc of, 439, 442

X

Xiphoid process, 178, 184, 187, 193, 195, 242–243, 245
of sternum, 183, 185
transverse section of, 324

Z

Zigzag line, 232, 270
Zinn, common tendinous ring of, 85–86, 88, 122
Zona orbicularis, 474, 530
Zonular fibers, 89–92
equatorial, 91
postequatorial, 91
preequatorial, 91
Zygapophysial joint, 22, 241
capsule of, 22–23, 159
Zygomatic arch, 6, 15–16, 48
Zygomatic bone, 1, 4, 6, 10, 83
frontal process of, 4
of newborn, 14
orbital surface of, 4
temporal process of, 4, 6
zygomaticofacial foramen of, 4, 6, 14
Zygomatic nerve (V_2), 52, 54, 122–123
zygomaticofacial branch of, 71, 123
zygomaticotemporal branch of, 71, 123
Zygomatic process, 14
of maxilla, 4, 10
of temporal bone, 6, 10
Zygomatic recess, 43
Zygomaticofacial artery, 3, 87
Zygomaticofacial foramen, 4, 6, 14
Zygomaticofacial nerve, 2, 52, 54, 71, 123
Zygomaticofacial vein, 3
Zygomatico-orbital artery, 3, 87
Zygomaticotemporal artery, 3
Zygomaticotemporal nerve, 2, 52, 54, 71, 123
Zygomaticotemporal vein, 3
Zygomaticus major muscle, 25, 48, 124, 151
Zygomaticus minor muscle, 25, 48, 124, 151

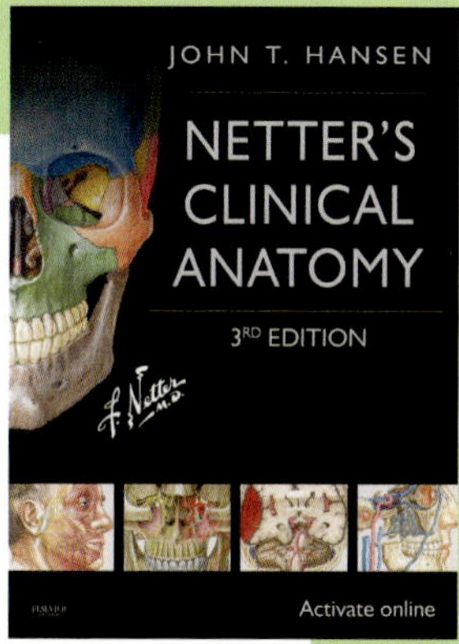

chapter 6

Lower Limb

1. INTRODUCTION
2. SURFACE ANATOMY
3. HIP
4. GLUTEAL REGION
5. THIGH
6. LEG
7. ANKLE AND FOOT
8. LOWER LIMB MUSCLE SUMMARY AND GAIT
9. LOWER LIMB ARTERY AND VEIN SUMMARY
10. LOWER LIMB NERVE SUMMARY
11. EMBRYOLOGY
CHALLENGE YOURSELF QUESTIONS

1. INTRODUCTION

As with the upper limb in Chapter 7, this chapter approaches our study of the lower limb by organizing its anatomical structures into functional compartments. The thigh and leg each are ... compartments ... into three functional compartments ... active muscles and neurovascular ... limb subserves the following ... features:

... body, and trans... leton across ...

- ... in the body ...
- **Popliteal fossa:** the region ... knee.
- **Gastrocnemius muscles:** the muscle mass that forms the calf.
- **Calcaneal (Achilles) tendon:** the prominent tendon of several calf muscles.
- ... **phenous vein:** drains blood from ... sal venous arch and posterior ... popliteal vein posterior to ...

... ins blood from ... and thigh ... to the ...

Challenge Yourself Questions

1. An elderly patient who has been minimally ambulatory is transported to the clinic with a swollen lower limb and evidence of a deep vein thrombosis. Your examination reveals a sizable clot in her small saphenous vein, and you are concerned that a thromboembolus might originate from this clot and pass to her heart and lungs. After it exits the small saphenous vein, the thromboembolus would next pass into which of the following veins on its journey to the heart?
   - A. Deep femoral
   - B. External iliac
   - C. Femoral
   - D. Great saphenous
   - E. Popliteal

2. An obese 48-year-old woman presents with a painful lump in her proximal thigh, just medial to the femoral vessels. Examination reveals the herniation of some abdominal viscera, which passes under the inguinal ligament. Through which of the following openings has this hernia passed to enter her thigh?
   - A. Deep inguinal ring
   - B. Femoral ring
   - C. Fossa ovalis
   - D. Obturator ca...
   - E. Superf...

4. A football player receives a blow to the lateral aspect of his weight-bearing right leg and immediately feels his knee give way. Under extreme pain, he is carried from the field and immediately examined by the team physician, who is able to move the player's right tibia forward excessively compared to the uninjured leg. Which of the following ligaments is injured?
   - A. Anterior cruciate
   - B. Fibular collateral
   - C. Posterior cruciate
   - D. Tibial collateral
   - E. Transverse

5. During a routine physical exam, the physician taps a patient's patellar ligament with ... hammer and elicits a knee-jerk ... of the following nerves ... reflex?
   - A. Com...
   - B. ...

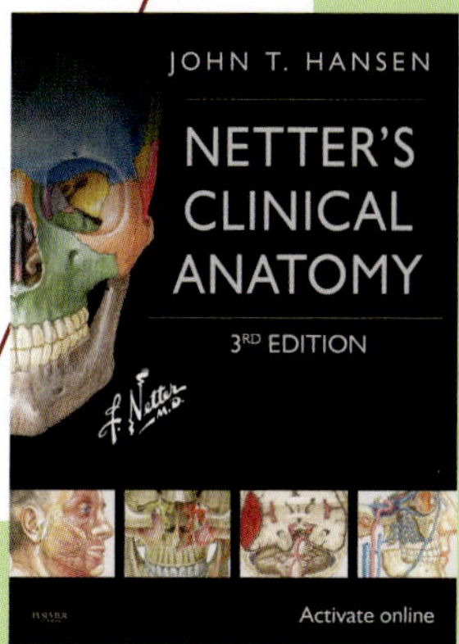

Sample page from Netter's Clinical Anatomy, 3rd Edition

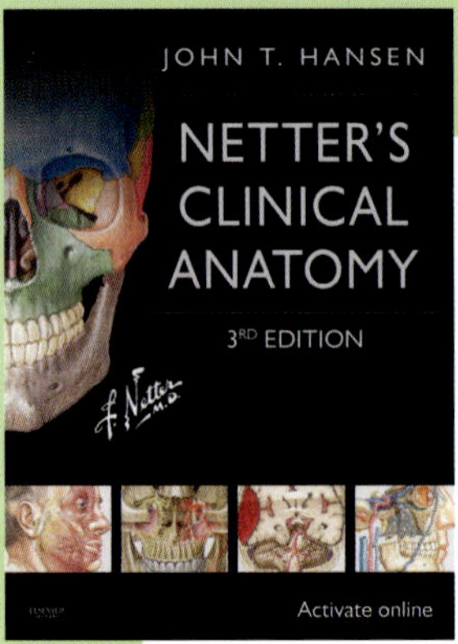

Sample page from Netter's Clinical Anatomy, 3rd Edition

Clinical Focus 2-6

Intervertebral Disc Herniation—cont'd

The most common sites for disc herniation in the cervical region are the C5-C6 and C6-C7 levels, resulting in shoulder and upper limb pain. In the lumbar region the primary sites are the L4-L5 and L5-S1 levels. Lumbar disc herniation is much more common than cervical herniation and results in pain over the sacro-iliac joint, hip, posterior thigh, and leg.

Intervertebral disc

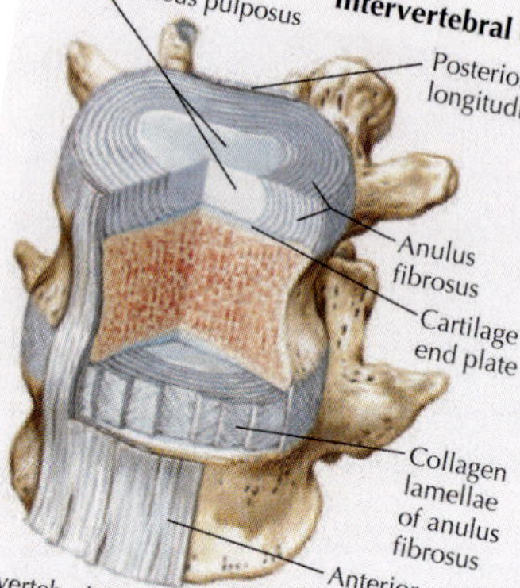

Intervertebral disc composed of central nuclear zone of collagen and hydrated proteoglycans surrounded by concentric lamellae of collagen fibers

Disc rupture and nuclear herniation

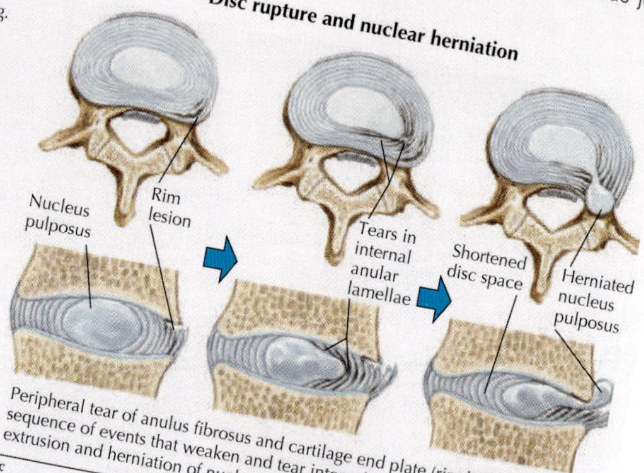

Peripheral tear of anulus fibrosus and cartilage end plate (rim lesion) initiates sequence of events that weaken and tear internal anular lamellae, allowing extrusion and herniation of nucleus pulposus.

Clinical features of herniated lumbar disc

Level of herniation	Pain	Numbness	Weakness	Atrophy	Reflexes
L4-L5 disc; 5th lumbar n. root	Over sacro-iliac joint, hip, lateral thigh, and leg	Lateral leg, first 3 toes	Dorsiflexion of great toe and foot; difficulty walking on heels; foot-drop may occur	Minor	Changes uncommon in knee and ankle jerks, but internal hamstring reflex diminished or absent
L5-S1 disc; 1st sacral n. root	Over sacro-iliac joint, hip, postero-lateral thigh, and leg to heel	Back of calf, lateral heel, foot to toe	Plantar-flexion of foot and great toe may be affected; difficulty walking on toes	Gastrocnemius and soleus	Ankle jerk diminished or absent

Sagittal MRI of an intervertebral disc herniation

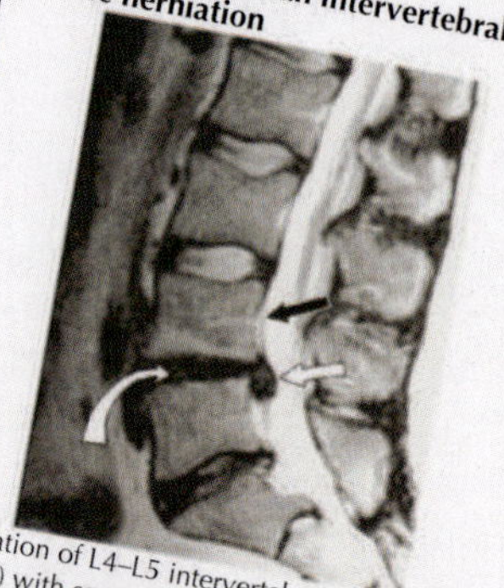

Herniation of L4–L5 intervertebral disc (*white arrows*) with some displacement of the posterior longitudinal ligament (*black arrow*). The two discs above this site show the normal hydrated appearance of the nucleus pulposus.

Reprinted with permission from Jackson S, Thomas R: Cross-Sectional Imaging Made Easy. Philadelphia, Churchill Livingstone, 2004.

Herniation of a lumbar disc

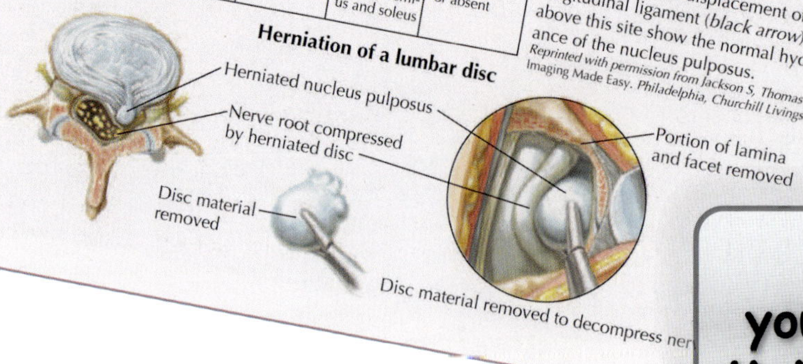

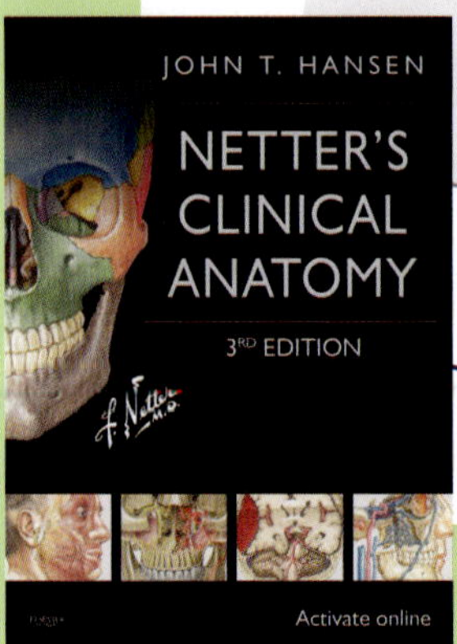

Sample page from Netter's Clinical Anatomy, 3rd Edition

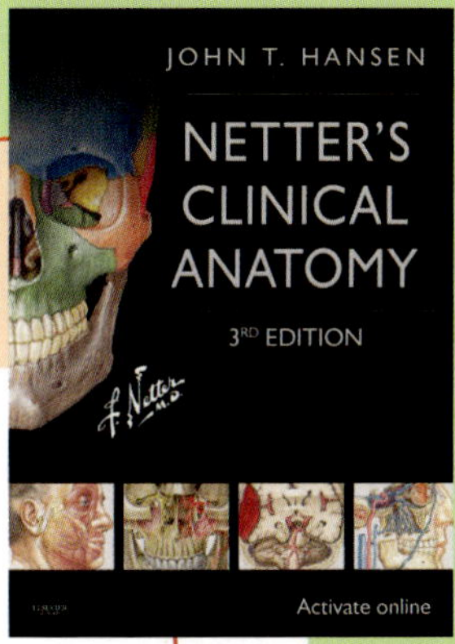

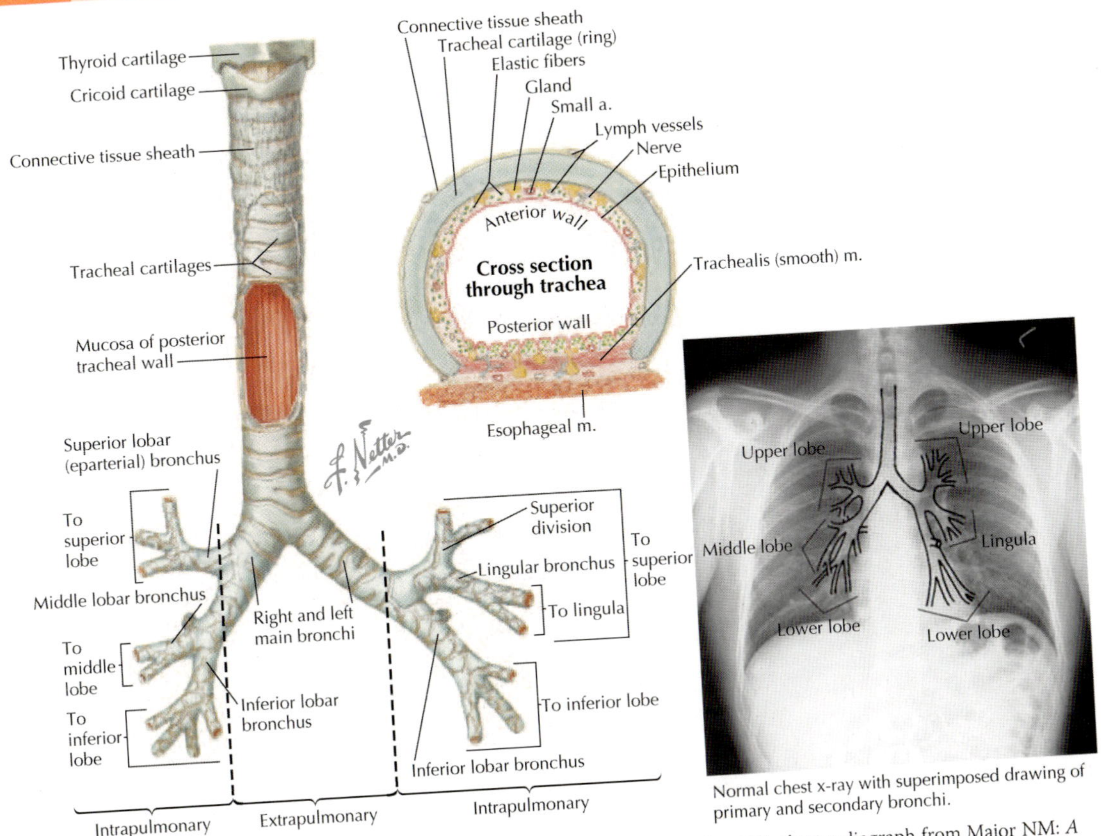

Normal chest x-ray with superimposed drawing of primary and secondary bronchi.

FIGURE 3-13 Trachea and Bronchi. (From *Atlas of human anatomy*, ed 6, Plate 199; chest radiograph from Major NM: *A practical approach to radiology*, Philadelphia, 2006, Saunders.)

TABLE 3-8 Features of the Trachea and Bronchi

STRUCTURE	CHARACTERISTICS
Trachea	Approximately 5 inches (10 cm) long and 1 inch in diameter; courses inferiorly anterior to esophagus and posterior to aortic arch
Cartilaginous rings	Are 16-20 C-shaped rings
Bronchus	Divides into right and left main (primary) bronchi at level of sternal angle of Louis
Right bronchus	Shorter, wider, and more vertical than left bronchus; aspirated foreign objects more likely to ...nto right bronchus
	...l, keel-like cartilage at ...ation of trachea
	... lobes of each lung (three ...ht, two on left)
	... bronchopulmonary ...ents (10 for each lung)

5. PERICARDIUM AND HEART

The Pericardium

The pericardium and heart lie within the **middle mediastinum.** The heart is enclosed within a fibroserous pericardial pouch that extends and blends into the adventitia of the great vessels that enter or leave the heart. The pericardium has a **fibrous outer layer** that is lined internally by a serous layer, the **parietal serous layer,** which then reflects onto the heart and becomes the **visceral serous layer,** which is the outer covering of the heart itself, also known as the **epicardium** (Fi... 3-14 and Table 3-9). These two serous layers for... a potential space known as the **pericardial s... (cavity).**

The Heart

The heart is essentially two muscular pumps... series. The two atria contract in unison, follov...

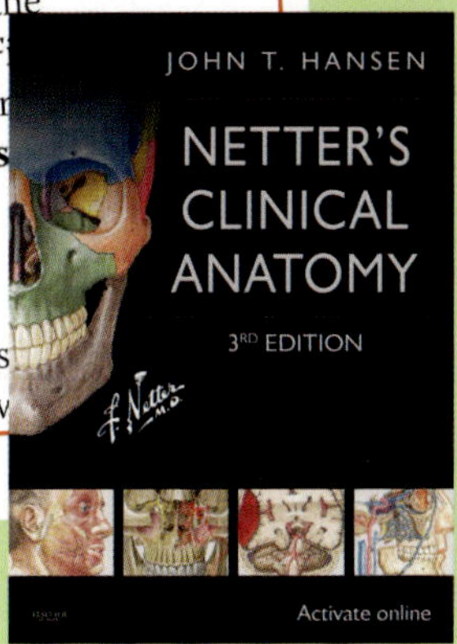

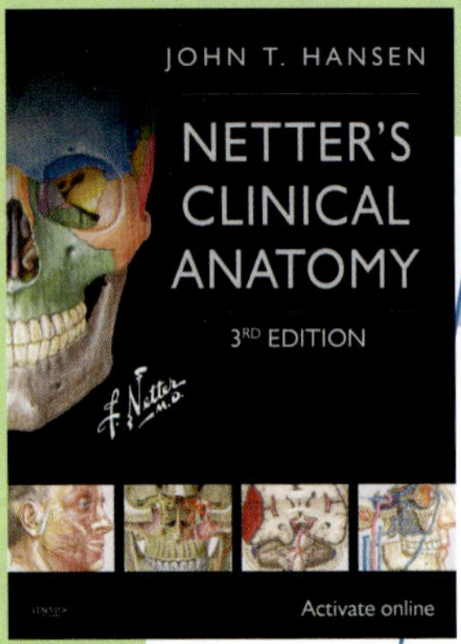

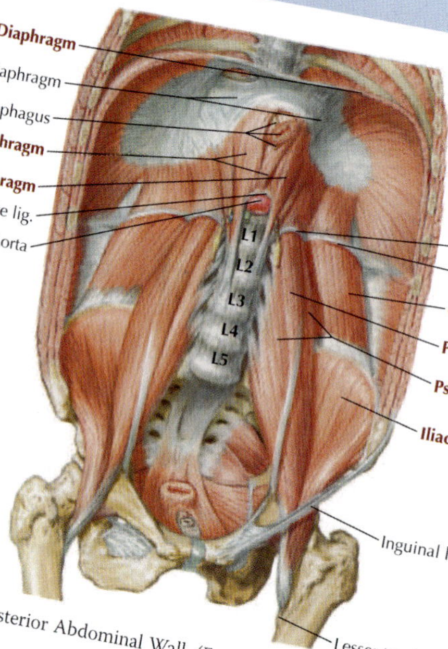

FIGURE 4-32 Muscles of Posterior Abdominal Wall. (From *Atlas of human anatomy*, ed 6, Plate 258.)

TABLE 4-10 Muscles of Posterior Abdominal Wall

MUSCLE	SUPERIOR ATTACHMENT (ORIGIN)	INFERIOR ATTACHMENT (INSERTION)	INNERVATION	ACTIONS
Psoas major	Transverse processes of lumbar vertebrae; sides of bodies of T12-L5 vertebrae, and intervening intervertebral discs	Lesser trochanter of femur	Lumbar plexus via ventral branches of L2-L4 nerves	Acting superiorly with iliacus, flexes hip; acting inferiorly, flexes vertebral column laterally; used to balance trunk in sitting position; acting inferiorly with iliacus, flexes trunk
Iliacus	Superior two thirds of iliac fossa, ala of sacrum, and anterior sacro-iliac ligaments	Lesser trochanter of femur and shaft inferior to it and to psoas major tendon	Femoral nerve (L2-L4)	Flexes hip and stabilizes hip joint; acts with psoas major
Quadratus lumborum	Medial half of inferior border of 12th rib and tips of lumbar transverse processes	Iliolumbar ligament and internal lip of iliac crest	Ventral branches of T12 and L1-L4 nerves	Extends and laterally flexes vertebral column; fixes 12th rib during inspiration
Diaphragm	Thoracic outlet: xiphoid, lower six costal cartilages, L1-L3 vertebrae	Converges into central tendon	Phrenic nerve (C3-C5)	Draws central tendon down and forward during inspiration

abdominal aorta. The **inferior vena cava** passes through the diaphragm at the T8 vertebral level to enter the right atrium of the heart. The right phreni... ve may accompany the IVC as it passes ... diaphragm, which it innervates. The ... asses through the diaphragm at the ... level, along with the anterior and ... l trunks and left gastric vessels. The ... hrough the diaphragm at the T12

vertebral level and is accompanied by the thor... duct and often the azygos vein ... superiorly.

Kidneys and Adrenal (Suprarenal) Glands

The kidneys and adrenal glands are ... neal organs that receive a rich arterial supply...

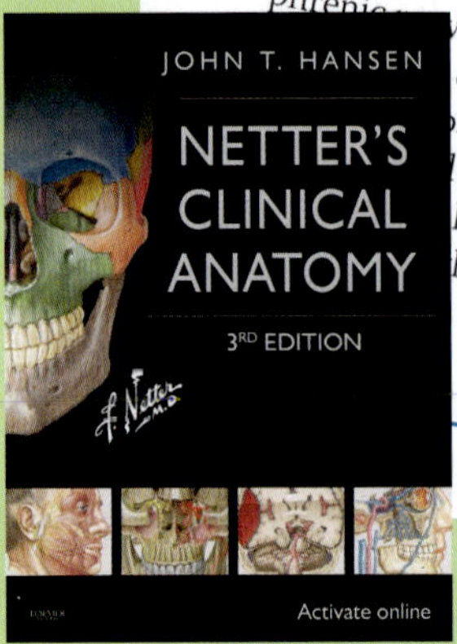

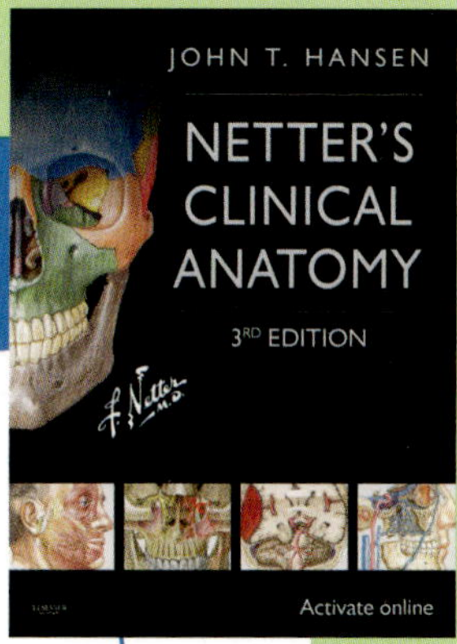

inguinal region, rectus sheath, and lateral thoracic wall. Most of its connections ultimately drain into the **axillary vein (4)** and then into the **subclavian vein**, **brachiocephalic veins**, which form the **superior vena cava**, and then into the **heart (6)**. The inferior epigastric veins (from the external iliac veins) enter the posterior rectus sheath and course cranially above the umbilicus as the superior epigastric veins and then anastomose with the internal thoracic veins that drain into the subclavian veins (Fig. 4-3).

The superficial veins can become enlarged during portal hypertension, when the venous flow through the liver is compromised. Important **portosystemic anastomoses** between the portal system and caval system can allow venous blood to gain access to the caval veins (both deep and superficial veins) to assist in returning blood to the heart.

Variations in the venous pattern and in the number of veins and their size are common, so it is best to understand the major venous channels and realize that smaller veins often are more variable.

Hepatic Portal System of Veins

The hepatic portal system of veins drains the abdominal GI tract and two of its accessory organs (pancreas and gallbladder) and the spleen (immune system organ) (Fig. 4-40). This blood then collects largely in the liver, where processing of absorbed GI contents takes place. (However, most fats are absorbed by the lymphatics and returned via the thoracic duct to the venous system in the neck, at the junction of the left internal jugular and left

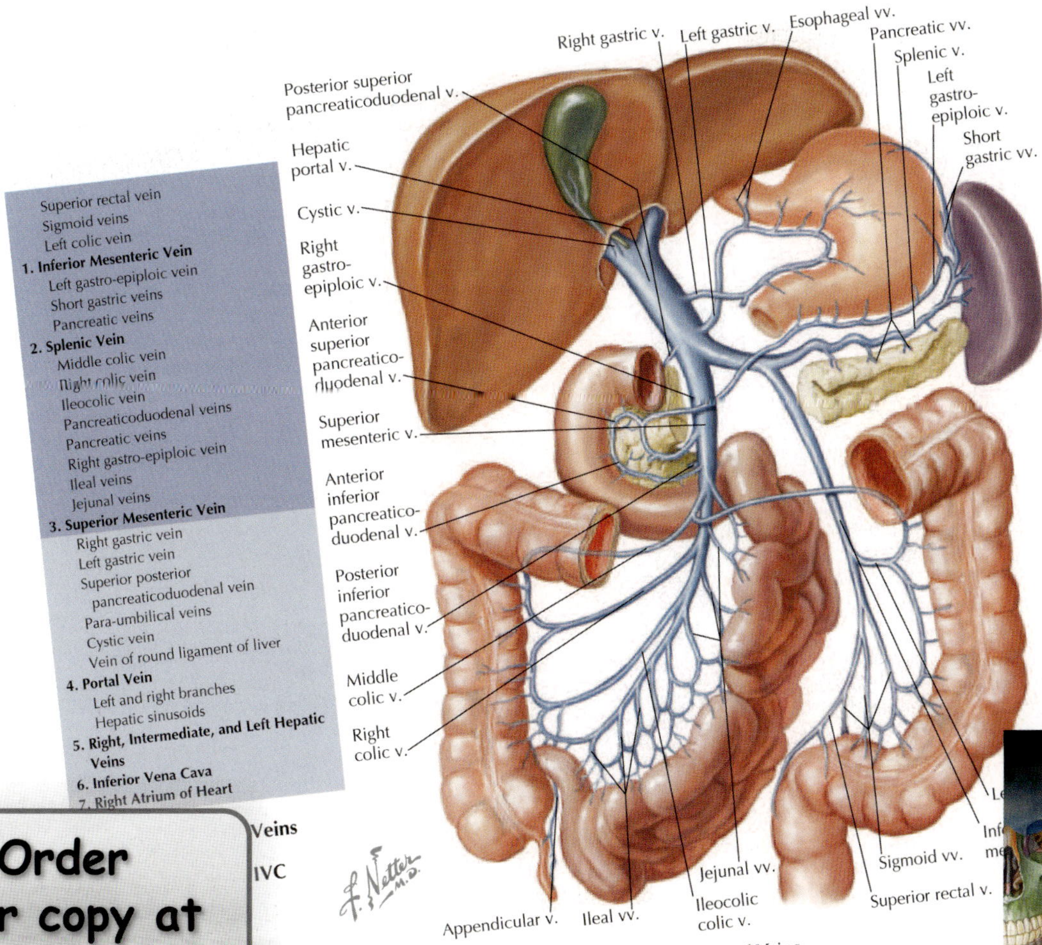

FIGURE 4-40 Hepatic Portal System of Veins.

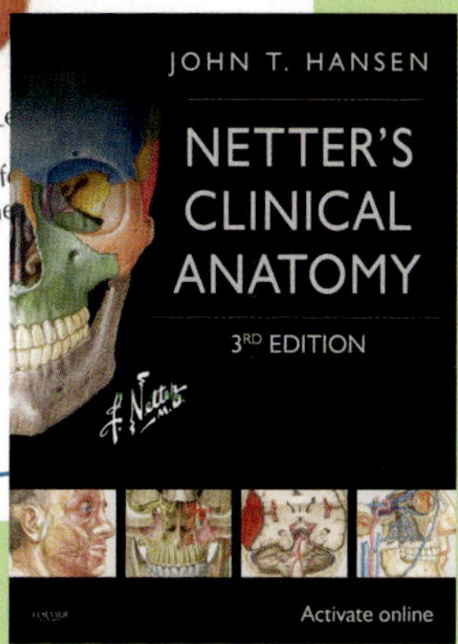

Sample page from Netter's Clinical Anatomy, 3rd Edition

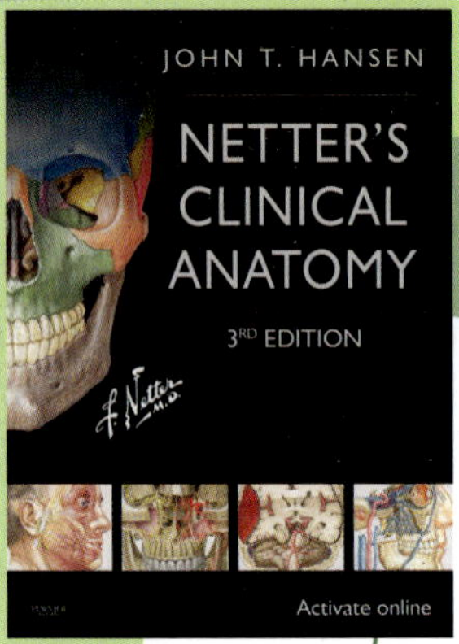

Clinical Focus 8-33

Nosebleed

A nosebleed, or **epistaxis,** is a common occurrence and often involves the richly vascularized region of the vestibule and the anteroinferior aspect of the nasal septum (Kiesselbach's area). Nosebleeds usually result from trauma to the septal branch of the superior labial artery from the facial artery.

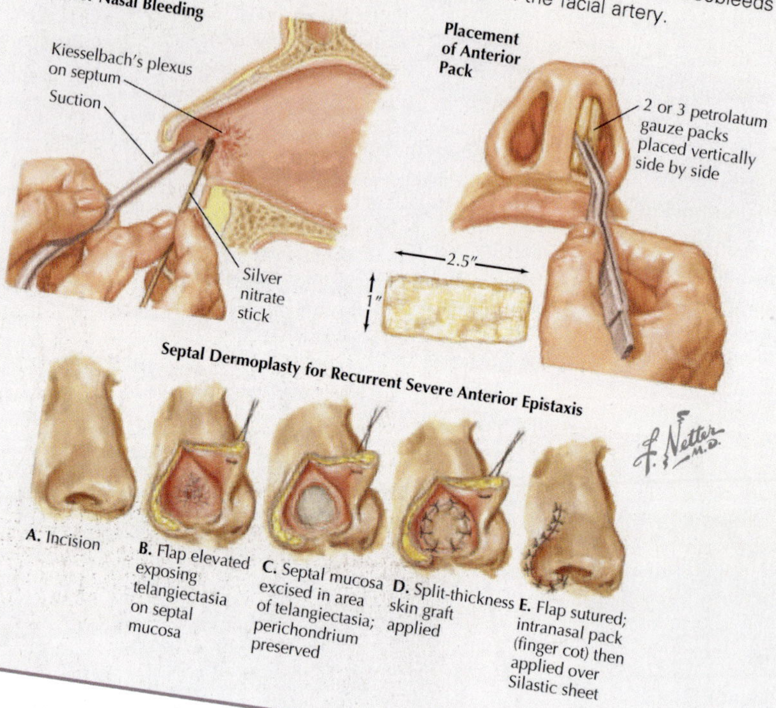

- **Frontal:** unpaired bone that contains the frontal sinus; forms part of the roof and septum of the cavity.
- **Vomer:** unpaired bone that contributes to the septum.
- **Nasal:** paired bones that form part of the anterior roof and lateral wall.
- **Maxilla:** paired bones that form the floor, septum, and lateral walls of the cavity.
- **Palatine:** paired bones that form the floor, septum, and lateral walls of the cavity.
- **Lacrimal:** bone that forms part of the lateral wall of the nasal cavity.
- **Inferior nasal concha:** paired bones that f... part of the lateral wall.

...ply and Innervation

... to the nasal cavities originates from ... major arteries (Fig. 8-33):

- **Ophthalmic:** anterior and posterior ethmoidal arteries
- **Maxillary:** sphenopalatine (terminal branch of the maxillary) and its septal branches, and the greater palatine arteries
- **Facial:** lateral nasal, septal branches, and superior labial artery

Corresponding veins drain the floor, lateral walls, and nasal septum, with most of the venous return passing into the **pterygoid plexus of veins** (Fig. 8-33). Some venous drainage also passes into the facial vein anteriorly and into the inf... thalmic veins superiorly.

The innervation of the nasal cavit... following (Fig. 8-34; see also Fig. 8-...

- **Olfactory:** CN I olfactory recep... sense of smell) in the olfactory... convey axons that pass from the ... part

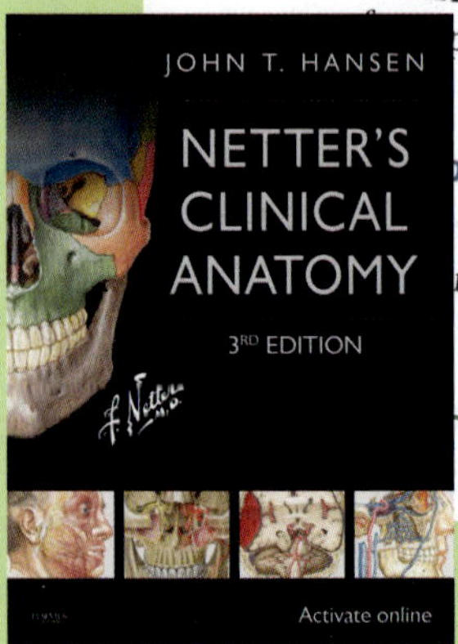